1 MONTH OF
FREE
READING

at
www.ForgottenBooks.com

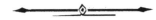

ISBN 978-0-260-86577-9
PIBN 10978086

LIST OF PLATES IN VOL. II

xi

LIST OF PLATES IN VOL. II

A SYSTEM OF SURGERY

THE BREAST

By W. SAMPSON HANDLEY, M.S.Lond., F.R.C.S.Eng.

ANATOMY OF THE BREAST

THE mamma is an organ developmentally arising from the skin, intercalated in the thickness of the subcutaneous fat, and probably representing a highly developed group of sebaceous follicles. It is firmly attached to the skin at the nipple, and is connected to it at numerous other points by fibrous septa called the suspensory ligaments of Astley Cooper. The size of the breast is no index to its secreting power, since prominent mammæ often consist mainly of fat.

Each mamma consists of from twelve to twenty lobes, which are really separate sector-shaped glands, packed closely together in one plane, their ducts converging upon the nipple, and opening by separate orifices upon its summit. The autonomy of each lobe is an important fact, since disease of one or more of the lobes is thereby hindered from spreading to the adjoining ones. In some cases of disease a sector-shaped tumour may be observed mapping out the limits of the affected lobe or lobes. It is possible sometimes to excise the diseased lobes of the breast without interfering with the healthy ones. The main duct of each lobe, before opening upon the nipple, is dilated to form a small reservoir or ampulla, $\frac{1}{4}$ to $\frac{1}{6}$ in. in diameter, the undue distension of which may give rise to galactocele, or, if lactation is not in progress, to a retention cyst containing serous fluid. Each lobe of the breast is composed of a number of lobules which bear to the main duct of the lobe the relation of a bunch of grapes to its stalk. A lobule of the breast consists of a small rounded packet of fibrous

b

THE BREAST

tissue, enclosing a small milk-duct surrounded by a group of acini or alveoli, the blind glandular recesses which discharge their secretions into the duct. A large amount of fibro-fatty tissue intervenes between the lobules, and serves to cushion and protect them. In microscopic sections the ducts are distinguished by their single lining of columnar epithelium, while the alveolar or secreting epithelium is cubical. The epithelium of the alveoli and ducts rests upon a basement membrane of flattened endothelial cells. In microscopic sections, breast tissue can be recognized by these characteristic groups of cubical-celled alveoli containing one or more columnar-celled ducts. The intervening fibrous and fatty tissue contains here and there the section of a larger duct, the whole presenting a characteristic histological picture.

Limits of the mamma.—Stiles showed that the outlying lobules of the breast extend as a thin marginal fringe in the subcutaneous fat considerably beyond the limits of the mammary prominence. Including these outlying portions, the vertical diameter of the breast extends from the lower border of the second rib to the sixth costal cartilage at the angle where it begins to sweep upwards to the sternum. Its horizontal diameter extends from a little within the edge of the sternum, opposite the fourth rib, to the fifth rib in the mid-axillary line. The lower and inner margin of the breast overlies the sixth costal cartilage midway between the angle and its sternal end, and is situated only about an inch from the dangerous area in breast cancer—the area of epigastric invasion.

In a majority of cases a tongue-shaped projection of breast tissue, known as the *axillary tail,* extends to the base of the axilla, under cover of the lower edge of the great pectoral. Frequently the axillary tail lies in almost direct contact with the lowest of the axillary lymphatic glands.

Relations to the underlying muscles.—Roughly speaking, the upper and inner two-thirds of the breast rests on the great pectoral muscle. The lower and outer third of the breast lies mainly on the serratus magnus—a fact often unwisely ignored in the operation for cancer. At its periphery the breast rests to a small extent below upon the aponeurosis of the external oblique and the origin of the rectus, externally upon some of the digitations of the external oblique. A portion of the breast, and especially its axillary tail, rests against the lower part of the inner wall of the axilla, and is separated from the axillary glands only by a fatty and ill-defined portion of the axillary fascia. The muscular relations of the breast are of great importance in the operation for breast cancer, for every muscle which directly touches the affected organ is very likely to be infected by microscopic secondary growths quite early in the case.

MAMMARY LYMPHATICS

Moreover, the thinner the muscular layer which separates the primary growth from the pleural cavity, the greater the probability of early pleural invasion. Thus, in outlying mammary growths the prognosis is worse than in the case of growths which are separated from the underlying ribs by the thickness of the great pectoral muscle. Portions of the glandular tissue of the breast are sometimes found beneath the pectoral fascia, in the substance of the great pectoral muscle.

Blood supply.—The arteries which supply the mammary gland are branches of the internal mammary, long thoracic, superior thoracic, and perforating branches from the second, third, and fourth intercostal arteries. It has been recently shown that the important perforating branches of the internal mammary artery for the most part turn round the margin of the breast and spread out upon its superficial aspect before penetrating its substance. Thus, the breast may be extensively stripped up from the pectoral muscle without interfering with its blood supply—a fact of surgical importance (*see* p. 40).

Lymphatic vessels.—The breast is richly supplied with lymphatic vessels. Each lobule possesses its own system of minute lymphatic capillaries which come into close relation with the acini. Many of the lymphatic vessels of the breast pass into, or communicate with, the pectoral lymphatic plexus, which lies in the pectoral fascia in immediate contact with the posterior surface of the mamma. On the anterior surface of the breast a plexus of large lymphatic vessels is present beneath the skin of the areola (subareolar plexus of Sappey). There can be no doubt that the normal lymph drainage of the breast - flows almost exclusively to the axillary glands of the same side. Large lymphatic trunks connect the pectoral lymphatic plexus and the subareolar plexus with the lower glands upon the internal wall of the axilla. It is, however, a mistake to regard the pectoral lymphatic plexus as an anatomical entity. It is in reality merely a conventional subdivision of the deep fascial lymphatic plexus (Fig. 251), whose network of intercommunicating channels forms a single system investing the entire body. The unity of this plexus is a fact of capital importance in the pathology of breast cancer, for it allows the indefinite spread of the process of permeation (*see* p. 60). This great plexus is divisible by the median plane of the body and by two horizontal planes, passing through the umbilicus and the clavicles respectively, into six " catchment areas," three on each side, which drain respectively into the cervical, the axillary, and the inguinal glands. Within each area a special set of trunk lymphatics arises from the plexus and converges on the corresponding set of glands. These trunk vessels are of such a size that fine particles, such as cancer cells, may be swept along them by the current, to lodge in the corresponding glands. But in the boundary zones of the catchment areas no trunk lymphatics are present. Here are found only narrow, tortuous channels, not navigable by floating cancer cells, and only to be penetrated by the slower process of permeation.

One lymphatic trunk deserves especial mention. It arises on the posterior aspect of the breast and pierces the great pectoral muscle to terminate in the subclavian lymphatic glands, without passing

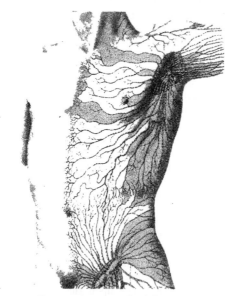

Fig. 251.—The trunks of the fascial plexus. The fine meshwork of vessels constituting the plexus itself is only partially indicated in this figure.

(*After Sappey's " Vaisseaux Lymphatiques."*)

first into the lower lymphatic glands of the axilla. Consequently, in breast cancer the subclavian glands may be found enlarged before the lower axillary glands have become affected.

The subclavian glands themselves are of great surgical importance. They are situated just below the clavicle, internally to the first part of the axillary artery and vein, and shielded in front by the great pectoral muscle and by the costo-coracoid membrane. Owing to their sheltered position they are very likely to escape removal at the hands of an inexpert operator for breast cancer. Their efferent vessels form the afferents of the supraclavicular glands, which are the next set to be involved in breast cancer.

It has been sometimes stated that efferent lymphatic vessels from the breast pass to the retrosternal chain of glands which accompanies the internal mammary artery. It is doubtless true that there is a mediate communication between the breast and these glands by way of the pectoral lymphatic plexus and of the perforating branches which run from that plexus to tho glands in question. But, fortunately, these perforating branches must be regarded not as true afferent lymphatics but as mere anastomotic channels of small diameter and sluggish stream, along which embolic transport of cancer cells cannot occur, though in a late stage of the disease they may be invaded by permeation. For, while invasion of the axillary glands is an early and almost constant event, cancer of the anterior mediastinal glands is only found in 6·5 per cent. of necropsies for breast cancer.

Lymphatic communication between the breasts.— It will be clear from the preceding description that the lymphatic systems of the two breasts communicate across the middle line indirectly, through the medium of the fine vessels of the fascial plexus. Cancer can thus only spread to the opposite breast in a late stage and after permeation has crossed the middle line, an event which is usually signalized by embolic invasion and enlargement of the opposite axillary glands. For sufficiently obvious reasons this embolic glandular enlargement precedes cancerous deposit in the opposite breast.

Lymphatic arrangements of the skin.—It was formerly thought that breast cancer spread in the plane of the skin along a hypothetical plexus described by Arnold, situated at the junction of the corium and subcutaneous tissue, and called the deep cutaneous plexus. Accordingly, the removal of a very large area of skin was considered imperative. In point of fact there is only one cutaneous lymphatic plexus, the subpapillary lymphatic plexus, and there is no evidence that permeation can spread to any extent along this plexus. The subpapillary plexus is drained by small vessels which run vertically downwards along the fibrous septa of the subcutaneous tissue to join the fascial plexus. Up-stream permeation of these small vessels accounts for the nodular invasion of the skin so often seen in the later stage of breast cancer.

From the muscles small tributaries reach the fascial plexus on its deep aspect. Up-stream permeation of these tributaries is responsible for the muscular nodules which may occur in a late stage of cancer in the pectorals, the serratus magnus, the deltoid, the rectus abdominis, the intercostals, or other muscles which lie within the area of permeation.

Development.—The breasts remain small and unimportant until puberty. Up to this age, and permanently in the male breast, the characteristic alveoli are absent, and the minute milk-ducts terminate in blind " end-sacs," lined by an epithelium which approximates in character to the columnar epithelium of the ducts. At puberty the alveoli are formed as hollow buds which grow outwards from the end-sacs into the surrounding tissues.

At two periods of life, normal activities of the mammary gland have been dignified by the name of mastitis.

1. During the first few days of life in either sex the breasts may become swollen, and a few drops of serous fluid or of true milk may be discharged from the nipple (*mastitis neonatorum*). This mastitis of new-born children, like the jaundice and the cutaneous hyperæmia which accompany it, is probably due to the first onslaught of bacteria upon the aseptic babe, the bacteria of the skin penetrating some distance along the ducts of the breast. It has no clinical importance and should be let alone; unwise and active treatment, such as massage, may prolong and aggravate the condition. A few rare cases are on record where infantile lactation has persisted for several weeks, and in one case for over three months.

2. With the onset of puberty, both in boys and in girls, the undeveloped breasts may become tender and swollen for some days or weeks (*mastitis adolescentium*). At the same time a scanty serous discharge exudes from the nipple, and the axillary glands become unduly palpable. No treatment is required for this condition, which derives its only importance from the parental anxiety it is apt to cause.

At puberty in the female, owing to the rapid development of the acini, and the deposition of fat between the growing lobes, the breast begins to assume its characteristic form and size. The onset of pregnancy leads to further marked changes in the gland, for the details of which a work on obstetrics should be consulted. Many new alveoli are formed, and the cell proliferation proceeds with such rapidity that until parturition initiates lactation the alveoli lose their lumen and consist of solid cords of cells; the breast becomes coarsely granular to the touch, the skin of the areola dark; and in the later months of pregnancy a watery fluid exudes from the nipple.

The establishment of lactation is accompanied by general congestion and swelling of the breasts, and sometimes by local tenderness and elevation of the temperature, and soreness in the axillæ. These activities may easily pass into acute mastitis.

Involution.—When lactation is over, the vascularity of the gland rapidly diminishes, and the lobules become much reduced in size and complexity by atrophy of their constituent alveoli. These changes make further progress at the climacteric. At this time also the fatty tissue of the breast often atrophies, while its fibrous tissue, increasing in amount, contracts upon and causes gradual atrophy or even complete disappearance of many of the glandular alveoli. The characteristic withered and flattened breast of old age is thus produced.

AMASTIA

DEVELOPMENTAL ABNORMALITIES

AMASTIA AND POLYMASTIA

In very rare cases one or both of the breasts are congenitally absent—a condition known as *amastia* or *amazia*. A rudimentary nipple is usually present. The condition is often associated with absence or rudimentary

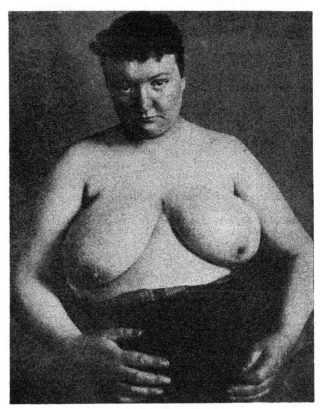

Fig. 252.—Hypertrophy of the breasts.
(*Beatson, Edin. Med. Journ., Dec.,* 1908.)

development of the sternal portion of the great pectoral muscle, and, less commonly, with other malformations.

Polymastia is a condition in which extra breasts or extra nipples are present, usually below the normal nipple. A supernumerary breast may or may not have a nipple, and is usually functionless, but may secrete milk during lactation. Polymastia is more frequent in men than in women. Mitchell Bruce, among 4,000 individuals examined, found 47 males and

14 females with supernumerary nipples. The accessory structures are most often found along a line leading from the axilla downwards and inwards to a point a few inches above the umbilicus. A case has been recorded in which five breasts were present, four of them functional. The fifth and lowest was median, and situated 5 in. above the umbilicus. Champneys has shown that during pregnancy the axillary sebaceous glands frequently become enlarged and lumpy, and that occasionally true milk may be expressed from the hypertrophied glands. Bryant has pointed out that certain cases of carcinoma resembling breast cancer, but primary in the axilla, may originate from such abnormal sebaceous glands.

HYPERPLASIA OR HYPERTROPHY OF THE BREASTS

This is a rare affection met with both in single and in married women, and is usually bilateral (Fig. 252). In the most marked cases the breasts within a few months may attain such an enormous size that they become a serious encumbrance, causing pain, dyspnœa, and palpitation. In Esterle's case, quoted by Rodman, they attained a combined weight of 30 lb. within little more than three months. In Delfis' case, occurring in a pregnant woman, the mammæ rested upon the thighs when the patient sat down. The disease comes on most frequently about puberty, or during pregnancy. The cases associated with pregnancy, though more rapid in their evolution, are favourable in this respect, that the hypertrophy may subside after parturition, whereas in other cases it is permanent and usually progressive. The enlargement depends upon a general overgrowth of the fibrous tissue of the mammæ, but in the cases associated with pregnancy true glandular hypertrophy may be present.

Treatment.—Pressure, mechanical support, and the administration of iodides may suffice in the milder cases, but the only treatment which has proved effective in well-marked examples is amputation of the breasts. The operation should not be undertaken during pregnancy.

GYNÆCOMASTIA

A unilateral or bilateral hypertrophic enlargement of the male breast to such a point that it resembles the virgin breast of the female is known as gynæcomastia. It may occur as part of a general tendency to the feminine type, in association with a high voice, and perhaps with developmental defects in the genital organs. It is said sometimes to follow removal of the testicles. It may be found in men of full sexual development. Histologically the breast resembles that of the virgin female.

Gynæcomastia probably predisposes to pathological changes. Thus, in a man, otherwise normal, who presented a slight degree of this condition, I observed bilateral chronic mastitis owing to the pressure of the braces upon the gland.

DISEASES OF THE NIPPLE AND AREOLA

RETRACTION OF THE NIPPLE

This condition is most often due to failure in the evolution of the child's rudimentary nipple towards the normal prominent adult type. The nipple may be merely flattened, or may be represented by a funnel-like concavity at the centre of the areola. This condition is of importance because it produces inability to suckle and favours sepsis at the orifices of the milk-ducts. It may thus become a cause of milk congestion, acute mastitis, and mammary abscess.

Acquired retraction of the nipple indicates a fibrotic process in the underlying breast tissue. It is an important sign of cancer, depending upon the reactive or inflammatory processes associated with the growth. Less commonly, retraction is associated with Paget's disease, or depends upon scarring, the result of an abscess or a shrivelled cyst. Some authors incorrectly state that it occurs in chronic mastitis.

SIMPLE ECZEMA OF THE NIPPLE

May arise in the course of or apart from pregnancy or lactation, and may be a cause of abscess of the breast. The *Staphylococcus pyogenes aureus* has been demonstrated in the discharge, and may also be present in the milk during lactation.

Treatment.—Various ointments may be tried. Boric, lead subacetate, and mild mercurial ointments are those most often used. If these fail and Paget's disease can be excluded, a trial of vaccine treatment should be made after bacterial examination.

When eczema of the nipple occurs during lactation it is best to wean the child, both on the mother's account, because a mammary abscess is a likely sequel, and for the child's sake, because the milk is likely to contain staphylococci. Only if the eczema is very slight in degree can sanction be given for continued suckling, through a nipple shield. In such circumstances no poisonous ointments must be prescribed.

Cracked nipple is the term applied to a fissured condition of the skin of the nipple, comparable to "chapped hands." It is usually associated with eczema of the nipple, and generally occurs during suckling. The treatment is the same as for eczema.

PAPILLOMA OF THE NIPPLE

This condition is sometimes met with, and the papilloma may attain a considerable size. Owing to the constant drag of the tumour on loose tissues, the larger examples of these tumours are pedunculated. In the course of years the pedicle may become long and attenuated, and pulsation may be felt in it. The tumour itself is usually globular, and its surface lobulated and warty. Owing to septic changes the tumour may exude an offensive serous discharge or may ulcerate.

Treatment.—A sessile wart of the areola should be excised. A pedunculated wart should be strangulated by tying a stout ligature round the base of its pedicle.

CARCINOMA OF THE NIPPLE

Carcinoma of the nipple is rare. It may be of the squamous-celled or spheroidal-celled type. In the latter case it probably originates in the sebaceous glands of the areola. Early ulceration takes place, and the disease then pursues a course similar to that of carcinoma of the mamma itself.

SEROUS DISCHARGE FROM THE NIPPLE

Serous discharge from the nipple may be due to duct papilloma or duct carcinoma. This is the commonest cause. It may occur in chronic mastitis, apart from duct papilloma—a fact easy to understand if it be remembered how frequently cysts are formed in chronic mastitis if duct obstruction prevents the exit of the serous secretion. (*see* Fig. 254). In any given case, however, it is practically impossible to exclude the presence of a small and impalpable duct papilloma, which may ultimately become carcinomatous. A serous discharge may occasionally persist for years, unaccompanied by any induration of the breast, but there is often a very slight sector-shaped induration of one or more of the lobes, only appreciable on very careful examination. Serous discharge is nearly always unilateral.

Treatment.—Mintz, in one of his cases, obtained a cure of three years' duration by giving large doses of potassium iodide. I have tried X-rays without success. In my opinion, persistent serous discharge is best treated by complete removal of the breast.

PAGET'S DISEASE OF THE NIPPLE

This affection is a unilateral chronic intractable eczema of the nipple, first described by Paget as preceding cancer of the mammary gland. The disease usually occurs in middle-aged or elderly women, very rarely in men. It begins with an eruption on the nipple and areola, which generally present a florid, intensely red, finely granulated surface like that of acute eczema or acute balanitis. The surface exudes a copious clear, yellowish discharge, and is the seat of tingling, itching, and burning sensations. In other cases the eruption resembles chronic eczema, with minute vesications, succeeded by moist, yellowish scabs or scales, and accompanied by viscid exudation. Sometimes it is dry, like psoriasis, with a few whitish scabs slowly desquamating. Within a period not usually exceeding two years, but possibly prolonged to ten years, a carcinomatous lump appears in the breast, often at a point remote from the nipple, and usually in discontinuity with the eczematous skin. (Fig. 253 and Plate 82.)

It should be stated here that eczema of the nipple, according to R. Williams, may persist as long as twenty years without the development of a cancer. Such rare cases may be explained by the facts of atrophic scirrhus (*see* p. 79), and they do not affect the broad statement that intractable eczema of the nipple is generally followed clinically by the development of cancer.

Histological appearances.—The description best borne out by my own observations is that originally given by Butlin. The mucous layer of the epidermis is much thickened from hyperplasia,

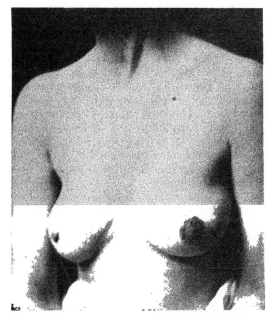

Fig. 253.—Paget's disease of the left nipple. A palpable carcinoma was present in the breast.

(*From a case under the writer's care at the Middlesex Hospital.*)

and its cells are vacuolated and swollen; the corium, the adjacent subcutaneous tissues, and the tissues round the ducts are infiltrated with small, round, lymphocyte-like cells. The galactophorous ducts are dilated and filled with epithelial cells and débris, while smaller ducts and acini may be filled with epithelium or may exhibit epithelial outgrowths into the surrounding tissues. In other cases fully developed carcinoma is seen at some part or other of the breast. The carcinoma may be a duct carcinoma, and Butlin has recorded a case in which squamous-celled carcinoma of the nipple was associated with chronic eczema, but the growth is usually acinous or spheroidal-celled, and accordingly the mass which it forms is unconnected at first with the eczematous areola, from which all induration is absent.

Pathology of Paget's disease.— Darier in 1889, supported by Wickham in 1890, declared that Paget's disease was due to infection of the skin by psorosperms, small parasitic algæ allied to the diatoms, frequently found in the liver of the rabbit and in certain fishes. Subsequent observers have shown that the supposed psorosperms in the skin of the areola are really vacuoles or secretion granules, or are appearances due to the degeneration of the epithelial cells. The psorosperm theory, abandoned by ·its originator, now finds very few supporters.

As far back as 1881, George Thin stated the view that in Paget's disease—or, as he called it, malignant papillary dermatitis—a carcinoma originating in the epithelium of the ducts near the nipple was the precursor of the changes in the skin of the areola. He believed the eczema to result from the irritant discharge of the carcinoma. Thin's view is probably true in some cases, but it is not applicable to most, for as a rule the carcinoma forms a lump in the breast isolated from the nipple by a considerable extent of clinically normal breast tissue, and is of acinous type.

Schambacher (1905) maintained that Paget's disease is a carcinoma originating within the epidermis and subsequently spreading along the milk-ducts. This view seems to be entirely negatived by the absence of any sign of neoplastic overgrowth in the eczematous skin.

My own views upon Paget's disease may be succinctly stated as follows : A carcinoma which may be either a duct carcinoma or one of acinous type originates in the breast. Frequently this carcinoma is of a somewhat atrophic variety, and it is known that an atrophic scirrhus may be present in the breast for years without producing any palpable lump. While still in the impalpable stage the carcinoma may permeate the lymphatics of the breast, many of which may be subsequently converted by fibrosis into solid strands of fibrous tissue. Considerable disturbance in the lymphatic circulation results, especially in the region of the nipple, which in middle-aged women is the most dependent part of the breast. Eczema of the nipple is merely a secondary manifestation of impaired lymphatic return from the skin of the areolar district, though it may precede by some years the stage in which the original carcinoma can be felt as a definite lump. Eczema as the result of lymphatic obstruction is frequently seen upon the sodden skin of the leg in elephantiasis, and even venous obstruction is competent to produce a like condition, as in the common case of varicose eczema. The swelling and vacuolation of the deeper layers of the epidermis of the areola and the round-celled infiltration of the derma are to be explained as the results of lymphatic obstruction.

Diagnosis.—If a lump presenting the characters of a carcinoma is already present in the breast, if the axillary glands are hard and enlarged, or if the nipple shows retraction or partial destruction, Paget's disease cannot be mistaken for simple eczema of the nipple. In cases where such signs are wanting, the failure of the usual appli. cations for eczema is the foundation upon which a diagnosis of Paget's disease must rest. While simple eczema of the nipple may be bilateral, Paget's disease is a unilateral affection.

Prognosis.—True Paget's disease is invariably associated with carcinoma, which usually manifests itself clinically within two years of the onset of the eczema. The prognosis is that of cancer of the breast in general, and is favourable only when early and complete operation is performed. Nevertheless, the form of cancer associated with Paget's disease often runs a prolonged course.

Treatment.—If dermatological treatment fails to cure the eczema, the case should be treated as one of cancer of the breast, even if no lump can be felt (*see* p. 82). In early cases it may not be thought necessary to ablate the pectoral muscles, but if this is not done it is extremely difficult to extirpate the highest axillary glands (subclavian glands). If the history of eczema is a long one it is safer to perform the complete operation for carcinoma (p. 89).

CHANCRE OF THE NIPPLE

Primary chancre of the nipple is rarely seen in the mother of a syphilitic infant, for either she is immunized by a previous attack of the disease, or, in accordance with Colles's law, the syphilitic fœtus has protected its mother without infecting her. On the other hand, a wet-nurse, or any woman, married or unmarried, who may casually hold the child to her breast, or who in any other way comes in contact with mucous patches on the lips, is liable to contract the disease.

A breast chancre is usually found on the areola at the base of the nipple, but may be situated on the skin of the breast. Though generally single, it may be multiple, and both breasts may be affected. It often fails to conform to the type of the characteristic Hunterian chancre. It may present itself as a non-indurated and apparently trivial fissure or excoriation, or as a minute, rounded and slightly elevated induration covered by reddened skin, which subsequently ulcerates at its centre. The ulcer gives rise to little discharge, and may be covered by a scab. In other cases the base becomes sloughy, and phagedæna may supervene. Sometimes the adjoining nipple becomes swollen and painful. Soon the axillary glands become enlarged and hard, but they are not tender nor do they lose their mobility. The further progress of the case is that of syphilis (*see* Vol. I., p. 729), and the appearance of secondary symptoms clears up any doubt as to the diagnosis, if a scraping has not already revealed the presence of the *Treponema pallidum* (*Spirochæte pallida*).

Chancre of the nipple would appear to be decreasing in frequency. Owing to its rarity it is apt to escape recognition.

DISEASES OF THE MAMMARY GLAND

ACUTE MASTITIS

Acute mastitis is usually associated with the function of lactation. This variety, therefore, will be first completely considered, and the rarer ones will be separately dealt with.

The acute mastitis of lactation has for its chief predisposing cause the condition known as milk engorgement, while its exciting cause is the entrance of suppurative organisms through a crack or abrasion of the nipple (*see* Cracked Nipple, p. 9), or along the milk-ducts. Acute mastitis may terminate by resolution, or may end in mammary abscess.

Milk engorgement.—During the earliest days of lactation the normal mammary hyperæmia may become excessive. This is specially likely if the milk secreted is unable to escape. Some of the mammary ducts from long disuse may be partially blocked by epithelial débris, and in this case the signs of engorgement may be restricted to the corresponding lobe or lobes of the breast. Diffuse engorgement of both breasts is usually associated with the sudden cessation of lactation, as upon the death or weaning of the child. Unilateral engorgement commonly depends upon congenital retraction of the corresponding nipple, with consequent inability to suckle on the affected side. The breast becomes swollen, hot, tense, and painful. Irregular branching areas of induration mark out the course of the distended milk-ducts, while the breast tissue itself takes on a coarse granular hardness. The superficial veins are prominent. The axillary glands may become tender and somewhat enlarged. Headache, slight pyrexia, and constipation are frequently present. If a portion only of the breast is affected, the swelling has a sector-shaped outline corresponding to the shape of the affected lobe or lobes. No sharp line of demarcation can be drawn between milk engorgement and acute parenchymatous mastitis terminating in mammary abscess, the one condition passing imperceptibly into the other.

It is important not to mistake mere engorgement or parenchymatous mastitis for suppurative inflammation of the breast. No incision should be made into the breast unless the signs of abscess are definite. The **treatment of milk engorgement** is to empty the breasts, to relieve pain and congestion, and to support the heavy breast by a sling or bandage. The first object is best attained by gentle massage directed from the periphery of the breast towards the nipple. Rodman recommends the use of a mixture of lanoline 1 part, and benzoated lard 7 parts, as a friction application, the mixture being melted on a water-bath each time it is used. Hot fomentations in the intervals of massage relieve pain and congestion, but are likely to increase the risk of suppuration, and in slight cases a cold evaporating lotion is better treatment. A mild purgative is given. If further lactation is not desired, glycerine of belladonna should be applied to the breast and a course of " white mixture " or potassium iodide ordered. Lastly, and perhaps most important, the nipple must be washed with boric lotions, and a mild mercurial ointment should be ordered if there is any crack or abrasion, provided that the breast is not being used for suckling. The breast must be relieved at intervals by the cautious use of the breast-pump.

If any crack or abrasion is present upon the nipple of an engorged breast, or if bacteria invade the milk-ducts, the engorgement passes by imperceptible degrees into a true bacterial inflammation or **acute mastitis.** T. H. C. Benians has recently found that, in a large proportion of cases, *Staphylococcus pyogenes aureus* is present in pure culture. In a certain number of cases, streptococci, and more rarely *Staphylococcus pyogenes albus*, are found, generally mixed with *S. pyogenes aureus.* Occasionally in puerperal septicæmia the microorganisms may gain access to the mammary gland by way of the blood, but mammary abscess is not a common complication of puerperal fever.

Cohn and Neumann find that staphylococci sometimes occur in the milk from normal breasts. If there is obstruction to the milkducts the bacteria rapidly increase in number, the imprisoned milk forming an ideal medium for the multiplication of the bacteria which are rarely absent from the region of the nipple. According to Benians the course of events is as follows : When suckling ceases, staphylococci multiply in the stagnant milk, and clotting ensues. The irritation caused by the milk-clot, the bacteria and their products, leads to invasion by leucocytes. If these cells are unable to destroy or to render inert the bacteria, a mammary abscess results.

The *Staphylococcus pyogenes aureus* is the usual cause of abscesses produced by obstruction to the flow of milk. In cases where a streptococcus is found a cracked nipple is usually present, and the infection spreads from the crack, along the lymphatics of the breast, without at first causing obstruction to the flow of milk.

Symptoms of acute mastitis.—The symptoms of milk engorgement are present in acute mastitis in a more pronounced degree ; the breast becomes more tense and prominent, and a local induration may become evident, especially in the lower part of the gland, while the pyrexia reaches 103° or 104°. Throbbing pain and often an erythematous blush are present. Such cases usually terminate in abscess, and fluctuation is soon to be detected over the indurated area, while one or more rigors may occur.

Treatment of acute mastitis.—Hot fomentations should be substituted for the cold applications suitable for milk engorgement, the infant should be weaned, and energetic measures taken to stop the secretion of milk. The breast should be carefully supported by a bandage, but any severe degree of pressure is too painful to be borne. A careful watch must be kept for signs of suppuration.

ACUTE MAMMARY ABSCESS

Though acute mammary abscess is usually connected with lactation, this is not invariably the case. Thus, infantile or adolescent mastitis, especially if meddlesome treatment be adopted, may not rarely terminate in abscess. At any age an injury of the breast, with or without the formation of a hæmatoma at the seat of injury, may lead to an abscess. Occasionally an apparently spontaneous abscess is met with in the adult virgin breast. Of 102 consecutive cases of mammary abscess observed by Bryant, 79 occurred during lactation, 2 during pregnancy, and 21 in patients who were neither lactating nor pregnant.

Abscesses of the breast are divided into three classes, according to their situation in the organ—(1) subareolar or supramammary abscess; (2) parenchymatous or deep or intramammary abscess; (3) retromammary abscess. The first two varieties are common, and usually either occur during the first month of lactation, or follow impairment of health by prolonged suckling, or the sudden cessation of lactation. Retraction of the nipple, which interferes with the due emptying of the breast by suckling, favours milk engorgement and abscess. The importance of cracks and abrasions upon the nipple has already been mentioned. Retromammary abscess is less closely associated with lactation.

1. In *subareolar abscess* pus forms immediately beneath the skin of the areola. Accordingly, redness of the skin is an early and prominent symptom, and fluctuation is very obvious. The abscess is smaller and causes less constitutional disturbance than the deeper varieties of suppuration.

2. *Intramammary abscess* is the most common and most important variety. Owing to the depth at which the pus forms, fluctuation may be absent, or difficult to elicit. Pus may burrow extensively through the gland in various directions before it approaches the skin. Meantime, constitutional disturbance is often severe, and the whole breast is involved in œdematous swelling. Later, when the abscess is beginning to point, the skin becomes red or mottled. After such an abscess, unless surgical treatment is careful and thorough, the breast may be left in a disorganized and useless condition, riddled by persistent sinuses, and sometimes shrunken and deformed by cicatrization.

3. *Retromammary abscess* is not common. It may arise from necrosis or tuberculosis of a rib, from tuberculosis of the sternum, from an infected hæmatoma, or from suppuration of the deeper portions of the breast. The collection of pus is usually large, and is situated between the great pectoral and the deep surface of the mamma. The breast is thrust prominently forward, and is found to be lying upon a fluctuating cushion of pus. The skin of the breast is not reddened. The abscess usually points at the lower and outer margin of the breast.

Prophylaxis of mammary abscess.—It is necessary to take precautions against cracks, fissures, or abrasions of the nipple, to keep the nipple and the child's mouth in as aseptic a condition as possible, and to maintain the patency of the milk-ducts. During pregnancy the nipple should be hardened by regularly rubbing it with alcohol (eau-de-Cologne or spirit). After suckling the nipple must be bathed with boric lotion and then carefully dried, and the infant's mouth cleansed with a rag dipped in the same lotion.

Treatment of mammary abscess.—The abscess, if *subareolar* or *intramammary*, must be opened at the earliest possible moment by a free incision, which, in order to avoid cutting the milk-ducts, should radiate from the nipple. The finger should be introduced into the cavity, and all septa found traversing it should be broken down so as to ensure free drainage. A rubber tube should be left in the cavity, and careful watch kept for burrowing or pocketing of pus in new directions. A dry gauze dressing, changed daily, may be applied.

If any signs of burrowing appear, a director must be passed in various directions, and the pockets must either be slit up along their whole length, or opened and drained by tubes at the most dependent points.

Constitutional and general treatment will vary according to the nature of the abscess. Lactation must be stopped either by the regular administration of white mixture, or of saline purgatives in other combinations, or by giving potassium iodide in doses of 5-10 gr.

thrice daily. At the same time glycerine of belladonna is applied to both breasts, which are then to be firmly bandaged over a layer of wool. If the patient is exhausted by long lactation a more tonic treatment is necessary. Saline purgatives must be replaced by iron and strychnine, and a generous diet prescribed, while a glass of burgundy with lunch and dinner may be of advantage after the flow of milk has ceased.

Retromammary abscess is best opened by an incision situated in the sulcus beneath the breast and at its lower and outer margin. Search should be made at the operation for bare bone, and for an opening communicating with the thoracic cavity.

Mammary abscess due to tubercle, actinomycosis, or syphilis will be referred to under the heads of those diseases. Abscess may result from hydatid disease of the breast.

Bier's hyperæmia in acute mastitis.—Bier recommends the treatment of acute mastitis in all its stages by a dome-shaped cupping glass, of a diameter about an inch smaller than the mammary gland itself, and with a margin curved to fit the chest wall. Air is cautiously withdrawn by a suction syringe; the breast protrudes into the bell and becomes blue and engorged. When the patient finally feels as if the breast would burst, the exhaustion of air should be stopped, for the entire procedure should be painless. Usually one or two ounces of milk escape. Abscesses and sinuses, which at first discharge blood and pus, yield only blood-stained serous fluid towards the end of the sitting. If pain is not relieved, an abscess must be suspected, and should be opened by a small incision, the patency of which must be maintained by a drainage-tube. Large incisions are said to be unnecessary when Bier's treatment is used. The glass is to be applied for forty-five minutes daily, suction for five minutes alternating with release of pressure for three minutes. When suppuration ceases the duration of the daily sitting may be lessened.

Vaccine treatment of acute mastitis.—The vaccine treatment of acute mastitis and mammary abscess is so recent that it is not yet possible to estimate its value. In acute mastitis where suppuration threatens, if a cracked nipple is present, a vaccine may be prepared from the organisms found in the crack, and by its prompt use the formation of an abscess may be averted. If streptococci are seen in a stained film, a stock vaccine may be used without waiting for a cultivation.

In cases of acute mastitis where no cracked nipple is present, the *Staphylococcus pyogenes aureus* is probably the infecting agent. It is accordingly reasonable to endeavour to avert suppuration by injections of a stock vaccine of this organism in doses of 400-500 millions at intervals of a week.

If suppuration has already occurred the pus must be let out by incision. The value of vaccine treatment during the acute stage is doubtful.

In cases where sinuses persist, usually as the result of inadequate surgical treatment, vaccine treatment appears to be of great value. The treatment should consist in the weekly injection of 400–800 millions of *S. aureus* in stock vaccine, controlled, if the case does not rapidly yield, by cultivations which may show the presence of other organisms. In such cases an autogenous vaccine is prepared for use.

CHRONIC MASTITIS

In women who have reached or passed middle life the breasts, or portions of them, are very liable to undergo certain fibroid changes, associated either with hypertrophy or with atrophy of the secreting epithelium. The condition is known as chronic mastitis or chronic lobular mastitis. According to the condition of the epithelium, two forms may be recognized—hypertrophic mastitis and atrophic mastitis. Chronic mastitis is a frequent precursor of breast cancer (*see* p. 50), and owes its chief importance to this fact and to its clinical resemblances to cancer.

Etiology.—Chronic mastitis may occur at any age after puberty. It is not very rare in young unmarried women, and its frequency probably increases up to a maximum at the menopause, the age near which a large majority of the cases occur. Some authors state that it is more common among married women, but my own experience indicates a greater frequency in the unmarried.

The onset of chronic mastitis is sometimes determined by a blow. Lenthal Cheatle has recently brought forward strong reasons to believe that the pressure of ill-fitting corsets, and more especially the impaling of the breast upon the upper end of a stay-bone, may induce local mastitis at the seat of pressure.

Chronic mastitis is most frequently seen in the axillary tail, and in the portion of the breast immediately adjoining, but may occur in any part of the breast.

It may be regarded as a morbid deviation in the normal physiological processes of evolution and involution which correspond with the sexual crises of a woman's life—puberty, menstruation, pregnancy, lactation, and the menopause. Apart from these physiological tides of tissue change, mild bacterial invasion and obstruction of the ducts may play a part, though Lenthal Cheatle's researches go to show that the disease is not dependent on bacterial infection.

Naked-eye anatomy of chronic mastitis.—A breast the seat of marked chronic mastitis, when cut across, is tough and "indiarubbery" in consistence, and has not the inelastic hardness of a typical carcinoma. Its colour is whitish or yellowish, with a trace of pink, but without the grey tones usually seen in a carcinoma. Small cysts containing clear or brownish fluid are sometimes a prominent feature. In some cases these cysts attain exceptional development and cause a considerable increase in the size of the breast. To this condition the name " cystic disease of the breast " has been given, but it differs in no essential respect from chronic mastitis (Fig. 254).

Histological changes.—In the hypertrophic form of chronic mastitis the lobules are much increased in size by proliferation of their constituent acini (Fig. 255). Though this is the most important change, it is not the earliest. The epithelial hypertrophy is preceded by changes in the lobular and peri-acinous connective tissue. The lobular connective tissue is swollen and increased in amount, and the connective-tissue sheath of each acinus becomes thickened and unduly cellular, and is the seat of a round-celled infiltration of varying degree. The elastic tissue around the ducts tends to disappear. Later the richly cellular peri-acinous connective tissue undergoes the usual transformation of young fibrous tissue, and changes into characteristic rings of homogeneous fibrous tissue almost free from nuclei. The interlobular tissue also undergoes a fibroid change, and much of the fat disappears.

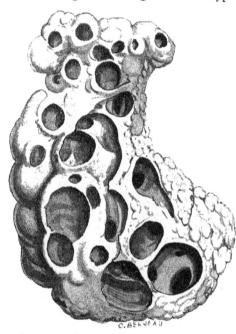

Fig. 254.—**Cystic chronic mastitis** (cystic disease of the breast).

(*From a specimen in the Middlesex Hospital Museum.*)

Atrophic chronic mastitis (fibroid breast) appears to be a late stage of the hypertrophic variety. In this form a microscopic section shows dense and old fibrous tissue, poor in nuclei. Embedded here and there in the fibrous tissue, islets of fat cells still remain. The lobules (groups of acini) which have escaped destruction are small, few in number, and widely scattered. The epithelium of the acini is far advanced in degeneration, and may be represented by a few shrunken cells, often lacking a central lumen, or merely by a little mass of débris (Figs. 256, 257).

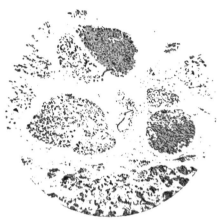

Fig. 255.—Hypertrophic mastitis. Note the increase in size of the lobules. At the lower margin of the figure the edge of an infiltrating carcinoma can be seen—a condition into which hypertrophic mastitis may readily pass.

Symptoms.—Many women present some degree of chronic mastitis without any corresponding symptoms. In other cases, however, pain is a prominent symptom—usually a dull ache, but occasionally very severe, lancinating or neuralgic in character, and very intractable. The pain may be worse, and the swelling more marked, during the menstrual periods. It is often aggravated by movements, and especially by the prolonged use of the arm or by jolting movements such as descending stairs.

Discharge from the nipple. — The frequent presence of tense cysts in chronic mastitis shows that there is considerable secretory pressure within the gland. It is, therefore, not surprising that a serous discharge from the nipple appears in certain cases in which

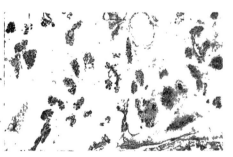

Fig. 256.—Microscopic appearances of atrophic mastitis. Note the atrophy of the lobules, the increase of fibrous tissue, and the disappearance of the interlobular fat.

obstruction of the ducts is incomplete. The discharge may be made to flow by pressure upon the affected portion of the gland. It emanates from the particular orifice upon the nipple which corresponds to the diseased lobe of the gland. Such cases are often very difficult to distinguish from early examples of duct papilloma. Fortunately the doubt in diagnosis makes no difference as regards treatment ; for it is a rule to which, in my opinion, there are no exceptions, that persistent serous discharge from the nipple in a woman of middle age should be the signal for excision of the breast.

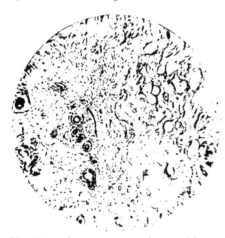

Physical signs.— There is a granular induration of the whole or part of the breast tissue, only vaguely felt when the breast is compressed between the flat hand and the pectoral muscle, but assuming the characters of a definite tumour when the breast is compressed laterally between the thumb and fingers. When cystic changes are present the cysts usually feel solid, and the breast feels more coarsely granular. Although it is often stated that retraction of the nipple and adhesion of the skin may occur in chronic mastitis, the presence of these signs should give rise to the gravest suspicion of malignant disease. Nor is adhesion of the breast to the pectoral fascia ever seen in chronic mastitis.

Fig. 257.—Advanced atrophic mastitis or fibroid breast. The lobular epithelium has almost disappeared, but a few dark rings indicate remains of epithelium. On the right is seen fat undergoing fibroid change.

Atrophic chronic mastitis involving the whole breast may reduce the gland to a firm, " rubbery," highly convex disc, with thick rounded edges, resembling in shape the end of a lemon, and not exceeding 2 in. in diameter. This condition is only found as the menopause is approached. It is due to fibrous change retracting all the lobes towards the nipple, their common point of attachment. It must be remembered that an abscess may leave a palpable fibrous area in the breast, adherent to the skin at the point where the abscess burst.

Sector-shaped indurations.—In many cases the area of induration is sector-shaped. In doubtful cases I have come to rely more upon this sector-shaped induration in the diagnosis of chronic mastitis than upon any other point. The breast is made up of a number of sector-shaped lobes which are practically independent organs, each opening upon the summit of the nipple by the separate orifice of its own proper duct. Very frequently chronic mastitis affects one of the lobes alone, or several adjoining ones, while the rest of the breast remains normal and unaffected.

It will be observed that these facts supply a most important means of distinction between chronic mastitis and malignant disease. It is a characteristic feature of carcinoma that it has little or no respect for anatomical boundaries. If a carcinoma starts at one point in the breast it will not remain confined strictly to the lobe in which it originated, but will infiltrate the surrounding tissues in a more or less centrifugal manner, producing a rounded lump which has no relation to the anatomical shape of the particular lobe in which the growth originated.

Sometimes the breast contains two or more non-contiguous sector-shaped areas of induration, while in other cases, of course, the whole breast presents an indefinite induration.

It must, however, be remembered, in respect to this important physical sign, that it does not exclude the possibility that an early carcinoma is present within the sector-shaped area. If, however, the area of induration is uniformly and finely granular, without any localized lump or induration, this unpleasant possibility may be excluded almost with certainty.

Chronic mastitis and fibro-adenoma.—Areas of chronic mastitis are not infrequently met with in the immediate neighbourhood of a fibro-adenoma, giving to the smooth surface of the tumour a rough, granular feeling. The pathology of such areas is not difficult to fathom if it be borne in mind that a fibro-adenoma often arises in connexion with, and necessarily obstructs, one of the ducts of the breast. The acini which open into this particular duct, having no outlet, undergo the usual changes of chronic mastitis. It is often exceedingly difficult to differentiate a fibro-adenoma, thus obscured by surrounding chronic mastitis, from a carcinoma. I have most frequently met with such fibro-adenomas in or near the axillary tail of the breast.

F. T. Paul has, moreover, shown that a fibro-adenoma may originate in an area of pre-existing chronic mastitis by the over-growth of the connective tissue of one particular lobule of the affected area. Thus fibro-adenoma may be either a cause or a consequence of chronic mastitis.

Chronic mastitis in duct papilloma.—In another condition chronic mastitis may arise from obstruction of the ducts, namely, duct papilloma. When a duct papilloma obstructs one of the large ducts near the nipple the corresponding lobe is often mapped out as a vague, sector-shaped induration. Pressure upon the indurated area often causes serous fluid to exude, or even squirt, from the affected duct, while pressure upon the normal portions of the breast has no effect.

Enlargement of the axillary glands.—It is not uncommon to find in chronic mastitis that the axillary glands are unduly palpable—that is to say, they are slightly but not much enlarged. The glands are firm and elastic, and sometimes tender. The slight degree of enlargement, the tenderness, and the absence of hardness help to distinguish them from secondary carcinomatous glands.

Bonney has drawn attention to the precarcinomatous changes which occur in lymphatic glands. When a cancer is present, e.g. in the breast, the axillary glands become enlarged, owing to the appearance of large and active germinal areas, to an increase in the number of lymphocytes, and to the appearance in the gland of large quantities of plasma cells. All these changes, according to Bonney, occur before any malignant cells have reached the gland. In a less degree he found the same changes in the axillary glands of ten breasts removed for chronic mastitis and proved microscopically to be free from cancer.

A consideration of these facts makes it seem likely that cases of chronic mastitis in which the glands are unduly palpable are more likely to end in cancer than are those in which this sign is absent. In such·cases removal of the breast may be the best course to pursue, but no general rule can be laid down.

Diagnosis.—The indurations of chronic mastitis are characterized by their vague definition when palpated by the flat hand, thus differing from both simple and malignant tumours. The sector-shape of the indurations is also characteristic when only part of the breast is involved. Moreover, as further distinctions from carcinoma, nipple retraction and adhesion to skin and fascia are absent. A carcinomatous lump in the breast is usually single, while the indurations of chronic mastitis are often multiple. The axillary glands are softish, elastic, possibly tender, and not much enlarged, while the glands in carcinoma are hard, painless, and often much increased in size. If a hardness is present in the area of ill-defined induration, it may be impossible to say without operation whether a carcinoma or a simple cyst is the cause (Fig. 258), for it must not be forgotten that a carcinoma may arise in a pre-existing area of mastitis.

Prognosis.—In young women, chronic mastitis is tractable and not dangerous ; but as the menopause is approached, a more guarded prognosis and a closer watch become necessary in view of the intimate relations between chronic mastitis and cancer.

Treatment.—In some cases of chronic mastitis, especially in young women, the usual medicinal treatment is satisfactory. The means employed comprise (*a*) pressure applied by means of strapping, or less effectively by bandages (massage is not advisable) ; (*b*) inhibition of the secretory activity of the epithelium by belladonna and iodides ; (c) the administration of drugs which promote the absorption of inflammatory infiltrations, especially mercury and the iodides. I am not aware that fibrolysin has been tried in mastitis, and the use of this drug for other conditions seems not absolutely free from danger. The old-fashioned emp. hydrarg. c. ammoniaco, renewed weekly, is a valuable application, but is liable to cause eczematous irritation of the skin. This risk can be minimized by antiseptic cleansing of the skin before the plaster is applied. Another method of using mercury is to apply Scott's ointment, diluted if necessary, and to secure pressure at the same time by means of strapping. Iodides may be applied locally in the form of the lin. pot. iod. c. sapone, a very clean and pleasant preparation, but not, in my belief, a very effective one. Belladonna may be used as the glycerinum or unguentum, combined, if necessary, with a mercurial ointment. It is especially valuable where pain is a prominent symptom.

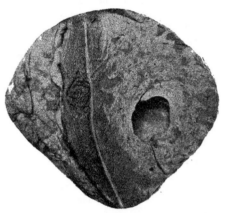

Fig. 258.—A breast, the seat of chronic mastitis and containing a single cyst. The case simulated a carcinoma, and the breast was therefore removed.

(*From St. Thomas's Hospital Museum.*)

But in numerous instances, more especially in climacteric mastitis, drug treatment seems to have no effect. In such cases, removal of the breast is often justifiable. F. T. Paul says :—" I am no advocate for the removal of the breast for mastitis in young women . . . but as regards the involution period, I strongly maintain that amputation is indicated in all cases of unyielding or very marked, and especially bilateral, chronic mastitis."

There can be no doubt that such a course is the safest. But removal of the breast, although not in itself a severe or dangerous operation, is a measure to which few women will consent unless the risk of cancer is immediate and great. Moreover, there are numerous clear cases of chronic mastitis in which cancer can be definitely excluded, even in women who have reached the cancer age. In such cases I do not advise operation.

Thus, deducting the cases where drug treatment is successful and those threatening or doubtful ones where operation is clearly indicated, there remains a considerable residue of cases for which hitherto no very hopeful treatment has been available.

In such cases, during the past few years, I have recommended a short course of X-rays as a sedative to epithelial activity and a prophylactic against cancer. So far, in none of the cases thus treated has cancer subsequently developed. But the number of cases treated is too small to make the evidence conclusive.

With regard to the clinically appreciable effects of X-rays in chronic mastitis, my experience is at present recent and restricted; but on more than one occasion after their use I have seen indurations of the breast clear up or become almost inappreciable. Sometimes, on the other hand, the induration remains unaltered.

The following is the first case in which I used X-rays for chronic mastitis :—

M. F., æt. 43, attended the Middlesex Hospital in March, 1906, complaining of pain and induration in the left breast. There was marked, though indefinite, induration of the breast, extending to its axillary tail. On October 3rd, 1906, I asked Mr. C. R. C. Lyster to give the breast six X-ray exposures of ten minutes each. The exposures were completed by October 17th. Up to October 15th the pain was aggravated, and on the 17th no palpable change could be detected in the breast. On October 31st, however, a striking change was manifest, for the left breast, instead of being more indurated than the right one, was distinctly softer. The patient, however, still complained of pain in the axillary tail of the left breast, and in this situation some induration remained. On October 31st I asked Mr. Lyster to give six exposures to the axilla, so as to reach the axillary tail, which is, of course, protected by the great pectoral when the arm is lying close to the chest. On December 10th, 1906, no lumpiness could be detected in either breast. The patient complained of pains in the arms and head, but not in the breasts. This patient was seen again in February, 1909, about three years after her first visit. The breasts, though somewhat fibroid, were quite free from localized indurations, and were practically normal. The cure may be presumed, therefore, to be a permanent one. The left breast is slightly smaller than the right.

Further experience has confirmed my belief in the value of X-rays in chronic mastitis.

TUBERCULOUS MASTITIS

Tuberculosis of the breast is rare, accounting for only about 1 per cent. of hospital admissions for mammary disease. More than half the cases occur between the ages of 25 and 35, and very few indeed after the menopause, though even old age is not exempt. The affection is usually unilateral. It may form the only discoverable tuberculous focus present in the body, but in 50 per cent. of cases it is secondary to tuberculosis elsewhere, as, for instance, in the supraclavicular or axillary glands, or in the lungs. Infection probably usually occurs through the blood-stream or by direct extension from the adjoining ribs or pleura. But it is not rare for tuberculosis of the cervical glands to extend downwards to the axillary glands, and a continuance of the same process of retrograde infection along the lymphatics to the breast may be responsible for some cases of mammary tubercle. It is also possible that direct infection along the ducts from the nipple may in some cases take place. In one recorded case the disease began as an ulceration of the nipple.

Morbid anatomy.—Miliary tubercles may be scattered through the breasts in cases of general tuberculosis, but this form of the disease possesses no separate importance. In tuberculous mastitis the breast in section presents multiple caseating foci, separated by fibrotic areas, and areas of healthy tissue. Later, these caseating areas tend to coalesce and break down, and one or more abscesses, lined by pale and flabby granulations and containing caseous pus, may be formed. These abscesses, after breaking through the skin, shrink into chromic sinuses, and in the latest stage the breast becomes a fibrous relic, riddled in all directions by tuberculous sinuses.

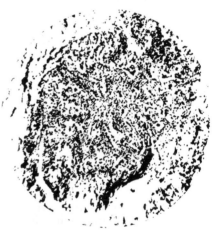

Fig. 259.—Tubercle of the breast. A lobule showing early tuberculous change occupies almost the whole field. The picture appears confused, but careful observation will show as characteristic points—(a) the quiet disappearance of the epithelium; (b) the formation of a ring of granulation tissue round each acinus; (c) the absence of giant cells, which appear later in the disease.

Microscopic anatomy.— In its earliest stage, tuberculosis of the breast presents itself microscopically in the form of dense masses of lymphocyte-like cells around the acini and along the course of the smaller ducts. The collection of round cells lies outside the layer of fibrous tissue which immediately surrounds the epithelium. Giant-cell systems may be absent. (Fig. 259.) As the areas of round cells increase in density the epithelial structures quietly atrophy and disappear, leaving a mass of tuberculous granulation tissue in which typical giant cells can now be recognized. This granulation tissue may undergo fibrosis or caseation, or from its liquefaction one or more abscesses of considerable size and lined by tuberculous granulations may be formed. The areas of fat intervening between the mammary lobules undergo fibrous degeneration.

If a large abscess is formed, the overlying skin may show the clinical appearance of *peau d'orange*, and as seen microscopically it may present the dermal thickening which indicates lymphatic obstruction.

Clinical features.—The first sign is the appearance in the breast of one or more vague indurations, indistinguishable from simple chronic mastitis. It is important to note that more than one indurated area is usually present in the affected breast. As the case progresses more massive indurations are formed, palpable with the flat hand, and suggestive of malignant disease. This similarity may be increased by the presence of enlarged tuberculous axillary glands, and by the adhesion of the mass to the skin and to the underlying fascia. The overlying skin may assume the characteristic orange-rind appearance. But soon after adhesion to the skin has occurred a soft central patch becomes evident in the indurated mass. The skin at this point becomes thin and reddened, and an abscess points and bursts, leaving a persistent sinus with pale flabby granulations at its entrance, discharging thin pus containing caseous débris.

Cold abscess of the breast presents itself as a cystic swelling with a tendency to become adherent to the skin. It is usually of tuberculous origin. *Tuberculous submammary abscess* is met with as the result of tubercle of the ribs, costal cartilages, or sternum.

Differential diagnosis.—In its earliest stage, tuberculosis of the breast cannot be distinguished from chronic mastitis. In the stage prior to softening and abscess-formation it may closely resemble carcinoma. The tuberculous patient is, however, generally under 35, and usually presents multiple indurations, while a carcinoma is commonly a single lump. The presence of a central area of softening in the mass and of reddening of the skin points to tuberculosis, and the diagnosis is confirmed if pus be withdrawn by a hypodermic syringe. In very rare cases, tuberculosis and carcinoma may coexist. Gumma of the breast may closely resemble tuberculosis (*see* p. 29). The diagnosis between chronic abscess and simple cyst is made by exploratory puncture if signs of pointing fail to give the clue. In duct papilloma, discharge from the nipple usually occurs at some time or other. Actinomycosis of the breast can only be differentiated by the detection of the ray fungus.

Prognosis.—Mammary tuberculosis has little tendency to

spontaneous cure, and, if untreated, will probably lead to multiple sinuses persisting for years. The continued discharge may undermine the health and lead to lardaceous disease. In the absence of other tuberculous lesions in the body, the prognosis after removal of the breast is good. The subsequent development of tuberculosis in the other breast is very rare, but 20 per cent. of patients who have suffered from mammary tuberculosis die ultimately of phthisis.

Treatment.—If a chronic abscess is the only sign of disease in the breast, it may suffice to open it, to scrape it, and to allow it to heal from the bottom. But if, as is usual, there are multiple foci, it is wiser to amputate the breast. The axillary glands, if markedly enlarged, should be removed at the same time. Partial resection of the breast is justifiable in young women if the disease is definitely confined to certain lobules.

No experience as to the effects of tuberculin in mammary tubercle is yet available. Unless it becomes possible to make the diagnosis earlier than at present, it seems unlikely that tuberculin treatment will supersede operation. It is stated that Bier's treatment by passive hyperæmia has given good results (see p. 18).

ACTINOMYCOSIS

Actinomycosis is one of the rarest mammary diseases. It may reach the breast primarily through a wound or abrasion, or secondarily by extension from the lungs and pleura, or by metastasis from other organs. In its early stage the disease presents itself as one or more areas of local induration indistinguishable from the vague indurations of chronic mastitis, or as a definite rounded tumour. The axillary glands are usually unaffected. Later, at various points over the indurated area, softening may be detected. The skin at these points becomes reddened, glazed, and thinned, and finally gives way. A number of discharging sinuses are left, burrowing in various directions through the shrunken breast, and exuding pus containing the characteristic and diagnostic "iodoform granules." The disease may spread by metastasis to other regions of the body.

Treatment.—In the early stage the free administration of potassium iodide in large doses is indicated. Later, if the disease is primary, complete excision of the affected breast is probably the best treatment. If the disease is well localized the affected part may be resected.

GUMMA OF THE BREAST

In the tertiary stage of syphilis, localized deposits of syphilitic granulation tissue may occur in the breast as in most other parts of the body. Gummata of the breast are, however, not common. They may be single or multiple, and are rarely found except in association

with active manifestations of the disease in other regions—a fact which
is of great assistance in diagnosis. A gumma presents itself as a firm
and even hard tumour, fixed in the breast, painless, palpable with
the flat hand, and sharply defined from the surrounding tissues. It
soon becomes adherent to the skin and to the underlying pectoral
fascia. The adherent skin may present the *peau d'orange* appearance.
Retraction of the nipple may be present if the tumour is subareolar.
Up to this stage the diagnosis from carcinoma depends chiefly upon
the history, and upon the presence of other syphilitic lesions. Soon,
however, the adherent skin over the tumour becomes thinned and
congested, and a central area of softening appears in the hard tumour.
The skin now gives way and a puriform discharge escapes. The ulcer
thus formed may present the characters of a typical gummatous ulcer
with a sloughy base. Occasionally a massive slough is thrown off,
and the ulcer spontaneously heals. The glands in the axilla do not,
as a rule, become enlarged unless secondary infection occurs through
the ulcer. Treatment is an important means of confirming a pro-
visional diagnosis of gumma. In rare cases, diffuse unilateral induration of the breast has been observed comparatively early in the
secondary stage of syphilis.

Treatment.—The only treatment required is the regular and
vigorous administration of potassium iodide, beginning with 5 or
10 gr. thrice daily, and increasing the dose to 20 or even 30 gr. The
induration rapidly and completely disappears. If the gumma is
ulcerated a mild mercurial ointment should be applied.

HÆMATOMA OF THE BREAST

This condition is not often seen, and is usually due to a blow.
The rapid appearance of a traumatic swelling, associated after a day or
two with cutaneous ecchymosis, and its disappearance within two or
three weeks, are characteristic points. The swelling may correspond
in outline to the sector-shape of a single mammary lobe, or of several
adjacent lobes. Hæmatoma may follow an operation for the removal
of a simple tumour, unless the cavity left is carefully obliterated.

Treatment.—The breast should be strapped, or at least supported in a sling, and manipulation must be avoided. In view of
the fact that trauma is a possible cause of malignant disease, a short
prophylactic course of X-rays may be advisable. If a swelling remains
after the lapse of some weeks, an exploratory incision must be made.

ELEPHANTIASIS

In tropical countries, in one case in 690 of elephantiasis, the
disease affects the breast. The breast becomes enormously and
uniformly enlarged, and the skin over it thick, leathery, and pitted

by enlarged gland orifices. The nipple may hang as low as the umbilicus, and may even reach the pubes.

These changes are preceded by attacks of acute lymphangitis, which lead to obliteration of many of the lymphatics of the breast. The enlargement of the organ and the thickening of the skin over it are results of lymphatic obstruction. The cutaneous appearances are exactly those of the " pigskin " familiar in cases of carcinoma.

Diagnosis.—In tropical countries, confusion may arise between elephantiasis and malignant disease of the breast. But in elephantiasis the breast is very greatly enlarged and no lump is present in it.

Treatment.—In early stages the breast must be supported by a sling. In view of recent work by Dufougeré, Foulerton, and myself, which tends to prove that elephantiasis depends upon a chronic infection by the *Staphylococcus pyogenes albus*, a vaccine of this organism should be tried to arrest the disease in its earlier stages. But in late cases amputation of the breast is indicated. It is unnecessary to remove the pectoral muscles or to clear out the axilla.

CYSTS OF THE BREAST

Cysts of the breast may be divided clinically into two main classes—(1) those arising in connexion with solid neoplasms (neoplastic cysts), and (2) those of obstructive or inflammatory origin where no new growth is present (simple cysts). It is difficult to be sure that a cyst, apparently simple, is not really neoplastic. When a cyst has been assigned to the neoplastic category the vital question still remains whether the solid tumour connected with it is innocent or malignant.

Cysts of the breast usually occur after the age of 40. They are not very common, forming less than 3 per cent. of cases of mammary tumour which come under hospital treatment.

The many varieties of cysts that occur in the breast may be classified as follows :—

1. Cysts arising from distension of the larger ducts. These cysts are usually single and situated near the nipple.

    i. Galactocele, or milk-cyst.

    ii. Simple subareolar cyst.

2. Multiple cysts arising from distension of the smaller ducts. These cysts are the result of chronic mastitis. The condition known as general cystic disease of the breast is simply an exaggerated form of cystic chronic mastitis (Fig. 254, p. 20).

3. Cysts due to the distension of lymphatic spaces.

4. Cysts arising in connexion with simple tumours.

    i. Cystic fibro-adenoma.

    ii. Cystic duct papilloma (Fig. 266).

5. Cysts arising in connexion with malignant tumours.
   i. Carcinoma with cystic degeneration, or arising in the
      wall of a pre-existing cyst.
   ii. Cystic forms of sarcoma.
6. Parasitic cysts due to the echinococcus.

In this section galactoceles, simple subareolar cysts, and hydatid cysts will be considered ; cysts of neoplastic origin will be dealt with in the section relating to the tumours with which they are associated.

GALACTOCELE

A galactocele is a rare mammary cyst containing milk in a more or less inspissated and altered condition. Arising from the obstruction of one of the large ducts or milk sinuses, these cysts are formed during lactation, though they may persist after it has ceased. In rare cases, galactoceles are said to occur in women who have never been pregnant, but some of these cases are probably tuberculous abscesses. The nature of the causative obstruction is not certainly known. Some authors maintain that it arises from excessive proliferation of the duct epithelium ; and blows, injuries, and surgical incisions near the nipple have been claimed as etiological factors.

Galactoceles are situated beneath or near the areola, and are, as a rule, single, though I have seen two in the same breast. They are of moderate size, rarely exceeding 3 in. in diameter ; but one enormous example, recorded by Scarpa, after two months' growth contained 10 pints of milk. The wall of the cyst, which in old examples may be of some thickness, is composed of fibrous tissue and lined by the stretched and atrophied epithelium of the duct. The contents may resemble colostrum, or normal inspissated milk, or may be a butter-like material.

Symptoms and signs.—Close to the areola there is present a rounded, painless, fluctuating swelling, which on pressure exudes a milky fluid through the nipple. It usually appears during the early weeks of lactation, and may increase in size during the act of suckling (Astley Cooper). In long-standing cases its contents become inspissated and its consistence doughy.

Diagnosis.—The commencement during lactation, and the exudation of milk from the nipple if the cyst be pressed, usually render diagnosis easy. A galactocele may, however, be mistaken for a chronic tuberculous abscess, for a simple subareolar cyst, or for a cyst connected with duct papilloma.

Treatment.—Unduly active treatment is to be deprecated. If the cyst reaches any size the child should be weaned, the cyst aspirated, and pressure applied to the breast by strapping. If these measures fail, the cyst is to be incised radially from the nipple, and either completely removed, or packed and allowed to heal from the bottom.

SIMPLE SUBAREOLAR CYST

Simple subareolar cyst is due to the obstruction of one of the large ducts near the nipple. These cysts are usually single, contain clear serous fluid, and seldom exceed 1 to 1½ in. in diameter. They are frequently associated with a vague induration of the corresponding lobe of the breast. Fluctuation is usually evident. Pain, tenderness. and enlargement of the axillary glands are generally absent. A discharge from the nipple is occasionally present, but if marked, and especially if blood-stained, it should arouse suspicion that the cyst is associated with duct papilloma.

Cysts exactly resembling the subareolar cyst may arise from the distension of ducts in the deeper parts of the breast ; they are usually associated with chronic mastitis.

Treatment.—Any suspicion of malignancy must lead to an immediate exploratory operation (*see* p. 86). If the cyst is certainly innocent, milder measures may be tried. The cyst may be aspirated and the breast subsequently strapped. A more effective method is to tap the cyst with a hypodermic needle, and to inject 5 to 10 minims of 1 per cent. solution of protargol, or the same quantity of pure phenol. The breast is subsequently manipulated to ensure that the fluid comes in contact with the whole interior of the cyst. If these measures fail, the cyst must be excised through an incision radiating from the nipple so as not to divide any of the ducts. In certain cases, Gaillard Thomas's operation (*see* p. 40) may be employed.

HYDATID DISEASE OF THE BREAST

This condition is of great rarity. A small, painless, hard lump forms in the breast, and is discovered by accident. When it reaches the size of an egg, fluctuation can usually be detected in it. Further slow increase in size during a period of years produces a prominent globular tumour as large as an orange, moving with the breast, still painless, and not adherent either to skin or fascia. The nipple is not retracted, nor are the axillary glands enlarged. If nothing is done, suppuration may ultimately occur, probably as a result of the death of the hydatid. Pain is felt in the swelling, the skin becomes reddened, and the tumour itself is larger and more prominent. The integument becomes thinned at one or several points, and sinuses form through which thin pus is discharged, containing daughter-cysts and hydatid membrane. In this way the whole of the hydatid may be discharged, and a spontaneous cure may result.

Diagnosis.—The presence of a globular, painless, fluctuating

d

single tumour, of slow growth, of considerable size, and presenting the other characters already referred to, raises a presumption of hydatid. A hydatid cyst does not give rise to discharge from the nipple—a point of distinction from cystic duct papilloma. A simple cyst rarely attains a size beyond that of an egg. The diagnosis can only be made con-elusive by an exploratory puncture. If the fluid withdrawn is free from albumin, and more especially if it contains hooklets, the diagnosis of hydatid is established.

Treatment.—The disease is practically free from risk to life. An incision radiating from the nipple is made down upon the cyst, which is enucleated entire. The cavity may be obliterated by suturing its walls together, and the skin sewn up. Of course, if suppuration is present, no attempt to secure primary union must be made.

Diagnosis of mammary cysts.—Cysts of the breast are often very tense, and consequently fluctuation is frequently absent, and diagnosis from a solid tumour may be impossible, especially if the cyst is deeply situated, without the aid of an exploring needle. The use of this instrument is free from objection, and is painless if a little ethyl chloride be used to freeze the skin. Microscopical examination decides whether the fluid is milky as in galactocele, serous as in duct papilloma, purulent as in tuberculous abscess or acute mammary abscess, containing hooklets as in hydatid cyst, or bloody as in malignant growth and in duct papilloma. Usually the microscopical examination is practically negative. If albumin is present in the fluid, non-suppurating hydatid cyst is of course excluded, and the diagnosis probably lies between two common types of cyst—the simple cyst associated with chronic mastitis, and the papilloma-bearing cyst. In the latter case there is usually a history of serous discharge from the nipple, often blood-stained.

This brief summary fails to take account of the cysts associated with malignant tumours, which, though rare, are of great importance. The question, " Is a malignant neoplasm also present ? " arises in every case of cyst. The size of the cyst is of great significance in settling this question. Simple cysts of the breast rarely exceed 1 to 2 in. in diameter. They are usually situated near the nipple, and do not rapidly increase in size. If the cyst is large and rapidly developed, a grave suspicion of malignant disease or of duct papilloma must be entertained, even though after aspiration no induration remains in the breast. I have a vivid recollection of removing by aspiration 15 oz. of fluid from a cyst, leaving the breast apparently quite soft and normal. Within six months the patient was dead from a most acute carcinoma, which developed so rapidly that operation was evidently useless. The rare cases of rapidly growing cystic adenoma are not numerous enough to impair the validity of the ruh:. Moreover, in view of the affinity of this tumour with sarcoma, excision of the breast is often the best treatment. For a large cyst of the breast, removal of the whole organ is the only procedure which gives anything like absolute security.

When a cyst is excised a microscopical examination of the cyst wall must on no account be omitted even when the characters of the excised cyst appear to be innocent.

TUMOURS OF THE BREAST

On its clinical side the subject of tumours of the breast is complex and difficult, while pathologically it is relatively simple, though its literature is puzzling owing to a redundant nomenclature.

The following list appears to contain all tumours primary in the breast. It might be lengthened by adding tumours of extraneous origin, such as secondary melanotic sarcoma, or angioma of the skin invading the breast, or by wrongly assuming that secondary accidents and degenerations, such as colloid change in carcinoma or cystic changes in fibro-adenoma, are fundamental characters.

A. INNOCENT TUMOURS.
    (a) Of *epithelial* origin, wholly or mainly.
        1. Duct papilloma.
        2. Pure adenoma.
    (b) Of *connective-tissue* origin, wholly or mainly.
        1. Fibro-adenoma.
        2. Soft fibro-adenoma.
        3. Fibroma (probably a fibro-adenoma from which epithe· lium has disappeared).
        4. Lipoma.
        5. Myxoma.

B. MALIGNANT TUMOURS.
    (a) Of *epithelial* origin.
        Carcinoma.
            i. Spheroidal-celled, originating in the acini.
            ii. Columnar-celled, originating in the ducts.
    (b) Of *connective-tissue* origin.
        Sarcoma, round-, spindle-, or mixed-celled, or containing cartilage (chondro-sarcoma) or bone.

Ernest Shaw has well summarized the relations of the mammary epithelium to tumour formation. He points out that the epithelium in a duct or acinus may grow (a) outwards, away from the lumen, or (b) inwards, into the lumen. In the former case the cells may in their growth either (*a*) imitate the normal gland tissue, forming new acini and ducts, accompanied by supporting connective tissue (adenoma), or (*b*) grow out in a disorderly manner, sometimes preserving for a time their tubular arrangement (adeno-carcinoma), but later penetrating the basement membrane and then infiltrating other tissues (carcinoma and duct carcinoma). If the cells grow into the lumen of a duct they may similarly (*a*) form a regularly organized simple papilloma (duct papilloma), or (*b*) form an irregular mass of cells which ultimately breaks through the wall of the duct and infiltrates the tissues beyond (duct carcinoma).

FIBRO-ADENOMA[1]

This simple tumour consists of an encapsuled mass of fibrous tissue containing tubes or spaces lined by epithelium. A large majority of the simple tumours of the breast are fibro-adenomas. When the term fibro-adenoma is used alone, the ordinary or hard fibro-adenoma is meant. This will be first described, and afterwards the rare soft variety will be considered. Fibro-adenomas may be single or multiple, and may present themselves in one breast or in both. They are very rare in the male breast. The smallest examples are of microscopic dimensions, while the largest may be 3 in. or more in diameter, enlarging the breast and forming a considerable part of its bulk. Usually they do not exceed the size of a hen's egg. They most commonly affect the neighbourhood of the nipple and the axillary tail of the breast. Their outline is sometimes obscured by a surrounding area of coarse granular induration due to local chronic mastitis, probably caused by obstruction of some of the ducts by the tumour.

Etiology.—Nothing certain is known with regard to the causation of these tumours. Among 100 cases of fibro-adenoma observed by Bryant, 27 were first discovered between puberty and the age of 20 ; 35 between 20 and 30 ; 22 between 30 and 40 ; 13 between 45 and 50 ; and 3 after 50. Forty-six of the patients were unmarried, 37 fruitfully married, and 15 married but sterile. In reference to these figures, it must be noted that a small tumour in the breast may remain undiscovered for years, and it is probable that nearly all fibro-adenomas arise between puberty and 30 years of age ; they do not occur before puberty. They sometimes respond by increased growth, after remaining stationary for years, to the stimulus of pregnancy. In a case of Erichsen's a fibro-adenoma the size of a walnut, after persisting unchanged for eighteen years, assumed the characters of a soft fibro-adenoma, and rapidly grew until in six months it weighed 5 lb. Such cases suggest the origin of sarcoma from fibro-adenoma, a question which will be again referred to.

[1] *See also* Vol. I., pp. 432 *et seq.*

Morbid anatomy.—Fibro-adenomas are always surrounded by a very definite capsule of fibrous tissue which is but loosely adherent to the surrounding breast substance. In shape the smaller examples are spheroid or ovoid, while the larger ones arc more or less lobulated (Fig. 260). On section the capsule is seen as a layer clearly defined from the whitish or pinkish-white substance of the tumour. Knobbed and foliated fibrous masses may protrude from the cut surface, or the tumour may be homogeneous, presenting a smooth section marked by whorls and bands of fibrous tissue, in which here and there a few small stellate chinks are just visible to the naked eye.

Microscopical anatomy.—Fibro-adenomas arise from local hypertrophy of the transparent fibrous tissue surrounding the epithelial tubes of the breast, called by Warren the periductal tissue, which develops at puberty. The epithelium in many cases of fibroadenoma appears to play a purely passive rôle, but sometimes the acini exhibit considerable proliferative activity. The microscopical varieties of fibro-adenoma are not clinically distinguishable.

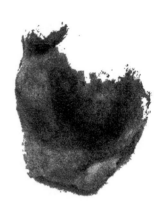

Fig. 260.—A typical fibro-adenoma after enucleation.

Origin and development of fibro-adenomas.—In the common form of fibro-adenoma, called by American authors *intracanalicular*, the growing fibrous tissue around a duct becomes convoluted and infolded into the interior of the duct in the form of blunt rounded processes, each of which is covered by atrophic epithelium representing the stretched epithelium of the duct. Secondary knobs and convolutions develop upon the ingrowing processes. The whole interior of the rounded tumour, within its fibrous capsule, is packed with these blunt polygonal processes. If in this stage the tumour is cut into, the closely packed lobulated masses come apart and protrude through the incision (Fig. 261, B). If an empty paper bag, squeezed together by the hands into a tight ball, be cut through with a knife, the appearance of a fibro-adenoma in section is closely simulated. Such a paper ball is structurally comparable to a fibroadenoma.

A microscopical section at this stage shows masses of fibrous tissue of polygonal outline separated by narrow epithelial-lined chinks.

The process resembles superficially what is seen in duct papilloma, but is really entirely different. In a fibro-adenoma the actively growing element is fibrous tissue, and the epithelium plays a merely passive rôle. In duct papilloma, on the contrary, the ingrowing papillæ present well-developed and actively growing epithelium, and the fibrous core of the papilla serves merely to nourish the active epithelium. A lack of appreciation of this distinction has led to endless confusion in works upon diseases of the breast. Discharge from the nipple—characteristic evidence of secretory activity of the epithelium in duct papilloma—does not occur in fibro-adenoma. The

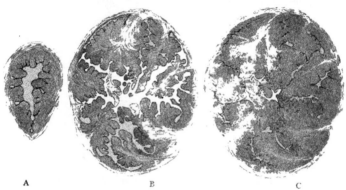

A   B   C

Fig. 261 (schematic).—Three stages in the history of the common intracanalicular fibro-adenoma. A, Ingrowth of the fibrous convolutions
into the duct. B, Their full development. C, Consolidation of the
tumour by fusion of the apposed processes. The chink-like spaces
so prominent in B have almost disappeared.

mutual pressure of the closely packed fibrous ingrowths in a fibro-adenoma ultimately leads to the atrophy and destruction of the thinned epithelium which covers them. The narrow intervening chinks now become bridged by newly organized fibrous tissue, and the lobulated processes are consolidated into a solid fibrous tumour in which, here and there, stellate spaces lined by unobliterated epithelium remain. In this stage a transverse section appears to the naked eye solid and homogeneous (Fig. 261, c).

In an old fibro-adenoma all traces of epithelium may become obliterated, and the tumour is then classified as a fibroma. A rarer variety of hard fibro-adenoma, called by American authors the *pericanalicular* fibro-adenoma, which is clinically indistinguishable from the common variety, presents active overgrowth of the fibrous tissue surrounding the acini and small ducts of one or more lobules of the

breast, but without bulging of fibrous prominences into the interior
of the affected epithelial channels. The ducts and acini remain un-
distorted, while the fibrous layer surrounding them undergoes a
concentric hypertrophy. Instead of irregular, flattened, chink-like
spaces lined by epithelium, this variety presents practically normal
epithelial tubes surrounded by masses of fibrous tissue arranged concentrically to the epithelial tubes. There is, however, no essential
difference between the two forms of fibro-adenoma just described,
for the same tumour may at different points present the characters
of both.

Symptoms and signs.—A fibro-adenoma of the ordinary or
hard variety presents itself as a firm, elastic, rounded lump, not
usually larger than an egg, palpable with the flat hand, and freely
movable in the breast tissues. There is no adhesion to skin or fascia,
nor enlargement of the axillary glands. Retraction of the nipple never
occurs. The smaller examples are more or less spherical in shape;
in the larger ones lobulation becomes evident. As a fibro-adenoma
enlarges, the subcutaneous tissues over it seem to undergo atrophy
from stretching, and the tumour becomes superficial, lying close
beneath the skin, across which enlarged veins may often be seen
coursing. The skin glides freely over the tumour; on stretching it
the lobulation of the tumour may become visually obvious.

As a rule, fibro-adenomas do not cause pain, except in neurotic
persons, or in those who are obsessed by the fear of cancer. Not
infrequently, however, they become tender during menstruation.
In exceptional cases, severe neuralgic pain in the breast may depend
upon the presence of a small fibro-adenoma.

Differential diagnosis.—A tense cyst in which fluctuation cannot be obtained closely simulates a fibro-adenoma. The
diagnosis is especially difficult if the swelling is deep in the breast.
Though exploratory puncture will often settle the diagnosis, it is not
imperative, since in either case an operation is usually necessary.

Considerable difficulty may arise when the fibro-adenoma is embedded in an area of indurated chronic mastitis. The rounded contours of the tumour are obscured, and its mobility sometimes seems
to be impaired. In such circumstances it may closely simulate a
carcinoma, and an exploratory incision may be the only means of
settling the diagnosis.

The simulation of fibro-adenoma by certain forms of carcinoma
is dealt with at p. 82. Here it need only be said that a tumour of
the breast, presenting the characters of a fibro-adenoma, should be
regarded with grave suspicion if it first appears after the age of 40.

Treatment.—Fibro-adenomas in young women under 30, if
small and not increasing, may be let alone, if the patient can

be kept under observation. But in view of the mental uneasiness caused by any lump in the breast, and of the possibility of malignant change, excision is the best treatment, and is imperative if the patient is approaching middle age. The tumour, grasped firmly in the left hand, is boldly cut down upon so as to expose its capsule by an incision radiating from the nipple. It can then easily be enucleated from its surroundings. The cavity left is washed out with 1-1,000 perchloride of mercury solution to destroy any mammary epithelium set free, and is obliterated by buried sutures approximating its sides. Unless this is done a hæmatoma is likely to appear.

Gaillard Thomas's method.—This is a convenient opportunity to describe the operation of Gaillard Thomas—a method of removing simple tumours of the breast which avoids a subsequent visible scar. The operation depends upon the fact that the important arteries of the breast enter at the upper margin, while its posterior surface has but few vascular connexions with the retromammary tissues. The incision follows the sulcus between the breast and the chest wall, along the outer and the lower margin of the breast. The edge of the breast being exposed, the gland is stripped upwards from the great pectoral, and is at the same time rotated so as to expose its posterior surface. The tumour is removed by a radial incision into the posterior surface of the organ, or if necessary a sector of the breast may be removed. The cavity left is obliterated by buried sutures, the breast turned down into position, and the skin incision sutured. The operation, though satisfactory unless the tumour is high up in the breast, and justifiable where æsthetic considerations are dominant, is not surgically desirable, and should never be used unless the tumour is quite certainly non-malignant. Such an extensive incision renders a subsequent operation for carcinoma on proper lines impossible.

SOFT FIBRO-ADENOMA

The rare soft variety of fibro-adenoma is distinguished by its rapid growth, soft or elastic consistence, and occurrence comparatively late in life.

A soft fibro-adenoma may originate from a hard one, or may be soft from the beginning. Erichsen states that these tumours are commonest between the ages of 35 and 40. They are rapidly growing but innocent tumours which may in a few months attain the size of a cocoa-nut. But even when the soft fibro-adenoma attains a large size it remains mobile and painless, and does not display any tendency to adhere to the skin or fascia, or to cause enlargement of the glands. If these signs develop the tumour must be classified as a sarcoma.

Soft adenoma differs from the hard variety in the nature of its stroma, which is not composed of dense fibrous tissue poor in nuclei, but is richly cellular. It may be made up of fusiform cells, sometimes mixed with more fully developed fibrous tissue. In other cases the tissue resembles myxomatous tissue, presenting stellate cells with abundant mucoid intercellular substance. This appearance is probably the result of mucoid degeneration of ordinary fibrous tissue.

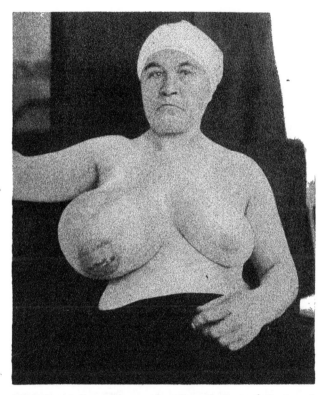

Fig. 262.—Soft, rapidly growing fibro-adenoma of the breast (so-called sero-cystic sarcoma of Brodie).

(*Beatson, Edin. Med. Journ., Nov.,* 1908.)

Small cysts often occur in soft fibro-adenomas. ' The embryonic nature of the fibrous stroma of these tumours indicates their close connexion with the sarcomas, and indeed they were formerly called adeno-sarcomas.

The case recorded by Beatson, and represented in Fig. 262, is a typical instance of a large fibro-adenoma of the soft variety. The patient was aged 50, and had noticed her right breast increasing in size for a period of two years. Pain was almost absent, and her health remained good. The tumour was situated in the upper hemisphere, so that the stretched-out and flattened nipple is seen upon its under surface. 'The superficial veins were large and distended. The breast felt very heavy, but was freely movable under the skin

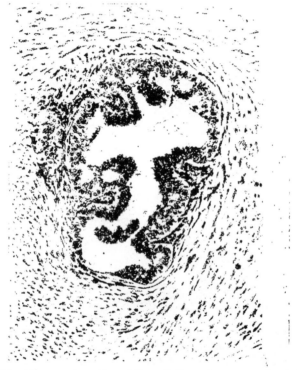

Fig. 263.—Microscopic section of the soft fibro-adenoma represented in Fig. 262. Note the cellular embryonic character of the stroma.

(*Beatson, Edin. Med. Journ., Nov.,* 1908.)

and upon the fascia. The tumour was smooth, elastic, and spherical, but with some irregularity of shape and tendency to lobulation. The breast was not tender, nor were the axillary glands enlarged. The mamma was removed, and the encapsuled tumour weighed 6½ lb. It was solid, but parts of it presented numerous cysts, while at other parts the stroma had undergone mucoid degeneration. On microscopical examination the stroma (*see* Fig. 263) was highly cellular, and its appearance, apart from the clinical history, would suggest sarcoma, except for the fact that epithelial structures usually disappear from a sarcoma of the breast.

Diagnosis.—Beatson points out that there are practically only three conditions which lead to the formation of really large tumours of the breast, i.e. soft fibro-adenoma (often cystic), hypertrophy, and sarcoma. Hypertrophy is bilateral, while the other conditions are unilateral. A sarcoma, if still encapsuled, cannot be distinguished from a soft fibro-adenoma. Only when a sarcoma begins to infiltrate, so that the breast becomes fixed and the skin involved, can the diagnosis be made.

Treatment.—Since soft fibro-adenoma is a large tumour to which the breast itself is merely a small appendage, amputation of the whole breast is usually preferable to enucleation. The pectorals need not be removed, nor the axilla opened.

Cystic Fibro-Adenoma

Most large soft fibro-adenomas contain cysts. If these are of any size the tumour is called a cystic fibro-adenoma. A cystic fibro-adenoma may be produced from fibro-adenoma by the collection of fluid in the epithelial-lined spaces and chinks which represent the distorted original duct. This must obviously take place before the stage of consolidation has begun. When the cystic tumour is cut into, fluid escapes and blunt foliated or lobulated masses are seen projecting into the interior of the cyst. Such a tumour must be clearly distinguished from cystic duct papilloma. Another form of cystic fibro-adenoma is due to partial or complete mucoid degeneration and liquefaction of the fibrous substance of the original tumour.

A perfect tangle of nomenclature has grown up around this form of tumour. Owing to the large size it rapidly reaches, and the cellular character of its stroma, it was formerly considered to be a sarcoma, and Brodie applied to it the name *sero-cystic sarcoma*. Johannes Müller called it *cysto-sarcoma*. French authors called it a *cystadenoma*, a correct term, but one which has led to confusion between this form of tumour and the cystic duct papilloma (papillary cystadenoma), an absolutely different condition. For this reason the term cystadenoma should be deleted from the nomenclature of breast tumours. Other names which have been applied to the cystic fibro-adenoma are *adenocele, cystoid glandular tumour,* and *cystic fibroma*. These obsolete terms are recorded, not to burden the student's memory, but as a key to the literature of the subject.

Clinical features.—The characters of cystic fibro-adenoma are those of the soft fibro-adenoma from which it originates, except that areas of definite fluctuation, corresponding to the cysts, may sometimes be felt.

Diagnosis.—A large tumour of the breast presenting fluctuat ing areas may be a cystic fibro-adenoma, a cystic duct papilloma, or a cystic sarcoma. The history or presence of serous discharge from the nipple distinguishes duct papilloma, while signs of infiltration will lead to the diagnosis of sarcoma.

Treatment.—The treatment is that of soft fibro-adenoma, and the prognosis is good.

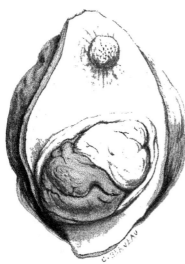

Fig. 264.—Fungating cystic adenoma of the breast. The edges of the skin are rolled back, not thinned and infiltrated as in sarcoma, and a mass of fibro-adenomatous tissue is protruding.

(From a specimen in the Middlesex Hospital Museum.)

FUNGATING CYSTIC FIBRO-ADENOMA (FUNGATING CYSTADENOMA)

In very rare cases of cystic fibro-adenoma the skin over the cystic portion of the tumour becomes thinned and gives way. Serous fluid escapes, and blunt lobulated and foliated masses of fibro-adenomatous tissue project through the opening (*see* Fig. 264). Septic and inflammatory changes may occur in the protruding mass, which becomes swollen and congested, and bleeds readily. In such circumstances the simulation of a fungating sarcoma is very close, though the tumour is really innocent. In these days of early treatment of breast tumours this condition is rarely seen.

Diagnosis.—A wedge of the protruding mass, ½ in. in depth, should be removed for microscopical examination. No anæsthetic will be necessary.

Treatment is that of soft fibro-adenoma.

PURE ADENOMA[1]

In a pure adenoma the tumour is almost entirely composed of epithelial tubes more or less closely simulating normal acini, and separated by a minimal amount of supporting fibrous tissue, in

[1] *See also* Vol. I., p. 431.

which, according to Ernest Shaw, no fat is present. Owing to the absence of fat, the lobular arrangement, so obvious in the normal breast, is obscured. Some of the gland tubes may be dilated into microscopic cysts, or may form irregular spaces encroached upon by convolutions of the epithelium. Regularly formed ducts are

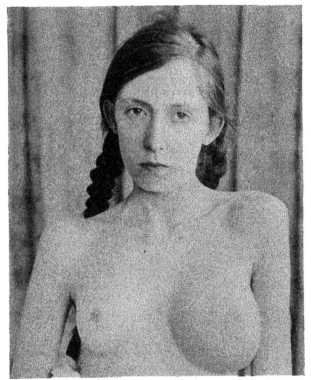

Fig. 265.—Pure adenoma of the breast in a young girl.

(From a case under the writer's care at the Bolingbroke Hospital.)

absent. The epithelium, though apparently so active, is everywhere confined within a basement membrane.

Simple adenoma is one of the rarest of breast tumours, so that in a large experience it may be observed not at all, or once only. It occurs at any age between puberty and the menopause. The case which is represented in Fig. 265 was observed by me in a young girl of 16.

Clinically, simple adenoma resembles a soft fibro-adenoma, though it does not seem to reach such a size. It does not adhere to the skin or fascia, but appears fixed in the breast. Enlarged veins may be seen coursing over it. In my own case, referred to on p. 45, the tumour appeared to constitute the whole breast, and but for its unilateral character a diagnosis of hypertrophy would have suggested itself.

Treatment.—Enucleation should be attempted unless the tumour is very large. In that case, amputation of the breast may be necessary.

DUCT PAPILLOMA OF THE BREAST (PAPILLARY CYST-ADENOMA, PROLIFEROUS CYSTS)[1]

This is a condition in which papillomatous elevations arise from the lining epithelium of the ducts. Serous discharge and often bleeding occur from the papillomatous masses. Thus the characteristic but not invariable feature of the disease is *a blood-stained serous discharge from the nipple.*

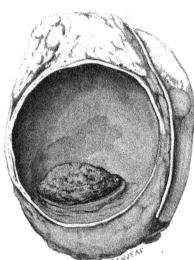

Fig. 266.—Cystic duct papilloma of the breast.

(From a specimen removed by the writer, and preserved in the Middlesex Hospital Museum.)

Duct obstruction and consequent distension with serous discharge frequently occur, and produce the cysts characteristic of certain forms of the disease. Duct papilloma is not malignant, but in the course of years frequently passes into duct carcinoma.

Etiology.—Duct papilloma appears to be unknown before puberty, and to be most frequent towards the end of active sexual life. It may, however, occur in old age, and has been recorded in the male breast. It occurs equally in the married and the unmarried.

Morbid anatomy.—Since the larger ducts converge upon the nipple, it is beneath or near the nipple that clinically appreciable duct papillomas are most often found. All the ducts may be affected, but very often the disease is confined to one or several of the mammary lobes.

[1] *See also* Vol. I., p. 453.

The acinous lobules of the affected lobe or lobes, if their ducts are obstructed, develop chronic mastitis, so that the affected lobe is sometimes mapped out as a sector-shaped area of granular induration even before the papillomas in its ducts have given rise to a tumour. The papillomas are soft in consistence and vary greatly in appearance. They may be broad-based and short, or attached inside the duct by a constricted narrow base, and giving off elongated processes. They may be closely set within the duct, or sparsely distributed over its surface. They may be minute and impalpable, or of considerable size. The amount of fluid secreted appears to vary considerably. Thus in some cases the duct is distended merely by the growth of the papillomas, and the tumour is practically a solid one. In other cases one or more large, freely fluctuating cysts make their appearance, e a c h containing only one or two papillomas (Fig. 266). The healthy lobes of the breast then appear merely as a small appendage to these cysts.

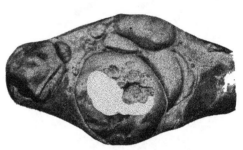

Fig. 267.—Section through a cystic duct papilloma.

(*St. Thomas's Hospital Museum.*)

The fluid in the cysts, or exuding from the nipple, is often clear and straw-coloured without cellular elements. If haemorrhage occurs the fluid takes on a shade of red. In the cysts it exhibits similar gradations, and in the older cysts it may assume a brownish opalescent appearance which is associated with the presence of cholesterin.

Microscopical appearances.—The ducts of the breast are lined with a single layer of columnar epithelium. As might be expected, therefore, duct papillomas are composed of vascular branching cores of fibrous tissue covered with epithelium of the columnar type (Fig. 268).

Clinical features.—Duct papilloma is usually painless. Pain may, however, occur upon the sudden cessation of serous discharge owing to the distension of the ducts by retained secretion. It may be felt at menstruation and at no other time. The patient's attention is attracted either by intermittent discharge, which may be redder and more profuse during menstruation, or by the discovery of a tumour. The evolution of the disease is very slow, and the discharge or tumour may be present for ten or more years before advice is sought. Suppuration of a duct papilloma, with protrusion of the growths through an orifice formed by the bursting of the abscess, has been recorded.

In all stages the tumour or tumours are freely movable in the breast, under the skin and upon the fascia. The axillary glands, though from irritation they may become easily palpable, are neither hard nor definitely enlarged. The nipple is not retracted nor is the breast shrunken. But it is evident that the physical signs of duct papilloma will vary very greatly with the number of lobes affected, with the size of the papillomas, with their degree of secretory power, and with the presence or absence of obstruction of the ducts.

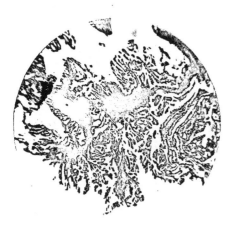

Fig. 268.—Typical duct papilloma. Its narrow base of attachment to the duct wall is seen upon the right of the figure. It presents a delicate branching framework of fibrous tissue, covered with a single layer of columnar epithelium. Note the absence of any sign of epithelial infiltration at the base of the papilla. × 10.

Early stage, tumour impalpable. — Intermittent blood-stained or serous discharge is present. One small segment of the breast, corresponding to the particular orifice upon the nipple from which the discharge issues, is vaguely indurated and granular, while the rest of the breast is soft and normal. Careful observation shows that the discharge comes exclusively from the particular orifice upon the nipple which corresponds to the affected lobe, and from none of the other orifices. Pressure upon the affected lobe increases the discharge, while pressure upon the non-indurated parts of the breast is found to have no effect. The papilloma itself is too small to be palpable.

Later stage, tumour palpable.—The papilloma has now become palpable as a small firm tumour situated beneath or near the nipple. In some cases the papillomas may attain a considerable size and may form a solid tumour, perhaps an inch in diameter. But the nipple is not retracted, nor is the lump fixed in the breast. The other signs are unaltered.

Cystic duct papilloma.—If a duct is blocked by the growth, serous discharge ceases. If the papillomas possess considerable secretory power, the retained secretion distends the duct behind the obstruction. One or more cysts of considerable size are thus produced, to which the remainder of the breast becomes a mere appendage. A large fluctuating swelling is present, perhaps 4 in. or more in diameter. The solid papillomas which it contains cannot now be felt, and the history of sanious discharge alone gives the clue to the diagnosis. Retraction of the nipple and adhesion to skin and fascia remain absent.

Fungating duct papilloma (*fungating papillary cystadenoma*). —In rare cases the skin over a duct papilloma may undergo a kind of pressure atrophy, and may give way, allowing the protrusion of the papillomatous masses. The same result may follow suppuration of a duct papilloma. Constricted by the margins of the skin opening, the protruding mass becomes congested and hæmorrhagic, and closely resembles a fungating sarcoma. It also simulates a fungating cystic adenoma. Malignancy may be excluded by the absence of fixation and gland enlargement. Microscopic examination of a portion of the fungating mass may decide its nature.

Treatment of duct papilloma.—The knowledge that a duct papilloma often becomes malignant should exert more influence upon its treatment. Duct papilloma is often a very circumscribed disease, affecting perhaps only one lobe of the breast. In these circumstances mere excision of the affected lobe is very tempting; but this policy is of doubtful wisdom. Since the eye is incompetent to map out the exact limits of the disease, and since early papillomas may be present in other ducts, it is much safer, in view of possible malignant degeneration, to excise the whole breast, even for early and limited duct papilloma. In young women, however, it may be justifiable to resect the affected lobe or lobes, leaving the remainder of the breast.

The axillary glands need not be removed. But the specimen should be carefully examined for carcinomatous change, and if this is found or suspected the axilla must be cleared out at a subsequent operation.

LIPOMA AND MYXOMA

Most so-called *lipomas* of the breast are really paramammary lipomas occurring in contact with the breast, but not forming part of it.

Myxoma of the breast is merely a pathological curiosity. It forms an encapsuled tumour resembling a fibro-adenoma.

CARCINOMA OF THE BREAST[1]

Etiology.—A carcinoma of the breast originates when the mammary epithelium, which is normally confined within its basement membrane, escapes into the tissue spaces of the breast, and continues to proliferate therein.

In females the breast comes second only to the uterus as a seat of election for malignant disease ; one case of malignant disease in every three affects the breast. On the contrary, only one case in every hundred of cancer in males is of mammary origin. The commonest sites of growth are in the upper and outer quadrant or beneath the nipple. Though no portion of the breast is exempt, the lower and inner quadrant is the part most rarely affected. In exceptional cases the growth begins in an outlying lobule situated beyond the visible limits of the breast. Campiche and Lazarus-Barlow find that the point of origin may be expressed in percentages as follows :—

Beneath nipple [2] . . 12·2	Upper and inner quadrant	16·7
In nipple . . . 7·6	Lower and outer ,, .	12·4
Upper and outer quadrant 44·9	Lower and inner ,, .	6·2

The proportion of married persons in the general female population above the age of 25 is about three out of four, and three out of four cancers of the breast are seen in married women. Thus the liability of married and unmarried women to cancer is about the same. Though a few striking family histories have been adduced, the influence of heredity in this and in other forms of cancer is unproven. Failure or inability to suckle at the breast, blows and injuries, a family history of tubercle, and a brunette complexion, have each been alleged as predisposing causes. A history of injury is present in about 10 per cent. of cases of carcinoma, but a relation of cause and effect has never been proved.

Age-incidence.—Carcinoma of the breast is unknown before puberty, and very rare before 35. Most commonly it begins in the years immediately following the ·menopause. It remains frequent up to the end of life, in proportion to the reduced number of persons living at the more advanced ages.

Chronic mastitis as a precursor of cancer.—The most important factor in the production of breast cancer appears to be chronic mastitis. Taking first the *clinical* evidence, Bryant found that out of 360 cases of cancer, mastitis had occurred at some antecedent period in 80. Gross found similar evidence in 71 of 365 cases of cancer. Sheild found evidence of past inflammatory trouble in only 10 per cent. of the St. George's Hospital cases, but he justly points out that

---

[1] *See also* Vol. I., pp. 561, 572.

[2] This table probably underestimates the frequency of growths beneath the nipple.

a focus of chronic mastitis much too small to be clinically appreciable may yet form an adequate nidus for a carcinoma. The clinical statistics, then, amount only to this—that there is evidence of past chronic mastitis in a large minority of cases of breast cancer.

The *pathological* evidence, however, in favour of chronic mastitis as a cause is very strong. Beadles, from the examination of the non-carcinomatous portions of 100 cancerous breasts at the Brompton Cancer Hospital, found without exception in each of these breasts such abnormal changes as undue proliferation of the acini and of the stroma, and cysts were of common occurrence. It must, however, be remarked that Lenthal Cheatle has found similar changes post mortem in apparently healthy breasts. F. T. Paul, as the result of prolonged observations, recorded in 1901 his belief that microscopical evidence of mastitis is present in nearly every breast affected with carcinoma. Later, Victor Bonney found traces of chronic mastitis in all the mammæ removed for early carcinoma which he had the opportunity of examining. Thus, pathological investigation shows chronic mastitis to be an almost universal precursor of carcinoma.

Fibro-adenoma and carcinoma.—General opinion favours the view that there is no connexion between fibro-adenoma and carcinoma. At first sight nothing could appear more innocent than a fibro-adenoma of the breast, persisting possibly for years without notable increase in size, and securely walled off from the normal tissues by its strong fibrous capsule. Yet, in my opinion, there can be no reasonable doubt that in a small proportion of cases malignant tumours may arise in or in connexion with these innocent neoplasms. Fibro-adenomas are often enveloped in an area of breast tissue exhibiting chronic mastitis which certainly may lead to cancer. It seems, then, probable that the irritative effect of a fibro-adenoma may be an important factor in inducing cancer in the surrounding breast tissue. This view is confirmed by the fact that the seat of election for breast cancer—the upper and outer quadrant, including the axillary tail—is also the seat of election for fibro-adenoma.

Is it possible, apart from the irritative effect of a fibro-adenoma upon the surrounding tissues, that the tumour itself may undergo a carcinomatous degeneration ? On various occasions I have observed in microscopical sections of breast cancer an intimate admixture of carcinomatous and fibro-adenomatous tissues, so that the histological appearances of these diverse tumours should be seen together on the same field of the microscope. Such observations, though suggestive, are not conclusive. There is, however, in the museum of St. Bartholomew's Hospital (3159c) an encapsuled acinous fibro-adenoma containing a central opaque area of spheroidal-celled carcinoma which is infiltrating the substance of the surrounding fibro-adenoma. This specimen is, so far as I know, unique, but there seems no doubt that it illustrates the possibility of the actual transformation of a simple fibro-adenoma into a malignant tumour.

Duct papilloma and malignant disease.—It is generally admitted that duct papilloma may give rise to duct carcinoma. The epithelium at the base of the papilloma may infiltrate the subjacent tissues; or the papilloma itself, by its continued growth, may erode the opposite wall of the duct and attack the tissues beyond, where its prominences lose their regular structure and infiltrate the tissues in an irregular and malignant way (see Fig. 282, p. 85).

Histological varieties of breast cancer.—Carcinoma of the breast presents itself histologically under two forms, spheroidal-celled carcinoma and columnar - celled carcinoma. The former variety—by far the more frequent — originates in the acini, the latter in the ducts of the breast. Some growths present both varieties of epithelium. Tumours originating in the nipple have received separate consideration.

Accounts of the histology of spheroidal-celled carcinoma have in the past been unnecessarily complicated because accidental or unimportant variations in the character of the growth have

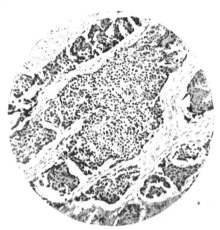

Fig. 269.—Rapidly growing (medullary) carcinoma of the breast, presenting large masses of epithelial cells with a minimum of supporting fibrous stroma. × 90.

been unduly emphasized. The very diverse appearances met with seem to depend mainly upon three variable factors—(a) the rate of multiplication of the epithelium; (b) the activity of stroma formation, i.e. the vigour of the reactive or defensive processes; (c) the degree of cohesion between the cancer cells. (Contrast Plates 83 and 84.)

Pathological basis of the clinical classification of breast cancers. — The three clinical varieties of cancer of the breast are medullary cancer, scirrhus and atrophic scirrhus.

If the epithelium proliferates very rapidly, a soft, bulky tumour is produced, rich in epithelium, and called a medullary carcinoma

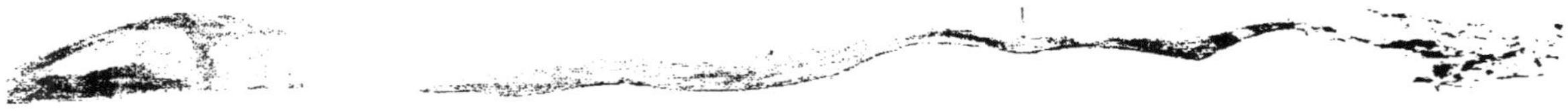

Naked-eye section, prepared by Rowntree's modification of the writer's translucent strip method, of a fibroid cancer of the breast removed by operation. The section passes at its right-hand end through the axillary tissues, and carcinomatous lymphatic glands are seen buried therein. The growth in the breast substance has caused retraction of the nipple. It is seen as a greyish area of fibrosis sending fibrotic prolongations in various directions. (Contrast Plate 84.) Along the lower edge of the section is seen the great pectoral muscle, on the upper edge the area of skin removed.

PLATE 83.

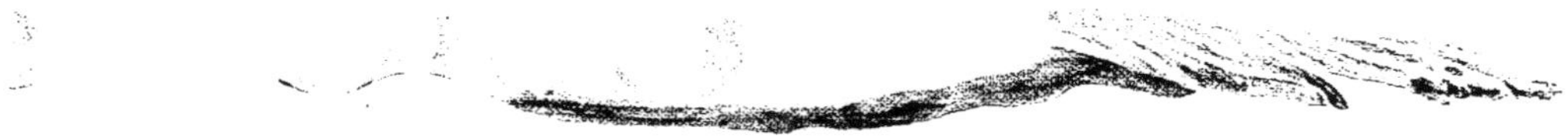

A similar section to that shown in Plate 83, from a soft or medullary cancer of the breast. The section passes at the left-hand end through the axillary tissues, in which numerous enlarged lymphatic glands are seen embedded. Along the lower edge of the section is seen the pectoralis major. The growth is pinkish in colour, and has not the scar-like appearance illustrated in Plate 83.

PLATE 84.

(Fig. 269). If, on the other hand, the proliferative power of the epithelium is low, while the fibrotic processes are active, the "atrophic scirrhus" of old age results. If these two opposing processes are balanced, a hard tumour of not inconsiderable size, the ordinary scirrhus, is produced. The name scirrhus is often reserved for those carcinomas where the epithelium has lost its tubular arrangement (Fig. 270). If the epithelium possesses sufficient power of cohesion to retain in some degree its arrangement in gland tubes, the name acinous carcinoma or adeno-carcinoma is applicable (Fig. 271).

It is important to recognize that all gradations occur between the forms of carcinoma which have just been named, and, moreover, that these gradations may occur in the same tumour. Thus, one part of a tumour may present a medullary appearance, while an older part shows a densely fibroid growth containing few epithelial cells. It must be remembered that a mass of cancer cells becomes increasingly fibrotic with age. But it is clinically convenient to classify the tumour according to its size and hardness, as medullary cancer, scirrhus, and atrophic scirrhus.

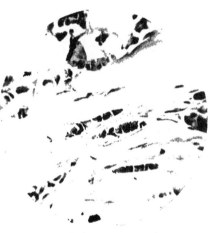

Fig. 270.—Typical appearance in chronic fibroid cancer of the breast. In a groundwork of dense fibrous tissue are embedded single lines of compressed and deformed cancerous epithelium. The terminal cells of the line are usually triangular in shape. × 160.

Diffuse carcinoma of the breast.—Cancer of the breast usually begins in one small district of the breast, if not at one microscopic point, and is correctly described as unicentric in origin. Cases are, however, met with where the whole breast or several of its lobes appear to undergo carcinomatous degeneration *en masse*, the disease lighting up simultaneously in every part of an extensive district. These cases may be described as multicentric carcinoma, diffuse scirrhus, or diffuse carcinoma. They include the most virulent forms of breast cancer, and the term diffuse carcinoma may perhaps be regarded as the pathological equivalent of the clinical term acute carcinoma or mastitis carcinomatosa (*see* p. 80).

Dissemination of Breast Cancer

It is of primary importance to know the mode and channels by which breast cancer spreads from the primary focus and gives rise to secondary deposits, for in the absence of this knowledge it is impossible to devise a scientific operation for the extirpation of the disease.

Until recently the subject of dissemination was enveloped in confusion and uncertainty. It was believed that the secondary deposits situated near the primary growth arose from particles carried along the lymphatics by the current ; while more distant deposits, such as those in the liver, were accounted for by the *embolic theory*. According to this theory, particles of the primary growth reach the blood by way of the axillary and supraclavicular glands, and are carried by the force of the circulation to remote districts where their cells proliferate and produce secondary nodules. Although, in 1889, Heidenhain found lymphatics filled with cancer cells extending from the breast to the pectoral fascia in two-thirds of the cancerous breasts he examined, this important observation remained isolated,

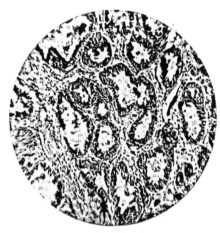

Fig. 271.— Columnar - celled adeno-carcinoma of the breast originating in the smaller ducts. Note the irregular shape of the gland-spaces. At other points in the growth infiltration had occurred, and the cancer cells had lost their gland-like arrangement. × 68.

and had no effect upon the general doctrine of dissemination. Stiles, whose work upon the surgical anatomy of the breast led to such great operative improvements, writing in 1889, continued to share the embolic view of dissemination.

Although it has been conclusively shown, especially by M. B. Schmidt, that cancer cells often obtain access to the blood-stream, upon a close examination the embolic theory presents many difficulties. Stephen Paget pointed out that, though embolism must be an impartial process to which all the organs are liable, certain organs are very prone and others relatively immune to secondary deposits of cancer. Thus, in pyæmia, a known embolic process, the frequency of splenic to hepatic abscess is as two to three. In breast cancer the frequency of splenic to hepatic metastases is only as one to fourteen. Again, the distribution of the secondary deposits is not the same, for instance, in cancer of the uterus as in cancer of the stomach, but varies according to the site of the primary growth. Yet embolism must be by its nature an impartial process. In cancers which affect the skeleton the secondary deposits are frequent in certain bones and very rare in others, although all the bones must be liable to embolism. These difficulties have never been convincingly met by the advocates of the embolic theory. In most cases, cancer cells which gain access to the blood-stream appear to undergo destruction. The details of the process, as seen in the lungs, have been demonstrated by M. B. Schmidt. The peculiarities of metastatic distribution, to be further referred to, show that blood embolism is a comparatively unimportant factor in dissemination.

PARIETAL AND VISCERAL DISSEMINATION

The secondary deposits in breast cancer may be considered under two headings—first, those in the parietes of the thorax, abdomen, and head, or in the limbs; second, the visceral deposits within the thorax, the abdomen, or the central nervous system.

Dissemination in the parietes.—In certain cases, widespread deposits are found in the bones or the subcutaneous tissues, while the internal organs are free from cancer. The escape of the internal organs in such cases is very difficult to explain if the seeds of the secondary deposits are distributed by the blood-stream. Moreover, on the embolic hypothesis, subcutaneous nodules might be expected to crop up at random anywhere upon the surface of the body. This is not the case. The subcutaneous nodules which are so frequently seen in breast cancer always make their earliest appearance close to the primary growth. Moreover, I have shown that they spread away from the (growth in a centrifugal manner) and occupy an area, roughly circular, which has for its centre the primary growth. In course of time and in exceptional cases, this circle may occupy the greater part of the surface of the body, and may spread to the limbs and head. But almost invariably the patient dies before subcutaneous deposits have made their appearance upon the distal portions of the limbs—the situation, of all others, where embolic particles might be expected to lodge. The arms below the deltoid insertion, and the lower limbs below the middle third of the thigh, appear invariably to remain free from nodules. The distal portions of the limbs enjoy an immunity from bone metastases as well as from subcutaneous

nodules. The following table shows the experience of the Middlesex
Hospital in this respect for a period of thirty years :—

TABLE SHOWING THE FREQUENCY OF CANCEROUS DEPOSIT OR SPONTANEOUS
FRACTURE IN 329 CASES OF MAMMARY CANCER AT THE MIDDLESEX
HOSPITAL, 1872-1901.

Bone		No. of cases	Percentage of total
Bones lying wholly or partially within the area liable to sub-cutaneous nodules .	Sternum	30	9·1
	Ribs	28	8·5
	Clavicle	5	1·5
	Spine	12	3·6
	Cranial bones	9	2·7
	Scapula	1	0·3
	Femur	14	4·2
	Os innominatum	—	—
	Humerus	9	2·7
Bones lying beyond the area liable to subcutaneous nodules.	Radius	—	—
	Ulna	—	—
	Tibia	1	0·3
	Fibula	—	—
	Patella	1	0·3
	Bones of hand	1	0·3
	Bones of foot	—	—

Owing to the impossibility of making a complete routine examination of the skeleton, it is probable that this table is incomplete, that
secondary deposits in the flat bones especially—bones which, owing
to their shape, are not liable to fracture as the result of secondary
growth—are more frequent than the table would indicate. But
advanced cancerous deposit in the bones of the forearm and leg would
certainly give rise frequently to spontaneous fracture, and would
thus attract the attention of the pathologist. The immunity of the
long bones of the forearm and leg must, therefore, be a real, not merely
an imaginary one.

The table includes two cases which form exceptions to the rule
just stated. In the first case, owing to ankylosis of the knee-joint,
cancer had extended to the tibia and patella by continuity from the
femur. In the second case, certain of the metacarpal bones were
fractured ; in this case, therefore, it appears probable that cancerous
embolism along the blood-vessels was the cause of the spontaneous
fracture. But it is a very striking fact, as indicating the inefficiency
of blood embolism in the causation of bone metastasis, that only
one case in thirty years showed bone deposit in the distal portions
of the limbs. Judging by the frequency of non-cancerous embolism
of the extremities, it is in these that bone deposits, according to the

embolic theory, should most frequently occur. It is noteworthy also that cancerous deposit in the femur, with the rarest exceptions, commences in the upper third of the bone. The intimate connexion of the periosteum with the deep fascia in the region of the great trochanter facilitates the invasion of the bone in the trochanteric region as soon as permeation has spread so far. Moreover, spontaneous fracture of the humerus occurs most frequently at the level of the deltoid insertion. As in the femur, fracture occurs most often at the point nearest the trunk at which the bone is subcutaneous, and consequently in close relationship with the fascial lymphatic plexus. Speaking generally, the liability of a bone to cancerous deposit or spontaneous fracture increases with its proximity to the site of the primary growth. All these peculiarities, difficult to explain on the embolic theory, show the working of a slow centrifugal process of spread from the primary focus. It may be especially mentioned that spontaneous fracture of the femur is three times more common upon the side of the primary growth in the breast than upon the opposite side.

A femur fractured owing to secondary cancerous deposit presents a characteristic skiagraphic picture in that the fracture is situated just below the great trochanter, while the trochanter itself presents an area of rarefaction owing to the replacement of bone by soft malignant tissue.

Perhaps the most extreme instance of secondary bone deposits is the case of which a plaster cast is preserved in the museum of St. Thomas's Hospital. The patient had a cancer of the right breast. At the time of death the skeleton was greatly distorted. The sternum and ribs sank until the former appeared to touch the vertebral column, the whole thorax being flattened out transversely. The pelvis exhibited a precisely similar modification. The right humerus and both femora were fractured. But the forearms and the legs preserved their normal shape. Thus even in this extreme case no support can be found for the embolic theory.

Taking centrifugal spread in the parietes as proved, the question arises, In what plane does the growth spread? On the assumption that the growth could spread along the skin to a considerable distance, many operators have advocated the ablation of very large areas of skin. My researches show that invasion of the skin is secondary to spread in the plane of the deep fascia. The skin nodules are isolated efflorescences springing up from below, and the (skin is not a highway for the spread of cancer.) The growth spreads in the plane of the deep fascia because in this layer is situated the main parietal lymphatic plexus, the fascial plexus. The results of operators who remove large areas of skin are less satisfactory than those of surgeons who remove less skin and a wider extent of deep fascia. In my own series of cases, although the skin removed is only a circle of four or five inches, but four instances of recurrence in the skin have come to notice.

Dissemination within the limits of the breast.—Langhans was the first to notice that the small lymphatics of the breast are invaded early and widely, far beyond the infiltrating edge of the primary growth. Stiles showed that the breast is a far more wide-spreading organ than it appears to be, and that for its complete removal, shown to be imperative by Langhans' observations, an extensive operation is necessary.

Extension of growth to the pectoral fascia.—Heidenhain, in 1889, showed that in two cases out of three, lymphatics filled with cancer cells are present upon the pectoral fascia. In opposition to Langhans, he maintained that the process is one of continuous growth along the vessels, not one of lymphatic embolism. Invasion of the lymphatics of the pectoral fascia precedes the clinical sign of adhesion of the growth to the fascia.

Embolism of the axillary glands.—Embolic invasion of the axillary glands along their afferent trunks almost invariably occurs as soon as the lymphatics of the pectoral fascia have been invaded. In the earliest stage a few cancer cells are seen lying in the subcapsular lymph sinus at the point of entry of the afferent lymphatics (Stiles). The cells slowly penetrate to the interior of the gland by infiltrating its lymph spaces, and ultimately reach the efferent lymphatics, along which they may be swept to the supraclavicular glands. At the same time they are infiltrating the capsule of the gland, which consequently loses its mobility upon the surrounding structures.

The lymphatic glands delay for a long time the further advance of the cancer cells, and there is evidence that they may destroy cancer cells brought to them, and that they only succumb to invasion after a prolonged resistance. It is important to note that widespread dissemination may occur in cases where, after death, the axillary glands are found to be free from cancer. In fact, the route which leads through the axillary glands is only a by-way of dissemination, and not the main avenue.

Invasion of the opposite axillary glands and of the opposite breast.—In a late stage of breast cancer, owing to extension of permeation across the middle line, enlargement of the opposite axillary glands often occurs. A little later, deposits of growth are noted in the opposite breast. Only in rare cases is such a deposit really a second primary growth. In a few cases the inguinal glands become enlarged, showing that permeation has extended below the level of the umbilicus into the region of the main tributaries of the inguinal glands. Embolic invasion of the inguinal glands then becomes a possibility.

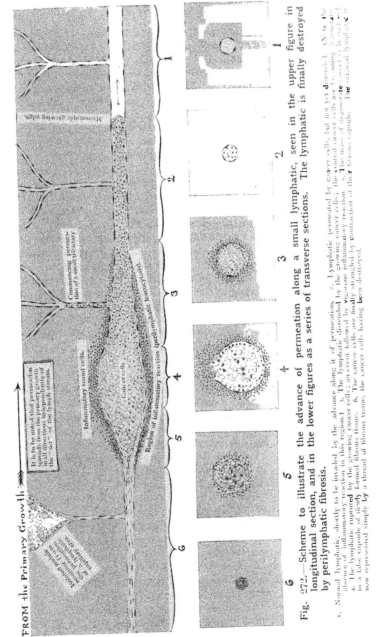

FROM the Primary Growth

It is to be noted that permeation spreads from the primary growth in all directions independently of the side of the lymph stream.

Microscopic growing edge.

Commencing permeation of a small tributary

Inflammatory round cells.

Cancer cells.

Region of inflammatory reaction (perilymphatic leucocytosis).

Fig. 272.—Scheme to illustrate the advance of permeation along a small lymphatic, seen in the upper figure in longitudinal section, and in the lower figures as a series of transverse sections. The lymphatic is finally destroyed by perilymphatic fibrosis.

1, Normal lymphatic, shortly to be invaded by the advance along it of permeation. 2, Lymphatic permeated by cancer cells, but not yet distended. (N te the absence of inflammatory reaction in this region.) 3, The lymphatic distended by the growing cancer cells; the central cancer cells are becoming degenerate. 4, The lymphatic ruptured by the growing cancer cells; an event followed by vigorous inflammatory reaction. 5, The mass of degenerate cancer cells becomes enclosed in a lobe capsule of newly formed fibrous tissue. 6, The cancer cells are finally strangled by contraction of their fibrous capsule. The original lymphatic is now represented simply by a thread of fibrous tissue, the cancer cells having been destroyed.

The permeation theory.—Although the force of the lymph stream carries cancer cells to the axillary glands, they are there filtered off and detained. If a reflux lymph stream carries them towards the opposite breast they are similarly filtered off and detained, near the middle line, in the meshwork of fine vessels which forms the only lymphatic communication between the opposite sides of the body. Thus the force of the lymph stream is ineffective as a means of *general* dissemination; it is effective only within the limits of the lymphatic area in which the primary focus is situated. In whatever direction the cancer cells attempt to leave that area, they find an effective filter blocking the way. But they do actually succeed in leaving it, as the facts of dissemination show. An illustration will make clear the method by which they overcome the obstacles to their spread into other lymphatic areas. Certain bacteria, which cannot be forced through a porcelain filter, will nevertheless, if left in it for a few days, grow through its pores and infect its outer surface. In the same way, cancer cells are able to traverse the lymphatic plexuses by actually growing along the fine vessels which compose them. This process, which I have called *permeation*, is the master-process of dissemination, for no barriers exist to stop its slow centrifugal progress. Permeation spreads in all directions with approximate equality, independently of the direction of the lymph stream, but keeping in the plane of the main lymphatic plexus until the pressure within its vessels forces the cancer cells up its minute tributaries to invade the adjacent layers. That is to say, in the case of the breast, the deep fascia will be extensively invaded over a circular area of which the primary growth is the centre, while a smaller circular area of the skin and of the subjacent muscles will show permeation or nodular deposits.

Perilymphatic fibrosis.—In view of its importance it may seem strange that the process of permeation so long eluded notice. In certain situations, such as the pleura, where it is sometimes visible to the naked eye, it had been described under the name *lymphangitis carcinomatosa*, but its importance remained unsuspected, and it was regarded as a pathological curiosity. Large areas of a tissue thickly sown with cancer nodules may be examined without finding any trace of permeation. Such nodules, it was therefore argued, must have resulted from embolism; and the argument appeared conclusive until I detected the crucial fact that a lymphatic along which cancer cells have pushed their way does not persist unchanged. The cancer cells by their continued growth distend and finally rupture the lymphatic. An inflammatory reaction is set up, abundant round-celled infiltration occurs round the liberated cylinder of cancer cells, the vitality of which has been much impaired by pressure, and a capsule of newly formed fibrous tissue contracts upon and strangles the degenerate cancer cells. Finally, the original lymphatic is replaced by a solid thread of fibrous tissue in which no cancer cells can be seen. This process may be called *perilymphatic fibrosis*. While it is taking place, cancer cells forced along the lymphatic capillaries may have originated nodular and apparently isolated deposits in the adjoining layers.

The tendency of a carcinoma to drag in towards itself the surrounding apparently healthy tissues is an inevitable consequence of the process of perilymphatic fibrosis, for the contraction of the new fibrous tissue threads, replacing the normal network of lymphatic vessels, leads to a general puckering and shrinkage of the affected zone. The process of perilymphatic fibrosis is especially interesting because it is an example of the local cure of cancer by natural processes (*see* p. 69). But the cure is local only, for the fibrotic process fails to overtake the spreading edge of permeation, which has meantime invaded new districts of the lymphatic system.

Owing to the regular centrifugal spread of permeation in an ever-widening circle away from the primary growth, three zones of cancerous infection can be distinguished around the obvious primary growth.

1. The inner zone of isolated or confluent *secondary nodules*. In this zone the permeated lymphatics have been destroyed.

2. A narrow zone in which *perilymphatic fibrosis* is actively progressing, and in which invasion of the layers adjacent to the main lymphatic plexus is seen in an early stage.

3. The *microscopic growing edge* or outer zone of fascial permeation. This zone is clinically inappreciable, for the infection is purely microscopic. The lymphatic vessels are choked by cancer cells, while infiltration is absent—that is to say, the interstices of the tissues are free from cancer cells. The microscopic growing edge is found in the plane of the deep fascia where the main lymphatic plexus is situated. The clinical importance of this fact cannot be over estimated.

The detection of the microscopic growing edge in the deep fascia is the primary fact upon which the permeation theory rests. It is a zone but a few millimetres wide, and it can only be detected by taking sections radiating from the growth far into apparently healthy tissues, and by examining these sections in their whole length. But this, the true growing edge of the cancer, though inappreciable by ordinary methods of examination, is just as definite and real as the visible spreading edge of a ringworm or of a tertiary syphilide. At first the microscopic growing edge forms a small circle immediately around the growth, but it constantly increases in size until it may attain a diameter of 2 ft., involving the scalp above, reaching the groins below, and enveloping the back.

Visceral dissemination.—Although the permeation theory of dissemination seems the only tenable one so far as the superficial metastases are concerned, it might appear at first sight necessary to invoke the embolic theory to explain secondary deposits in the viscera. Careful investigation shows that this is not the case. The visceral metastases in breast cancer mainly arise from permeation along the numerous fine anastomoses which, piercing the parietes, connect the lymphatic plexus of the deep fascia with the subendothelial lymphatic plexuses of the pleura and the peritoneum, and with the mediastinal and portal glands. But as soon as the subserous plexus is reached, permeation is relegated to a subsidiary position, for the cancer cells soon erode the over-lying endothelium and escape into the serous cavities. Under the influence of muscular movements and of gravity, the cancer cells become widely diffused throughout the invaded cavity, and implant themselves upon the serous surfaces of the various organs. Here they grow and originate secondary deposits. This mode of cancerous dissemination

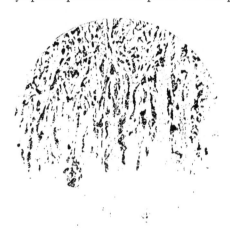

Fig. 273.—Infiltration in breast cancer. Narrow columns of cancer cells are growing along the cellular interspaces. × 20. Cf. Fig. 274.

may be called *transcœlomic implantation.* It only occurs very late in the disease, but once initiated it rapidly leads to the death of the patient.

In accordance with this view is the fact that the thorax and the abdomen may be invaded independently. That is to say, after death secondary deposits may be found only in the thorax and not in the abdomen, or only in the abdomen and not in the thorax—a fact for which the embolic theory fails to account. Moreover, as might be expected, the presence of serous (non-cancerous) adhesions is found to delay dissemination by hindering transcœlomic implantation. The secondary deposits, too, in the serous cavities show a preference for the serous surfaces of the viscera, and, owing to the action of gravity, tend to affect the lower limits of the serous cavities, especially the pelvis.

Epigastric invasion of the abdomen.—According to the researches of Stiles, the lower and inner margin of the breast overlies the sixth costal cartilage—that is to say, this part of the mammary circumference is distant only about an inch from the epigastric angle. In the epigastric angle the deep fascia is separated from the subperitoneal fat and the peritoneum only by a single layer of fibrous tissue, the linea alba. As soon as fascial permeation has spread an inch beyond the margin of the breast, cancer cells are thus brought into close proximity with the peritoneal cavity, and they have only to infiltrate the linea alba and pass through the loose subserous fat before reaching it. This mode of abdominal invasion, which I have traced microscopically in all its stages, may be called *epigastric invasion*. Reaching the peritoneum by this route, the cancer cells first implant themselves upon the convex upper surface of the liver, close to the falciform ligament. Other cancer cells may fall into the pelvis and give rise to deposits filling the pouch of Douglas, or to secondary ovarian growths. Epigastric invasion probably occurs sooner or later in at least one case in three. It is especially likely to supervene early in cancers

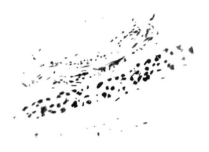

Fig. 274.—A permeated lymphatic in longitudinal section. The endothelium of the lymphatic is visible outside the mass of cancer cells which fills it. Above it is seen a normal blood-vessel. Infiltration of the tissues is absent. × 150. Cf. Fig. 273.

(*From Handley's "Cancer of the Breast and its Operative Treatment."*)

affecting the lower and inner quadrant. It may be suspected when epigastric pain and tenderness are present, even apart from hepatic enlargement and jaundice, and may be diagnosed with confidence if subcutaneous nodules are present in the epigastric region.

Other modes of invasion of the abdomen.—The retroperitoneal abdominal organs, especially the liver, kidneys, and suprarenals, or the lumbar spine may be attacked by the downward extension of permeation through the diaphragm from pleural deposits. This may be called retroperitoneal invasion of the abdomen. In rare cases the peritoneal cavity may be reached, when the pleura is already cancerous, by cancerous infiltration of the anterior portion of the diaphragm (diaphrenic invasion).

Invasion of the thorax.—Breast cancer may reach the interior of the thorax in several ways. (*a*) Permeation may extend, by means of lymphatic anastomoses piercing the anterior end of the intercostal spaces, to the anterior mediastinal glands, and thus to the other thoracic glands and to the pleura. Fortunately this is not common, for cancerous anterior mediastinal glands are found in only 6·5 per cent. of necropsies on breast cancer. (*b*) The pleural cavity may be invaded by direct infiltration of the chest wall beneath the primary growth. (*c*) Cancerous supraclavicular glands may become adherent to the dome of the pleura. Subsequently, cancer cells infiltrate the pleura and escape into the pleural cavity.

Thoracic dissemination may be delayed or prevented by the presence of old pleural adhesions.

Secondary deposits in the brain.—Secondary deposits occur in the brain in about 4 per cent. of cases, and in the dura mater with about the same frequency. They may be due to blood invasion, but often they result from upward permeation along the cervical lymphatics from enlarged supraclavicular glands.

Permeation and infiltration contrasted.—Some recent writers have used the terms permeation and infiltration indiscriminately, and it will be well to lay down clearly the differences between these two modes of spread of carcinoma, and to indicate their relative importance.

INFILTRATION (Fig. 273)	PERMEATION (Fig. 274)
In point of time, the earliest disseminative process.	In point of time, begins after infiltration.
Best seen at the edge of the primary growth, as defined by the naked eye.	Best seen at the *microscopic growing edge*, which, in advanced cases, may be situated in apparently normal tissues, 6 in. or more from the apparent edge of the primary growth.
The cancer cells are spreading along the tissue interspaces, e.g. between fat cells, or between adjoining fibrous bundles. (*See* Fig. 273.)	The lymphatic vessels, not the lymphatic spaces, are filled up and choked by solid cords of cancer cells. The tissue interspaces are free from cancer cells. (*See* Fig. 274.)
If infiltrating cancer cells intrude into a capillary lymphatic vessel the process of infiltration merges into that of permeation.	If a permeated lymphatic ruptures, the cancer cells set free may infiltrate the surrounding tissues. Thus permeation may lead to infiltration.

Infiltration is a very slow process, because of the resistance offered to the passage of cancer cells through the cramped and tortuous tissue interspaces.

Infiltration, on account of its slowness, is of relative unimportance as a factor in general dissemination.

Permeation is a more rapid process than infiltration, because the cancer cells are growing with little resistance along the open lumen of the lymphatic vessels.

Permeation may carry cancer cells to a very considerable distance from the primary tumour, and is capable of traversing the minute anastomotic lymphatic plexuses. It is accordingly the principal factor in general dissemination.

Summary.—It will be clear from what has been said that the processes concerned in dissemination are mainly three in number—(a) permeation, (b) infiltration, (c) transcœlomic implantation. To these must be added, as playing subsidiary parts—(d) lymphatic embolism, which leads only to gland deposits, and (e) blood embolism, which is usually ineffective owing to the inability of the cancer cells to colonize the blood-stream.

Effects of lymphatic obstruction in breast cancer.

—Certain of the later manifestations of breast cancer do not depend upon actual cancerous growth, but upon interference with the return of lymph from the affected part owing to obstruction of its lymphatics by permeation and perilymphatic fibrosis. The changes due to lymphatic obstruction are seen in the skin, the arms, and the serous cavities, and need brief separate consideration in each of these situations.

"Pig-skin," or "peau d'orange."—One of the most characteristic signs of cancer of the breast in a somewhat advanced, though perhaps still operable, stage is the appearance known as pig-skin or *peau d'orange*. In this condition the orifices of the sebaceous glands, normally just visible, become enlarged and deepened, to form obvious dotted depressions, sometimes blackened and emphasized by ingrained dirt. The affected skin is obviously thick and leathery, and has lost its suppleness. It overlies the carcinoma, and is usually adherent to it, but later the surrounding skin may be involved to a considerable distance (Fig. 275). It is sometimes erroneously stated that orange-rind integument is seen only in carcinoma. Although due to cancer in nearly all cases, it may occur in syphilis, in tubercle, in cold abscess of the breast, and in elephantiasis.

Pathology.—It has been taught until recently that *peau d'orange* depends upon the anchorage of the breast to the overlying skin by means of the fibrous bands called the ligaments of Astley Cooper, and that it is produced by the contraction of these ligaments following their invasion by growth. This view appears to hold an element of truth, but, since an identical appearance may be seen upon the skin in elephantiasis, the explanation is incorrect. Leitch has shown convincingly that the appearance is produced by swelling of the skin due to lymphatic stasis, i.e. ·by lymphatic œdema. Where the skin is transfixed by hair-follicles it is unable to swell, and at these points

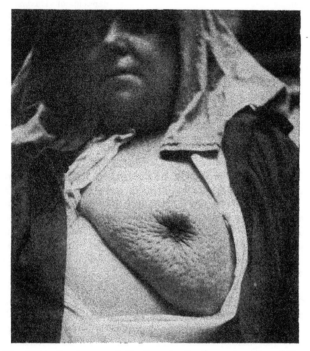

Fig. 275.—Carcinoma of the breast, showing retraction of the nipple, and marked and extensive *peau d'orange*.

obvious pits are seen, comparable to the buttoned depressions in a stuffed arm-chair. The occurrence of the lymphatic obstruction is explained by the facts of permeation (*see* p. 60).

Cancerous pachydermia (cancer en cuirasse).—In certain cases of breast cancer the skin over and round the tumour becomes hypertrophied, leathery, and thickened. The condition just described as pig-skin is the earliest sign of this pachydermatous change. Usually the skin retains its normal colour and does not pit on pressure. In the late stage of the affection, cancerous nodules, which may ulcerate,

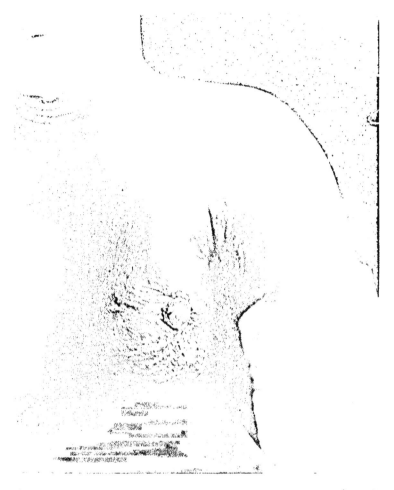

inoma of the breast of atrophic type, showing early " cancer en cuirasse."
breast and skin are firmly fixed to the thorax. Lymphatic œdema of the
is present as high as the clavicle and beyond the middle line in front.
(*See* p. 66.)

*From a case under the care of Mr. A. B. Mitchell of Belfast, to whom the author is indebted for the
beautiful coloured photograph here reproduced.)*

PLATE 81.

appear here and there in the affected area, and the skin, previously leathery, now becomes hard and brawny, purplish or red in colour, and perhaps covered by rough desquamating crusts. Cancerous pachydermia first appears over the primary growth and spreads from it in all directions, involving an increasing and roughly circular area which ultimately includes the whole of the front of the chest, and encroaches on the abdomen, neck, and back. It is usually associated with "brawny arm," and in its latest stages both arms may be swollen (Fig. 276 and Plate 81).

In an extreme instance of cancerous pachydermia recorded by Velpeau, the skin was affected from the umbilicus to the larynx, and from the loins to the occiput. The thickened skin was sown with scirrhous ulcers and closely-set cancerous bosses. The arms were tripled in bulk. and as hard as marble. The respiration resembled that of a person whose chest is gripped in a vice, and the arms and head were immovable, while pain in the arms was constant and terrible, so that the sufferer longed for death. In such cases, asphyxia may be the actual cause of death.

The condition I have just described was regarded until recently as due to cancerous invasion of the skin, and this view is correct as regards the later stages. But if the thickened skin be examined in the early stage of leathery hypertrophy no cancer cells can be found in it, and I have shown that the condition is one of lymphatic œdema, the changes being identical with those met with in the skin of elephantiasis. The altered skin of the breast may sometimes attain a thickness of 6 mm. before any cancer cells can be detected in it.

The factor which causes lymphatic obstruction is cancerous permeation and subsequent fibrotic obliteration of the underlying fascial lymphatic plexus and its tributaries. The name *cancerous pachydermia* is thus the most appropriate which can be found. The name *cancer en cuirasse* should be reserved for the later stage of cancerous pachydermia in which the skin shows nodular or diffuse cancerous infiltration.

The "brawny arm" of breast cancer.—In a late stage of breast cancer the corresponding arm often becomes swollen and œdematous. At first the œdema pits on pressure, but it soon becomes solid and brawny. The arm is the seat of an unbearable heavy dragging pain, and may attain a size twice or three times its normal volume. The skin is tense and shiny. Muscular power is gradually lost, until complete paralysis results. This condition has been ascribed to venous obstruction, a view shown to be incorrect by the absence of œdema after resection of the axillary veins. It has been said to be due to obstruction of the lymphatic trunks by growth outside or within them. If this were the case it should invariably occur in an early stage of the disease, for cancerous infiltration of the axillary glands must necessarily obstruct the trunks which lead to them. In point

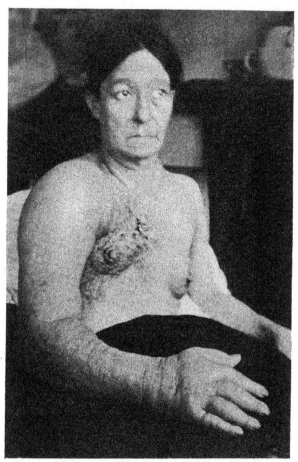

Fig. 276.—Carcinoma of the breast in a late stage, showing cancer *en cuirasse* and an extreme degree of lymphatic swelling of the arm. The swelling extends to the shoulder, and on this account the case is not a suitable one for lymphangioplasty.

of fact, lymphatic œdema of the arm is a consequence of the spread of permeation to the lymphatic plexuses about the shoulder, and of the subsequent conversion of the permeated vessels into solid cords of fibrous tissue. The arm is thus completely cut off from the lymphatic circulation. No collateral circulation can be established, and the limb necessarily falls into a condition of lymphatic œdema.

The treatment of this condition is discussed at p. 95.

Serous effusions in breast cancer.—The collection of fluid in the serous cavities is a sign that the patient has at most but a few months to live. Sometimes pleuritic effusion appears only a day or two before death, and in such cases it is due to terminal heart-failure. But generally it appears to depend upon lymphatic obstruction, and more especially upon permeation of the subpleural lymphatic plexus, which may be completely injected with cancer cells (so-called lymphangitis carcinomatosa). This condition is recognizable post mortem by the naked eye. The pressure of enlarged cancerous glands must also be regarded as a cause of pleuritic effusion. Similar factors are at work in causing ascites, and the distension of the abdomen may be extreme. It is thus obvious that lymphatic obstruction is often the proximal cause of death in breast cancer.

Serous effusions causing distress should be treated by aspiration, but sometimes the interference is not worth while.

Natural regression or repair in breast cancer.—The close observation of breast cancer has shown that occasionally, in cases running their natural course, and in the absence of all treatment, subcutaneous secondary deposits may shrink and disappear, enlarged glands may become impalpable, cancerous ulcers may completely heal, and osseous union may take place in bones fractured as the result of secondary deposits.

One case recorded by Pearce Gould presented numerous thoracic sub-cutaneous nodules, enlarged and hard glands above the clavicles and in the axillæ, spontaneous fracture of the left femur, and great dyspnœa and emaciation. All the deposits spontaneously disappeared within a few months, and the patient remained well for at least three years, when she was lost sight of.

The most probable explanation of these facts is that certain pro-cesses of repair, which in exceptional cases may become clinically manifest by the disappearance of massive secondary deposits, are a normal part of the cancer process. In a mass of cancer cells, owing to nutritional difficulties, the central portions sooner or later become fibrotic and degenerate, a fact clinically shown by the almost invariable ulceration which occurs in primary growths and by the umbilication found in secondary deposits in the liver. The process of repair tends to spread from the centre of the mass to its circumference, and its ultimate outcome, unless the death of the patient intervenes, is the replacement of the mass of cancer cells by a fibrous scar. Thus in chronic cases the older secondary deposits may be reduced to fibroid masses in which no epithelium can be detected. But the fibrosis and cure of the older deposits does not interfere with the process of dissemination or delay the fatal event.

Degeneration in carcinoma. — The improvised vascular arrangements of a carcinoma frequently prove insufficient to meet the needs of the rapidly growing cell masses which fill the meshes of the stroma. Since these masses are themselves avascular, there comes a time when the central cells of each alveolus, cut off from their base of supply, degenerate and die. They may necrose, or liquefy, or change into colloid material. In some cancers these changes are only recognizable by the microscope; in others large visible areas of the tumour are affected.

Necrotic changes.—The greyish appearance which most carcinomas present on section is probably due to early necrotic changes. In more marked instances, areas of necrotic material are seen as greyish dots upon the cut surface, and exude as plugs resembling sebum when the tumour is compressed. Microscopically, necrotic cells fail to stain, and present a granular homogeneous appearance. Here and there cell outlines may still be recognizable.

Liquefaction.—In some carcinomas each fully developed alveolus presents histologically a central cystic cavity, often containing many leucocytes. Occasionally, larger cysts containing clear serous fluid may be formed.

Colloid degeneration.—Colloid is a material closely allied to mucus, formed by the degeneration of the epithelium of a carcinoma. At first the stroma does not share this change, but remains unaltered, enclosing spaces filled with clear jelly-like colloid material. In naked-eye specimens, unaltered vessels and areas of tissue which have escaped degeneration may be seen embedded in a translucent mass of colloid. Colloid degeneration can usually only be diagnosed when the breast is cut across, and it has little clinical importance. In the specimens I have seen, the cancer has been usually rather movable and of slow growth, and the patient beyond middle age. The signs dependent upon contraction, such as retraction of the nipple, are usually absent.

Calcareous degeneration has been recorded in the more fibroid forms of carcinoma.

Pathological classification of the signs of breast cancer.—The signs of breast cancer may be divided into classes :—

    A. Those dependent upon the presence of the primary growth, and upon its infiltrative tendencies (fixity of the tumour in the breast, adhesion to skin and fascia).

    B. Those dependent upon permeation and subsequent fibrosis of the lymphatics of the surrounding districts (dimpling of

the skin, shrinking of the breast, elevation and retraction
of the nipple).

c. Those dependent upon lymphatic obstruction (orange-rind
skin, brawny arm, serous effusions).

D. Those dependent on fibrosis and failure of nutrition in the
central parts of the older deposits (ulceration of primary
growth, ulceration or umbilication of the older secondary
deposits).

E. Those dependent upon the formation of satellite or metastatic nodules—

  1. In the lymphatic glands, from lymphatic embolism.
  2. In continuity with the primary growth, as terminal out-
  crops of long lines of lymphatic permeation.
  3. In the viscera and serous membranes, from invasion of the
  serous cavities and subsequent transcœlomic implantation.
  4. Those resulting from blood embolism.

Symptoms and signs.—It is unfortunate that in the earliest
stage of breast cancer the signs are equivocal. Most of the classical
signs are not produced by the growth itself, but by the fibrotic processes which are the reaction of the organism to the invading epithelium. Thus they are only available when the disease has already
made a certain amount of progress. A patient with cancer may
appear well nourished and in excellent general health. The so-called
cancerous cachexia is a late sign, often produced by septic absorption
from an ulcerated primary growth, or due to the habitual use of
morphia.

First sign noticed by the patient.—In four-fifths of the cases
of mammary cancer the patient is led to seek advice because she finds
a lump in the breast. In a few of these cases an occasional sharp
twinge of pain has led to the detection of the lump, but as a rule pain
and discomfort have been conspicuous by their absence. It is rare
to find a cancer in a patient whose only complaint is of mammary
pain. If the patient comes complaining of severe pain and a cancer
is found, the growth is usually so far advanced as to be inoperable.
The patient may have recognized and concealed its existence for a
long period, perhaps for years, or, if exceptionally unobservant, she
may not have noticed the lump. Occasionally a lump in the axilla
may be noticed by the patient before she detects anything wrong
with the breast. Discharge or bleeding from the nipple, retraction
of the nipple, discoloration or puckering of the skin, contraction or
ulceration of the breast, swelling of the arm, pain in the spine, hip, or
abdomen, fracture of the femur, an abdominal swelling, or signs of
paraplegia—each of these conditions may be exceptionally the reason

assigned by the patient for seeking advice. Many of these signs imply an advanced degree of dissemination, so that the disease is hopeless when first seen. The causes of this regrettable fact are feelings of delicacy, dread of operation, and the insidious and painless course of the disease in its earlier stages.

The signs of breast cancer will now be separately described, one by one, in the order of their appearance. The order is, however, far from being constant.

Presence of a lump in the breast. — The primary growth usually forms a definite localized lump in the breast, characteristic-ally single, of stony hardness, palpable with the flat hand, and fixed in the substance of the breast. In the early stage the small lump may be mobile and indistinguishable from an innocent tumour, and all other signs of carcinoma may be absent. It is the surgeon's ideal to detect and remove the carcinoma in this stage, and in all such doubtful cases the diagnosis should be completed without delay by an exploratory operation, especially if the patient is over 30.

Dimpling or retraction of the skin.—This is one of the ear-liest signs of the carcinomatous nature of a small lump in the breast, and perhaps the most valuable. Dimpling is sometimes obvious to the eye (Fig. 277), but careful manipulation and close observation are necessary to appreciate the slighter degrees, which are of great value and significance. The finger and thumb placed firmly upon the skin on opposite sides of the growth are to be slowly approximated. In carcinoma the convex fold of skin which is thrown up by this manoeuvre presents upon its summit a slight and very shallow cir-cular depression; or a definite fold may fail to make its appearance, and may be replaced by a number of ill-defined wrinkles.

Another method of demonstrating retraction is to push the whole breast in the direction of the area of skin to be tested. Owing to its attachments to the underlying tumour a local depression appears upon this area of skin.

Adhesion of the skin.—In the earlier stages of dimpling the skin still moves over the subjacent growth; but later, actual adhesion becomes manifest over the centre of the growth. The *pig-skin* or *peau d'orange* appearance is now usually seen (*see* Fig. 275 and p. 65).

Adhesion to the pectoral fascia.—Early cancerous growths move freely with the breast over the subjacent pectoral fascia; but in a comparatively early stage, especially if the growth is deeply situated in the breast, signs of fixation of the growth to the fascia become manifest. Careful attention to detail is necessary to demon-strate this sign. Either by the patient's voluntary contraction of the great pectoral, or better by passively elevating the arm, the fibres of this muscle are made taut. The growth is grasped in the hand

and is moved to and fro in a direction parallel to the fibres of the muscle. Partial or complete fixation may thus be detected. Movements at right angles to the fibres is, of course, present even when the growth is completely fixed to the muscle. Deep growths become fixed to the muscle before adhesion to the skin is evident, while in superficial ones the reverse is the case.

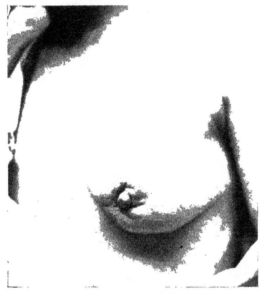

Fig. 277.—Absence of retraction of the nipple in advanced breast cancer. Note the presence of *peau d'orange,* and of extensive puckering and adhesion of the skin.

Local flattening of the contour of the breast. — Lenthal Cheatle has drawn attention to local flattening of the curved contours of the breast, when the organ is viewed in profile, as a sign of carcinoma.

Enlargement of the axillary glands. — This sign is often present by the time the patient seeks advice. The prognosis is more favourable in cases where the cancer has not yet affected the glands. The glands on the same side as the tumour become unduly palpable, hard, and inelastic. A little later they are definitely enlarged, hard, and mobile, but not tender. Only in inoperable cases do they become fixed to the skin or to the thoracic wall. To examine the axilla the arm is slightly abducted, and the fingers, made into a cone, are pressed upwards as high as possible along the outer wall of the axilla. The palmar surfaces are then pressed against the inner wall, and are slowly drawn downwards still firmly pressed against it. If enlarged glands are present they will be felt to slip past the descending finger-tips.

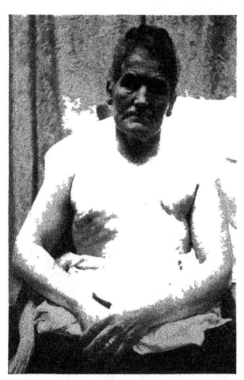

Meantime the pectorals must be relaxed, the patient allowing the arm to hang loosely by her side.

Retraction and elevation of the nipple.—Retraction of the nipple occurs in one case out of four, and when present usually indicates proximity of the primary growth to the nipple. The nipple is first flattened, and then indrawn, so that a conical depression replaces an elevation (Fig. 275). The absence of retraction (Fig. 277) possesses no significance unless the growth is near the nipple, nor is its presence significant unless the nipple has previously been normal. In cases of

Fig. 278.—Case of true primary carcinoma of each breast. The carcinoma on the patient's right side developed twelve years after the removal of a carcinoma of the left breast.

atrophic scirrhus, retraction of the nipple may precede the appearance of a tumour, and may be the earliest change noted.

The whole breast is often drawn up towards the pectoral fascia, so that the nipple is situated on a higher level than that of the sound side. This sign is a consequence of extensive perilymphatic fibrosis in the lymphatics of the breast.

The foregoing signs may all be present in cases which are still favourable ones for operation. Those now to be described indicate, that the case, though perhaps still suitable for operation, is an unfavourable one.

Shrinkage of the breast.—The whole breast in fibrotic growths becomes flattened and smaller than its fellow, owing to the conversion of its permeated lymphatic vessels into a network of threads of fibrous tissue.

Ulceration of the growth.—Adhesion of the skin is soon followed by discoloration, infiltration, and ulceration. The ulcer has a sloughy, irregular base and thickened rampart-like edges, and the skin around it is puckered and indrawn. On the average, ulceration begins two and a half years from the time when the disease is first noticed. Unless the ulcer is kept aseptic by local applications it gives rise to a thin offensive discharge, sloughs form upon its surface, and serious hæmorrhage may occur. Many cancers are inoperable by the time ulceration begins, but this is by no means invariably the case.

Pain in the breast.—It is an unfortunate fact that, as in cancer generally, pain is not an early symptom of cancer of the breast. As a rule the onset of serious pain coincides with the appearance of ulceration, but in rare cases pain may be absent almost throughout. It is usually described as pricking, throbbing, or stabbing in character. The really severe pains of breast cancer occur in the inoperable stages, and are then associated either with supraclavicular deposits pressing upon the brachial plexus, with lymphatic œdema of the arm, or with spinal deposits, or other deposits in the bones.

Nodular invasion of the surrounding skin is a very unfavourable sign, and if the nodules extend more than 2 in. from the primary growth the case should be looked upon as inoperable, for the area of fascial permeation will be too large for removal.

Enlargement of the supraclavicular glands is regarded by some authorities as placing a case in the inoperable category. But if the glands are still mobile, operation should, in my opinion, be advised.

The conditions which render a case of breast cancer inoperable are detailed at p. 88.

Diagnosis.—It is desirable that breast cancer should be operated upon before the signs of adhesion and contraction have manifested themselves—that is to say, before the disease is clinically recognizable. This object can only be attained by exploring all doubtful tumours of the breast occurring in patients over 30 years of age.

The conditions which most closely simulate breast cancer are chronic mastitis, a deep cyst, especially if surrounded by an area of chronic mastitis, a fibro-adenoma situated in an area of chronic mastitis, a gumma of the breast, and tuberculosis.

The diagnosis between *chronic mastitis* and cancer may here be summed up in tabular form :—

CHRONIC MASTITIS	CARCINOMA
A mobile induration uniformly and finely granular, only vaguely palpable with the flat hand.	A definite lump fixed in the breast and easily palpable with the flat hand.
Indurations often multiple.	A single lump.
Indurations sector-shaped, mapping out the limits of one or more lobes of the breast.	The lump is more or less rounded, and does not respect the anatomical boundaries which separate adjoining lobes.
Indurated areas often tender and may be the seat of pain.	Lump neither painful nor tender.
The indurated areas do not adhere to skin or to fascia.	Lump usually (but not necessarily) shows signs of adhesion to skin or fascia, or both.
Axillary glands only slightly enlarged, often distinctly tender, not hard.	Axillary glands often (but not necessarily) enlarged, hard and not tender.
Nipple not retracted.	Nipple may be retracted.
Skin normal.	Skin may present the orange-rind appearance.

Diagnosis is, however, complicated by the fact that a carcinoma may arise in an area of chronic mastitis. A local lump in the midst of a sector-shaped area of granular induration may be a cyst, a fibro-adenoma, or an early carcinoma. Multiple rounded and movable lumps will probably prove to be *cysts ;* a single and fixed one is' often a carcinoma, and imperatively demands exploration. Only in cases where the indurations are vague, sector-shaped, and uniformly and finely granular can a carcinoma be excluded with certainty. In the large class of doubtful cases, experience alone can decide, and less harm is done by exploring unnecessarily than by awaiting the full development of a carcinoma. Nevertheless, routine operations in chronic mastitis are much to be deprecated.

A cyst deeply situated in the breast of a stout patient may simulate a carcinoma most closely, especially if surrounded by chronic mastitis. It is exceptional to obtain fluctuation in a deep cyst. The absence of enlarged axillary glands and of adhesion to skin or fascia, while suggesting that the tumour may be a cyst, does not exclude carcinoma. It is true that the puncture of the tumour by a trocar and cannula will settle whether a cyst is present ; but the surgeon's anxiety is merely transferred from the tumour to the surrounding breast tissue, since a carcinoma not infrequently arises in the breast tissue near a cyst. In the absence of unequivocal signs of cancer, certainty can only be reached by exploration and histological examination.

The remarks made respecting a deep cyst apply also to a *fibro-adenoma* deeply situated and surrounded by an area of chronic mastitis which partially fixes it in the breast. The diagnosis from cancer then becomes impossible, and exploration is imperative. Signs of contraction and adhesion are absent. Puncture with a trocar shows that the tumour is solid. All the means of diagnosis, save actual exploration, fail to exclude carcinoma.

Gummatous and tuberculous mastitis, which in their early stages simulate ordinary chronic mastitis, may later produce one or more indurated fixed lumps in the breast. Adhesion to skin and fascia may occur, and orange-rind skin may be present. Moreover, in tubercle, and even sometimes in gummatous mastitis, the axillary glands may be enlarged, hard, and not tender. At this period the resemblance to carcinoma is very close. Usually, however, in syphilis a careful search will detect tertiary lesions other than those in the breast, and the rapid effect of treatment with iodide will clear up all doubts. Tuberculosis usually occurs in younger people than does carcinoma, but sometimes the diagnosis is impossible before operation. In the later stages of both gumma and tubercle the diagnostic feature is a central area of softening in the midst of the indurated mass, and still later the discoloration of the skin which heralds the bursting of an abscess.

Fibrotic changes in the breast resulting from a former abscess may be accompanied by some of the signs of cancer, and especially by adhesion of the skin and shrinkage of the affected breast. The history of suppuration, the presence of a scar upon the skin, and the absence of an underlying tumour will suffice to prevent a mistake.

In the rare cases in which a *simple tumour* of the breast penetrates the skin (fungating cystic adenoma, fungating duct papilloma), malignant disease is closely simulated. Microscopical examination of a large piece of the fungating tissue is the best solution of the difficulty. In fungating simple tumours it may be possible to pass a probe some distance within the cystic cavity.

The diagnosis between a hard cancer and a *sarcoma* is easy, owing to the absence in sarcoma of the signs dependent upon contraction, and the large size, softness, and rapid growth of the tumour. But a soft cancer and a sarcoma may be quite indistinguishable save on microscopical examination. In sarcoma, however, the axillary glands are only exceptionally infected.

Prognosis.—The prognosis in breast cancer is difficult. The questions requiring answer are mainly two. If the growth runs its natural course, how long has the patient to live ? After operation, what is the chance that the growth will not return ?

Upon the first point very little that is helpful can be said, and the widest experience is liable to err. If the growth is of recent and rapid development, and the patient young, life will probably terminate within a few months. In fibroid cancers of slow development the expectation of life is two to four years. But a cancer may remain active for forty years without killing its possessor, as in a case which I have seen.

A prognosis of non-recurrence after operation can be given with fair confidence if the growth has not acquired adhesions to skin or fascia, nor caused axillary enlargement, always provided that a complete operation is performed. These are the cases detected by exploratory operation. In cases where diagnosis is possible without exploration the chances are in favour of recurrence, and it is best to state that time alone will settle the question. In cases still operable, but presenting advanced symptoms, such as ulceration, operation should not be pressed, and the probability of internal recurrence should be mentioned. But apparently advanced cases sometimes do well, and in cases which seem early some disappointments will nevertheless occur.

The percentage of patients who are permanently cured by operation has steadily increased of late years as operative methods have improved. Future advances depend upon the earlier recognition of the disease, increasing knowledge of its pathology, and the abandonment of restricted or badly planned (though extensive) operations.

Halsted's results show that when the modern complete operation is performed before the axillary glands have become involved, two out of three patients are permanently cured; while when the axillary glands are already infected at the time of operation, three out of four patients ultimately die of their disease. Time alone can show the effect of recent modifications of operative methods.

At least 20 per cent. of patients who survive the operation three years die of later recurrence.

Unusual varieties of breast cancer.—Breast cancer is so variable in its manifestations that it is impossible to furnish a description which suits all cases. Certain special forms need separate consideration.

Medullary or soft carcinoma. — The hardness of a typical scirrhus is due to the fibrotic processes which are associated with it. If the proliferative activity of the cancerous epithelium outstrips these defensive fibrotic processes, a large lobulated growth of relatively soft consistence is rapidly formed. The axillary glands become enlarged and may soon attain the size of chestnuts, and the skin becomes extensively adherent and assumes the orange-rind appearance. Ulceration supervenes, and a fungating mass of malignant tissue protrudes, from which large sloughs may separate. Sepsis, repeated bleeding, and dissemination lead rapidly to death. To growths of this character the name medullary carcinoma was formerly applied, as indicating their soft, marrowy consistence. They occur more especially in young women, and are of bad prognosis. Many of the cases which clinically present the features to be described as characteristic of sarcoma are nevertheless found on microscopical examination to be carcinomas of this type.

Atrophic scirrhus.—Cases are not uncommon in which the struggle between the cancer and the individual is prolonged and doubtful. Such appears to be the true explanation of cases of atrophic scirrhus. In the most marked form of atrophic scirrhus a puckered scar, to which the skin may be attached, slowly forms in the breast. The whole breast becomes somewhat shrunken and the nipple indrawn, but no definite tumour makes its appearance.

The disease in this form is usually painless, and the patient's attention is attracted only by local puckering and adhesion of the skin. Frequently the patient attaches no importance to these signs, and it is only when she consults a medical man for some other condition that the lesion of the breast is discovered. The condition may persist for many years without obvious change until the patient dies of some other disease, but if she survives long enough it is likely that local malignant ulceration or dissemination resulting from permeation will terminate the case.

In less extreme cases of atrophic scirrhus the primary focus, after attaining the dimensions of a definite tumour, subsequently shrinks and disappears, or leaves only a mass of dense fibrous tissue, in the central portion of which no trace of malignant epithelium can be found. The breast is reduced to a small fibrous relic resembling the male breast. Complete fibrosis of the primary growth does not necessarily or usually prevent dissemination, which, however, in these cases is very slow, attacking rather the skin, subcutaneous tissue, and bones than the internal organs.

Some authorities state that cases of atrophic scirrhus should not be operated upon—an opinion which probably dates from the time when nearly every operation upon breast cancer was an incomplete one. If any part of the growth is left behind, it is quite likely that it may be stimulated to vigorous activity by the operative interference. But there is now a reasonable hope of complete operative eradication of the disease, and, even if this end is not attained, the inhibitory action of X-rays may be called in to assist the effect of the operation. I hold, therefore, that cases of atrophic scirrhus, except in very old or very feeble patients, should be operated upon. No one can tell when an atrophic scirrhus may blossom forth into a carcinoma with active powers of dissemination.

In deciding whether to operate upon an atrophic scirrhus an especially careful general examination must be made, for the growth may have been present for years and dissemination may have made progress before the mammary signs led the patient to seek advice. Sometimes a spontaneous fracture of the femur, a deposit in the spine, or the presence of an abdominal, pelvic, or hepatic tumour may be the first obvious sign of an atrophic carcinoma of the breast, or of a tumour of some size embedded in a voluminous mamma. If a tumour is detected in a woman of middle age, whatever its situation, the breasts must be carefully examined for signs of carcinoma.

Peripheral carcinoma.—A carcinoma of the breast may commence in some outlying lobule apparently quite separate from the main body of the gland. The possibility that these outlying growths may begin in a supernumerary mamma must not be overlooked.

The prognosis of peripheral carcinoma is worse than that of the more central variety. A peripheral growth is likely to be separated from the pleural cavity by a relatively thin protective layer of muscles, as compared, for instance, with a growth which overlies the great pectoral. Consequently the growth early becomes adherent to the chest wall, and therefore inoperable. Moreover, operations for peripheral carcinoma in the past have nearly always violated the rule, deduced by the writer from the permeation theory, that the primary growth must form the centre of the field of operation and of the area of tissue removed. The observance of this rule is of cardinal importance in these outlying growths.

The case of peripheral scirrhus represented in Fig. 279 was that of a female aged about 65. Situated accurately in the middle line, just above the ensiform cartilage, at the point to which the lower contours of the mammæ converge, was an irregular ulcer, about an inch in average diameter, with a sloughy base, and hard, irregular, raised edges surrounded by subcutaneous induration. The whole mass, which could be covered by a florin, was firmly adherent to the underlying sternum, which, however, was not exposed in the floor of the ulcer. The situation of the lesion suggested a gumma. This, however, was excluded by the absence of suppuration, by the fact that bone was not exposed, by the absence of a syphilitic history, and above all by the presence in *both* axillæ of hard enlarged glands of the type familiar in carcinoma. The median situation of the growth had led to simultaneous invasion of the axillary glands on both sides.

·   **Acute cancer of the breast** (*mastitis carcinomatosa, brawny cancer*). — The most acute form of breast cancer is found only in women below middle age, and usually of florid aspect. It is accompanied by an erythematous blush of the skin over the tumour. It generally develops during lactation, though it may also occur in virgins. All the signs of inflammation are present. The whole breast is swollen and prominent. The skin is red and hot, and mav be swollen and œdematous, sometimes presenting the typical *peau d'orange* appearance. The nipple may be either retracted, or swollen and œdematous. A large tumour rapidly involves the entire breast and becomes firmly fixed to skin and fascia. Within a few weeks the

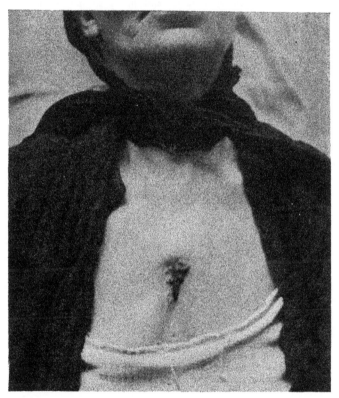

Fig. 279.—Ulcerated scirrhous carcinoma situated in the angle between the two breasts, in the middle line.

chest wall may present the appearance of advanced cancer *en cuirasse*. The thickened and rigid skin, now immobile upon the chest wall, is covered with cancerous bosses. General dissemination rapidly takes place, and within a period of from six weeks to three months after the onset of the disease the patient is dead. Operation in these cases is useless. The cutaneous œdema may lead to the erroneous diagnosis of mastitis or mammary abscess.

g

In some cases of acute cancer, swollen white cords, radiating from the nipple, may be seen upon the surface of the skin. It is usually believed that they are the larger superficial lymphatics distended by lymph. The intermediate skin is swollen from lymphatic œdema.

Diagnosis.—Not infrequently acute cancer of the breast has been mistaken for mammary abscess, and has been incised under this

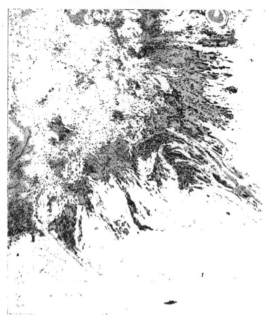

Fig. 280.—Edge of an actively infiltrating cancer of the breast under a low magnification (× 5). Note the narrow dark columns of cancer cells penetrating the interstices of the surrounding tissues. Cf. Fig. 281.

impression. Although œdema of the skin may be present over a pointing abscess, it is rarely extensive. In acute cancer the lymphatic œdema of the skin is coextensive with the breast, and, moreover, the affected area is uniformly and firmly adherent to the underlying breast, and often indurated from commencing cancerous infiltration. The breast, too, is firmly fixed to the chest wall, which is not the case in acute mastitis.

Impalpable carcinoma of the breast.—It is an important fact that in rare cases a carcinoma may be present in the breast for a long period, and even for many years, without giving rise to any palpable tumour. Sometimes in these cases enlargement of the axillary glands and the later signs of dissemination remain absent, and the description "atrophic scirrhus" is appropriate (*see* p. 79). In other cases, however, though the primary growth remains of microscopic size, enlargement of the axillary glands occurs, and the glands may even reach the size of chestnuts. These cases were formerly described as primary cancer of the axillary glands. In such cases, if the glands are

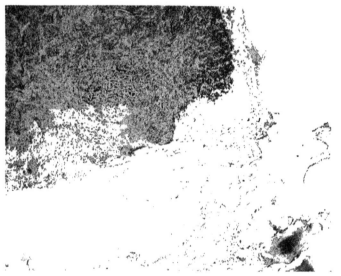

Fig. 281.—The edge of a mobile (non-infiltrating) carcinoma of the breast under a low magnification (× 5). The growth was surrounded by a capsule of fibrous tissue almost as definite as that of a fibro-adenoma. Cf. Fig. 280.

cancerous and no other primary focus can be found, the breast should be removed, and, as in a case of which Dr. Macnaughton Jones informs me, thorough microscopical examination may reveal a minute mammary carcinoma. Halsted has met with two similar cases. The facts of impalpable carcinoma have an important bearing upon the pathology of Paget's disease of the nipple (*see* p. 10).

In certain cases which simulate impalpable carcinoma, a primary growth originating at the axillary edge of the breast may be mistaken for an enlarged axillary gland.

Mobile carcinoma of the breast.—It is too often assumed that a carcinoma of the breast is always firmly fixed in the organ. This is indeed the case if the growth is an actively infiltrating one. But certain exceptional carcinomas of the ordinary spheroidal type are sluggish in this respect, and they consequently acquire a fibrous capsule, sometimes almost as definite as that of a fibro-adenoma. The capsule may be complete, even upon histological examination (Fig. 281), and in such cases the tumour is mobile and may even be enucleated without much difficulty. Thus, after removal of the tumour, and still more easily before operation, it may be mistaken for a fibro-adenoma. An apparent fibro-adenoma first appearing after the age of 40 is more likely than not to be a carcinoma.

Although these cases are exceptional, they lead to conclusions of the greatest importance : (1) In women approaching the cancer age, all rounded tumours of the breast, even those which appear quite innocent, should be dealt with promptly by operation. (2) All tumours of the breast after removal must be submitted to microscopical examination.

Duct cancer of the breast (*columnar-celled carcinoma*).— Histologically this disease is divisible into two forms—(1) carcinoma originating in the large ducts ; (2) carcinoma beginning in the small ducts. In the former variety (Fig. 283) the breast is riddled with caseous areas which are the greatly dilated ducts filled with the caseous débris of cancerous epithelium, or with richly plicated papillomatous outgrowths, or with hæmorrhagic débris. Outside these spaces there is irregular cancerous infiltration of the tissue spaces of the breast. Such cases appear to originate as innocent duct papillomas which have undergone malignant degeneration (Fig. 282). The growths are of slow development and of relatively good prognosis. They are slow in becoming adherent to their surroundings and in affecting the axillary glands. They develop usually beneath the nipple, and in women over middle age. Retraction of the nipple is usually absent.

The other variety of duct carcinoma—that originating in the small ducts—has not yet been clinically differentiated from the ordinary spheroidal-celled or acinous carcinoma. The histological picture is that of small, irregularly proliferating spaces lined with columnar cells. These spaces infiltrate the breast tissue and convert the regular pattern of its lobular structure into a confused and irregular maze. The picture presented recalls that of a columnar-celled adeno-carcinoma of the intestine (Fig. 271).

Not infrequently this variety of duct cancer is accompanied by cancerous changes in the acini also, and it may be difficult to say whether the growth is a columnar- or a spheroidal-celled carcinoma.

Clinical history.—In cases of carcinoma of the breast, if there is a history of serous discharge from the nipple of some years' standing, the disease will almost certainly prove to be a duct cancer ; if Paget's disease of the nipple has been present, it is not unlikely that the disease may be of the columnar-celled variety. But the distinction between columnar- and spheroidal-celled cancer is not one of great clinical importance, since in either case the treatment is the same. It is, however, essential to recognize clearly that the absence of signs of contraction and adhesion is not inconsistent with the presence of a carcinoma of the duct variety.

Carcinoma of the male breast.—The male breast is liable to most of the diseases which affect the female breast. Chronic mastitis, adenoma, sarcoma, duct papilloma, and other conditions occur as rarities in the male. But the only disease whose comparative frequency gives it importance is carcinoma, which may be of the spheroidal- or the columnar- or the squamous-celled variety. The disease appears later in men than in women, and in nine cases collected by C. R. Keyser

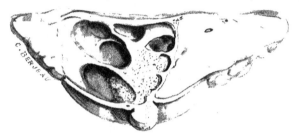

Fig. 282.—Cystic duct papilloma passing into duct carcinoma. The papillomatous growths beneath the nipple are commencing to infiltrate the surrounding tissues.

(From a case under the writer's care. The specimen is preserved in the Middlesex Hospital Museum.)

the average age was 61 years. J. R. Lunn has recorded a case of duct cancer in a man of 91, and this appears to be the oldest age on record in this connexion. Of 100 breast cancers, only one occurs in a male. A history of definite injury is common, The disease begins as a button-like induration, at first mobile, situated beneath or near the nipple. Later, adhesion to skin or fascia develops, the axillary glands become enlarged, and, by the time the growth has reached the size of a walnut, ulceration sets in. In more than half the cases the tumour is ulcerated when the surgeon first sees it. This may be accounted for by the absence of pain prior to ulceration, and the freedom of men from dread of this particular disease.

In all its essential features, cancer of the male breast is identical with the same disease in the female. It requires treatment on the same lines and by an equally free operation. There can be little doubt, however, that operations for cancer of the male breast have been unduly restricted, the small size of the breast and of the primary lesion seeming to invite a limited excision.

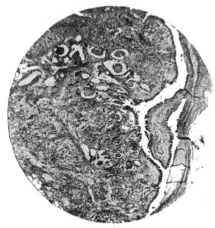

Fig. 283.—Duct papilloma and duct car-cinoma in the same microscopic field. A large duct crosses the field vertically. From its right wall a small duct papilloma projects into the lumen. From its left wall is seen an outgrowth of columnar-celled carcinoma which is infiltrating the surrounding tissues. × 20.

Exploratory incision prior to operation. — Some surgeons believe it to be dangerous to incise a doubtful carcinoma before removing it, on account of the danger of liberating cancer cells which may become implanted upon the field of operation. The risk is a very small one if precautions are taken; but, of course, a carcinoma should not be incised if the diagnosis is certain. In case of doubt a small incision is made down upon the growth and its enucleation is attempted. If the effort is unsuccessful an incision is made into, but not through, the central portion of the growth. If, after inspection, or removal of a small piece, malignancy is diagnosed, the wound is stuffed with a small swab, the deeper portion of which has been dipped in pure phenol, and the small wound is tightly sewn up over the swab. The instruments, towels, swabs, and gloves so far used are discarded, and the operation for carcinoma is begun.

Naked-eye characters of an incised carcinoma. — The tumour may creak under the knife, but more commonly cuts like a piece of potato. It cannot be shelled out of its bed, save in rare instances, and it exhibits radiating fibrous processes firmly anchored amid the surrounding fat. In colour it is greyish or pinkish-grey, in this respect and in its consistency contrasting with the leathery toughness and yellowish tinge of chronic mastitis, and with the whitish enucleable fibro-adenoma. Upon the greyish surface of a carcinoma, yellow dots representing areas of necrosis are frequently visible. An opaque fluid (cancer juice) can be scraped from the cut surface, which becomes characteristically concave as soon as the section is made.

Rapid microscopical examination.—If naked-eye inspection does not resolve doubts as to the nature of the tumour, it is, I think, better as a general rule to sew up the wound and defer the operation for a few days until a paraffin section of the excised piece has been made. But if a skilled pathologist is available an immediate examination should be made in the theatre by one of the rapid freezing methods, perhaps the best of which is Leitch's. The method is not to be relied upon unless the observer has had long practice in the examination of frozen sections—a fact acknowledged by its pioneer, Ernest H. Shaw. Few pathologists possess the necessary experience, and for this reason the method, though ideal, is at present not generally applicable.

Principles of the operation for breast cancer.—While many technical variations are possible in the operation for breast cancer, especially as regards the planning of the skin incision, certain general principles determined by the mode of spread of the disease must be held inviolable. The aim of the operation is not merely to "amputate the breast," though this is in all cases necessary, but *to remove intact the permeated area of the lymph-vascular system which surrounds the primary growth, in one piece with the lymphatic glands which may have been embolically invaded along the trunk lymphatics of the permeated area.* To attain this object certain points must be specially borne in mind.

1. *The area of the operation must be concentric with the growth.* Only when the growth itself is central must the nipple be taken as the central point of the area of skin and subjacent tissue to be ablated.

2. The area of tissue removed must approximate to a circle in shape, in view of the centrifugal spread of permeation.

3. Since permeation spreads primarily by way of the deep fascial lymphatic plexus, the ablation of tissue must be most extensive in the plane of the deep fascia, and the area of fascia removed must be a circle.

4. Smaller circular areas of skin and of muscle also require removal, on account of the secondary invasion of these layers from the permeated fascial plexus.

5. The skin incision, subject to the preceding condition, should afford convenient access, and should not be so placed that the scar will lie along the anterior axillary fold, since in this situation it will tend to bind the arm to the side.

It may here be repeated that the very extensive ablation of skin carried out by some surgeons, based upon erroneous ideas concerning dissemination, is not found in practice to improve the results of the operation.

6. During the operation, precautions should be taken against the possibility of epigastric invasion of the abdomen.

Choice of cases for operation.—Now that the immediate risk of operation is under 2 per cent., it is unfair to refuse operation unless the case is evidently hopeless. Apparently advanced cases sometimes do well, and, even if internal recurrence takes place, the patient may be saved the distress of an ulcerated growth. In early cases operation should be urged, in later cases offered.

Except in rare instances as a palliative measure for the removal of a foul ulcerated mass, operation should be refused—

(a) When the primary growth has become attached to the bony thorax.

(b) In the presence of cancer *en cuirasse*, or of subcutaneous nodules or skin infiltration situated more than 2 in. from the primary growth.

(c) If there is a fixed mass of growth in the axilla, evidently adherent to its walls.

(d) If there is marked œdema of the arm.

(e) If the supraclavicular glands are enlarged, hard, and fixed.

(f) If there is evidence of visceral or bone metastases.

(g) If there is incurable constitutional disease—tuberculosis or diabetes, for example—likely to be fatal in a few years at most, or to lead to a postoperative fatality.

(h) In the acute forms of carcinoma.

Examination prior to operation.—Remember to examine the spine for angular curvature, the epigastric parietes for nodules, and the pelvis for deposits in the ovaries and in Douglas's pouch, in addition to the usual preoperative medical examination.

Preparation of the patient.—Since massage of the mammary region must tend to favour dissemination, no compress should be employed. The axilla should be dry-shaved overnight, and the whole field painted with iodine a few hours before operation, and again upon the table.

During the operation the arm must not be forcibly stretched upwards so as to injure the brachial plexus. The whole operative field must, as far as is possible, be covered up with relays of hot towels. The best anæsthetic is C.E mixture, accompanied by a feeble stream of oxygen. Pure ether is inadvisable because by inducing very free hæmorrhage it may be the indirect cause of postoperative shock.

Technique of the operation (Handley's method).— The skin incision is only just deep enough to open up the subcutaneous fat without extending through it into the neighbourhood of the deep fascia. It consists of three parts :—

1. A ring incision, as first practised by Mitchell Banks, 4 to 5 in.

in diameter, accurately centred on the growth and surrounding it at a safe distance, slightly tailing off into incision No. 2 above, and into No. 3 below.

2. A curvilinear incision for giving access to the axilla. The axilla is opened by turning forward a flap, consisting of skin and a thin layer of subcutaneous fat, whose base lies along the anterior axillary fold. The axillary incision begins at the lower edge of the great pectoral, close to its insertion. It ends, also at the lower edge of the great pectoral, by joining the annular incision, No. 1. It crosses the base of the axilla, and marks out a shallow semilunar flap of skin, whose convexity lies in the vault of the axilla not far from the edge of the latissimus dorsi. It affords perfect access to the axilla, and good drainage afterwards.

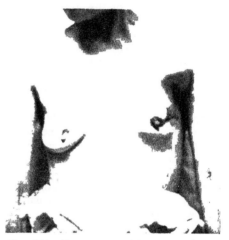

Fig. 284.—Recurrence of breast carcinoma following an inadequate operation. A portion only of the breast has been removed, and the axilla has not been cleared. Recurrence has taken place in the subclavian glands, and a mass of growth is seen pushing the pectorals forward.

3. A linear incision coming off from the lower and inner part of the annular incision and passing downwards for about 2 in. along the linea alba. Its object is to give access for the removal of the deep fascia over the upper part of the abdominal wall. Without it this important step in the operation cannot be properly carried out.

Elevation of the skin flaps.—The skin flaps are next undermined in the mid-plane of the subcutaneous fat until there is exposed an area of the deeper subcutaneous fat, forming a circle 10 to 12 in. in diameter, with the primary growth at its centre. The exact anatomical limits of this dissection will, of course, vary with the situation of the growth in the breast. The assistant retracts the skin flaps as they are formed, and subsequently keeps them carefully wrapped in hot towels frequently renewed. Neglect of this precaution is likely to be followed by ulceration of the edges of the flaps.

At this period of the operation no attempt should be made to apply artery forceps to every small bleeding-point. Spouting vessels in the deep surface of the skin flap should be clamped, but bleeding from the exposed surface of subcutaneous fat is sufficiently checked by the pressure of large flat swabs, for nearly all the exposed vessels will again be divided at a deeper level.

Delimitation of the area of deep fascia to be removed. —An annular incision, marking out the 10-in. circle of deep fascia to be removed, is now carried down to the muscles through the deeper subcutaneous fat close to the base of the skin flaps, which are meanwhile strongly retracted by the assistant.

Elevation of deep fascia from the underlying muscles. —The circular area of deeper subcutaneous fat and deep fascia, in which lies embedded the presumably permeated area of the fascial lymphatic plexus, is now dissected from the subjacent muscles for some distance from its circumference towards its centre, so as to form a wide marginal fringe of the main mass, consisting of breast, pectoral muscles, and axillary contents, which is to be subsequently removed. The fringe of deep fascia is to be raised up all round the field of operation until the knife reaches either the margin of the great pectoral muscle, the margin of the axillary outlet, or the edge of the breast, as the case may be.

The amount of dissection required varies in different parts of the field of operation. At the upper limit of the field of operation hardly any freeing of the fascia will be required, since in this region it will come away with the great pectoral when that muscle is divided below its clavicular origin. Towards the middle line the fascia will usually require dissecting up from the inner margin of the opposite great pectoral and from the sternum. In doing this the perforating branches of the internal mammary artery on the side *opposite* to the growth are often divided, and must be secured. The division of these branches necessarily implies also division of the lymphatics which run with them from the pectoral lymphatic plexus to the anterior mediastinal glands, and thus additional security against thoracic invasion is obtained. (The corresponding perforating branches on the same side as the growth are divided later during the detachment of the great pectoral.)

As regards the lower limit of the field of operation, it will be found that a 10-in. circle of deep fascia with the growth at its centre will usually extend well down over the epigastric region of the abdomen. In this part of the field of operation the anterior layer of the rectus sheath on both sides of the middle line should be raised up, and removed with the deep fascia. In order to accomplish this, the linea alba must be split from below upwards in the coronal plane. It is particularly in the epigastric region that wide and careful removal of the deep fascia is most imperatively called for, so as to prevent the access of cancer cells to the peritoneal cavity. In this part of the field of operation numerous small blood-vessels emerging from the rectus muscle will probably need attention.

Towards the outer side of the field of operation the fascia must be dissected up from over the anterior edge of the latissimus and from the serratus magnus. Higher up, especially if the growth lies in the outer portion of the breast, the fascia over the inner margin of the deltoid muscle and about the posterior margin of the axillary outlet must be raised if it falls within the circle marked out for removal, although the requisite dissection is difficult and tedious.

Division of muscles.—If the growth is an early one, or is situated low down in the breast, it is probably safe to leave the uppermost fibres of the pectoralis major near the margin of the deltoid muscle. With this exception the whole of the great pectoral needs removal, as Halsted first pointed out. It is split below its clavicular attachment; next, a finger is inserted beneath the muscle from above, so as to put its fibres on the stretch, and its chondral and sternal attachments are rapidly divided from above downwards close to their origin. The muscle is lifted from the chest and turned outwards, and the external anterior thoracic nerve and the vessels which run with it are divided where they pierce the costo-coracoid membrane.

The pectoralis minor now comes into view, and is best removed, except in early cases. It is divided at its costal origin.

The pectoral muscles are now cut across at their insertions respectively into the humerus and the coracoid process, and the whole mass of tissue is allowed to fall over towards the axilla.

Removal of axillary contents.—The costo-coracoid membrane, now freely exposed, is cautiously divided just below the clavicle, and the fat at the extreme apex of the axilla is thus brought into view. It now becomes easy to reach the highest axillary glands—subclavian in the strict sense of the word—which so easily escape notice unless they are carefully looked for. The axillary vein is sought for in this situation, and is carefully cleared from above downwards. As this dissection proceeds, the subscapular vein and other axillary tributaries come into view, and are secured and divided. The subscapular nerves are exposed, isolated, and preserved. The inner and posterior walls of the axilla are cleaned from above downwards, preserving the nerve of Bell, and the mass of tissues is now retained only where the lower and outer part of the breast overlies the serratus magnus. The digitations of this muscle, which lie in direct contact with the deep surface of the breast, should be divided at their origin from the ribs. The whole mass of tissues is now freed and removed by the division, farther back towards the scapula, of these same digitations of the serratus magnus. A superficial layer of the digitations of the external oblique, which arise from the fifth and sixth ribs, should also be removed.

The parts removed form a single circular biconvex-lens-like mass with thin extensive fascial edges. To its outer side a pyramidal mass of axillary fat and glands is attached. The mass shows a central circular patch of ablated skin on its superficial aspect. On its deep aspect are seen the pectorals, and portions of the serratus magnus and of the anterior layer of the rectus sheath.

Hæmostasis and drainage.—Any bleeding-points which have escaped ligature or forcipressure are now attended to. Two small drainage-tubes are inserted through punctures in the extreme base of the skin flaps, one in the epigastric angle, the other at the posterior margin of the axilla. These tubes are removed at the first dressing, twenty-four hours later.

Sutures.—Trial is now made to secure the best coaptation of the edges of the incision. The problem varies in each case according to the situation of the growth in the breast, and to the degree of laxity of the skin. The most striking indirect advantage of the operation now becomes evident. The wide removal of the deep fascia so mobilizes and frees the surrounding skin that even after the removal of a 5-in. circle of integument the edges of the incision can usually be brought together, without the use of tension stitches, by a single continuous suture of fine catgut. Tension in the skin flaps—the principal cause of prolonged shock, of pain and discomfort to the patient, of impaired circulation in the skin flaps, and of delayed union and ulceration in the sutured incision—is thus entirely avoided.

Often it will be found best to bring the edges together in triradiate fashion, in other cases as a sinuous line. In growths of the upper and outer quadrant some difficulty may be met with in covering the raw area, and in these cases the axillary flap of skin may be pulled inwards to assist in covering the thoracic gap.

Removal of the supraclavicular glands. — The posterior triangle should be opened up, and the supraclavicular glands removed if these glands are palpably enlarged, or in any event if the subclavian glands at the apex of the axilla are cancerous, or if the primary growth is situated in the upper hemisphere of the breast. My experience as regards recurrence shows that the posterior triangle should be cleared much oftener than is at present the practice in this country, and that Halsted and Rodman are right in advocating the frequent if not the invariable performance of this dissection.

After-treatment.—It is my practice to confine the arm to the side until the incision is healed, leaving the forearm and hand free to move. Some operators prefer to fix the upper arm in an abducted position to prevent subsequent binding of the arm to the side—a danger which, in my experience, need not be feared if, after the healing of the incision, a course of massage is applied to the skin of the thorax. The abducted position tends to increase tension in the flaps, and thus to interfere with healing.

In every case, as soon as the wound is healed, a prophylactic course of X-rays must be applied to the thorax, axilla, and supraclavicular region—a precaution which I believe to be imperative. Four cases only of recurrence in the skin have come under notice in my series of operations, of which three were those of patients who had not undergone a prophylactic course of X-rays (the percentage of my patients who escape a prophylactic X-ray course is a very small one).

After the operation for breast cancer a prolonged course of open-air treatment should be advised. If the patient will not consent to this, she should, at any rate, live as much in the open air as possible. A sea voyage may be of advantage.

Plastic operations in cancer of the breast.—Much ingenuity has been expended by surgeons in devising plastic flaps to fill the gap left after removal of a cancer of the breast (Jackson's, Tansini's). These operations are unnecessary, for, if an adequate area of the deep fascia be removed, and if ablation of the skin be not pushed to the point of unnecessary sacrifice, difficulty in bringing the flaps together is rare ; it is only met with in thin women with ill-developed chests. Immediate skin-grafting by Thiersch's method is the best solution of the difficulty.

Plastic methods are not only unnecessary, they are also dangerous, for the tissues utilized to form the flap are frequently situated within the area of possible cancerous infection.

Cause of death in breast cancer.—Although dissemination is the rule, a cancer of the breast may run its course without producing secondary deposits. The disease makes slow progress until the viscera are attacked. When visceral involvement declares itself, the patient has usually but a few months to live.

The patient may die from general dissemination, from exhaustion, from septic absorption, from deposits in the brain, from pleural and pericardial effusions, from ascites, from paraplegia due to spinal deposits, and in rare cases as the direct result of bleeding from the ulcerated growth. Intercurrent diseases, especially pneumonia and erysipelas, are responsible for a certain number of deaths. The average duration of life after the appearance of the growth is stated by Campiche and Lazarus-Barlow to be about four years.

Treatment of inoperable breast cancer. — In cases where complete removal of the growth is impossible, all that remains is to make the patient as comfortable as possible, and to endeavour to delay the march of the disease.

X-rays in inoperable carcinoma.—The principal use of X-rays in breast cancer is as a prophylactic against postoperative recurrence. But even in advanced cases they are often an effective means of relieving pain. I have known pain in the back and thorax completely disappear for a time after one application of the rays, although the patient was utterly sceptical of the value of the treatment. In some cases, however, especially when pain is due to pressure upon deep-seated nerves, the rays are powerless.

Apart from their analgesic properties, X-rays promote the fibrosis and superficial healing of deposits in the skin and subcutaneous tissues. Upon visceral and other deep deposits they have no influence, nor do they appear to delay the course of dissemination.

Open-air treatment.—I have a strong impression that the disease runs a slower course in rural than in urban patients. Moreover, I have observed that a sea voyage or a stay in the country sometimes retards its progress. The resemblance of the reactive or defensive processes in cancer to those seen in tuberculosis also strongly suggests the advisability of systematic open-air treatment in the more chronic cases of inoperable cancer. Experience has convinced me of its value in checking the disease.

Drug treatment.—It was formerly the practice to resort to morphia as soon as pain began to interfere with sleep. This practice is much to be deprecated, for the drug soon impairs the personality of its habitués, and interferes with the action of the stomach, bowels, and kidneys, thus accentuating the toxic or cachectic condition which may be already present. Phenacetin at night, alone or combined with caffeine, will generally give sufficient relief to allow of sleep. Aspirin may be tried, but my own experience of it is disappointing. Cannabis indica may also be used. The aim should be to defer the use of morphia until the last stage of the disease. The drug will then exert its maximum effect, unimpeded by the toleration of habit, at the time when it is most urgently needed.

Oöphorectomy in inoperable breast cancer. — The sudden cessation of menstruation produced by the removal of the ovaries is known to exert a powerful influence on general metabolism, and to bring about regressive and fibrotic processes in the uterus, the breasts, and perhaps in other tissues. Since carcinoma tissue is imperfectly organized, and very subject to degeneration from malnutrition of its cells, it is not surprising that the shock of an artificial menopause falls with especial force upon it. As a result the primary growth and large secondary deposits may shrink and disappear, and the patient may regain her health and activity. But the disturbing effect of the menopause upon the patient's general health rarely extends beyond two or three years. In the same way the carcinoma appears to recover from the shock, and reasserts itself after the lapse of a few years only. And in some cases the progress of the growth is not even temporarily disturbed by the operation.

Oöphorectomy should be reserved for inoperable cases in women who are still actively menstruating, and who are anxious for prolongation of life. Owing to the uncertainty of its action the operation should not be urged, though in suitable cases it may fairly be offered.

Beatson, who introduced this method of treatment, regards cases of acute carcinoma and cases where metastatic growths are already in evidence as unsuitable for oöphorectomy. It should be stated that he advises a subsequent course of thyroid extract. His experience shows no case of permanent cure. Though in one instance the disease remained in abeyance for six years, in another for four, and in several for two years, in a majority of cases it reasserted itself within twelve months. In any given case the results of the operation cannot be predicted, but in a large number of cases the general health is improved, pain is relieved, and there is a slackening in the progress and activity of the disease. The operation is probably more beneficial before the menopause, but, in Beatson's opinion, is not contra-indicated in older women.

Treatment of lymphatic œdema of the arm.—In slight and early cases, where the œdema still pits on pressure, habitual elevation of the arm, either during the night or for several hours daily, will afford relief for some time. Later on, in properly selected cases, the writer's operation of lymphangioplasty affords great relief at a very small risk; but it is, of course, a palliative only, and does not delay the progress of the growth. In suitable cases the following benefits may be expected: (a) Complete relief from pain within twenty-four hours unless the pain is partially due to some cause, such as nerve pressure, independent of the œdema. (b) A marked and rapid fall in the tissue tension of the whole area drained by the threads, so that the arm becomes soft and flabby. (c) Rapid subsidence of the swelling, commencing immediately in the hand, and extending to the forearm within twenty-four hours. At first the upper arm is unaffected, or its diameters may even slightly increase; but within a week or two the diameters of the upper arm also are markedly lessened. The subsidence is usually permanent, unless and until pleural effusion supervenes to interfere with drainage. These effects are at first dependent upon the adoption of proper postural after-treatment, but, after a few months, elevation of the arm may be entirely abandoned without marked increase of swelling. (*d*) Return of power to the paralysed arm, provided that the paralysis is of recent date. Thus, one of my patients, whose arm was totally paralysed, was subsequently able to write me a letter. (*e*) An improvement in the general condition, dependent partly upon relief from pain and insomnia, and partly upon the abandonment of sedatives.

Technique of lymphangioplasty for brawny arm.—The special materials necessary are a set of suitable probes, lymphangio-

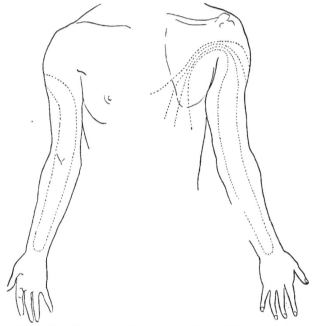

Fig. 285.—Diagram of the course of the silk threads in lymphangioplasty (front and back of arm).

plasty forceps with jaws specially designed to take a firm grip of either end of the probe, and a supply of No. 12 tubular silk. The tissues of the arm are drained by two long **U**-shaped lines of silk, each line composed of two threads of No. 12 tubular silk (Fig. 285). One of these lines drains the front of the arm, the other the back. The bend of each **U** lies immediately above the wrist, and its two limbs occupy respectively the radial and ulnar side of the limb. Thus, along the whole length of the limb are found four double lines of silk, spaced out round the limb as nearly as possible at quadrant intervals. Towards the shoulder the lines of silk on the flexor aspect curve outwards around the deltoid muscle, and converge to meet the ascending threads from the posterior aspect at a point near the posterior border of the deltoid. From this point the silk threads again radiate in the subcutaneous tissue of the back, terminating by free ends in the subcutaneous tissues of the scapular region. It is perhaps still better to lead some of them to the scapular region of the opposite side, and others to the lumbar region of the same side, if there is any sign of the œdema extending from the arm to the trunk.

The operation is done as follows : Take a double line of silk, rather more than twice as long as the arm, and mark its mid-point by clipping on it a pair of artery forceps. Wrap up one half of its length in gauze. Thread the two ends of the other half through the eye of a long probe. Make an incision ½ in. long through the skin at the middle of the front of the forearm, just above the wrist-joint. Thrust the probe in the desired line upwards in the subcutaneous tissues well away from the skin towards the region of the elbow, as high as is convenient, and cut down upon its point. Withdraw the probe through the incision last made, and draw the silk after it as far as it will come. Introduce the probe through the incision from which it has just emerged, thrust it upwards again in the selected line, and repeat the foregoing steps until the point selected for the convergence of the threads is reached. Here an incision 1 in. long is made, through which the probe with its two silk threads is drawn out. The other half of the silk loop is now led upwards in the selected line along the other border of the flexor surface. The limb is turned over and the extensor loop of silk is similarly introduced. When this has been done, eight free ends of silk are hanging out from the incision of convergence at the posterior border of the deltoid. Two at a time, these are tucked away in various directions in the subcutaneous tissues of the back by the following manœuvre : Clip a forceps on the selected pair of silk threads just where it emerges from the topmost incision. Take a long probe, cut off the ends of the two threads so that they are 4 in. shorter than the probe, and thread them into the eye. Thrust the probe downwards from the incision in the desired direction until the probe unthreads itself. Withdraw the probe carefully, leaving the two silk threads to occupy its track. Complete the operation by sewing up the incisions with horsehair.

The principal difficulties of the operation are connected with the maintenance of the silk in an aseptic condition. Owing to the large area dealt with, extending on to the back, the necessary changes in the posture of the arm, and the length of the silk threads, accidental contact may very easily occur between the silk and the surface of

h

the skin, the edges of the incisions, or surrounding objects. The silk ends not actually dealt with at the moment must be kept wrapped in sterile gauze, which is also useful to protect them from the edges of the incisions as they are being drawn in after the probe. If necessary, all the threads can be withdrawn by reopening the two incisions just above the wrist. I have never been obliged to do this. There is no need to fix the upper ends of the threads by knotting them together, for the silk soon becomes adherent to the tissues along its whole length.

Lastly, it is necessary to state that severe lymphatic œdema of the arm does not usually develop until within a few months of the patient's death from her disease. A long period of survival after the operation must not, as a rule, be expected. The aim of the operation is not the prolongation of that period, but its conversion from one of torture into one of comparative comfort.

Cases unsuitable for lymphangioplasty.—The operation of capillary drainage by silk threads is contra-indicated in cases where a general anæsthetic cannot be borne, and in cases where the threads would have to pass through cancerous tissue. It is also inadvisable to operate if there is growth present about the shoulder, or if the pain is mainly axillary, or is a lancinating pain shooting down the arm. In the presence of pleural effusion or secondary growths the operation is hardly worth doing, for its effects at best will be transient.

Amputation of the arm, or interscapulo-thoracic amputation, is the only resource in cases unsuitable for lymphangioplasty.

Treatment of cancerous ulcers.—Ulceration of the growth is due primarily to necrosis of the central portions of the growth from nutritional failure. But, unless care be taken, the ulcer becomes the seat of septic processes and the source of an offensive discharge. These distressing evils can be prevented or mitigated by careful attention to the antiseptic dressing of the ulcer. Strong antiseptics such as 10-volume hydrogen peroxide at full strength, acetone, or zinc chloride 40 gr. to the ounce, may be applied once or oftener if the ulcer is foul. The separation of sloughs may be hastened by hot fomentations. Subsequently the ulcer is dressed daily with mild unirritating applications, such, for instance, as boric lint, boric ointment, or lint wrung out of sanitas, or solution of cyllin 10–20 minims to the pint.

SARCOMA OF THE BREAST

Etiology.—It is doubtful whether injury plays a definite part in the origin of carcinoma, but there can be little doubt that sarcoma of the breast is occasionally of traumatic origin (Coley); that is to say, the sarcoma develops at the site of, and within a short interval after, a single definite blow. Bland-Sutton has drawn attention to the possible medico-legal importance of this fact.

Fibro-adenoma and sarcoma.—A fibro-adenoma, after persisting for years without marked change, may take on rapid growth, and may in a few months form a large tumour to which the name soft fibro-adenoma is applied. As a rule, when the breast is removed, the tumour is still found to be encapsuled, and it does not recur.

In other cases a small tumour present for some time in the breast begins to grow rapidly, and a large hemispherical mass is produced which soon fungates through the skin. On removal an unencapsuled sarcoma is found to be infiltrating the breast. If we remember, in conjunction with these facts, that the microscopic appearances of a soft fibro-adenoma resemble very closely those of a sarcoma, we may explain the statement made by various authorities that a fibro-adenoma may become a malignant tumour of the sarcomatous type,

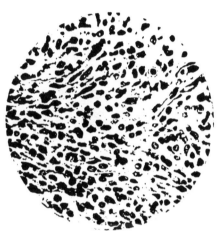

Fig. 286.—Spindle-celled sarcoma of the breast. × 250. Note the complete disappearance of the normal glandular elements of the breast. This is characteristic of sarcoma.

and that the soft fibro-adenoma is either an intermediate form or an intermediate stage in the conversion. These statements, though not generally accepted, are, in my opinion, correct.[1]

The routine histological examination of tumours of the breast has shown that sarcoma of the breast is much less frequent than it was formerly thought to be. Though some authors say that one malignant tumour of the breast in fifty is a true sarcoma, this is probably an over-statement. Many cases which present the clinical signs of sarcoma turn out to be soft carcinomas, others to be cystic adenomas. Sarcoma of the male breast is excessively rare.

Age-incidence.—Though it may occur at any age from childhood upwards, Rodman finds that sarcoma, like carcinoma, is a disease of middle life, and that half the cases occur between the ages of 40 and 50.

[1] But *see* Vol. I., p. 433.

Clinical signs.—A typical sarcoma of the breast is a rapidly growing tumour which soon attains a large size. In contrast to carcinoma, the growth of the tumour is not accompanied by any shrinkage or contraction of the tissues. The swelling formed is a

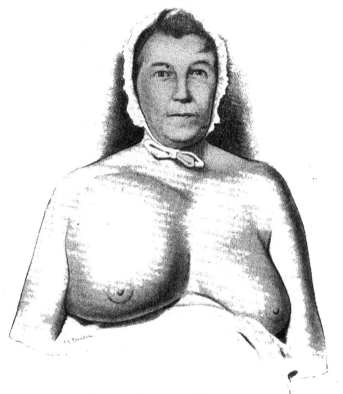

Fig. 287.—Sarcoma of the breast.
(*Beatson, Edin. Med. Journ., Jan.,* 1909.)

large, prominent, hemispherical mass, soon involving the whole breast. Large veins course over its surface, and pulsation may be present in it. The axillary glands usually remain of normal size. Soon the skin adheres to the tumour over a wide area, and the breast becomes adherent to the pectoral fascia. At the summit of the swelling the skin becomes thinned and reddened, and finally gives way like a rubber sheet under tension, exposing a vascular area of tumour tissue.

Through the opening thus formed a vascular mass of growth, often sloughy in appearance, rapidly protrudes (Fig. 288), and the patient frequently succumbs to hæmorrhage and exhaustion before dissemination has taken place. In some cases, however, numerous secondary deposits are found in the internal organs, the bones, and the lymphatic glands.

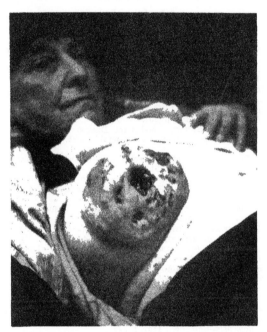

Fig. 288.—Fungating sarcoma of the breast.

CHONDRO-SARCOMA OF THE BREAST

In rare cases, sarcomas of the breast may contain areas of cartilage. Such chondro-sarcomas sometimes undergo calcification, or true bone with well-marked Haversian systems may be formed in them. The patients are middle-aged or old; the tumours are characterized by their stony hardness, but portions of them may be soft and fluctuating owing to the liquefaction of areas of cartilage. These tumours may quickly recur after operation, and may become disseminated. Calcified cartilage has been detected in the secondary deposits (Bland-Sutton).

In a case of chondro-sarcoma recently under my care a duct papilloma had been excised from the breast five years previously.

Treatment of sarcoma.—Sarcoma of the breast requires an operation similar to that for carcinoma of the breast. A margin of at least an inch must be left around the adherent area of skin, and grafting will in many cases be required.

Most of the photomicrographs illustrating this article were kindly taken by Mr. R. W. Annison, M.R.C.S., from the writer's specimens.

BIBLIOGRAPHY

Banks, Sir Mitchell, "Removal of Axillary Glands in Breast Cancer," *Brit. Med. Journ.,* 1882, ii. 1138.

Beatson, Sir G. T., "Sarcoma of the Female Mamma," *Edin. Med. Journ.,* Jan., 1909.

Benians, T. H. C., "The Use of Vaccines in Acute Mastitis," *Brit. Med. Journ.,* April 15, 1911.

Bland-Sutton, John, "Secondary (Metastatic) Carcinoma of Ovaries," *Brit. Med. Journ.,* May 26, 1906; *Arch: of Middx. Hosp.,* 1910, xix. 98.

Boyd, Stanley, "On Oöphorectomy in Treatment of Cancer of Breast," *Brit. Med. Journ..* Feb. 4, 1889, p. 257.

Campiche and Lazarus-Barlow, "Malignant Disease of Breast: a Statistical Study from Records of Middlesex Hospital," *Arch. of Middx. Hosp.,* 1905, vol. v.

Cheatle, G. Lenthal, "A Clinical Lecture on Chronic Traumatic Mastitis," *Brit. Med. Journ.,* March 4, 1911.

Coley, W. B., "Injury as a Causative Factor in Cancer," *Ann. of Surg.,* May, 1911.

Gould, Sir A. Pearce, "Cases illustrating Repair in Cancer of Breast," *Clin. Journ.,* May 9, 1900.

Halsted, Prof. W. S., "Removal of Breast and Axillary Tissues in Breast Cancer," *Ann. of Surg.,* Nov., 1894.

Handley, W. Sampson, "Centrifugal Spread of Mammary Carcinoma of Parietes, and its Bearing on Operative Treatment," *Arch. of Middx. Hosp.,* 1904, vol. iii. *Cancer of Breast and its Operative Treatment.* London, 1906.

Heidenhain, "Ueber die Ursachen der localen Krebsrecidive nach Amputatio Mammæ," *Arch. f. klin. Chir.,* 1889, S. 97.

Leitch, Archibald, *Brit. Med. Journ.,* May 22, 1909. (A rapid staining method for use during operations.)

Lockwood, C. B., "An Address on Carcinoma of Breast," *Brit. Med. Journ.,* Jan. 27, 1906.

Moore, Charles, "Influence of Inadequate Operations on Theory of Cancer," *Trans. Roy. Med.-Chir. Soc.,* 1867, i. 245.

Osler, Sir William, "Medical Aspects of Breast Cancer," *Brit. Med. Journ.,* Jan. 6, 1906.

Paget, Sir James, "On Disease of Mammary Areola preceding Cancer of Mammary Gland," *St. Bart.'s Hosp. Repts.,* x. 87.

Paget, Stephen, "Distribution of Secondary Growths in Cancer of Breast," *Lancet,* March 23, 1889.

Rodman, Prof. W. L., *Diseases of the Breast.* 1908.

Sappey, *Vaisseaux Lymphatiques.*

Schmidt, M. B., *Die Verbreitungswege der Karzinome.* Jena, 1903.

Shaw, Ernest H., "Tumours of the Breast," *St. Bart.'s Hosp. Journ.,* May, 1904; "The Immediate Microscopic Diagnosis of Tumours at the Time of Operation," *Lancet,* Sept. 24, 1910.

Stiles, Harold, "On Dissemination of Cancer of Breast," *Brit. Med. Journ.,* 1889, i. 1452; "Contributions to Surgical Anatomy of Breast," *Edin. Med. Journ..* 1892; article in Burghard's *System of Operative Surgery.*

Török and Wittelshofer, "Statistics bearing on Dissemination in Breast Cancer," *Arch. f. klin. Chir.,* 1881, xxv. 873.

Velpeau, "Diseases of the Breast," *Sydenham Soc. Trans.*

Williams, Roger, *Diseases of the Breast.*

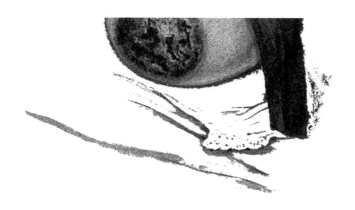

Paget's disease of the nipple. The nipple has been entirely destroyed;
its place and that of the areola are taken by an intensely red, raw, and
"weeping" surface which extends considerably beyond the original limits
of the areola. A carcinoma was present in the breast.

(From a case under the author's care at the Middlesex Hospital.)

PLATE 82.

THE SPLEEN

By C. GORDON WATSON, F.R.C.S.

SPLENECTOMY

Effects of removal of the spleen. — The spleen can be removed without causing any serious physiological disturbance.

Its removal causes a transitory diminution in the number of the red, and a temporary increase in the number of the white, blood-corpuscles. This deficiency is made up by an increased activity on the part of the lymphatic glands, of the bone marrow, and perhaps also of the thyroid gland, inasmuch as thyroid hypertrophy has in some instances followed excision of the spleen. The temporary anæmia which usually follows excision may in part be accounted for by the actual volume of blood removed with the spleen.

In the initial leucocytosis an increase of the polymorphonuclears usually occurs. Later on, and coincidently with the lymphatic enlargement, there is a definite lymphocytosis, which has been known to continue, in patients under observation, for as long as three years after removal of the spleen. Eosinophilia may be observed, either transitory, or immediate and persisting for some years after operation. Warthin has shown by animal experiments that lymphatic enlargement occurs as a compensatory substitute for the spleen in the sheep and goat. The pain which is often complained of along the bones of the limbs after splenectomy suggests that the bone marrow takes a part in compensation.

In some instances, after convalescence from splenectomy there has been a gradual onset of progressive emaciation, with general weakness, headache, thirst, drowsiness, and irritability, and sometimes with pyrexia, rapid pulse and respiration. In two cases, recorded by Ballance, in which this condition arose, ultimate complete recovery followed the administration of extract of sheep's spleen and bone marrow, and finally arsenic. Possibly this train of symptoms was dependent on the loss of an internal secretion, and it may be that the bone-marrow, lymph-glands, and perhaps the thyroid, were unable at once to meet the demands made upon them so suddenly to

103

compensate for the loss of the spleen. In other cases an element of sepsis may afford a reasonable explanation of the symptoms. The condition described is certainly not a common sequela of the operation.

Splenectomy should not be lightly undertaken. The mortality is high. The chief dangers are shock and hæmorrhage. The size of the spleen and the presence of adhesions may present serious difficulties.

G. B. Johnston has collected 708 cases of splenectomy, showing a mortality of 27·4 per cent. If the cases of removal for injuries are excluded (150 with 51 deaths), the mortality is 13·2 per cent.

Although the spleen has been removed for a great variety of conditions, the cases in which splenectomy is either desirable or suitable are in the main limited to (1) injuries or ruptures which endanger life from hæmorrhage; (2) strangulation of a normal or diseased spleen, due to torsion of the pedicle; (3) hypertrophy combined with excessive mobility, when causing troublesome symptoms; (4) primary malignant disease, if recognized early; (5) malarial hypertrophy, when the size of the spleen is a menace to the patient's life; and (6) some cases of splenic anæmia.

The operation.—The most convenient incision is a vertical one along the outer border of the left rectus. When the diagnosis is uncertain a median incision is usually employed, and if necessary the left rectus is subsequently divided transversely. In the case of very large tumours, and especially in women, in whom the subcostal arch is less divergent than in the male, the median incision is probably the most suitable, as it allows of a longer incision than can be secured in the linea semilunaris. Some surgeons adopt an oblique incision parallel to the costal arch.

If adhesions exist, they must be dealt with before any attempt is made to ligature the pedicle. If adhesions are extensive between the spleen and neighbouring viscera, it will often be advisable to abandon the operation. Adhesions between the spleen and the parietal peritoneum are best dealt with by gentle pressure with swabs on holders. Omental adhesions must be carefully transfixed and ligatured.

Before the pedicle is ligatured the spleen should, if possible, be delivered outside the abdomen. The pedicle is most easily approached when the spleen is rotated so that the posterior surface looks forward. The vessels should be separately ligatured with stout silk, and divided at some distance from the ligatures. The greatest care must be taken to avoid undue tension or torsion on the large splenic veins. Some surgeons have by design included the tail of the pancreas in the ligatures, to lend support and security to the vascular stump.

It must be remembered that the splenic artery breaks up into from five to seven branches when it reaches the spleen, and that the vasa brevia are branches of the splenic artery to the greater curvature of the stomach, running in the gastro-splenic omentum. These, together with the gastro-epiploica sinistra (the large vessel supplying the cardiac end of the greater curvature of the stomach), should be avoided, if possible, when separating the spleen from the stomach by division of the gastro-splenic omentum. The splenic artery ends by crossing the upper end of the left kidney, and its terminal branches pass through the lieno-renal ligament to reach the hilum, so that the close relationship of the spleen to the kidney must be remembered when the pedicle is dealt with.

In some instances dragging on the pedicle has produced alarming symptoms of collapse, probably due to injury of the splenic nerve plexus, which arises from the solar plexus and runs with the splenic vessels.

The capsule of the spleen is normally very thin, and the splenic tissue very friable, so that rough handling of the viscus is to be avoided.

RUPTURE—PROLAPSE—TORSION

RUPTURE OF THE SPLEEN

In severe injuries to the abdomen (e.g. when a cart-wheel passes over the thorax or abdomen) the spleen may be torn, severely lacerated, or even severed from its vascular pedicle. Such a case generally presents associated injuries to the liver or other viscera, with or without injuries to the bones of the thoracic wall, and seldom comes within the range of surgical interference. In other instances a crush or blow upon the abdomen may produce an injury to the spleen without damage to other viscera, and be followed by grave internal hæmorrhage which demands prompt operative treatment. In a few instances a similar result has followed a fall without any direct blow upon the abdomen.

When the spleen is enlarged, as in malaria, even slight injuries have been known to produce rupture of the capsule and severe internal hæmorrhage (p. 111), and spontaneous rupture of the spleen sometimes occurs in enteric fever and in splenic infarction.

Diagnosis.—Traumatic splenic rupture can seldom be diagnosed with certainty, but may be assumed when signs of internal hæmorrhage are associated with injury in the splenic region, especially if at the same time the natural splenic dullness is increased. Deepening pallor, restlessness, great thirst, acute abdominal pain, and faintness are combined with a pulse which diminishes in volume as it increases in rate until it becomes running and almost imperceptible. Abdominal rigidity is soon general, but is locally exaggerated and accompanied by tenderness in the left subcostal region. If the hæmorrhage is abundant, a shifting dullness in the flanks soon follows—a valuable sign when obtained. If, when the signs of fluid are increasing, the dullness in the right flank can be made to shift by a change of position, while that in the left remains constant, an injury to the spleen is strongly suggested. In many cases of severe abdominal injury it it is quite impossible at first to arrive at any certain diagnosis, and it may be difficult to decide whether a patient is suffering only from severe shock, or from collapse due to a concealed hæmorrhage.[1]

Treatment.—In all cases of suspected injury of the spleen, exploratory laparotomy is imperative if there are signs of internal hæmorrhage. The question whether laparotomy should be immediate, or whether reaction from the shock and collapse incident to the injury should be awaited, can only be decided by the circumstances of the individual case.

Speaking generally, *delay is dangerous.* Frequently, by slowing of the heart's action and temporary clotting, natural arrest of hæmorrhage occurs, and encourages the surgeon to hope that by masterly inactivity he may allow the arrest to become permanent without subjecting the patient to the additional danger of operation ; too often, however, recovery from shock leads to a recurrent and not seldom fatal flood of hæmorrhage.

On the other hand, cases occur in which, after the initial hæmorrhage has ceased, recovery without recurrence follows.

There are two specimens in the Museum of St. Bartholomew's Hospital which demonstrate repair of the spleen after rupture from injury. One (Fig. 289) is the spleen of a woman aged 30, who, falling 30 ft. from a window, fractured her femur and died ten days later, but without symptoms of abdominal injury. At the autopsy it was apparent that the spleen had been torn across, and a firm white scar had formed ($\frac{1}{4}$ in. thick), uniting the lacerated surfaces. There was also an encapsuled collection of blood (partly fluid) around the spleen, and the subperitoneal tissue in the neighbourhood was stained with blood pigment.

The other specimen (2308B) was removed post mortem from a woman aged 39, who was run over by an omnibus and died sixty hours later. The spleen had been torn on the outer surface near the upper extremity, and the rent was closed by a firm clot.

Doubtless similar specimens are to be met with elsewhere.

Each case must be judged on its merits. Some cases are hopeless from the first, but in most the collapse resulting from the loss of blood opens a loophole for recovery, although, as already stated, a recurrence of hæmorrhage usually follows. Occasionally the spleen may be injured and yet no symptoms of hæmorrhage occur for many hours or even days after the accident. Possibly in some of these cases the

---

[1] *See* Vol. I., p. 305.

bleeding first occurs beneath the capsule, and intraperitoneal hæmorrhage only follows a subsequent rupture from the tension of the blood effused beneath the capsule ; in others a temporary clot may occur,

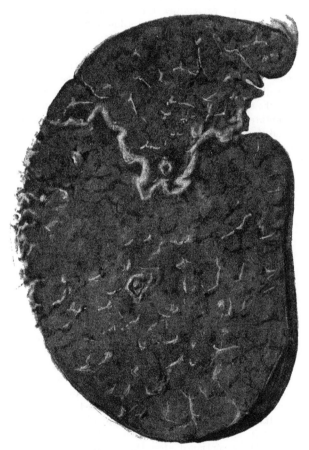

Fig. 289.—Rupture of the spleen ; spontaneous cure. The site of the injury is occupied by a firm white scar, measuring ½ in. across.

(*Specimen* 2308A, *St. Bartholomew's Hospital Museum.*)

and yield subsequently to a recurrent or secondary hæmorrhage. If the patient survive the hæmorrhage and no operation be performed he may yet succumb to peritonitis, which has often been known to follow large effusions of blood into the peritoneal cavity.

In hospital practice, and in private practice when surgical aid is obtainable, preparation for an operation should be made as soon as a diagnosis is established. Meantime, absolute rest and freedom from any disturbance must be enforced. The foot of the bed should be raised, and the extremities firmly bandaged. If operation be decided on, continuous subcutaneous saline infusion should be commenced as soon as the abdomen has been opened. For this purpose the rubber bags designed by Arbuthnot Lane are very efficient. As some uncertainty as to the nature and extent of the injuries in these cases must always exist, it is advisable to open the abdomen freely in the middle line above the umbilicus so that the liver and kidneys as well as the spleen can be examined. If it be found that the spleen only is ruptured, further procedure will depend on the extent of the injury, and it may then be necessary to make an incision in the left linea semilunaris.

In most cases splenectomy (p. 103) is advisable. In cases of minor injury, packing with gauze may suffice to arrest bleeding, but this method is not free from risk of subsequent hæmorrhage, and may be followed by infection, suppuration, and a septic sinus. In extreme cases, however, when the collapse is so great that excision seems out of the question, it may be employed.[1]

Attempts to suture tears in the spleen have usually failed, and time devoted to this procedure will be more profitably spent in ligaturing the splenic vessels and excising the damaged viscus. If suture be employed, the linked mattress-suture should be used, as less liable to " cut out " than other forms of suture.

Immediately the splenic origin of the hæmorrhage is ascertained an assistant should secure and digitally compress the splenic vessels until the surgeon is prepared to ligature these and remove the organ. At the conclusion of the operation all blood-clot should be removed from the abdomen, and the peritoneal cavity flushed out with hot saline solution (115–120° Fahr.). The abdominal flushing can be commenced as soon as the abdomen is opened, and carried on continuously by an assistant while the surgeon proceeds with the operation. As a rule, drainage is unnecessary. As much saline solution as possible should be left in the peritoneal cavity. Rectal or subcutaneous infusion should be continued after the operation, and regulated by the condition of the pulse.

Complications.—Sepsis is the complication most to be feared. Pneumonia and empyema frequently follow operation, and may be

[1] D'Arcy Power successfully plugged the splenic area in the case of a boy who was kicked by a horse and who developed symptoms of severe hæmorrhage two days after the injury. Encouraged by this success, he employed the same method on the next occasion that he operated for ruptured spleen, but unfortunately the hæmorrhage recurred and death resulted.

explained, in some cases at any rate, by associated injuries to the lung and thoracic wall. In other cases, subphrenic abscess, faecal fistula, and secondary haemorrhage have occurred. All these complications may follow injury to the spleen without operation.

Other possible complications which require brief mention are— (1) recurrent haemorrhage, which may either result from the slipping of a ligature or arise from points of adhesion as the blood-pressure increases after recovery from collapse ; (2) secondary haemorrhage from sepsis ; (3) the obscure train of symptoms already mentioned (p. 103) ; (4) thrombosis of the splenic vein, which may extend to the mesenteric veins and so give rise to grave abdominal symptoms.

PROLAPSE OF THE SPLEEN

(MOVABLE, WANDERING, ECTOPIC SPLEEN)

This condition is rare in men, and more frequent in women who have borne children. Although abnormal mobility of an otherwise natural spleen may occur, particularly in cases of general enteroptosis, prolapse is usually associated with hypertrophy. When the phrenico-colic ligament, which normally suspends the spleen beneath the diaphragm, is stretched or torn the spleen readily prolapses, and is then very imperfectly supported by the splenic vessels, the gastro-splenic omentum, and the licno-renal ligament.

A movable spleen, if not greatly enlarged, may give rise to no symptoms at all. Great mobility, especially if combined with considerable hypertrophy, induces severe spasms of pain closely simulating those of movable kidney.[1] Owing to the close connexion between the spleen and the stomach through the gastro-splenic omentum, gastric disturbances are not uncommon.

In extreme cases the spleen may be found to occupy the left iliac fossa, or to have crossed to the right of the middle line, and it has been found impacted in the pelvis.

The loss of the normal splenic dullness, the absence of colon resonance in front of the wandering viscus, its superficial position, and its notched border should serve in most cases to distinguish it from a movable kidney.

Treatment.—A well-fitting abdominal belt may in some instances prevent the pain and discomfort which sometimes result from a prolapsed spleen. In severe cases, especially in idiopathic or malarial hypertrophy, excision (p. 103) may be justifiable if the patient is so inconvenienced as to be unable to follow his employment or to enjoy active exercise. In a few cases the operation of **splenopexy**

[1] I. Macdonald and W. A. Mackay record an operation in a case of movable and twisted spleen which was mistaken for movable kidney.

has been performed. An incision is made through the parietal peritoneum under the left cupola of the diaphragm, and the peritoneum freed from the parietes until the spleen can be passed through the parietal peritoneum and couched in such a way as to lie in contact with the diaphragm over the area from which the peritoneum has been stripped and to which it should become adherent. It should be kept in position by suturing the stripped peritoneum together round the pedicle of the spleen. If firm adhesions quickly form, and the spleen is not greatly enlarged, this operation may be successful, but if not, the weight of the spleen, the stretched pedicle, and the constant movement of the diaphragm are factors which militate against fixation. Absolute rest on the back should be enforced for at least a month after the operation.

TORSION OF THE SPLEEN

The movable or wandering spleen, especially if enlarged, is very liable to become twisted on its vascular pedicle and to undergo strangulation through obstruction to the blood supply and, ultimately, gangrene with thrombosis of the splenic vessels. The condition is analogous to the twisting of the pedicle of an ovarian cyst or a retained testis, and the symptoms are very similar—acute abdominal pain and vomiting, and later, if unrelieved, general peritonitis.

The strangulation may come on gradually, or quite suddenly, and, if a movable spleen has not been previously recognized, may so closely resemble acute perforation of a viscus or intestinal obstruction as to escape diagnosis before laparotomy.

Treatment.—The only satisfactory method of treatment is that of splenectomy. Splenopexy, or simple relief of the strangulation, is liable to be followed by recurrence. It will be remembered that normally the spleen is slung beneath the arch of the diaphragm by the phrenico-colic ligament, and closely connected to the greater curvature of the stomach by the gastro-splenic omentum, and to the left kidney by the licno-renal ligament. The tail of the pancreas lies in contact with the hilum of the spleen just below the point of entry of the large vessels. All these points should be borne in mind in dealing with torsion of a prolapsed spleen.

HYPERTROPHY

IDIOPATHIC AND MALARIAL HYPERTROPHY

Chronic splenic enlargement without obvious cause is not common in this country, but White Hopkinson states that in Southern China and the Malay States it occurs in about 90 per cent. of the population. Some cases may be explained by past acute infective disease or by latent malarial infection. Others are probably due to unrecognized syphilis. Such an enlarged spleen is liable to prolapse, and therefore to cause not only inconvenience but danger from torsion of the pedicle, intestinal obstruction, or pressure on other organs.

Chronic malaria is by far the commonest cause. A malarial spleen (ague-cake) may attain an enormous size and become a veritable burden to the owner. The soft and moderately enlarged spleen of acute malaria usually yields to medical treatment. The hypertrophied spleen of chronic malaria may exist for many years without giving rise to symptoms. Excessive hypertrophy, combined with abnormal mobility, leads to considerable risk of rupture following on slight injury.

Death has been known to ensue in a few minutes after "turning in bed," a "flick with a cane," a "dig in the ribs" (Battle). The late Surg.-Gen. Coull-Mackenzie states that 68·9 per cent. of cases of rupture of malarial spleen ended fatally within half an hour. A not uncommon method of assassination in Southern China is by a blow in the abdomen with a cruciform iron instrument known as a "larang" (Crawford). Rupture of a malarial spleen may be compared to that of an aneurysm; rupture of a normal spleen to that of a large artery (Battle).

Treatment.—The large spleen of chronic malaria is often accompanied by extreme anæmia, and for this reason, as also for extreme mobility and torsion, or to avoid the risk of torsion or rupture, has been frequently removed. According to Jonnesco, "to remove the spleen is to remove the breeding place."

Statistics show that the mortality of the operation is high both for malarial and for so-called idiopathic hypertrophy, but Johnston's table indicates that the mortality is much lower when the hypertrophy is accompanied by increased mobility. This fact is probably accounted for by the comparative ease with which a movable spleen, even though of considerable size, can be delivered outside the abdomen. The rate of mortality for so-called idiopathic hypertrophy and simple malarial enlargement (in the absence of ectopia or torsion) is not encouraging to the surgeon.

Vanverts states that of 39 splenectomies for malarial hypertrophy with adhesions 28 died, whereas out of 35 for hypertrophy without adhesions only 2 succumbed.

Operation is only indicated when the condition is complicated by excessive mobility, and when by reason of the patient's occupation there is danger of rupture or torsion.

HYPERTROPHY IN SPLENIC ANÆMIA

This is a disease of young adult life, and should be distinguished from the anæmias of infancy, which are often associated with splenic enlargement. It can be distinguished from leukæmia by the blood count, and from Hodgkin's disease by the absence of glandular enlargement. For an account of this disease the reader is referred to the medical textbooks.

Briefly, the spleen enlarges *pari passu* with progressive anæmia, diarrhœa, vomiting, and intestinal hæmorrhage. No enlargement of the lymphatic glands occurs, and death usually results from exhaustion. The first change in the blood is a diminution of hæmoglobin, and to a lesser degree of red corpuscles. Later the diminution of red corpuscles and hæmoglobin becomes extreme, and small, imperfectly formed, and nucleated red cells may be found. The coagulability of the blood is also diminished. The white corpuscles are, as a rule, both actually and relatively fewer. The differential count should show no marked changes, and myelocytes are absent. The spleen is always enlarged, often to five or ten times its usual size. Atrophy and sclerosis of the Malpighian bodies has been noted by Banti—a point of differentiation from leukæmia. It is important not to mistake for splenic anæmia the enlarged spleen which may accompany portal hepatic cirrhosis.

Treatment.—Osler advises operation in chronic cases with recurrent attacks of hæmorrhage (intestinal). Sippey regards the disease as fatal unless relieved by surgical interference. Of the 61 cases collected by Johnston, 49 recovered after operation. Medical treatment in the past has been very unsuccessful in checking the progress of the disease. If we assume that the enlargement of the spleen is the essential feature of the disease, splenectomy seems to offer the best chance of cure.

HYPERTROPHY IN BANTI'S DISEASE

This disease is characterized by a progressive enlargement of the spleen due to overgrowth of its connective tissue, with atrophy of the pulp and Malpighian bodies. In the later stages the hypertrophy is associated with an atrophic cirrhosis of the liver. The disease closely resembles splenic anæmia, and some authorities regard it as a late stage of that affection.

Banti's cases showed an increase in the marrow of the long bones and a return to the red or fœtal conditions. There are extreme anæmia, cachexia, and wasting.

Many cases of this disease have been cured by excision of the spleen. Hagen records 16 cases of splenectomy for Banti's disease, with 13 recoveries. Two of the patients were in excellent health 8 and 6½ years respectively after operation (Collins Warren and Harvey Cushing).

Failing operation, the disease progresses steadily to a fatal issue.

ε HYPERTROPHY IN LEUKÆMIA

The distinction between splenic leukæmia and splenic anæmia can only be made by a differential blood examination. The characteristic change in the blood is the presence of myelocytes and a great increase in the total number of white corpuscles.

Treatment.—In Johnston's table only 6 out of 49 cases of splenectomy for leukæmia survived operation. This heavy mortality would suffice to contra-indicate operation, apart from the fact that enlargement of the spleen is only one manifestation of a general disease, and that its removal, although relieving the abdomen of a heavy burden, is unlikely to check the progress of the disease should the patient survive the operation.

INFLAMMATIONS

ABSCESS

In general blood infections the spleen is frequently the seat of acute congestion. The circulation in the large capillaries and veins is slow, and the walls of the vessels are very pervious, so that microorganisms are readily deposited from the blood-current. Abscess of the spleen may occur in the course of acute infective diseases, or in any general pyæmia. It not uncommonly results from the breaking down of a septic infarct, e.g. in infective endocarditis, and sometimes follows on injuries, the abscess probably resulting from the breaking down of a hæmatoma.

The pneumococcus has been found in some cases of acute splenic abscess (Fig. 290), and J. P. Maxwell has recorded 2 cases of splenic abscess in South China in which he found the amœba of dysentery.

Chronic suppuration may be due to tuberculosis, actinomycosis, or hydatid disease, or result from the breaking down of a gumma or a septic infarct.

A splenic abscess may rupture and invade the general peritoneal cavity, the subphrenic space, the stomach, or the colon, or may burst through the diaphragm and cause an empyema.

Perisplenitis and adhesions readily form. The area of splenic dullness increases, and, when adhesions form with the abdominal wall, localized swelling and œdema may occur.

Diagnosis.—The diagnosis of splenic abscess is based on the general signs and symptoms of suppuration—a septic temperature, leucocytosis, etc.—and the local signs of pain, tenderness, and swelling in the situation of the spleen. The condition may generally be distinguished from renal suppuration by the absence of colon resonance between the tumour and the anterior abdominal wall.

ɪ

Treatment.—The treatment follows general surgical principles. In several cases the spleen has been excised, but in the majority of

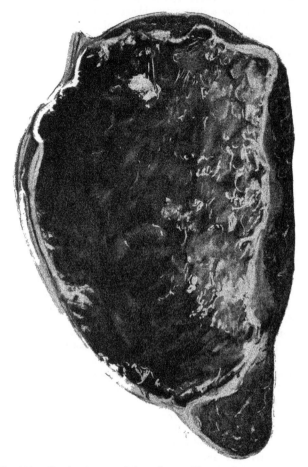

Fig. 290.—Single abscess of the spleen. The specimen was removed from a man æt. 49, who died with pneumonia. It weighed 50 oz. unopened, was adherent to the diaphragm, and contained a reddish-brown turbid fluid. The right lung was consolidated, and contained an abscess with similar contents.

(*Specimen* 2295L, *St. Bartholomew's Hospital Museum.*)

cases the operation would be not only difficult, but dangerous owing to the adhesions and the risk of rupture of the abscess and infection of the peritoneal cavity. Splenotomy with free drainage, if possible by an incision below the costal arch, or, after resection of a portion of a rib or ribs, below the level of the base of the lung, should be adopted in most cases. If no adhesions exist between the spleen and the anterior abdominal wall, the greatest care must be taken to avoid infection of the general peritoneal cavity. Before the abscess is opened, the surrounding area must be carefully packed with gauze, and, when the pus has been evacuated, the abscess wall should be sutured to the parietes. Or the operation may, if the case is not urgent, be performed in two stages: after the spleen has been exposed and the abscess localized, the wound is packed until the spleen becomes adherent, and the abscess is not opened till about two days later.

INFARCTS

Infarction of the spleen consequent on infective endocarditis or some other general infection does not come within the scope of surgery.

Occasionally infarction may follow thrombosis of the splenic or portal vein, and under such conditions the infarct may rupture and give rise to hæmorrhage or general peritonitis (Collins Warren).

In the Museum of St. Bartholomew's Hospital there is a specimen (1914c) illustrating a chronic gastric ulcer in the cardiac region, with thrombosis of the splenic vein and an infarct of the spleen. The patient succumbed after severe hæmatemesis. In this case the thrombosis and infarction undoubtedly followed the ulceration, spreading from one of the gastric vessels which join the splenic vein. Thrombosis of the splenic vein is not uncommonly met with in infarction of the spleen, and also in cases of torsion of the spleen, and may lead to severe hæmatemesis. This is illustrated by a specimen (St. Bartholomew's Museum, 2271B) of a large pancreatic cyst which produced fatal hæmatemesis owing to pressure on and subsequent thrombosis of the splenic vein.

An infarcted spleen may rupture spontaneously or from slight violence. A case is recorded by Collins Warren of rupture of an infarcted spleen simulating an acute perforation of a gastric ulcer, for which laparotomy was performed. A quantity of blood was found in the peritoneal cavity, and a large rent in the spleen. The spleen was removed, but the patient succumbed. At the autopsy the portal and splenic veins were found thrombosed. Warren says: " It would seem highly probable that distension of the capsule nearly to the bursting-point by the cutting off of the egress of the blood by thrombosis of the splenic vein had prepared the way for rupture of the capsule by slight violence."

Should an infarct of the spleen break down and result in an abscess it may require to be dealt with on the lines already laid down (p. 114).

TUBERCULOSIS

In generalized tuberculosis the spleen is very commonly affected. Occasionally primary caseous tubercle develops in the spleen and may require to be treated surgically, either by excision when exten-

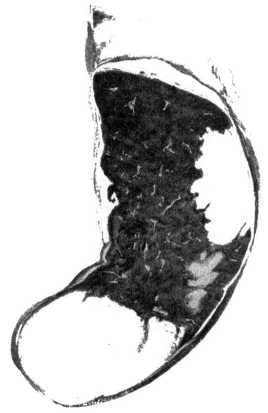

Fig. 291.—Actinomycosis of the spleen. From a woman æt. 35, who also had extensive actinomycosis of the liver. The upper pole of the spleen is seen to be adherent to the diaphragm and liver.

(*Specimen* 2306c, *St. Bartholomew's Hospital Museum.*)

sively involved, or by splenotomy, scraping, and drainage if adhesions are extensive or if the deposit of tubercle is limited to a single focus and the spleen not greatly implicated.

ACTINOMYCOSIS

Actinomycosis is sometimes met with in the spleen (Fig. 291), though far less frequently than in the liver. Should the condition be recognized before adhesions have formed, and before suppuration

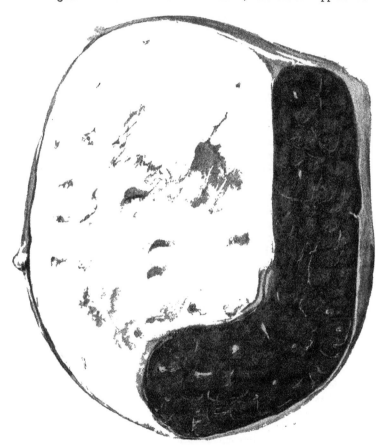

Fig. 292.—Gumma of the spleen.

has spread to the abdominal wall, excision of the spleen is indicated. Usually it will only be possible to deal with the case on lines appropriate to chronic suppuration. Surgical treatment should be supplemented by large doses of iodide of potassium, increased up to 200 gr. per diem, and a vaccine treatment may be tried.

GUMMA

Large gummata are sometimes met with in the spleen (Fig. 292), and are not easily diagnosed without an exploratory operation. The spleen has been excised on several occasions for this condition, when the gumma has failed to respond to antisyphilitic remedies.

Some cases of chronic hypertrophy of the spleen are regarded as syphilitic, and it is advisable to administer iodide of potassium in all cases of hypertrophy of uncertain origin.

NEOPLASMS

HYDATID CYST OF SPLEEN

Cases of solitary hydatid cyst of the spleen are rare. These growths may attain an enormous size, and have been mistaken for ovarian cysts (Plate 85).

Not infrequently the cyst becomes calcified and obsolete.

When suppuration ensues, adhesions readily form, and rupture is liable to take place, especially in the case of large cysts. Often there are no symptoms other than that of a tumour, although, if the cyst is large and the spleen mobile, there may be symptoms of pressure or traction on the stomach or other viscera.

Fluctuation or hydatid thrill may sometimes be obtained.

Treatment.—Exploratory puncture should never be employed. If the cyst is of moderate size and adhesions are limited, splenectomy is advisable, but considerable caution is necessary to avoid rupture in dealing with adhesions.

In most cases it is safest to fix the cyst wall to the parietes, and to incise and drain.

Single *blood cysts*, *serous cysts*, *lymph cysts*, and a few rare instances of *dermoid cysts* have been met with in the spleen.

CAVERNOUS ANGIOMA

A few cases of this rare disease have been recorded for which the spleen has been successfully removed (Hoge).

The spleen to the naked eye is dark, soft, and highly vascular. Microscopically the capillary system is lost, and the blood collects in a number of freely intercommunicating spaces closely resembling in structure the corpus cavernosum of the penis. The walls of these spaces consist of thin connective tissue with an epithelial lining.

SARCOMA

The spleen, though sometimes attacked by secondary deposits both of carcinoma and of sarcoma, is very seldom the seat of primary sarcoma (Fig. 293).

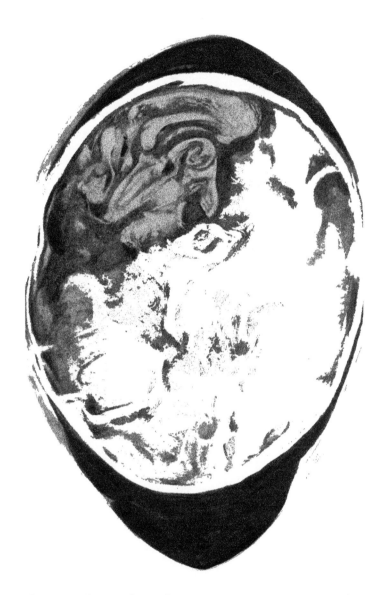

Large hydatid cyst of the spleen. From a woman aged 54, who died of acute bronchitis in an asylum. There were no symptoms to draw attention to the spleen. No other hydatid cysts were found post mortem.

(*Specimen* 2360B, *St. Bartholomew's Hospital Museum.*)

PLATE 85.

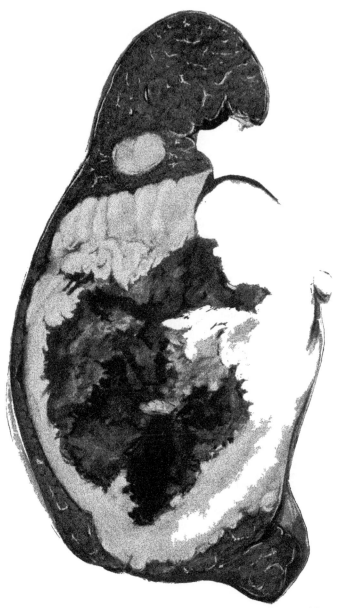

Fig. 293.—Primary round-celled sarcoma of spleen. Removed from
a woman æt. 49, who had suffered for a week with pain eight
months prior to operation, and since then had been much subject to vomiting. She made a good recovery from the operation.

(*Specimen* 2304D, *St. Bartholomew's Hospital Museum.*)

A sarcoma arising in the spleen will grow rapidly and give rise to a hard, irregular tumour. Metastasis will occur early, and wasting with cachexia may be the only symptoms to attract attention. Pain is not likely to occur in the early stages unless the tumour is on the surface and the peritoneum is involved. In some cases a leucocytosis together with eosinophilia has been noted.

The **diagnosis** of sarcoma will usually be made by a process of exclusion. Splenic anæmia, leukæmia, and malarial enlargement can be excluded by the absence of the characteristic changes in the blood, or by the history of the case.

Prognosis and treatment.—If recognized early, and if splenectomy is performed before metastases have formed, the prognosis may be not unfavourable. Johnston has collected 12 cases of splenectomy for sarcoma, with 9 recoveries from the operation. It is probable that if the after-histories of these cases were traced it would be found that death from recurrence had ultimately resulted.[1]

BIBLIOGRAPHY

Ballance, *Lancet*, 1896, i. 484.
Battle, Annual Oration Med. Soc. of London, 1910.
Bessel-Hagen, *Arch. f. klin. Chir.*, 1900, vol. lxii.
Crawford, D. G., *Ind. Med. Gaz.*, 1902 and 1906.
Emery, D'Este, *Lancet*, 1907, i. 1896.
Hoge, *Med. Rev.*, Sept., 1895, and *Ann. of Surg.*, 1897, vol. xxv.
Johnston, G. B., *Ann. of Surg.*, July, 1908, p. 50.
Jonnesco, *Gaz. des Hôp.*, Oct. 27, 1898.
Lewis, *Amer. Journ. of Med. Sci.*, 1908, cxxxvi. 157.
Macdonald, I., and W. A. Mackay, *Lancet*, 1909, ii. 917.
Maxwell, *J. P.*, *Lancet*, 1909, vol. ii.
Osler, *Amer. Journ. of Med. Sci.*, Oct., 1900, p. 54.
Power, D'Arcy, *Clin. Journ.*, Nov. 28, 1906, and *St. Bart.'s Hosp. Repts.*, xliv. 101.
Sendler, "Traumatic Splenic Abscess," *Deuts. Zeitschr. f. Chir.*, 1893, Bd. xxxvi., Heft 5.
Sippey, *Amer. Journ. of Med. Sci.*, 1899, pp. 428, 570.
Vanverts, *De la Splénectomie*, Thèse de Paris, 1897.
Warren, Collins, *Ann. of Surg.*, May, 1901.
Warthin, *Contributions to Medical Research*, p. 234. 1903.

[1] In a case of round-celled sarcoma of the spleen, weighing 66 oz., successfully removed by D'Arcy Power (Fig. 293), death occurred six months later.

MALFORMATIONS OF THE FACE, LIPS, AND PALATE

BY CYRIL A. R. NITCH, M.S.LOND., F.R.C.S.

Development of the face and lips.—At a very early stage of development the stomodæum appears as a depression between the yolk-sac and the anterior extremity of the embryo. The depression becomes deepened by the outgrowth of the heart immediately

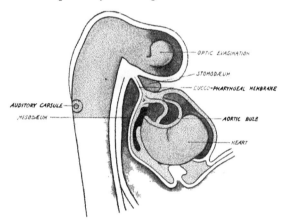

Fig. 294.—Reconstruction of the anterior portion of an embryo of 2·15 mm.

(After His and McMurrich.)

below it, and by the ventral bend that takes place at the anterior extremity of the brain, until its floor, lined by ectoderm, comes in contact with the entoderm of the mesodæum. These two layers are known as the bucco-pharyngeal membrane (Fig. 294). They fuse together, atrophy, and disappear, so that by the end of the third week the stomodæum and mesodæum are continuous with one another. During the same week, five processes—one mesial (the fronto-nasal) and four lateral (the two maxillary and the two mandibular)—bud out from the base of the primitive cerebral capsule around the margins of the stomodæum, and, by their growth and ultimate coalescence, enclose the cavity, which is now termed the oro-nasal cavity, and complete the facial portion of the head at the end of the second month (Fig. 295).

The mesial or fronto-nasal process which bounds the upper part of the oro-nasal cavity becomes elevated on either side of the mid-line to form two marked protuberances, the globular processes.

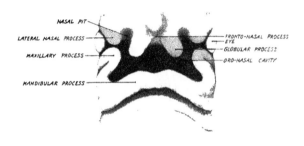

Fig. 295.—Face of an embryo of 8 mm.
(After His and McMurrich.)

Simultaneously with the formation of the globular processes, two oval depressions or grooves, the nasal pits, appear externally to them, and thus separate the lower end of the fronto-nasal process into three parts—a mesial nasal process with its globular processes, and two lateral nasal processes.

These processes are in reality the anterior extremities of three vertical septa that grow down from the base of the primitive cerebral capsule; they are kept apart by the gradual deepening of the nasal pits, and ultimately form the septal and lateral walls of the nasal cavities. The portion of the mesial nasal process which intervenes between the two globular processes is divided into an upper triangular and a lower quadrilateral area by a transverse ridge which later becomes moulded into the tip of the nose. The upper triangular area becomes the dorsum of the nose, the lower quadrilateral portion the columella, i.e. the septum between the anterior nares. By the elevation of this median portion to form the external nasal organ, the globular processes are enabled to fuse together to form the middle third of the upper lip (philtrum) and the premaxilla. Imperfect union in this situation leads to that rare malformation, median hare-lip. While these changes are taking place above, the mandibular processes below have united (in the fifth week) to form the mandible, lower lip, and chin. All that is now required to complete the face

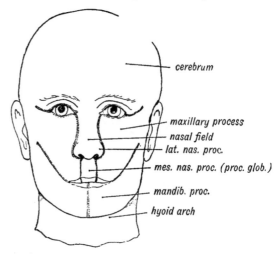

Fig. 296.—Showing the parts of the face formed from the nasal, maxillary, and mandibular processes.

(*From Keith's " Human Embryology and Morphology."*)

is the closure of the gap between the mandibular bars and the lateral nasal and fronto-nasal processes.

This is effected by a bud-like projection known as the maxillary process, which springs from the upper border of the base' of the mandibular bar on each side, and sweeps inwards and forwards beneath the eye and the nasal groove, thereby separating them from the oral cavity. Above, it blends with the lateral nasal process to complete the ala of the nose ; anteriorly, with the globular process to complete the upper lip ; and below, with the mandibular bar to diminish the size of the oral aperture. Therefore, failure of union between the maxillary and either of these three processes results in facial cleft, lateral hare-lip, or macrostoma. (Fig. 296.) Conversely, fusion of the maxillary and mandibular processes beyond the normal degree leads to microstoma.

Development of the palate.—If the interior of the oro-
nasal cavity be examined in a fœtus of seven weeks (Fig. 297), the
olfactory chambers will be seen opening into it, by the primitive
choanæ, between the maxillary processes and the shelf-like projection
from the posterior part of the mesial nasal (globular) process in which
the premaxilla is developed. Laterally, two horizontal plates will be
noticed springing from the inner aspect of the maxillary processes.
These, the palatal plates, grow inwards beneath the nasal septum,

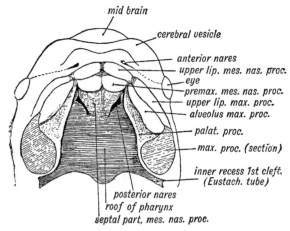

Fig. 297.—Showing the ingrowth of the palatal plates of the
two maxillary processes early in the second month. The
openings erroneously indicated as " posterior nares " are
the primitive choanæ. (*After Kollmann.*)

(*From Keith's " Human Embryology and Morphology."*)

and, fusing from before backwards, first with the premaxilla, and
later with each other, complete the hard and soft palates and separate
the nose from the mouth. From this it will be understood that
partial cleft palate is due to defective fusion of the palatal processes
with each other; that complete cleft palate follows non-union of a
palatal plate with the premaxillary process in front and the opposite
palatal plate behind; and that, in complete cleft palate and hare-lip,
the line of cleavage passes between the maxillary and palatine processes externally, and the globular, premaxillary, and palatine
processes mesially. As the process of fusion spreads from before
backwards, partial cleft palate occurs with greater frequency than
complete cleft palate, and a complete cleft is not always accompanied by hare-lip. Similarly, partial or complete hare-lip is not

necessarily associated with cleft palate, for, as Fig. 297 clearly shows, the upper lip is completed by the union of the maxillary and globular processes, whilst the palate is fashioned from the three horizontal plates which grow inwards from these processes.

The foetal palate has a very high arch, for the palatal plates develop in an upward as well as a horizontal direction, in the endeavour, as it were, to meet the nasal septum, with which they eventually fuse. This peculiarity of growth accounts for the frequent combination of a high arch with cleft palate, and in such cases is of great value to the surgeon if a " flap-sliding " operation is undertaken, for, when the

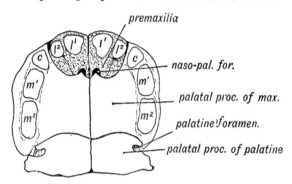

Fig. 298.—Showing the hard palate at birth. The premaxillary part is formed from the mesial nasal processes ; the remainder by the palatal plates of the maxillary processes.

(*From Keith's " Human Embryology and Morphology.*")

flaps are separated from the bone, they fall into a horizontal plane and so naturally approach one another.

Development of the premaxilla.—The premaxillary bones are ossified from two centres which appear side by side in the premaxillary process on the deep aspect of the mesial nasal process ; later, these bifurcate and give origin to the four incisor bones. (Fig. 298.) As a rule, all four upper incisor teeth are developed on this process, each bone forming the socket for one tooth ; but, according to Keith, the lateral incisor may occasionally appear on that part of the alveolus which is developed from the maxillary process.

In the majority of mammals the premaxilla is highly developed and forms the prognathion or snout. This characteristic is well simulated in the infant in those cases in which a cleft in the hard palate bifurcates at the naso-palatine foramen into two branches, that pass forwards and outwards between the premaxillary and palatine processes. In such cases the premaxilla, having no lateral attachments to fix it, is pushed forward by the palatine processes as they approach each other, and at the same time undergoes excessive development from lack of restraint (*see* Fig. 305).

MALFORMATIONS

MACROSTOMA

Macrostoma, or buccal cleft, is due either to failure of union of the posterior portions of the maxillary and mandibular processes, or, after union has taken place, to arrested growth caused by the pressure of amniotic bands. (Fig. 299.) The condition varies from a slight defect at the angle of the mouth to a cleft which may extend nearly to the auricle ; though usually bilateral, it may be unilateral, and in either case is not infrequently associated with other congenital defects, such as oblique facial cleft and accessory auricles. As usually seen, the defect is limited to a slight increase in the size of the oral aperture, and, beyond its unsightly appearance, gives rise to no inconvenience ; but in severe

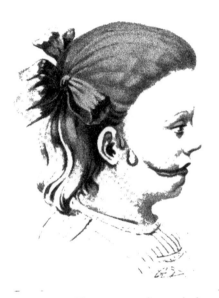

Fig. 299.—Macrostoma with auricular appendages.

cases the constant escape of saliva, and the defective nutrition that results from the inability of the child to retain food in the mouth, render an operation imperative.

Treatment.—The edges of the cleft should be pared with a sharp scalpel, and then united with an inner muco-mucous layer of catgut and an outer cutaneous layer of fine salmon-gut sutures. The only detail requiring attention is the identification of Stenson's duct before paring the edges of the cleft.

MICROSTOMA

Microstoma, or congenital atresia oris, is, as its name implies, the very reverse of macrostoma. This rare defect is the result of an excessive degree of fusion between the maxillary and mandibular processes, and may take place to such an extent as to leave an opening which will only admit a small probe. It must not be confused with acquired stenosis following cicatricial contraction after burns, syphilitic ulceration, lupus, etc.

Treatment.— When necessary, the oral aperture may be elongated by incising the cheek at the angles of the mouth and suturing the mucous membrane to the skin.

FACIAL CLEFT

This is such a rare malformation that a passing reference to it will suffice. As already stated in the account of the development of the face, it is due to partial or total failure of union between the maxillary process below and the lateral nasal and globular processes above. Another, and possibly more accurate, explanation of the

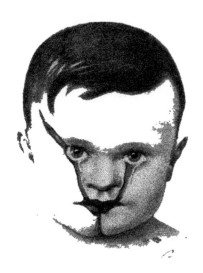

Fig. 300.—Mandibular cleft and two varieties of facial cleft.

cause of facial, buccal, mandibular, and auricular clefts is offered by Ballantyne, who infers that they are due to the presence of amniotic adhesions and bands formed during morbid conditions of development, rather than to defective union of normal elements. The cleft, commencing in the red margin of the upper lip just externally to the philtrum, may extend to the middle of the lower eyelid, thence to the outer canthus, and, very rarely, into the temporal region. It may be bilateral and asymmetrical, as shown in Fig. 300, and usually involves only the soft parts.

Treatment.—Simple clefts may be closed by suture after paring the edges, but clefts involving the orbit generally require a complicated plastic operation.

FISTULA OF THE LIP

The opening of a fistulous track, lined with mucous membrane and directed upwards towards the ala of the nose, is sometimes seen on the red margin of the upper lip, close to the philtrum. Its presence is probably due to defective fusion of the soft parts, and serves to emphasize a lucky escape from hare-lip. In some instances similar good fortune is shown in a more definite manner by the presence of a well-marked groove at the site of union of the globular and maxillary processes. Congenital fistulæ of the lower lip situated on either side of the mid-line have also been described. Their method of formation is obscure.

Treatment is only required if the fistula gives rise to a copious discharge, or repeatedly becomes inflamed from retention of its secretion. In such a case, or more applications of the galvano - cautery will suffice to close it.

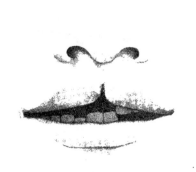

Fig. 301.—**H. H. Clutton's** case of median hare-lip and cleft alveolus.

(This and the next two figures are from drawings in the Museum in St. Thomas's Hospital Medical School.)

MANDIBULAR CLEFT

This defect usually involves both the bone and the soft parts, and is situated in the middle line of the lower jaw at the point where the two mandibular processes should have united (Fig. 300). It is the rarest congenital malformation of the face, and seldom occurs alone, being usually associated with various forms of facial cleft, or with a cleft of the tongue and the floor of the mouth.

Treatment.—The cleft may be closed by one of the methods employed in the treatment of hare-lip.

HARE-LIP

Hare-lip is the commonest malformation of the face, and, according to Stone, occurs in one out of every 2,400 infants. Though isolated

examples occur in families, heredity usually plays a powerful part
in its causation, and in such instances the tendency is generally
transmitted by the
mother. Two ana-
tomical varieties are
met with, the me-
dian and the lateral.

MEDIAN HARE-LIP

One of the rarest
of malformations in
the human being, this
occurs as a natural
characteristic in the
animal from which
it derives its name.
Being due to persist-
ence of the notch
between the two
globular processes
(Fig. 295), it can

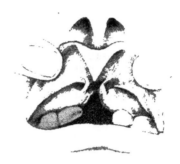

Fig. 302.—Same case as in Fig. 301.

never extend quite
to the columella of
the nose, for this is
developed by the
elevation of the
(mesial) fronto-nasal
bud. In the classi-
cal example de-
picted in Figs. 301
and 302 it will be
seen to involve the
lip for a little less
than half its depth.

True median hare-
lip must not be con-
fused with another
rare median defect
of the upper lip in
which the cleft,
though anatomically
median, is embryo-

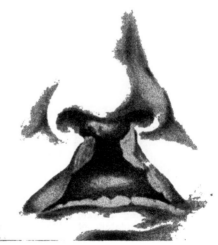

Fig. 303.—Median defect of upper lip due to
imperfect development of the premaxilla.

logically due to a bilateral hare-lip complicated by an entire absence
of the lower end of the fronto-nasal process and the premaxillary

bone. In such a case the nose is extremely flattened owing to absence of the columella and the lower end of the nasal septum, and for the same reason its alæ form the anterior boundary of an oro-nasal cavity (Fig. 303).

Treatment.—In slight cases the defect is readily corrected by Nélaton's operation (p. 138), but when the cleft is at all deep the methods advocated by Rose (p. 138) or Mirault (p. 139) give the best result.

LATERAL HARE-LIP

This, the most usual form of hare-lip, may be unilateral or bilateral, may involve the soft parts only, or be complicated by a cleft alveolus or complete cleft palate. The defect is more common in boys than in girls; when unilateral, it occurs more often on the left side, and may be accompanied by cleft alveolus or cleft palate, while the bilateral variety rarely occurs without a corresponding cleft in the alveolus and palate. In both varieties the defect varies from a slight indentation in the red margin of the lip to a deep fissure which extends into the nostril.

In the slighter grades a narrow shining strip of skin having the appearance of scar tissue is sometimes seen extending between the apex of the indentation and the nostril. As microscopical examination has proved that none of the elements of scar tissue are present in these strips, their appearance can only be accounted for by the disturbance in the normal process of development and by delayed union.

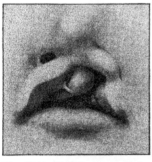

Fig. 304.—Unilateral complete hare-lip, showing forward and outward rotation of the premaxilla and flattening of the ala nasi.

(*From a patient at the Evelina Hospital.*)

Unilateral, or **single hare-lip** as it is generally called, is unfortunately more often a deep than a shallow cleft, only separated from the nostril by a narrow strip of skin representing the remains of the upper lip. When the fissure extends completely into the nostril the alveolus is invariably cleft as well, and not infrequently the defect in it extends backwards into the hard and soft palates.

The margins of the cleft are often unequal in length, and the nostril of the same side is broadened and flattened. When the cleft extends into the nose the flattening is more marked, and frequently the outer margin of the fissure is directly continuous with the ala nasi. The deformity is further increased by the presence of a cleft in the alveolus, for in such cases the inner or premaxillary portion of the bone projects forwards in advance of the outer margin of the cleft, and, owing to the loss of its lateral attachment, looks obliquely upwards and towards the unaffected side; the apex of the nose and the root of the columella are carried with it, and the ala nasi forms a flat and almost tense band of tissue bridging over the upper extremity of the cleft (Fig. 304).

Bilateral hare-lip, like the unilateral form, may be partial or complete, but more often the cleft on one side is partial, involving only a portion of the lip, and on the opposite side is total, extending

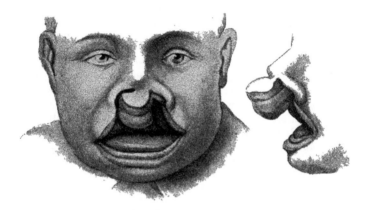

Fig. 305.—Bilateral complete hare-lip. The profile shows protrusion and upward rotation of the premaxilla.

through the whole depth of the lip, and generally through the alveolus and the hard and soft palates as well. When the clefts are total on both sides and extend to the bone, the premaxilla or os incisivum, no longer kept in position by its lateral attachments to the hard palate, is pushed forwards and upwards by excessive growth of that part of the nasal septum formed from the premaxillary process, and in severe cases projects beyond the tip of the nose, giving the child the characteristic prognathous appearance (Fig. 305). Frequently the pedicle by which the premaxilla is attached to the nasal septum is so narrow that considerable lateral movement of the process is permitted. The skin and subcutaneous tissue corresponding to the median portion (philtrum) of the upper lip is smaller than usual and possesses no lower free margin, being firmly attached to the subjacent bone, and blending laterally and below with the mucous membrane enveloping the premaxilla. The nose is flattened, and the antero-posterior length of its columella is shortened in proportion to the degree of projection of the premaxilla. The teeth of the premaxilla are liable to many variations from the normal; they are generally irregular in position and obliquely directed; in the majority of cases only two, the central incisors, are present, but occasionally there are four or more.

Site of the cleft.—In true median hare-lip the cleft lies between the two globular processes, outgrowths of the mesial nasal process, while in lateral hare-lip it is placed between the globular process on the inner side and the maxillary process on the outer side —not between the globular process and the lateral nasal process, as suggested by Albrecht, for it is now well known that the latter process takes no part in the formation of the lip. The much-discussed position of the cleft in the alveolus is described under Cleft Palate (p. 146).

Treatment of Hare-Lip

Obviously the only method of treating such an unsightly defect is by an operative procedure, having for its object the closure of the cleft and the restoration of the red margin of the lip. The only detail on which opinions have differed is the **age at which the operation should be performed.** This depends to a certain extent (1) upon the size and nature of the defect and the condition of the child, and (2) upon the skill of the operator, the rapidity with which he works, and his familiarity with the method he proposes to employ. No surgeon should approach the task in a light-hearted manner, for, no matter how slight the defect, its accurate closure requires a certain degree of skill only to be acquired by practice, as the tyro will readily confess when he sees the result of his work, six months or a year later. Speaking generally, the best time for operation is during the second month, for by then the infant has become accustomed to its nurse, is familiar with its surroundings, sleeps for the greater part of the day, and, in the event of the size of the cleft or the condition of the mother having rendered bottle or spoon feeding necessary, should be free from gastro-intestinal disturbances. But if the child is undeveloped or badly nourished, the operation must be postponed until the patient's condition has materially improved, for the mere remedy of the defect at an early age is unlikely to have a marked effect upon its general health.

In slight cases the child can generally suckle without difficulty, so that if the mother can nurse it properly it is wiser to defer the operation until the time for weaning arrives; for, if the lip is sutured at an earlier date, lactation is necessarily interfered with for at least a week, and may have to be discontinued altogether. When the cleft is large, natural feeding can, and should, be carried out by means of a glass nipple-shield to which is fitted a large rubber teat that fills the gap in the lip. After the operation the child should still be fed with maternal milk, drawn off with a pump, until such time as it can be put to the breast again.

In cases of *bilateral cleft*, natural feeding is, of course, impossible. In such circumstances the child must be spoon-fed, and operated upon as soon as the surgeon judges that its condition will permit; afterwards it can be brought up on the bottle in the usual manner. Another reason for operating on bilateral hare-lip at an early age is the urgent necessity of replacing the premaxilla, and counteracting its forward growth by the pressure which is brought to bear upon it by the united lip. It is surprising what a marked effect this procedure has in inhibiting the prognathic tendency, especially if the mother or nurse be instructed to assist it by frequently and regularly applying pressure until the protrusion is reduced.

When hare-lip coexists with cleft palate, and when the early operation upon the palate (Lane's or Brophy's) is contemplated, the closure of the gap in the lip must be deferred until healing of the palate is complete. As the ultimate appearance of the lip will depend in great measure upon the neatness of the scar, it is of the utmost importance that primary union should be secured. In order to attain this desirable end, no operation should be undertaken until the child is in a satisfactory state of health, and the mouth, the nose, and the aural cavities have been examined and found to be free from any septic condition.

Preparation for the operation.—When the surgeon has to deal with a healthy, well-nourished infant, no special preparation is necessary, other than the administration of a small dose of castor oil two days beforehand; in fact, the less the normal routine and surroundings of the child are disturbed, the better it will bear the operation. But when the infant is peevish, ill-nourished, and the subject of gastro-intestinal catarrh from improper feeding, the operation may have to be delayed for a month or longer. If the child is being suckled and does not thrive as well as it should do, it must either be weaned at once or its nourishment augmented by two or more bottle-feeds daily. Though the quality and quantity of a feed must be varied to a slight extent for different babies, the following formula is a very useful one on which to base its composition :—

At two months

Milk	.	.	.	.	.	.	.	. $\mathfrak{z}$ 1½
Whey	.	.	.	.	.	.	.	. $\mathfrak{z}$ 1½
Cream	.	.	.	.	.	.	.	. $\mathfrak{z}$ 1
Sugar	.	.	.	.	.	.	.	. 1 eggspoonful ?

The addition of cream is important as a fattening agent, and Barbadoes sugar is preferable to the Demerara or crystallized variety on account of its better laxative properties. The milk should be sterilized or pasteurized as a routine, for it is practically impossible to obtain bacteriologically pure milk, no matter how healthy the cow or how carefully the milk is collected and conveyed. The addition of sodium citrate, in the proportion of one grain to the ounce of milk, is often of great assistance in diminishing the size of the curd and rendering the milk more digestible. Patent foods and tinned milks should never be given. The child's condition can always be greatly improved by daily inunction with cod-liver oil after a warm bath, the unpleasant odour and greasy nature of the oil being compensated for by its beneficial effect. The room in which the operation is performed should be well heated, and the infant should be well wrapped up. Young babies being very susceptible to shock, every precaution should be taken to guard against it.

Position of the patient.—The position of the infant during operation depends mainly on the individual habit of the operator : some prefer the upright position, the child then being wrapped in a blanket, with the arms and legs secured, and seated on a firm cushion placed upon the nurse's lap ; others go to the opposite extreme and favour the supine position with the head hanging over the end of the table. As a matter of fact, any position will do, provided it be so arranged that blood cannot trickle into the pharynx. Perhaps the most satisfactory position is a semi-reclining one, with the head tilted to one side and steadied by an assistant so that blood can readily escape and the surgeon can obtain a good view of the lip.

The operation.—In order to avoid repetition, the general principles of the operation will be described first, and later a few of the most useful and practical methods of closing the defect will be given. For a full account of the numerous methods and modifications that have been suggested and employed, the reader is referred to a manual of operative surgery.

The choice of the anæsthetic naturally depends upon the anæsthetist, but, as a general rule, chloroform, given on a mask to commence with, and continued with a Junker's inhaler, is very satisfactory provided that special care be taken not to push the anæsthesia beyond the "contracted-pupil" stage. The operation should never be performed without an anæsthetic. Before it is begun, the nose and mouth should be cleared of mucus, and the lips washed with ether soap.

The main principles that underlie a successful and ornamental issue are (1) the free liberation of the lip, the cheek, the ala of the nose, and occasionally of its columella, from the underlying bone ; (2) the shaping of the nostril ; (3) the paring of the margins of the cleft or the cutting of a good-sized flap or flaps; (4) the accurate suturing of the raw surfaces.

1. The *free liberation of the lip* is the first and most important step in the operation, for unless this be thoroughly and systematically carried out, coaptation without tension will be impossible. In unilateral cases the lip on the outer side of the cleft should be raised with the fingers, and the mucous membrane divided with a sharp knife at its junction with the gum. The handle of the scalpel is then used to detach the lip and cheek from the bone, care being taken to stop the dissection short of the infra-orbital foramen lest the infra-orbital nerve be damaged. If the ala of the nose is flattened in the slightest degree, it must be freed from the subjacent bone at the same time. Provided the tissues are torn and not cut from the maxilla, the hæmorrhage is very slight and can easily be controlled by pressure. When the outer portion of the lip has been sufficiently mobilized, the inner margin and the columella of the nose, if at all displaced, are freed in a similar manner.

2. The next step consists in so *shaping the nostril* as to make it harmonize with that of the opposite side. Needless to say, this is only necessary when the hare-lip is a complete one, as the contour of the nose is seldom altered in the partial variety. To commence with, a straight, sharp needle threaded with a salmon-gut suture is entered at the lower end of the naso-labial groove, and carried inwards and downwards to emerge at the junction of the nostril with the outer margin of the cleft. It is then passed in an upward direction from the inner margin of the cleft, through the base of the nasal septum, into the opposite nostril. The parts are now approximated, and, if the deformity has been properly corrected, the ends of the suture are secured with split shot after the edges of the lip have been pared.

In many cases this simple procedure produces the desired result, but occasionally the cartilage of the ala becomes so folded upon itself as partially to block the aperture. In such cases a large V-shaped piece may be excised, as depicted in Fig. 306, or a flap of mucous membrane can be turned up and the redundant cartilage bodily removed; or a portion of the ala may be excised (by an incision that follows the naso-labial groove), and re-attached to the lip and cheek with a few fine sutures. Though the rectification of the ala nasi appears simple enough in theory, in practice a perfect result is seldom obtained.

Fig. 306. Method of rectifying infolded ala by excision of V-shaped piece of mucous membrane and cartilage.

3. The *paring of the margins of the cleft* or the *shaping of flaps* is accomplished with a pointed, sharp, narrow-bladed scalpel, in

preference to a tenotome, which is either unduly pliant or unnecessarily thick in the back.   The red border of the lip being seized with
fine rat-tooth forceps at the point where its horizontal portion merges
into the vertical border of the cleft, the scalpel is entered exactly at
the junction of the skin and mucous membrane, plunged through
the whole thickness of the lip, and carried with a gentle sawing motion
upwards towards the nostril, or even into it if necessary.   The incision
should be kept just external to the vermilion border of the lip, and
should never be allowed to encroach upon it, otherwise when the
operation is completed the result will be marred by the presence of a
patch of red mucous membrane in the line of the scar.

If the operator intends to turn down two flaps of mucous membrane,
as in Fig. 308, it is of the utmost importance that the incision, at its
lower end, should lie exactly between the mucous membrane and the
skin, otherwise the vermilion border of the lip will be interrupted
by a white line formed by the included skin.   In some cases it may
be necessary to deepen the lip.   This is accomplished by curving
the upper part of the incision outwards well into the skin, so that
the raw surface presents a concavity towards the cleft, as in Fig. 308 ;
but at its lower extremity it must still follow the junction of the
mucous membrane and the skin, or the unsightly patch of skin will
again appear in the vermilion border.   The hæmorrhage that follows
division of the coronary arteries in the margin of the lip is controlled
temporarily either by an assistant seizing the lip between his fingers
or with a pair of narrow-bladed artery forceps, and permanently
when the sutures are inserted.

In cases of bilateral hare-lip the alæ nasi and the lips are
thoroughly freed, and the edges of the latter denuded or shaped into
flaps in the manner already described.   The suture that was employed
for restoring the shape of the nostril in the unilateral case should
perforate the base of the nasal septum as before, and then be passed
through the nostril from within outwards, and made to emerge at a
point in the naso-labial groove exactly corresponding to its point of
entry on the opposite side.   Before cutting the labial flaps, it is
advisable to freshen the edges of the skin covering the premaxilla in
order to obtain a better idea of the size and thickness of the flaps
necessary effectively to close the defect.   As it is important to preserve as much of this premaxillary tab of skin as possible, and also to
shape it in such a way that it will dovetail nicely between the labial
flaps, its inferior margin should be cut to resemble a wide V (Fig. 314).
If the premaxilla is unduly prominent, it should be returned to its
normal position at the same time, either by simply pushing it back or,
if this is not successful, by the operative procedure described later.

4. The fourth and last stage of the operation consists of *so suturing*

the raw surfaces that the edges of the vermilion border are brought into accurate apposition and form a continuous line. To obtain this desirable end, the first suture should enter the lip exactly at the junction of its red border with the skin on one side, and emerge at a corresponding point on the opposite side. When the method of closing the defect depends upon apposition of two inverted flaps, as in Fig. 308, it is important to see that they project below the margin of the lip in the form of a well-marked papilla, otherwise the cicatricial contraction that follows healing will leave an unsightly notch in the red margin. The remaining sutures are then passed deeply into the substance of the lip, but they must not penetrate the mucous membrane. Finally, the whole lip is everted and the mucous membrane on its deep aspect is united by a few fine sutures. Fine silkworm-gut, technically designated " ophthalmic," forms the best suture material, being pliant, non-irritating, and easily removable. Hare-lip pins are now obsolete.

Dressing the wound.—In ordinary circumstances the wound is better left uncovered, so that it may be frequently and easily cleaned with a damp sponge. The doubtful advantages that accrue from the use of a strip of gauze, soaked in collodion or Whitehead's varnish, and fixed by a dumb-bell-shaped piece of strapping so applied as to relieve tension, are neutralized by the ease with which particles of food, or mucus from the nose and mouth, collect beneath the dressing and infect the wound. Before the child leaves the operating table, the depression beneath the lower lip should be well painted with thick collodion. This, by contracting as it dries, produces an amount of eversion of the lip just sufficient to leave an airway into the mouth and so minimize the danger of asphyxiation, for, immediately after closing the cleft, the upper lip is somewhat tightly stretched across the alveolus, possesses little if any movement, and, by the increase in its depth (i.e. height), is in close contact with the floppy, redundant lower lip, which is sucked against it at everv inspiration until consciousness returns.

After-treatment.—For the first few days after the operation the child must be nursed and coaxed as much as possible in order to reduce the amount of its crying to a minimum, otherwise some, or possibly all, of the sutures may tear out. In the event of such a catastrophe, the surgeon must wait until the raw surfaces are covered with healthy granulations, and then readjust them with the aid of sutures and adhesive strapping. Feeding is best carried out with a small spoon, or a drinking-cup provided with a long piece of india-rubber tubing, until such time as the child can be put to the breast again. In cases of incomplete cleft of slight degree this may be permissible in three or four days, but in the severer grades eight to ten days must elapse before suckling can be allowed with safety. The stitches may be removed by degrees, commencing on the third day, or all may be left until the seventh or eighth day. Either method gives satisfactory results, provided common sense is employed in carrying it out. When removing stitches it is always advisable to stupefy the child with chloroform, lest a sudden movement or a violent fit of crying make the wound gape.

Operations for Single Hare-Lip

Nélaton's operation.—As a primary operation this method is only applicable to defects of very limited extent, and for this reason can seldom be employed. It is more often of value in correcting an

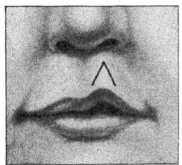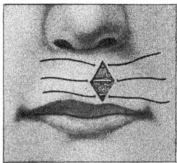

Fig. 307.—Nélaton's operation.

indentation of the lip, the result of cicatricial contraction after some other form of operation (Fig. 307).

An inverted **V**-shaped incision is made through the whole thickness of the lip above and around the margin of the cleft. The skin and mucous membrane is then pulled downwards until the wound becomes diamond-shaped, when its edges are approximated with a few horizontally placed sutures.

Rose's operation.—As this method only yields good results when the two sides of the cleft are more or less symmetrical, its application is somewhat limited. It is described here because it illustrates two of the points that were emphasized in discussing the operative procedure in general, viz. (1) that the height of the lip may be increased by curving the vertical incisions outwards, and (2) that the incisions forming the flaps must be placed exactly between the skin and the red border of the lip.

Two curved incisions with their concavities directed towards each other are carried from the apex of the cleft to the junction of the skin and the red border of the lip, on each side of the defect (Fig. 308). The points at which these incisions terminate must be selected with care, for, if they are placed too far apart, the "Cupid's bow" curve of the lip will be too exaggerated when suturing is completed; and if they are too close to the margins of the cleft, the red border will be horizontal at the completion of the operation, and notched upwards when cicatricial contraction has taken place. From the termination of the first incision a second incision is carried inwards and upwards exactly between the vermilion border and the skin, to emerge about the middle of the cleft and form two long flaps of mucous membrane. These are inverted, and when the raw surfaces are sutured a well-marked projection is formed

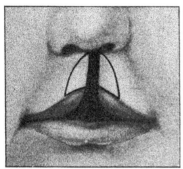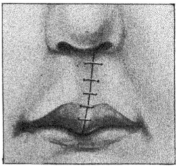

Fig. 308.—Rose's operation.

at the margin of the lip. If the flaps are too long, the redundant portions can always be removed before suturing is completed.

Mirault's operation.—This operation is employed when the two sides of the cleft are of unequal length, differently curved, or widely divergent. To obtain a good result a certain degree of mathematical accuracy is required in paring the edge and shaping the flap.

On the more oblique side of the cleft (Fig. 309) a point, A, is selected at, or just below, the centre of the curve; A' represents a point in the normal line of the lip perpendicularly below A; C is situated at the junction of the horizontal and vertical borders of the steeper side of the cleft; B marks the termination of the flap incision. The distance between B and C must equal the distance between A and A'. The oblique side of the cleft is pared by the concave incisions D A, E A, leaving a projection at A. On the opposite side, a flap B D C is formed. This is turned down and applied to the raw surface opposite, so that the projection at A fits into the angle formed at B. The redundant tissue at the apex

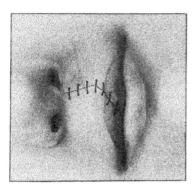

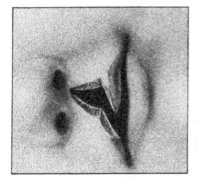

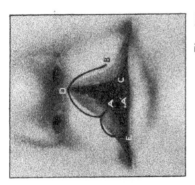

Fig. 309.—Stages of Mirault's operation. (For references, see text.)

of the flap B D C is removed by an oblique incision so placed that the edges of the red border come into accurate apposition. This incision should not be made until the flap has been laid in position.

Edmund Owen's operation, though resembling that of Mirault to a certain extent, differs from it materially in that the flap which is brought across the fissure is large and fleshy instead of thin and attenuated. The method is particularly applicable to the closure of large and deep clefts with asymmetrical sides, and in good hands gives most excellent results.

The mucous membrane on the smaller side of the cleft and lip is removed nearly as far as the angle of the mouth (Fig. 310). On the opposite side a large flap is cut, with its apex at the top of the cleft. The incision by which this flap is formed is, near its extremity, carried parallel to the normal line of the lip for a short distance, so as to diminish the tendency to puckering that takes place at this point when the sutures are inserted. The large flap thus formed is then turned down, forming the mucous border of the restored lip, and the raw surface on the opposite side of the cleft is adjusted in such a way that it fits into the angle made by the inversion of the flap. The direction of the scar is shown in Fig. 311.

To obtain a good cosmetic result in this, as in every other

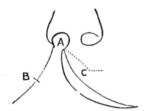

Fig. 310.—Edmund Owen's operation. Mucous membrane removed from whole length of outer margin of cleft ; large thick flap cut from inner margin.

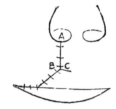

Fig. 311.—Edmund Owen's operation. Flap from left side adjusted along right half of lip.

(This and the preceding figure are from Owen's "Cleft Palate and Hare-Lip.")

operation for hare-lip, it is essential that the lip and cheeks be freely separated from the underlying bone. " The great advantage of this method," to quote Owen, "is that the resulting and inevitable scar does not traverse the mucous membrane in the line of the scar in the skin, but, being deflected outwards, may escape attention as it gradually tails out to the free border, which it may reach at a slight distance from the corner of the mouth."

Rectification of the maxillary arch.—When one side of the alveolar margin is unduly prominent and cannot be reduced by pressure, the deformity can be corrected by a wire mattress-suture inserted in the manner depicted in Fig. 312, after

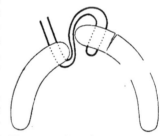

Fig. 312.—Showing method of rectifying prominent maxillary arch.

dividing the bone at a convenient spot between two tooth-germs.

Operations for Double Hare-Lip

When double hare-lip is complicated by an unduly prominent premaxilla, the operation upon the cleft must not be commenced until the prognathion has been reduced or completely removed. The opinions of surgeons as to the best course to adopt have differed in the past, and doubtless will continue to do so in the future. When the prognathion is ill developed, obliquely directed, and rotated forwards at a right angle to the alveolar margin, there can be no two opinions as to the best course to pursue : it should be resected, but the tab of skin covering it should not be sacrificed, for, small though it may be, it will be of use in the reconstruction either of the columella or of the lip. On the other hand, when the premaxilla is well shaped, firmly attached, and only slightly in advance of the alveolar margin, it should be preserved and utilized in closing the defect, for the very fact of attaching the margins of the cleft to it will prevent its becoming prominent, and, if the operation be performed within the first two months of life, may even lead to its recession between the maxillæ. It is in the intermediate type of this deformity, when it becomes necessary to fracture the vomer before the premaxilla can be replaced, that the difficulty in deciding upon the best line of treatment arises. If the premaxilla is preserved, its pedicle must be divided before it can be forced into position, and the mobility thus acquired may persist in afterlife, rendering it useless for mastication, and a continual source of annoyance to its possessor. Again, as the bone is replaced by rotating it through the arc of a circle the centre of which is at the seat of fracture of the pedicle, the incisor teeth, apart from their tendency to erupt irregularly, may also point backwards instead of downwards, and so be worse than useless. On the other hand, if this bone be removed, a permanent gap is left in the alveolar margin, and the width and forward curve of the maxillary arch do not fully develop. In consequence, the lower jaw projects considerably in advance of the upper, the flat, tense, reconstructed upper lip is underhung by the well-developed lower lip, and the child starts life with a profile that is as unsightly as it is characteristic (Fig. 313). Therefore, taking everything into consideration, it is of the highest importance to preserve this portion of bone whenever possible, for there is always the possibility of fibrous union taking place between it and the maxillæ ; and even if, in spite of this, the bone still remains mobile, it can always be excised after the permanent teeth have developed, and the gap filled in with an obturator fitted by a skilled dental surgeon.

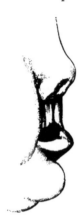

Fig. 313.—Characteristic profile after excision of the premaxilla and suture of the lips. (*Holmes.*)

Operation for replacement of the premaxilla (von Bardeleben's modification of Blandin's method).—The muco-periosteum on the free edge of the nasal septum is incised in an antero-posterior direction about half an inch behind the premaxilla. The length of the incision corresponds to the distance that the premaxilla projects beyond the alveolus. The muco-periosteum is then freely separated from each side of the vomer, and the bone divided by a vertical cut made with a pair of scissors. The premaxilla can now be pushed back with ease, and, if necessary, trimmed until it fits into the cleft. Though it is maintained in position by the plastic operation that is immediately performed upon the lip, it is sometimes

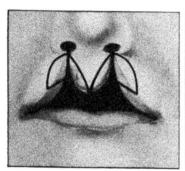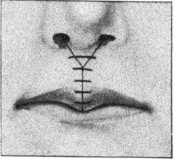

Fig. 314.—Rose's operation for double hare-lip.

necessary to fix it to the maxillæ with a couple of chromicized catgut sutures.

Operations for bilateral hare-lip. *Rose's method.*—When the premaxillary bone is in proper position, the skin over it is freed and pared laterally to resemble the letter **V**. Flaps are then cut from each margin of the cleft, inverted, and sutured above to the premaxillary skin, and below to each other, as depicted in Fig. 314. In most cases this method yields an excellent cosmetic result, but if the upper lip is shallow and skimpy, or the clefts are very wide, Hagedorn's method is more suitable.

Hagedorn's method.—After freshening the edges of the skin over the premaxilla, as in Fig. 315, a flap is cut by the incisions 4, 2; 2, 3, from the outer margin of the cleft on each side, with its base at the junction of the horizontal and vertical portions of the vermilion border. These two flaps are inverted, and pulled upon so as to straighten them out. An incision, 1, *a'*, is now made downwards and outwards into the lip, commencing a short distance above the level of the lateral angle *a*, on the premaxillary tab of skin. This incision, when opened up, gives additional height to the lip and, when the parts are approximated, receives the angular projection *a*. When the suturing is completed as far as the vermilion border, the redùndant portions of the flaps are removed, care being taken to leave a projection long enough to compensate for cicatricial contraction.

Summary of the choice of operation.—As no one operation is applicable to every variety of hare-lip, and as every exponent of this particular branch of surgery is naturally biased in favour of the methods with which he himself has obtained the best results, the following indications, made with due regard to these facts, are given as suggestions rather than as a series of rules :—

1. *Unilateral hare-lip.*—For partial clefts with equal sides, employ Rose's method; for partial clefts with unequal sides, Mirault's method; and for complete clefts, Edmund Owen's method.

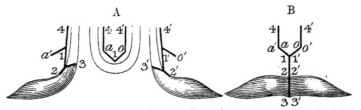

Fig. 315.—Hagedorn's operation for bilateral hare-lip. The unshaded part of the margin of the cleft corresponds to the portion of the flap removed when suturing is nearly completed.

2. *Notching of the lip* following any of the above operations may be remedied by Nélaton's operation.

3. *Bilateral hare-lip.*—For narrow clefts, or clefts with a large premaxilla, employ Rose's method. For wide clefts, with uneven sides and a small premaxilla, employ Hagedorn's method.

CLEFT PALATE

Varieties.—Clinically, two varieties of cleft palate are recognized—*partial*, in which the cleft is limited to a portion or the whole of the soft palate, or to the soft palate and a portion of the hard palate ; and *total*, when the defect extends through the alveolus as well as through the hard and soft palates. The latter form is frequently complicated by unilateral or bilateral hare-lip.

Anatomically, the different varieties are classified with greater accuracy as follows :—

1. *Tripartite palate.*—The three palatal elements are widely separated by an elongated Y-shaped fissure, the limbs of which meet at the posterior inferior angle of the nasal septum (Fig. 316). In this variety the central element is formed by the premaxilla and the

lower margin of the nasal septum, and the lateral elements by the alveolar margin, the hard palate, and the soft palate. Tripartite palate is generally complicated by complete bilateral hare-lip and excessive protrusion of the premaxilla.

2. *Bipartite palate.*—In this variety, owing to the union of the premaxilla with the maxilla on one side, the cleft is single and lies between the premaxilla and the opposite maxilla, extending from the alveolus to the naso-palatine foramen, and posterior to this (in

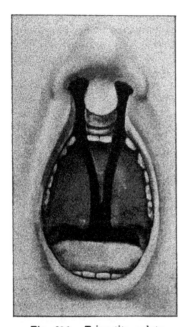 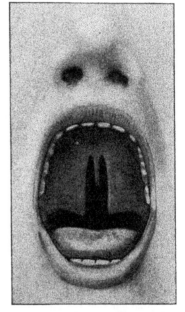

Fig. 316.—Tripartite palate.   Fig. 317.—Intermaxillary cleft.

the middle line) between the two halves of the hard and soft palates (Fig. 318). Theoretically, the cleft should bend outwards in its course between the naso-palatine foramen and the alveolar margin, but as a matter of fact the divergence from the mid-line is very slight, as the premaxillary portion of the alveolar arch is always rotated forwards, upwards, and away from the cleft. The maxillary element with which the premaxilla fails to unite is usually the left one; but why this should be, no satisfactory explanation is forthcoming. The nasal septum, instead of being free, as in the tripartite palate, is generally adherent for a part or the whole of its length to the right

k

margin of the cleft, and in such cases is also sharply deflected towards the left.

3. *Intermaxillary cleft.*—As this form of cleft is due to failure of union between the palatal plates, it is situated in the middle line, involves either the soft palate alone, or both soft and hard palates, and never extends farther forwards than the naso-palatine foramen (Fig. 317). Though the nasal septum may be free, it is more often attached to the right margin of the cleft, as in the bipartite palate.

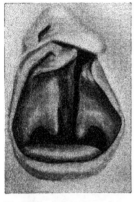

Fig. 318.—Bipartite palate. The nasal septum is adherent to the right margin of the cleft, and is sharply deflected to the left, forming a well-marked " spur."

(From a case at the Evelina Hospital.)

4. *Premaxillary clefts.*—One variety of this malformation is due to arrested union between the premaxilla and the maxilla. The cleft extends from the alveolar margin to the naso-palatine foramen ; posterior to this, the hard and soft palates are complete and well formed. The cleft, though generally unilateral, may be bilateral. The second variety, a very rare one, is associated with median hare-lip, the cleft lying in the middle line between the two halves of the premaxilla. (*See* Fig. 302.) The third form is rather a gap in the lip and palate than a cleft, for it is due to suppression of the globular processes from which the philtrum of the lip and the two halves of the premaxilla are developed. (*See* Fig. 303.)

Line of the cleft, and relationship to it of the incisor teeth.—Because clinicians repeatedly pointed out that the cleft is usually situated between the mesial and lateral incisor teeth, Albrecht formulated the theory that each half of the premaxilla is developed in two parts—the mesial, with the central incisor, from the mesial nasal process ; and the lateral, with the lateral incisor, from the lateral nasal process. Consequently, he and many others believed that the line of cleavage passes between these two portions of the premaxilla, and not between the premaxilla and the maxilla. The presence of a separate incisive bone for each tooth strengthened this theory. However, Kölliker and His have conclusively proved that the lateral nasal process takes no part in the formation of either the premaxilla or the lip, and that, though an incisive bone for each tooth is found, these bones are not developed separately, but are formed by cleavage of the single ossific centre in each half of the premaxilla long after the cleft formation in the palate has taken place. (*See* under Development of the Premaxilla, p. 125.) Consequently, it is now generally acknowledged that the cleft passes between the premaxilla and the maxilla, or, in other words, is meso-exognathic. The varying relationship of the incisor teeth to the margins of the cleft is thus explained by Arthur Keith : " The germ of the lateral incisor, although carried by the mesial nasal process, is laid down in the cleft between the maxillary and premaxillary

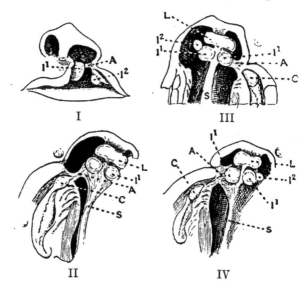

Fig. 319.—Four specimens of cleft palate, showing various degrees in the development of the bond between the premaxillary, maxillary, and lateral nasal processes.

A, The bond or bridge of tissue crossing the cleft ; 1^1, central incisor sac ; 1^2, lateral incisor sac ; c, canine sac ; L, median part of upper lip ; s, septum of nose.

(*From Keith's " Congenital Malformations of the Palate."*)

(mesial-nasal) processes. In cases of cleft palate the processes move apart under the strain of growth during the middle and later months of fœtal life. Three fates may then overtake the bud of the lateral incisor : it may be destroyed, it may remain attached to the pre-maxillary process, but more frequently it moves outwards attached to the maxillary process. I have seen it stranded on the bridge of tissue between the processes, or loosely attached at one side of the fissure or the other." (Fig. 319.)

Symptoms.—In early life the patient is often quite unable to suck owing to its inability to create a vacuum in the mouth, while the attempt to swallow fluids is followed by their regurgitation and escape through the nose. During the early months, death may take place from malnutrition ; and in addition there exists, at all ages, a very real danger from inflammation of the mucous membranes caused by the lodgment and decomposition of secretions and food-stuffs in the oro-nasal cavities. These inflammatory changes may set up chronic nasal catarrh, chronic pharyngitis, œdema of the mucous membrane of the Eustachian tubes and subsequent deafness, gastro-intestinal disturbances, bronchitis and pneumonia.

As age advances, the difficulties of deglutition persist ; and when speech commences, it is imperfect, indistinct, and nasal in tone.

The act of phonation is in reality an exceedingly complicated process, demanding for its proper performance a sounding-box that can be rendered air-tight, and a compressing force. The sounding-box is formed by the bony walls of the buccal cavity ; the escape from it of air is prevented by the closure of the lips and the elevation of the soft palate ; and its shape is altered by the movement of the tongue and cheeks. The compressing force comes from the chest. The presence of a cleft in the palate has little effect upon the vowel sounds, as in enunciating them some of the expired air is normally allowed to pass through the nose, but it interferes greatly with the pronunciation of the majority of consonants, for their production depends upon the complete closure of the naso-pharynx, and the more or less sudden escape of compressed air from the buccal cavity through the orifice of the mouth. Thus the letters D and T are pronounced by allowing the compressed air to escape with an explosive effect through an opening between the tip of the tongue and the anterior part of the hard palate ; the sibilant S is sounded by forcing air through a chink between the tongue and the palate just behind the incisor teeth. In normal circumstances the naso-pharynx is separated from the oral pharynx during phonation by the elevation of the soft palate until it comes in contact with a ridge of tissue, the ridge of Passavant, formed on the posterior and lateral walls of the pharynx by the contraction of the superior constrictor muscles. When the palate is cleft, this closure cannot be effected, so that labial, lingual, and palatal consonants such as P, D, T, S, C, and K cannot be pronounced. The subject of the defect is by long practice frequently able to overcome a few of these difficulties by forming some of the closed sounds in the larynx and by making others in a different part of the mouth. In this he is often materially assisted by the presence of hypertrophied turbinate bones and adenoids which offer an obstacle to the escape of air through the nose, and in the latter case also add to the projection formed by the ridge of Passavant.

Treatment of Cleft Palate

The number of cases in which the partial or total closure of the cleft by suture cannot be attempted must be very small indeed, but occasionally the surgeon meets with one in which the gap is so wide and the available tissue so scanty, either as a result of the magnitude of the deformity or of cicatricial contraction after an operation that has failed, that he has to consider seriously the advisability of having a suitable obturator fitted rather than subject the child to an operative procedure which, from the nature of the cleft or of the tissues bounding it, is doomed to failure from the outset.

Though the use of an obturator gives the best result in connexion with a cleft in the hard palate alone, its employment for this purpose is seldom required, for such clefts can nearly always be closed by operation. At the present time such an instrument is rarely employed, and then only for irremediable defects in the soft palate, when its function is to close the naso-pharynx and so improve a defective articulation. The appliance consists of a dental plate (held in position by the permanent molars), to which is attached either a soft elastic balloon (Schlitsky) that fills the *naso-pharynx* and adapts itself to the changes in shape that occur therein during the act of phonation, or a flexible indiarubber velum (Moriarty) that hangs down in *front* of the soft palate, and is blown against the posterior wall of the pharynx when the air is compressed in the buccal cavity. Except in rare cases, when any means are justified in securing an improvement in phonation and deglutition, mechanical devices should only be used as a complement to surgical treatment.

Age at which the operation should be performed. —This important consideration has been, and still is, the subject of much argument. Surgeons experienced in the treatment of cleft palate may be divided into two classes: those who favour operation within the first three months of life, and those who defer treatment until the third to the sixth year. Both bring forward analogies, arguments, and proofs in favour of their contentions, and each school criticizes severely the methods advocated by the other. In discussing the advantages and disadvantages of the early and late operations, it should always be remembered that the cleft is only one manifestation of a developmental error that has involved not only the soft parts but also the bony walls of the oral and nasal cavities, so that the mechanical closure of the cleft at an early age, no matter how perfect it be, seldom confers upon the patient a normal speaking apparatus. The same consideration applies with even greater force to the result of the late operation, for the child who passes the first few years of his life with a cleft palate cannot even be taught to articulate clearly, and when the defect is remedied his speech is so little better that the phonetic lesson must be commenced all over again.

The advocates of the early operation close the cleft by the methods of Arbuthnot Lane or Brophy; those who favour the late operation employ Langenbeck's method.

In order to obtain the best phonetic result, two factors are essential: (1) that the soft palate should be well formed and freely movable, and (2) that the child should not have learned to talk before the closure of the cleft is brought about. Brophy's method is the only one that fulfils both these requirements. Unfortunately, the operation is a severe one, is only applicable in selected cases, and in some unsuccessful ones has been followed by extensive necrosis of the maxillæ and sloughing of the soft parts. It is owing to the danger of necrosis that this ingenious operation has not received more general support amongst English surgeons. Arbuthnot Lane's method complies with one of the essentials, in that the cleft is closed long before the child commences to talk; but, owing to the extensive flaps that must be fashioned, the resulting soft palate is seldom mobile, and phonation suffers in consequence. Similarly, Langenbeck's method fails in one of the necessary requirements, inasmuch as it can seldom be performed until after speech has commenced; but it undoubtedly possesses the great advantage of leaving the patient with a well-shaped, freely movable soft palate, which, so far as the phonetic result of the operation is concerned, is an absolute necessity.

Taking these various facts into consideration, and disregarding the ideal operation of Brophy for the reasons already mentioned, my opinion is that *Langenbeck's operation, performed between the ages of two and three years*, or earlier if the size of the cleft and the thickness of the tissues permit, gives the best result in the majority of cases. Coexisting hare-lip should be operated upon at the age of three months. When Lane's method is employed, however, the treatment of the defect in the lip should invariably be deferred until some weeks after the palate has been successfully closed.

Preparation of the patient.—It is always advisable to place the patient, a week before the operation, under the care of the nurse who is to look after it, so that it may become accustomed to its surroundings and have any irregularities in its diet corrected. If the bowels are acting regularly there is no necessity to upset the child by administering an aperient, but if there be constipation a small dose of castor oil should be given twenty-four hours before operating. When the time comes, the child should be warmly wrapped up, and placed upon a warm- (not a hot-) water pillow, on a high table, with its head hanging over the edge, so that the operator, who is seated, may obtain a good view of the palate. The mouth is kept open with two of Lane's spring gags, one on each side, and the tongue is drawn forwards by a suture passing through its tip.

During the operation, sterilized marine sponges, being soft and highly absorbent, are preferable to woollen swabs for mopping up the blood and saliva. The only special instruments required are: two pairs of long dissecting forceps, one toothed and one plain; one stout, narrow-bladed scalpel; one cleft-palate knife with a long thin handle, a narrow pointed blade, and a cutting edge not more than a quarter of an inch in length; two pairs of curved and bent elevators; a pair of rectangular scissors; and Lane's needle-holder and cleft-palate needles. In addition to the foregoing, there are required for Brophy's operation a pair of large curved needles on strong shafts, shaped somewhat like the needles employed in the repair of a ruptured perineum.

Early operation for cleft palate.—The *advantages* of the early operation are—

1. The young infant, with few exceptions, is healthy.
2. Its digestion has not been impaired by experimental feeding.
3. Repair of its tissues takes place with great rapidity.
4. The absence of teeth renders its mouth free from pathogenic and putrefactive micro-organisms, and so minimizes the danger of sloughing.
5. The absence of teeth also permits of the fashioning of large flaps.
6. Hæmorrhage is very slight, and the vessels, being so small, seldom require ligation.
7. The baby seldom vomits after the anæsthetic, and takes its food with gusto within a few hours of the completion of the operation.
8. It generally sleeps for the greater part of the day.

The *disadvantages* are—

1. The field of operation is small, and the tissues are very friable.
2. The soft palate formed by Lane's method becomes a rigid piece of cicatricial tissue if the muscular layer is encroached on when cutting the flaps.

Brophy's operation.—The performance of this operation is practically impossible after the third month, owing to the ossification of the maxillæ, and, according to its originator, is best carried out about the third week. In this country it has the support and approval of no less an authority than Edmund Owen, who regards it as the ideal operation for cleft palate. (Figs. 320 and 321.)

The subjoined account is taken from Brophy's paper, read at the
Third International Dental Congress, Paris, 1900 :—

" Pare the edges of the cleft and trim the opposing edges of boue as well
it will secure a sufficient exudate, so essential to a perfect union, to make

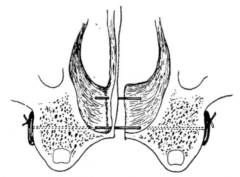

Fig. 320.—Brophy's operation : Sutures passed.

the operation successful in this respect at least. . . . The knife will easily cut
through the soft bone of the hard palate as well as the alveolar processes
of young patients.   Then raise the cheek, and well back toward the posterior
extremity of the hard palate, just back of the malar process and high enough
to escape all danger of not being above the palate bone, insert a large braided

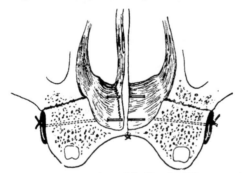

Fig. 321.—Brophy's operation : Maxillæ forcibly approximated
and sutures secured over lead buttons.

silk suture, carrying it through the substance of the bone to the central
fissure by means of one of the strong needles, with the opposite needle carrying
a corresponding suture through the opposite side. We then have two silk
suture loops carried to the centre of the cleft, and passing one loop through
the other enables us to carry the one loop through both of the maxillary
bones. The silk is more easily introduced by the needle than wire, but a
silver wire should always be substituted for it and drawn through to take

its place. The wire should be No. 20, and may be doubled in case the condition of the parts and the tension upon the tissues necessary to approximate them seem to require it. Nearer the front portion of the maxilla insert another wire, carrying it through the substance of the bone above the palatal plate, and through the outer side in a position corresponding to the place of entrance. Thus we will have one wire passing over the palate in front of the malar process of the bone, and another behind it.

" The next step is to make lead plates (No. 17 American gauge) to fit the convexity of the buccal surface of the bones. Have them provided with eye-holes, through which are passed the protruded ends of the wire on each side. Twist these together—that is, the right end of the posterior with the right end of the anterior wire, and the same on the left side. These form heavy tension sutures, and the parts when once approximated by their use cannot be separated, *as the sutures do not cut out.* If the cleft is a very wide one and we are not able to close it by twisting the wires together upon the lead plates, force may be exerted by the thumb and fingers, or by means of a forceps designed for that purpose. If by such force the edges of the cleft do not approximate, then there is a further step to be taken which will obviate these difficulties. After the cheek is well raised, divide the mucous membrane and the bone through the malar process. Carry the knife in a horizontal direction, and, when well inserted, sweep the handle forward and backward. In this way a maximum amount of bone and a minimum amount of mucous membrane will be divided. This done on either side, the bone can readily be moved toward the median line. The wire sutures passing through the lead button may now be again twisted, and the cleft of the hard palate be closed by approximation of the two sides. The incision of the mucous membrane must be made as small as possible, as this membrane must serve to retain the bones in proximity, or to hold them nearly together. If, after the parts are approximated, they are kept antiseptically clean, or as nearly so as possible, they will unite kindly, and the palate will be formed so that its full function will be established. Separation of the bones is attended with very little hæmorrhage, and the parts do not, as a rule, cause more inconvenience to the patient than the ordinary operation of lifting the hard palate, according to the practice of Sir William Fergusson. Should hæmorrhage require attention it is easily controlled by the application of sponges wrung out of water at about 170° F. These hot sponges, held in contact with the bleeding surfaces a very few minutes, will be all that is required. The germs of the teeth are sometimes disturbed, and I have found occasionally certain teeth imperfectly developed when erupted. The palatal arch is in some cases contracted, but this will not be permanent, for, if the operation is performed early enough, when development is complete, the teeth of the upper jaw occlude naturally with those of the lower jaw. It is a well-known fact that the alveolar processes develop with the teeth, and this seems to be a pronounced factor in the formation of the jaw and the guiding of the teeth into their proper position. After the approximation of the edges in the manner that I have described, the parts should be thoroughly dried, the edges of the cleft carefully examined, and, if need be, some fine silk sutures inserted here and there to ensure the perfect coaptation of the parts. These coaptation sutures, formerly used by me in the closure of the hard palate in young children, are now seldom employed."

Arbuthnot Lane's operation.—As the method now to be described aims at the closure of the cleft by large flaps composed of muco-periosteum in the case of the hard palate, and mucous membrane and submucous tissue in the case of the soft palate, it is essential that it be performed before the milk teeth erupt, or the size of the flaps will be seriously curtailed.   Though Lane advises the performance of the operation within a few days of birth, I have found by experience that from six weeks to three months is the most suitable age.   In spite of the apparent severity of the procedure, hæmorrhage is inappreciable in amount and there is little if any shock.   The cosmetic result, even with extensive clefts, is as good as can be desired. There are very few clefts that cannot be closed at one operation, and, what is more important still, the closure is permanent.   There is only one place where gaping is liable to occur, and that is at the junction of the hard and soft palates, but the aperture is usually so small that it can easily be closed a few weeks later by a simple plastic operation.

So excellent is the result of this operation, as far as it concerns the closure of the cleft, that in a series of upwards of forty cases, operated upon between six weeks and five months of age, I am able to record only two real failures, and in both of these the malnutrition of the infant was the predisposing factor.

General principles of the operation.—The following description is quoted from Arbuthnot Lane's article on the Treatment of Cleft Palate in the *Lancet* of January 4th, 1908 :—

" Practically the flap formation employed to close in the hard and soft palates resolves itself into two methods.   If the soft parts overlying the edges of the cleft are thick and vascular, a flap is cut from the mucous membrane, submucous tissue, and periosteum of one side, having its attachment or base along the free margin of the cleft.   The palatine vascular supply (the great or anterior palatine artery) is divided while the flap is being reflected inwards, and it depends for its blood supply on vessels entering its attached margin.   The mucous membrane, submucous tissue, and periosteum are raised from the opposing margin of the cleft by an elevator, an incision being made along the length of the edge of the cleft.   The reflected flap, with its scanty supply of blood derived from small vessels in its attached margin, is then placed beneath the elevated flap, the blood supply of which is ample, and it is fixed in position by a double row of sutures.   In this way two extensive raw surfaces well supplied with blood and uninfluenced by any tension whatever are retained in accurate apposition.   If, on the other hand, the cleft is too broad to admit of its safe and perfect closure in this manner, one flap, comprising all the mucous membrane, submucous tissue, and periosteum on one side, is raised, except at the point of entry of the posterior palatine vessels, while the soft parts on the opposite side are raised in a flap from which the posterior palatine supply has been excluded, and which turns on a base formed by the margin of the cleft.   Here we have a mobile, well-vascularized flap, which can be thrown as a bridge in any direction and can be superimposed on the flap of the opposite side, the closure being necessarily rendered complete by flaps from the edges of a hare-lip. . . .   As time goes on, the damage done to the temporary teeth by the separation of the superjacent mucous membrane becomes steadily greater. Still, this is a matter of no moment as compared with the importance of the early closure of the cleft, since the milk teeth are often unsatisfactory in cases of cleft palate, apart from operative interference, while the permanent teeth escape damage from it if undertaken sufficiently early in life."

The application of these methods will now be described briefly ; for further details the reader must consult the original paper.

Fig. 322 represents the roof of an infant's mouth with *a broad cleft of nearly the whole palate*, in which the nasal septum occupies a median position. The incision A B commences at the anterior limit of the cleft, and runs forwards and outwards across the alveolus to its outer surface. From its termination, the incision B C D is made to pass along the outer side of the alveolus, and then through the mucous membrane of the soft palate, to terminate at the anterior pillar of the fauces. From this point, D, a third incision is made along the posterior free border of the soft palate as far as the tip of the uvula, E. The flap A B C D E thus outlined is dissected up, and when reflected will hinge upon the margin of the cleft, A E. The anterior half, A B C, of this flap consists of muco-periosteum. When cutting it, care must be taken not to allow the portion reflected from the alveolus to be too thick. The posterior half, C D E, should consist of mucous membrane and submucous tissue only, and should leave the muscles of the soft palate exposed, but uninjured. The reader will now readily perceive the advantage that accrues from performing this operation before the teeth erupt, for the incision B C can then be made on the *outer* side of the alveolus, and thereby the width of the flap increased by a quarter to half an inch.

On the opposite side of the cleft, an incision, A Z, is carried forwards and outwards to terminate on the alveolus, as in the diagram, or beyond it if necessary. A second incision, A F, is then made along the margin of the cleft, and the muco-periosteum between Z, A, and F is raised from the bone. During this procedure due care must be taken to avoid injuring the anterior palatine artery. The point of the uvula, H, is now seized with toothed forceps and pulled towards the operator, so as to expose the upper or *nasal* surface of the soft palate. Along this nasal surface of the soft palate an incision is carried (through the mucous membrane and submucous tissue only) from F, the point at which the incision along the margin of the cleft terminated, to G, just below the posterior pillar of the fauces. The free edge of the soft palate is then incised from G to H, as on the opposite side. The flap F G H, thus marked out, is dissected up with a short-bladed scalpel, and reflected inwards so as to hinge upon its attached margin, F H, at the border of the cleft. The last step consists in freeing the nasal surface of the soft palate from the posterior margin of the hard

palate from F to K. All that now remains is to take the large flap
A B C D E, turn it inwards, tuck it under the raised muco-periosteum
Z A F in front, and cover it behind with the flap F G H, as in Fig. 323.

Sutures are then inserted, as shown in Fig. 323, first along the line
B C D, uniting the free edge of the reflected flap to the raised flap and
to the raw surface on the nasal aspect of the soft palate ; next, along
the line D H G, uniting the free edges of the soft palate ; and lastly, a
third row, A F G, uniting the reflected flap to the free edge of the raised
flap, A F, and to the edge, F G, of the flap that has been turned inwards

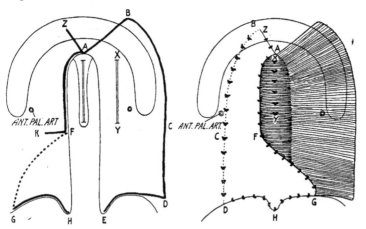

Figs. 322 and 323.—Arbuthnot Lane's operation (*see* text).

from the nasal surface of the soft palate. When the nasal septum
occupies the middle line, as in Fig. 322, the reflected flap may be fixed
to it by an additional row of sutures (A X, Fig. 323), provided that the
mucous membrane is removed from the edge of the septum and from
the surface of the reflected flap along the area of apposition. Though
this row of sutures is not essential, it constitutes a refinement which
gives additional security to, and increases the blood supply of, the
reflected flap.

The remaining diagrams, illustrating the application of these
methods to different varieties of clefts, need but a brief description,
as the principles underlying the operations are the same in every case.

Fig. 324 illustrates *a complete cleft in which the nasal septum is
adherent to the right margin.* The reflected flap should always be
formed from the side of the cleft to which the septum is adherent,
as it obtains an additional supply of blood, from the septal vessels
at its attached border, along the margin of the cleft. If the cleft is

very wide, the raised flap F A Z can be converted into a mobile flap
by continuing the incision from z to y, and bent inwards to cover the
large reflected flap (Fig. 325). In raising this flap the operator
must avoid carrying the dissection too far in a backward direction,
or he will divide the anterior palatine artery, a vessel that must be
preserved.

Figs. 326 and 327 represent the method of closing *a cleft involving the soft palate and a portion of the hard palate.* The flap

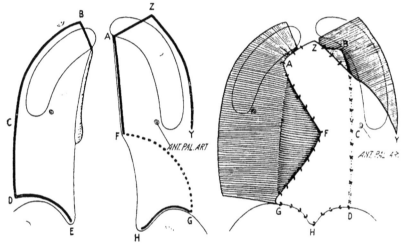

Figs. 324 and 325.—These and the six following diagrams illustrate the
application of Arbuthnot Lane's method to different varieties of
cleft (*see* text for each).

A G H is cut from the nasal surface of the soft palate, and is then
reflected inwards and superimposed upon the reflected flap A B C D, as
in Fig. 327.

Fig. 328 depicts a large cleft with a mesial nasal septum. If it be
considered impossible to close this at one operation by the method
already described, it can be closed in two stages by another method.

First stage.—Flaps A B C D and E F G H are outlined and freed,
care being taken to avoid injuring the great palatine arteries. The
flap I J K L, attached at K L, is turned backwards and sutured to the
nasal septum along its line of contact, after the mucous membrane
on both flap and septum has been removed along this line. The two
large lateral flaps are then pivoted inwards and their anterior extremities are sutured together as in Fig. 329.

Second stage.—This is deferred until the raw surface left after

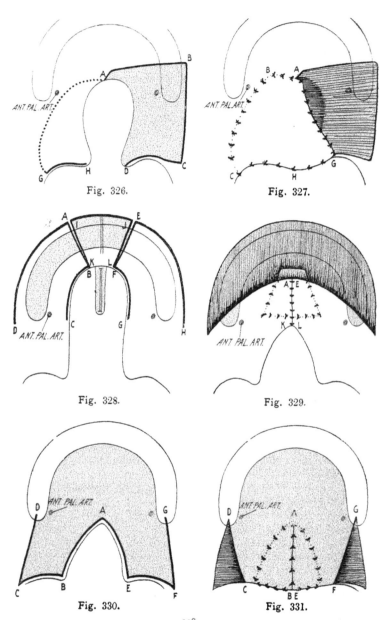

Fig. 326.

Fig. 327.

Fig. 328.

Fig. 329.

Fig. 330.

Fig. 331.

the first operation has completely healed. Flaps A B C D and A E F G (Fig. 330), composed of mucous membrane and submucous tissue only, are raised, displaced inwards, and sutured to each other along their inner margins. A row of sutures is also placed between the flap on each side and the subjacent edge of the cleft, indicated by the dotted line in Fig. 331.

Although a considerable area of raw surface is exposed after any of the foregoing operations, it is surprising how rapidly it becomes covered by mucous membrane and how slight is the scarring. Sloughing of the flaps seldom occurs, and union becomes quite firm in about five days.

The **late operation** should be performed at about the third year. In several instances, where the cleft has been narrow, I have obtained good results in cases ranging between fifteen months and two years of age, but in the majority it is seldom wise to attempt the operation before the child is at least two and a half years old.

Advantages :—

1. The cleft narrows as age advances.
2. The tissues are thicker and less friable than in the young infant.
3. There is less danger of postoperative pneumonia.
4. The co-operation of the child may be invoked during the healing process, so that it refrains from crying or talking, and from pressing its tongue against the palate.
5. If the operation is successful the appearance of the palate and the mobility of the soft palate are unsurpassable.

Disadvantages :—

1. Coincidently with the appearance of the teeth, the bacteria and the putrefactive organisms that normally inhabit the mouth increase in number and variety.
2. In consequence, the danger of sloughing is very great.
3. The amount of tissue available for union depends upon the thickness of the flap alone.
4. If there is the least tension the coaptation sutures commence to tear out very shortly after the operation.
5. Owing to these drawbacks the percentage of failures is greater than the percentage of successes.

The operation (Langenbeck's).—The uvula being seized with toothed forceps, both edges of the cleft are carefully and thoroughly pared. Two lateral incisions (Fig. 332) are then made midway between the alveolus and the margins of the cleft ; they should commence in front of its anterior limit, and extend backwards as far as is necessary to relieve tension when the two halves of the soft palate are approximated. The mucous membrane of the hard palate, between the lateral incision and the edge of the cleft on each side, is then thoroughly separated with a curved elevator. One blade of a pair of rectangular

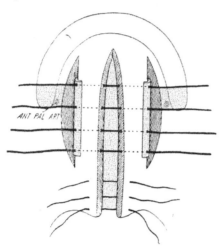

scissors is now introduced between the muco-periosteum and the bone, and pushed gently backwards until the posterior border of the hard palate is reached. The scissors are then rotated until the other blade lies in the naso-pharynx above the soft palate, which is divided at its attachment to the hard palate (Fig. 333). When this step is completed, should the two halves of the soft palate fail to meet, the lateral relieving incisions must be extended backwards. Sutures of silver wire, fine salmon-gut, or silk are then inserted from behind

Fig. 332.—Langenbeck's operation : Flaps transfixed by silver wires held in position by aluminium plates.

forwards, and the suture line and raw lateral surfaces are given a coating of Whitehead's varnish.

To relieve tension after the sutures have been tied, some surgeons pack the lateral incisions with gauze in order to push the flaps inwards; but, owing to the decomposition of the exudate absorbed by the gauze, this is not a satisfactory method. C. H. Mayo ties the flaps together with a piece of tape, which is then rotated so that the knot projects into the nasal cavity. Of late I have transfixed the flaps with two or four strands of fine silver wire,

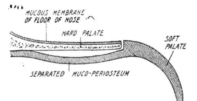

Fig. 333.—Langenbeck's operation : The soft palate and the muco-periosteum of the hard palate have been completely separated from the bone.

and fastened the ends over an aluminium plate which is bent over their lateral edges (Fig. 332). The advantages of this method, apart from the relief of tension, are the support given to the flaps by the wire and the accurate apposition of their approximated edges.

After-treatment.—The mouth should be sprayed daily with a mild antiseptic and alkaline lotion, but no attempt should be made to inspect the wound lest the child struggle and cry. Liquid nourishment in small quantities at a time should be given with a spoon for the first week, after which the amount may be increased. A baby must be nursed and soothed to prevent it from crying, and an older child must be forbidden to talk. The stitches should not be removed until the tenth day, and during the process it is always advisable to make the child drowsy with an anæsthetic. No matter how perfect the cosmetic result, no operation for cleft palate can be called successful unless the speech be improved. Consequently it behoves the surgeon to urge the necessity of lessons in elocution by a competent teacher as soon as possible, for without such lessons many patients will be unintelligible and few will articulate clearly. In some the result of careful training is so excellent that the ordinary observer would not suspect the presence of a congenital defect. It is always advisable to see the patient some three months after the operation ; if then the soft palate appears unduly tense, increased flexibility and a corresponding improvement in the speech will be obtained by teaching the mother or the nurse to massage and exert pressure upon it with the finger.

BIBLIOGRAPHY

Brophy, *Proceedings Third International Dental Congress*, Paris, 1900.
Keith, Arthur, "On Congenital Malformations of the Palate, Face, and Neck," *Brit. Med. Journ.*, 1909, ii. 312.
Lane, W. Arbuthnot, "The Modern Treatment of Cleft Palate," *Lancet*, Jan. 4, 1908.
Owen, Edmund, *Cleft Palate and Hare-Lip*. London, 1904.

THE TONGUE

By W. H. CLAYTON-GREENE, B.A., M.B., B.C.Cantab., F.R.C.S.Eng.

Development.—The tongue is developed from two separate elements in the floor of the primitive pharynx. The *buccal* or anterior portion arises during the third week (Keith) from the 1st branchial bar and interbranchial space, by the development of the tuberculum impar (Fig. 334), a median elevation. It was at one time held, as the name suggests, that there was a single unpaired

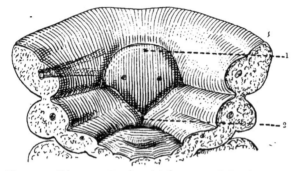

Fig. 334.—Diagram showing development of the tongue.
1, Tuberculum impar ; 2, posterior portion of tongue, developed from 2nd and 3rd arches.

element entering into the formation of this part, but it has been shown that right and left elevations arise and fuse to form the tubercle. This early evidence of bilateral origin more clearly explains the rare conditions of bifid tongue and median cysts sometimes found.

This portion, developed from the mandibular arch, is innervated by the special nerve of this part, the 5th, while the chorda tympani, a sensory nerve to the 1st branchial cleft, also supplies it.

The *pharyngeal* portion is developed from the fused ends of the 2nd and 3rd arches (Fig. 334). The glosso-pharyngeal—the nerve of the 3rd arch—supplies this part.

Between the anterior and posterior portions there is found at one period a well-marked **V**-shaped groove, which ultimately is occupied by some of the circumvallate papillæ. Farther from the hypoblastic covering in the middle line a downgrowth of epithelium takes place which forms the median tubular portion of the thyroid gland, and which normally is responsible for the production of the small median depression at the apex of the **V**, called the foramen cæcum (Fig. 334*a*). Under normal conditions this duct or canal, the thyro-glossal duct, should disappear, but it may persist, and cysts may arise in

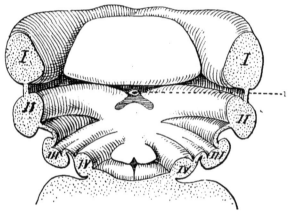

Fig. 334*a*.—A more advanced stage of development of the tongue.

1, Foramen cæcum.

any part of its course. Such cysts, thyro-glossal in origin, are sometimes met with in the substance of the tongue.

The muscles of the tongue arise in a curious way from the three posterior head segments. They grow forward into the fundament of the tongue, carrying with them their appropriate nerve, the 12th cranial or hypoglossal.

General anatomy of the tongue.—The *body* of the tongue is composed of striated muscle, of which the genio-hyo-glossus and the hyo-glossus are the largest extrinsic muscles.

The *dorsum* is covered with a peculiar mucous membrane, and is divisible into two areas which correspond closely with the two portions developed respectively from the tuberculum impar—the lingual portion; and that which arises from the 2nd and 3rd arches, the pharyngeal part—these two portions being separated by the **V**-shaped groove mentioned above, along which lie the circumvallate papillæ.

The anterior or lingual portion is covered with mucous membrane beset with filiform and fungiform papillæ, the former being delicate papillomatous processes of connective tissue covered with epithelium. When this epithelium proliferates and desquamates in excess, and especially when bacteria and food particles collect in the spaces between the papillæ, the condition described as "furred tongue" arises. In the middle line a slight fissure may be seen, which in some pathological conditions becomes peculiarly exaggerated.

The posterior or pharyngeal portion is beset with small nodular masses, each surrounding a central pit, visible to the naked eye. These nodules are masses of lymphoid tissue, and in the aggregate are termed the lingual tonsil.

The circumvallate papillæ, which are placed at the junction of the two parts, are actively concerned in the sense of taste ; they are curious flat-topped elevations surrounded by a trench in which the taste-buds are embedded. The V-shaped groove along which these papillæ lie is termed the sulcus terminalis, and at its apex the foramen cæcum may be occasionally found. At its extreme posterior part the dorsum linguæ is attached by a median fold to the epiglottis, the glosso-epiglottidean fold, while laterally it is connected to the pharynx by the pharyngo-epiglottidean folds, which together with the glosso-epiglottidean folds form the boundaries of the two lateral depressions, the valleculæ.

The *inferior surface* is free from papillæ, but shows a median band, the frænum linguæ, connecting the mucous membrane of the tongue with that of the floor of the mouth ; and close to the latter, on either side of the frænum, the openings of Wharton's duct, the duct of the submaxillary gland, can be seen.

On either side of the frænum the large ranine veins are clearly visible, while placed still farther laterally are the plicæ fimbriatæ—folds which correspond to the under-tongue of the lemurs, and which mark fairly accurately the course of the ranine arteries.

The *lateral margins* possess papillæ similar to those found on the anterior part of the dorsum, while just in front of the anterior palatine fold—a band which descends to the tongue in front of the tonsil and contains the fibres of the palato-glossus—a number of vertical ridges are situated, the folia linguæ, which are studded with taste-buds and represent the papillæ foliatæ of the rabbit.

The **muscular mass** of the tongue is divisible into two main groups, the extrinsic muscles, which reach the tongue from surrounding bones and structures, and the intrinsic or linguales, which are confined to its substance. Except the palato-glossus, which probably derives its nerve supply from the spinal accessory by means of the **pharyn**geal plexus, the muscles are supplied by the hypoglossal nerve.

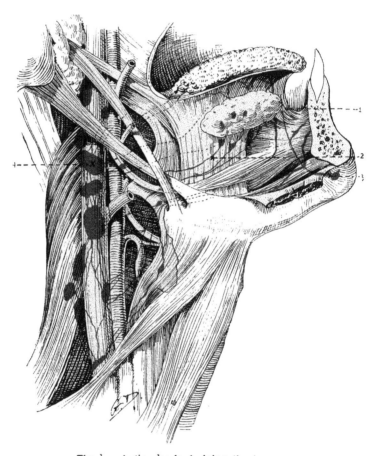

The lymphatic glands draining the tongue.

1, Submaxillary gland and its lymph-nodes. 2, Gland on hyo-glossus. 3, Submental group.
4, Deep cervical chain.

PLATE 86.

Glands of the tongue.—There are a number of small racemose glands situated in the posterior part of the tongue, and a few are found in relation to the circumvallate papillæ.

The most important, however, are the apical glands of Blandin and Nuhn, which are situated on the inferior surface, a little distance from the apex.

They are mixed serous and mucous glands, and they open by means of three or four small ducts on either side of the upper attachment of the frænum.

Arteries.—The main artery of the tongue is the lingual, a branch of the external carotid, which reaches the organ by passing under cover of the hyo-glossus muscle, its terminal branches being the sublingual, to the sublingual gland, and the ranine, peculiar to the tongue. There is no free anastomosis between the vessels of the two sides. The posterior portion is supplied by the dorsalis linguæ branch of the lingual, reinforced by the tonsillar branch of the facial.

Veins.—The veins do not follow closely the course of the arteries. There are two venæ comites which run with the lingual artery beneath the hyo-glossus, but they are small, the greater part of the blood being conveyed back by the ranine veins, two large vessels situated one on either side of the frænum, immediately beneath the mucous membrane. These veins pass backwards over the hyo-glossus and usually join with the venæ comites to form a common trunk which receives the dorsalis linguæ vein before joining the internal jugular.

Nerves.—The anterior two-thirds of the mucous membrane is supplied by the lingual branch of the inferior maxillary division of the 5th nerve, accompanied by the chorda tympani, which may convey special taste-fibres to the former, but more probably is concerned with supplying the lateral margin of the tongue. The posterior third is supplied by the glosso-pharyngeal, which is generally considered the special nerve of taste. A few fibres are also derived from the superior pharyngeal branch of the vagus. The nerve supply of the muscles has been described.

Lymphatics (Plate 86).—In modern surgery the course of the lymphatic vessels, influencing as it does the spread of malignant disease, is of the utmost importance.

In the tongue itself there are two main sets of lymph-channels, the rich submucous network, and the scantier intramuscular vessels; in the case of the former, it is to be noted that there is communication between the lymph-vessels of the two sides across the middle line. From these vessels the lymph passes to the glands, the muscular lymphatics uniting early with the submucous; and it is possible to define four distinct sets for the purposes of description, as follows:—

1. The *apical set* pass from the submucous network on to the genio-hyo-glossus; some of the vessels pierce the genio-hyoid and terminate in the submental glands and the inferior cervical glands. This latter fact is of supreme importance, since in malignant disease of the tip of the tongue both the submental and submaxillary regions may escape, the infection being carried directly to the glands which lie along the internal jugular vein at the point where it is crossed by the omo-hyoid muscle.

2. The *lateral set* descend from the sides of the tongue and terminate mainly in the submaxillary lymph-glands; these are situated not only in relation to the submaxillary salivary gland, but are actually embedded in its substance—a condition which necessitates removal of the gland in malignant disease. A few lymphatic channels pass directly to the superior deep cervical glands. The lymph from the submaxillary region passes into these cervical glands, one of which, situated at the level of the bifurcation of the carotid, is especially important, and is often described as the principal gland of the tongue.

3. The *basal set* arise in the submucous tissue and lymphoid follicles of the posterior part and pass deeply to the superior deep cervical glands.

4. The *median set* arise from the submucous network in the middle line in front of the circumvallate papillæ. The vessels pass deeply between the genio-hyo-glossi, and finally, after piercing this muscle and the hyo-glossus, end in the submaxillary glands.

A point of special importance is to be noted in connexion with this median set, namely, that according to Piersol they may pass to either side of the middle line, thus accounting for infection of the glands of the neck on the side opposite to that upon which a cancerous ulcer is found.

The lymphatics from the floor of the mouth have a termination similar to the termination of those of the tongue.

Occasional glands will be found embedded in the substance of the hyo-glossus.

Methods of examination of the tongue.—In examining the tongue for the many surgical diseases which attack it, both inspection and palpation are necessary. In the case of the former a good light is essential, and the patient should preferably be sitting opposite to the surgeon. If daylight should not be available, or if swelling of the tongue should impair the view, a laryngeal mirror will afford great assistance, especially in cases of deep hæmorrhage, or, better still, a small portable lamp which can be sterilized may be introduced directly into the mouth; an old cystoscope acts admirably.

A metal or glass tongue-depressor should be at hand, and lip-retractors are required in a difficult case.

If the tongue be foul and covered with fur or adherent sloughs, these should be gently wiped away with cotton-wool swabs steeped in weak carbolic acid (1–60), or the surface of the tongue can be dried by pressing a strip of white blotting-paper over it—a proceeding which brings out more clearly some of the pathological conditions met with.

Palpation is of special value in detecting the characteristic induration of malignant disease, the nodular hardness of a primary chancre, and the local tenderness of an abscess; it is advisable to protect the finger with a glove or finger-stall.

Histological and bacteriological examination supplement the former procedures. These methods are specially required in the case of doubtful ulcers, of which a piece—not too small—should be removed and examined microscopically. If too small a piece is removed the examination will be very unsatisfactory, and an effort should be made to obtain some of the adjacent apparently healthy tissue, since this will show in a more convincing manner the spread of any malignant epithelial cells.

Bacteriological investigation is required in some of the parasitic diseases, diphtheria and thrush, and abscess.

Stress must be laid on the following points :—

1. It is not easy to obtain fluctuation in many cases of abscess.

2. The ulceration which occurs around a calculus impacted in Wharton's duct is easily mistaken for malignant ulceration.

3. Inflammatory conditions in the submaxillary gland may be confused with acute glossitis.

4. When an ulcer is acutely tender it should be painted with some 1 per cent. cocaine solution before palpation is practised.

MALFORMATIONS

ABSENCE OF THE TONGUE]

Several cases of so-called absence of the tongue have been recorded, but in each instance the case seems to have been one of suppressed development of the tuberculum impar rather than actual absence of the organ. In such cases the anterior portion of the organ is small and rudimentary, and is moreover firmly fixed to the floor of the mouth, rendering free movement impossible. The base is always present and apparently normal. In a case seen by me the above condition was associated with arrested development of the lower jaw, the whole bone being small and underhung. As in other recorded cases of the deformity, the speech was intelligible.

BIFID TONGUE

This very rare condition arises from the incomplete fusion of the two parts which form the tuberculum impar, and represents a developmental error occurring at a very early date, the form being comparable to the forked tongue of the reptilia. The malformation may be associated with hare-lip or cleft palate.

Treatment is comparatively simple in those cases that require it. The edges of the cleft are pared, and the raw surfaces united with sutures.

ANKYLOGLOSSIA

Abnormal fixation of the tongue occurs as either a congenital or an acquired deformity. The congenital variety, when not associated with a rudimentary condition of the organ, results from intra-uterine inflammatory changes, or from imperfect destruction of embryonic structures such as the pharyngeal membrane, or possibly as the result of imperfect innervation and movement. The amount of control of the frænum upon the tongue being largely influenced by movement of the organ, as shown by the fact that some cases of acquired tongue-swallowing are due to stretching of this anchoring band, it is possible that, as in the case of joints, some interference with the normal range of movement that should obtain during embryonic life is responsible for the short and adherent frænum.

Cases such as the one described by Lapie, where there were large adhesions between the tongue and the palate—a form described by French writers as superior ankyloglossia—suggest either some inflammatory source for the adhesions, or the persistence of some membrane ; while in the more common variety—the inferior ankyloglossia, which is the more complete when the tongue is very rudimentary—it would seem probable that lack of motive power is an important factor in producing this result.

In this inferior form we can recognize two varieties—the complete, which is properly considered above under the heading of congenital absence, and the more common partial form. In point of fact, partial ankyloglossia is uncommon, as insisted on by Butlin, who deprecates the number of unnecessary operations often performed for a condition which will tend to rectify itself. The routine section of the frænum is to be unhesitatingly condemned. Children of rather weak mental development, who learn to speak late, are often subjected to the operation of "cutting the tongue-tie," in the hope that it will help the development of speech. This idea is entirely erroneous, since, given the requisite mental power, speech is quite possible in the most severe forms of ankyloglossia.

Should, however, a case present itself in which the frænum is obviously too short, and especially if the child's feeding is interfered with, the operation becomes necessary.

Treatment.—The tongue is raised with the index and middle fingers of the left hand, the frænal band is rendered tense, and is nicked with a pair of scissors close to the jaw, so as to avoid injuring the ranine vessels. The wound must not be enlarged by tearing up the tongue with the finger. If the child is put to the breast or given a teat to suck, the movement of the tongue thus induced will help to prevent recurrence.

This operation is by no means free from danger. A case of fatal hæmorrhage is quoted by Reboul, while macroglossia developed in cases recorded by Burton, Sédillot, and Dollinger. If the tongue is carelessly stripped up after the band has been divided, an ugly wound is left which may form a troublesome ulcer, or cause so much cicatrization that the tongue becomes more fixed than it was at first. For serious hæmorrhage following division of the frænum a suture should be passed through the tip of the tongue, a strip of gauze dusted with iodoform should be gently packed into the sublingual region on to the bleeding area, and the tongue then pulled out by the suture, which in turn is fixed by a bandage or piece of strapping to the chin; thus the bleeding area is fairly firmly compressed. If this method fails to arrest the bleeding, an anæsthetic must be given and an attempt made to secure the bleeding-point; it will be found more satisfactory to under-run the vessel with a curved needle threaded with catgut than to attempt to seize it with forceps in the friable tissues of a young child. The cautery must not be used.

ACQUIRED ANKYLOGLOSSIA

This condition is the result of extensive destruction of the organ following sloughing in smallpox, or mercurial or caustic poisoning; occasionally it is due to widespread syphilitic damage, or to operative procedures of various kinds.

TONGUE-SWALLOWING

Excessive mobility of the tongue usually results from extreme length and looseness of the frænum, which therefore fails to control the movements of the organ; the tongue itself is unduly long. Fairbairn records a case of suffocation, and Hennig mentions a case where the child died in a paroxysm of whooping-cough, apparently from sucking the tongue into the pharynx.

A similar but less marked condition sometimes occurs in patients under the influence of anæsthetics, and after removal of portions of the tongue it is one of the complications to be specially treated.

If the child be seen in a state of suffocation arising from this cause, the finger should be introduced into the mouth and the tongue hooked forward. The condition is likely to recur; but the constant sucking of a teat will help to prevent it.

INJURIES

WOUNDS

Injuries to the tongue, rarely the cause of serious hæmorrhage, are usually penetrating wounds produced by foreign bodies such as pipe-stems and fish-bones, but are specially important in that an abscess of the tongue may follow and the foreign body may be retained in the tongue substance. Many instances are recorded where pipe-stems or teeth have been removed from the tongue some time after an accident, comparatively few symptoms having arisen during the interval.

Occasionally, severe or even fatal hæmorrhage may occur, as in the case published by Bransby Cooper, where the pipe-stem penetrated through the tongue into the carotid artery, and the patient, a sailor, died from bleeding.

The tongue may be severely bitten in the convulsions of epilepsy, eclampsia, or tetanus, or as the result of blows or falls on the chin, and the bleeding may be serious. In ordinary circumstances the tongue is rarely severely bitten during mastication, but if the 5th nerve is paralysed considerable damage may be done.

Treatment.—The chief indications in treatment are—first, to control any hæmorrhage; and second, to make certain that no foreign body is left behind in the muscular substance.

When the tongue is bitten it is usually the anterior part that suffers, a part easily accessible and amenable to simple treatment.

On the other hand, in punctured wounds the lesion may be far back; and if, as Butlin points out, there be free arterial hæmorrhage owing to the fact that the vessels lie deeply, there will be a deep wound in which a foreign body may be hidden, and in which it may be very difficult indeed to secure the bleeding-point.

For the temporary arrest of severe hæmorrhage the manœuvre recommended by Heath should be adopted. The forefinger is passed to the back of the tongue, and the whole organ is hooked forward with the hyoid bone, the lingual arteries being thus put on the stretch.

In the slighter forms, where the hæmorrhage is mainly venous, it will be sufficient to approximate the edges of the wound with catgut or black silk; the stitches should not be tied too tightly, as the tissues swell up considerably, but they must arrest the bleeding.

In severe hæmorrhage an anæsthetic must be given; the mouth should be widely opened, the tongue drawn out by two stitches passed through it near the tip, the wound enlarged if necessary, and a search made for the bleeding-point. This is a difficult matter even when skilled assistance is at hand, and without it the operator is severely handicapped.

It may be wise, owing to the severity of the hæmorrhage, to perform laryngotomy and to plug the pharynx before attempting to deal with the bleeding. I strongly recommend this in a difficult case, as I have invariably practised it before any extensive operation on the mouth or jaws, and am very much impressed with its value.

A good deal of difficulty will be experienced, even under the best conditions, in applying a ligature to the bleeding vessel, as the tongue tissue is friable and readily tears away in the pressure-forceps. If this occurs, it is better at once to under-run the vessel with a silk ligature by means of a curved needle ; even though some of the lingual tissue is included and may slough, the procedure is a satisfactory one. The hæmorrhage having been arrested, search must be made for a foreign body, and the edges of the wound may be drawn together, but it must not be closed completely.

Cases may be met with where the above directions will fail, necessitating ligature of the lingual artery, or even of the external carotid in the neck, but they will be infinitely rare.

In secondary hæmorrhage the same treatment should be carried out, though the sloughing condition of the tissues may make ligation of the vessel a matter of the greatest difficulty, and the operator will do well to under-run it with a silk ligature at once. It will rarely be necessary to tie the main vessels in the neck.

The **after-treatment** of wounds of the tongue consists in promoting oral asepsis with mouth-washes, of which carbolic acid 1-40, hydrogen peroxide 1-4, are the most effective. Fluids only must be taken, and if there is much swelling and pain the patient should be fed per rectum. A careful watch must be kept for œdema of the glottis, a complication necessitating tracheotomy, also for secondary hæmorrhage and for abscess.

Gunshot wounds are to be treated on the same main lines as punctured wounds ; they are very liable to be followed by secondary hæmorrhage and abscess, and therefore should not be closed completely.

Stings of the tongue are to be regarded as poisoned wounds. Generally speaking, the treatment should be similar to that employed for scalds, but there is some danger of onset of œdema of the glottis.

BURNS AND SCALDS

The degree of severity of these injuries varies, here as in other parts of the body, from slight erosion to deep destruction.

Slight burns which result from cigarettes or other causes merely lead to superficial destruction of the papillæ, but are very painful from the exposure of the sensory nerve filaments. Sometimes a slight burn is the starting-point of an ulcer, and in some cases the condition has progressed from one of trivial injury to epithelioma. For this reason Butlin warns against the use of the cautery in simple diseases of the tongue.

In the corrosions produced by strong mineral acids and caustic alkalis the back of the tongue suffers more than the anterior part ; indeed, it is not uncommon for the tongue to escape, the œsophagus and stomach receiving the chief damage. When affected, the mucous covering of the tongue is destroyed and peels off as a superficial slough, and the whole organ swells as in parenchymatous glossitis. Corrosive sublimate produces a characteristic white, shrivelled appearance.

Severe scalds are most usually met with in children who have attempted to drink out of a boiling kettle, the steam rather than the water producing the injury. The effects are often very severe, the tongue becoming enormously swollen and covered with blebs ; in fact, a state of acute glossitis is set up.

In all the above conditions, so long as the trouble remains limited to the tongue there is little need for anxiety, but unfortunately, especially in scalds, owing to the coexistent damage to the epiglottic region and the upper respiratory tract, œdema glottidis and pneumonia may follow.

General treatment.—According to the severity of the burn or scald, solid food must be prohibited, and the patient should be fed on fluids, even rectally in the more serious injuries. Ice may be sucked, and in adults the painful areas may be painted with a 1 per cent. solution of cocaine ; chlorate of potash mouth-washes are of value from the first ; later, when the pain is less, astringent lotions should be substituted.

The blebs which form rarely require treatment.

A careful watch must be kept for signs of œdema of the glottis, as shown by stridor and dyspnœa. In adults scarification may be of value occasionally, but in children it is wiser to perform tracheotomy than to try what is always a difficult operation, even in adults.

INFLAMMATORY DISEASES—ACUTE

Acute inflammatory lingual diseases are here dealt with according to the following scheme :—

1. Superficial. { Local. { Nervous. { Diffuse. { Membranous.
2. Deep.
3. Unilateral.
4. Inflammation of the lingual tonsil.
5. Abscess.
6. Gangrene.

1. ACUTE SUPERFICIAL GLOSSITIS

Is seen to follow most burns or injuries of the tongue of slight extent, and tends in these cases to be local or patchy, readily yielding to mild remedies such as mouth-washes or emollient applications of borax, borax and honey, or Listerine.

The diffuse form occurs in two main types, the nervous and the membranous.

The nervous variety, which is often unilateral, is associated with trigeminal neuralgia or, in some cases, with facial paralysis. There is an outbreak of vesicles on the tongue, which becomes red and tender. The associated nervous affections justify us in regarding the condition as related to herpes zoster. There is no special treatment ; sedative mouth-washes, tonics, and antipyrin or phenacetin should be tried.

Membranous glossitis may occur as part of a generalized diphtheria, the disease then not being confined to the tongue. The tongue and the submaxillary lymphatic glands are swollen. Wharton published a case of primary diphtheria of the tongue—a very rare condition.

Pseudo-diphtheria.—True diphtheria can only be diagnosed if the typical Klebs-Löffler bacillus be found, other forms being classed under the heading of pseudo-diphtheria. Membranous glossitis is occasionally met with in children who are suffering from measles and who are the subjects of impetigo and eczema. The membrane contains desquamated epithelium and streptococci or staphylococci.

Hutchinson has described under the name *pellicular glossitis* a more chronic form which occurs in smokers.

Treatment of acute superficial glossitis is simple. A purge is given and the patient is put upon a liberal though fluid diet. Ice may be sucked if there is much pain, and 10-15 grains of chlorate of potash should be administered to an adult until a drachm has been taken. This drug, given internally, is of very great value in the inflammatory or ulcerated conditions of the tongue and mouth, but must be given with caution, especially in children, as it is liable to produce hæmaturia. Weak solutions of cocaine may be applied occasionally for pain, or a mouth-wash of Listerine used as an alternative. When the acute stage subsides, astringent lotions—alum, 10 gr. to the ounce, or zinc sulphate, 2 gr. to the ounce—should be substituted. Occasionally a solution of bicarbonate of soda, 30 gr. to the drachm, will be found more serviceable than the other lotions.

In the membranous forms the tongue should be swabbed with 1-1,000 perchloride of mercury, and, if the Klebs-Löffler bacillus is isolated, antitoxin should be given.

2. DEEP OR PARENCHYMATOUS GLOSSITIS

This is a comparatively rare condition and affects adults, males rather than females. The disease comes on with pain and stiffness in the tongue, the pain often being referred to the neck and ear; the tongue swells progressively until in extreme cases it cannot be retained in the mouth, but is protruded, indented and cut by the teeth which have pressed into it. The swelling is hard and tender. The dorsum of the tongue is covered with a thick white fur and there is profuse salivation, the glands in the neck are swollen and tender, and the temperature and general condition are indicative of an acute septic intoxication.

Etiology.—This affection is said to be more common in cold and damp weather. Over-indulgence in alcohol appears to have a predisposing influence, but the most important factor is undoubtedly a septic state of the mouth and teeth. Of the many organisms which normally inhabit the mouth, the staphylococci and the streptococci seem to be the most important agents in exciting the condition.

The staphylococcal form is the less acute and tends to be more localized. The streptococcal variety, on the other hand, is associated with extreme swelling of the tongue, which may pass back to the aryteno-epiglottidean folds, and of the glands in the neck. Sabrazès and Bousquet quote a fatal case secondary to puerperal fever, and Syme records two cases that occurred in workmen engaged in cleaning out a sewer. Mercurial glossitis will be considered later.

Course.—The disease runs on to resolution in the milder forms, but some permanent thickening and stiffness may be left for months after the acute process has subsided. In other cases, suppuration follows, a deep abscess being formed, which is not easily detected. Occasionally, sloughing and even gangrene may occur, and the tongue may be extensively destroyed and become fixed to the floor of the mouth.

The risk of œdema of the glottis and of septic pneumonia is very great in the streptococcal variety.

After the acute stage has subsided, some permanent thickening of the tongue substance may be left—one variety of the "*glossites profondes chroniques*" of the French, a condition easily mistaken for one of the manifestations of syphilis.

Treatment must be active from the start. It should begin with a calomel purge; hot mouth-washes of 1–60 carbolic acid should be prescribed, and leeches applied to the submaxillary region. If the swelling be great, as in the streptococcal type, free incisions should be made into the dorsum of the tongue two-thirds of an inch on either side of the middle line, and one-third of an inch deep (Butlin).

They should be made freely with a curved bistoury. The relief is almost immediate, and severe bleeding is rare.

Modern treatment naturally suggests the use of vaccines, especially in the streptococcal infections.

The diet in parenchymatous glossitis should be the same as in the superficial form (p. 173).

MERCURIAL GLOSSITIS

This affection is still occasionally seen, though much more rarely than formerly. It is distinguished from the preceding by the history, by the general *œdematous* state of the tongue, which is softer than in true parenchymatous glossitis, and by the accompanying affection of the gums, which are tender, swollen, and vascular. The fetor is very great, and the salivation even more profuse. There is considerable tendency to sloughing.

Treatment consists in stopping all mercury, giving 2 drachms of sulphate of magnesia at once, and 10–15 gr. of chlorate of potash every four hours up to a drachm. Leeches may be applied to the submaxillary region, and ice should be sucked. Incision may be, but rarely is, required. When the acute symptoms disappear, salvarsan is of value, and tonics are demanded. On no account should iodide of.potash be given.

It must be borne in mind that small doses of mercury may produce this condition in susceptible subjects. Cases are recorded of acute inflammation of the tongue having followed the repeated administration of blue pill or calomel for purposes other than the treatment of syphilis.

3. UNILATERAL INFLAMMATION

A unilateral condition, hemiglossitis, is described but is very rare. It is never very acute, and should be treated.on the same main lines as the above ; incisions are not required.

A form of *indurative glossitis*, rather chronic in nature, is sometimes caused by the impaction of a salivary calculus in Wharton's duct. .

4. INFLAMMATION OF THE LINGUAL TONSIL

This condition results from an infection of the lymphoid follicles which, collected together at the base of the tongue, form the mass described as the lingual tonsil. In some cases there is a general infection of the throat and base of the tongue, the faucial tonsils being the parts chiefly. affected, in others the process seems confined to the lingual base. The trouble is common in the dry days of summer, especially in towns, and is probably due to irritation set up by inhaled bacteria and particles of horse-dung. Anæmia and constant use of the voice seem to be predisposing causes.

The **symptoms** are practically those of a quinsy; there is special pain on swallowing, together with an unpleasant feeling of suffocation, and, from the situation of the inflammatory process, there is considerable risk of laryngeal obstruction. On examination with the laryngeal mirror the base of the tongue is seen to be swollen and congested.

In many cases the acute symptoms subside, leaving, however, a mass of swollen lymphoid tissue, the crypts of which are often distended with inspissated secretion; in others an abscess forms, which is not always confined to a follicle (follicular abscess), but may burrow into the tongue substance and form a purulent collection of considerable size.

Treatment.—In the milder forms a mercurial purge, and mouth-washes of chlorate of potash, followed by 10-gr. doses of salicylate of quinine every four hours, will effect a cure. In the more severe cases, if an abscess forms, it must be opened carefully with a curved knife, the patient sitting with the head hanging down so that the risk of the pus finding its way into the larynx is avoided.

At a later date, if concretions form in the epithelial crypts, they should be removed, and the walls of the crypt and follicle destroyed by the cautery; or if there is general hypertrophy of the whole lymphoid mass it may be removed by a special tonsillotome.

5. ABSCESS

A lingual abscess may be acute or chronic, and owe its origin to a number of different causes. It may follow wounds of the tongue, especially those in which a foreign body becomes included in the lingual substance; it may be due to infection from carious teeth, without any very obvious breach in the integrity of the mucous membrane; or it may result from the acute infections previously described under the head of Glossitis.

Acute abscess is characterized by a gradual onset, accompanied by pain in the tongue and often also in the ear. On examination, a tender swelling can be felt in the substance of the tongue, but fluctuation can seldom if ever be detected.

Chronic abscess is much rarer than the acute, and is due to organisms of low virulence which do not excite a violent inflammatory reaction; it is not necessarily tuberculous, but it may follow the secondary infection of a tubercular or gummatous area. The development is very slow and is unaccompanied by any marked pain, and the condition is very likely to be mistaken for a gumma.

Treatment consists in incision, care being taken that the pus has free exit from the mouth. Attention should be given to any exciting cause, and mouth-washes should be employed.

6. GANGRENE OF THE TONGUE

Is a rare complication. It has followed an acute glossitis, the inflammatory reaction having been so severe that thrombosis has ensued. Syphilis has been responsible for its production in several instances, possibly favoured by the injudicious administration of mercury.

Cancrum oris may spread to the tongue, and lead to considerable destruction of the tissues. In one case seen by me, after ligature of both lingual arteries, one half of the tongue then being excised for cancer, the remaining half became gangrenous.

Treatment.—The general treatment consists in keeping the mouth as clean as possible, and assisting the separation of the dead material. Frequent washing of the mouth with carbolic or permanganate lotions should be enjoined, while occasional applications of chlorate of potash or iodoform powder are of great service. The former is somewhat painful, and the latter must be very sparingly used, and care should be taken that the patient does not swallow the drug.

INFLAMMATORY DISEASES—CHRONIC

In considering the following affections of the tongue we are justified in grouping them under the above heading, since the pathological findings support their inflammatory origin, and they may, therefore, fittingly be described as the varying expressions and results of a chronic superficial glossitis.

In the following descriptions Butlin's classification is adopted :—
1. Erythema migrans.
2. Dyspeptic tongue.
3. Furrows and wrinkles.
4. Glossodynia exfoliativa.
5. Herpes.
6. Leucoplakia.
7. Black tongue.

1. ERYTHEMA MIGRANS

Synonyms. — Wandering rash ; geographical tongue ; superficial excoriation (Müller).

Erythema migrans is a rare affection and appears to be almost entirely confined to the earlier years of childhood, occurring in children of impaired general health and nutrition who are nervous and often subject to skin eruptions. It has no special sex predilection.

m

Small circular or oval patches appear on the dorsum of the tongue, always in front of the sulcus terminalis. At first the size of a pea, these patches gradually enlarge, forming smooth red areas from which the filiform papillæ have been shed, the fungiform occasionally standing out the more prominently in consequence. The margin of these patches is distinctly redder than the centre, is sharply defined and limited by a whitish or yellowish border, a very characteristic feature. The patches are usually multiple, and may extend from the dorsum of the tongue on to its under-surface, the result being that the organ has the appearance of being cut up into irregular areas not unlike those present on a map—hence the term " geographical tongue."

The affection is exceedingly chronic, and does not respond to treatment. According to Parrot, each patch or ring has a life-history of seven days, spreading to the periphery and gradually disappearing, after which a fresh one makes its appearance. Nothing definite is known of its etiology. Parasites, syphilitic and other, have been the causes accredited by many writers, but there is no evidence to warrant these assumptions. It is essentially an inflammatory condition; according to Vanlair and Johnstone, a primary affection of the derma, " a subacute papillitis," possibly in some obscure way under the influence of nervous irritation or change. Few symptoms are complained of; indeed, in many cases the condition is discovered during the routine examination of the child; but in some instances there have been salivation and itching. Vanlair found the affected areas were hyperæsthetic.

Diagnosis.—Erythema migrans must be distinguished from mucous tubercles by the greater elevation of the latter, by their general grey appearance, and by the presence of other well-marked signs of syphilis elsewhere.

Treatment has no marked effect. Attempts should be made to improve the general health of the child with tonics and cod-liver oil, while slightly astringent mouth-washes of alum and tannin may be ordered. In all cases the teeth should be carefully examined, and treated if necessary.

2. DYSPEPTIC TONGUE

Among dyspeptic subjects, affections of the tongue are extremely common, as is natural, since to some extent the appearance of the tongue may be taken as a reflection of the condition of the gastric and intestinal mucous membranes. A great variety of conditions have been described, but in the present section attention is drawn only to the more important varieties, ulcers being considered later.

The dyspeptic tongue is usually enlarged, its surface smooth, more sensitive and redder than normal; the surface epithelium has been shed, and the sensitive papillæ are exposed.

In some instances the pain complained of is of a severe burning character; in appearance the tongue seems raw, though in actual fact the "raw" areas are covered by a thin layer of epithelium. These areas are very liable to suffer from slight traumatism which would not affect the normal organ, and the patient has recurring attacks of acute soreness and excoriation.

Pathologically the tongue appears to be the seat of a chronic superficial inflammation, though here the response is peculiar when compared with the other varieties of this affection, in that its sensitiveness is increased and the epithelium has no tendency to proliferate.

Gouty subjects are especially liable to this condition.

Treatment.—Suitable measures must be taken to deal with the dyspepsia, or gout if it be present, and the teeth must be carefully attended to, since collections of tartar, sharp edges, or carious stumps will, if allowed to remain, render any treatment abortive.

Mouth-washes of chlorate of potash or other non-irritating antiseptics should be employed, and the tongue should be painted occasionally with chromic acid, 10 gr. to the ounce. If there is much pain a half-per-cent. solution of cocaine may be applied, or a cocaine ointment may be ordered. Carbolic acid (1–80) will sometimes succeed when the other drugs fail.

3. FURROWS

The tongue is sometimes found cut up by a number of deep grooves or furrows. Some, but not all of these, are the result of chronic inflammatory changes, either simple or specific, the grooves resulting from the scarring in the submucosa; the syphilitic varieties will be considered later. In other cases, as, for example, the "fern-leaf pattern" tongue, the inflammatory origin is not so clear, and we are forced to the conclusion that such a condition is only one of the natural varieties of configuration in which the depth of the natural grooves or sulci is exaggerated. The natural grooves are usually longitudinal, the acquired transverse.

When, however, fissures or cracks result from chronic inflammation, they are apt to be a source of anxiety to the patient from the pain they cause, and to the surgeon from their tendency, if remaining unhealed for a long time, to become the seat of cancer.

Treatment.—The mouth must be kept clean with ordinary mouth-washes, and chromic acid applied to the bottom of the fissure by means of a small camel's-hair brush. Ointments are very useful.

4. GLOSSODYNIA EXFOLIATIVA

In this condition violent pain is complained of in the tongue out of all proportion to the local change, which is very similar to that occurring in the preceding variety. It appears to be a neuralgia of the lingual nerves associated with a thinning of the epithelium' which may be compared with the trophic changes occurring in some forms of trigeminal neuralgia. Anæmic women are more subject to it than men.

Treatment.—The application of nitrate of silver or the actual cautery is sometimes of service. Da Costa mentions a case in which the chewing of a piece of tarred rope relieved the pain.

5. HERPES

Attacks the tongue as it does other parts of the body, the resulting eruptions having all the usual features of the herpetic type. There is a formation in the epidermis of multiple vesicles which are surrounded by inflammatory zones. In some cases the vesicular formation proceeds to such an extent that the term *hydroa* has been given to it. The ordinary course of the disease is for the vesicle to rupture, sometimes becoming pustular first, and to leave an ulcer covered with a pellicle which consists chiefly of desquamated epithelium.

Healing usually takes place under appropriate treatment, but occasionally the ulcer persists or even spreads.

The amount of pain attending the eruption varies enormously; in some cases it is violent, comparable to the pain in herpes zoster.

The disease is presumably of nervous origin, with a remarkable tendency to recurrence, this recurrence being favoured in susceptible subjects by excess in the use of tobacco or alcohol, or by exposure to cold. There is no evidence to connect the disease with syphilis, although it is often associated with herpetic eruptions on the penis. Dyspeptic subjects are said to suffer from it. It must not be confused with the pustules of impetigo.

Treatment.—A sharp mercurial purge should be given, and careful dieting and complete abstinence from stimulants must be enjoined. Arsenic may be tried. According to Butlin there are two classes of case—one in which a mouth-wash of carbolic acid, spirits of chloroform, myrrh, and eau-de-Cologne will bring about speedy resolution; another in which an ointment with a basis of lanolin and vaseline, to which are added cocaine and a weak antiseptic such as boric acid, will give the best result.

6. LEUCOPLAKIA

Synonyms.—Leucokeratosis; ichthyosis; psoriasis linguæ; smoker's patch.

We now come to the most common form of chronic superficial

glossitis—a form which, as the above names imply, presents itself in a number of different guises.

Pathology.—As the result of some irritation—and it by no means follows that the irritant is of the same intensity and nature in every case—a chronic inflammation ensues in the mucous membrane of the tongue; the papillæ disappear, a corneous change takes place in the epidermis, and there is a development of scar tissue in the derma. Changes occur chiefly in the Malpighian layer, where the cells become vacuolated and multiplied and loaded with eleidin granules.

It is most important to recognize that the features of a chronic inflammation are present in the true derma—a phase which is rightly regarded as indicating a want of stability, a precancerous stage in fact, together with abnormal and misdirected activity on the part of the epithelial cells of the epidermis. For a time at least matters are more or less equally balanced, and the barrier of dermal tissue keeps the epithelial cells in check, but, weakened by the effects of inflammation and subjected to greater strain by the active changes in the epithelium, the barrier gives way, the epithelial cells, sometimes preceded by a round-celled infiltration, pass beyond their normal limits into the subjacent derma, and a nucleus of cancer is formed.

Etiology.—Smoking, syphilis, and gout are the three conditions mainly accused as being contributory, if not actual causative agents, but, while they may be all or severally responsible for the production of chronic superficial glossitis, it is now generally acknowledged that the disease depends upon some inherent susceptibility or weakness of the superficial tissues of the tongue. Just as some patients are liable to skin eruptions and desquamations, so others are subject to superficial glossal changes, without any of the three causes mentioned above contributing to them in the least degree.

Although syphilis produces a chronic inflammatory change in the superficial layers of the tongue, and in this respect paves the way for the development of a leucoplakial state, it cannot be too firmly insisted on that leucoplakia *per se* is not a syphilitic manifestation.

Smoking, especially if a short hot pipe is used, undoubtedly produces localized areas of inflammation which are known as smoker's patches, and which are classed clinically under the head of leucoplakia. This must be allowed as an important but not the sole cause of the condition. Hartzell has reported a case in a girl of only 11, but it is very rare before the age of 26–30.

Almost any persistent cause of lingual irritation, such as long-continued drinking of crude spirits, or the presence of chronically infected teeth or teeth-sockets, may act as potent etiological agents. Most frequently several causes are at work simultaneously.

Clinical appearance.—The appearance of the organ varies with the stage of the disease and with the response of the tissues. One of the earliest phases, which can be well studied in a smoker's patch, is the development of a smooth, red, slightly raised area on the dorsum of the tongue. In cases where the epithelium has not proliferated to any extent, or where it has been shed, this stage may persist for some time, and involve smaller or larger areas of the dorsum linguæ; to this condition, in which the papillæ have been removed, the term " red glazed tongue " has been applied. In others, and perhaps the majority, the patch slowly becomes covered with a layer of thickened epithelium, which gives it the appearance of having been covered with white paint that has " hardened, dried, and cracked " (Butlin).

The patches may be multiple, or the whole surface may be uniformly affected; the process tends to spread on to the buccal mucous membrane, or it may begin there and spread to the tongue. The thickened epithelium may form a definite plate of a warty nature. Cracks and fissures are apt to appear, and a spreading ulceration which soon becomes malignant is often associated with it.

Symptoms.—There is little pain, hence many patients do not ask for advice until an advanced stage is reached. Occasionally, " hardness and dryness " of the tongue is complained of, while, if fissures and cracks are present, highly seasoned food or hot dishes may cause a sharp smarting, or even severe pain. Taste is not impaired.

Course.—The disease is extremely chronic, and when well advanced a cure is very doubtful. There are recurrent attacks of inflammation, and slowly but surely in a large number of cases the inflammatory stages pass into malignant ulceration.

Drugs have little effect in advanced cases, and antisyphilitic remedies, far from being of benefit, are often actually injurious. When there is a well-marked history of syphilis, or if other stigmata of the disease be present, mercury and iodide may be tried, but they should not be given indiscriminately. Very marked results are obtained by the use of salvarsan.

The prognosis is always unfavourable.

Treatment is mainly directed to removing any source of irritation, such as carious teeth or ill-fitting tooth-plates. Smoking must be prohibited. Tobacco-chewing is especially to be condemned. Spirits, strong wines, highly spiced or hot foods, should not be taken.

Mouth-washes of chlorate of potash, and paints of chromic acid 1-2 gr. to the ounce, salicylic or lactic acid, will be successful only in the early cases. When the tongue is harsh and dry, it should be wiped dry with a clean, soft cloth, and a little ointment (*see* p. 180) rubbed in night and morning. No caustics should be employed;

there is no doubt that their repeated application has led to increase of the inflammation and has precipitated the development of cancer.

Operation (Fig. 335).—Any local thickened plaque or wart should be excised at once, since it is probable that a cancerous

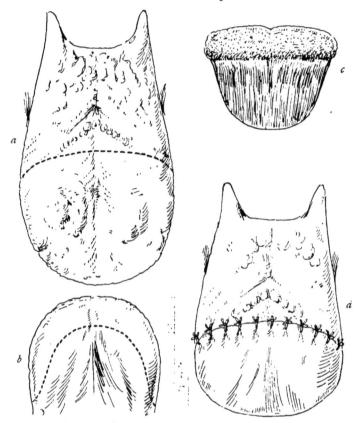

Fig. 335.—Partial removal of tongue for chronic ulceration and fissuring.

An incision across the dorsum and the under-surface of the tongue is made as shown in *a* and *b*, and a ventral flap turned back as in *c*, which shows the end of the stump. This flap is brought over the muscular stump and sutured to the cut mucous membrane on the dorsum, *d*.
(*After Butlin: Burghard's "System of Operative Surgery."*)

change has already begun. Butlin was averse to interference unless definite warty conditions were present, but Morestin has published some cases of excision of large leucoplakial areas with a fair amount of success. He excised the affected areas with scissors, and united the edges with sutures. In any case a very careful watch should be kept, and, if there is the slightest suspicion that cancer has supervened, half or the whole of the organ should be excised.

Radium is not beneficial, as a rule, in cases of leucoplakia. There may be a temporary improvement, but the disease returns worse than before.

7. BLACK OR HAIRY TONGUE (NIGRITIES)

Is a rare condition due to the overgrowth of the filiform papillæ. The affected area is usually found on the dorsum just in front of the circumvallate papillæ. No hairs are present, but the long hypertrophied papillæ give the appearance of wet hair. The colour is apparently due to bacterial action, or to stains from smoke or particles of food. The disease causes no symptoms and is frequently discovered accidentally. A mouth-wash and a salicylic paint should be ordered. Mechanical cleansing by gentle scraping with a curved piece of whalebone or similar instrument is often useful.

ULCERS

Under this heading we consider the various morbid conditions which lead to ulceration of the tongue, and some of the distinguishing features which characterize the individual type. Butlin's valuable classification of the different varieties has been followed, but it would be well to make clear at the outset that a state of ulceration is merely a further stage of the changes considered in the preceding section.

SIMPLE ULCERS

Ulcers of this type usually result from long-standing, neglected chronic superficial glossitis. As has been pointed out previously, there is a gradual transformation of the vascular submucosa into scar tissue, with the inevitable result that the vitality of the part is impaired owing to its imperfect nutrition. The relative avascularity of the fibrosed tissue interferes with the integrity of the surface epithelium, and further has an injurious effect upon the healing of any area that has been damaged ; and, as might be expected, although in many cases a certain amount of improvement may be encouraged by appropriate treatment, there is always an unfortunate tendency for the recently healed ulcer to break down again and again.

Such ulcers are generally situated in the centre of the tongue and are fissured or stellate in shape, with callous edges. Sometimes by a process of actual sloughing they extend laterally and deepen. . The amount of pain they produce varies greatly, and, no doubt, depends upon the depth of the ulcer and also the state of the sensory nerve filaments of the papillæ. Any irritant food sets up a burning pain which lasts for some time, especially if the fissure is a deep one and particles of food become lodged in its depth.

The general lines of **treatment** are the same as for leucoplakia (*see* above), but in addition the floor of the ulcer must be carefully cleansed and local treatment in the shape of chromic acid paint, 5-10 gr. to the ounce, undertaken regularly night and morning. This application is certainly one of the best, for, in addition to its marked healing properties, it allays the pain and irritability of the ulcer. The local treatment must be undertaken with great patience and discrimination if a good result is to accrue, and it is safe to say that no two cases react alike to the applications.

In some patients a weak carbolic lotion, 1-80, will succeed when the chromic acid fails; in others more good will follow the use of a little iodoform powder, tannic acid, or chlorate of potash. Dilute glycerine of tannic acid is of great service in many of the ulcerated conditions of the tongue. Nitrate of silver, except in very dilute solution (1-500), should never be used.

Again, it must be borne in mind that, even when these ulcers and fissures occur in syphilitic subjects, the mere exhibition of mercury and iodides is insufficient to effect a cure ; nay, more, by their powerful action on the oral mucous membrane they may make things worse— a point to be kept carefully in mind in treating syphilitic ulcers in the mouth. In such cases the local treatment should be as advised above. Chromic acid is of great value in many of the specific lesions of the mouth.

In cases where the ulcer resists all treatment or relapses frequently, especially if the edges become indurated, it should be excised by means of elliptical incisions, and the edges of the wound should be brought together by silk sutures after ligation with catgut of any vessels that require it. The stitches should be removed in four days.

DYSPEPTIC ULCERS

Arise in severe or exaggerated forms of dyspeptic glossitis in which the surface excoriations break down into true ulcers. They are usually situated near the tip, and appear as small, circular, punched-out multiple ulcers, with a red areola, associated with a general redness or beefiness of the anterior part of the tongue, the posterior part being covered with a thick, unhealthy fur. Some patients seem possessed of an idiosyncrasy in regard to certain articles of food, which have a regular tendency to produce such ulceration.

The general **treatment** is the same as for dyspeptic tongue, but here local treatment with nitrate of silver is very beneficial.

HERPETIC ULCERS

While herpetic glossitis is chiefly the property of the adult, herpetic
ulcers, in which the herpetic vesicles pustulate and ulcerate, are
more commonly met with in unhealthy children between the ages of
6 months and 3 years. The child is thin and often ill nourished, the
bowels act sluggishly, the mouth is hot and full of·saliva, and the
breath offensive. The teeth are often covered with tartar or are
decayed. The ulcers, which are multiple, are covered with the membranous pellicle described above ; they affect the anterior portion of
the tongue, also its under-surface, and the adjacent buccal mucous
membrane.

The glands in the submaxillary region may be swollen.

Treatment.—Give a dose of salts, castor oil, or rhubarb, and
keep the bowels acting regularly. Put the patient on a plain diet,
including fruit but avoiding pastry. Chlorate of potash in 4–5 gr.
doses may be given every four hours for two days, but it must be
used with care as it often has an irritant action on the kidneys. The
tongue should be kept clean with a piece of soft Turkey sponge soaked
in boric-acid solution or a solution of bicarbonate of soda ; later, more
stimulating lotions such as alum or chromic acid may be needed.

Mercury in all forms must be avoided. It may produce a gangrenous stomatitis in these subjects.

TRAUMATIC ULCERS

"Dental ulcers" are wounds that remain unhealed owing to persistent irritation. They result from rough, broken, or irregular teeth,
which are often carious, or from ill-fitting tooth-plates. Sometimes
a broken pipe-stem may be responsible.

They vary enormously in depth and appearance, but are usually
situated on the sides or the tip. In more recent cases there is a shallow
erosion—sometimes, however, acutely inflamed—surrounded by œdematous tissue, and associated with glandular enlargement. Such a
syndrome points to an acute bacterial infection superadded to the
trauma. In most cases, however, the ulcer is chronic, perhaps covered
with a slough, the edges becoming progressively indurated the longer
the ulcer is left untreated.

Patients who suffer from such ulcers are usually in bad health.
The tongue is covered with fur, the breath is foul, and there is often
a marked condition of pyorrhœa alveolaris.

The **diagnosis** may be very difficult in old and neglected cases,
and the observer must always keep in mind the possibility of an ulcer
of this appearance being tuberculous, syphilitic, or cancerous. The
general points which influence the differential diagnosis will be con-

sidered under the appropriate headings to avoid repetition, but we must here draw attention to the tendency of such ulcers, if neglected, to become ultimately carcinomatous.

In making a differential diagnosis the finding of some local cause is exceedingly important; only recently I saw a patient who had a chronic ulcer which had been diagnosed as malignant. On inquiry it was found that the patient wore an ill-fitting tooth-plate which pressed against the ulcer, but, as it was not always worn, its importance in producing the condition had been overlooked; when this was remedied the ulcer speedily healed under the application of chromic acid.

Treatment consists primarily in removing the source of irritation, and in applying local remedies such as chromic acid, and ordering an antiseptic mouth-wash. In most cases the response to treatment is prompt. There is one point, however, which requires special attention. While these ulcers are truly traumatic in their incipient stages, they become " infected " ulcers, as shown by their liability to undergo acute inflammatory changes, and by the glandular enlargement which accompanies them. As has been pointed out, a condition of pyorrhœa is often associated with them, which, by constantly reinfecting the ulcer, renders local treatment futile. Such cases are eminently suitable for vaccine treatment, which in pyorrhœa has succeeded admirably in the hands of Goadby; if this be undertaken, together with the remedies advised above, healing of the ulcer will be speedy and complete.

In cases where treatment is resisted or where the surgeon suspects a commencing malignant change, a piece (or better still, the whole) of the ulcer should be excised and submitted to microscopic examination. If a malignant change has supervened, the radical operation for lingual carcinoma should be performed.

ULCER OF THE FRÆNUM

This condition occurs in children affected with whooping-cough, and is due to the tongue being forced up against the incisor teeth in the violent expiratory efforts of the coughing. It has been incorrectly stated that this ulceration is the cause and not the effect of whooping-cough. Sometimes these ulcers are associated with small papillomatous growths on either side of the frænum—Riga's disease. The ulceration subsides as the cough disappears.

MERCURIAL ULCERS

In ulcers resulting from the injudicious administration of mercury an unclean state of the mouth is a very important contributory factor. Patients whose mouths are kept scrupulously clean are able to tolerate mercury better, and are much less liable to stomatitis and ulceration, than those whose mouths are septic and unhealthy.

The ulcers are multiple, shallow, and irregular in outline, surrounded by a red area, but not so defined as the dyspeptic variety ; they may lead to extensive sloughing. The tongue as a whole is swollen, showing indentations from the teeth at its sides, the breath is foul, there is profuse salivation, the gums are swollen, spongy, and retracted from the teeth, which are loose in their sockets. Such a picture is seldom difficult of diagnosis.

Treatment.—Give a saline purge, and prescribe chlorate of potash, 10 gr. every four hours for two days (*see* above). Order astringent mouth-washes, sulphate of iron, or acetic alum (E. Lane). Nitrate of silver is of value, and for the salivation belladonna may be prescribed.

Tuberculous, syphilitic, and malignant ulcers will be considered specially in the sections on Tuberculosis (*see* below), Syphilitic Diseases (p. 191), and Malignant Tumours (p. 204).

TUBERCULOSIS

The present advanced state of our knowledge of the manifestations of tuberculous disease attacking the tongue is largely due to Butlin's writings, and his descriptions and opinions are closely followed in the ensuing section. In the past many of these cases were mistaken for malignant disease, and no doubt in a few instances they were successfully subjected to operative treatment and a permanent cure of cancer was claimed.

The systematic examination of all ulcers and tumours removed has shown us that the tongue, like other tissues of the body, is subject to tuberculous invasion, and in the diagnosis of difficult cases it has given us valuable information, and occasionally unpleasant surprises.

Tuberculosis attacks the tongue either as a primary infection of the subepithelial tissues, the bacilli reaching the part from the blood-stream or by means of infected food ; or as a secondary complication of tuberculous disease of the lung or alimentary canal, the tongue then being infected by the sputum. When we think of the rarity of tuberculous disease in this region, as compared with its frequency elsewhere, and the constant exposure of the lingual surface to infected sputum in tuberculous subjects, we are forced to the conclusion that the tongue possesses special powers of resistance ; probably, unless there is some breach in the surface epithelium, secondary infection of the organ does not occur.

The diagnosis of the tuberculous nature of a lingual ulcer is facilitated by the discovery of signs of pulmonary disease.

All authorities do not accept the occurrence of primary tuberculosis, and it has been held, with some reason, that in the reported cases a localized patch of pulmonary tubercle has been overlooked.

Pathology.—The microscopic appearances of lingual tubercle are peculiar. It is rare to find the system of tubercles at all well marked, while even the giant cells are scarce. Again, careful staining will often fail to reveal tubercle bacilli.

In many cases the arrangement of the proliferating endothelial cells is atypical, and in the form which is described as "infiltrating tubercle" they may be mistaken for epithelial cells, and a diagnosis of new growth (endothelioma) may be made. In doubtful cases it may be necessary to inoculate a guinea-pig with the suspected material.

The various tubercular lesions may be grouped under the following headings :—

1. *Nodes.*—Small nodular masses varying in size from a pin's head to a nut, multiple in cases of generalized miliary tubercle, or single in the locally infected cases. These nodules consist of tuberculous granulations, covered at first with normal epithelium, which with the increase in the size of the tubercle is liable to break down and leave an ulcerated surface.

The centre of the tuberculoma may undergo caseation.

2. *Fissures,* which are really fissured ulcers, probably originally simple ones that have become infected with tubercle, are very difficult to diagnose. When the edges of the cleft are separated, it is found to be much deeper than was expected, and to be lined with swollen granulations, with perhaps caseating margins. The material scraped from the surface may be shown to contain tubercle bacilli. Occasionally the margins of these fissures are covered with protruding growths of a papillary nature, to which the name *tuberculous papilloma* has been applied.

3. *Ulcers.*—The appearance of true tuberculous ulcers is very varied, no doubt because in but a very few instances, and then for a short time only, is the infection "unmixed." Sooner or later a tuberculous ulcer in a cavity such as the mouth is liable to contamination with the various bacteria and mycelia regularly found there, and thus becomes modified in appearance. This fact explains why some ulcers are covered with a foul slough, and others are surrounded by an indurated zone suggesting cancer.

It is a feature of the pure tuberculous process here, as elsewhere, that there is complete absence of induration.

4. The *lupoid ulcer,* which has been described by Butlin and Leloir, is exceedingly rare, and is caused either by extension of the lupoid ulceration into the interior of the mouth, or by contagion due to the drawing of the tongue over the infected lips. In appearance

the lupoid ulcer is a crusted sore without surrounding inflammation ; when the crust is removed a nodular or mammillated area is exposed, with perhaps some small caseous foci, the general colour being bluish-pink.

The true ulcer, as has been explained above, occurs in very many different forms. The pure tuberculous ulcer is oval in shape, with a pale, flabby, anæmic surface, the granulations having a glistening, watery appearance ; the edges are sloping, not everted or indurated, and rarely undermined. The anterior part of the dorsum is the usual situation of the ulcer, the margins being often involved. Occasionally, caseous areas may be seen. There is no surrounding inflammation. The above type represents the unmixed tuberculous infection ; there are also dozens of different varieties, some with induration, some with surrounding inflammation and œdema, others with a large foul sloughing surface, but no useful end is served by trying to classify these diverse appearances. Suffice it to say that in a doubtful case a careful clinical examination of the lungs and a microscopical examination of the ulcer will be required to make the diagnosis clear.

The adjacent set of lymphatic glands which drain the affected area are enlarged.

Symptoms.—Tuberculous manifestations are usually painful when ulceration has occurred ; indeed, in some cases there is excruciating pain, and the misery of tuberculous disease in this situation may be compared to that which results from tuberculous infection of the bladder. There is a tendency to profuse salivation, and in neglected cases the mouth becomes exceedingly foul.

Prognosis.—Most authorities agree in giving a very gloomy prognosis. Butlin asserts that the disease is usually fatal in from one to two years, and he goes on to say that " the patient is to be regarded as fortunate if he is relieved by rapidly progressive tuberculosis of the internal organs before the ulcer of the tongue has become larger and painful." Pouzergues and Ducrot take a more hopeful view.

If a primary lesion can be removed, or if an early secondary infection can be radically treated and the pulmonary disease checked by appropriate remedies, there is some hope of the picture being a little brighter in future.

Treatment.—The main line of treatment is operative. All tuberculous manifestations should be freely excised, unless pulmonary disease or other constitutional debility is a contra-indication. The question of the wisdom of operating in the presence of active pulmonary tubercle must be left to the discretion of individual surgeons ; but if by performing a comparatively simple operation we are able to prevent the pain and suffering which the progress of the ulcer entails, we are entirely justified in pursuing that course. Even in the presence of the infected sputum, healing does occur. The enlarged glands should also be removed.

Cases which are not submitted to operation should be treated like those of chronic glossitis or simple ulcer (q.v.). Soothing, weak astringent mouth-washes are to be preferred, and caustics are to be avoided.

It may be necessary to give all food finely minced so that its prolonged presence in the mouth for mastication may not be needed.

Cocaine and orthoform are useful applications, but the first must, of course, be used with care.

An application to the ulcer of iodoform 1 gr., morphia $\frac{1}{6}$-$\frac{1}{2}$ gr., borax 3 gr., by means of a soft brush, is advisable after the surface has been gently cleaned with cotton-wool. A bismuth ointment is sometimes valuable as an alternative.

SYPHILITIC DISEASES

The tongue may be attacked by syphilis in any of the three recognized periods of the disease, and the frequency with which the organ suffers makes it a valuable signpost in cases of doubtful syphilis. As in other parts of the body, these syphilitic manifestations copy, often in a very accurate manner, the appearances produced by other pathological conditions, so that the possibility of a lesion of the tongue being syphilitic must always receive due consideration. At the same time it will not be out of place to quote Butlin's warning in this respect : " Nothing leads to greater errors in diagnosis and treatment than the tendency to see syphilis in every form of obscure affection of the tongue, or to persist in a diagnosis of syphilis when a short and vigorous administration of antisyphilitic remedies has proved of no service."

CHANCRE

The initial lesion of syphilis is occasionally found on the tongue. Fournier discovered it here 53 times in 642 cases of extragenital chancre. The infection is conveyed by direct personal contact, or indirectly by the use of cups, pipes, glass-blowing and other instruments, contaminated by infected persons. As a rule the chancre is situated on the anterior part of the tongue, and, as in the case of the genital affection, may or may not show well-marked ulceration.

The **pathology** of the lesion is the same here as elsewhere ; there is extensive proliferation of the fixed connective-tissue cells of the subepithelial layer, some infiltration of leucocytes, and thickening of the arteries and veins. As these changes cease fairly abruptly at the margin, the chancre feels like a hard nodular mass embedded in the normal supple tongue. The amount of ulceration present probably depends upon the extent to which the epithelium is affected, upon the degree of "mixed" infection that has occurred, and upon the presence or absence of trauma.

The smooth chancre appears as a firm, hard, well-defined nodule, aptly compared in shape and feel to a nux vomica seed embedded in the tongue. The ulcerated form has a characteristic appearance like the bowl of a spoon, the induration being accompanied by more infiltration than in the preceding variety, and by pain and salivation. A fissured chancre has been described.

Within ten days of the appearance of the primary lesion the sub-maxillary and submental lymphatic glands will be found enlarged; and, as so often happens in the glandular enlargement associated with an extragenital chancre, the degree of swelling is considerable, and relatively greater than that of inguinal adenitis in genital chancres.

The characteristic induration, the glandular enlargement, and the short history of the lesion make the **diagnosis** easy; in a doubtful case it may be necessary to try Wassermann's reaction, or even to wait for symptoms of the generalized disease, before a definite opinion can be given.

Active **treatment** of the disease must be undertaken as soon as the diagnosis has been made; a mercurial mouth-wash should be ordered, and a little iodoform powder may be applied occasionally to the ulcerated varieties.

The infectious character of the disease in this and in the secondary stages should be pointed out to the patient.

I may add that *soft chancre of the tongue* has been described by Emery, Sabouraud, and Fournier.

SECONDARY STAGE

In this stage, mucous nodules or patches are met with which present the characteristic pathological features of syphilitic lesions, arising from localized proliferation of the connective-tissue cells, the resulting elevation being covered with thickened epithelium.

The proliferation of the connective-tissue cells extends over a wider area than in the primary lesion, and does not proceed to the same degree of development, the resulting papule or projection only just standing out from the surface of the tongue.

Influenced, no doubt, by the agencies referred to above, the surface of the patch may ulcerate, even deeply, and the so-called secondary ulcer may be formed. These patches may be met with anywhere on the tongue or fauces, but they are more common on the dorsum in front of the circumvallate papillæ; they are also found on the under-surface.

In their course they arise as small nodular elevations the size of a pea, and gradually extend to the size and shape of an almond. The surface epithelium, being thickened, takes on a greyish-white appearance ; the edge is sharply defined and, unless ulceration has occurred, there is no surrounding redness. If the epithelium is shed, a smooth, red, elevated surface is left behind ; but in their usual position on the dorsum the patches are exceedingly liable to become fissured or ulcerated, and accordingly modified in appearance.

The **diagnosis** has to be made from leucoma, but the mucous patches are not so pearly-white as those of leucoma, while ulceration, if present, extends more deeply in the syphilitic lesions. Other symptoms, too, of generalized syphilis will be present.

Constitutional **treatment** of the disease is required, but for local application Butlin found that chromic acid, 10 gr. to the ounce, has a wonderful action, far superior to that of any mercurial remedies applied locally.

In this as in all forms of syphilitic or other ulceration the lines of treatment laid down for superficial glossitis should be carried out rigidly.

Tanturri has described an affection of the lymphoid follicles at the base of the tongue, a syphilitic hypertrophy of the adenoid tissue.

TERTIARY STAGE

In the third stage the tongue is more deeply affected. The pathological changes again concern the fixed connective-tissue cells, which are stimulated to proliferate, either locally or generally.

In the local form the aggregation of mononuclear cells leads to the development of a nodular mass, and the tendency of these newly formed cells to necrose from imperfect nutrition causes the formation of the central slough or dead core of the gumma. When the process is more widely diffused this tendency to local degeneration is not marked, but special complications attend and follow this connective-tissue overgrowth.

Fournier describes two main varieties, *superficial sclerosing glossitis* and *deep* or *parenchymatous glossitis :* in both the essential pathological change is the same ; it is only the extension of the process into the deeper parts of the tongue in the latter form which causes any difference.

In the superficial form the main change is in the connective tissue subjacent to the epithelium, and leads to the development of flat plate-like masses beneath the epithelium. The latter is soon affected ; proliferating abnormally at first under the stimulus of the infection, its nutrition becomes impaired as the inevitable contraction of the newly formed connective tissue supervenes, and there is a ready tendency to ulceration. Further, in its contraction the fibrous tissue causes disfigurement of the tongue surface, and the formation of the

n

clefts and fissures seen on the surface of the syphilitic tongue. Sometimes the arrangement is quite regular, the indurated surface of the tongue being cut up by lines which divide it into perfect quadrilateral areas ; in others the arrangement is very irregular.

In the parenchymatous form the cellular hyperplasia affects the deeper parts of the organ, and gives rise, in fact, to a general cirrhosis. In the early stages, when the connective-tissue cells are actively proliferating, the tongue is swollen, often extremely so, indented laterally by the teeth, and may be eroded and ulcerated. In the extreme cases, which are rare, however, a condition of *syphilitic macroglossia* is set up.

Sooner or later the period of active cell-formation is replaced by the period of fibrous contraction or sclerosis ; the tongue becomes shrunken and distorted as in the superficial variety, but to a much greater extent. As in the case of the cirrhotic liver, the surface is mammillated and lobulated, the lobules being separated from one another by deep fissures ; there is deep induration, not unlike that of cancer, but more generalized. Ulcers, often intractable, sometimes malignant, are apt to form in the depths of these fissures.

Gummata may develop either superficially or deeply. The superficial variety, often multiple, is characterized by its appearance on parts of the tongue which are not irritated, and by its breaking down and forming a gummatous ulcer early. The deep gummata arise frequently in the centre of the tongue, in the " avascular area," though they may be found at the sides.

Men are much more liable to this manifestation of syphilis than women. The gummata develop as round or oval deep-seated tumours, which may cause great difficulty in diagnosis, simulating as they do new growths or abscesses. When they break down, which they are somewhat slow to do, they may lead to great destruction of the tongue substance, and appear as indolent, painless, gummatous ulcers.

The gummatous ulcer is characterized by its ragged borders, somewhat undermined edges, and sloughy surface ; if of long standing it may show induration ; the glands are not enlarged unless some other infection is superadded. The painlessness and slow development of the ulcer are two points of most importance in the diagnosis, but in many doubtful cases iodide and mercury must be administered before a suspicion can be converted into a certainty.

Tertiary affections of the tongue, as Butlin points out, are prone to attack the dorsum.

The general treatment of tertiary syphilis must be undertaken, and locally the ulcers are to be cleansed with washes and painted with chromic acid, 10 gr. to the ounce. In some obstinate cases, iodipin, given either hypodermically or by the mouth, is of very great service; and it may be stated generally that the oral and lingual manifestations of syphilis are rapidly benefited by a course of salvarsan.

CYSTS AND TUMOURS

DERMOID CYSTS

The group of cystic tumours in the tongue to which the term dermoid may be applied consists of three main varieties, depending upon the particular developmental irregularity responsible for their formation.

In this consideration we must take into account the changes which occur in the developing neck. In the middle line of the neck, where the lateral folds meet one another in the process of fusion, portions of the epidermis may become unnaturally included in the underlying mesoblast, and may later develop into the type of cyst called by

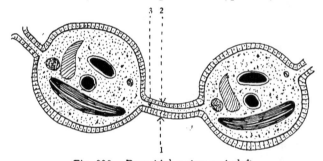

Fig. 336.—Branchial arches and cleft.

1, External cleft depression; 2, internal cleft depression; 3, cleft membrane

Bland-Sutton *sequestration dermoid ;* such dermoids may be met with embedded in the substance of the tongue.

Again, if the process of obliteration of the branchial depressions by the opercular folds of the cervical sinus be imperfectly carried out, embryonic remains may later develop into cystic tumours. Between each branchial bar and the next there is a depression or cleft recess, limited by the cleft membrane—the outer part, or external cleft depression, being lined by epiblast; the inner, or internal cleft depression, by hypoblast (Fig. 336). Dermoid cysts arising in connexion with the external cleft depression present all the usual characteristics of a dermoid cyst, being filled with pultaceous sebaceous matter and having typically epidermal walls, upon which hairs may be found. Cysts arising from the inner cleft depression, markedly rare, appear rather in the form of pharyngeal diverticula, or more rarely as cystic tumours containing glairy fluid, and in most cases some connexion with the pharyngeal wall can be discovered.

Strictly speaking, such dermoids as these do not occur primarily in the tongue, being generally found in the submaxillary region, from which, by extension, they may invade the lingual substance.

The third variety is the one which develops in connexion with the median thyroid rudiment (Fig. 337); such cysts or, it may be, solid tumours occur deeply in the posterior part of the tongue; this form is called by Bland-Sutton a "*tubulo-dermoid.*"

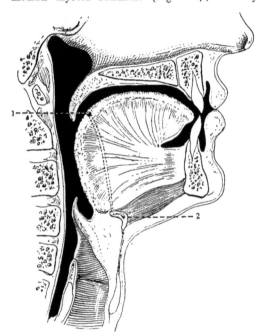

Fig. 337.—Diagram showing position occupied by thyroid tumours and cysts in the base of the tongue, indicated by the double dotted line.

1, Foramen cæcum; 2, hyoid bone.

SEQUESTRATION DERMOIDS

These cysts usually occur in the anterior part of the tongue, in the middle line, and are then situated between the two genio - hyo - glossi; sometimes they are laterally placed, but this is owing to their irregular extension, or more probably to the cysts having arisen in a branchial recess. Such cysts grow slowly and protrude either into the mouth or into the submental region; in advanced cases a very large swelling may be formed which renders closure of the mouth impossible. The swelling has a curious doughy feel, pits on pressure, and in some cases is of a yellowish colour.

If the cyst has been allowed to rupture, or has been incompletely removed, dermoid *fistulæ* form, and discharge the sebaceous débris and hairs found in these cavities; the cavity usually becomes infected, and the contents may be horridly fetid.

In a case under my care, a French boy complained of this offensive discharge, but at first nothing could be detected on examination of the mouth. Closer inspection, however, showed a few fine hairs projecting from the side of a fistula in the position of the submaxillary papilla. A probe passed into a deep cavity let out a quantity of very offensive sebaceous matter; an attempt was made to destroy the cyst wall, and this failing, the cyst was completely dissected out after division of the mandible.

Treatment.—Dermoid cysts must be excised, either through the open mouth or, if large, by an incision below the jaw (Regnoli's incision, p. 226). As a rule they shell out easily by blunt dissection, though they are usually adherent to the hyoid bone at one point.

Sometimes great difficulties from surrounding inflammation are encountered, rendering a laryngotomy or a tracheotomy necessary; while, if the cyst has ruptured, the dissection of the sinus is a matter of the greatest trouble, and may, as in the case recorded above, necessitate division of the jaw at the symphysis. The whole cyst wall or fistulous track must be removed, or the operation will be a failure. The cavity should be plugged with iodoform gauze, kept clean, and allowed to heal up from the bottom.

Lateral dermoids are treated in the same way.

TUBULO-DERMOIDS, THYRO-DERMOIDS, OR THYRO-GLOSSAL DERMOIDS

These growths are found at the back of the tongue, in the region of the foramen cæcum, or deeply embedded in the posterior part of the tongue substance. When situated near the surface they are more often solid than when placed more deeply. As in the case of the thyroid gland itself we meet with adenomas in which there is no cystic change, and with others in which the whole tumour undergoes a cystic transformation, so in the thyroid tumour of the tongue it is a mere chance which variety will occur.

These cystic tumours are generally regarded as retention-cysts of the thyro-glossal duct, and as such are infinitely commoner below than above the hyoid bone; in actual fact, however, we are hardly justified in putting this interpretation on their origin, since there is no evidence to show that the thyro-glossal duct was ever a functional canal for the purpose of conveying secretion into the mouth; it is rather the track of the developing thyroid, and would be better called the thyro-glossal tract, along the course of which aberrant thyroid particles may develop into cysts or tumours. The thyro-glossal tract, indicated in Fig. 338 by a thick black line, passes from the foramen cæcum, through the base of the tongue, to the hyoid bone. It usually runs behind, but occasionally in front of this bone, and in rare instances through it. Thence it extends down in front of the thyroid cartilage.

When these thyroid tumours develop at the base of the tongue they are often solid and consist of vascular thyroid tissue exceedingly prone to bleed; severe and even fatal hæmorrhage has occurred spontaneously or as the result of incautious puncture. Cystic change may occur, and this is no doubt the origin of the so-called blood cysts of the tongue.

Treatment.— Thyro-glossal cysts should be completely excised; this entails a dissection of the tubular canal, which may be found extending from the thyroid gland up to, or even beyond, the hyoid bone. Incomplete removal is always followed by recurrence. Although it is rarely necessary to continue the dissection beyond the hyoid bone into the tongue substance, the operator must be prepared to do this, even dividing the hyoid bone if necessary.

No treatment should be undertaken in the case of the solid thyroid tumours at the base of the tongue, unless they are the cause of trouble. Not only is an operation for their removal attended by a considerable amount of danger, but in some cases these tumours consist of the only functional thyroid tissue which the patient possesses, and removal of them has been followed by cachexia strumipriva. If, however, they give rise to serious hæmorrhage from ulceration, or difficulty in swallowing or breathing, they must be removed. When projecting from the surface, and especially if somewhat pedunculated, they may be snared off with a cautery wire.

The more deeply situated tumours must be dissected out. Rose's

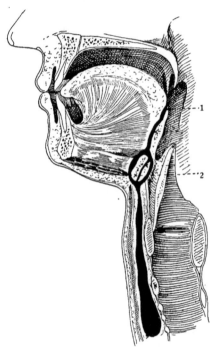

Fig. 338.—Diagram showing " thyro-glossal tract."

1, Thyro-glossal tract; 2, hyoid bone.

position (p. 219), the head hanging over the table, may be sufficient in some cases, but in others the upright position with division of the mandible will give better access. Again, a preliminary laryngotomy may be advisable. In every case, care must be taken to check all hæmorrhage and to bring the edges of the cavity together with deep sutures.

After-treatment as in operations for cancer must be carried out.

Other cystic conditions which have been described are *mucous cysts*, from distension of the mucous glands, and *parasitic cysts*, from the deposit of the *Cysticercus cellulosæ* or of echinococcus parasites.

MACROGLOSSIA, OR ENLARGEMENT OF THE TONGUE

The several causes of enlargement of the tongue fall conveniently under the following headings :—

    1. Lymphangiomatous.
    2. Muscular.
    3. Inflammatory.
    4. Syphilitic.
    5. Mercurial.

1. LYMPHANGIOMATOUS ENLARGEMENT

This, the most usual form of macroglossia, is caused by a dilatation of the lymphatic spaces, with subsequent thickening and induration of the lingual tissues. The condition is usually congenital, but it is not invariably present at birth ; in some cases, indeed, it is not noticed until several years after.

Pathology.—The normal lymph spaces of the tongue (the anterior three-fourths) are increased in size and in number. This change has generally been ascribed to some obstruction to the efferent lymphatics of the tongue, so that the existing spaces become distended. It is not by any means clear that this is the sole cause, and from the progressive spread of the disease it has been suggested, with a considerable amount of reason, that there is an actual overgrowth of the lymph spaces and tissues in the tongue substance, constituting an actual lymphangioma or new growth. Hutchinson suggested the term "infective lymphangioma," analogous to lupus lymphaticus, to explain its progressive course, but it is simpler to regard the condition as comparable to nævoid or angiomatous growths of the veins and capillaries, affecting in this instance the lymph- rather than the blood-vascular system.

Virchow compared the disease with elephantiasis, and the similarity is great ; at the same time, the occurrence of macroglossia among the sufferers from elephantiasis Arabum is exceedingly rare.

Precisely the same pathological phenomena will be observed if the lymphatic tissues of a part enlarge to such an extent that the existing lymphatic vessels are unable adequately to drain the region, as if those vessels were the site of an obstruction preventing them from draining in normal circumstances.

In some cases a definite injury has preceded the development of macroglossia. Stone records a case of this kind.

The microscopic appearances have been carefully described by Butlin, to whom we are indebted for the following accurate account :—

" If a vertical section be made of a simple lymphangioma, the lymphatic spaces immediately beneath the epithelium are dilated ; by further enlargement the lymph space bulges towards the surface, thinning the epithelium by pressure until only a layer of corneous epithelium covers the surface. The contents of the space are lymph-serous fluid containing numerous white corpuscles.

" By extension between the muscular fibres and fusion of the lymph spaces large cysts are formed, so that the portion of the substance of the tongue invaded has a honeycombed look. Around these dilated lymphatic spaces three changes take place, and it is in accordance with the relative proportions in which each occurs that the differences found in advanced cases are due. These are—(a) dilatation and new formation of blood-vessels ; (b) inflammatory changes with formation of fibrous tissue ; (c) new growth of lymphadenomatous tissue.

" (a) The capillary loops between the vesicles in the simple form develop into arteries, thin-walled, coiled, and of a considerable size. The veins also increase in number and become dilated. Then the blood-vessels rupture into the large lymphatic spaces, which become distended, partly by blood-clot, partly by circulating blood. In this way is produced the cavernous form of macroglossia (Barker, Hutchinson, jun.).

" (b) The dilatation of the lymph space is accompanied by inflammation. Small round cells infiltrate the connective tissues, and tough fibrous tissue increases and slowly surrounds the spaces. The inflammation is subject to sharp fluctuations, a marked increase accompanying the extravasation of blood ; then it subsides, but to recur again and again. With each attack there is a further formation of fibrous tissue, which permanently enlarges the portion of the tongue affected, and gives the enlarged tongue a tough or almost wooden feeling, varying with the amount of œdema in the fibrous tissue.

" The fibrous tissue presses aside the muscular fibres and causes them to degenerate, so that, whilst the tongue enlarges, the amount of muscular substance is being continually reduced, until it disappears altogether from the affected portion of the tongue. The section shows simply fibrous tissue with a variable number of spaces containing either lymph or blood.

" (c) Small round cells collect in the connective tissue between the muscular fibres, amongst the lymph spaces ; and between the cells retiform tissue may be met with. These small round cells are not replaced by fibrous tissue, but a new growth goes on slowly until lymphadenomatous masses are produced. A macroglossia may even terminate by the development of a small round-celled or lympho-sarcoma."

Clinical features.—The first symptom which attracts attention is an increase in the sensitiveness of the organ, accompanied

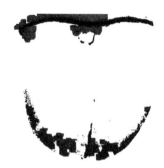

Lymphangioma of dorsum of the tongue, which was beset with clear vesicles, between which were scarlet capillary loops and blood-filled vesicles. A few of the vesicles were filled with opaque, white material. The condition was associated with a capillary nævus involving the lower lip and about half an inch of skin surface parallel to the muco-cutaneous margin, and extending across the alveolar margin to the under surface of the tongue, where there were some dilated veins.

(*E. Rock Carling's case.*)

PLATE 87.

by the development of minute cysts or "blisters," which readily rupture. (Plate 87.) At first only a portion of the tongue is affected, but the process spreads until the whole organ is attacked. From time to time there are outbreaks of acute inflammation, which leave the tongue larger and firmer than before.

At first the tongue is concealed within the mouth, and shows, on inspection, general enlargement with hypertrophy of the papillæ; gradually, however, with the increasing size there is difficulty in retaining it within the oral boundaries, the saliva dribbles away, and the tongue protrudes, its surface, from exposure to the air, becoming hard, brown, cracked and fissured. Progressively the bones of the oral cavity become affected; and in some cases, even after proper treatment of the affected organ, closure of the jaws may be impossible.

Treatment consists in freely removing part of the organ by means of a **V**-shaped cut, and suturing the edges of the wound together. A sufficient amount should be removed to allow the tongue to lie easily within the mouth; and at the same time the operator must bear in mind that he is dealing with a form of new growth, and he should therefore endeavour to cut wide of the morbid tissue, otherwise recurrence in the stump is likely to ensue. The operation is attended by profuse bleeding, and steps must be taken to deal promptly with the hæmorrhage.

In the case of very young children it may be wise to postpone the operation for some years, as its performance has been fatal. The child should be spoon fed—it cannot suck—until sufficiently strong to stand what may be a formidable surgical procedure, and then subjected to the operation.

2. MUSCULAR MACROGLOSSIA

A true muscular hypertrophy, in which there is an increase in number and size (Helbing) of the muscular fibres, is occasionally seen. Such a condition may occur in a normal individual, the "lingua vituli"; more usually it is met with in cretins and congenital idiots. In some cases the enlargement may be unilateral. It may be associated with abnormal enlargement of other parts of the body, and is therefore part of a gigantism or increased growth of the individual, probably the effect of some obscure nervous influence.

Treatment.—The activity of the treatment must depend upon the amount of inconvenience resulting from the deformity. Treatment is not to be undertaken so readily as in the former variety, since the progress of the growth is slow and there are none of the characteristic features of a "new growth" present. Occasionally the two forms are combined, in which case early radical treatment is indicated.

If operation becomes advisable in the pure muscular variety, it should consist in removal of a wedge-shaped piece of tongue, rather than in ligation of the lingual arteries—a method which is neither certain nor safe.

3, 4, 5. INFLAMMATORY, SYPHILITIC, AND MERCURIAL ENLARGEMENTS

Inflammatory enlargement is merely the result of an acute glossitis, after which a large indurated area may be left.

Syphilitic hypertrophy has been considered in connexion with syphilitic parenchymatous glossitis (p. 194). The condition calls for no special treatment.

With regard to mercurial enlargement, it should be remembered that excessive use of mercury in syphilis tends to exaggerate any existing hypertrophy, and that the drug may even produce an inflammatory enlargement by its own action.

INNOCENT TUMOURS

The tongue is rarely the seat of a simple growth—a marked contrast to its ready tendency to undergo malignant change. Innocent tumours of many varieties have been described, such as *lipomas*, recognized by their yellowish colour when superficial ; *fibromas ; chondromas ;* localized or general *lymphangiomas ; neuro-fibromas ; myomas* of both striped and unstriped types ; *amyloid masses* in the subjects of chronic bronchitis and emphysema ; and even *osseous tumours* and those of a *teratoid* nature. Many of these growths are of the greatest rarity, and may be regarded as being more of pathological interest than of clinical importance. In general they will be treated by removal if the tumour appears to be a source of discomfort or danger

VASCULAR TUMOURS

On the other hand, the vascular tumours are not only a good deal commoner than the preceding, but since they may be the source of dangerous hæmorrhage they must be specially considered.

Among the vascular tumours, examples of *arterio-venous aneurysm* have been met with, as the result of injury. They have occurred usually on the floor of the mouth, and have been treated by ligation of the lingual arteries. A few instances of *cirsoid aneurysm* have been recorded ; one half of the tongue, in the published cases, being occupied by large tortuous arteries which bled violently as the result of injury.

NÆVI

Nævi, both capillary and cavernous, are much more common. The *capillary* form may be congenital in origin, or may appear later, possibly as the result of injury. Capillary nævi bleed readily and profusely, and in this respect are similar to the small but dangerous capillary hæmorrhoids described by Allingham.

The *cavernous* nævi, usually found on the anterior part of the tongue, may attain some size, and may be associated with a similar state of the lip and cheek. They are quite painless, and as a rule circumscribed, but they have an unfortunate tendency to increase in size, and are liable to bleed profusely if injured. A cavernous nævus is recognized by its dark colour and soft consistence, in addition to the enlargement of the vessels in the neighbourhood.

Treatment.—Nævi should receive active treatment, as there is always a risk of severe bleeding, which cannot in all cases be readily controlled. Capillary or even small cavernous nævi should be treated by the galvano-cautery—the point, at a dull-red heat, being thrust deeply into the spongy tumour. The application must be repeated until the blood spaces are finally obliterated. Electrolysis is often of use in these cases.

In more extensive and diffuse cases excision is indicated, by means of a wedge-shaped cut placed well outside the line of the nævus, care being taken to secure the larger vessels as they are cut. As a preliminary measure, one or both lingual arteries may require ligation.

VARICOSE VEINS

May be met with in the tongue as in other parts of the body ; some degree of varicosity is usually associated with nævi. As a rule no treatment is required, especially when the posterior part of the organ is affected, as there is little danger here of injury and bleeding. In the anterior part, if increasing in size they should be treated as nævi, of which very often they form a part.

PAPILLOMAS

These growths are found chiefly on the dorsum, and are in many cases congenital. They may be single or multiple.

Irritation unquestionably plays a part in the production of a certain number of papillomas. One variety, found on the side of the frænum from contact with the incisor teeth in whooping-cough, appears to follow the development of an ulcer which is commonly present in this situation.

Tongues which are the seat of chronic superficial glossitis are prone to develop large sessile papillomas, which must be regarded as examples of local irritative hypertrophy.

Warty growths also occur in syphilis.

Treatment.—Papillomas should be excised or, if small, destroyed completely by the galvano-cautery. The inflammatory papillomas are unquestionably liable to become cancerous; indeed, it is sometimes impossible to distinguish clinically between the simple tumour and one that has already undergone a malignant change. They should be removed by elliptical incisions which pass deeply into the tongue, and the edges of the wound should be sutured.

MALIGNANT TUMOURS

SARCOMA [1]

Primary sarcoma of the tongue is rarely met with, and probably many of the recorded cases do not properly fall under this heading. Microscopically the tumour may consist of round or spindle cells, and in most cases there is a very well-marked history of injury or prolonged irritation.

The degree of malignancy in the recorded cases varies so enormously that it is, perhaps, too early yet to speak with decision of the diagnosis and treatment of sarcoma of the tongue.

In some cases the growth appears distinctly encapsuled, as do sarcomas elsewhere in the body; in other cases the tongue is extensively invaded and the growth soon spreads to the lymphatic glands.

Lympho-sarcomatous tumours originating in the lymphoid tissue at the base of the tongue have been described, and seem to form the most malignant variety. The large round-celled tumour grows much more slowly, while slowest of all is the fibro-sarcoma, that pathological cross-breed, midway between the fibroma and the malignant growth.

With regard to **treatment,** we may repeat what has been said above in connexion with simple tumours. All new growths of the tongue should be removed. If the rate of growth of a tumour suggest a sarcomatous nature, or if there be recurrence after removal of a doubtful tumour, an attempt should be made to extirpate the disease by cutting widely into the healthy tissues beyond the limits of the growth. Glandular involvement, which has been a not infrequent concomitant in reported cases, will be a contra-indication to operative treatment, unless there be a good prospect of getting wide of the disease.

ENDOTHELIOMA, OR ENDOTHELIAL SARCOMA [1]

Tumours of this nature starting in the lymph spaces or blood-vessels of the tongue have been described by Eve and others. They appear to vary much in malignancy, in some instances growing slowly and causing a local invasion only. At the present time much uncertainty exists as to the exact nature of some of the tumours which have been described as endotheliomas. Here, as

[1] *See also* Vol. I., p 498.

elsewhere, there appears to be a growing tendency on the part of pathologists to classify as endotheliomas many of the growths which have been hitherto accepted as carcinomas. Only one instance of the kind has come under my notice : a nodular tumour, unaccompanied by marked ulceration, occupying the posterior part of the right side of the tongue in a man of 60, was removed locally and submitted to microscopical examination ; the report stated that the structure was very unlike carcinoma, and that the condition was one of endothelial sarcoma. The patient refused the extensive operation that was proposed.

More information is still required on this subject, the chief difficulty at present being our inability to distinguish with certainty by microscopical examination between connective-tissue and epithelial cells.

CARCINOMA [1]

Few parts of the body are so susceptible to malignant change as the tongue, and in no position is its occurrence more distressing to the patient, or more trying to the surgeon, although at first sight it would appear more favourable to radical treatment than growths in many other situations.

Of all cases of cancer in the male sex, about 8 per cent. are cases of cancer of the tongue, according to the figures given by Butlin and Jessett ; while on comparing the relative frequency of the disease in the two sexes, allowing for some slight variations, the figures work out at 85 per cent. males to 15 per cent. females. This greater frequency in the male sex is no doubt due to the fact that the precancerous states induced by irritation and disease are commoner in the male than in the female.

Although the " cancerous " age may be taken as beginning at 40, cases of very malignant cancer have been recorded in quite young subjects—Variot has recorded a case in a boy of 11, Billroth in a patient of 18 ; while out of 290 cases recorded by Barker, in 8 the ages of the patients lay between 20 and 30. Nor does old age confer immunity, although after 70 the incidence of the disease is rare. O. Weber has observed a fatal case in a centenarian.

Etiology. Predisposing causes.—Whatever the future may have to show as to the cause of cancer, in no situation do the predisposing causes of irritation and inflammation play such an important part in encouraging the disease as in the tongue ; and until our knowledge of the actual cause becomes more exact we must devote our attention specially to those factors which influence the incidence of a cancerous change.

It is now universally acknowledged that the chronic conditions of

[1] See also Vol. I., p. 535.

leucoplakia, and syphilitic fissuring, and unhealed ulceration are liable to become malignant. A tongue which for years has been in an unhealthy state, and in which there has been an irregular proliferation of epithelial and connective-tissue elements, is exactly the kind of soil in which the cancer cell grows and flourishes. This "precancerous condition," as it has been called, has attracted wide attention, and it is now recognized that chronic patches, inflammatory papillomas, or indurated fissures which do not subside under appropriate treatment should be dealt with surgically. We are as yet ignorant of the cause which converts these wavering tissues into actual cancer, but we know that the irritation of carious teeth and ill-fitting tooth-plates and the incautious use of caustics have a very serious effect. Butlin's dictum with regard to caustics should be quoted in full: " If there be one thing more harmful than another in the treatment of a simple indolent sore and affections of the tongue in persons over 30 years of age, it is the application of a strong caustic."

Smoking has always been credited with a considerable degree of importance in the production of cancer of the tongue, and it may act by first producing a condition of leucoplakia, then by additional irritation urging that on to a cancerous stage. It is probably the kind of smoking indulged in that is of special importance ; " hot smoking " with short pipes, and especially rough-stemmed pipes, such as clays, is more dangerous than other forms.

Syphilis is another predisposing cause, not only from its tendency to produce chronic inflammatory conditions, but from its liability to leave thin, unstable scars or fissures which readily become the seat of carcinoma.

The position with regard to our present knowledge of the etiology of cancer may be summed up as follows : There exists under normal circumstances a " balance of power " between the epithelial and connective tissues of the body, possibly between individual cells also ; in parts which are the subject of chronic inflammatory processes, or subjected to prolonged irritation, that balance is disturbed, either in the shape of abnormal activity conferred on one cell element, the epithelial, or a diminished control on the part of another, the connective-tissue. Then comes the actual exciting cause, which we have yet to discover, whether a parasite or some peculiar inherited property possessed by the cells ; it is here that the border-line which separates the precancerous from the cancerous stage is passed, a border-line indistinguishable by the clinical eye and not always clearly defined to the pathological. From now onwards it is an unequal fight. The cancerous epithelial cells are pitted against the resistant power of the connective-tissue cells, and the victory is nearly always with the former. In order that in future our treatment may be successful, we must operate at the earliest possible moment; by surgical activity in the unstable precancerous stage we may hope to avert a malignant catastrophe, while by extensive operations along modern lines when the disease has declared itself we may hope to improve results which in the past have been indeed deplorable.

Pathology.—Most cancers of the tongue are squamous-celled epitheliomas, due to the downgrowth of epithelial columns from the surface. Steiner has recorded a case of columnar carcinoma. Starting from the surface, the cells penetrate between the muscular fibres in a series of vertical columns which tend to anastomose and to develop cell-nests; it is the presence of a number of these cell-nests, due to a corneous degeneration of the central cells of the tubular down-growth, which conclusively denotes a cancer on section. This spread is accompanied by an active proliferation of round connective-tissue cells at the periphery, a reaction which we must regard as in part protective, a poor attempt to limit the relentless growth. It is the connective-tissue proliferation which produces the " infiltration " of the tongue substance, and is also responsible for the fixation of the organ that occurs at a later date.

The superficial cells of the growth degenerate partly from lack of nutrition, partly as the result of the action of the connective-tissue cells, and thus give rise to surface ulceration. Those cases where the growth appears as a nodule in the tongue substance are examples of delay of the degeneration and consequent ulceration.

In some instances the growth and spread of the epithelial cells is extraordinarily rapid, and the term medullary carcinoma is applied. In others the process is slow and is accompanied by the develop-ment of mature fibrous tissue from the active connective-tissue cells surrounding the downgrowth of epithelium ; this form is sometimes referred to as the scirrhous type. The importance of these varieties in course and prognosis will be considered later.

Glandular infection.—Sooner or later the cancer cells detached from the primary focus find their way into the lymphatic channels and reach the glands which drain the region. These have been already described. The glands, when attacked, increase in size, and at first appear as hard movable masses, tending later to fuse and to undergo two special changes peculiar to secondary cancer of the tongue, mouth, and lip, namely, cystic degeneration and suppuration. The cystic change is mainly the result of necrosis of the central cells ; suppuration is due to a bacterial infection which accompanies the cancer cells to their destination in the glands.

Clinical appearance and classification.—Cancer of the tongue appears in a number of different forms, the variation being due, first, to the primary condition of the organ in which the growth has started; secondly, to peculiarities in the growth itself; thirdly, to the amount of resistance that it encounters on its way.

1. **Papillary form.** — Two varieties are seen : (1) The small indurated papillomatous cancer, which has started in a plaque or neglected leucoplakial patch, and is only recognized by its induration. Very often a deep fissure can be seen traversing the papillary area. (2) The large fungating cauliflower-growth. I have seen two marked cases of this form. The appearance at first sight did not suggest a cancer, but rather a benign papilloma. There was, however, a history of rapid growth, and the mass was much larger and whiter than is usual with the simple papilloma. In both instances there was a curious absence of induration. The diagnosis of cancer was confirmed by microscopical examination, but in each instance there was rapid and fatal recurrence after operation. I regard this type as exceptionally malignant.

2. **Nodular form.** — The nodular type is somewhat rare. It appears as a hard nodule or plaque which seems situated in the tongue substance, closely simulating a primary chancre. There is little or no ulceration, because the degenerative process is not marked. In a case of this kind under my care I was very doubtful of the diagnosis until I had removed the mass and submitted it to microscopical examination. On squeezing the mass before excision, I made caseous matter ooze from a small opening on the surface, and thought I had to deal with a chronic inflammatory mass, possibly caused by a foreign body. The pathologist's report left no room for doubt.

3. **Ulcerous form.** — This is the common variety, but here again the ulcer may present itself in a number of different guises, depending upon the rate at which it spreads, the presence or absence of an active bacterial infection, or upon the particular type of ulcer, such as a dental ulcer, on which the cancerous process has been grafted.

The chief characteristics of the typical cancerous ulcer are as follows : It is usually situated at the side of the tongue, very commonly at the posterior part, and the tongue, being fixed by the infiltration, is protruded with difficulty. In advanced cases the patient may not be able to open his mouth widely. There is an abundance of saliva, which runs away when the mouth is opened.

The surface of the ulcer is usually foul and covered with food, bacteria, and epithelial débris ; the edges are raised, and for a distance of a quarter of an inch or more the thickened epithelium of the margin stands out as a white or yellowish-white band from the surrounding normal cuticle. This peripheral thickening of the epithelium is present in epitheliomas of the lip, and is an important detail.

On passing the finger over and round the ulcer the edges feel hard and indurated, like cartilage, while a mass can be detected in the tongue substance continuous with the ulcer. The surface bleeds readily on examination.

If the mouth has been kept clean, and especially if, with the idea of cleaning up a dental ulcer, washes have been ordered or iodide of potash prescribed, the appearance may be different.

The surface of a foul ulcer readily cleans under proper treatment, and sloughs and offensive smell may both be absent.

4. **The fissured form** commences in the cracks or clefts left after chronic glossitis, syphilis, and more rarely tuberculosis. Fissured cancer is uncommon, and is difficult to diagnose in the early stages; the chief features being the callous character of the ulcer and the induration of its edges.

5. **Indurative form** ("wooden tongue").—The whole tongue becomes peculiarly fixed, shrunken, and hard, often as the result of previous inflammatory changes. The amount of ulceration present may be quite slight, and may be overlooked when situated at the posterior part.

An attempt has thus been made to describe the chief clinical varieties of the disease; and it may be well to emphasize again the fact that ulceration, although usual, does not invariably accompany the development of cancer.

6. **Double epithelioma.**—Diffuse and hypertrophic forms have been described.

Situation.—Any part of the tongue may be attacked, but the disease is much commoner in the anterior two-thirds. The sides of the tongue, more liable to irritation, are also more liable to cancer. I have seen a great many cases at the junction of the anterior faucial pillar with the side of the tongue.

Cancers at the back of the tongue are easily overlooked; they spread rapidly and deeply, and are difficult to deal with.

Epithelioma may affect the tongue from surrounding structures, such as the floor of the mouth, tonsil, and lip, but these will be considered under their respective headings.

Symptoms.—Pain, salivation, bleeding, inability to open the mouth, are some of the symptoms which cause a patient to seek relief. Pain often referred to the ear is common in cancers at the back of the tongue. The pain in the ear is generally regarded as referred from the lingual to the auriculo-temporal, but it may well be connected with the course of the glosso-pharyngeal or vagus, especially the latter, since similar auricular pain is common in cancer of the larynx. Sometimes pain is curiously absent, and the patient comes dissatisfied with the non-healing of an ulcer, or delays seeking advice until a large fungating mass involves the tongue. Salivation is usually present and troublesome.

Inability to open the mouth is a late symptom and due to the infiltration spreading back into the tonsillar region ; rarely it is due to reflex pain.

Hæmorrhage in the early stages is always slight, and, even when the growth is advanced, serious hæmorrhage in the primary focus is rare, though it is more common and fatal from the secondary deposits.

Course.—The disease, when once established, progresses steadily to a fatal termination within one or two years, unless arrested by operative treatment. In some cases, death has occurred as early as five months from the first appearance of the disease.

To the gradual but definite spread of the lingual growth there is added, sooner or later, the glandular infection. No exact period can be laid down before which it may be safe to assume that the glands have escaped ; it is again a question of resistance and virulence. The natural resistance which the tissues are able to offer to the spread of the growth may prevent lymphatic permeation for several months ; on the other hand, a growth of high malignancy fostered on a fertile soil may spread with appalling celerity to the glands and involve them extensively. Nor, again, are we able accurately to determine the state of the glands on clinical examination. In the early stages of their infection the small shotty glands are quite out of reach of the examining finger.

It is true that a growth accompanied by sloughing and ulceration will give rise early to inflammatory glandular enlargement, an enlargement which may subside after the growth has been removed, but we cannot with any safety rely on this to help us, for cancer cells may have settled in the glands at the same time as the bacteria, and, if the glands are left, these cells will, by their progressive development, ultimately render an operation for their removal imperative—an operation which perhaps has been most unwisely deferred.

In all cases in which cancer in the tongue is proved we must assume infection of the glands.

If the case is seen too late for operative treatment, there is nothing to look forward to but a horrible, lingering agony, to which the final complication comes as a great relief. Progressively, the ulcer increases in size ; food is taken only with difficulty ; pain, fetor, and salivation combine to render the patient unbearable to himself and to those who surround him ; the glands enlarge, break down and ulcerate ; and death is happily ushered in by a fatal hæmorrhage or a low form of pneumonia. Probably few have watched the final struggles of these exhausted patients, and only those who have can realize the extent of the misery which the disease entails. It is well that this should be fully appreciated before a decision is arrived at that a case is inoperable, since, even if only the primary growth can be dealt with, death from glandular recurrence is infinitely less painful.

The rapid spread of lingual carcinoma has been explained by Heidenhain as due to the contractions of the lingual muscles, which are constantly forcing on the cancer cells; but, apart from the glands, dissemination to a wide extent is uncommon, probably because the patient dies from the lingual or glandular disease before extensive metastases can form.

Diagnosis.—A certain diagnosis in cases of early carcinoma of the tongue is impossible without the aid of microscopical examination. In the more advanced cases, the pain, induration, thickened epithelial margin, fixation, and glandular enlargement, all indicate malignant disease. The chief difficulty will be experienced in distinguishing between carcinoma on the one hand, and a chronic ulcer from irritation, gummatous ulcer, and perhaps more rarely tuberculosis, on the other. A careful examination should be made of the mouth, to see whether a local cause, such as a rough carious tooth or an ill-fitting tooth-plate, exists. Careful inquiries into the history should be made, and the lungs should be thoroughly examined. If this investigation does not throw any light upon the case, no time should be wasted before making a careful microscopical examination of the margin of the growth; for this purpose it may be sufficient to snip off a small piece after the part has been painted with a 5 per cent. solution of cocaine, but I am of the opinion that it is far wiser to cut out a fair piece of growth and adjoining tissue. I have so frequently seen the futility of trying to form an opinion from a small piece of shrunken tissue. A mere scraping of the growth is, in my view, insufficient, even though it show a number of cell-nests; in order to be certain we must study the epithelial changes in relation to the adjoining connective tissues.

It has been argued that such an examination tends to disseminate the growth, and to excite it into abnormal activity. Personally I place no reliance on this statement, since, once it has been decided to examine a doubtful growth, a radical operation can be undertaken almost at once if the preparation of the section is hurried. I should regret it extremely if I had performed one of the extensive modern operations for cancer of the tongue on insufficient grounds.

On the other hand, no time should be wasted in trying potassium iodide, unless indeed the clinical condition of the ulcer and the past history should strongly favour syphilis. It is, unfortunately, a common line of treatment to combine the administration of iodide of potash with the application of antiseptic lotions to the ulcer. Under this combination cancerous ulcers will improve, the fetor and pain diminish, and even the induration will subside to some extent. Lulled into a state of false security, patient and surgeon allow valuable time to elapse, and then, when the true state of affairs is realized, the ulcer is probably much more advanced, and less favourable for treatment than it was at first.

If there is an obvious source of irritation, let it be removed, and let the ulcer be treated with a mild antiseptic and occasional touches of chromic acid ; strong caustics are never to be applied. If there is no obvious improvement in ten days, remove a piece of the margin for examination as suggested above.

Tuberculosis should be less frequently confused with cancer, as it is much rarer and occurs in younger subjects, who are generally sufferers from pulmonary tubercle ; Nedopil, however, cut out several tuberculous ulcers under the impression that they were cancerous. As this is a recognized treatment for tuberculous ulcers, no harm is done, provided nothing very extensive is attempted. In a case of my own, in a man of 65, a large ulcer sprang from the side of the tongue, crossed the mouth, and involved the lower jaw extensively. There were hard, enlarged glands in the submaxillary triangle. All who saw him agreed that the condition was malignant, and the general appearance certainly favoured this diagnosis. I removed the growth and the glands at one sitting, and he did very well, recovering completely ; but further microscopical examination showed that the growth and glands were tuberculous.

Prognosis.—Unless a lingual cancer is operated upon, death is certain. Unfortunately, the operative results still leave much to be desired. They will be considered later.

Treatment.—Cases of carcinoma which come for treatment fall into four main groups :—

1. The condition is inoperable ; it is not reasonable to attempt to remove even the primary growth ; palliative measures alone must be employed.

2. The condition is too advanced to permit of complete extirpation, but local removal of the primary focus may be attempted, with the view of prolonging life and averting some of the horrible terminal complications. This applies especially to carcinoma situated in the posterior part of the tongue.

3. There is a good or reasonable chance of clearing away the disease. Here each case must be judged on its merits, and the opinion of different surgeons will vary as to what may be considered operable or otherwise. No absolute rules can be laid down. Extensive and fixed glandular metastases will contra-indicate a complete operation. Extensive local spread may do the same, but with the knowledge of the certain fatal issue and its attendant sufferings we should be ready to operate on all but the most hopeless.

4. The disease is very early; the diagnosis may be doubtful, and glandular metastases are not obvious.

The results of operative treatment up to the present have not been very encouraging, largely owing to the fact that the lymphatic spread has only recently been emphasized and appreciated. The trend of modern surgical opinion is towards a free removal of the tongue and a complete removal of the lymphatic areas that drain it.

As a preliminary to any operative treatment, some effort should be made to get the mouth into as clean a state as possible. Absolute asepsis cannot be attained, but obviously carious teeth should be removed or filled, the others should be scaled, and a week may be spent in frequent irrigation of the oral cavity. The best solutions for this purpose are weak permanganate of potash, carbolic acid 1–100, bicarbonate of soda 30 gr. to the ounce, or peroxide of hydrogen 5 vols. I recommend carbolic acid; it is cleanly and sedative, though slightly painful at first. A solution of bicarbonate of soda to alternate with the carbolic is distinctly useful, as it is a solvent of the mucus and allays acid fermentation better than do acid antiseptics. Similar solutions may be used after the operation. Formamint lozenges are valuable.

I advise patients to brush the teeth three times a day, and to wash the mouth out well every hour or half-hour while they are in the house. At the same time it is not necessary to confine a patient to the house for the whole week; he should be encouraged to go out and occupy his mind as far as possible with things around him. These days of waiting may be usefully employed in training him to the use of the nasal or stomach tube, and in accustoming him to swallow from the rubber tube attached to the " feeder."

If the disease is advanced, the patient should rest in bed, and be fed with stimulating foods, strong soups, some alcohol, and possibly nutrient enemas.

If he is old and enfeebled, injections of glucose (6 per cent.) and normal saline should be given per rectum, one pint every four hours during the two days that precede the operation. Glucose, when so administered, has a powerful stimulating effect.

I have had no experience of the use of antistreptococcic serum, and cannot appreciate its value unless it is known that the wound is infected with the particular group of streptococci from which the serum was prepared. The blind administration of these serums seems unscientific and unsatisfactory; it would be much better, in my opinion, to take a few cultures from the mouth beforehand, and to prepare a vaccine for any obvious growths of streptococci and staphylococci.

OPERATIVE METHODS

In a discussion concerning the various operative procedures for cancer of the tongue the following points have to be especially considered :—

1. A preliminary laryngotomy or tracheotomy.
2. The preliminary ligation of the blood-vessels.
3. The relative order in which the growth and the glands should be attacked.
4. The amount of lingual tissue to be removed.

1. Should a preliminary laryngotomy or tracheotomy be done?—The objects which have induced operators to perform this initial step have been : first, to prevent blood trickling down into the lungs during the performance of the operation ; secondly, to prevent suffocation from the falling-back of the stump of the tongue subsequently ; thirdly, to prevent septic pneumonia— the pharynx being plugged for some days, the patient is allowed to breathe only through the artificial opening.

The answer to the question must, to a large extent, depend upon the nature of the operation to be attempted. If the more formidable lateral operation of Kocher is selected, a preliminary opening of the trachea may be an advantage, as a large wound is left in the mouth and neck from which discharges may infect the lungs unless the wounded area is kept carefully plugged. There are, however, other less objectionable measures at our disposal, and there is at present a strong opinion against the performance of tracheotomy.

In the milder procedure of Whitehead, when only one half of the organ is removed by the intrabuccal method, even a preliminary laryngotomy is not always required. Nor is it necessary in the cases where the median method of Syme is chosen, since here the patient's head is propped up, the jaw is divided in the middle line, and all the blood escapes externally.

Again, when the vessels are secured during the dissection of the glands, the final stage of the removal of the tongue is accomplished without any bleeding at all, and in these circumstances laryngotomy is not required.

Where the more extensive operations are attempted, especially those designed to remove growths situated posteriorly, I am strongly of the opinion that a laryngotomy should be performed, the entrance to the larynx being firmly plugged with a soft marine sponge. There is no doubt that this preliminary step enables the operator to act with greater deliberation and confidence.

Laryngotomy should be preferred to tracheotomy on account of its greater simplicity and its freedom from complications ; but if the operator makes his opening in the air-passage with the idea of preventing the patient from breathing air which has passed over the oral wound before it is clean, then tracheotomy and not laryngotomy should be performed. A laryngotomy tube is not tolerated for any length of time, and I advise its removal either at the end of the operation or not later than the following day.

The introduction into the practice of surgery of nasal anæsthesia by means of tubes introduced into the larynx through the nares, and of the administration of ether by the intravenous method, may do much to render these preliminary operations unnecessary. Intravenous anæsthesia has much to recommend it, especially for extensive operations on the mouth.

2. **Preliminary ligation of the blood-vessels.**—Dawbarn of Philadelphia has written very forcibly on the subject of preliminary or temporary ligation of the blood-vessels before attempting an extensive removal of the tongue, and before operations on the mouth and jaws. There is no doubt that this control is largely to the surgeon's and the patient's advantage, though, again, the performance of this step must depend upon the particular procedure to be attempted.

If the surgeon decides to attack the glands in the neck before the disease in the mouth, usually, when the glandular involvement is advanced, the external carotid and its branches, the lingual and facial, are exposed in the course of the dissection, on one or occasionally on both sides, and deliberately ligatured, the carotid being secured between the lingual and superior thyroid branches. The removal of the tongue may conclude the operation, as mentioned below; or this final procedure may be deferred. The objection to this is that there is considerable chance of the tongue becoming gangrenous when its blood supply has thus been cut off.

The old operation of ligature of the lingual artery, beneath the hyo-glossus, should remain only as a dissecting-room exercise, and should cease to occupy any place in the surgery of lingual cancer. In cases where it was desired to perform an extensive removal of the tongue the operation failed in its object, as the vessel was often cut through on the proximal side of the ligature, and in any case the dorsalis linguæ branch was frequently not controlled.

Ligation of the external carotid and its branches ensures occlusion not only of the lingual but also of the facial, which gives branches to the tonsillar region.

Temporary closure of the common carotid is practised by Crile in his extensive " block dissection " of the neck, and will be considered later, but it is not recommended, as the consequences of closing the vessel, even for a short time, have been very serious.

3. **Relative order in which growths and glands should be removed, and the question of removing the glands from the opposite side of the neck.**—There is much difference of opinion on these points, and I will briefly review the chief arguments for and against the various procedures.

By primary removal of the lingual growth the mouth can be got healthy and clean, the patient relieved of pain, and when he has recovered from this operation the glands can be removed by a systematic dissection.

As an objection it is urged that such an operation does not remove all the infected tissue, since, if we are to operate here on the same lines as are practised in the surgery of the mamma, the growth and lymphatics should be removed in continuity.

This is certainly a sound objection, but it has been met with the statements (1) that lymphatic infection in lingual cancer is by embolism and not permeation, and that the portions of the lymph system left between the tongue and the glands do not contain cancer cells ; (2) that the operation is much more severe if both glands and growth are removed in continuity—the cellular tissue of the neck is put into free communication with the mouth, and various septic complications are likely to arise.

If the first of these two statements is correct—and we have no evidence in its favour—there is good ground for separating the two operations. Personally, however, from the study of sections, I think there is considerable danger of leaving some portion of the growth behind, and pathological opinion favours the idea that this disease spreads by permeation and not by embolism.

Lenthal Cheatle has been kind enough to show me some of the work he has done in connexion with lingual cancer. The sections are entirely convincing, and they show a steady spread of the growth by permeation between the muscular fibres of the hyo-glossus in lateral cancer, of the genio-hyo-glossus in median cancer. Recurrence after operation results, in my opinion, from such infected areas being left in the portion of the tongue attached to the hyoid bone, from which situation, as it were from a primary focus, the growth is disseminated towards the glands. The tendency of the growth will be to spread away from the mouth, and this accounts for the fact that recurrence in the mouth is rare.

With such evidence before me, and as the result of my own experience, I have no hesitation in saying that the soundest operation consists in removing glands and tongue simultaneously through a wide incision in the neck. Particulars of the operation will be given later. It is a dangerous procedure, however, when both sides must be attacked ; but when only one side is attempted it is very satisfactory and the wound heals well, if care has been taken in preparing the mouth.

Many surgeons are of opinion that, having in mind the risks and dangers of the operation mentioned above, the needs of the case are adequately met by removing the tongue first by means of an intrabuccal operation, the glands being dissected out by a routine dissection in ten days' time. Such a procedure may pass as satisfactory in early cases, or if it is the intention of the surgeon to perform a palliative operation. In most cases, however, it must be regarded as incomplete.

If the operation *must* be performed in two stages, especially in advanced cases, it would seem better to dissect the triangles of the neck, ligating the external carotid on one or both sides, and then in a week or so to remove the tongue very freely by some intrabuccal method.

There is still another detail for consideration, and that is whether the glands should be removed from both sides of the neck. As before stated, the tendency in modern surgery is to progress to more radical methods, but at the same time these methods should be checked by pathological and clinical observations.

It will be seen from the description of the lymphatics of the tongue (p. 165) that certain vessels near the middle line communicate with the glands on both sides. The same occurs in the case of the lymphvessels at the tip. In cancers situated near the middle line or tip of the tongue, *both* triangles, therefore, should be attacked.

Cancer of the posterior third of the tongue also leads to rapid bilateral glandular infection, and in these cases the glands must be removed from both sides as a routine.

Out of 27 cases of lingual cancer carefully examined post mortem by Dr. Kettle, pathologist to the Cancer Hospital, the glands were affected on both sides of the neck in 11. Out of 6 cases of cancer in the floor of the mouth, both sides of the neck were attacked in 5. Obviously, therefore, in cancer situated in the floor of the mouth that is presumably near the middle line, the glands on both sides must be removed. With regard to other cases of lingual cancer, when but a small part of the side of the tongue is affected it will be sufficient to remove the glands on the affected side only, but *they must, of course, be removed even if the disease is met with at an early stage, and although they may show no obvious infection.*

In more extensive cases both sides must be operated upon.

In clearing away the glands in the anterior triangles of the neck it must be remembered that, in order efficiently to remove those embedded in the substance of the submaxillary salivary gland, this latter must be sacrificed. It is also well to remember that at least one of this submaxillary group is actually on the face at the anterior border of the masseter.

One. point in the figures supplied by Kettle is very striking, and that is the rarity of anything like general dissemination. Out of 33 cases, distant dissemination was noticed only in 5 :—

Axilla and bronchial glands	1
Spleen	1
Lung	1
Lung and pleura, 4th rib	1
Cutaneous. nodules over clavicle	1

It may be argued that patients with lingual cancer die before the period of general dissemination is reached, these cases thus differing from cases of mammary cancer ; but it is certainly striking that in 40 per cent. of fatal cases the glands on both sides of the neck are affected, and it suggests the lines on which further research is needed and along which operations should proceed.

4. **The amount of lingual tissue to be removed.**— By the ordinary intrabuccal operation of Whitehead only that portion of the tongue that is covered with mucous membrane, or little more, is removed ; and, as Cheatle very truly says, the tongue does not merely consist of the part that is visible in the mouth, but of a considerable extrabuccal portion extending to the hyoid bone. It would be regarded as an example of the most imperfect surgery if a surgeon were locally to excise a carcinoma of the breast or a carcinoma of the cervix uteri ; and so, in cases of lingual cancer, the entire half of the tongue must be removed down to the hyoid bone in cases where the growth is situated laterally, the entire organ when situated centrally.

As can be seen from Plate 88, the growth spreads along the lymph spaces in the hyo-glossus and genio-hyo-glossus muscles, inferior lingualis, and stylo-glossus, and therefore *every part of the affected muscle must be cleared away* in as systematic a manner as the great pectoral is removed in carcinoma mammæ.

There is a further important detail : Cheatle's specimens show the presence of glands between the fibres of the hyo-glossus, and dissemination of cancer cells in the lymph spaces of the submucosa for a considerable distance away from the primary focus, and such evidence proves the risk of partial operations in any but very early cases.

In cancer of the tip of the tongue the spread of the disease, as shown in the diagram of the lymphatics (Plate 86), is through the genio-hyoids, and *these muscles, together with the fascia covering them, must be removed.*

It has been urged that in all cases the whole tongue should be excised, but I am quite unable to agree with this suggestion. As has been shown, the tendency of the growth is to spread along

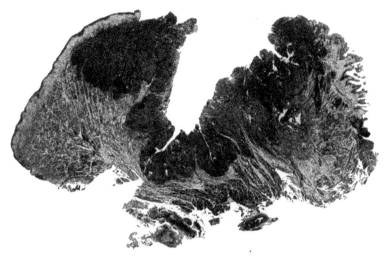

Fig. 1.—Section of tongue showing cancerous growth invading the genio-hyo-glossus.

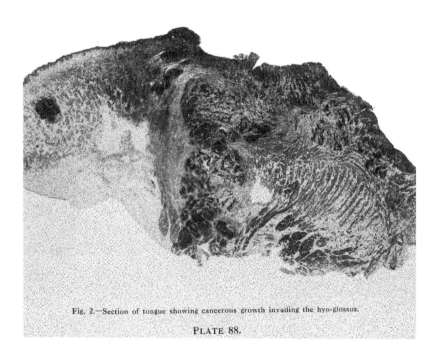

Fig. 2.—Section of tongue showing cancerous growth invading the hyo-glossus.

PLATE 88.

the muscles on the affected side ; indeed, *the septum appears to exercise a limiting influence.* Recurrence on the opposite side of the tongue is very rare, and the more extensive operation of complete removal should be reserved for those cases in which it is obvious that both sides are involved, or in which there is disease of the opposite half demanding removal.

Large ulcerating and infiltrating growths will require complete removal, and so will most of the growths situated in the posterior part.

THE OPERATIONS FOR LINGUAL CANCER

1. **Whitehead's intrabuccal operation and its modifications.**—This method consists in removing the whole or half of the tongue through the oral cavity, any of the preliminary steps mentioned previously, such as laryngotomy or ligation of the external carotid or lingual, being performed according to the opinion of the operator.

In cases where sufficient room cannot be obtained by the introduction of the gag, the cheek may be split back towards the masseter on the affected side. If it is desired to follow out the recommendations given above, and remove the muscular tissue down to the hyoid bone, this additional step will be found to give easy access. I have no hesitation in recommending it, as we must no longer consider the question of deformity, but endeavour to remove the disease completely. By such an operation as this, with subsequent dissection of the glands, the requirements of the early case are met.

Position of the patient.—This must depend upon whether a preliminary laryngotomy has been performed or not. If this has been done, and the back of the pharynx has been firmly plugged, the position of the patient is only of importance to the operator ; the head may be raised or turned on the side, whichever appears the more convenient.

When no laryngotomy has been done, even if the large vessels have been tied, there is always a risk of blood trickling down the larynx into the lungs and favouring the development, later, of septic pneumonia. There are two positions in which the patient may be placed which will tend to prevent this :—

i. *Rose's position.*—A sandbag is placed under the shoulders, and the head is allowed to hang back over the end of the table so that the mouth and throat are on a lower level than the trachea ; in this position little blood, even when the bleeding is free, can pass into the lungs. Unfortunately the position causes great congestion of the veins and venous bleeding.

ii. *The lateral position.*—The patient lies on his side with the head unsupported by a pillow and turned forwards and downwards towards the surgeon ; in this position the blood tends to run out of the angle of the mouth. Special gags which do not interfere with this position will be required.

Gags.—The surgeon will with advantage take some care in the selection of his gags for these cases. Nothing is more annoying, even dangerous occasionally, than the slipping of the gag or the inability to expose the parts thoroughly. Butlin recommends Coleman's gag ; Jacobson, Hewitt's modification of Mason's gag. Lane's or Wingrave's is a useful instrument when the head is turned on the side, as there are no handles to get in the way. A pair of large lip and cheek retractors should be at hand.

When only half the tongue is to be removed, the gag is placed on the side opposite to that affected, but a second gag is often required.

Sponges.—Although marine sponges have been abandoned for modern surgical work in the abdomen, they have a distinct field of usefulness in operations on the mouth and throat, and are strongly recommended. It will be found, however, that the coarse Turkey sponge is much more serviceable than the finer sponges usually employed, as it absorbs blood better and does not get so slimy. One dozen small swabs, to be used on holders, and three or four larger ones, each firmly secured by a stout silk thread, should be in readiness. These are wrung out of weak carbolic (1–100), and are placed in charge of a nurse, who rinses and returns them clean to the surgeon as he requires them.

The anæsthetic.—When anæsthesia has been induced, the administration may be continued either through the laryngotomy tube or the nose, as the case may be. Chloroform is the best anæsthetic. The laryngeal reflex should not be lost. Intubation anæsthesia is largely employed in America.

Operation.—The mouth being widely opened, two stout threads are passed through the tip of the tongue, one on each side of the middle line. A further thread may with advantage be passed through the base of the organ close to the epiglottis, of course wide of the disease. This step is especially advantageous when the whole tongue is to be removed, and is usually required at the completion of the operation, to prevent the stump falling back and occluding the larynx ; as a preliminary measure it will facilitate the protrusion of the tongue and also the dragging of the bleeding-point into view in the event of hæmorrhage.

The tongue is now pulled well forwards by means of the ligatures, and the surgeon cuts through the tongue along the middle line of the dorsum from base to tip by means of a knife (Fig. 339). This incision is deepened, by cutting, blunt dissection, or tearing, to the hyoid bone. The mucous membrane is then cut through with scissors, around the affected half, from the frænum anteriorly, to the anterior pillar of the fauces posteriorly. If necessary, this latter structure is divided. As much mucous membrane as possible should be left, as it falls into position and covers the raw surfaces, but the first essential is to cut wide of the growth.

If the disease is situated near the anterior part of the tongue, it is advisable to draw one or two incisors, so that the scissors can be dipped down behind the jaw close to the bone.

The affected half is now free internally and laterally, so that by

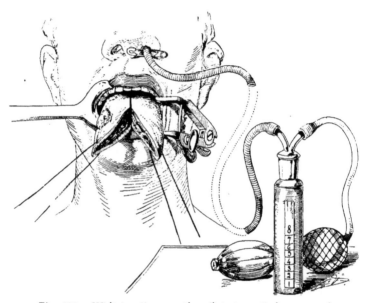

Fig. 339.—Whitehead's operation (intrabuccal) for removal of half the tongue. (*After Fowler.*)

traction on the suture it can be dragged well out of the mouth. By a series of short scissor-cuts, beginning in front, the deep attachments to the hyoid bone are severed ; this dissection should be very thorough, every effort being made to remove the muscular fibres right down to the hyoid. The half of the tongue will now be attached posteriorly only, and contains the lingual arteries still intact. If these have not been secured previously, they may be exposed before division, as follows : A number of short snips are made through the posterior attachments of the organ, with separation of the muscular fibres : near the middle line the artery will start into view as a bluish cord, and can then be secured with forceps or, better, ligatured by means of an aneurysm-needle, before the final severance of the affected portion. It is well worth while to spend a little time securing the vessel, for the lingual tissue is extremely friable, and as the tongue is brought forward under tension the forceps may be dragged off and troublesome bleeding may ensue; if this does occur, the fingers should be passed back beyond the epiglottis and the base of the tongue should be hooked forward, after the method recommended by Heath—a step which, while it checks the bleeding, temporarily enables the stump to be brought well into view.

Cathcart (quoted by Jacobson) secures the artery in the following way : After the ordinary steps have been taken and the tongue, well freed, has been dragged out of the mouth, "the anterior border of the hyo-glossus is defined by a few vertical strokes of the director; this instrument is next insinuated beneath the muscle, the tissues being separated with the point before it is pushed in. The muscle is next carefully cut through on the director for about two-thirds of its extent (this incision should be close to the hyoid), and the fibres retracting leave the artery exposed at the bottom of the wound, covered only with a little connective tissue; it can be under-run with a ligature carried by an aneurysm-needle and leisurely tied." Whitehead relied mainly on twisting the artery, but it is wiser to ligature it with silk or chromicized catgut.

If the whole tongue is to be removed, it may be split, provided that the split does not pass through diseased tissue, and each half may be dealt with as recommended above; or each side may be freed without the median incision, and the arteries secured by the methods previously recommended. In any case when the whole organ is excised a stout ligature should be left through the stump close to the epiglottis to enable the surgeon to pull it forward in case of hæmorrhage, and also to prevent the falling back of the stump and consequent obstruction to respiration.

After the diseased tissues have been freely removed, any vessels which still bleed should be clamped, and tied if possible, but the friable tissue and the depth of the wound may make this procedure difficult. Any mucous membrane that is left should be used to cover over the raw surface, being fixed in position by catgut sutures; if only half the tongue has been excised, the anterior part may be folded back and used to cover the raw surface near the median line. Such a step checks the oozing and accelerates the healing of the wound.

If, in spite of the above precautions, bleeding still continues, gauze strips should be packed on to the raw surface.

Whitehead swabs the wound over with a special varnish, made by substituting for the spirit used in Friar's balsam a saturated solution of iodoform in turpentine or ether. Iodoform powder may be used instead. I recommend the use of antiseptics, especially of iodoform and carbolic, for these cases.

The gag is removed, and the suture through the lingual base is fixed to the cheek by a piece of strapping.

The after-treatment will be considered later.

2. **Kocher's submaxillary method.** — By this method, which was introduced by Professor Kocher in 1880, an attempt was made to remove the lymphatic glands, salivary glands, and tongue in

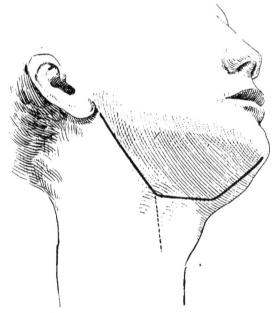

Fig. 340.—Lines of incision for modified Kocher's operation.

continuity, without cutting across infected lymphatic spaces ; further, a preliminary tracheotomy was performed, and the pharynx was kept plugged for some days until all danger of septic pneumonia was past. Although founded on a sound scientific basis, the method has not been very successful, and Kocher himself has abandoned it for the procedure usually described as Syme's operation (p. 225).

Cheatle's modification.—Lenthal Cheatle has described to me an operation which is a modification of Kocher's method, and which is believed to be an advance on many of the operations practised.

No preliminary tracheotomy or laryngotomy is done. A free incision .is made from the mastoid process to the symphysis, curving down below the hyoid, and a vertical or oblique incision is added below (Fig. 340). The dissection is then carried out from below upwards, all glands, fat, and fascia being dissected away from the main vessels. The facial and lingual arteries are tied near their origin. The interval between the posterior belly of the digastric and the mylo-hyoid is now sought for, and these muscles are retracted, the former backwards and downwards, and the latter forwards, its fibres being divided if necessary. The base of the tongue at its attachment to the hyoid is exposed, and the hyo-glossus is divided along its whole hyoid attachment close to the bone; continuing anteriorly, the genio-hyo-glossus is cut close to the jaw—a difficult step—and the median interval between the muscles is sought for. The genio-hyoid fibres of the genio-hyo-glossus are very rarely invaded and may be left. If only one half is to be removed, the mouth is now gagged open as in Whitehead's method, and the remaining attachments of the organ are divided as in that operation, the posterior division going back to the styloid process. Turning again to the neck, it will now be possible to remove the tongue and the other structures freed by dis-section in continuity, the separation being effected by a few touches of the knife. The wound is left widely open.

If the whole organ is to be removed, similar steps are taken on the opposite sides to free the deep attachments and to secure the main vessels; the oral mucous membrane is divided by the intra-buccal method, and the whole mass is extracted from the side first attacked.

Author's modification.—I have recently practised a modifica-tion of this operation for cases of cancer limited to one half of the tongue, with satisfactory results. The main points of difference are these :—

i. The three flaps fashioned by the skin incisions are turned upwards, backwards, and forwards, and consist of skin only, very little subcutaneous fat being left.

ii. The external carotid is ligatured as well as the lingual and facial arteries in the course of the dissection.

iii. The dissection is carried right on to the face, above the lower border of the mandible, so that the glands in the parotid and mas-seteric regions are removed.

iv. Everything except the main vessels and muscles is removed within the triangular area bounded by these flaps.

v. The attachment of the tongue to the hyoid bone is cut through.

vi. Before the final step of removing the tongue is attempted, the sterno-mastoid is stitched to the digastric and the hyoid muscles, so as to cover up the carotid and jugular vein, and the skin wound is partially closed.

vii. Half the tongue is excised from the mouth after White-head's method, the division of the muscles previously mentioned making it an easy matter to complete a free removal. There is no bleeding.

viii. I make it a point that the mouth and neck wounds should freely communicate with one another, so that I feel more certain that no "intervening" tissue has been left behind. The wound is packed with iodoform gauze.

ix. Enlarged glands on the opposite side are removed at a second operation.

I am quite satisfied with the procedure in cases where only half the tongue has to be excised. It seems sound and adequate ; there is no trouble with the wound in the neck, if sufficient care has been exercised in cleaning the mouth beforehand ; and I have not found that it puts the recuperative power of patients to any severe test. On the other hand, if both sides of the neck have to be attacked in more advanced cases, and the whole tongue has to be excised, the risk is very much greater ; but, in my opinion, it remains the best procedure for dealing with carcinoma of the tongue.

Whether the mortality which follows its employment will be so high as to render it unjustifiable remains as yet to be seen. Cheatle lays considerable stress on leaving the wounds widely open so that free drainage is obtained. He does not dissect the glands below the omo-hyoid at the time of the main operation, but defers that step, if required, until a later date.

The great dangers of the operation, apart from septic pneumonia, are sloughing, cellulitis, and secondary hæmorrhage ; but covering the wound surface with sterile vaseline, as suggested by Upcott of Hull for. operations on the tonsil, might possibly be of service in preventing cellular infection. I have been very pleasantly surprised to find how kindly these neck wounds heal, but I spend seven or eight days in preliminary cleaning of the mouth.

3. **Syme's operation.**—This operation is practically identical with that now performed by Professor Kocher. It consists essentially in dividing the soft tissues in the middle line from the lip to the hyoid bone, and sawing through the mandible so as to gain access to the mouth and hyoid regions. Kocher operates with the patient in the Trendelenburg position, but the operation can be efficiently performed if the head and shoulders are raised and held forwards as in operations upon the tonsils and throat.

If it be desired, lateral incisions may be carried outwards from the lower termination of the vertical incisions, and flaps can be dissected up, thus enabling the operator to remove the salivary and lymph-glands of the submaxillary triangle at the same time.

The actual operation is performed as follows : The anæsthetic having been administered (a preliminary laryngotomy or tracheotomy is not required), the surgeon divides the soft parts of the chin as far down as the hyoid bone. The vessels being secured, the jaw is drilled, without previous separation of the periosteum, below the teeth a quarter of an .inch on either side of the middle line, and is then sawn through. The two halves are forcibly retracted, the tongue is well drawn out by a loop of strong silk, the mucous membrane snipped through between the tongue and the alveolar 'process, and the anterior pillars of the fauces are divided. The genio-hyo-glossi and genio-hyoids (one side only if only half the tongue is to be removed) are now cut through, and the tissues of the floor of the mouth separated as deeply as necessary with scissors or bistoury aided by the finger, any vessels that require it being tied with silk. The tongue being thus freed laterally and below as far back as is needful, the transverse section is made one half at a time, the lingual arteries being secured as recommended above.

Bleeding is checked, the wound is treated by Whitehead's method, and the two halves of the jaw are united by wire ; the skin incision is sewn up, but a large drain is inserted into its lower end above the hyoid bone.

There is no doubt that this operation gives an easy access to the diseased organ, and it is especially valuable when the growth extends far back. At the same time, it is open to the objections that the lymphatic glands are not thoroughly removed, that there is some risk of cancer contamination of the wound, and that the jaw is liable to necrose near the saw-cut. In cases where the disease lies anteriorly and extends to the bone, the surgeon can by a simple modification remove growth and bone in continuity.

Regnoli's operation, which consists in an exposure of the tongue by a transverse incision below the jaw, with transverse division of the muscles attached to the hyoid, is rarely practised. It is most suitable in cases where the disease attacks the anterior part of the tongue and floor of the mouth.

Carless, quoted by Jacobson, recommends transhyoid pharyngotomy when the disease is far back, the anterior part of the tongue being saved.

When the growth affects the posterior part of the tongue or spreads back to the palate and tonsil a favourable result can be obtained but rarely, and very complicated and dangerous procedures, such as Langenbeck's method of slitting the cheek and dividing the jaw, will be required if complete extirpation is to be attempted. The results of those operations rarely justify their performance, and it must be admitted that cancer of the tongue far back is most unfavourable for·surgical treatment.

When the jaw is involved anteriorly, the outlook, though less hopeless, is distinctly unfavourable. An attempt should be made to remove the growth and the affected bone by some of the methods mentioned above; and it is often possible to leave a bridge of healthy bone from the lower border of the horizontal ramus, with the effect of contributing to the patient's comfort.

Whatever operation is performed, it is always advisable to pass a suture through the stump of the tongue, and to bring the suture out of the mouth and fasten it to the cheek or ear.

After-treatment in operations for lingual cancer.— For the first twenty-four hours, or longer in severe cases, the patient must be kept lying on the side or even on the face, with the head low, so that the discharges can trickle out of the mouth on to a pad of gauze or wool. A special nurse should always be in attendance, and should watch for bleeding (usually venous oozing) and for obstruction to respiration. Bleeding as a complication will be considered later.

If the breathing becomes obstructed, the stump of the tongue should be pulled forwards by means of the attached string; and if that fails, a finger should be passed to the base of the tongue, the pharynx cleaned, and the stump hooked forwards. These manœuvres usually succeed. Morphia, $\frac{1}{4}$–$\frac{1}{2}$ gr., should be given, and the patient should be fed by nutrient enemata and disturbed as little as possible.

If the weather is cold, screens or curtains should be placed round the bed, and a bronchitis kettle charged with some antiseptic, such as tinct. benz. co. or guaiacol carbonate, should be used to keep the air warm and moist. This is not intended to imply that every patient is to be kept in an atmosphere saturated with steam, but to suggest that there are very definite uses still for the steam-kettle. If the steaming is overdone there is a greater risk of pneumonia. Should the patient show signs of collapse after the operation, enemata of hot saline (103° F.) with strong coffee and brandy should be given.

During the first twenty-four hours the patient should not be disturbed; the mouth may be swabbed out occasionally with some weak permanganate of potash if there is any tendency to the collection of clots and mucus; but on the whole the quieter he is left the better, for frequent and unnecessary manipulations are decidedly harmful.

Small pieces of ice may be given to him if the mouth is dry and thirst is intense.

At the end of the twenty-four hours any gauze plugging that

has been introduced should be removed, and the routine treatment of the mouth undertaken. This consists in frequent irrigations and swabbings with weak antiseptics, preferably weak carbolic or permanganate of potash, alternated with a solution of bicarbonate of soda to get rid of the clinging mucus. A large irrigator fixed to the wall near the head of the bed, and fitted with a glass vaginal douche nozzle controlled by a tap or clip, allows the nurse, and afterwards the patient, to wash out the oral cavity very thoroughly; of course, provision must be made for free exit of the fluid.

The patient should be propped up in the sitting position for dressing and inspection of the mouth, which should be done in a good light, and in the less severe cases he may remain sitting up after the first twenty-four hours; in the more severe the recumbent posture must be maintained for two or more days.

Dawbarn insists on the need for keeping these patients in the Trendelenburg position until they are able to swallow, so preventing them from inhaling septic matter from the wound. This position is very uncomfortable for the patient, and, if the wound can be kept decently clean, is unnecessary; but if the wound is foul, owing to the loss of control of the epiglottis there is a real danger of septic particles finding their way down the larynx and trachea, and the position must be maintained.

Every two hours during the day, and every four during the night, the nurse on duty should gently wipe away blood and débris with a small, soft sponge moistened in antiseptic. The patient should be encouraged to irrigate his own mouth every hour during the day. Adherent blood-clot can be removed with forceps, but when sloughs appear the greatest care should be exercised in detaching them, as their removal may be followed by hæmorrhage. If the case goes well the patient should be got up in a chair on the third day. It will often be advisable to keep the patient recumbent for a longer period, and to delay his getting up if old and enfeebled, but the special points to attend to are frequent irrigations and the preservation of local cleanliness as far as it is possible to obtain it.

Feeding.—For the first twenty-four or forty-eight hours, food should be given rectally; after that, in many cases the patient is able to swallow, and the food is given by a feeder, to the spout of which is attached a rubber tube that can be passed well to the back of the throat. It is well to make a trial with some water first, in case the food should regurgitate and soil the wound.

All food given should be carefully sterilized until healthy granulations have covered the raw surface.

In the more severe cases the patient must be fed through nasal or œsophageal tubes until the power of swallowing is regained. Great care should be exercised in the feeding, and absolute cleanliness is essential.

Complications.—**Hæmorrhage** may occur shortly after the patient has been returned to bed, and is commoner after the more severe operations. It may be due to the slipping of a ligature, or to the opening up of veins which had ceased to bleed during the operation. Such a complication must be carefully watched for, since a sudden hæmorrhage of this kind may choke the patient, or by trickling down the trachea favour the development of septic pneumonia. If the bleeding is free, the mouth should be widely opened, clots swabbed out with a sponge, and a strip of gauze packed on to the bleeding area. If thought advisable, forceps may be applied and the vessel ligated.

True secondary hæmorrhage is rare, in spite of the often septic state of the wound ; even when extensive operations are done upon the neck, which is thrown into communication with the mouth, it is rare for the ligated vessels to bleed. The precaution should always be taken, in these cases, to tie the vessels a little distance, from half an inch to an inch, away from the main trunk ; if the external carotid is tied, it should not be secured too close to the common vessel.

Should this secondary bleeding occur, it is usually encountered when the sloughs separate, is rarely serious, and readily yields to treatment. The mouth should be opened widely, washed out and swabbed ; if the bleeding-point can be seen, it should be caught with forceps and a ligature applied. Failing this, it is often sufficient to pack a strip of gauze firmly down towards the bleeding-spot and get the patient to close his mouth upon it. As a temporary, even as a permanent, measure this is wonderfully efficient ; in the only case of secondary hæmorrhage under my care, this method of treatment was followed by the complete arrest of the bleeding.

Sloughing and cellulitis.—After extensive operations, especially where the mouth has been unusually septic beforehand, cellulitis may occur. It should be treated by free incisions and carbolic fomentations. As a preventive measure, few sutures should be employed in the large neck wounds, as they favour the retention of discharges. Frequent irrigations are the surest way of dealing with these infected wounds. I have no experience of antistreptococcic serum, but recommend the preparation and use of a vaccine.

This complication, following on a long and exhausting operation, is a very serious one, likely to lead to a fatal issue.

Septic pneumonia is responsible for the fatal termination of a large number of cases. More can be done to prevent it than to treat it when it has supervened. Local cleanliness, avoidance of hæmorrhage, and the adoption of a position of the patient favouring the free removal of discharges are to be strongly advocated. In very septic states, inhalations of guaiacol carbonate are of distinct value.

When signs of pneumonia have developed, every effort should be made to support the patient's strength with nourishing food and stimulants. A localized abscess or gangrene of the lung will probably require treatment, should the patient survive.

Removal of the glands.—If the intrabuccal method of

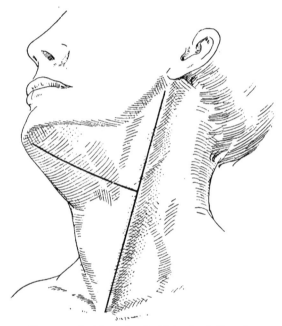

Fig. 341.—Incisions for Butlin's gland dissection.

.Whitehead is selected, whether the glands appear enlarged or not, a complete dissection should be made of the anterior triangle of the neck within ten days of the removal of the tongue. The indications for attacking both sides have been given already.

Butlin's method (Fig. 341).—The best method for removing the glands in early cases is that described by Butlin. Three flaps of skin, with very little subcutaneous fat, are dissected back, and then, starting from below upwards, everything is cleaned away in one sheet except the muscles and the large vessels. The submaxillary gland and the lower portion of the parotid gland should be removed deliberately. This point is especially important, as there are a number of lymphatic glands situated among the glandular alveoli in both instances. The wound should be freely drained. Healing is, as a rule, by first intention, and the results are excellent ; some saliva may escape from the posterior angle of the wound, but this soon ceases to run. I use two drains. The operator should bear in mind that the lymph-vessels from the tip of the tongue pass directly to the glands of the internal jugular vein.

Maitland's operation is somewhat more radical, and is suited to more advanced cases. The skin incisions are similar, except that the lower vertical incision is carried back along the clavicle. Maitland is careful not to leave the subcutaneous fat behind in the submental and submaxillary regions, as the glands here are very superficial. He begins his dissection posteriorly and above after reflection of his flaps, and insists on the removal of the lower part of the parotid and the whole of the submaxillary gland. Next he dissects the anterior triangle from below, dividing the sterno-mastoid, and then, working upwards, he approaches the region already attacked, finally severing the sterno-mastoid at its upper attachment. If necessary, he removes the internal jugular vein subsequently ; he does not recommend securing it before, as the veins become congested, and there is then a great deal of venous oozing. This is a very radical operation, and efficient ; it gives easy access to the upper deep cervical glands, which are reached with difficulty when the sterno-mastoid is preserved, and it is not open to the same objection as Crile's dissection, which entails temporary compression of the common carotid.

Block dissection, as practised by Crile, should be reserved for the most advanced cases. It is an operation of the greatest magnitude, and consists in removing the glands, the sterno-mastoid, and the internal jugular vein in one solid mass from below upwards. A clamp is placed on the common carotid artery. The main skin incisions are similar to those employed by Butlin.

Cases so advanced as to require these extremely radical measures are regarded by most surgeons as inoperable.

General conclusions with regard to operations for lingual cancer.—1. For very early cases the removal of the tongue by Whitehead's method, and dissection of the glands in ten days' time, may be adequate, but it is inferior to Butlin's.

2. For more advanced cases, with definite enlargement of the glands, Cheatle's modification of Kocher's operation is to be preferred. On the whole, I recommend this as the routine operation for all cases that permit of its being done.

3. If in these advanced cases a two-stage operation is decided upon, the glands should be attacked first, the external carotid or its branches should be tied, and the tongue should be excised later.

4. In all advanced cases, and in those specially mentioned above, the glands on the side opposite to the disease should be removed subsequently.

Results. Mortality.—Whitehead reports 101 cases with only 3 operative deaths. Butlin gives two tables, 11 out of 98 in the first series, 9 out of 99 in the second; the mortality in the second series would be lower but for the severe procedures practised in advanced cases. **Recurrence** has been the rule, the successful cases being 28 in the first series, 32 in the second. These are better figures than most surgeons can quote. If our results are to improve, we must operate early, and even more extensively than has been the custom in the past.

Some of the procedures described are still in the experimental stage, and very careful observations will be required to decide whether the simpler and less dangerous method of Whitehead is to be preferred, in spite of its incompleteness, or whether, by improvements in operative technique, we can so lower the mortality of the extensive and scientific modern operations as to make them more generally applicable.

Palliative treatment.—For the unfortunate patients who seek surgical advice when the growth has extended too far for radical treatment, little can be done beyond an attempt to relieve the more distressing symptoms—pain, salivation, and fetor. How far a surgeon is justified in removing a fungating cancer merely for the relief of the local condition must be left to his discretion, and the prospects of the case must be clearly explained to the patient.

Pain can be mitigated by local applications of cocaine and morphia, and the lingual nerve may be divided—a measure which is said to check the salivation. Ligature of the lingual arteries has little effect.

For the fetor no application is better than iodoform, but the odour of this drug is so disagreeable to some patients that carbolic acid, peroxide, thymol, or creosote may be used instead. Atropin, $\frac{1}{200}-\frac{1}{50}$ gr., combined with morphia, may be given liberally to ease the final stages of one of the most distressing diseases to which man is subject.

Radium treatment.—The emanations of radium contain certain rays, a, β, γ, which have a powerful action on the tissues of the body, the γ rays being very potent in restraining cell-activity, and so are of value in the treatment of cancer, nævi, etc. Radium should never be employed by anyone unfamiliar with its application and effects, but in suitable cases it is of decided assistance to the surgeon.

As in the case of nævi elsewhere, its action is prompt and

remarkable in bringing about a complete destruction of the nævoid tissue.

In cancer it should never be regarded as an alternative to operation if operation is feasible, but by its use an unfavourable growth will often improve so that an operation may be attempted; while, after an operation has been performed successfully, I am firmly of the opinion that the application of radium has some effect in preventing recurrence.

Radium may ease the pain in inoperable cases, but its curative effects on the cancer cell are much less marked in lingual cancer than in cancer situated elsewhere.

BIBLIOGRAPHY

Burton, *Lancet,* 1897, i. 241.
Butlin, *Diseases of the Tongue.* 1900.
Cooper, Bransby, *Guy's Hosp. Repts.,* 1837, ii. 404.
Da Costa, Keen's *Surgery,* iii. 666–9.
Dawbarn, *Treatment of Certain Malignant Growths by Excision of the External Carotids.* 1903.
Ducrot, Thèse de Paris, No. 355, 1879.
Duplay and **Reclus,** *Traité de Chir.,* 1898, v. 144.
Eve, *Proc. Roy. Soc. Med.,* 1910.
Fairbairn, *Med. Times,* 1845, xii. 392.
Fayrer, *Clin. Surg. in India,* p. 485. 1866.
Fournier, "Leçons sur les Syphilides tertiares de la Langue," École de Médecine, Paris, 1877.
Goadby, K. W., "Treatment of Pyorrhœa Alveolaris by Vaccines," *Brit. Journ. Dent. Sci.,* London, 1905, xlviii. 562, 963
Helbing, *Jahrbuch für Kinderheilkunde,* 1896, xl. 442.
Hennig, *ibid.,* 1877, xxi. 290.
Jacobson and **Rowlands,** *Operative Surgery,* i. 588. 1907.
Johnstone, *Laryngoscope,* St. Louis, 1908, xviii. 286–92.
Keith, Prof. A., *Human Embryology and Morphology,* p. 42. 1904.
Lapie, *Bull. de l'Acad. Roy. de Chir.,* Paris, 1857, iii. 16.
Levy, R., "Tuberculosis of the Mouth," *Amer. Laryngol., Rhinol. and Otol. Soc.,* St. Louis, 1907, pp. 253–63.
Maitland, *Austral. Med. Gaz.,* Oct., 1906.
Morestin, "Leucoplasie linguale étendue traitée par la Décortication," *Bull. de la Soc. Franç. de Derm. et de Syph.,* 1908, xix. 65.
Morrison, R., "The Diagnosis of some of the Common Ulcers of the Mouth," *Brit. Dent. Journ.,* 1907, xxviii. 1211–4.
Parrot, *Progrès Méd.,* Paris, 1881, p. 191.
Piersol, *Human Anatomy,* p. 954.
Pouzergues, Thèse de Paris, No. 229, 1873.
Reboul, Assoc. Franç. pour l'Avancement des Sciences, *Gaz. Hebd. de Méd. et de Chir.,* 1897, p. 786.
Sabrazès et **Bousquet,** *Presse Méd.,* 1897, p. 209.
Stone, W. G., "Lymphangioma of the Tongue," *Trans. Clin. Soc.,* 1907, xl. 280.
Tanturri, *Giorn. Ital. delle Mal. Vener. e della Pelle,* 1872, iv.
Upcott, "Operations on the Tonsil," *Lancet.*
Vanlair, *Rev. Mens. de Méd. et de Chir.,* Paris, 1880, p. 54.
Warren, J. C., "Cancer of the Mouth and Tongue," *Amer. Surg.,* Philadelphia, 1908, xlviii. 481–514.
Wharton, *Med. News,* Philadelphia, 1895, lxvi. 406.

THE SALIVARY GLANDS AND FLOOR OF THE MOUTH

By IVOR BACK, M.A., M.B., B.C.CANTAB.,
F.R.C.S.ENG.

INJURIES OF THE SALIVARY GLANDS

THE PAROTID GLAND

ANY of the salivary glands may be involved in an injury, but it is the parotid which is most frequently damaged in this way, on account of its comparatively exposed situation. The injury may be inflicted wilfully, as by stabbing or gunshot wounds, or accidentally, as during the course of a surgical operation. Armstrong of Montreal has recorded a case in which he accidentally injured the submaxillary gland while attempting to enucleate an overlying tuberculous gland. A fistula resulted which only closed after two further operations, in which the fistulous track was excised and the edges were approximated by deep sutures. Injuries involving the submaxillary or sublingual gland are of far less serious import than those in which the parotid is concerned, because if a permanent fistula results the gland can be excised completely with comparative ease and slight resulting disfigurement. But the parotid gland is so intimately connected with important structures that such a proceeding is rarely justifiable in its case unless the surgeon is dealing with a malignant new growth whose presence will inevitably cause the death of the patient. Injuries to the parotid may be subdivided according to whether the gland substance itself is injured, or its duct only.

INJURIES OF THE PAROTID GLAND SUBSTANCE

The tissue of the parotid gland is frequently incised during the course of surgical operations in the neck, but primary union nearly always follows if the wound is closed with deep stitches, and a salivary fistula from this cause is uncommon.

Treatment.—In dealing with an external wound of the parotid gland substance, the first duty of the surgeon is to exclude the presence

234

of injury to the important structures which traverse the gland, particularly the facial nerve. The trunk of the transverse facial artery or some of its branches may be severed, so that there is likely to be severe hæmorrhage. This must, of course, be arrested, and the wound sewn up. The important point to observe is that the sutures must pass down into the depths of the wound so that all the divided tissue is included ; otherwise, pockets may form which will prevent healing. If the edges are jagged the contused portions must be cut away. A firm bandage should then be applied. The patient should be kept on a simple diet which does not demand mastication, and talking should be forbidden until the wound is healed.

Injuries of the Parotid Duct (Stenson's Duct)

Stenson's duct is liable to injury in vertical wounds of the face which cross its course at right angles. The wound may or may not perforate the cheek and form an opening into the mouth. The prognosis is better in the former case, since if primary union of the divided ends does not occur (and, in spite of the statements of König, it rarely does occur) there is a possibility that the resulting fistula may become an internal one, and a spontaneous cure be thus effected.

When the wound has been cleaned and the hæmorrhage arrested, the divided ends of the duct will be seen protruding from the cut surfaces. The circumference of the duct is so small that partial division of it is rare.

Treatment. — König believes that many such injuries have remained unrecognized, and that primary union of the duct has occurred spontaneously. He maintains, therefore, that it is the duty of the surgeon to unite the divided ends with fine catgut sutures, and close the external wound. If any wound is present in the mucous membrane it should be left open. He lays stress on the importance of the after-treatment described in connexion with wounds of the parotid gland itself (*see* above). This operation is one of extreme difficulty in view of the diminutive circumference of the duct, and, in my opinion, primary union rarely, if ever, occurs. Moreover, if it fails, an external fistula is bound to ensue if the original wound was a non-penetrating one. A better chance of obtaining a successful result is ensured by converting a non-penetrating wound into a penetrating one by incising the mucous membrane. The external wound is then accurately closed. In the case of a wound which originally penetrated the mouth, closure of the external wound is all that is necessary. In a certain proportion of cases the external wound remains closed, and an internal fistula is formed, which, as far as functional activity is concerned, will answer all the purposes of the normal orifice of the duct.

SALIVARY FISTULÆ

The term salivary fistula is here taken to indicate an external fistula through which the secretion is discharged on to the surface of the cheek. Internal fistulæ exist, and are sometimes congenital. Bochdalek described one in which the opening into Wharton's duct was eleven lines behind the sublingual caruncle. But the condition does not present any surgical interest, since it causes the patient no inconvenience.

An external fistula, on the other hand, may render his existence miserable. The constant discharge of saliva, aggravated as it is at meal-times, may render him objectionable to his fellow-men, so that he is compelled to satisfy his hunger in solitude. Further, the orifice of the fistula is often surrounded by an eczematous area from the constant irritation of the fluid dribbling over the cheek. It has been said that the continual loss of salivary fluid may impair the health of the patient. It is hard to believe this, though it is known that the amount excreted may assume large proportions. Two classical experiments prove this. Duphenix collected from a salivary fistula 70 grammes of fluid in fifteen minutes, and a patient of Jobert's discharged " several cupfuls " in twenty-four hours.

A persistent salivary fistula usually results from one of the injuries already described. It may have been originally neglected or inadequately treated ; or attempts to obtain primary union may have been made and have failed. The principal conditions which militate against primary union are sepsis occurring in the original wound, or severe contusion of its edges. In the case of an injury to Stenson's duct, primary union of the wound, even though its edges were clean-cut and it remained aseptic throughout, must be regarded as the exception rather than the rule, and an obstinate fistula often results.

Salivary fistulæ are also caused occasionally by ulcerative processes invading the tissues of the cheek, e.g. rodent ulcer, lupus, and actinomycosis.

Treatment.—For practical purposes, salivary fistulæ may be, divided into two main classes, the second of which is again divisible.

1. Gland fistulæ, communicating with the gland substance. ˙
2. Duct fistulæ, communicating with the duct (i) as it lies over the masseter muscle (masseteric), (ii) as it lies in front of the anterior border of the masseter (buccal).

1. **Gland fistulæ.**—The treatment is usually rewarded with success, though patience is demanded on the part of the patient, and perseverance on that of the surgeon. Cauterization with a silver-nitrate stick should first be given a prolonged trial. It should

be done every alternate day, and a fairly firm bandage applied.
Küttner states that the actual cautery is more efficacious. If
these measures fail after a reasonably long trial, the whole fistulous
track should be excised, and the edges brought together with *deep*
sutures which include all the exposed tissue ; in other words, after excision of the track, the resulting wound must be treated in the same
way as a primary wound of the gland. Care must, of course, be taken
not to cut any branches of the facial nerve during the operation.

2. Duct fistulæ.—The cure of a duct fistula is a much more
tedious and difficult business. The variety of procedures which have
been advocated from time to time, and the ingenuity which has been
expended in devising them, furnish evidence that there is no royal
road to success.

The several methods which have been described come under two
main headings—(*a*) those in which an attempt is made to restore the
natural aqueduct, and (*b*) those in which an attempt is made to convert
an external into an internal fistula. If their respective merits are
regarded from an academic point of view, there can be no doubt
that the former is preferable, since it aims at restoring a natural state
of affairs ; but, practically, the chances of success by this method are
so small, that I am of opinion that the second is the method of choice
for the treatment of duct fistulæ.

Armstrong of Montreal gives a clear account of the method of
Nicoladoni, who is the chief exponent of the first method. He writes :
" Nicoladoni has successfully joined the ends of the divided duct
after removing the scar tissue. When there is a considerable gap,
he incises the cheek, picks up the proximal end of the peripheral portion,
and frees it from the buccinator up to the caruncle ; then, by making
a crescentic incision through the buccal mucosa in front of the caruncle,
he is able to displace the duct orifice as much as 1·5 cm. towards the
gland, and so approximate the ends of the divided duct that he can
unite them through an external incision." It is obvious that this
method is ideal if it can succeed. But, since it rarely does so
even in a primary wound of the duct, how much less is the chance
of its doing so in an old-standing injury, when the ends have become
widely separated and the peripheral portion of the duct has usually
ceased to be permeable !

The simplest method of converting an external into an internal
fistula is that described and employed by Deguise in France and Pearce
Gould in this country. It consists in passing a strong suture (either
silk or silver wire) from the fistula through the buccal mucous membrane
in two places, one 0·5 cm. behind the other (Fig. 342). The ends which
now protrude in the mouth are tied very tightly. The tissue enclosed
necroses, and thus an internal opening is formed. The external

fistula then closes of its own accord. But, to make assurance doubly
sure, the edges of the fistula may be pared and united with one or two
fishing-gut sutures. This method has obvious limitations. It cannot,
for instance, be used in a masseteric fistula, since it would be necessary
to include the muscle in the ligature, and this is not feasible.

Kaufmann has devised a modification of this method. The cheek
is perforated opposite the fistula, and a small rubber tube 3 mm.

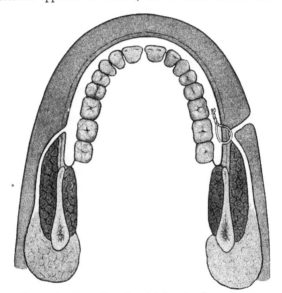

Fig. 342.—Operation for fistula of salivary duct.

thick is drawn through so that it projects both internally and externally. At the end of a week it is cut down on both sides so that
it is flush with skin and mucous membrane. In another week it is
removed entirely. He claims that the saliva will now flow into the
mouth through the artificial orifice, and that the external fistula will
close, especially if it is cauterized from time to time, or its edges are
approximated by suture. The technique is extremely simple. One
practical point must be observed : the tube must fit tightly in the
perforation in the mucous membrane, or it will not remain in position.

This method has one advantage over Deguise's. By making the
track of the tube oblique, so that it enters the mouth in front of the
masseter, it is applicable to masseteric fistulæ, whereas Deguise's
method can only be applied to the buccal variety with any prospect
of success.

None of the methods of dealing with a salivary fistula described can be regarded as infallible; and if, after a patient trial, a cure is not effected, the question of arresting the salivary secretion altogether must be considered. Two methods of doing this have been described. Bramann has ligatured the duct on the proximal side of the fistula in three cases, and in two of them the result was satisfactory. But he allows that a certain amount of risk is attached to it; for instance, the gland may become swollen from retention of its products, and abscess-formation may develop secondarily. The other alternative is to dissect out as much of the gland as possible, taking care not to damage the facial nerve. This will necessarily lead to some disfigurement, but that is preferable to the distressing phenomena associated with a persistent salivary fistula.

DISEASES OF THE SALIVARY GLANDS

INFLAMMATION

Etiology.—The etiology of sialo-adenitis is still a vexed question. It used to be held that the salivary glands were liable to infection apart from any exciting or predisposing condition; but recent researches have modified our ideas upon the matter. It is now agreed that there are few, if any, inflammatory conditions of the salivary glands which are not primarily due to an ascending infection from the mouth along the duct.

The etiology of sialo-adenitis as it is understood to-day may be compared with that of appendicitis. The appendix is normally inhabited by the *Bacillus coli communis*. If stagnation occurs in it as the result of kinking, or the presence of a stercolith, its resistance to infection is diminished, and the bacillus at once becomes a toxic instead of a benign organism, and acute appendicitis is the direct outcome. In the same way the mouth is normally inhabited by a number of mixed micro-organisms. As long as the salivary glands function adequately, these organisms are inert; but if there is any diminution of the salivary activity, as occurs in pyrexia or after laparotomy (Pawlow has experimentally proved that this is a constant phenomenon in dogs), an ascending infection along the ducts immediately follows.

Ginner has tabulated the results of bacteriological examination in 52 cases of suppurative parotitis, as follows:—

Staphylococcus aureus.	. 28	Pneumobacillus	. .	. 1
Staphylococcus albus .	. 2	Micrococcus tetragenus	.	. 2
Pneumococcus . :	. 11	Bacillus typhosus .	.	. 2
Streptococcus . .	. 5	Elongated bacillus (unclassifiable)		1

This table may be regarded as evidence in favour of the view that sialo-adenitis is nearly always, if not always, an ascending infection, since most of the micro-organisms mentioned, except the last, have been found in an apparently healthy oral cavity. Epidemic parotitis, the organism of which has not been definitely isolated, is alone inexplicable upon this hypothesis, but even in this case there is generally a prodromal stage of stomatitis, which is, at any rate, presumptive evidence in favour of the view that it is an ascending infection. It must be confessed, however, that the secondary implication of the testis, which is so characteristic a feature of the disease, cannot be explained on such simple grounds. It must, on our present knowledge, be regarded as an infection by way of the blood-stream. We are, therefore, compelled to recognize two forms of acute sialo-adenitis.

1. PRIMARY ACUTE SIALO-ADENITIS

Epidemic parotitis is a highly infectious disorder, attacking adolescents. It is said that males are more commonly attacked than females.

The incubation period is long (sixteen to twenty-one days or more, even up to six weeks). The onset is characterized by pyrexia, generally not higher than 101°, and pain below the ear. In a day or two, one parotid gland begins to swell, and its outline becomes obvious. The skin over it is tense and œdematous. A day or two later the gland on the opposite side follows suit. The course of the disease is generally benign. The temperature falls in a week, and the swelling then begins to recede gradually. It usually disappears completely in a month, but sometimes induration remains for a longer period.

The **treatment** is simple. The patient should be kept in bed, and a cold compress be applied to the swollen gland. Occasionally, suppuration occurs in the parotid ; an abscess must be incised as soon as its presence is diagnosed.

One of the most interesting features of the disease from a surgical point of view is the inflammation of the testis which sometimes is a complication. The treatment of the orchitis is identical with that of the parotitis. Atrophy of the affected testis, even if spontaneous resolution occurs, supervenes, according to Kocher, in one-third of the cases ; and if the orchitis has been bilateral, sterility often results. Other glands may be similarly affected ; they are the pancreas, the lachrymal glands, and, in the female, the ovary and mamma.

2. SECONDARY ACUTE SIALO-ADENITIS

This differs from the primary form in running a more acute course ; in fact, suppuration is the rule.

The predisposing conditions may be divided into three main classes :—

i. Abnormal conditions of the oral cavity, particularly all forms of stomatitis.

ii. Acute diseases, such as typhus, variola, pneumonia, typhoid, and pyæmia. Less acute disorders have also been known to cause it. In carcinoma it is not uncommon, and in a case of Klippel's it was a complication of tabes. Carr has recorded an attack of acute gangrenous parotitis, as a terminal event, in a case of granular kidney.

iii. Abdominal disease. Attention was first directed to the association of acute parotitis with abdominal disease in cases in which ovariotomy had been performed. In view of the observation that epidemic parotitis was often followed by orchitis and oöphoritis, it was at first presumed that there was some sympathetic connexion between the two sets of organs, and that one responded reflexly to disease or injury of the other. Stephen Paget collected 101 cases of parotitis following upon disease of the abdomen or pelvis ; and of these " 50 were due to injury, disease, or temporary derangement of the genital organs," a percentage which lent colour to the hypothesis. This view is not generally held now. After laparotomy, as in pyrexia, the mouth is dry and there is diminished salivary secretion, so that the glands are in a state which renders them particularly liable to infection. Further investigation has shown that the abdominal cases which are most constantly followed by parotitis are those in which rectal feeding is necessary, such as gastric ulcer. In patients who are being rectally fed the mouth readily becomes septic, in spite of the most skilful care and attention, and the infection spreads up to the glands along the ducts.

Secondary acute inflammation is confined almost entirely to the parotid. When it occurs after laparotomy, the swelling of the parotid begins about the end of the first week. In connexion with other diseases no definite date can be stated. The lower pole of the parotid generally enlarges first, but soon the swelling involves the whole gland, so that the side of the face is broadened and the ear is pushed out. The skin over the parotid is at first tense, but later becomes red and œdematous, with dilated veins running over the swelling. Great pain is experienced by the patient because the gland is covered by dense, unyielding fascia, and the tension of the parts is considerable. General malaise is complained of, and the temperature is always raised ; it may reach 105°.

Treatment. — Spontaneous subsidence may begin about the fourth day from the onset of symptoms; but this is an unusual termination. In the majority of cases suppuration supervenes. It is very difficult to decide in any given case whether an abscess is

q

present or not. Owing to the denseness of the fascia over the parotid, the ordinary signs of an abscess, a red, fluctuating swelling, may be entirely absent. In my opinion, an incision should be made into the swelling in every case in which the symptoms have steadily increased in severity or have even persisted without abatement for five days or longer. In making the incision, regard should be had to the course of the facial nerve. Even if no abscess is found, the tension will be relieved by division of the deep fascia. If a localized abscess is discovered, it should be drained by means of a rubber tube, and hot fomentations should be applied. In other cases no definite abscess can be found, but the whole gland is disintegrated and infiltrated with pus (this was the state of the gland in Carr's case, already quoted). In these circumstances the prognosis is extremely grave, and a fatal termination must be expected.

If relief is not afforded by early surgical interference, a parotid abscess may travel and point in several directions. Most commonly it makes its way backwards and discharges its contents through the external auditory meatus; or it may burrow behind the pharynx and œsophagus, and extend into the mediastinum.

Beveridge has recorded a case in which a parotid abscess travelled upwards behind the zygoma, and pointed in the temporal fossa. Other untoward results which have been observed are complete destruction of the facial nerve and thrombosis of the jugular vein and lateral sinus, with extension of the septic process to the interior of the cranium.

SUBACUTE AND CHRONIC INFLAMMATION OF THE SALIVARY GLANDS

This condition is very rare apart from inflammation of the duct; in fact, to Küttner alone we owe our knowledge of it. According to him, it is only found in the submaxillary glands, which become enlarged so as to form an oval swelling. This tends to enlarge in size, and to become adherent to surrounding tissues; for this reason Küttner advises enucleation of the affected glands. When examined microscopically they are found to contain foci of granulation tissue and small abscesses. The chief point of clinical interest is the difficulty of diagnosing the condition from a sarcoma or a gumma.

INFLAMMATION OF THE SALIVARY DUCTS

The salivary ducts are liable to inflammation from the same causes which produce parotitis, i.e. septic conditions of the mouth. The condition is peculiarly prone to occur in any form of xerostomia.

A series of cases of this nature has been reported by Raymond Johnson. The patients sought advice on account of a swelling of one parotid gland, which was painful and became larger at mealtimes.

Some of them had discovered for themselves that pressure on the swelling caused a discharge of watery fluid into the mouth, with a temporary relief of the symptoms.

On examination, the orifice of the duct of the affected gland was found red and inflamed, and, in some cases, stood up like a papilla. Pressure on the swelling caused first the extrusion of a plug of mucus from the duct, followed by a flow of watery saliva. In the way of **treatment,** relief is obtained by the application of dry heat externally, with frequent use of hot mouth-washes combined with the periodical passage of a probe along the duct. Raymond Johnson followed up the history of his cases and found that the swelling usually took some months to disappear; and in certain instances reappeared at intervals, although the attacks tended to decrease in severity. In his opinion, the enlargement of the gland is due entirely to obstruction, and not to any secondary inflammation in it. In some cases it is certain that if an inflamed duct becomes stenosed by fibrosis, the enlargement of the gland is then very chronic, if not absolutely persistent. The only measure that is of any avail is to slit up the fibrosed duct into the buccal cavity.

SALIVARY CALCULI

The genesis of a salivary calculus is so intimately connected with inflammation of the duct, that the condition may well be considered at this juncture. The mode of formation is analogous to that of calculi in other parts—the gall-bladder, for instance. As the result of the sialo-ductitis a plug of mucus containing bacteria is retained within the duct, and forms a nucleus for the successive deposits of inorganic salts, principally the phosphate and carbonate of lime.

Calculi are more often found in the ducts of the sublingual and submaxillary glands than in that of the parotid. This is only what might be expected, seeing that their secretion is viscid and highly charged with salts, while that of the parotid is more watery. They are greyish-white in colour, and generally ovoid in shape, like the stone of an olive. Their surface is usually roughened.

A salivary calculus may exist for a considerable time without giving rise to symptoms; but as the stone gradually enlarges, it will eventually obstruct the duct more completely. When this occurs, periodic enlargements of the affected gland will be noticed, particularly at mealtimes, owing to the obstruction to the discharge of the secretion. The patient complains of pain, occasionally of a quite acute nature, so that French writers have given the name " *coliques salivaires* " to these attacks.

Suppuration may occur round the stone, as it lies in the duct; a circumstance which can be diagnosed by the periodic discharge of pus into the mouth. More rarely, the stone may ulcerate through the wall of the duct either into the mouth or, in the case of a stone in Stenson's duct, externally, giving rise to a salivary fistula.

Calculi may also be situated in the substance of one of the salivary glands. In this position they are nearly always small and multiple, and each calculus is surrounded by a small abscess. In such a case the gland is chronically enlarged and tender, and there is a more or less constant escape of pus into the mouth.

The diagnosis is not a matter of difficulty in the absence of secondary septic changes. In most cases, the calculus can easily be felt as a hard body through the mucous membrane, on bimanual examination. But if acute inflammation has supervened, the true cause may easily be overlooked, and the case treated as one of septic adenitis due to an ascending infection. To avoid this error, an attempt should always be made to probe the affected duct. Alsberg states that an X-ray examination is of material assistance.

Treatment. — If the stone lies in the duct, this is easy. All that is necessary is to slit up the mucous membrane and remove the calculus with forceps. Antiseptic mouth-washes should be prescribed. The symptoms will rapidly abate, even in cases in which sepsis has supervened. Calculi in the gland are not so easily dealt with. If the affected gland is the submaxillary, it is best to enucleate it entirely ; but in the case of the parotid this is not feasible. Here an incision must be made and the calculi extracted, care being taken of the facial nerve. A gland fistula may result ; this must be subsequently treated in the manner already described.

ACTINOMYCOSIS, TUBERCULOSIS, SYPHILIS, MIKULICZ'S DISEASE

The infective granulomata very rarely attack the salivary glands. **Actinomycosis** has not been recorded as a primary infection, but any of the salivary glands may become implicated by a direct extension from the disease when it starts in the face or jaw.

Tuberculosis is also exceedingly rare ; only about a dozen cases have been recorded in all. The main clinical interest lies in the difficulty of diagnosing the condition from subacute septic inflammation. Too much reliance should not be placed on the tuberculin reaction. The only positive method of diagnosis is microscopical examination of a portion of the enlarged gland removed by operation. The clinical history closely resembles that of tuberculosis of lymphatic glands, i.e. the enlargement is chronic, but cold abscess formation is prone to occur. Treatment consists in draining the abscess or in partial removal of the parotid or total excision of the submaxillary gland, according to the pathological condition present, and its position.

Syphilis attacking the salivary glands is also rare, the whole of medical literature affording only some twenty-five cases. It is a late manifestation, gumma formation or interstitial fibrosis being the usual manifestation. Neumann has, however, reported five cases occurring in the first year of the disease. It used to be said that the diagnosis was only possible in the presence of other manifestations of syphilis, but it can now be made absolute with the aid of the Wassermann reaction. No special treatment, other than general antisyphilitic remedies, is required.

Mikulicz's disease is a rare condition, which has been described as a clinical entity by von Mikulicz of Breslau. It consists of a symmetrical enlargement of the salivary and lachrymal glands. Other glands, according to subsequent observers, may also be involved, e.g. the labial and buccal glands, and the gland of Blandin and Nuhn.

The enlargement begins in early adult life, without apparent cause, and is steadily progressive ; the parotid may enlarge to the size of a man's fist. The swellings are firm or elastic to the touch, but do not fluctuate, nor are they tender. Disfigurement and inconvenience due to the local enlargement are common, but life is not endangered. Arsenic and potassium iodide have produced improvement in some cases, in others the disfigurement has been sufficient to call for extirpation of the affected glands. There is no tendency to recurrence.

The **pathology** of the condition is extremely obscure. Microscopically the glands show an infiltration of round cells. Mikulicz himself regards it as being " a new formation of lymphadenoid tissue which is spread round the acini as centres, and leads to the destruction of the specific gland tissue." Tietze's view is that it is an " adenoid proliferation of the lachrymal and salivary glands." Other authorities lean to the view that it is a chronic infective process. In no case has any relation to syphilis or tubercle been demonstrated.

CYSTS OF THE SALIVARY DUCTS AND GLANDS

CYSTS OF THE DUCTS

Retention cysts are known to occur in connexion with both salivary ducts and glands. Cysts in Stenson's or Wharton's duct may result from definite obstruction due to a calculus or to cicatricial fibrosis of the orifice ; but they are occasionally found when there is no appreciable obstruction to the outflow of secretion, as evidenced by a discharge of salivary fluid from the duct when an irritant fluid such as vinegar is placed in the mouth. In such a case, it must be supposed that the cyst is a collection of fluid in a congenital dilatation of the duct, just as a saphenous varix is a congenital dilatation of the vein rather than an enlargement due to obstruction. The cyst may become septic owing to an ascending infection from the mouth ; and the condition will then closely resemble that described in connexion with a salivary calculus. In certain cases phosphate and carbonate of lime are deposited on the walls of the cyst, and the diagnosis from a salivary calculus is hardly possible.

In an uncomplicated case the **diagnosis** should be easy. An ovoid tumour can be seen lying in the position of the duct, with its long axis parallel to the line of the duct. If it is picked up between the fingers it will be felt to contain fluid. Firm pressure will expel its contents, and the walls will fall into apposition.

The most efficient **treatment** is to make an incision in the mucous membrane and dissect the cyst out entirely. The wound in the mucous membrane should be left open.

Cysts of the Glands

More rarely, retention cysts form in the salivary glands themselves. They commence as such in one or more of the smaller ducts. If multiple they coalesce and tend eventually to form a cyst of considerable size. In the early stages it is not easy to make certain of their presence, but later they tend to come to the surface and form a superficial fluctuating swelling. Even then it is not easy to diagnose them from salivary tumours which have undergone cystic degeneration ; the only reliable method being to withdraw a portion of the contents with an aspirating syringe, and subject it to a microscopical examination.

Treatment.—If the cyst is situated in the submaxillary gland, it is best to enucleate the gland entirely. In the case of the parotid, attempts should be made to obliterate the cyst by periodic injections of tincture of iodine or of a concentrated solution of carbolic acid. But if these fail, as they often do, it is justifiable to undertake an operation for the excision of the cyst.

Ranula

Ranula is considered by some authorities to be a retention cyst of the sublingual gland or of one of the ducts of Rivini, and a short account of it will therefore be given at this point.

A ranula is a cystic swelling in the floor of the mouth, to one or other side of the frænum. It may extend across the middle line, and is then constricted by the frænum linguæ. Several observers have reported a bilateral ranula, but this condition must be regarded as one of great rarity.

It presents as a rounded, bluish-grey, translucent, fluctuating swelling, with vessels of the mucous membrane stretched over it. It contains a slimy, colourless material like the white of egg. It causes no symptoms other than the inconvenience due to the presence of an abnormal swelling in the mouth, which may interfere with mastication and render articulation imperfect.

The **etiology** of a ranula is much disputed. According to von Hippel, it is a sublingual gland cyst, starting in the smaller excretory ducts, entirely analogous to the salivary-gland cysts already described. Neumann regards it as an epithelial cyst derived from a tubule of one of Bochdalek's glands; while von Recklinghausen inclines to the view that it is a cyst derived from the gland of Blandin and Nuhn, either by simple retention or by degeneration of the retained products of its secretion.

A dermoid cyst in the floor of the mouth may resemble a ranula very closely. A sublingual dermoid is usually adherent to the mandible or to the hyoid bone, and this is the only point on which reliance can be placed in the differential diagnosis.

Treatment. — The only really efficient treatment is to dissect out the cyst entirely after incising the overlying mucous membrane. If this is not possible, the next best method is to cut away the whole of the anterior wall and to allow the cavity so formed to cicatrize up slowly.

Some authorities advise removing a ranula through a submental incision, especially if the cyst is a big one and projects downwards and forwards towards the mylo-hyoid. But there is little advantage in this. The exposure afforded is no better than that obtained by the intrabuccal method; and, from an æsthetic point of view, a scar in the mylo-hyoid region should always be avoided if possible.

TUMOURS OF THE SALIVARY GLANDS

Tumours of the salivary glands may be classified as follows :—

A. Tumours of *epithelial origin*—
    Innocent: Adenoma.
    Malignant: Carcinoma (a) Adeno-carcinoma.
                   (b) Scirrhus.

B. Tumours of *connective-tissue origin*—
    Innocent: Angioma.
            Fibroma.
            Chondroma.
            Lipoma.
    Malignant: (1) Pure sarcoma—
                        (a) Round-celled.
                        (b) Spindle-celled.
                        (c) Melanotic (Billroth and Kaufmann).
              (2) Mixed sarcoma—
                      (a) Chondro-sarcoma.
                      (b) Fibro-sarcoma.
                      (c) Myxo-sarcoma.
                      (d) Angio-sarcoma or perithelioma.

C. *Mixed* tumours.

A. Tumours of Epithelial Origin

A pure **adenoma** of the salivary glands is so rare (Nasse has reported four cases) that it demands only passing mention. It grows slowly, and on section resembles the normal structure of the gland atypically arranged. It is possible that several of the cases described as hypertrophy of the parotid were in reality adenomas.

Carcinoma attacks the salivary glands, usually the parotid, in two forms, the medullary or adeno-carcinoma, and the scirrhus. **Adeno-carcinoma** may occur at any age, but generally does so in early adult life. A rapidly growing tumour develops. It is firm and elastic in consistence. Ulceration of the overlying skin and subsequent fungation are common features if the condition is allowed to progress. Facial paralysis, of varying degrees, is usual, according to whether the main trunk of the nerve or some of its branches are involved. **Scirrhus** in this region is closely analogous to the mammary form. It attacks elderly patients, grows slowly, forms a densely hard tumour, and the overlying skin soon becomes fixed to the growth and puckered. Metastatic deposits are found in the lymphatic glands in both varieties. The sublingual gland may also be the seat of carcinoma. In fact, some authorities believe that all carcinomas of the floor of the mouth are derived from this source. The prognosis with regard to life is bad in either case, but worse in the medullary form. The diagnosis can only be made with certainty by removing a portion of the growth and subjecting it to microscopical examination.

As soon as the diagnosis is certain, no time should be lost in enucleating the affected gland completely, if this is still feasible. It can rarely be done if the surface is already ulcerated. In this case the outlook is very bad indeed, but improvement is sometimes produced by the application of X-rays or of radium, or by zinc ionization.

B. Tumours of Connective-Tissue Origin

The innocent tumours of this class are exceedingly rare. Clinically, their characteristics do not differ from those presented when they occur in other parts of the body. An accurate diagnosis is rarely arrived at before the tumour is removed and examined histologically.

Sarcoma.—Many forms of sarcoma have been described, as the table of classification shows. Pure sarcomas, whether round- or spindle-celled, form rapidly growing ill-defined tumours which are difficult to distinguish from subacute inflammation. The mixed forms, particularly the fibro-sarcomas, are more often encapsuled and present as localized swellings, which can be enucleated in their capsule from their surroundings. It is said that if this is done completely they do not tend to recur. I am sceptical of the truth of this statement.

Melanotic sarcoma of the parotid has been described by Kaufmann and Billroth. The pigment is said to be excessive. It is difficult to understand whence it is derived.

When the presence of sarcoma has been diagnosed, the affected gland should be removed in its entirety. A fibro-sarcoma may, however, be shelled out with its capsule, as has already been said. It should be noted that the true sarcomatous nature of these tumours has been called in question. Coley has reported a cure of a small round-celled sarcoma of the parotid by the injection of his fluid (*Ann. Surg.*, *Philadelphia*, 1902).

C. MIXED TUMOURS

This class of tumour, of which specimens are shown in Figs. 343 and 344, is the most interesting from the pathological, as well as the most important from the clinical point of view, since it is the commonest neoplastic affection of the salivary glands.

A mixed tumour forms a localized well-defined outgrowth from the gland. The direction of its greatest prominence will depend upon the portion of the gland from which it takes origin. In the parotid this is usually the anterior inferior angle, and the growth tends to extend down into the neck. Occasionally the growth starts on the deep aspect, and it will then extend inwards towards the pharyngeal wall. In the submaxillary gland it usually springs from its superficial surface, and forms a swelling in the submental region. The sublingual gland is rarely if ever attacked.

As a rule, these tumours occur in middle life. Preceding inflammation or injury is said to dispose to them. Their form is as variable as their consistence, and depends upon the relative amount of the several connective-tissue elements contained. Most often they are firm, rounded or ovoid, and irregular on the surface. They are movable on the deep structures, if they spring from the superficial aspect of the gland, and the overlying skin is not attached to them. If left, they tend to enlarge progressively ; but they are not malignant in the true sense of the word—that is, they do not endanger the life of their possessor, do not cause metastasis, and do not recur if completely removed.

Mixed tumours cause few **symptoms,** unless they are allowed to grow to a great size. They may then be painful, and facial paralysis may be observed. In the case of parotid tumours, deafness due to occlusion of the external auditory meatus may be noticed. Excess of salivary secretion is more common than diminution. One curious feature with regard to their growth must be mentioned. Often, after slowly increasing in size for years, they suddenly enlarge rapidly, and many patients then seek advice for the first time. This is an indication that the tumour has taken on the true characteristics of malignancy, and the prognosis is then correspondingly grave.

The **histological appearances** of mixed tumours are exceedingly variable. Their name is derived from the fact that on microscopical examination both epithelial and connective-tissue elements are seen. Representatives of various types of connective tissue

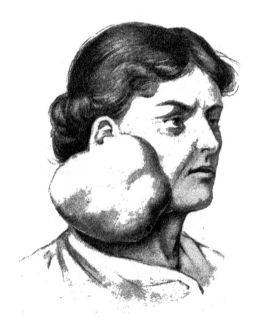

Fig. 343.—Mixed tumour of the parotid gland.

are found, particularly fibrous, myxomatous, and cartilaginous, and epithelial cells are seen arranged in columns or in groups. Some of these show a tendency to cell-nest formation, others to colloid degeneration. Much discussion has taken place as to the origin of these cells. Ribbert holds that they are genuine epithelial cells, derived from the normal cells of the gland. He supports his argument by the assertion that prickle processes can be demonstrated between adjacent cells and that the separate groups are bounded by a membrana propria. Volkmann and others assert that the cells cannot be shown to resemble any definite epithelial type, and that they must therefore be regarded as of endothelial origin. Most pathologists are agreed that the connective-tissue elements are derived from errors of development; thus, the cartilage comes from displaced remnants of the bronchial arches or of the cartilages of the ear. But Ribbert has also described a special mixed tumour of the submaxillary gland which he calls a cylindroma. He says that in this both epithelial

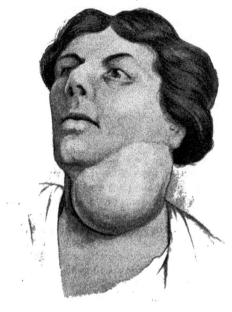

Fig. 344.—Mixed tumour of the submaxillary gland.

and connective-tissue elements are derived from the original structure of the gland itself.

The **diagnosis** of these tumours is not easy. Reliance cannot be placed on any one sign alone; it is, however, safe to assume that any hard, irregular, movable tumour in the region of one of the salivary glands which has persisted for some time is probably a mixed tumour. The diagnosis can only be clinched with the aid of the microscope.

Treatment.—This consists in removing the tumour at the earliest possible opportunity. It is said that a mixed parotid tumour can be shelled out, and that if this is done completely there is little, if any, chance of recurrence. This, however, is not the experience of all surgeons. Butlin, in an interesting paper in the *Lancet* (1904), admitted that recurrence had taken place in several cases in which he thought he had completely removed the primary growth. Further, the recurrent tumour was in nearly all cases more rapidly growing than the primary one. The probable explanation is that an apparently complete enucleation is rarely so in fact. Processes of the growth, so small as to be inappreciable to the finger, invade the capsule, and are left behind. Under the influence of the altered tissue tension resulting from the operation, they take on a new and rapid growth, and, when seen on a subsequent occasion, are often found to be inoperable. It is therefore essential in all cases to remove the whole capsule with the growth. In view of these facts it would seem reasonable to remove the entire submaxillary gland when this is the situation of a mixed tumour.

When enucleating a parotid tumour, care must, of course, be taken not to injure the facial nerve. It is better not to search directly for the nerve, but merely to avoid wounding any branches which happen to become exposed during the operation.

Operative technique.—Mention has been made in connexion with malignant tumours of complete removal of the parotid and submaxillary glands. A brief account of the technique of these operations will therefore be added.

The **parotid** is best exposed by a **T**-shaped incision, the vertical part extending from an inch above the zygoma down directly in front of the tragus to a point an inch below the angle of the jaw. A second incision is made extending forwards from this at right angles about half an inch below the zygoma. Two flaps of skin can thus be dissected up, and the gland exposed. The external carotid artery should be found at the bottom of the wound and divided between two ligatures. No hard-and-fast rule can be laid down about the actual enucleation of the gland, but it is generally best to begin below and work upwards. The greatest difficulty will be experienced in removing the posterior deep part which extends down to the spine of the sphenoid. If all vessels are tied as they are met, and the field of operation thus kept bloodless, the gland can nearly always be removed entire by the exercise of patience and care. The facial nerve must of necessity be sacrificed. The lymphatic glands which drain the parotid should, if possible, be taken away at the same operation.

The extirpation of the **submaxillary** gland is a more simple procedure. An incision is made parallel to and below the mandible, curving slightly downwards in the centre. After exposing the gland the facial artery should be sought for at its lower border, and tied between two ligatures. When this is done, the gland can be enucleated without danger or difficulty.

THE ŒSOPHAGUS

By H. M. RIGBY, M.S.Lond., F.R.C.S.Eng.

Anatomy.—The œsophagus extends from the lower border of the cricoid cartilage to the cardiac end of the stomach. Its upper extremity (Quain) is opposite the disc between the sixth and seventh cervical vertebræ. In its course downwards it follows a somewhat sinuous direction, and has two distinct curves to the left side. The first curve to the left extends from its origin to the root of the neck. As the superior mediastinum is reached, the œsophagus tends to regain the mid-line, which it attains in the posterior mediastinum about the level of the fifth dorsal vertebra. From this point it again deviates to the left side. It passes through a special opening in the diaphragm, and ends in the stomach opposite the lower border of the tenth dorsal vertebra. Its length is 9–10 in.

It is especially prone to disease in three portions. These are—

1. The upper end, in the region of the cricoid cartilage and larynx, one of the narrowest parts of the œsophagus. It is situated opposite the seventh cervical vertebra. and is, in the adult, 6–7 in. from the incisor teeth. This is a very frequent site of growths and ulcerations. The œsophagus is much flattened antero-posteriorly in this part owing to the close apposition of the cartilage of the larynx and the vertebræ.

2. That part of the œsophagus in the neighbourhood of the bifurcation of the trachea, and in close relation with the left bronchus. The trachea bifurcates just above the body of the fifth dorsal vertebra, and the left bronchus crosses in front of the œsophagus at the level of this vertebra, i.e. about 11 in. from the incisor teeth. This part of the œsophagus is also a favourite position for malignant growths. Its close relation to such structures as the trachea, aorta, pleuræ. and pericardium lends additional importance to the occurrence of growths in this situation.

3. The lower end, at its junction with the stomach, 15–16 in. from the incisor teeth. Here the lumen of the œsophagus undergoes marked narrowing, and the structure of its mucous lining manifests

an abrupt change into that of the stomach. This is again a favourite
position for stricture from ulcer or malignant growths.

According to Bryant, the average diameter of the œsophagus is
⅖ in., but at its commencement the diameter is ½ in. The transverse
exceeds the antero-posterior diameter. In the dead subject the
lumen is small and the mucous membrane thrown into folds. The
appearances as seen in life are very different. Viewed with the
œsophagoscope, the œsophagus is an open tube, its lumen enlarging
and diminishing with each respiratory movement.

Anatomical relations in the neck.—The deep situation
of the œsophagus in the neck renders its exposure difficult. Its most
important relations, laterally, are the carotid artery and jugular veins.
The posterior surface of the left lateral lobe of the thyroid is in
relation with its anterior surface. The left recurrent laryngeal nerve
has close relation to its wall. The trachea lies directly in front, the
vertebræ, prevertebral muscles, and fasciæ behind.

Operation for exposure in the neck (Fig. 345).—The
œsophagus can be satisfactorily exposed by an incision along the
anterior margin of the sterno-mastoid muscle on the left side, low
down in the neck. The great vessels are identified and drawn outwards with the sterno-mastoid muscle. The trachea and left lateral
lobe of the thyroid are displaced inwards. The superior and middle
thyroid veins are divided or avoided. The inferior thyroid artery
and recurrent laryngeal nerve should be avoided. The œsophageal
wall will then be exposed after a little blunt dissection.

Anatomical relations in the thorax.—The œsophagus
traverses the superior and posterior mediastina. It is situated immediately behind the lower part of the trachea and the left bronchus,
the latter structure crossing it from right to left. It then lies in close
relation to the posterior surface of the pericardium and the diaphragm.
It passes through a special aperture in the diaphragm, and enters the
cardiac end of the stomach about 1½ in. below this opening.

It has close relation with both pleuræ. The arch of the aorta
crosses in front of it from right to left. The descending thoracic
aorta first lies to its left side and then passes behind it, and finally
reaches its right side at a point 3 in. above the diaphragm.

Behind the œsophagus are the vertebral column and left longus colli
muscle; the thoracic duct in the superior mediastinum; the vertebral
portions of the right intercostal arteries and the vena azygos minor.

The vagus nerves have close relation to its wall, forming the
"plexus gulæ."

Operation for exposure in the thorax.—The œsophagus
may be exposed in the thoracic part of its course by removing portions
of the ribs between the angles and the transverse processes of the

corresponding vertebræ. Portions of three ribs are divided, and a flap composed of the bones and soft parts is raised up. This operation —posterior mediastinal thoracotomy—has been described and practised

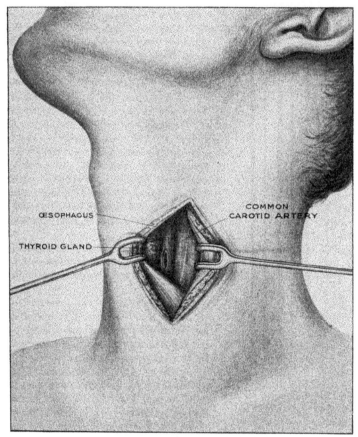

Fig. 345.—Structures exposed in the operation of cervical œsophagotomy.

by Bryant. The position at which the operation is carried out depends on the site of the lesion in the œsophagus.

METHODS OF EXAMINATION

1. **Inspection and palpation.**—These can only be of value when the cervical portion of the œsophagus is affected. Tumours

of the wall may reveal a swelling to the left side of the trachea. A pouch may form an easily recognizable tumour. Enlarged glands secondary to œsophageal disease may be present.

2. **Percussion.**—This method is seldom of assistance. A large pouch in the neck may give rise to a tympanitic note, or a greatly dilated œsophagus may possibly occasion altered resonance over the posterior thoracic wall.

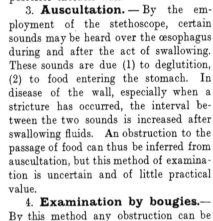

3. **Auscultation.** — By the employment of the stethoscope, certain sounds may be heard over the œsophagus during and after the act of swallowing. These sounds are due (1) to deglutition, (2) to food entering the stomach. In disease of the wall, especially when a stricture has occurred, the interval between the two sounds is increased after swallowing fluids. An obstruction to the passage of food can thus be inferred from auscultation, but this method of examination is uncertain and of little practical value.

4. **Examination by bougies.**— By this method any obstruction can be located, and its extent and permeability determined.

As a preliminary the presence of aneurysm must be carefully excluded, for the sac of an aneurysm pressing on the œsophageal wall might be penetrated by the injudicious use of a bougie.

Again, in advanced carcinoma of the œsophagus the instrument must be carefully passed ; otherwise the ulcerated wall may be perforated or violent hæmorrhage excited by the point of the bougie.

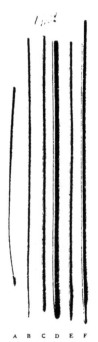

A B C D E F

Fig. 346.—Bougies for examination of œsophagus.

A, Bougie with metal acorn tip; B, graduated conical bougie ; C, D, cylindrical bougies; E, conical bougie ; F, bulbous-ended bougie.

With these exceptions, bougie examination becomes a matter of routine in cases of dysphagia. The instruments used are generally solid flexible cylindrical or oval bougies, which are either conical in shape or have a bulbous end. They are composed of silk web or elastic gum, and are easily malleable when warmed. They are usually 22 in. in length, and vary in size from No. 7 to No. 24, English catheter gauge. (*See* Fig. 346.)

The introduction of an œsophageal bougie is a simple procedure, though at first decidedly unpleasant to the patient. When the larynx is reached, violent expiratory efforts with a closed glottis are generally excited, often followed by retching as the stomach is entered. However, tolerance is surprisingly soon established by custom.

In passing a bougie the surgeon should stand facing the patient. The instrument should be dipped into a basin of warm water, lubricated with oil or vaseline, and curved so as to pass easily over the base of the tongue. The patient is then directed to extend the neck and open the mouth. A gag is unnecessary, and any introduction of fingers or instruments to depress the tongue should be avoided, inasmuch as it only excites retching and additional discomfort. The point of the bougie is now pushed over the dorsum of the tongue and gently on down the posterior pharyngeal wall, past the region of the larynx, where it is generally arrested by spasm of the inferior constrictor and the narrowness of this part of the œsophagus. With slight gentle pressure forwards, the point then enters and passes down the œsophagus to the site of the obstruction. Any further manipulations must now be carried out with gentleness. If the wall of the œsophagus is ulcerated, considerable pain may be caused by the contact of the bougie. Hæmorrhage may occur, and even perforation of the wall has resulted from violent efforts to overcome an obstruction. If the bougie will not readily pass, smaller ones should be tried. Should the obstruction prove impassable, the further methods of examination to be presently described should be employed. If there be a stricture through which a bougie can be made to pass, its extent and diameter can be estimated by means of a bougie with an acorn-shaped extremity (Fig. 346, A).

5. **X-ray examination.**—This method depends upon the introduction of certain substances which are known to be impervious to the X-rays. Sounds containing metallic cores of lead or mercury are passed down the œsophagus and held in position while the X-rays are passed through the thorax and focused on a screen. More frequently, in the place of sounds, certain preparations of bismuth or iron are administered by the mouth. Bismuth oxychloride, subnitrate, or oxide is given in the form of a cachet or suppository paste, or in suspension. For this purpose the oxychloride is preferable to the subnitrate.

This method of examination is very valuable in the recognition of strictures and pouches of the œsophagus.

The patient is made to stand or sit with the arms raised and the hands resting on the top of the head. The thorax is so placed that the rays traverse it in the oblique direction, usually from right to left. By this means the shadows formed by the vertebral column and heart and great vessels are avoided. The rays are focused on a screen placed behind the patient, who is directed to swallow the prepared bismuth ; the shadow formed by this substance as it passes down the œsophagus can be easily seen. If a stricture be present, the bismuth collects at its site and may form a dark mass of considerable size which reproduces the shape of the œsophagus at the site of the constriction. If the existence of a pouch be suspected the patient is directed to take some bread - and - milk or mashed potatoes with which the bismuth salts are mixed.[1]

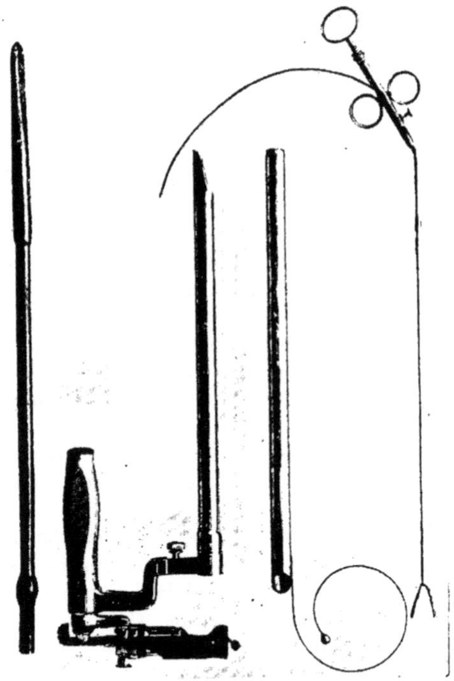

6. **Direct examination.**—By the employment of the œsophagoscope a direct examination of the interior of the œsophagus can be undertaken. Foreign bodies can be seen, and their nature, shape, and position be determined ; morbid growths and ulcerations can also be investigated. The instrument devised by Killian and modified by Brüning has many advantages. Its essential parts are shown in Fig. 347.

Fig. 347.—Instruments used in œsophagoscopy.

A, Brüning's electroscope with œsophageal tube ; B, extending œsophageal tube ; C, elastic gum obturator ; D, œsophagus forceps.

The important features of this instrument are the ingenious method of illumination and the ease with which an instrument can be manipulated within the tube.

Œsophagoscopy may be performed under either local or general anæsthesia. As a rule it is far better to employ ageneral anæsthetic ; the examination may take some time, and the necessarily constrained position, with the head extended, is.very trying to the patient.

[1] *See also* Vol. I., p. 648.

The patient may be placed in the following positions during the passage of the instrument, viz. : (1) Sitting on a stool with the neck extended and head thrown well back ; (2) recumbent with the head hanging well down over the end of the operating table ; (3) lying on the side with the neck again fully extended.

The tube is to be warmed and oiled ; it may then be introduced with a pilot bougie inserted through its lumen, but it is far safer and more satisfactory to pass the instrument by direct vision with the illuminating apparatus attached.   This method obviates the risk of perforating an ulcer just below the cricoid, or of pushing on an impacted foreign body ; it also permits the examination of the pharynx during the passage of the tube.

While the patient's head is held well extended by an assistant, the surgeon with his left hand passes the tube over the dorsum of the tongue until he sees the posterior pharyngeal wall ; he then tilts the handle upwards and continues the introduction until the upward movement is checked by the upper incisor teeth.   The assistant now slightly inclines the head towards the left shoulder, without rotating or tilting the neck, and the surgeon slips the tube into the right angle of the mouth and passes it onwards down the œsophagus.   The whole manœuvre is carried out by direct vision through the tube.

MALFORMATIONS

The following rare malformations may occur (Whipham and Fagge) :—

Congenital absence of the entire œsophagus.

Bifurcation of the œsophagus with union of the two divisions towards the lower end.

Congenital atresia, often associated with œsophago-tracheal fistula.

Pressure pouches.

Strictures due to the pressure of a valve-like fold of mucous membrane.   ·

Congenital stenosis of the lower end of the œsophagus.

Only two of these conditions need be considered here, viz. congenital atresia and congenital stenosis.

CONGENITAL ATRESIA.   TRACHEO-ŒSOPHAGEAL FISTULA

This malformation has more of a developmental than a surgical interest, and little can be done to remedy it.

Loss of continuity of the œsophagus with the pharynx, in these cases, occurs near the lower end of the trachea.   There is normally a narrowing of the œsophagus about 2¾ in. below its origin, marking the origin of the pulmonary diverticulum.   In congenital atresia the pharynx and upper end of the œsophagus terminate blindly just above this region, while the œsophagus ends above by opening into either the trachea or one of the bronchi.

Keith and Spicer show that the trachea and bronchi are derived directly from the foregut through subdivision of the channel by the tracheo-œsophageal septum. The fistula formed between the œsophagus and trachea in the above-mentioned deformity is the result of failure in union of the lateral ridges which unite to form this septum.

Shattock points out that this does not depend on a failure of communication between the stomodæum and the anterior blind end of the mesenteron, as the pharynx is itself developed from the mesenteron. He suggests that the atresia is a secondary process due to kinking of the wall of the mesenteron during the development of the lower part of the trachea and lungs.

In rare cases the upper part of the canal communicates with the trachea. The lower portion may end blindly above without communication with the air-passages, or it may be simply represented by a fibrous cord. The two portions may be connected by a narrow fibrous cord (Lotheissen).

The symptoms produced by this deformity are those of complete œsophageal obstruction ; all food taken is immediately vomited, and the infant rapidly dies of inanition.

The condition can be diagnosed by the passage of a bougie. The only possible treatment is gastrostomy, with a view to dealing with the obstruction later. The prognosis, however, is generally quite hopeless (Keith and Spicer).

Strictures due to a valve-like folding of the mucous membrane occur either just below the pharynx or near the lower end of the œsophagus.

Stenosis of the Lower End of the Œsophagus

Whipham and Fagge record a case of tubular fibrous stricture of the lower end of the œsophagus in a girl of $4\frac{1}{2}$ years. They could only find records of six similar cases.

DIVERTICULA [1]

Diverticula of the œsophagus occur : (1) At or about the junction of the pharynx with the œsophagus ; (2) in the middle third of the œsophagus in close relation with the bifurcation of the trachea and left bronchus ; (3) in the lower part of the œsophagus above the diaphragm.

---

[1] This account of the condition is largely based on an excellent paper by Halsted.

From an etiological point of view these pouches are classified as follows :—

1. Pressure diverticula.
2. Traction diverticula.
3. Traction-pressure diverticula.

According to Halsted they occur in the following situations, viz. (a) in the pharynx ; (b) at the pharyngo-œsophageal junction ; (c) at the upper margin of the left bronchus (epibronchial) ; (d) just above the diaphragm (epiphrenic).

1. PRESSURE DIVERTICULA

The commonest and most interesting are those found at the junction of the œsophagus and pharynx. They give rise to flask-shaped pouches communicating with the lower end of the pharynx by a narrow opening which has a constant position on the posterior pharyngeal wall at the lower border of the inferior constrictor muscle. Like other diverticula in the alimentary canal, they really consist of herniated pouches of mucous membrane protruding between the fasciculi of the muscular wall. The muscle fibres generally end more or less abruptly at the neck of the sac, and the main part of the wall of the pouch is composed of mucous membrane covered with an envelope of thickened fibrous connective tissue. As this pouch enlarges it takes the path of least resistance, and therefore tends to protrude on either side of the œsophagus, more commonly the left. It may extend gradually downwards, and its neck become so elongated that the fundus of the sac reaches the mediastinum. It may give rise to a well-marked swelling in the posterior triangle of the neck. The gradual enlargement of the pouch is due to food being forced into its interior from above by the contraction of the constrictor muscle of the pharynx.

The etiology of these diverticula has been much discussed. They are said to be congenital, but there is no actual proof of this statement. At the lower border of the pharynx, where it joins with the œsophagus, there is said to be a natural deficiency of muscular support, the so-called " Lannier " triangle (Mayo).

Probably, as Keith suggests, they are generally produced as follows : In the act of deglutition the bolus of food is rapidly thrown to the lower and narrowest part of the pharynx, when it is immediately grasped and driven downwards by the forcible contraction of the lower constrictor muscles. The food is squeezed between the broad resisting base of the cricoid in front and the upper end of the œsophagus behind. The posterior part naturally presents a weak resistance, owing to the peculiar arrangement of its muscle fibres, and so a small protrusion may readily occur. A slight protrusion, once formed, can be easily enlarged by intake of food at each act of deglutition.

There are undoubtedly other explanations for this condition, as Halsted points out. Injury to the œsophageal wall in this region has been followed by pouch formations, and the association of congenital stricture of the upper part of the œsophagus with a diverticulum has been recorded. (*See* Fig. 348.)

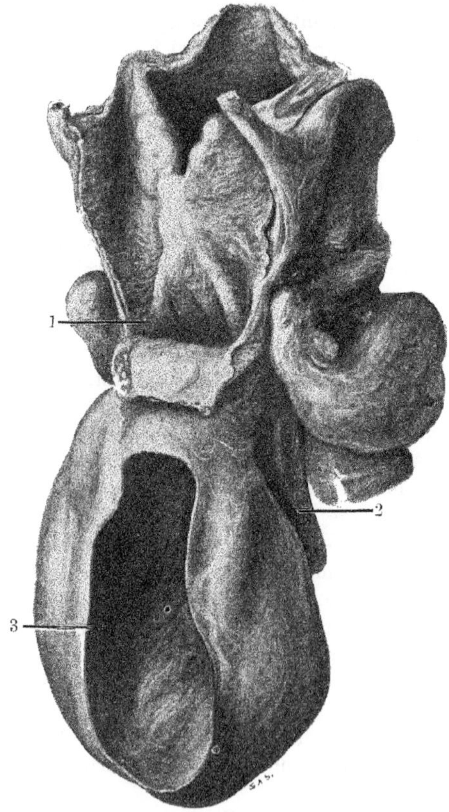

Pressure diverticula generally occur in elderly male patients. They often give a history of long-standing dysphagia, and the first symptoms are merely those indicative of stenosis of the œsophagus, for a long period unaccompanied by loss of weight or deterioration in health. Later the following symptoms arise : If solid food be taken, a feeling of discomfort and pressure is experienced in the neck, as if a foreign body were present. Regurgitations of portions of food occur sometimes shortly after eating, but occasionally at long intervals, even twelve hours after a meal. Ejection of gas may accompany the evacuation of the food by the mouth. The food is undigested, and not at all suggestive of stomach contents ; and when the pouch gets filled, further passage of food down the œsophagus may be

Fig. 348.—Pressure diverticulum at pharyngo-œsophageal junction.

1, Neck of pouch ; 2, œsophagus ; 3, pouch. (*Royal College of Surgeons Museum.*)

completely arrested. The œsophagus becomes pushed to one side, and the pouch comes to lie more directly in a line with the lower part of the pharynx. Pressure on the filled pouch in the neck may be followed by rejection of some portion of the contained food. The spitting up of quantities of mucus has been noticed in one case.

Examination of the neck may reveal a swelling on the left side, below the cricoid cartilage, but this sign is often absent. It is said to be present in one-third of the cases reported.

If a bougie be passed it generally enters the pouch, and, if made of metal, its point may be felt in the posterior triangle of the neck. The simultaneous passage of two bougies, one of which enters the pouch and the other the stomach, is sometimes possible.

The presence of a pouch has in several cases been clearly illustrated by X-ray examination after the administration of a bismuth meal. A pouch filled with this throws a dense shadow on the screen and clearly demonstrates its outline.

The double opening should be easily seen by the use of the œsophagoscope.

Mayo refers to a method of diagnosis employed by Plummer. A silk thread is swallowed in sufficient quantities to pass through the stomach into the intestine. A bulbous-ended œsophagus probe is threaded on the silk and passed down. When it can be passed no farther, the string is tightened. If a diverticulum be present, the bulbous end is pulled upwards to the mouth of the diverticulum. If a stricture only be present, the position of the probe is not altered.

2. TRACTION DIVERTICULA

These are of less surgical importance, as they generally remain of small size and may not give rise to any symptoms. They usually occur in the middle and lower portion of the œsophagus. As their name implies, they are generally caused by traction on the œsophagus wall (Rokitansky). This may be due to inflammation of glands or to fibrous contraction following inflammation in the peri-œsophageal tissues.

The structure of the wall of the pouch is similar to that of a pressure diverticulum. The diverticulum is horizontal, or the opening may be on a lower level than the pouch itself: hence food rarely tends to collect, and results of pressure do not occur.

The pouches are situated on the anterior wall of the œsophagus, just below the bifurcation of the trachea (Fig. 349).

The chief danger associated with traction diverticula is the possibility of perforation of their wall by foreign bodies, leading to hæmorrhage or mediastinal infection. Fistulous communication with the air-passages has also been noted.

3. TRACTION-PRESSURE DIVERTICULA

These are formed as the result of the passage of food into traction diverticula. They are rarely encountered, for the reasons given above.

Treatment of diverticula.—The treatment of œsophageal pouches consists in their removal by dissection, with closure of the neck by suture.[1]

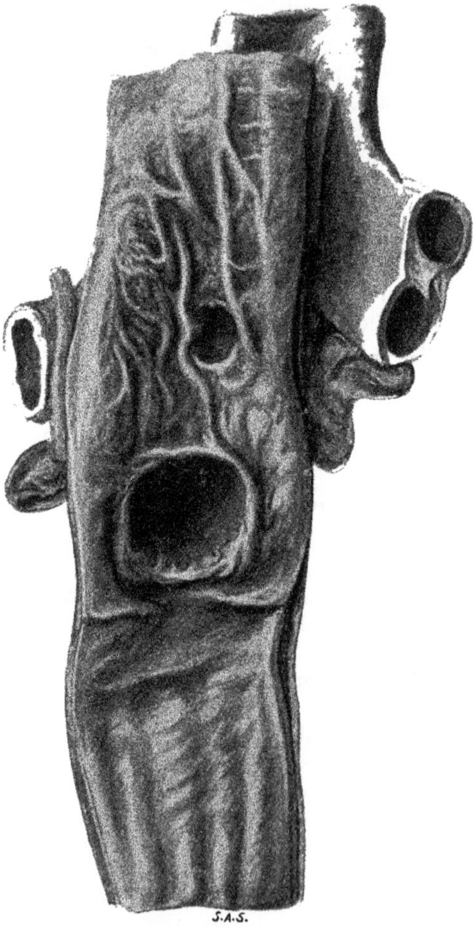

Fig. 349.—Traction diverticulum on the anterior surface below the bifurcation of the trachea.

(*London Hospital Pathological Department.*)

After a preliminary cleansing of the patient's mouth, the pouch is emptied, then exposed by an incision along the anterior margin of the sterno - mastoid muscle, and dissected out with the least possible disturbance of the surrounding tissues. It may be either cut away and its neck secured by tiers of sutures, or it may, if small, be invaginated into the œsophagus. The chief risk is subsequent leakage and formation of a fistula. Free drainage should always be employed, and rectal feeding administered for the first three days after operation. The fistula, if it occurs, tends to close naturally in a few weeks. This operation is not accompanied by much shock, and it has been successfully performed in elderly patients.

[1] The operation is well described in Jacobson's " Operations of Surgery," and full reference is there given to Butlin's and Maurice Richardson's well-known papers on the subject.

The results of operative treatment in 60 cases have been tabulated by Dervil Stetten as follows:—

Of 60 cases, 50 were cured and 10 died, a mortality of 16·6 per cent.

Of 48 cases in which the sac was excised without preliminary gastrostomy, 9 ended in death, a mortality of 18·7 per cent.

Of 5 cases in which a preliminary gastrostomy had been performed, 1 ended fatally, a mortality of 20 per cent.

All the patients operated on by the other methods recovered. In 4 cases invagination of the sac was employed. In 2 the sac was excised in two stages, and in 1 case the mucosa of the sac was destroyed.

Primary union of the œsophagus wound occurred in 21 of the 50 cases that recovered. In the others leakage occurred.

No recurrences were reported.

RUPTURE

Rupture of the œsophagus has resulted from over-distension of its wall, previously weakened by disease. In a few cases in which a rupture was found post mortem, no evidence of disease was present.

Bowles and Turner describe the case of a woman aged 62, in whom rupture of the œsophagus occurred after a severe attack of vomiting. West, Andrews, Williams, and others have noted similar cases.

Rupture of the œsophagus may be a result of severe injuries to the thorax or upper abdomen. In the absence of disease or injury a rupture is an extremely rare event; I could only find one doubtful case in the pathological records of the London Hospital during the last twenty years.

It has been suggested that some degenerative change in the œsophageal wall, so-called " œsophago-malacia," precedes, and may be the direct cause of, the rupture.

Rolleston points out that simple ulceration and rupture are generally found in the lower part of the œsophagus. In all the recorded cases the rupture appears to have been situated in the neighbourhood of the cardiac end. The tear is longitudinal, generally of small extent, from $\frac{1}{2}$ to 1 in. in length, and is complete, so that the œsophageal contents can escape into the posterior mediastinum. The accident appears to be more common in males than in females. Possibly chronic alcoholism may be a predisposing factor.

The **symptoms** generally occurred in association with or immediately after a severe attack of vomiting. Extreme pain referred to the lower part of the thorax, both back and front, was usually present. In some of the cases hæmatemesis followed, but generally vomiting ceased after the rupture. Attempts to swallow were followed by severe pain referred to the lower part of the thorax. The pulse was either slow and tense, owing to irritation of the vagi, or small and quick if much shock was present. In the early stage no definite physical signs were noted; later the implication of the mediastinum or pleura gave rise to signs of spreading suppuration in the neck or thorax.

Subcutaneous emphysema was noted in some of the cases re-ported.

Diagnosis has always been most difficult; it must be well-nigh impossible, indeed, in the absence of previous history pointing to disease of the œsophagus.

Surgical treatment by exposing the œsophagus through the posterior mediastinum appears to be the only possible course to adopt. The diagnostic difficulty and the rapidly fatal termination of these cases account for the absence of surgical intervention up to the present time.

INJURIES

The œsophagus, on account of its protected position, is not fre-quently injured. Its wall may, however, be penetrated from without or from within, in either the cervical or the thoracic portion of its course.

1. INJURIES FROM WITHOUT

(a) *Wounds of the cervical portion* are more common, and include incised and stab wounds and injuries by a bullet.

The œsophagus is not usually injured in self-inflicted wounds of the neck. These are generally placed obliquely at the upper part of the neck, and open the pharynx above the thyroid cartilage. The rare cases of incised wounds of the œsophagus are generally com-plicated by extensive injury to the trachea.

Stab wounds of the neck may penetrate the œsophagus with but little injury to the surrounding parts.

Bullet wounds of the œsophagus in the neck generally inflict severe injury on the surrounding structures.

The œsophagus has been wounded in rough attempts to perform tracheotomy, and in the performance of surgical operations such as thyroidectomy (Berry).[1]

(b) *Wounds of the thoracic portion* are uncommon. They are generally caused by stab or gunshot wounds. Penetration of the œsophagus here generally implies injury to the thoracic viscera, and is most dangerous owing to the certain risk of infection of the sur-rounding tissues, mediastina, pleura, or pericardium.

2. INJURIES FROM WITHIN

These include wounds of the wall inflicted by the passage of foreign bodies, bougies or other instruments. If a pathological condition of the wall is present or ulceration has occurred, penetration may be

[1] "Diseases of the Thyroid Gland," p. 304.

the result of but slight violence. The infliction of damage during the passage of bougies to relieve a stricture is not uncommon.

The œsophagus has been wounded by "sword swallowers."

Symptoms and signs of injury.—The symptoms of œsophageal wounds may be masked by those of injury to the surrounding structures.

Dysphagia accompanied by vomiting of blood suggests implication of the œsophagus; attempts to swallow may cause severe pain. If there is an external wound the presence of food or saliva in the discharge points to a wound of the œsophageal wall. In the cervical portion the diagnosis is generally obvious.

Treatment.— If possible, an attempt should be made to suture the wound in the wall of the œsophagus. Free drainage is essential.

FOREIGN BODIES

In children the objects most frequently swallowed by accident are metal toys, pins, and coins. In adults, bones of meat or fish, and other constituents of food too hastily swallowed, may lodge; or an ill-fitting tooth-plate, especially when worn at night, is very liable to become detached and slip down the œsophagus (Figs. 350, 352).

A proportion of these foreign bodies pass down the œsophagus into the stomach, and are voided in the fæces without causing trouble. Impaction of a foreign body in the œsophagus is always a source of great danger. Those with sharp or jagged edges are very liable to cause ulceration or even penetration of the œsophageal wall. Decomposition of retained particles of food as a result of the obstruction is an additional source of danger.

Foreign bodies tend to lodge opposite the three narrow portions of the œsophagus. By far the commonest site, however, is the upper part, between the cricoid cartilage and the tracheal bifurcation. Fortunately, foreign bodies seldom become impacted in the lower half of the œsophagus, though this may occur if they have been pushed down by instruments used for their extraction. In children, foreign bodies generally lodge about the level of the episternal notch. In hospital practice the impaction of coins at this level is a matter of common occurrence.

The **symptoms** produced vary considerably. Unless secondary complications arise, but little discomfort may be present. The severity of the symptoms is determined by the site of the impaction and the shape and position of the foreign body.

If it be impacted at the upper part of the œsophagus, the larynx may be irritated or actually compressed so that urgent dyspnoeic symptoms are excited. But if, as is usually the case, the foreign body be fixed near the upper end but below the cricoid, then respiratory symptoms are absent. There is more or less dysphagia, and generally solid food cannot be swallowed. Occasionally the œsophagus is so completely obstructed that even fluids are regurgitated ; on the other hand, in certain cases, semi-solid food can be swallowed with ease. Constant vomiting may be excited by the lodgment of a foreign body in the upper part of the œsophagus. This was present in a case under my care. In another case the impaction of a tooth-plate in the cervical portion of the œsophagus (Fig. 350) gave rise to severe pain even when saliva was swallowed. Pain referred to the sternum in front, or between the scapulæ posteriorly, may be caused by impaction of a foreign body in the lower part of the œsophagus.

When ulceration has occurred, vomiting of mucus streaked with blood may be present.

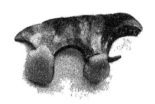

Fig. 350.—Tooth plate removed by the author by cervical œsophagotomy. It had lodged opposite the seventh cervical vertebra.

Foreign bodies may remain lodged in the œsophagus for years and cause but little trouble. They may, however, soon after impaction, occasion complications accompanied by symptoms of great urgency.

The secondary **complications** are—

1. Ulceration of the œsophageal wall at the site of impaction.
2. Formation of a submucous abscess.
3. Perforation of the wall of the œsophagus.
4. Peri-œsophageal inflammation and suppuration in the neck or thorax.
5. Erosion of the trachea or bronchi, with formation of fistulæ.
6. Perforation of large vessels.
7. Inflammation or suppuration in the pleuræ or pericardium.
8. Formation of a cicatricial stricture due to ulceration.

The symptoms caused by these complications are those either of hæmorrhage or of septic involvement of the neck or mediastina.

Perforation of the œsophageal wall causes severe pain, accompanied by rise of temperature and general malaise. Cervical emphysema generally ensues later. When a large vessel is involved, hæmorrhage may be slight at first ; it is recurrent, generally ingravescent, and a final severe bleeding may bring about a fatal issue.

Perforation of the aorta by impacted coins and other foreign bodies led to a fatal issue from hæmorrhage in five cases recently reported by Turner.

Involvement of the air-passages, pleuræ, etc., gives rise to characteristic signs and symptoms.

Diagnosis.—In most cases the diagnosis of the presence of a foreign body impacted in the œsophagus is a matter of no great difficulty. A history of the swallowing of the article in question is often obtainable, but in the case of children this may be entirely absent. Sudden onset of dysphagia in a child without another cause is suggestive of the presence of a foreign body, and routine examination as a rule clears up the diagnosis.

In *children* the first step, whenever possible, is to make an examination by the X-rays. It is not advisable to start the examination by the passage of bougies, as this requires a general anæsthetic, and may do harm by displacing the foreign body downwards. If the X-ray examination reveals a shadow it will, as before stated, generally be situated near the upper border of the sternum. The position and size of the body can by this means, as a rule, be determined with accuracy. Occasionally a coin, if impacted in the upper part of the œsophagus, can be palpated in the neck.

In *adults* it is also advisable to employ the X-rays as the preliminary step in the examination. As a general rule, foreign bodies can easily be detected in the œsophagus of an adult by this means. The rays must be caused to pass obliquely through the patient, especially if impaction has occurred low down, to avoid the shadow caused by the vertebræ, heart, and great vessels. Metallic bodies are generally recognized with ease, but small portions of vulcanite tooth-plates with teeth attached may form so faint a shadow that their detection is a matter of great difficulty. In these cases it is a good plan to administer bismuth emulsion, which adheres to the plate. The radiograph plate should be examined in the wet state, immediately after its development.

When X-rays are not available, a bougie, preferably a flexible one with a cylindrical metal tip, should be passed down. The presence of a foreign body and the site of impaction are then determined.

The œsophagoscope is invaluable for the detection and direct examination of foreign bodies in the œsophagus. It is advisable always to examine with this instrument under general anæsthesia, therefore its employment is better deferred until attempts at extraction have been decided upon. In one case, where a small tooth-plate was impacted at the lower part of the œsophagus, I was able through an œsophagoscope tube to move it from its position and push it down into the stomach. In other cases, removal through or with the tube may be possible.

Treatment.—The methods employed for the removal of foreign bodies from the œsophagus are as follows :—

1. Displacement downwards into the stomach by means of bougies.
2. Extraction by means of instruments through the mouth.
3. Extraction by means of instruments through an opening made in the œsophagus or stomach.

1. **Displacement downwards** should only be attempted in the case of smooth bodies, and sometimes when impaction takes place in the lower part of the tube.

2. In the majority of cases, **extraction by means of instruments through the mouth** is the method of choice, and is generally practicable. Incision of the œsophagus or stomach should only be considered when this has failed. The fact that most foreign bodies tend to become impacted in the upper part of the œsophagus facilitates their removal by the mouth.

In children, instrumental treatment should always be carried out under an anæsthetic. In adults this is not always necessary. If the foreign body be a small one, such as a pin, fish-bone, etc., it may be extracted by means of the well-known expanding probang of Fergusson, or by means of forceps (Fig. 351, A, B, C, F).

If the patient be a child, and a coin or other article be impacted in the upper part of the œsophagus, attempts at extraction are made. An anæsthetic is given, and the instrument passed down through the mouth. Coins can generally be removed by means of a coin-catcher or forceps, preferably the former (Fig. 351, D, E). This instrument is composed of steel, and the handle and stem should be made in one piece. At the extremity a ring of steel, bent at its middle to an acute angle, is soldered to the stem. The ring should not be hinged, but securely fastened to the stem. Many accidents have happened as the result of faulty construction of this instrument.

I always employ the X-rays during the introduction of the coin-catcher. The child is placed flat on the back on a couch beneath which the X-ray lamp is placed. The coin-catcher is gently passed down the œsophagus until an obstruction is felt; the room is then darkened and the X-ray light switched on, a hand-screen being placed over the front of the neck and thorax. The end of the coin-catcher and its relation to the foreign body can be clearly seen, and further manipulations can be performed with exactness. If, however, as must often happen, the X-rays are not available, the coin-catcher is passed under anæsthesia, and the coin can generally be extracted

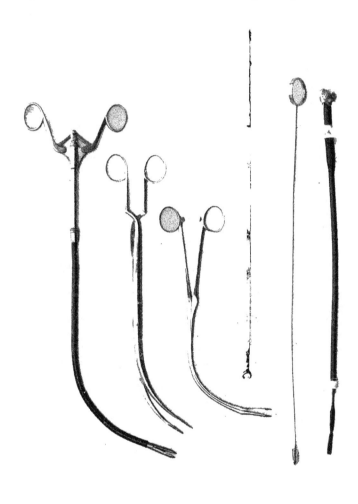

Fig. 351.—Instruments used in removing foreign bodies from the œsophagus.

A, Œsophageal forceps; B, C, laryngeal forceps; D, E, coin-catchers; F, Fergusson's probang.

without much difficulty. The end of the instrument must be passed with great gentleness until below the foreign body, and then pulled upwards. When the coin reaches the narrow portion at the cricoid a hitch is generally felt, but with a little manœuvring this can be overcome. If the foreign body be of angular shape, the coin-catcher is not of much use, and various forceps (Fig. 351, A, B, C) should be used for the extraction. The use of X-rays is invaluable, again, for this latter procedure.

Treatment for an adult should be conducted on the same lines.

If careful attempts at extraction have failed by these means, and the foreign body is firmly impacted owing to its irregular shape or sharp edges, it may be possible to alter its position, or even to extract it, by means of the œsophagoscope. Von Hacker considers that extraction by means of this instrument is generally practicable. It is hardly possible to extract any but small bodies through the largest tube of this instrument, but it is an easy matter to grasp them with forceps introduced through the tube, or even to cut them up with an instrument suitable for the purpose.

3. **Extraction through an incision in the wall of the œsophagus.**—The indications for this are—

i. When the foreign body cannot be displaced and extracted through the mouth.

ii. When evidence of ulceration of the wall of the œsophagus is present.

iii. When symptoms of perforation of the wall of the œsophagus are present.

iv. When complications, such as hæmorrhage or septic infection of the surrounding tissues or thoracic viscera, have supervened.

Cervical œsophagotomy is indicated, as a rule, for the removal of sharp, jagged bodies, such as a tooth-plate, impacted in the upper part of the œsophagus. It is possible by this means to remove, by the introduction of suitable forceps, a body situated as low down as the position of the bronchi (Bennet May). On one occasion I removed a tooth-plate which was impacted opposite the 3rd dorsal vertebra (Fig. 352).

Richardson says that a length of œsophagus 6 in. below the cricoid is accessible by this route. In certain cases it is necessary to cut up the foreign body to facilitate its extraction. In the case of a toy bicycle impacted in the œsophagus, and removed by me, this manœuvre had to be carried out before extraction was possible (Plate 89). This procedure was also necessary in a case recorded by Lawson.

The operation of cervical œsophagotomy is not difficult, but is attended with some danger owing to the risk of septic infection of

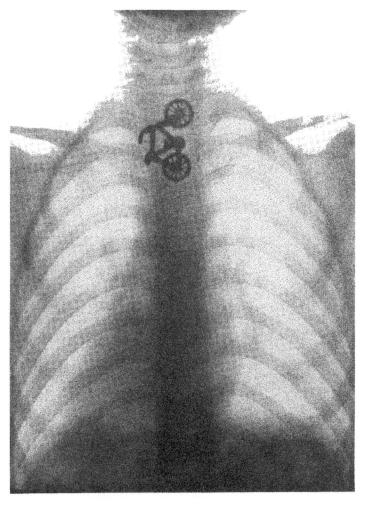

Toy bicycle impacted in the œsophagus. Removed by the author
by cervical œsophagotomy. The machine had to be cut in two by
forceps before extraction was possible.

PLATE 89.

the tissue planes in the neck. The dissection to expose the œsophagus should be made with accuracy, and with as little tearing of the tissues as possible. The opening made in the œsophagus wall can usually be closed by absorbable sutures, and free drainage must be permitted ; in fact, the wound may be entirely left open for this purpose. In most cases a fistula occurs and persists for a short time, especially if ulceration be present, but, as a rule, it closes spontaneously; Rectal feeding is advisable for three days after this operation.

If the foreign body be impacted in the œsophagus at its lower part, it may be extracted from below after gastrotomy. According to Richardson, 3 in. of the lower end of the œsophagus is accessible for this purpose.

The most difficult problem to deal with is impaction of a body in that part of the œsophagus inaccessible from above or from below. For these difficult cases, Bryant has

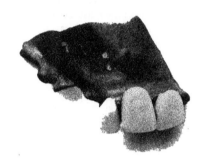

Fig. 352.—Tooth-plate removed by the author by cervical œsophagotomy. It had lodged opposite the 3rd dorsal vertebra.

devised and carried out the operation of mediastinal œsophagotomy. He approaches the œsophagus from the right side, in the case of a foreign body situated below the aortic arch, by resecting portions of three ribs close to the spine. The posterior mediastinum is opened up and the œsophagus incised. In this operation there is great risk of infection, and it has seldom been carried out in this country. Fortunately, impaction of a foreign body rarely takes place in that portion of the œsophagus which is inaccessible from above or below. It may be possible, by means of forceps introduced through the tube of an œsophagoscope, as in a case mentioned above, to displace a body impacted in this position downwards until it comes within reach of the cardiac orifice.

Gastrotomy is indicated for the removal of bodies situated 13 in. or more below the incisor teeth. The stomach is opened and attempts are made to dilate the cardiac orifice by the finger or a suitable instrument.

Careful traction of the stomach downwards with flexion of the spine renders the cardiac orifice easier of access (Bryant).

Mortality of œsophagotomy for foreign bodies.—Tillman quotes G. Fischer—in 108 cases a mortality of 26 per cent.—and Egloff—in 135 cases a mortality of 24·8 per cent.

OBSTRUCTION

The conditions which lead to a narrowing of the œsophagus, giving rise to dysphagia, are as follows :—

I. INTRINSIC, originating in the œsophageal wall.

    1. *Spasm* of the muscle coat. Œsophago-spasm. Cardio-spasm. Globus hystericus.

    2. *Cicatricial contracture*, consequent upon ulceration of the mucous membrane.

        Causes—(a) Wounds.

            (b) Burns.

            (c) Syphilis.

            (d) Tuberculosis.

            (e) Typhoid fever.

            (f) Peptic ulcers.

    3. *New growths.*

        (a) Innocent.

        (b) Malignant.

II. EXTRINSIC. Pressure on, or invasion of, the wall of the œsophagus from without.

    1. Aneurysms.

    2. Tumours. Enlarged glands, new growths.

    3. Abscess.

INTRINSIC OBSTRUCTION

SPASM OF THE MUSCLE COAT

A diffuse dilatation of the wall of the œsophagus associated with contraction of the cardiac opening, or cardio-spasm, occurs in young adults of both sexes. The etiology of this somewhat rare condition has given rise to much discussion, and its treatment to the exhibition of much mechanical ingenuity.

Pathology.—The specimen of which Fig. 353 is a drawing shows the pathological changes usually present. The muscular coat of the entire wall of the œsophagus is hypertrophied, whilst, in the lower three-fourths of its extent, marked dilatation has taken place. The mucous coat is also greatly thickened, and scattered over its surface are numerous shallow ulcers. At the cardiac orifice the muscular hypertrophy is most noticeable; the lumen is here greatly diminished, and the mucous membrane is thrown into longitudinal folds. There is, however, no ulceration seen in this part. Such marked changes are found in the chronic forms of the disease.

Etiology.—It is doubtful whether a true primary dilatation occurs irrespectively of obstruction to the cardiac orifice. In most cases the dilatation and hypertrophy are probably secondary to a narrowing of the cardia dependent on muscular spasm, which may be of nervous origin, and has been said to follow emotional disturbances (Sippey). This spasm may be secondary to inflammation or actual ulceration of the mucous membrane, but very often stands alone. In a case reported by Ledderhose it appeared to be caused by the presence of a polypus. Malignant growths at the cardia are often associated with spasmodic contraction of the muscular coat, but the obstruction is then dependent chiefly upon the presence of the growth itself.

Cardio-spasm is, however, frequently independent of any pathological change in the mucous membrane, and many theories have been suggested to explain this fact. Some authorities hold that an alteration in the nerve muscular mechanism exists. Degeneration of the vagi nerve fibres which supply this part of the œsophagus has been demonstrated by Kraus. According to Rosenheim, the condition is due to primary action of the muscle wall, associated with disturbance of innervation. Klebs found fatty degeneration of the muscular wall. Fleimer believes that the dilatation is due to some developmental anomaly. Mikulicz, Meltzer, and Leichtenstern agree that spasm of the cardia is the cause of the dilatation, but are unable to explain the spasm.

Young adults of both sexes may be the subjects of this curious condition, though females of hysterical tendencies are, perhaps, more frequently affected. The clinical course of the disease is suggestive of a congenital origin.

The **symptoms** may be of long duration, and the intermittent form sometimes lasts over many years. The onset may be either sudden or gradual.

The most important symptom is *dysphagia*. The onset is sometimes acute, and for some time the patient is quite unable to swallow either solids or fluids. A stage of remission follows, with recurrence of symptoms after a variable period. The dysphagia due to mechanical obstruction differs in that it is gradual and progressive. Nothnagel points out as a characteristic sign that solid food may sometimes pass down more easily than liquids. Dysphagia is accompanied by a feeling of pressure in the thorax, and sometimes by burning pains

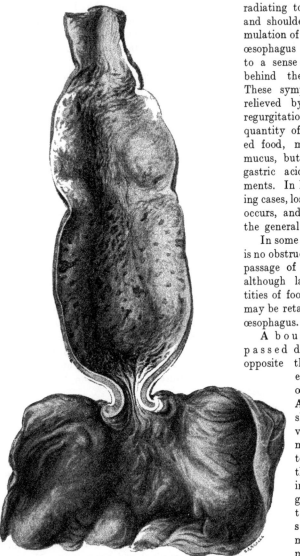

Fig. 353.—Diffuse dilatation of the œsophagus with
cardio-spasm.

(London Hospital Pathological Department.)

radiating to the neck and shoulders. Accumulation of food in the œsophagus gives rise to a sense of fullness behind the sternum. These symptoms are relieved by effortless regurgitation of a large quantity of undigested food, mixed with mucus, but free from gastric acids or ferments. In long-standing cases, loss of weight occurs, and failure of the general health.

In some cases there is no obstruction to the passage of a bougie, although large quantities of food or liquid may be retained in the œsophagus.

A bougie, when passed down, stops opposite the cardiac end of the œsophagus. After a short interval its point may be felt to engage in the opening and be gripped by the constricting muscle. It may then be passed through into the stomach by a little pressure. If this happens, the diagnosis of spasmodic stricture may be confidently made. More often the bougie will not pass, nor even engage the stricture. Keen points out that the tube can be abnormally moved about in the dilated œsophagus.

Examination with the œsophagoscope should then be undertaken. In the recorded eases the cardia has been seen constricted, and the mucous membrane heaped up in longitudinal folds so as to give a rosette-like appearance. The surface of the mucosa may be pale, or intensely red, or even ulcerated.

The œsophageal dilatation can be demonstrated by the X-rays on the fluorescent screen after the administration of bismuth in food. A fusiform shadow is seen in a typical case ; by this means the presence of a diverticulum may be excluded.

Examination by auscultation shows retardation or absence of the second swallowing sound.

Among other methods of examination may be mentioned the two-tube test of Rumpel, and the passage of a rubber-coated sound connected to a eudiometer as suggested by Strauss.

The **prognosis** is unfavourable.

Treatment is difficult, and may only relieve temporarily. The indications are to attempt to overcome the spasm by means of medicines and the passage of sounds. If emaciation be present, hollow sounds for feeding purposes should be passed if possible.

The œsophagoscope may assist the passage of sounds. Rectal feeding is sometimes necessary in the acute attacks, whilst for extreme cases gastrostomy may become necessary. If dilatation has occurred, the passage of bougies gives only temporary relief (Sippey).

Rolleston refers to cases successfully treated by Sippey, who employed a rubber-bag dilator.

Mikulicz recommends that the stomach be opened and the cardia dilated by means of special rubber-coated forceps. He quotes six successful cases.

Rosenheim in two cases successfully dilated a cardiac spasmodic stricture by introducing rubber bags which were then filled with air or water.

FIBROUS STRICTURE OF THE ŒSOPHAGUS

Etiology.—Fibrous cicatricial stricture occurs as a late result of ulceration of the mucous membrane.

This ulceration is generally due to the swallowing of *corrosive fluids* or of *boiling water*, but occasionally follows the impaction of a *foreign body*, whilst rarely it is *tuberculous* or *syphilitic* in origin.

Pathology.—The formation of the stricture depends entirely on the position, extent, and degree of the burn or injury inflicted on the wall of the œsophagus.

As regards position, naturally the brunt of the injury falls upon the narrower portions of the tube, viz. (1) at its origin ; (2) opposite the bifurcation of the trachea ; (3) at the cardiac end.

The burns may be sharply localized to any one of these positions, or may extend over the entire wall, causing greater destruction of tissue opposite the narrower portions.

The degree of the burn and the amount of tissue destruction depend on the nature of the fluid and the rapidity with which it enters the stomach.

The stricture resulting from a localized burn may be only superficial, giving rise to an annular or linear narrowing. This is not common. More extensive and deep burns cause considerable tubular narrowing with marked fibrous thickening of the entire wall of the œsophagus. Even the peri-œsophageal tissues are sometimes involved, and their contraction may distort the wall of the œsophagus and lead to a deviation from its natural position. The œsophageal wall above the stricture may be dilated and thinned, but this is not often seen. More commonly a thickening involving the muscular and outer coat is present and extends above and below the stricture. In my experience this is more commonly seen in tubular strictures. (In superficial annular strictures dilatation *above* the narrowing is more likely to occur.)

The œsophagus at the site of the stricture, and above and below, is generally transformed into a tough, unyielding tube (Fig. 354). Progressive contraction of the cicatrized area gradually occurs, leading to a dense and resistant stricture. The mucosa is usually destroyed, but the submucous tissue contains large numbers of plasma cells and everywhere shows formation of new connective tissue. The circular muscular fibres are generally much hypertrophied.

Sometimes ulceration of the mucous membrane occurs in the dilated wall above the stricture as the result of the lodgment and decomposition of retained particles of food. Pouches of the wall very rarely take place.

The **diagnosis** of fibrous strictures of the œsophagus due to the action of a corrosive is not difficult. The patient complains of a gradually increasing dysphagia, commencing at variable periods after the injury. The symptoms immediately following the burn are chiefly pain and inability to swallow any but liquid food. This condition improves after a few days, when more and more solid food can be taken. After a week or two the symptoms of a progressive dysphagia supervene. The dysphagia is painless and ingravescent, and, unless treatment be adopted, gradually becomes absolute. The diagnosis is confirmed, after the usual routine examination to exclude other causes of œsophageal stenosis, by the introduction of the œsophagoscope and the passage of bougies. If the patient is able to swallow fluids, a solution of bismuth given by the mouth and the employ- ment of X-rays may give valuable information as to the site and extent of the stricture.

Treatment. 1. **By mechanical dilatation.** —This treatment should be attempted at first in all permeable fibrous stric- tures of the œsophagus. A medium-sized flexible gum-elastic bougie with conical tip is passed down the œsophagus, and very gentle attempts are made to engage its point in the stricture. If any difficulty is experienced, a smaller- sized bougie must be tried. If that fails, a filiform bougie or catgut whip should be used. A stiff graduated bougie (Fig. 355, B) will sometimes be found the most useful in- strument in locating and engaging the mouth of the stricture. The whip may be used alone, or be di- rected to the stricture through a hollow bougie which is first passed down to the site of the obstruc- tion. If the bougie and whip

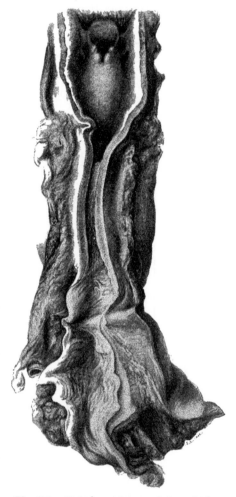

Fig. 354.—Tubular stricture of the middle third of the œsophagus resulting from the action of a corrosive.
(*London Hospital Pathological Department.*)

fail to enter the stricture, the œsophagoscope should be passed down and attempts made to see the opening. If it be impossible to find the

opening by this means, or to pass any bougie, then further operative treatment must be considered.

If a bougie passes through the stricture, dilatation can be pro-
ceeded with.

Dilatation can be effected either (a) by passing bougies in gradually increasing sizes at intervals of several days (intermittent dilatation), or (b) by inserting and leaving in position suitable catheters through which the patient can be fed (continuous dilatation).

In children and in other cases in which much difficulty or distress is occasioned by the passage of the bougie, the latter method will be found 'most serviceable.

(a) *Intermittent dilatation.*—The bougie is passed and left in position for a few minutes ; a larger size is then introduced and kept in for a similar period ; this is removed, and after a couple of days' interval a further trial is made with a bougie of slightly larger calibre. By this means gradual dilatation is effected.

Special forms of bougies have been invented in order to overcome the difficulty of gradual dilatation. The so-called " railway " bougie (Fig. 355, A) consists of a hollow gum-elastic bougie, which is passed over a small solid bougie already intro-

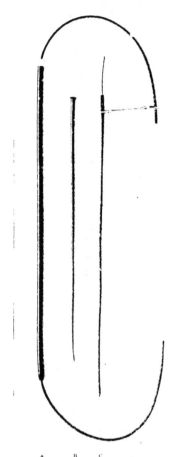

Fig. 355.—Bougies for dilating the
œsophagus.

A, " Railway " bougie ; B, graduated bougie ; C, rubber
tube stretched on whalebone. (*Von Hacker.*)

duced through the stricture as a guide. By the successive passage
of larger ones the stricture can sometimes be rapidly dilated.

Von Hacker has invented an ingenious method of dilating tight and difficult strictures. The instrument (Fig. 355, C), consisting of a rubber drainage-tube stretched on a central guide of whalebone or other stiff material, is inserted into the stricture. When the guide is withdrawn the tube shortens and retracts, with corresponding expansion of its circumference. This rubber tube is left in the stricture for some time, and thus the stricture is uniformly dilated. The guide must be well oiled to obviate difficulty in withdrawal. In my experience this method is unsatisfactory for very tight strictures. A straight, rigid guide is difficult to introduce and to engage in the opening of the stricture.

(b) *Continuous dilatation.* —A hollow tube with a funnel-shaped upper end is passed down by means of an introducer and left *in situ.* Symonds's well-known tubes are of the greatest value and the best for this purpose (Fig. 356, A to D). They are especially useful when there is much difficulty in passing bougies, and if the patient is in urgent need of nourishment. When multiple strictures are present, as is not infrequent, a short Symonds's tube will dilate the upper,

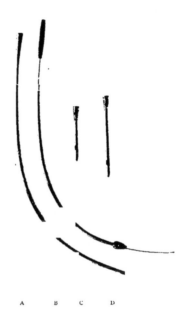

Fig. 356.—Symonds's tubes.

A, Symonds's long tube; B, introducer; C, D, Symonds's short tubes.

and perhaps more constricted, portion, and so permit later access to the lower part of the œsophagus. These tubes may be left in for a week or ten days at a time.

In strictures in the upper part of the œsophagus the long, upper, funnel-shaped end is apt to irritate the larynx. In a case of mine this was obviated by cutting down the funnel. The tube is kept *in situ* by silk which comes out of the mouth or nose and is fixed to the auricle. It is a good plan, if the silk is passed out of the mouth, to thread upon it a piece of small rubber drainage-tube. This prevents the possibility of the silk being bitten through if an anæsthetic has been given.

2. **Palliative measures.**—If no instrument can be passed through
the stricture, then a temporary *gastrostomy* should be made, to permit
feeding and to afford rest to the œsophagus. After a few days, further
attempts at dilatation may be successful. If, however, after a suitable
period, bougies cannot be passed down, the procedure adopted by
Abbe, Dunham, and others is worth a trial. This consists of making
the patient swallow one end of a string of silk (Dunham), or of a piece
to which a shot has been attached (Abbe). The silk passes down
into the stomach, and is found and brought out through a gastrotomy
opening. Abbe employs the string to act as a saw and so divide the
constricted portions : when this is done a bougie is fastened to the
upper end and pulled down from below.

When the stricture is placed low down in the œsophagus it can
sometimes be dilated from below, through the opening in the stomach,
by the passage of suitable forceps or dilators, or even the finger. Considerable difficulty is often experienced in this manœuvre, but successful
cases have been reported by Kendal Franks and others.

Cutting instruments after the pattern of urethrotomes have been
devised for the division of impassable œsophageal strictures (*internal
œsophagotomy*). These are always dangerous owing to the risk of
their cutting through the wall and leading to mediastinal infection.
They are condemned by most surgeons.

Electrolysis of the stricture has been attempted in a few cases
(Franks), but the method has little value.

Finally, mention may be made of operations which are planned
to divide the strictures from without (*external œsophagotomy*), or even
to excise the stenosed portion. Such operations are indicated when
an impassable stricture of small extent is situated in the upper portion
of the œsophagus.

The œsophagus is exposed as for œsophagotomy, and the extent
of the stricture determined. If possible the wall is opened below
the stricture, and the latter divided from below upwards ; bougies
are then passed, and dilatation effected. The opening in the wall
is now carefully closed, and free drainage provided. This gives most
satisfactory results, but unfortunately is seldom practicable. The
stricture is often found to extend into the thorax, so that the incision
has to be made either directly over the stenosed portion or above it.
It is better in these cases to open the œsophagus above and attempt
to find the upper opening of the stricture. This can then be enlarged
by a cutting instrument or by the passage of a probe or stiff bougie.

In exceptional cases, excision of the entire segment has been
successfully carried out (Kendal Franks). The skin of the neck has
been employed to make good the portion which has been removed
(von Hacker).

Recently, attempts have been made to bring a segregated loop of jejunum up under the skin, and by anastomosing it with the œsophagus above the stricture, and with the stomach below, to reconstitute a gullet.

Non-Malignant Tumours

These comprise polypi, fibromas, myomas, lipomas, warts, and retention cysts (mucous glands). All of them are so rare as to be of little surgical interest.

The polypi are perhaps the least uncommon. They usually occur in the upper part of the œsophagus in elderly males. They are fibromas, and generally contain fat in their structure. The tumour may develop a long stalk, and cases have been published in which the polypi protruded into the pharynx and could be seen through the mouth. The pedicle is generally attached to the anterior wall of the œsophagus below the cricoid. They may give rise to no symptoms, but if large may cause dysphagia, and if protruded upwards may induce attacks of dyspnœa and alteration in the voice.

They are treated by removal, after division of the stalk, by means of a suitable snare.

Polypi have been removed through the mouth. The tumour is ejected and held in position, the pedicle ligatured and cut through. If this be found impossible, it should be removed through an œsophagotomy opening. If situated in the lower portion of the œsophagus (an uncommon site) it is possible that the tumour might be removed with the help of the œsophagoscope (von Hacker).

Malignant Tumours

Carcinoma of the Œsophagus

It has been estimated that about 5 per cent. of all carcinomas arise in the mucous membrane of the œsophagus. The growth most commonly begins in the epithelium, and is a typical squamous-celled carcinoma. Less frequently the epithelium of the glands in the mucous membrane undergoes carcinomatous change and develops a tumour composed of cylindrical cells (Franke). In 30 cases of malignant disease of the œsophagus, Perry and Shaw found 28 squamous-celled epitheliomas and 2 sarcomas. A colloid growth is occasionally met with.

In its early stages the carcinoma is limited to the mucous membrane, and involves only a small portion of the wall of the tube ; it tends to spread along the surface of the mucous membrane, either transversely, so as to involve the whole circumference in an annular form (Fig. 357), or longitudinally, giving rise to a growth of large extent (Fig. 358). The former condition is more commonly found.

As the growth extends, it infiltrates the outer coats and may penetrate the muscular wall and invade the peri-œsophageal tissues.

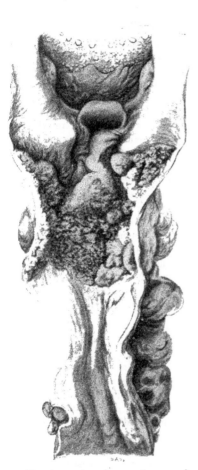

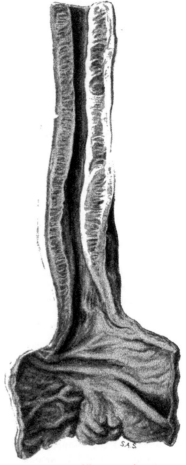

Fig. 357.—Annular carcinoma of   Fig. 358.—Diffuse carcinoma
  upper end of œsophagus.   of œsophagus.

(Royal College of Surgeons Museum.)   *(Royal College of Surgeons Museum.)*

A primary growth in one part of the œsophagus has been found
to be associated with other growths lower down, suggesting the
possibility of a secondary implantation.

Metastatic growths from œsophageal carcinoma have been recorded, but are of rare occurrence.

Glandular deposits are frequently noted. The lower deep cervical glands on either side are affected when the primary growth is situated in the upper part of the œsophagus. Growths in the thoracic portion lead to involvement of the mediastinal glands.

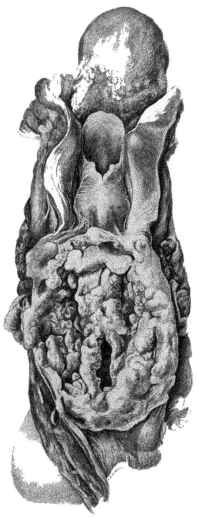

As the growth extends outwards into the muscular wall it may finally penetrate to those structures in close relation to the œsophagus. Peri-œsophageal adhesions and infiltration lead to implication of nerves, viz. the vagi, recurrent laryngeal, and sympathetic. Perforation of the large vessels in the thorax, or of those portions of the air-passages in close relation to the œsophagus, have been noted in many cases (*see* Fig. 359). Less commonly the pleura and lungs are involved.

Perforation of the lung leads to gangrene and cavity formation, with possible secondary erosion of branches of the pulmonary artery.

In 70 cases of perforation into the air-passages collected by Zenker and von Ziemssen (Kraus), 26 involved the right or left bronchus, 21 the trachea. In 23 cases the lungs were invaded ; the right lung was three times more commonly affected than the left.

The pleural cavity is seldom penetrated. The posterior

Fig. 359.—Extensive carcinoma of œsophagus opening into trachea.

(London Hospital Pathological Department.)

mediastinum on the right side may be invaded, and a case of extensive subcutaneous emphysema has been recorded as the result of this occurrence.

An œsophageal cancer sometimes extends to the pericardium.

A carcinomatous ulcer, situated at the upper or lower end of the œsophagus, may spread to the pharynx or stomach respectively. At the upper end the ulcer may extend (a) forwards over the cricoid, and involve the arytenoids or larynx, or (b) backwards, and become adherent to, or even erode, the vertebræ.

Growths at the cardiac end have been seen to spread for some distance into the wall of the stomach. Carcinoma of the cardiac end of the stomach spreads to the œsophagus. Of 26 cases of malignant disease of the cardiac end of the stomach, in 16 it had invaded the œsophagus for some distance (Fawcett).

It would appear that the growth is sometimes determined by some previous change in the epithelium, such as scarring due to old ulceration from various causes. The common location of the growth in the narrow portion of the wall suggests that irritation may be a factor in its development. It has frequently been noted that œsophageal carcinoma is associated with raised plaques of thickened epithelium scattered over other portions of the mucous membrane. They appear to be analogous with leucoplakia of the tongue, and their association with carcinomatous change is most significant of the presence of some chronic irritation.

Sex- and age-incidence. — Carcinoma of the œsophagus is essentially a disease of the male sex. It is estimated that about 80 per cent. of the cases occur in males. A family history of carcinoma was found in 6 per cent. (Rolleston). It is a disease of later life, and but seldom met with before the age of 40. In the female sex it is found to occur at a somewhat earlier period (Rolleston). Its greater frequency in the male sex has been attributed to the greater liability to irritation from tobacco, alcohol, etc., and possibly to the more frequent occurrence of syphilitic lesions.

Distribution. — Carcinoma tends to arise in certain well-defined areas of the œsophageal wall. It affects the narrow portions of the tube, namely, the origin, the neighbourhood of the tracheal bifurcation, and the lower end.

The relative frequency with which carcinoma involves any one of these portions has been a matter of dispute. Mackenzie (1875) maintained that the upper portion of the œsophagus was affected in 40 per cent. of all cases. Other authorities (von Hacker, Butlin, Rolleston) favoured the lower portion and the part in relation to the tracheal bifurcation. Von Hacker (Kraus) in 100 cases found that 40 per cent. arose at the tracheal bifurcation, and 30 per cent. at the lower end, whilst only 10 per cent. involved the upper portion. Von Bergmann maintains that the region of the bifurcation of the trachea is the most common situation of cancer. Butlin points out that the lower half of the œsophagus is much more commonly affected than the upper. Rolleston (Clifford Allbutt) noted that in women the upper portion was more commonly affected. Keen ("Textbook") states that in 68 per cent. the carcinoma is situated in the lower portion of the œsophagus, between the hilus of the lung and the cardia.

Of 214 cases quoted by Rawling, only 24 occurred in the cervical region, whilst 163 were in the thoracic portion of the œsophagus. Sauerbruch in 186 cases found that 26 were at the commencement, 43 at the bifurcation of the trachea, and 117 at the cardiac end.

Symptoms.—A gradual onset of dysphagia associated with loss of flesh and strength, occurring in an elderly male patient, is generally indicative of the presence of a carcinomatous obstruction in the œsophagus.

The dysphagia occasionally comes on suddenly. As a rule, pain is absent until the disease is advanced, but even in the early stages complaints may be made of a feeling of tightness in the throat or of vague feelings of discomfort in the chest when food is swallowed. Loss of body-weight and strength are comparatively early symptoms. The dysphagia is at first slight, but later is slowly progressive. A difficulty in swallowing dry, solid food is first experienced, then semi-solid food cannot be taken into the stomach without some delay ; later still, only liquids or very finely divided substances can pass down. At a still later stage, fluids tend to regurgitate unless taken slowly ; and in the final stages, even fluids cannot pass the site of the obstruction. Pain, as previously mentioned, is not an early symptom ; when it occurs it is generally coincident with the taking of food. It is often referred to the sternum when the stricture is in the lower half of the œsophagus ; thence it radiates to the back of the shoulders, or even up to the throat. If the growth is in the upper part the pain is referred to the neck on each side. In growths at the cardiac end, pain may be entirely absent.

In the later stages, symptoms arise which depend on the position of the growth and its spread to neighbouring structures. An ulcerating growth at the upper part generally leads to much laryngeal irritation, distressing cough, or expectoration of frothy mucus associated with fetor.

Severe bleeding is rare, unless a large vessel becomes involved, but blood-stained, foul-smelling mucus is brought up in late ulcerating growths situated at any part of the tube. The breath acquires an offensive fetor.

In some cases the voice becomes altered and develops the character suggestive of paralysis of a vocal cord.

In long-standing cases, symptoms of encroachment on the air-passages by the growth may develop.

The **diagnosis** is made (1) by a consideration of the above-mentioned symptoms, (2) by certain routine methods of examination conducted in a methodical manner in order to exclude the many other causes of dysphagia.

Careful inspection and palpation of the neck should be undertaken to eliminate tumours originating either in the lymphatic glands, the thyroid gland, or the vertèbræ. Increased fixation or undue bulkiness of the œsophagus can be noted. Rarely, the presence of a pharyngeal diverticulum may be discovered by this means.

Evidence òf alteration of the pupils should be noted, or inequality of the palpebral fissure. Signs of venous obstruction, or increased hyperæmia of one side of the face, are suggestive.

External examination of the thorax should next be undertaken, and the condition of the heart and lungs carefully noted. The upper abdomen should then be palpated for the presence of a possible tumour.

The methods employed in the internal examination of the œsophagus have been previously described. They include—

(1) Examination by sounding ; (2) the employment of X-rays and fluorescent screen after the administration of bismuth by the mouth ; (3) examination with the laryngoscope and the œsophagoscope.

1. Examination with bougies.—This method is most commonly employed, and is of great practical value. By its means the site, extent, and permeability of an œsophageal stenosis can be estimated. In careful hands the risks of this procedure are slight. The chief dangers are—(a) perforation of the wall of the œsophagus, already thinned by an ulcerating growth ; (b) rupture of a sac in cases of aortic aneurysm.

The former danger can be minimized, in cases where the growth appears to be of long duration, by employing a soft stomach-tube in place of the usual gum-elastic or whalebone sound. Careful consideration of the symptoms and physical signs should render the latter risk an unlikely one.

Gum-elastic sounds, either oval or round, should be used, or Symonds's whalebone sound with olive-shaped end. The sound is passed as described at p. 257.

If an obstruction be felt, no attempt should be made to push the instrument forcibly past the constricted part. A smaller-sized bougie should be used, and gradually smaller ones inserted until one is felt to pass the site of the obstruction.

By the employment of Symonds's sounds the length of the con-. stricted portion can be measured.

2. Examination with X-rays.—Radiography after the administration of bismuth is now extensively employed in this condition. Its chief value is to exclude the presence of a pouch or foreign body.

The presence of the stricture can be shown by the stoppage of the bismuth, given either as a suppository or as an emulsion. If in the latter form, it will be seen to collect and form an oblong opaque shadow, somewhat cone-shaped, with the base uppermost. The apex of the cone points into the mouth of the stricture, through which the solution may be seen to drop down slowly into the stomach. In early growths, when slight stenosis exists, the method is of little value. I have observed a case in which bismuth solution passed into the stomach, but sounds could not be made to pass the site of the growth.

In doubtful cases of aneurysm the method is of great value, as the use of sounds is contra-indicated. The presence of the aneurysm may be demonstrated by a pulsating shadow, and a stricture by the dense opacity produced by the retained bismuth.

3. **Direct inspection with the œsophagoscope.**—This method gives the most exact information as to the character and extent of an œsophageal growth. By its means portions of the tumour can be removed for microscopical examination, and local applications can be made or radium applied. The employment of this instrument, however, is not to be advised as a routine method of examination in general practice. The introduction of an œsophagoscope, even under anæsthesia, is a proceeding which entails certain risks and requires technical experience. The diagnosis of an œsophageal carcinoma can generally be confidently made without its use. It is invaluable in cases in which the diagnosis of a malignant growth is doubtful, or in which treatment by radium, or some other local application, is thought advisable. As seen through the œsophagoscope, a carcinoma of the mucous membrane of the wall can be easily recognized. In the very early stages only a slight swelling may be seen, but in the average case the raised ragged edge of the growth and the ulcerating surface are quite distinctive. The fixation of the œsophageal wall at the site of the growth is a noticeable feature, and the natural rhythmic respiratory movements, which are always present in the healthy œsophagus, are absent.

·**Examination with the laryngoscope** will only reveal a growth situated at the commencement of the œsophagus. This instrument, however, should be employed in every case in order to investigate the condition of the vocal cords.

Treatment.—Operations for the removal of carcinoma of the œsophagus have up to the present time met with but little success. Excision of growths in the cervical portion have only been tem-porarily successful. Records of 15 cases treated by cervical œsophagectomy have been collected by Quervain, and these include the well-known cases operated on by Czerny, Mikulicz, and Garré.

The results are gloomy : 5 patients died as the result of the operation, and no case survived for longer than thirteen months.

In Czerny's case the upper end of the lower segment of the œsophagus was fixed to the margins of the skin wound, and the patient was fed by means of a tube.

The field of this operation is a limited one ; it is only suitable for small growths situated in the upper part of the œsophagus. The risks of infection are great, and it is generally found impossible to restore the continuity of the œsophageal wall after thorough excision of the growth.

In the majority of cases, carcinoma invades the thoracic portion of the œsophagus, and the dangers and difficulty of attempting its removal by operation can be easily understood.

The operation of **thoracic œsophagectomy** is one of great difficulty and of peculiar danger owing to the effect of the atmospheric pressure on the lungs. In order to overcome the evil results of the atmospheric pressure, various forms of apparatus have been devised. (*See* under Respiratory System, Vol. III., p. 266.) Although by these means one risk of this operation has been minimized, yet the anatomical difficulties of extirpating a growth in this portion of the œsophagus are still present. The wall of the œsophagus, unlike that of the intestine, cannot be freely excised with any prospect of a successful union of the divided ends. An end-to-end anastomosis by suture is rarely feasible. If sutures are used, they have a tendency to cut out owing to tension and the constant movement in the thorax. The absence of omentum and, more important still, of a serous coat on the œsophageal wall, are conditions prejudicial to satisfactory union.

The total number of reported operations on the œsophagus by thoracotomy is 39 (Meyer). In 21 cases, resection of a growth was carried out; in 9 cases, exploratory thoracotomy was satisfactorily performed. There were no cases of recovery after resection. This operation will probably only be practicable in the lower portion of the œsophagus. A cone-shaped portion of the stomach wall is drawn up into the thorax and anastomosed to the œsophagus on the proximal side of the growth. This operation, known as *œsophago-gastrostomy*, has been performed by Sauerbruch and, in dogs, by Willy Meyer, who thinks that the operation may have a future if carried out in two stages and conducted in the " positive differential pressure chamber." In the first stage, thoracotomy is performed, and the cone-shaped portion of the stomach brought up and transferred into the thorax through an opening in the diaphragm. In the second stage, two or three weeks later, the growth is resected and the œsophago-gastrostomy completed.

Meyer says that the stomach can only be pulled up for 3–4 in. into the thorax.

For tumours situated in the middle and upper portions, Meyer recommends excision of the growth, when possible, with closure by inversion of the divided ends and gastrostomy. The upper end may be sutured to the skin, and an attempt made later to unite it by various means with the gastric opening. This has been done by the use of an instrument or the employment of a portion of the small intestine (Roux, Kocher, Tuffier, Kümmell).

Sauerbruch considers that growths at the lower end of the œsophagus are most favourable for removal. They form late metastases, and do not spread locally with rapidity. He recommends that, if the tumours be small, the end of the œsophagus should be invaginated into the stomach and resected later. He prefers the use of the Murphy buttons to sutures.

Janeway and Green advocate removal of the major portion of the stomach in cases of growth involving both the lower portion of the œsophagus and the cardiac end of the stomach. Through an abdominal incision the stomach is loosened from its mesenteric attachments. The thorax is opened, and the stomach brought up through an opening in the diaphragm. The pylorus is then divided. The œsophagus is cut across above the growth, and the ends of the œsophagus and pylorus are united by suture. The pylorus is then secured to the opening in the diaphragm. This operation has been carried out with success in dogs.

Palliative measures.—Short of removal of the growth, the indications are to prevent starvation of the patient (which will inevitably ensue) and to add to his comfort.

The increasing dysphagia may be relieved by—

1. The passage of sounds or bougies from time to time.
2. The introduction of feeding-tubes.
3. Application of radium.
4. Cervical œsophagostomy.
5. Gastrostomy.

1. The **periodical passage of sounds** in order to dilate a malignant stricture has some value, but it is not advisable as a routine practice. The passage of the sound may cause bleeding, and no doubt in some cases hastens the spread of an ulcerating growth. The relief obtained is at best only temporary, and swelling of the mucous membrane, induced by the sounding, may increase the dysphagia.

2. **Permanent intubation of the œsophagus** by means of Symonds's funnel-shaped feeding-tubes passed through the stricture has been widely employed. The tubes are introduced by means of

an instrument inserted into the funnel-shaped upper extremity. They may be left *in situ* for several months. A piece of silk fastened to the upper end is brought out of the mouth, and secured to the auricle or cheek. The patient is able to swallow and enjoy nourishment. This procedure is not suitable for strictures in the upper part of the œsophagus, as the tube is apt to irritate the larynx. The disadvantages are that the tubes get very foul, may require to be frequently changed, and sometimes tend to stimulate the spread of an ulcerating growth. Jacobson recommends their employment so long as the patient can swallow sufficient food by this means.

In discussing this method of treatment, Symonds summarizes as follows :—

(a) In cricoid obstruction the long rubber tube gives good results.

(b) In disease of the central portion of the œsophagus the short tube is advised, though if pulmonary symptoms arise the long tube is substituted for it.

(c) In disease of the cardiac orifice, gastrostomy is preferable to intubation.

Success has recently followed the use of a permanent feeding-tube devised by William Hill and consisting of a malleable silver stilette of small diameter surrounded by a rubber tube. This is passed through the stricture with the aid of the œsophagoscope. It can be used even when the obstruction is at the lowest portion of the œsophagus. The upper end is fixed to the teeth. It is surprising how soon food can be swallowed *beside* this tube, and its presence is generally well tolerated.

3. **Radium** has been employed recently in carcinoma of the œsophagus, with some hopeful results. A small tube containing radium is passed down by means of the œsophagoscope, and left for some hours within the stricture. In some cases ulceration and fungation of the growth have disappeared, and the lumen has markedly increased so that feeding-tubes can be inserted (Hill, Finzi).

4. The operation of **cervical œsophagostomy,** whereby an opening is made in the œsophagus in the neck, has little to recommend it. It can only be employed when the growth is at the upper end of the œsophagus. The reasons against it are thus epitomized by Fagge :—

(1) The greater difficulty and danger of the operation.

(2) The difficulty of making the opening sufficiently below the growth to prevent later involvements.

(3) Discomfort from the flow of saliva over the wound, and risk of local infection of the cellular tissues from this source.

5. Treatment by **gastrostomy** is indicated when intubation has proved unsatisfactory.

Comparatively recent technical improvements have greatly increased the value of this operation. The disheartening results previously experienced through leakage of stomach contents can now be avoided.

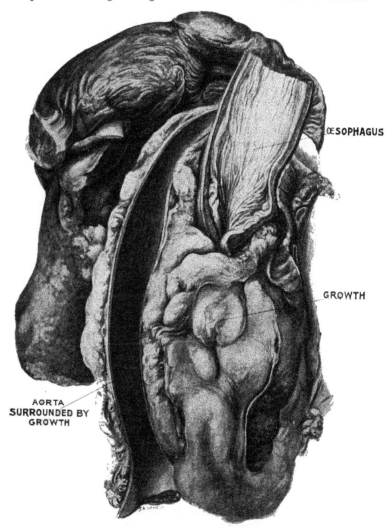

Fig 360.—Obstruction to the œsophagus caused by a mediastinal growth.

(*London Hospital Pathological Department.*)

By any of the modern methods in use a perfectly dry wound can be guaranteed. The results would be better still if only the operation were performed before the patient is in a state of starvation, as is only too often the case.

Leakage of stomach contents after a gastrostomy operation is prevented by the formation of a valvular opening, which is constructed by one of the following methods :—

(1) Inversion of a cone-shaped portion of the anterior wall of the stomach round a rubber feeding-tube, inserted through a small opening, and fixed by absorbable sutures. The cone-shaped portion is inverted, and secured either by rows of purse-string sutures, after the method of Senn or Abbe, or by means of layers of transverse sutures inserted on the Lembert principle (Kader's operation).

(2) The tube is passed through a small opening in the anterior wall of the stomach, and some inches of the tube are secured in a groove formed by two ridges of the wall sutured over it (Witzel's method).

In each of the above methods the stomach wall is secured to the abdominal wall by sutures.

(3) The principle adopted by Frank and modified by other surgeons (viz. Kocher, Albert and Cheyne) depends on drawing up a cone-shaped portion of the stomach wall, which is fixed at its base to the opening in the abdominal parietes. The cone is then passed beneath the skin, or through the rectus muscle, and its summit fixed to the edges of a second smaller opening made either above or to one side of the original incision. By this means a subcutaneous œsophagus composed of stomach wall is formed. The opening into the stomach is finally completed a few days later.

All the above methods of operation are valuable. In my experience the operation devised by Senn has given extremely good results. Leakage can be certainly avoided, the operation is very simple, and the patient can be fed immediately.

Sarcoma of the Œsophagus

Primary growths of this nature are very rare, but have been reported. They are either spindle- or round-celled, and are sometimes pedunculated (Albrecht). They are more commonly situated at the entrance of the œsophagus, or near the bifurcation of the trachea (Bergmann). The primary growth may lead to secondary bony metastases (Rolleston). One primary lympho-sarcoma has been reported.

Secondary sarcomatous growth in the œsophagus is generally an extension from neighbouring bones or soft structures in the neck or thorax. The employment of the œsophagoscope is necessary for the correct diagnosis of this condition.

EXTRINSIC CAUSES OF OBSTRUCTION

In any part of its course the œsophagus may be pressed upon or invaded by a tumour or swelling arising in neighbouring tissues. Such obstruction may be due to aneurysm, enlarged glands, new growths, or abscess, and is more apt to occur within the thorax than in the neck. An example of obstruction caused by a mediastinal new growth is seen in Fig. 360. For a description of extrinsic forms of obstruction the reader must be referred to other parts of this System or to text-books of Medicine.

BIBLIOGRAPHY

MALFORMATIONS

Ballantyne's *Antenatal Pathology*, ii. 462. 1904.
Keith, *Textbook of Embryology.*
Keith and **Spicer,** *Journ. Anat. and Phys.*, xli. 53.
Lotheissen, in Bergmann's *Surgery.*
Shattock, *Trans. Path. Soc.*, 1890, xli. 87.
Spicer, *Lancet*, 1907, i. 157.
Whipham and **Fagge,** *Lancet*, 1905, i. 22.

DIVERTICULA

Butlin, *Brit. Med. Journ.*, July 11, 1903.
Halsted, *Ann. of Surg.*, 1904.
Jacobson and **Rowlands,** *Operations of Surgery*, 5th edit.
Keith, Lectures at the R.C.S., *Brit. Med. Journ.*, 1910, i. 376.
Lanner, *Beitr. z. Anat. des Œsophagus.*
Mayo, *Ann. of Surg.*, July, 1910.
Pathologie und Therapie, Leipzig, 1877, vii., Abteilung i.
Richardson, Maurice, *Ann. of Surg.*, 1900.
Robertson, *Results of Operations for Pouches.*
Stetten, *Ann. of Surg.*, 1910. (With complete bibliography.)
Wien. med. Jahrb., 1883, S. 364.
Zenken and **von Ziemssen,** *Krankheiten des Œsophagus.*
Zesas, *Deuts. Zeits. f. Clin.*, 1906, lxxxii. (42 cases, 8 deaths; fistulæ formed in all but 6 cases.)
von Ziemssen, *Handbuch der Speiseröhre.*

RUPTURE

Bowles and **Turner,** *Med. Clin. Trans.*, 1899, lxxxiii. 241-255.
Rolleston, *Trans. Path. Soc.*, 1893, xlv. 58.
West and **Andrews,** *Trans. Path. Soc.*, 1896, xlviii. 73-77.
Williams, *Trans. Path. Soc.*, 1846, i. 151.

FOREIGN BODIES

Allen, *N.Y. Med. Journ.*, 1895, lxii. 203-10.
Black, *Amer. Med.*, Philadelphia, 1905, ix. 155.
Bryant, *Operative Surg.*, ii. 1288.
Burghard, *Syst. of Op. Surg.*, vol. ii. ; Fagge, p. 273. Ref. to Killian, *Zeits. f. Ohrenheilk.*, 1908, i. 120.
Church, " Œsophagotomy," *St. Bart.'s Hosp. Repts.*, xix. 67.
Fullerton, " Œsophagotomy," *Brit. Med. Journ.*, 1904.
von Hacker, Bergmann's *Syst. of Surg.*, vol. iv.; *Deuts. med. Woch.*, 1905, xxxi. 1535.
Jacobson, " Œsophagotomy," *Operations of Surgery*, i. 724.

King, *N.Y. Med. Record*, 1900, lviii. 643–5.
Lawson, " Œsophagotomy for Tooth-Plate," *Clin. Soc. Trans.*, xviii. 292.
Lediard, *Clin. Soc. Trans.*, xviii. 297.
Littlewood, "Four Cases of Tooth-Plates," *Lancet*, Aug. 12, 1905.
MacIntyre, *Journ. of Laryng.*, London, 1902, xvii. 467–74.
May, Bennett, Jackson's *Operative Surg.*, i. 724.
Richardson, " Accessibility in Neck," *Lancet*, 1887, ii. 707.
Richardson, *Lancet*, 1907, vol. ii.
Rigby, *Ann. of Surg.*, 1907.
Scott, *Cleveland Med. Journ.*, 1902, i. 147–53.
Tillman's *Textbook*, vol. ii.
Turner, *Lancet*, May, 1910.

OBSTRUCTION

Goldman, *Lancet*, 1906, i. 21.
Keith, *Lancet*, 1903, i. 639.
Kraus, in Nothnagel's *Pathologie und Therapie.*
Lockwood, *Brit. Med. Journ.*, 1903, i. 1367.
Mikulicz, in Keen's *Surgery.*
Sippey, *Ann. of Surg.*, 1906, xliii. 859, 945.
Strauss, *Berl. klin. Woch.*, 1904, No. 49.

STRING-METHOD GASTROTOMY

Abbe, *Ann. of Surg.*, 1897, xxv. 359.
Campbell, *Trans. Assoc. Amer. Surg.*, 1883, i. 517.
Coombes, *Internat. Clin.*, 1904, iv. 172–80.
Dunham, *Ann. of Surg.*, 1901, xxxiv. 822.
Franks, *Ann. of Surg.*, 1890, xii. 321–9.
Johnson, G. R., *N.Y. Med. Times*, 1900, xxviii. 166.
Lilienthal, *N.Y. Med. Journ.*, 1894, lix. 496.
Mansell-Moullin C., *Clin. Journ.*, 1894, iv. 288–91.

TREATMENT OF STRICTURE

Dunham, *N.Y. State Journ. of Med.*, 1903, iii. 93–5.
Johns Hopkins Hosp. Bull., 1905, xvi. 147.
Mayo, *Internat. Clin.*, 1900, iv. 43, 54.

OPERATIVE TREATMENT

Abbe, *Ann. of Surg.*, 1894, xix. 88.
Franks, *Brit. Med. Journ.*, 1894, ii. 973 ; *Ann. of Surg.*, 1894, xix. 385, 398.
von Hacker, Bergmann's *Syst. of Surg.*, vol. iv.
Thomas, *Liverpool Med. Clin. Journ.*, 1902, xxii. 50–3.

TUMOURS]

Fagge, Burghard's *Syst. of Op. Surg.*, ii. 279.
Fawcett, *Trans. Path. Soc.*, 1905, lvi. 259.
Frank, *Virchow's Arch.*, 1903, clxxiv. 563.
Hill, *Med. Soc. Trans.*, Feb. 13, 1911.
Janeway and Green, *Ann. of Surg.*, July, 1910.
Meyer, *Ann. of Surg.*, July, 1909.
Perry and Shaw, *Guy's Hosp. Repts.*, 1891, xxxiii. 137.
Quervain, *Arch. f. klin. Chir.*, 1899, S. 858.
Rawling, *Clin. Journ.*, March 2, 1910.
Sauerbruch, *Beitr. klin. Chir.*, 1905, xlvi. 405 : *Journ. Amer. Med. Assoc.*, ii. 803t
Symonds, *Lancet*, 1902, ii. 353.

THE STOMACH AND DUODENUM

By JAMES SHERREN, F.R.C.S.Eng.

Anatomy and physiology.—Although the stomach and duodenum are anatomically separate, it is advisable, for surgical reasons, to consider them together. From an embryological standpoint they are closely related, and they are liable to similar diseases.

The stomach and the duodenum, as far as the entrance of the common bile-duct, are developed from the foregut and receive their blood supply from the cœliac axis, while the duodenum below this point is developed from the midgut and, like it, is supplied by the superior mesenteric artery.

Our conception of the size and shape of the *stomach* has altered during the last few years owing to the frequency of direct operative examinations, to the introduction of X-rays, and to improved methods of anatomical investigation. Formerly regarded as a bag or sac into which the food dropped, it is now known to resemble more closely the intestine, and to be normally in a state of contraction.

From the anatomical, embryological, physiological, and pathological standpoints the stomach can be divided into two portions, pyloric and cardiac, which are in health functionally separated by a band of transverse muscle, the mid-gastric sphincter (Figs. 361, 362). The cardiac portion lies to the left of the right margin of the cardiac orifice, its boundary being marked by a notch on the lesser curvature. At this point the stomach turns almost at a right angle to run horizontally to the right, as the pyloric portion.

X-ray examination of the normal stomach after the ingestion of a bismuth meal reveals the same condition. Systematic work in this method of examination was first done in this country by Hertz, on whose early observations the following account is based. When food is swallowed it is received into the cardiac reservoir, from which it is passed on into the pyloric portion. Fresh food swallowed passes to the centre of the mass already there, the action of the ptyalin in this way being allowed to continue unchecked by the gastric juice. Very little active movement takes place in the cardiac part of the stomach. The pressure here has been shown by Sick to be only 6 to 8 cm. of water, with slight and irregular variations. The musculature of the pyloric portion of the stomach is thick and is the seat of peristaltic waves which occur at intervals of about fifteen to twenty seconds, beginning about thirty minutes after a meal. In the early stages of digestion the pylorus is closed and a central reflux of food occurs, the mass being pushed backwards and forwards and thoroughly triturated and mixed with the gastric juice. As digestion proceeds, the pressure in this part of the stomach varies from 20 to 60 cm. of

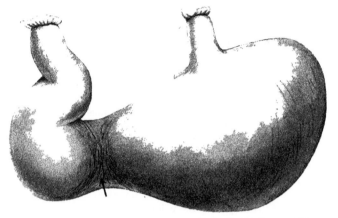

Fig. 361.—Mid-gastric sphincter, as depicted by Sir Everard Home. (*After Keith.*)

water. Recent work by Barclay and Hertz's later observations have thrown some doubt on the separation into two compartments as seen on X-ray examination.

Since Beaumont's time it has been considered that the acidity of the gastric contents causes relaxation of the pylorus. But it is more probable that the pylorus relaxes with each peristaltic wave which sweeps over the pyloric portion of the stomach, unless inhibited by reflexes set up by the presence of free acid in the first portion of the duodenum (Pavlov). The presence in the stomach of solid particles, or of fluids warmer or colder than the body temperature, also causes closure of the pylorus.

The time at which the food leaves the stomach varies with its nature; carbohydrates pass out first, then fats and proteins. The cardiac portion of the stomach is empty before the pyloric; about six hours after a full meal, or three and a half to four after a light meal, the whole stomach should be empty.

The capacity of the stomach varies according to the amount and kind of food habitually taken. Its average capacity, according to Sidney Martin, is 35 to 40 fluid oz.

The function of the stomach is to prepare food for absorption, and so prevent injury to the intestine. It renders meals possible, to a certain extent it sterilizes the food, corrects it to the body temperature, and reduces it to a fluid mixed with gastric juice.

The *duodenum* is that portion of the small intestine between the pylorus and the duodeno-jejunal junction. For the purposes of descriptive anatomy it has been divided into three or four parts. The first or superior portion extends to the neck of the gall-bladder, the second or descending ends opposite the third or fourth lumbar vertebra, and turns sharply to the left as the third portion, which runs across the spine and then ascends to the left side of the first or second lumbar vertebra. The left ascending portion is sometimes called the fourth part. The more important division surgically is into the part above (supra-ampullary) and that below (infra-ampullary) the entrance of the common bile-duct. The supra-ampullary portion is affected by the diseases that attack the stomach, whilst diseases of the infra-ampullary are rare and resemble those of the remainder of the small intestine.

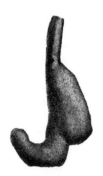

Fig. 362.—Stomach of a full-term fœtus, showing subdivision into cardiac and pyloric portions. (*After Cunningham.*)

This differentiation, according to Keith, is seen as early as the third month, when the fundus buds out from the dorsal border of the stomach

At the level of the junction of the first and second lumbar vertebræ, the gut turns directly forward at the duodeno-jejunal flexure to become the jejunum. The anatomy of this region is of great importance in connexion with the operation of gastro-jejunostomy (p. 406). The duodeno-jejunal junction is held in position by a band of fibres containing unstriped muscle attached to the left crus of the diaphragm; this is enclosed in a peritoneal fold which is usually small, but occasionally, as pointed out by Mayo, may extend several inches along the jejunum. Murphy has shown that in the process of development a loop of jejunum may be left posterior to the peritoneum. This may extend as low as the brim of the pelvis, and then, passing backwards and upwards, may enter the peritoneal cavity through its posterior wall, just below the level at which the duodenum crosses the aorta. The whole of the small intestine has been found in a secondary sac bounded by omentum and mesocolon (Malcolm).

When the jejunum is turned over to the right, folds of peritoneum are seen running from the duodenum and jejunum to the parietal peritoneum. . Of these, the inferior and superior, bounding small recesses with their openings directed upwards and downwards respectively, are most often seen. Hernias may occur in this situation, and may not only complicate the operation of gastro-jejunostomy, but render it entirely impracticable, as in a case of chronic duodenal ulcer recently under my care. A. E. Barker has placed on record a similar case.

Blood-supply of stomach and duodenum.—The stomach and supra-ampullary part of the duodenum are supplied with blood from the branches of the cœliac axis.

The remainder of the duodenum is supplied from the superior mesenteric artery by means of its inferior pancreatico-duodenal branch. The superior mesenteric vessels have an important relation to the third portion of the duodenum, in that they cross its middle and by the pressure produced in certain conditions have been said to cause acute dilatation of the stomach (p. 324).

The veins of the stomach and duodenum pass to the portal system.

Lymphatics.—Knowledge of the lymphatic system of the stomach is essential to the correct surgery of malignant disease. The present operation of partial gastrectomy is based upon the researches of Cunéo, published in 1900. His results have been confirmed and extended by Dobson and Jamieson, on whose work the following account is based.

The lymphatics arise around the glands in the mucous membrane, and form submucous, muscular, and subserous plexuses continuous throughout the whole of the stomach and communicating with those of the duodenum and œsophagus. From the subserous plexuses the vessels pass out to enter the lymphatic glands into which they drain. Although no barrier could be demonstrated by injection experiments between the areas drained by the several sets of glands, yet one lymphatic territory becomes fully injected before the fluid spreads over into a neighbouring one.

The groups of lymphatic glands are placed along the course of the principal blood-vessels, and, as elsewhere, they drain the corresponding areas.

The main groups of glands are the following (Fig. 363) :—

1. The *coronary set* lie along the descending branch of the coronary artery and are divided into two groups, upper and lower. The lower glands lie close to the lesser curvature and rarely extend farther to the right than the mid-point between œsophagus and pylorus ; they increase in size and number as they approach the cardia. The upper group lie in the falx coronata with the stem of the artery. The *paracardial* are outlying members of this group, and lie around the cardia, sometimes extending to the left of the cardiac orifice ; occasion-

ally there are one or two glands on the bare area of the stomach. On tracing the upper coronary glands backwards they become continuous with the glands around the cœliac axis.

2. The *cœliac glands*, situated at the upper border of the pancreas, have been divided into three groups, the middle (around the cœliac axis), left (on the splenic), and right (on the stem of the hepatic artery) suprapancreatic. To the left suprapancreatic group (splenic) belong the glands occasionally present in the gastro-splenic omentum. The

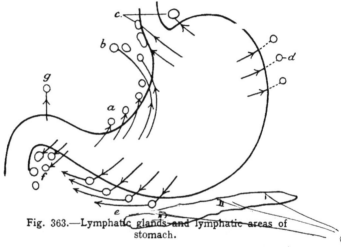

Fig. 363.—Lymphatic glands and lymphatic areas of stomach.

a, Lower coronary glands ; *b*, upper coronary glands ; *c*, paracardial glands ; *d*, outlying glands of left suprapancreatic group : *e*, right gastro-epiploic glands ; *f*, subpyloric glands ; *g*, suprapyloric gland.

efferents from the suprapancreatic glands pass to the receptaculum chyli and communicate freely with the superior mesenteric glands.

3. The *right gastro-epiploic group* of glands lie below the artery of the same name. They are from four to seven in number, and rarely extend to the left farther than the middle of the greater curvature, though they have a tendency to stray downwards between the layers of the great omentum. The vessels from these glands pass to the subpyloric group.

4. The *subpyloric glands* are situated to the right of the pylorus, in the angle between the first and second parts of the duodenum, in front of the head of the pancreas and in close relation to the bifurcation of the gastro-duodenal artery. They receive lymphatic vessels from the pylorus and duodenum and the efferent vessels from the right gastro-epiploic glands. Their efferents pass to the suprapancreatic and superior mesenteric glands.

The stomach is divided into *three lymphatic areas*, viz. the lesser curvature, the greater curvature, and the fundus. The lymphatics from the lesser curvature and its immediate neighbourhood pass into the lower coronary group of glands. Occasionally a vessel passes by this group to end in the upper coronary set (Fig. 387, p. 382). In addition, vessels from the upper part of the pyloric canal run upwards into the lesser omentum, sometimes into one or two suprapyloric glands whose efferents with the uninterrupted vessels pass downwards to end in the right suprapancreatic glands. Occasionally a vessel passes behind the duodenum to end in a gland behind the pancreas close to the common bile-duct.

The vessels from the fundus close to the cardia pass to the paracardial glands, and thence to the upper coronary set. Those from the remainder of the fundus down to a point in the greater curvature immediately below the œsophagus pass to the splenic glands. The right portion of the greater curvature drains into the right gastro-epiploic glands.

Nerves of the stomach.—The stomach receives fibres from both vagi and also through the solar plexuses from the 7th, 8th, and 9th dorsal nerves.

Bacteriology.—According to Miller and to Harvey Cushing, the healthy stomach, when empty, contains no micro-organisms. In the duodenum the number of micro-organisms is small, but they become more numerous lower down in the intestine. This is in accordance with surgical experience. Operations upon the alimentary canal in the upper abdomen as a whole have a lower death-rate than those in the lower.

These facts are of the utmost surgical importance. It is possible to render the stomach and upper part of the small intestine sterile, and thus to lessen the danger of extensive operations in this region, in cases in which there is no obstruction. If, however, the stomach and duodenum are prevented from emptying themselves, their contents teem with organisms.

Clinical examination.—In the investigation of suspected disease the history should be taken with the greatest care, and the patient allowed, as far as possible, to tell his own tale, being guided skilfully along the necessary channels. It is important to elicit the initial symptom, the first alteration from normal which attracted the attention of the patient. Was the onset sudden or gradual ? In some cases, pain is the first and most important symptom throughout, both in acute and in chronic cases ; in others, the sudden vomiting of a large quantity of blood when in apparent health, the passage of blood by the rectum, loss of appetite, or a continuous and inexplicable loss of weight, or anæmia. In a few of the cases of perforation of a gastric or duodenal ulcer, the sudden onset of symptoms of an abdominal catastrophe is the first indication of alimentary disease.

The course of the disease must be as carefully investigated, and the occurrence of complications inquired for. In some cases, particularly in chronic ulcers of the duodenum, and less often in chronic gastric ulcers, the symptoms intermit and there are periods of perfect health.

It must never be forgotten that "dyspepsia" may be caused by disease of neighbouring organs, particularly the gall-bladder and bile-ducts, and appendix, by direct involvement or reflexly. It should also be remembered that although for anatomical reasons the digestive tract is split up into separately named portions, physiologically it is a whole, each part of which is dependent for its efficient working on the health of the others. Hedblom and Cannon have shown experimentally on cats that irritation of the colon or cæcum retards the discharge of food from the stomach.

Pain and tenderness.—It is universal knowledge that pain in the epigastric region after food is a symptom of interference with the normal functions of the stomach. The causation of this pain in disease of the stomach and duodenum, however, is a matter for discussion. Considerable research on the sensibility of the viscera has been carried out since Lennander's pioneer work appeared in 1901. The stomach and intestines are insensitive to those stimuli which cause pain when applied to the surface of the body; they can be cut or burnt without the patient evincing any sign of discomfort. It is evident, therefore, that the afferent nerves of the stomach require for their excitation stimuli different from those of the skin. The parietal peritoneum was considered by Lennander to be sensitive; this has been shown by Ramström to be due to the rich plexus of nerves in the subserous tissue. These nerves are branches of those which supply the muscles of the abdominal wall, and are beset with Pacinian corpuscles. The sensibility of this layer is that form named by Head and the present writer "deep."

According to Lennander and his followers, visceral pain is due in all cases to stimulation of the parietal peritoneum as the result of direct pressure, traction upon mesenteries, or inflammation. That other factors must come into play is evident. The most severe abdominal pain is associated with irregular muscular contractions in hollow organs, due to irritation or obstruction (colic). In these cases it is difficult to believe that it is due to pressure on the parietal peritoneum or traction on mesenteries, and observation upon exposed portions of intestine in breaches of surface of the abdominal wall has proved this view to be incorrect.

Henry Head and the present writer showed that ice-water and

water at 50° C., introduced directly through gastrostomy or colostomy openings, gave rise to sensations of cold and warmth. We considered this showed that the sensibility of the viscera resembled protopathic sensibility elsewhere. The sensation produced was never localized inside the abdomen, but usually in the umbilical region. James Mackenzie does not accept these conclusions, and explains the feeling of cold as due to vaso-constriction in the vessels of the skin of the abdomen reflexly produced. Hertz came to the conclusion that "the œsophagus and anal canal are almost always sensitive to heat and cold, the stomach rarely if ever, and the colon to a limited extent in a very small number of cases." Whatever the explanation of the recognition of ice and hot water, most of the pain complained of in diseases of the organs with which we are dealing is reflected and not direct.

Pain resulting from disease of the stomach is most often complained of in the epigastric region, particularly on the left side, also posteriorly at the lower angle of the left scapula. It is frequently associated with tenderness (hyperalgesia), both superficial (cutaneous) and deep, and with increase of reflexes or muscular rigidity.

Cutaneous hyperalgesia is occasionally met with. Its exact surgical significance is unknown. It is most often associated with ulcer of the stomach in women, rarely in men, and has also been observed in cases of hæmorrhagic gastritis. Usually left-sided, it may extend as a band around the body in the region of the 7th, 8th, and 9th thoracic segments, or be present only in front or behind. It is certainly absent in perforation of the stomach or duodenum.

Following Head, it has been the teaching at the London Hospital that the presence of *deep tenderness* indicates an affection of the peritoneum. Although deep tenderness is seen in its most exquisite form in cases of recent perforative peritonitis, marked deep tenderness is often present without peritonitis. The muscular and subserous layers of the abdominal wall are supplied from the same nerves. Head and the writer have shown that the afferent fibres running with motor nerves, when stimulated as the result of pressure, cause pain, and the painful contractions of muscles are also well known. I believe that deep tenderness is often "reflected"; but in peritonitis the nerves themselves are directly affected by the inflammation of the parietal peritoneum. Stimulation of these nerves subserving deep sensibility is the cause of the widespread muscular rigidity in diffuse peritonitis.

The *localized rigidity* which may be manifest in a segment of the rectus in many cases of stomach disease is due to increased briskness of the reflex, and does not indicate peritonitis. It is not present on gentle handling, and is associated with deep tenderness; on the other hand, the rigidity accompanying the deep tenderness in peritonitis is permanent and will be felt with the gentlest handling.

To recapitulate, pain and hyperalgesia, both superficial and deep, and muscular rigidity, in disease of the stomach and duodenum unaccompanied by peritoneal irritation, are reflex, due to the heightened excitability of certain segments of the spinal cord receiving abnormal impulses from the affected viscus.

The important points to elicit with regard to the pain are— (1) Its character, position, and spread. (2) Its relation to food; the time at which it appears; does it waken the patient at night? (3) Is it relieved by vomiting, or by taking food, drugs, or fluid? (4) Is it accompanied by or relieved by flatulence?

Vomiting.—Vomiting is nearly always met with during the course of any surgical disease of the stomach or duodenum. But, while rarely absent at some time during the course of gastric disease, it is only present as a late complication in certain diseases of the duodenum.

The important points to investigate are—(1) Its frequency. (2) Its relation to food. (3) Does it relieve pain? (4) Its colour, odour, etc. (5) Does it contain blood?

(*See also* under Examination of the Vomit, p. 310.)

Hæmorrhage.—Bleeding more or less severe probably occurs in all diseases accompanied by a breach of surface of the mucous membrane. Blood may be vomited (hæmatemesis) or passed per rectum (melæna). If a large amount is poured out it may be vomited at once and is easily recognized; if poured out in small quantity it is altered in colour and becomes coagulated in tiny brownish-red masses resembling coffee-grounds. Death may result before the appearance of any blood externally, but this is very unusual. While the presence of any large amount of blood is obvious, smaller amounts should not be overlooked, for their importance is great.

Appetite.—Information with regard to appetite is important. In some cases of carcinoma of the stomach, loss of appetite or repugnance to the sight of food is the first sign of the disease. In duodenal ulcer the appetite may be good and the patient may say that he eats more during the attack of pain than at any other time; or, as in some cases of gastric ulcer, the appetite is good, but fear of the consequent pain restrains the patient from satisfying it.

Jaundice.—This is a rare complication and arises as the result of obstruction to the biliary passages from pressure or involvement in new growth, adhesions or contraction of an ulcer, or direct spread from the duodenum. It is more often met with in diseases of the duodenum than in diseases of the stomach, where it is usually a late result of carcinoma. It may be an important symptom in the

u

differential diagnosis between affections of the gall-bladder and those of the stomach or duodenum.

Physical examination.—Special examinations are necessary in many cases of stomach disease. These should not supersede the routine methods employed to investigate disease in other parts of the abdomen.

The age and general appearance of the patient must be taken into consideration. The condition of the teeth must be carefully looked to; it may be found that the symptoms can be accounted for on dental grounds, but in any case no operation on the stomach or intestines should be done, unless in an emergency, until septic stumps have been removed and the mouth rendered as sterile as possible.

For the physical examination the patient should be lying comfortably on a couch with the shoulders a little raised; the whole of the abdomen and the lower part of the thorax must be uncovered, for many tumours have been overlooked through neglecting this precaution.

The hand should never be placed on the abdomen until inspection has been thorough. Note should be made of the general condition of the abdomen and of obvious signs of tumour, localized bulgings, visible peristalsis, skin cracks, etc.; then special attention directed to the epigastric and left hypochondriac regions, where tumours may be seen descending on respiration which cannot be detected in any other way. The narrow upper abdomen so often present in enteroptosis should not be overlooked. In many cases it is associated with a floating tenth rib, which Stiller considers a stigma of gastric neurosis.

Palpation should first be directed towards eliciting the presence of areas of tenderness, superficial or deep, or of muscular rigidity. Search must then be made for a tumour; its position, mobility, and respiratory movement must be investigated, and, when doubt exists, re-examined after inflation of the stomach and occasionally the colon (P. 308). Splashing may be obtained, but is only of importance when found in districts other than those occupied by the normal stomach or when occurring more than three hours after a meal. Peristalsis may sometimes be elicited by gently flicking the abdomen. The size of the liver should be noted. The right kidney should always be examined, and if there is any suspicion of gastroptosis the patient should be seen in the erect position.

The supraclavicular region on the left side must be palpated for evidence of glandular enlargement.

Percussion and auscultation.—It may be possible to mark out by percussion the position of the greater curvature, but it is occasionally difficult to distinguish between the note given by the colon and that given by the stomach. Percussion must be light and should be systematically done from below upwards. The lower border of the normal stomach does not reach the umbilicus. It is possible to mark out by percussion the adjacent areas of liver and lung, but this is of little importance in disease of the stomach. The abdomen should be percussed for evidence of free fluid ; but a considerable amount may be present without any marked increase of dullness being perceptible in the flanks.

Auscultation-percussion often gives more aid than percussion alone. The stethoscope is placed about the centre of the gastric area, and light scratching movements are made on the abdominal wall, beginning near the stethoscope and working outwards ; as soon as the borders of the stomach are reached the sounds change in character. Hertz in his recent investigations has found that the area so obtained did not show any resemblance to the true shape of the stomach as seen by X-ray examination after a bismuth meal.

Auscultation alone may detect bubbling sounds or friction. It has been stated that delay in the time occupied in the passage of food from the mouth to the stomach may be of diagnostic importance in early cases of carcinoma or obstruction at the cardiac end of the stomach. Hertz has recently investigated this with the aid of X-rays, and has come to the conclusion that great variation exists in the time at which the sound is heard. It was formerly considered due to the food entering the stomach, but Hertz has shown that it does not occur until the œsophagus is empty. It can usually be heard about four seconds after swallowing, but may be delayed as long as ten seconds in normal individuals, so that little reliance can be placed upon it as a diagnostic sign.

When the symptoms are indefinite, examination must be made for signs of *tabes*. Cases have been recorded in which gastric crises were treated by gastro-jejunostomy.

There are five **special methods of examination** which are of use—(1) Illumination and examination of the stomach. (2) Inflation of the stomach. (3) X-ray examination. (4) Examination of stomach contents. (5) Examination of fæces.

1. Illumination.—It seems that the difficult problem of inspection of the interior of the stomach by means of an instrument passed by the mouth will shortly be solved.

Many attempts have been made since the introduction of the cystoscope to perfect an instrument with which the stomach could be similarly examined. Mikulicz in 1881 appears to have been the first to use the gastroscope which was constructed by Leiter with his help. The great difficulties of construction and of introduction prevented its general use, and intragastric examination remained in abeyance until the adoption of direct examination of the œsophagus and trachea stimulated to further research. Chevalier Jackson of Pittsburg introduced in 1907 the direct examination of the stomach through a straight tube, and by its means has diagnosed many surgical conditions.

The Souttar-Thompson gastroscope was a great advance and showed that the greater part of the stomach could be investigated by indirect vision. I believe, however, that the use of an indirect-vision gastroscope of this type is more dangerous than exploratory laparotomy in the hands of a competent surgeon.

The Hill-Herschell gastroscope, which combines both direct and indirect methods, is a great improvement, and has already been used with success in the differential diagnosis between multiple hæmorrhagic erosions and chronic ulceration.

2. Inflation.—Inflation with air is useful in the diagnosis of gastroptosis, dilated stomach, or hour-glass stomach, and in showing the relationship of certain tumours to the stomach. In the latter case dilatation of the colon is sometimes also employed.

This method was first adopted in England by Samuel Fenwick. It must be used with care in selected cases, and never employed when evidence of active ulceration is present. Fatal accidents after inflation have occurred from rupture of the stomach and from hæmatemesis in cases with active disease.

The stomach may be inflated in two ways—with air through a stomach-tube to which a Higginson syringe is attached, or by CO_2 evolved from the intragastric mixing of tartaric acid and sodium bicarbonate. The former method is the more accurate, and is absolutely under the control of the observer, its only disadvantage being that it involves the passage of a stomach-tube. It should be used in all cases in which the patient permits this manœuvre. On the other hand, inflation with CO_2 is easier and involves less manipulation. A little less than a teaspoonful of tartaric acid dissolved in about 2 oz. of water is administered; a teaspoonful of bicarbonate of soda dissolved in half a tumbler of water is then given slowly until the desired degree of inflation is reached. The outline of the stomach in many cases becomes visible, or is easily mapped out by light percussion.

3. X-ray examination.—Examination of the stomach by means of a screen after the ingestion of a bismuth meal is of aid in the diagnosis of obscure cases, and may demonstrate the shape, size, and position of the viscus, the presence of gastroptosis, dilatation, hour-glass deformity, or cardiac stricture. (Fig. 364.)

From 1 to 2 oz. of bismuth carbonate is given in bread-and-milk or arrowroot, and the patient screened at intervals according to the nature of the case.

4. Examination of stomach contents.—Chemical examination of the contents of the stomach should be made in every case, and the amounts of total and free HCl estimated. The contents of the stomach should be obtained by means of the stomach-tube after a test meal. Examination of the vomit, useful for certain purposes, does not supply the necessary information (p. 310).

Attempts have been made to estimate the motor power of the stomach, apart from examination of the stomach contents, after a

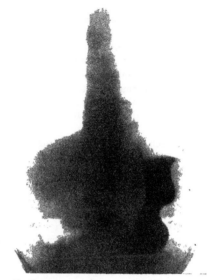

Fig. 364.—Radiograph of an hour-glass stomach after a bismuth meal. (*Schall.*)

test meal. The salol test of Ewald is based upon the fact that salol is decomposed into carbolic and salicylic acids in an alkaline medium, the latter appearing in the urine as salicyluric acid normally in about an hour. The test is not altogether reliable, as the salol may be decomposed in the stomach owing to the presence of alkaline mucus. or delayed in the intestine owing to acid fermentation. A similar test is made with iodipin. One gram of iodipin is given in a capsule immediately after a meal ; normally, iodine can be detected in the saliva in forty-five minutes. Attempts have also been made to estimate the acidity of the gastric contents without the passage of the stomach-tube. In Günzburg's method a tablet of 0·2 grm. of potassium iodide is inserted into a thin rubber tube, the ends folded, and the packet tied with three threads of fibrin hardened in alcohol. One is swallowed three-quarters of an hour after an Ewald test meal, and the saliva tested for KI at intervals of fifteen minutes till the reaction is obtained, normally in an hour to an hour and a quarter.

Another test of a similar character is the "desmoid" test of Sahli. It is based on the assumption that catgut in the raw state is soluble in the stomach. A pill is made of 0·5 grm. of methylene blue and enclosed in a rubber sac made by twisting up the pill in a thin piece of rubber tissue and tying the neck with thin catgut. The pill is given with or just after the midday meal, and the urine examined five, seven, and eighteen or twenty hours after. Its excretion is recognized by the bluish colour given to the urine. If this be absent, the chromogen alone may be occasionally though rarely present ; it may be demonstrated by the appearance of a greenish-blue colour when the urine is boiled with one-fifth its volume of glacial acetic acid. If it be found within eighteen or twenty hours the test is called positive. Opinions differ as to the value of these tests ; the information obtained is approximate only ; they should not be used when it is possible to give a test meal.

The fasting stomach should be empty or nearly so. Motor insufficiency is present if, on the morning after a light evening meal, or six hours after a test meal (Leube) of a quarter of a pound of minced meat and bread, food can still be extracted from the stomach by the tube.

After the stomach-tube has been passed in the morning in the fasting stomach, Ewald's test breakfast (a slice of stale bread or toast and a pint of weak tea) should be given, following gastric lavage if necessary. It is withdrawn by the stomach-tube an hour later. The general appearance is noted, and total acidity and free HCl estimated.

Examination of the vomit.—The quantity vomited should be noted as an indication of dilated stomach, as also the characteristic yeasty smell, and presence of food known to have been taken by the patient some days previously. The presence of blood in large quantities is obvious ; in smaller quantities it may be difficult to discover or may demonstrate itself as coffee-grounds vomit. The presence of traces of blood may be proved by the detection of hæmin crystals, by spectroscopic examination, or by the benzidin test. Pus is occasionally found in the vomit from communication with an empyema of the gall-bladder, rupture of an abscess of the gastric wall, or of a perigastric abscess into the stomach cavity. The presence of bile in the vomit is important in cases of duodenal stricture and in regurgitant vomiting following gastro-enterostomy ; it is detected by Gmelin's test.

Fæcal vomit is found in cases of gastro-colic fistula.

Microscopical examination of the vomit may reveal, in addition to fragments of undigested food, various micro-organisms. The most important are the Oppler-Boas bacillus, sarcinæ, and yeast fungi. These are usually found in cases of dilatation of the stomach. The Oppler-Boas bacillus is said to be constantly present in advanced cases of cancer of the stomach, and is a cause of lactic-acid fermentation ; it is usually absent in non-malignant disease of the stomach. It is a long, non-motile bacillus, frequently joined end to end to form threads.

Sarcinæ occur in the form of colonies of cocci arranged in squares, said to resemble bales of cotton ; they are rarely found in advanced cases of carcinoma of the stomach.

5. **Examination of the fæces.**—After the exclusion of other causes of hæmorrhage, especially hæmorrhoids, the discovery of occult blood in the fæces may be useful in the diagnosis of duodenal ulcer and of cancer of the stomach. It may be recognized spectroscopically, by the formation of hæmin crystals, or by Adler's benzidin test. Extreme care in preliminary dieting is unnecessary, as well-cooked meat does not interfere with the test. (For methods of examination, the reader is referred to Hutchison and Rainy's "Clinical Methods," 5th edition, 1912.)

MALFORMATIONS AND MISPLACEMENTS, ETC.

Congenital malformations and misplacements of the stomach and duodenum are rare. Stenosis may occur at the pylorus, in the descending portion of the duodenum, or at the junction of the cardiac and pyloric portions of the stomach (congenital hour-glass stomach) ; occasionally diverticuli are present.

Acquired malformations almost invariably result from contraction of fibrous tissue or from new growth.

Congenital misplacement may be present in situs transversus or in hernia, while the acquired variety may be part of a generalized enteroptosis or may occur as the rare volvulus.

CONGENITAL ATRESIA OF THE PYLORUS

Cases have been described in which the pyloric end of the stomach terminated blindly, or in which only an exceedingly fine communication existed between the stomach and the first part of the duodenum. In these cases no thickening is found around the pylorus. In all the recorded instances the disease has run a rapidly fatal course. Frequent vomiting from birth should direct attention to the possibility of this condition. Hitherto no case has been diagnosed. Gastro-duodenostomy or gastro-jejunostomy should be performed.

CONGENITAL STRICTURE AND OCCLUSION OF THE DUODENUM

These are rare conditions. Out of 13 cases of congenital occlusion or stenosis of the intestines (other than those in connexion with the rectum) collected by Barnard from the records of the London Hospital, in no instance was the duodenum affected.

Out of 185 cases of congenital occlusion of the intestines collected by Kuliga, 46 were of the duodenum. Schlegel, quoted by Braun, states that occlusion occurs in the duodenum in 32·5 per cent. of the cases.

There may be a septum, with or without a perforation in its centre, running across the bowel, composed of the muscular as well as of the mucous and submucous coats. The interruption of the duodenum may be complete.

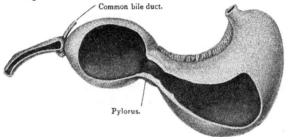

Fig. 365.—Congenital occlusion of duodenum, in a child a few days old. (*Roe and Shaw's case.*)

(*Royal College of Surgeons Museum.*)

The occlusion is usually situated in the region of the ampulla of Vater (Fig. 365), and is in many cases associated with malformations of other structures. Occlusion is more common than stenosis; in 57 cases collected by Cordes, it was present in 48.

Occlusion or stenosis is occasionally present at the junction of the duodenum and jejunum (5 out of 57 cases, Cordes).

As a rule, vomiting occurs soon after birth, its character depending on the position of the atresia or stenosis, but in the case of stenosis the symptoms may be delayed, one case having been recorded in a girl of 13 (Shaw and Baldauf).

Treatment.—If the condition is recognized, gastro-jejunostomy offers the only hope of saving life.

ACQUIRED STRICTURE OF THE DUODENUM

This condition is usually the result of chronic ulceration, and in the later stages may bring about dilatation of the stomach. A stricture may also result from affections of the pancreas, or from adhesions due to gall-stones.

The superior mesenteric vessels crossing the third portion of the duodenum have been credited with the causation of duodenal obstruction (p. 324). Hour-glass duodenum has been recorded as a late result of duodenal ulcer.

Symptoms of duodenal stenosis.—The disease is usually chronic ; when produced by pressure of vessels or lodgment of a gall-stone it may be acute.

The chronic forms must be divided into two groups—those in which the stenosis is above, and those in which it is below, the entrance of the common bile-duct. The diagnosis of the former, which is the more common, has never been made before operation, as the symptoms are identical with those of stenosis of the pylorus ; but X-ray examination after a bismuth meal might possibly reveal its seat. When the stricture is below the entrance of the common bile-duct the symptoms are characteristic : there is dilatation of both the stomach and the duodenum, and bile and pancreatic juices pass readily into the stomach and are vomited. The reaction of the gastric contents is neutral or alkaline. The motions may be colourless, or nearly so.

Treatment.—Stricture of the duodenum should be treated so as to restore as far as possible the normal condition of parts either by duodenoplasty or by Finney's operation (p. 418). Where this is impossible from the presence of adhesions, or inadvisable from the presence of an ulcer, posterior gastro-jejunostomy should be performed, as near the pylorus as possible.

GASTRIC DIVERTICULA

These are rare, and usually arise as the result of gastric ulcer, rarely of carcinoma. They belong to the " traction " group of diverticula, and are the result of the adhesion of the stomach to the abdominal wall, liver, or pancreas.

Diagnosis is usually impossible. If the pouch is so shaped or situated as to permit lodgment of food, it may cause symptoms due to its distension or inflammation. This condition usually occurs in women, and should be thought of when, with stomach symptoms in a woman, there is a tumour adherent to the abdominal wall in the left epigastric region.

Treatment should consist of excision of the diverticulum, accompanied by gastro-enterostomy if necessary.

Two cases are recorded, in both of which the patients recovered after operation (Kolaczek, Silbermark).

DUODENAL DIVERTICULA

Diverticula of the duodenum are usually situated close to the biliary papilla, are small and formed of the mucous coat only (Fig. 366).

They were held by Letulle to be a congenital abnormality, but are now usually considered to be acquired. Arthur Keith states that they are not uncommon in old people, especially in those who are the subjects of enteroptosis. In 3 of the 12 cases that he studied there were two pouches, the orifices being to the right and left of the common bile-duct.

INFANTILE STENOSIS OF THE PYLORUS (CONGENITAL HYPERTROPHIC STENOSIS)

This is a condition producing symptoms in the early weeks of life characterized by propulsive vomiting associated with a definite pyloric tumour. Among its many names, "infantile" stenosis is

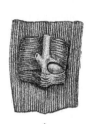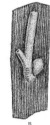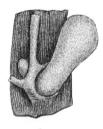

A   B   C

Fig. 366.—Duodenal pouches. (*Keith.*)

A, An early stage; B, a small pouch to the right of the common bile-duct; C, pouches on each side of the duct.

preferable, as its causation is not certain, and the name often applied to it—congenital hypertrophic stenosis—is therefore misleading.

Although the first case of this disease was recorded in 1788 by Hezekiah Bardsley (Osler) as "scirrhus of the pylorus," it is only of recent years that the condition has been readily recognized, largely owing to the work of John Thomson. It must certainly be regarded as uncommon. In spite of the considerable attention directed to it within the last few years, up to May, 1905, Scudder and Quinby had collected only 115 cases. During the years 1899-1908 only 6 cases were met with at the London Hospital, and no case was operated upon. Coutts had met with only 1 case during the last twelve years at the East London Children's Hospital, and during this time the condition had been found there in only 3 post-mortems.

Etiology.—A considerable difference of opinion exists with regard to causation. There are two principal theories—(1) that the condition is primary and due to congenital overgrowth of muscle; (2) that it is secondary to pyloric spasm. Cantley and Dent uphold the former theory; Robert Hutchison and John Thomson the latter, which receives the greater amount of support. In favour of its secondary origin is the fact that it has never been met with in the foetus. Keith states that there is not a single specimen in museums of a stenosis of pylorus of this nature obtained from young or new-born infants.

It has been suggested, as explaining differences in the result of treatment (p. 318), that there are two groups of cases, one a true congenital condition, the other the result of pyloric spasm.

Infantile stenosis is more frequently met with in male than in female children (80 per cent. males); of the 6 cases at the London Hospital, 5 were males.

The stomach is large and has thickened walls. The pyloric region feels firm, and on section shows a marked thickening due to hyperplasia of the circular muscular fibres, sharply limited on the duodenal side, but extending for some distance into the pyloric antrum. (Fig. 367.) The pyloric canal may be completely blocked to the passage of fluid, although a probe may pass readily. The mucous membrane in the pyloric region is thrown into longitudinal folds (Fig. 368). As Cantley and Dent have pointed out, "A single longitudinal reduplication of the mucous membrane, much more marked than any other fold, forms a conspicuous feature in many of the specimens. This prominent fold may be compared to the verumontanum of the male urethra. Indeed, these stomachs in appearance commonly resemble the dissected-out bladder and prostate."

A chronic gastritis often complicates these cases, and aids in the production of the obstruction.

Symptoms.—These are characteristic. The child is perfectly healthy at birth, and in most cases is breast-fed for about a fortnight and does well. Then vomiting unaccountably commences, perhaps as early as three days or as late as six weeks after birth. It is forcible, projectile, contains mucus, and occurs sometimes after every feed, at others after three or four have been retained. Bile is never present in the vomit. The food is changed; apparent improvement occurs in many cases for a few hours or a day, but relapse inevitably occurs. Considerable delay in the adoption of proper treatment is often occasioned by this intermission. The child loses weight and becomes constipated.

If the abdomen is examined shortly after a meal, peristalsis may be noticed passing across the epigastric region from left to right, and a definite tumour lying transversely—the hypertrophied pyloric portion of the stomach—may be felt. The remainder of the abdomen is sunken. In some cases tetany develops.

Diagnosis.—The history of vomiting coming on a few days or weeks after birth, its projectile character, the presence of visible peristalsis and a palpable tumour, make a clinical picture which is unmistakable.

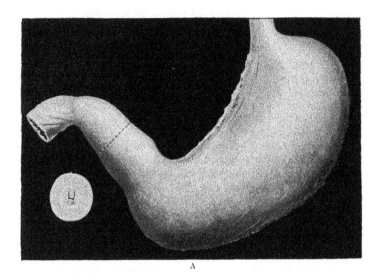

A

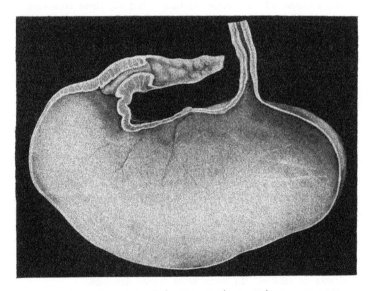

Fig. 367.—Infantile pyloric stenosis.

A, External appearance, with section in pyloric region showing great increase in muscular coat;
B, section showing increase of muscular coat in the pyloric antrum.

(London Hospital Museum and Pathological Institute.)

Willcox and Miller have shown that the condition may be diagnosed from acid dyspepsia with pyloric spasm by examination of the stomach contents. In infantile stenosis the total acidity and active HCl are low, mucus is present in considerable amount, and ferment activity is high. In pyloric spasm, on the other hand, the total acidity is high, mucus is absent, and the ferment activity is low. They also point out that acid dyspepsia presents neither visible peristalsis nor tumour, and that it occurs in infants of 3 months or older.

Prognosis.—This is largely determined by the time at which the condition is recognized and treatment adopted. If untreated or treated late, it is inevitably fatal.

Of the 6 cases, all under the age of 6 months, treated by medical means at the London Hospital, all died. Neurath has recorded 41 cases in infants less than a year old, all of whom died under medical treatment. Cautley and Dent state that, unless operated upon, all die before reaching the age of 4 months. Robert Hutchison records a death-rate of 78 per cent. in a series of 64 cases medically treated at Great Ormond Street Children's Hospital. Thomson has

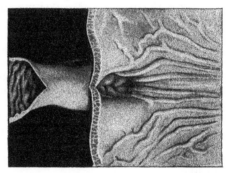

Fig. 368.—Infantile pyloric stenosis. Stomach opened to show the longitudinal folds of mucous membrane in pyloric portion.

(*London Hospital Museum.*)

had 41 cases under his care : 27 were submitted to operation, with 8 recoveries: in 13 not operated upon there were 4 recoveries. Still has had 42 cases with 36 complete histories : of 14 which were operated upon, 8 recovered ; whilst of the 22 who were medically treated, 11 recovered. On the other hand. Robert Hutchison has seen 20 cases of undoubted infantile stenosis in his private practice : of these 17 were treated at home, and all recovered without operation ; 3 were sent into hospital, and 2 died. Bloch has reported 12 cases : 8 patients recovered after medical treatment, 2 died after operation, and 2 were moribund when first seen. Heubner records 19 recoveries out of 21 cases treated medically.

There can be no doubt that the prognosis is grave, and that spontaneous cure rarely if ever occurs ; if the condition be recognized and treated at an early stage, recovery will take place in the majority of cases. This opinion is supported by Deaver and Ashurst, who state it as their belief that " in the immense majority of cases, medical treatment promptly instituted and energetically applied will be successful in curing the patient."

The ultimate condition of these children remains for further investigation. Maylard, Robson, and others have recorded cases of chronic gastric disease in young adults due to congenital narrowness of the pylorus, with dilatation of the stomach, and cases have come under my notice in which symptoms of dilatation of the stomach in early adult life were associated with a history of difficulty in feeding in infancy. The relation of these cases to the disease under discussion has yet to be fully worked out.

Treatment.—Opinions differ as to the advisability of surgical treatment at any stage of the disease. All, however, are agreed that lavage and appropriate feeding should be adopted in the early stages.

Robert Hutchison considers that " operation is never in any sense justified in these cases," and Carpenter states that medical treatment has proved " eminently satisfactory." On the other hand, Fisk holds that all cases should be submitted to surgical treatment after a week or ten days' careful feeding. It has been stated by Harold Stiles that the cases which get well are cases of pyloric spasm without congenital hypertrophy, and that the treatment of the true stenosis is surgical.

In one patient under my observation in whom all the symptoms—propulsive vomiting, visible peristalsis, and the presence of a tumour—were those of congenital stenosis, recovery followed lavage continued for over three months, and now at the age of 5 the boy is in good health.

The stomach should be washed out daily, and small feeds of peptonized milk given. Gastric lavage is easily carried out through a No. 12 rubber catheter attached to a glass funnel. If vomiting is severe, normal saline enemata of 2 to 3 oz. should be given two or three times a day. Lavage with suitable feeding must be continued often for three, four, or five months. At first there is no gain in weight and the child may appear to be going downhill. Hutchison states that this should not prevent continuance of lavage.

This treatment must be persisted in until the necessity for surgical intervention arises or the stomach is repeatedly found free from curds.

If, in spite of lavage, *weight* is steadily lost and the quantity of curd returned shows no diminution, operation should be undertaken. Since surgical treatment was first advocated by Schwyzer, in 1896, various operations have been performed, among others pyloroplasty, pylorodiosis (pyloric dilatation), and gastro-enterostomy. If operation be indicated, some form of pyloroplasty is undoubtedly the ideal procedure. The death-rate of all methods of operative treatment is high—taken as a whole, certainly not less than 40 per cent.

A considerable number of the cases of pylorodiosis have relapsed.

Nicoll's operation, which has hitherto given the best results with the lowest death-rate, is performed as follows : A **V**-shaped incision is made in the pylorus down to the mucosa ; the pylorus is then forcibly stretched by forceps introduced through a separate incision in the stomach wall, and the pyloric incision sewn up in a **Y**-shaped manner. No relapse has followed this operation.

Some such operation as this should be performed when surgical intervention becomes necessary ; if it be impossible, then gastro-jejunostomy should be done.

HERNIA OF STOMACH

The stomach in rare instances has been found in both congenital and acquired umbilical hernias, especially the former, in postoperative ventral hernias, and more rarely still as a content of the sac in inguinal and femoral hernias. It is, however, most often found in hernia of the diaphragm ; thus, in 59 cases collected by Lawford Knaggs, the stomach was present in almost all, but in only 9 cases was it the sole content.

In most cases the condition is present at birth, and observed in infants who are stillborn or who do not survive long. In others the opening is congenital, but the protrusion of the stomach occurs later ; in a few the opening is the result of accident. A part, usually the pyloric portion, or the whole of the stomach may be involved.

In a few cases in which adult life has been reached, gastric symptoms, such as discomfort after food, flatulence, or even pain, are present and, if the patient is a middle-aged male, may lead to suspicion of a chronic gastric or duodenal ulcer ; in other cases, acute dilatation or volvulus of the stomach may supervene. It may be complicated by tetany, as in a case recorded by Russell Reynolds. It is a condition that should be borne in mind in obscure gastric cases. The position of the heart and the abnormal area of resonance will point to the correct diagnosis, which will be confirmed by X-ray examination after a bismuth meal.

GASTROPTOSIS

In this condition the stomach is displaced downwards, alone, or more usually in association with the right kidney, or all the abdominal viscera. It is commonly met with in women, and may cause symptoms owing to its interference with the motor power of the stomach.

Etiology.—The principal factor in the production of gastroptosis is loss of tone in the abdominal muscles, which may be due to many causes. In the few cases in which the stomach alone is prolapsed the condition may be congenital, or perhaps is sometimes secondary to atonic dilatation of the stomach.

The stomach is usually somewhat dilated. It may assume an almost horseshoe shape, allowing the pancreas to appear above the lesser curvature, or in rare cases the pylorus itself may descend and the stomach become vertical.

Symptoms are absent in many cases, and when present resemble those of atonic dilatation of the stomach. It should be remembered that they do not depend upon the abnormally low position of the stomach, but upon motor insufficiency from general ill-health or from pyloric obstruction.

The patients are usually thin, and often the subjects of neurasthenia. The chief complaint is usually of a feeling of fullness after meals, often necessitating loosening of the clothes. Vomiting is unusual, but nausea and retching are common. In many cases pain is complained of directly food enters the stomach.

Diagnosis.—Examination of the patient readily leads to correct diagnosis. Inspection of the abdomen when the patient is standing will usually reveal the prominent lower belly characteristic of enteroptosis. If the stomach has descended, the low position of the lesser curvature is readily seen, often immediately above the umbilicus, moving up and down with respiration.

Treatment.—Surgical treatment is only called for in the rare cases in which obstruction due to kinking is present at the pylorus, and is not remedied by medical means, such as rest in bed with the foot of the bed raised, combined with abdominal massage and, if there is evidence of retention of food, gastric lavage for at least three weeks. On the resumption of the erect position a well-fitting abdominal belt should be worn.

Many operative procedures have been advised and adopted since Duret sutured the anterior gastric wall to the peritoneum in 1894. Of operations designed to remedy the position of the stomach the best is undoubtedly Sir Frederic Eve's modification of Beyea's operation. The stomach is raised to the under surface of the liver by sutures passed through the attachment of the lesser omentum to these organs. Beyea reports 26 operations; all the patients except 3 are quite well. In my opinion, however, operations of this nature are not more successful than non-operative treatment, and in cases with marked obstruction have failed to relieve the symptoms entirely.

Other surgeons, among whom are Deaver and Mayo Robson, prefer gastro-jejunostomy for the rare cases which need operation. But it is in atonic stomachs such as these that the operation is liable to be followed by regurgitant vomiting. For the emphatically rare cases in which operative measures are indicated, I believe Finney's gastro-duodenostomy gives the best results, and I have used it with perfect success.

GASTRIC VOLVULUS

In gastric volvulus the stomach may become twisted in one of three directions : (1) Around its transverse axis; (2) around an antero-posterior axis; (3) around an axis at right angles to its greater curvature.

This is an extremely rare condition, of which the recorded cases number 20. Deaver and Ashurst have collected 13, and individual cases have been recorded by Jiano, Knaggs, Hermes, Türmoos, Payer, Niosi, and Delangre.

Until the normal relations of the stomach have been altered in some way, volvulus is impossible. It may arise in gastroptosis, and has occurred (Knaggs) in association with diaphragmatic hernia ; in 3 cases it complicated hour-glass contraction of the stomach in which the pyloric pouch was large; cases have been recorded following injury, in others the symptoms have appeared suddenly during apparent health. In most of the cases the stomach became twisted around its transverse axis, the transverse colon passing upwards and backwards. As a result of this, both orifices of the stomach are usually obstructed.

Symptoms.—The onset is sudden, with pain in the epigastric region, followed by collapse. As a rule the patient does not vomit, but only regurgitates food which enters the œsophagus. A tense, resonant swelling rapidly forms in the epigastric region. The signs resemble in many respects those of acute dilatation of the stomach, but diagnosis can be made by the absence of vomiting and by the impossibility of passing a tube from the œsophagus into the stomach.

Treatment.—Operation should be undertaken at once. In most cases, as soon as the abdomen is opened the stomach presents as a tense cyst which usually needs puncture before the type to which the volvulus belongs can be determined or the volvulus reduced. The opening should be sutured and the volvulus reduced. In the usual type of case (1) the posterior gastric wall presents.

The operations recorded number 14, with 3 recoveries.

HOUR-GLASS STOMACH (SEGMENTED STOMACH—Wölfer)

In this condition the stomach is divided into cavities, as a rule two, but occasionally three or even four. It is more often met with in women than in men ; among 154 cases collected by Schomerus, 128 were in women.

Etiology.—Its chief cause is gastric ulcer (Fig. 369) ; more rarely it results from cancer (Fig. 370) ; very rarely indeed it may be congenital. A " saddle-shaped " ulcer of the lesser curvature usually produces the condition, but perigastric adhesions as the result of the ulcer may constrict the stomach or bind it to the abdominal

v

wall or liver so that diverticula are formed. Out of 45 cases operated upon and reported by Mayo Robson and Moynihan, 37 were
the result of ulcer or perigastritis. Hour-glass stomach is met with
as a complication of gastric ulcer in from 3·3 per cent. (W. J. Mayo,
in 925 operations) to 9 per cent. (Moynihan, in 198 operations) of the
cases. I believe that Mayo's figures represent the truer proportion.

Perigastric adhesions other than those due to ulcer may cause
the condition. It may be the result of the healing of ulcers after

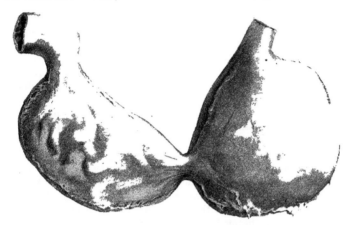

Fig. 369.—Hour-glass stomach, due to cicatrization of a saddle-
shaped lesser-curvature ulcer.

(London Hospital Pathological Institute.)

corrosive poisoning; I have recently operated upon such a case.
Cases have also been described as due to syphilis of the stomach.

Undoubtedly, though extremely rarely, the condition may arise
congenitally, for Delamere and Dieulafé, and Gardiner, have recorded
cases, and according to Martin there is a specimen in the McGill
Museum. As the stomach in the early stage of development consists
of a tubular pyloric portion and a cardiac pouch, a continuance of
the fœtal condition would account for these cases. (Fig. 362.)

The constriction is generally single and situated towards the
pyloric end of the stomach, and, as a rule, the greater curvature is
drawn up towards the lesser. The cardiac pouch is usually larger
than the pyloric. When, however, as not infrequently happens,
pyloric obstruction coexists, the pyloric pouch may be as large as
the cardiac. The recognition of this fact is important, for the
pyloric pouch may be mistaken at operation for the whole stomach,
and a gastro-jejunostomy performed on it with a fatal result; well-

known surgeons, among whom are Bier, Czerny, and Hartmann, have fallen into this error, and recorded their experience for the sake of others. It may also become the seat of a volvulus.

Symptoms.—These resemble very closely those of pyloric stenosis and follow in many cases on the history of a gastric ulcer. The physical signs may render a diagnosis possible before operation. These depend upon—(1) inflating the stomach; (2) the introduction of fluid; (3) examination by X-rays after a bismuth meal.

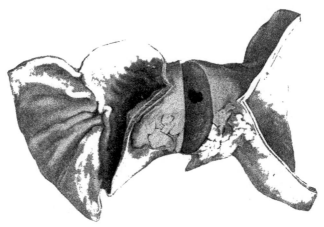

Fig. 370.—Hour-glass stomach from malignant growth.
A portion of the cardiac pouch has been removed.
(London Hospital Museum.)

1. On inflating with CO_2 or air, the upper pouch may be seen to become dilated, and this is followed, if the abdomen be watched for a few minutes, by the pyloric pouch.

2. If a measured quantity of liquid has been passed into the stomach through a tube, a large portion of it cannot be recovered. Moreover, during lavage, after the fluid has returned clear there may be a gush of cloudy fluid with gastric contents.

It may be impossible to obtain any fluid even when splashing occurs, the fluid having passed into the pyloric pouch (sign of paradoxical dilatation).

On passing in a quantity of fluid the cardiac pouch may become distended first; this gradually subsides, to be followed by another swelling due to fluid in the pyloric pouch.

3. X-ray examination after a bismuth meal should be carried out in all suspected cases, and is the only reliable means of diagnosis (Fig. 364).

In rare cases the constriction is close to the cardia, and the symptoms resemble those of œsophageal obstruction.

Free HCl is usually absent and the total acidity of the gastric contents low.

It is important to consider every case of dilated stomach as a possible hour-glass stomach, so as to avoid the fatal error of performing gastro-jejunostomy on a dilated pyloric pouch. In every stomach-operation, the whole of the stomach must be examined to prevent such errors in treatment.

Treatment.—This consists in providing free exit for the stomach contents. Gastro-jejunostomy should be done in every case. Where there is a large cardiac pouch with a small pyloric one, this operation will suffice, but if pyloric stenosis is also present it is not enough ; gastroplasty should be combined with it, or, as suggested by von Hacker in 1895, and by Weir and Foote in 1896, a separate gastro-jejunostomy done on each pouch. This, I believe, will be more frequently done in the future. To avoid the risk of hernia between the stomach at the constriction and the jejunum between the two openings, the gut should be united to the stomach.

Where more than two pouches exist they should be connected by gastro-gastrostomy, and then gastro-jejunostomy performed on the largest pouch.

Other operations have been proposed, such as gastroplasty or a gastro-gastrostomy alone ; but Paterson has shown that these are associated with 25 to 30 per cent. of relapses.

If the condition be due to malignant disease, partial gastrectomy should be performed.

Results.—Veyrassat has collected all the cases recorded to August, 1908. There are 181. Of these, 73 were treated by gastro-jejunostomy ; 72 per cent. were cured, and only 2·7 per cent. failed. Of the 14 deaths, 6 were due to the anastomosis being done to the pyloric pouch.

ACUTE DILATATION OF THE STOMACH

This condition is by no means uncommon. Its diagnosis is of the utmost importance to the surgeon, following as it sometimes does abdominal operations, with an inevitably fatal result unless recognized early. There is no doubt that many cases recorded as " postoperative ileus " were of this nature.

Although its recognition dates from the description given in the *Guy's Hospital Reports* of 1872–3 by Hilton Fagge, Rokitansky in 1842 had drawn attention to one of the features connected with it —compression of the third part of the duodenum by the mesentery and superior mesenteric artery as a cause of intestinal obstruction due to external pressure. Albrecht in 1899 was able to collect 19 cases only; by 1902, Campbell Thomson published the records of 44 cases, including 5 in which he had made the post-mortem examination. Since then many more cases have been published, Nicholls in 1908 analysing 225 collected cases.

Etiology.—The condition may arise after operations performed on any part of the body, but most often follows those upon the abdomen. It may complicate other diseases, appear after injury, or in rare cases arise primarily as the result of indiscretion in diet.

It may be met with at any age, the youngest recorded being 9 months, the oldest 75 years, but it is most common in youth and early adult life.

Of the 225 cases collected by Nicholls, 47 per cent. followed operation, and of these 69 per cent. were abdominal, most often on the biliary tract, next in frequency on the kidney, then on the appendix. Dilatation may follow injury (in 17 out of 217 cases collected by Laffer, the injury in 5 being abdominal). In 40 cases it complicated some other disease—most often pneumonia or typhoid. In 11 cases spinal curvature was present.

Many opinions have been advanced as to its cause : (1) Obstruction of the duodenum by the superior mesenteric artery (Rokitansky, Albrecht) ; (2) excessive secretion (Fagge, Henry Morris) ; (3) paralysis (Campbell Thomson) ; (4) compression of the third portion of the duodenum by the paralysed dilated stomach (Box and Wallace) ; (5) septic intoxication.

The condition probably consists primarily of a paralytic dilatation of the stomach. This is the conclusion arrived at by most modern writers on the subject. It may in a certain number of cases be kept up or complicated by mesenteric compression, but out of 120 cases in Laffer's series, in only 27 was it of this type.

It is stated by Stavely that a chronic dilatation of the duodenum or stomach may result from pressure of the mesenteric vessels. In one case retrocolic gastro-duodenostomy was performed for this condition.

Morbid anatomy.—The post-mortem appearances in all the recorded cases are similar. The stomach is dilated into a huge V-shaped tube which may fill the whole abdomen. There is usually a sharp kink at the lesser curvature. The dilatation rarely affects the stomach alone, but may, as previously stated, stop short at the point at which the superior mesenteric vessels cross the duodenum, and in one instance (Bäumler) there was a localized constriction here with a well-marked circular area of necrosis in the intima of the gut. But in some cases the dilatation extends lower and involves the jejunum to a greater or less degree.

The walls of the stomach are thin, and the mucous membrane shows hæmorrhages. As noted by Fagge, whitish striæ are frequently observed on its peritoneal surface, the result of distension.

If an abdominal operation has been performed, there is usually no trace of peritonitis.

Symptoms.—The onset is, as a rule, sudden, in the postoperative cases occurring from twelve to forty-eight hours after the operation, usually about twenty-four; it has been delayed to the second week. Epigastric pain and a feeling of distension are first complained of, and are followed by the vomiting of large quantities of fluid with very little effort but with no relief. The fluid is usually greenish-grey, turbid, and seldom offensive. As the disease advances, thirst becomes intolerable, the pulse rapid, respiration embarrassed, and there is great restlessness. Tetany has been observed.

On examination, the great abdominal tympanitic distension is evident, chiefly on the left and in the middle line. Splashing is readily obtained, and peristalsis very rarely seen. If the stomach-tube is passed there is an abundant escape of gas and a large quantity of fluid is evacuated, but the stomach refills after a short time.

Diagnosis.—Early recognition is important, particularly in the postoperative cases where complications due to the anæsthetic or to the operation may be more in the mind of the surgeon. It may be confused with postanæsthetic vomiting, but this does not persist; or it may appear for the first time twenty-four hours after operation. In the recorded cases the postanæsthetic vomiting had ceased. Early peritonitis following abdominal operations may be suspected, but the symptoms of the two conditions differ entirely. The temporary relief following the evacuation of gas and fluid by a stomach-tube should lead to the correct diagnosis.

Prognosis.—The death-rate of recorded cases is 63 per cent., most of the deaths occurring within the first week.

Treatment.—As soon as it is even suspected that this condition is supervening, the stomach-tube should be passed and lavage employed. The recumbent position with the foot of the bed raised should be adopted. It has been recommended that in persistent cases the patient should lie on the face or assume the knee-elbow position.

If these measures fail, what is to be done? Operation has been carried out in 14 cases with 2 recoveries, and in 1 of these (Macevitt) after the abdomen was opened—the diagnosis not having been made before operation—the operator contented himself with passing a stomach-tube. In the second, a kink at the duodeno-jejunal flexure was relieved by suturing the jejunum to the transverse meso-colon (Petit). Gastrotomy has failed to relieve in 5 instances. Gastrojejunostomy has been recommended as applicable, but should never, in my opinion, be done. In the 2 recorded cases (Kehr, Körte), death ensued. The condition has arisen after and in spite of gastro-

jejunostomy, and, if not relieved by lavage and position, is unlikely to be cured by this operation.

I am of opinion that operation is not indicated. In the early
cases, life will be saved by lavage; in those that are overlooked, no
surgical treatment will be of any avail.

CHRONIC DILATATION OF THE STOMACH

These cases fall into two groups :—

1. Those in which the dilatation is the result of mechanical
   obstruction in the region of the pylorus—obstructive.
2. Those in which the enlargement of the stomach is the
   result of weakness of its walls—atonic dilatation.

The former variety possesses most interest; it is doubtful if the
second form should ever be treated surgically.

It must always be remembered that gastric dilatation is not a
disease, but a symptom.

1. Obstructive Dilatation

These cases, again, fall into two groups, each of which is further
subdivided into those due to malignant growth and those the result
of simple causes. The groups are—

(1) Those in which the cause is in the wall of the stomach or
    duodenum.
(2) Those in which it is external to them.

    i. (a) Malignant disease of the stomach or duodenum.
       (b) Ulcers of the stomach or duodenum and their sequelæ.
           Simple tumours; infantile hypertrophic stenosis;
           fibrous stricture; gastroptosis.
    ii. (a) Malignant disease of the pancreas, gall-bladder, and
            biliary passages.
        (b) Non-malignant disease of gall-bladder and bile-ducts.
            Perigastritis; mobile kidney; aneurysm.

Carcinoma of the stomach frequently arises in the pyloric region,
and is one of the common causes of obstructive dilatation of the
stomach (p. 380). The onset of symptoms of interference with gastric
motility in a previously healthy adult should always direct attention
to this possibility.

Gastric dilatation may be due to the presence of a chronic ulcer
of the pyloric region of the stomach, to the contraction of scar tissue
formed as the result of its healing, to perigastric adhesions, or to ulcer
of the first part of the duodenum. The last-named is the most
common simple cause. The obstruction is sometimes due to spasm of
the pylorus brought about by the irritation of the ulcer, but in such
cases the dilatation is rarely great, and seldom in itself calls for

surgical assistance, though it may be advisable to deal with the ulcer by surgical means.

Dilatation may be due to a simple polypus playing the part of a ball valve (p. 377).

Infantile stenosis of pylorus is considered on p. 314. In some cases, recovery from this condition is followed by definite symptoms of secondary dilatation of the stomach later. Maylard has called attention to a group of cases of simple narrowing of the pylorus which may be congenital.

Simple fibrous stricture of the pylorus is occasionally the cause of obstructive dilatation. Mansell-Moullin has called attention to this fact, and describes the condition found at operation as follows : " It simply seemed as if the circular muscular fibres had disappeared and had been replaced by tough or unyielding fibrous tissue." He goes on to say : " The most probable explanation is that the fibrous degeneration is the outcome of long-continued spasmodic contraction caused by persistent dyspepsia."

I have operated upon three such cases in which at operation neither adhesion nor trace of scarring was present.

Gastroptosis may cause obstructive dilatation by producing a kink at the pylorus (p. 320).

Malignant growths of the pancreas, gall-bladder, or bile-ducts may produce, among other symptoms, those of dilatation of the stomach.

Perigastric adhesions, which are due most often to chronic gastric ulcer or, less frequently, to gall-stones and their sequelæ, a distended gall-bladder, or the obstruction caused by the ulceration of a gall-stone into the duodenum or stomach, may cause symptoms of gastric dilatation.

Mobile kidney, by its traction on the duodenum, is an unusual but very definite cause.

Dilatation due to pressure of a simple tumour external to the stomach is an extremely rare occurrence. It has been recorded as the result of pressure by an aneurysm.

2. Atonic Dilatation

This is a condition in which, owing to weakness of the stomach-walls, the gastric contents are not passed rapidly enough into the duodenum. Amenable to medical treatment in its early stages, it is but rarely that it becomes so extreme that surgery has to be called in to its aid.

Symptoms.—In the early stages the symptoms are indefinite and consist of gastric discomfort or a sense of fullness after meals.

If at this stage gastric motility were estimated by any of the methods mentioned on p. 309, it would be found deficient.

In many of the simple cases there is a previous history of duodenal or gastric ulcer, or of dyspepsia.

Later the symptoms become characteristic : food is retained in the stomach and vomited at irregular intervals of two or three days— the vomit consists of large quantities of sour-smelling fluid, containing perhaps fragments of food taken several days before ; there are associated thirst, wasting, and constipation, and the patient presents the dry, harsh skin seen when the tissues are deprived of water. At this stage, too, free HCl is usually absent and the total acidity low, whether the dilatation be due to simple or malignant causes.

Tetany may complicate gastric dilatation from any cause, but as a rule it is only seen in simple cases. Attention has been particularly directed to this by Mayo Robson, who in 1898 pointed out the necessity for surgical treatment of the gastric dilatation when this complication has supervened. Its recognition is important as, probably of toxic origin, it is a serious complication and fatal in a large proportion of cases unless treated by operation. In its fully developed form it is uncommon (McKendrick in 1907 was able to collect 63 cases), but lesser degrees are far from rare. Patients complain not infrequently of formication or numbness, or of heaviness in the limbs, followed by cramps.

Examination.—The enlarged stomach may be distinctly seen, reaching in some cases as low as the pubes, and peristalsis may be noticed crossing from left to right, or it may be elicited by gently flicking the abdomen. The area of stomach-resonance is increased, and splashing sounds may be obtained over an area not usually occupied by the stomach at a time when it should be empty. When any doubt exists as to the presence of dilatation, the stomach should be distended with air or gas. The abdomen should be carefully examined for evidences of tumour, mobile kidney, or gastroptosis, and the possibility of hour-glass contraction considered.

Diagnosis.—There are two essential points to consider in the diagnosis of gastric dilatation—(1) the discovery of the dilatation ; (2) the discovery of its causation.

(1) Diagnosis has to be made from—

(a) Gastroptosis.—In these patients, usually women, the history is one of vague indigestion and could only be mistaken for that of a very early stage of gastric dilatation. It is more often confused with the early symptoms of carcinoma. Distension of the stomach will show the gastroptosis, and passage of the stomach-tube will demonstrate any motor insufficiency ; if this is present it may require surgical treatment.

(*b*) Hour-glass stomach.—It is rarely possible to distinguish this by its *symptoms* from pyloric obstruction, which not infrequently coexists; but its possible presence should always be borne in mind, and its diagnosis attempted, in order to prevent errors in operative treatment. Certain symptoms (p. 323) noticed on the passage of a stomach-tube may facilitate the diagnosis; in other cases, X-ray examination after the ingestion of bismuth will reveal the condition.

(2) An attempt must be made to discover the nature of the dilatation or its causation. Chief reliance has to be placed on a careful anamnesis. A history of preceding abdominal disease, pointing to gastric or duodenal ulcer, is obtained in many of the simple cases. The rapid onset of the symptoms of dilatation in an adult who has had no previous gastric trouble will point very strongly to malignant disease.

Examination of the stomach contents after a test meal may be of service in the differential diagnosis.

A history of biliary trouble would point to the condition being secondary to disease of the biliary passages; one of difficult feeding in infancy or of lifelong dyspepsia followed by dilatation of the stomach would suggest a congenital origin.

Prognosis.—Obstructive dilatation is a disease of grave prognosis unless treated surgically; but if treated on modern surgical lines the death-rate is small and the ultimate recovery in the majority of cases perfect. In cases in which tetany has developed the death-rate under medical treatment has been from 70 to 90 per cent. Under surgical treatment the prognosis even of the cases with tetany has been greatly improved; thus, McKendrick has collected 24 such cases with only 3 deaths.

Treatment of chronic dilatation.—*Obstructive* dilatation of the stomach should be surgically treated; it is useless attempting to cure the condition by lavage.

The exact operation necessary will depend on its causation. The choice lies in the majority of cases between gastro-jejunostomy and gastro-duodenostomy (Finney's method). Operations such as pylorodiosis or pyloroplasty are followed by relapse in many cases, and should not be considered.

In cases in which the dilatation is due to mobility of the right kidney, this organ should be fixed before resorting to further treatment. In cases due to disease of the gall-bladder, the removal of gall-stones and division of adhesions may suffice to cure.

If the obstruction is due to congenital narrowing of the pylorus or to the "fibrous" variety of stricture, gastro-duodenostomy by Finney's method is the best operation, restoring the condition of the parts as nearly as possible to normal. When, owing to the presence of active ulceration or of many adhesions around the pylorus, this is inadmissible, posterior no-loop gastro-jejunostomy should be performed, the anastomosis being made to the pyloric portion of the stomach.

The result of surgical treatment on these lines is most gratifying; the death-rate in large numbers of cases does not exceed 5 per cent., and in the hands of those who are doing much work of this kind is less than 2 per cent.

Advanced cases of *atonic* dilatation may in rare instances need surgical treatment, but this must only be carried out after the failure of prolonged medical treatment, rest in bed, and lavage. As first pointed out by Mikulicz, and again by Paul and the present writer, gastro-jejunostomy in this condition is frequently followed by the establishment of a vicious circle.

In these cases a mechanical factor is added, namely, kinking of the pylorus. Finney's operation, followed by medical treatment, will give relief, and should be carried out.

Attempts have been made to treat the condition by folding the wall of the stomach so as to make it smaller (gastroplication). This is useless, for the size of the stomach matters not at all; the patient is suffering from weakness of the stomach wall, with or without obstruction, and in neither case can good result.

INJURIES

The stomach or duodenum may be injured by violence applied from without, in abdominal contusions and wounds; or from within, as the result of the passage of instruments, over-distension, or the action of swallowed corrosive fluids or foreign bodies.

RUPTURE OF THE STOMACH

Uncomplicated rupture of the stomach is an accident of extreme rarity. The cases may be divided into two groups, the "spontaneous" and the traumatic. In both the rupture may be complete, involving all the layers of the stomach-wall, or incomplete: the latter can be subdivided into those involving the serous coat only; those involving serous and muscular coats—the interstitial, usually due to external injuries; and those causing rupture of mucosa, generally the result of internal violence.

Spontaneous Rupture of the Stomach

This heading should cover only cases of rupture of a presumably healthy organ, occurring apart from external violence. It has been customary to include ruptures due to lavage and distension with air, but these fall more appropriately into the next group. It is an exceedingly rare condition, for not more than 10 cases have been recorded, all of which terminated fatally. The rupture is usually at the lesser curvature, and generally occurs as the result of spontaneous over-distension ; in at least 3 of the cases it followed vomiting.

It is impossible to diagnose more than the occurrence of a perforative lesion in the upper abdomen. Operation should be undertaken at once, the rent in the stomach closed by a continuous stitch of thin chromic catgut taking up all the coats, followed by a continuous Lembert stitch of silk, Pagenstecher, or linen thread.

TRAUMATIC RUPTURE OF THE STOMACH

These fall into two groups, due to—(1) direct violence, (2) indirect violence.

1. *Direct Violence*

The violence may affect the stomach (*a*) from without, as in abdominal contusions, or (*b*) from within, the result of over-distension or of the passage of instruments.

(*a*) *Complete* rupture of the stomach from external violence is rare ; rupture of the stomach apart from injury to other viscera is rarer still. Among 270 cases admitted to the London Hospital for abdominal contusion in the ten years 1899–1908, the stomach was ruptured in 5, and in 1 only of these was it ruptured alone, and even then the right kidney was "bruised." Gastric ruptures usually occur in "run-over" accidents, the wheel passing over the epigastric and umbilical regions. Another and rarer cause is localized injury to the epigastric region, such as by a kick from a horse ; in this variety the stomach is more likely to suffer alone. In both it is unlikely to be injured unless full.

Ruptures from external violence are usually situated in the region of the greater curvature.

Treatment.—After any abdominal contusion the patient should be placed in bed and carefully watched, the pulse and temperature being taken hourly. No morphia should be given until the question of operation has been settled, and then only if the patient has to be moved to hospital or nursing-home.

If the abdomen is rigid, or contains free fluid or gas, operation should be immediate. If the signs are inconclusive, operation should be undertaken as soon as it is seen that the patient is getting worse or not rallying from the shock.

The rent should be sutured and extravasated fluid carefully sponged away. The employment of drainage will depend upon the extent of peritoneal soiling or existent peritonitis. If peritonitis is present, the usual treatment for this condition must be adopted (p. 569).

Prognosis.—This is extremely grave ; all the cases treated at the London Hospital have died. According to Deaver and Ashurst, only 4 operations for traumatic rupture of the stomach have been recorded, and all resulted in death. I have operated upon 2 cases, one of which was complicated by complete rupture of the transverse portion of the duodenum ; the patient lived four days after closure of both rents, and at the autopsy no cause for death was found. In the other the right kidney was also ruptured, and hæmopericardium was found post mortem.

Diagnosis.—It is unusual for this to be made before operation. It is unwise to make any attempt at definite diagnosis by such means as inflation with air. The important point is to decide that exploration is necessary.

As the result of external violence the stomach may be *partially ruptured*, its serous, muscular, or mucous coats, alone or together, being torn ; in some cases a hæmatoma develops in the gastric wall, and may be absorbed, or may form a cyst which may become infected, and result in an interstitial abscess. This may rupture into the stomach, the pus be vomited, and recovery ensue; or into the peritoneal cavity; or, after adhesions have formed externally, may discharge, producing a gastric fistula.

The gradual formation of a swelling in the epigastric region following an injury should lead to the suspicion of a partial rupture of stomach and to exploration. Pseudopancreatic cyst (Jordan Lloyd) must be considered in diagnosis.

An injury of the mucous membrane may lead to the formation of the so-called " traumatic ulcer " of the stomach, characterized by the usual symptoms, but as a rule healing rapidly. In a few cases such " ulcers " become chronic and have given rise to perforation, hæmatemesis, hour-glass stomach, or gastric dilatation.

The treatment of this condition is identical with that of non-traumatic ulcer (p. 350).

(*b*) Rupture, *complete or partial,* may follow distension of the stomach by fluid used for lavage, or gas used in distending the stomach for diagnostic purposes. These cases are rare. One example only has occurred at the London Hospital in the last ten years, in a patient with dilated stomach the result of pyloric carcinoma. During lavage there was a sudden onset of abdominal pain and collapse. At operation five hours later a rupture at the lesser curvature was found. The patient died sixteen hours after operation.

Ruptures from over-distension occur most frequently at the lesser curvature, very occasionally at the site of an ulcer, simple or malignant. Ruptures may also be produced by the passage of instruments, such as the gastroscope, for exploratory purposes.

If sudden pain and collapse follow the passage of a stomach-tube or diagnostic instrument, thus raising the suspicion that this accident has occurred, immediate operation must be undertaken.

2. *Indirect Violence*

Cases have been recorded in which gastric hæmorrhage has followed falls on the back or the buttocks, or after lifting heavy weights. It is just possible that lesions of the mucous membrane may account for these cases ; from their nature they do not lead to post-mortem examination. Bleeding after indirect injury comes, in most cases, from œsophageal varices due to cirrhosis of the liver. All the cases of this nature that have come under my observation, in which there was no history of previous gastric trouble, appeared to be due to this cause, but I have known severe hæmatemesis follow indirect violence due both to falls and to strains, in patients with chronic gastric ulcer.

Injury may be the exciting cause leading to the perforation of a gastric or duodenal ulcer ; several cases have come under my care in which perforation occurred at the time the patient was straining to lift a heavy weight ; in two cases in which a duodenal ulcer perforated, the patient had had no previous gastric symptoms. The onset of sudden pain and acute abdominal symptoms in circumstances such as these should lead to a suspicion of perforation and to immediate operation.

RUPTURE OF THE DUODENUM

While rupture of the stomach is extremely rare, rupture of the duodenum is still rarer.

Thus, out of 270 cases of contused abdomen admitted into the London Hospital between the years 1899–1908 there were 19 cases of ruptured gut, and in these the duodenum was affected twice only. In one case already mentioned the stomach also was ruptured ; in the second case no operation was performed.

Berry and Giuseppi found records of only 132 cases of traumatic intestinal rupture in ten London hospitals from 1893–1907 ; the duodenum was affected in 23 and the duodeno-jejunal flexure in 3. Meerwein, in publishing (1907) an account of a case under his care, collected all the published cases of traumatic rupture of duodenum, 64 in number. These include only 2 of those collected by Berry and Giuseppi.

The transverse portion of the duodenum usually suffers, the rent being most often at right angles to the long axis of the gut. As in ruptures of the stomach, the lesion may be complete or incomplete ; the latter is rare, but Berry records an instance in a boy of 15 in whom " a clot of blood as large as a hen's egg lay between the peritoneal and the muscular coats and completely blocked the second part of the duodenum." The rupture may be retroperitoneal. This occurred in 4 out of the 23 cases collected by Berry and Giuseppi.

As in other parts of the alimentary canal, partial rupture may be recovered from and lead to obstructive symptoms later. Meerwein records 2 cases in which spontaneous recovery occurred, but biliary obstruction in one, and dilated stomach in the other, necessitated operation.

Diagnosis.—It will be impossible to make a definite diagnosis of the portion of the gut injured before operation. Rupture of the duodenum should be suspected in all cases of injury to the upper abdomen. Retroperitoneal injury should be suspected when symptoms of sepsis follow an injury to the upper abdomen.

Treatment.—The general rules which govern operation after abdominal contusions are to be followed. Rupture of the duodenum should always be borne in mind, and its whole extent carefully examined. It was overlooked at operation in 7 of Berry and Giuseppi's cases, and in 7 of the 29 cases recorded by Meerwein in which operation was performed.

If the rent involves, as is usual, the anterior wall of the duodenum only, it should be closed in two layers, the inner with fine chromic gut through all the coats, buried by fine silk Lembert stitches. If the rent is complete, gastro-jejunostomy will be the best course to pursue after closure of both ends of the gut. End-to-end suture of the second or third parts of the duodenum is unlikely to be successful on account of the absence of peritoneum from its posterior surface.

Prognosis.—This is extremely grave. Complete rupture, unless treated by operation, is inevitably fatal. Death followed in all the cases recorded by Berry and Giuseppi, and in all but 2 of the 29 recorded by Meerwein in which operation was performed. In only 1 case in this country (Godwin's), operated on in 1905, has recovery followed, although a patient whom Moynihan treated by closure of both ends and gastro-jejunostomy lived 104 days after operation, and died as the result of the lodgment of the Murphy's button used.

WOUNDS OF THE STOMACH

The stomach may be injured in penetrating abdominal wounds, the result of stabs with sharp implements or of gunshots.

STAB WOUNDS

Wounds of the stomach are rare in civil life. Thus, in 125 patients with penetrating wounds of the abdomen treated at the London Hospital between 1899 and 1908, in no instance was the stomach injured. Among 75 cases of wounds of the stomach collected by Siegel, 4 were the result of stabs. Even when the stomach is wounded, the case is often complicated by simultaneous injury to other organs.

The stomach may be injured alone in stabs in the epigastric region, and it is important to remember that stab wounds of the lower chest are not infrequently complicated by injury to the stomach.

Symptoms.—These will depend to a certain extent upon the contents of the stomach at the time of the infliction of the injury, and the size of the wound. Sudden leakage of gastric contents into the peritoneal cavity will be followed by the usual signs accompanying perforation of an abdominal viscus. In a few cases the escape of gastric contents from the wound, their presence upon the instrument inflicting the injury, or hæmatemesis may render the diagnosis certain. But it must be remembered that the stomach may be wounded and no symptoms be present at an early stage, also that hæmatemesis may occur from bruising or laceration of the mucous membrane of the stomach without penetration.

Treatment.—If it is certain from the symptoms that the wound is a penetrating one, it should be opened up and a careful examination made, remembering, if a wound is found on the anterior surface of the stomach, that the posterior surface may have been simultaneously damaged. The wound in the stomach should be closed by a continuous stitch of fine chromic gut through all its coats, this being buried by a Lembert stitch of silk, Pagenstecher, or linen thread. Any extravasated contents should be gently wiped away. If there is extensive soiling of the peritoneum, a tube should be put in above the pubes; if general peritonitis is present, the appropriate treatment should be adopted.

Prognosis.—If operation is carried out within the first twenty-four hours the prognosis is good; recovery took place in 8 of the 9 recorded cases.

GUNSHOT WOUNDS

It is rare for the stomach to be injured alone in wounds of this nature. Thus, out of 126 cases collected by Forgue and Jeanbrau, in which the lesion was verified post mortem or by operation, in only 32 did it suffer alone. In about 10 per cent. of these cases only one perforation existed; and in 3 cases the bullet lodged in the stomach.

In wounds in war, from modern rifles, the bullet usually passes through the body unless turned aside by bone. On the other hand, in the gunshot injuries of civil life the wounds are large and the bullet usually remains in the body.

Symptoms.—The most important are shock and hæmatemesis.

Diagnosis.—This may be possible from the presence of the above symptoms, but all penetrating abdominal wounds in civil life must be explored even if symptoms are absent.

Treatment.—The abdomen should be opened through a median incision, and the stomach carefully examined. After suture of a wound on the anterior surface, the posterior surface should be exposed by making a wide opening in the gastro-colic omentum. In every case search should be made for injury to other organs. If the diaphragm be simultaneously wounded, the pleural cavity should be drained. It is only in cases in which the fact of perforation is doubtful that the bullet wound itself should come into the incision. .

FOREIGN BODIES IN THE STOMACH AND DUODENUM

The patients are usually children, hysterical girls, insane people, and jugglers. Occasionally a foreign body such as a tooth-plate or a piece of bone is swallowed by sane adults.

The majority of foreign bodies swallowed pass out of the stomach, and are discharged naturally a few days later. A few, depending on their size and shape, may lodge in the stomach, or in rare cases in the duodenum. The foreign body may remain in the stomach for years without giving rise to symptoms, or it may perforate acutely, or cause ulceration, subacute perforation, perigastric abscess, or gastric fistula.

In children and the insane no history may be obtainable, and the onset of vomiting and pain causes attention to be directed to the stomach. The finding of a foreign body in the vomit may lead to a diagnosis of the cause of the symptoms.

The foreign body may be composed of hair, the so-called hair-ball. In these cases the patient or friends may fail to connect the habit of hair-biting with the abdominal signs, and the surgeon may omit to consider this possibility, but in all obscure abdominal tumours in women it should be remembered. These tumours are rarely found in men, and are uncommon in the insane. In 42 cases collected by Butterworth, 39 were females.

The quantity of hair present varies : in one case operated upon successfully by Swain, it weighed 5 lb. 3 oz. The mass can usually be felt through the abdominal wall. When small it occupies the pyloric region, but as it increases in size it forms a cast of the stomach which may in rare cases extend into the œsophagus or into the duodenum (Fig. 371). Symptoms may be absent, and the abdominal tumour be discovered by accident. As a rule, however, pain and vomiting are present after food. The tongue is foul, and the patient is usually anæmic.

Fenwick states that the average duration of the disease in these cases is about fifteen years. All end fatally, unless operated upon, from ulceration and perforation of the stomach and its sequelæ, or from exhaustion.

Concretions formed of vegetable fibres are occasionally found,

w'

usually in patients who have chewed roots which have reputed medicinal properties; and gastroliths in patients who have drunk varnish in their craving for alcoholic liquor. The gastrolith is usually composed of shellac. According to Fenwick, only 4 cases have been recorded.

Treatment.—This will depend on the form, consistence, and size of the article swallowed. Rounded objects, coins, buttons, etc., usually give rise to no trouble; tooth-plates and pencils rarely pass. If it is thought that the foreign body is likely to pass, a diet of porridge

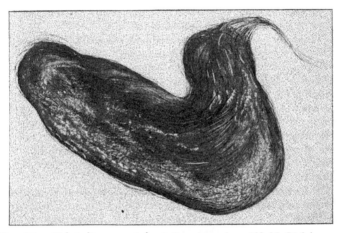

Fig. 371.—Hair-ball removed from the stomach. (*H. M. Rigby's case.*
(*London Hospital Museum.*)

or mashed potatoes should be given, but no purgatives. The patient should be X-rayed, and the exact location of the foreign body determined. It must be remembered that its weight may displace the stomach, and it may be necessary to use X-rays after bismuth emulsion has been taken. If the foreign body is giving rise to no symptoms, no hurry is necessary.

If natural discharge is impossible, from the size, shape, or number of foreign bodies, or if symptoms are produced, immediate operation should be resorted to.

In most cases it will be necessary to open the stomach after packing off the peritoneal cavity with gauze. The incision in the stomach should be transverse to its long axis, and, after removal of the foreign body, should be closed with a continuous stitch of fine chromic gut through all its coats, and this buried with a continuous Lembert stitch of fine silk. It may be possible to remove the foreign body, after the abdomen has been opened, by means of forceps such as Brüning's or Bilton Pollard's.

If the foreign body is in the duodenum, an attempt should be made to push it back into the stomach and extract it from there ; only if this fails should the opening be made in the duodenum.

Prognosis.—This is extremely good. Out of 20 cases published since 1900, and collected by Deaver and Ashurst, in which operation was performed, there was only 1 death.

INJURY BY CAUSTIC FLUIDS

Mineral acids and alkalis, swallowed by accident or with suicidal intent, cause serious injury to the stomach. In many of these cases surgical treatment is sooner or later necessary to remedy the resulting contraction-deformities of the stomach.[1]

The cardiac end and pyloric portion of the stomach suffer most, and in some cases the latter is alone injured.

The stomach is markedly affected if a large quantity of corrosive fluid has been swallowed and the stomach is empty. Vomiting is incessant,. and the vomit contains blood and is often foul-smelling. In two cases the smell was so offensive that I was asked to see the patients as examples of gastro-colic fistulæ. Thirst is marked, restlessness is extreme, and many patients succumb in the early stages to lung complications.

Perforation may take place. This is stated to occur most frequently after alkalis, an unusual form of corrosive poisoning in London. Of the 12 cases of perforation recorded in the footnote below, 11 occurred after hydrochloric acid, being nearly half the fatal cases.

Treatment.—After the appropriate antidote has been given, rectal feeding must be employed and no food given by the mouth. If there are ulcerated surfaces in the mouth and pharynx, these should be kept clean by mild antiseptic solutions.

After a few days, feeding should be cautiously begun. Small quantities of albumin water should be first tried, and, if this causes no pain or vomiting, Benger's or Allenburys' food may be given. If at the end of about a week it is found that the introduction of food causes pain and vomiting, operation should be performed without delay. In most cases jejunostomy will be necessary, but if the lesion proves to be confined to the pyloric portion of the stomach, gastrojejunostomy should be performed.

[1] Cases of caustic-swallowing admitted to London Hospital in the decennium 1899–1908—total, 189. Deaths within a few days, 35—of these 12 died of gastric perforation (11 HCl, 1 carbolic); and 8 cases required operations for mechanical disabilities within a few months, viz. 4 for pyloric stenosis, 3 for œsophageal stricture, and 1 for both. There is no doubt that 8 out of 154 greatly understates the frequency of late surgical complications.

In less severe cases it not infrequently happens that, after five or six weeks, signs of cardiac or pyloric obstruction develop. The appropriate operation should be done—in the former case gastrostomy, in the latter gastro-jejunostomy. It sometimes happens that hour-glass stomach develops. This should be treated on the usual lines (p. 324). Gastro-jejunostomy will suffice in most cases, as the pyloric pouch is small.

GASTRIC AND DUODENAL ULCERS

The stomach, and the duodenum as far as the entrance of the common bile-duct, are frequently the seat of ulcers, which are identical so far as their anatomical features are concerned, and probably caused in a similar manner; it is customary to classify them as acute and chronic.

GASTRIC ULCER

Etiology.—Gastric ulcer is an extremely common condition. Brinton's statement that a " peptic " ulcer, open or healed, was present in 5 per cent. of all autopsies has been confirmed by Welch and Greenhough and Joslin. It is more common in northern climates, and in England than in Europe.

Sex and age.—It was at one time customary to consider gastric ulcer essentially a disease of women. In the cases diagnosed *clinically* the proportion is about 75 females to 25 males. But since the development of the surgery of the stomach our ideas have undergone a change, for in many cases, diagnosed clinically as gastric ulcer, particularly in young women, no ulcer was found; for these Hale White suggests the name gastrostaxis; according to Sir Bertrand Dawson, some of them proved to be septic gastritis. If these cases are excluded, it is found that the frequency is only slightly greater in women than in men.

During the ten years 1899–1908, 343 patients with gastric ulcer in whom the diagnosis was confirmed by operation or post mortem were treated in the London Hospital; of these 199 were women and 144 men. Perforation had occurred in 136 of these cases, 92 of which were those of women. This about corresponds with the figures given by Brinton for perforated ulcers— twice as common in women as in men. Of the chronic ulcers operated upon for causes other than perforation, the numbers were almost equal: women 107, men 100. Of 28 patients with perforated ulcer personally operated upon up to December, 1911, 13 were men; but of the patients operated upon for chronic ulcer, 97 in number, in all of whom a definite ulcer was demonstrated, 60 were men. In addition, I have explored the stomach in 11 patients, all women with symptoms of gastric ulcer, and found no gastric lesion; such cases have by some been described as " medical ulcers."

It is safe to say that acute perforating ulcer is more usually met with in women, but that the chronic ulcer needing surgical treatment is more common in men.

Gastric ulcer is a disease of adult life; although isolated cases have been recorded in children and in old people, yet the majority occur between the ages of 20 and 45. Among the London Hospital cases of perforated gastric ulcer the youngest patient was 3 years, the oldest was 81 ; but the condition has been recorded in a centenarian, and in infants of 45 hours, 2 months, and 1 year respectively.

Mayo Robson states that in women 75 per cent. of the cases are found before the age of 20, whilst in men only 25 per cent. occur so early ; these figures agree with those at the London Hospital. Perforation occurs later in men than in women ; for example, in 92 consecutive cases of perforated gastric ulcer in women at the London Hospital, 55 occurred between the ages 15-20, whilst of 44 in men only 6 occurred during this period, 14 between 25 and 35, and 13 between 35 and 45. In women the greatest number of chronic cases are treated between the ages 25-35 (43 out of 107), in men between 35-45 (42 out of 100). It is evident, therefore, that chronic gastric ulcer is most often met with in adult life, in men later than in women.

Immediate etiology.—In discussing the causation of gastric ulcer, gastric erosions and acute and chronic ulcers must be considered together.

Certain observations, experimental and clinical, stand out prominently. It has been found possible to produce gastric ulcers experimentally by methods which will lead to ulceration in other parts of the body, as the result of injury to the mucous membrane, injury to nerves, embolism and thrombosis, and local infection ; but as a rule the ulcers so produced heal rapidly.

Bolton has shown that gastric ulcers are due to the action of the gastric juice upon devitalized gastric mucous membrane. By injecting into guinea-pigs gastrotoxic serum prepared by injecting the gastric cells of the guinea-pig into the rabbit, areas of necrosis and punched-out ulcers were produced. The formation of these could be prevented by neutralizing the gastric juice with 20 c.c. of a 1 per cent. solution of bicarbonate of soda. Hyperacidity of the gastric juice alone would not produce ulcers, but any excess of hydrochloric acid increased the lesion produced by the injection of gastrotoxic serum. The injection of hepatotoxin, enterotoxin, and hæmolysin also produced necrotic patches in the mucous membrane of the stomach indistinguishable from those produced by gastrotoxin.' A chronic ulcer could not be produced either by repeated injections of gastrotoxin, by increasing the percentage of hydrochloric acid, or by feeding on infected food ; but motor insufficiency of the stomach delayed healing for at least twice the normal time, and when the ulcer healed the mucous membrane was of a lower type than normal. Turck has been able to produce gastric and duodenal ulcers in dogs by feeding them for prolonged periods on food containing cultures of the colon bacillus. When the feeding was stopped the ulcers healed.

There are certain pathological and clinical data bearing on the subject.

C. H. Miller has stated that lymphoid follicles are grouped chiefly at the lesser curvature and in the pyloric region, and tend to disappear between the ages of 45–50; that as the result of infection they may become swollen and eroded, leading in many cases to hæmatemesis. In examining the non-ulcerated portions of the stomach in cases of gastric ulcer, he found a great increase in the amount of lymphoid tissue present, an enlargement of the individual follicles, and a thickening of the submucous layer. He believed that these changes might be a factor in the non-healing of an acute ulcer which was due to a follicular erosion.

Erosions and ulcers of the stomach and duodenum are found in many acute diseases—in erysipelas, septicæmia, local septic infections, genito-urinary affections, burns, etc. During the years 1907, 1908, and 1909, 26 acute ulcers were found in the stomach and 4 in the duodenum in autopsies performed at the London Hospital on patients dying from causes other than gastric.

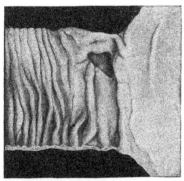

Fig. 372.—Acute duodenal ulcer found post mortem in a child of 3½ who died of gangrene of the leg following a crush.

In these 26 cases the cause of death was as follows: Suppurative appendicitis, 12; pylephlebitis, 2; gangrene of the foot, 2; chronic nephritis, 2; ulcerative endocarditis, 2; intestinal obstruction, 2; carcinoma of gall-bladder, 2; puerperal septicæmia, lobar pneumonia, and mitral stenosis, 1 each. (*See* Fig. 372.)

Hort considers that gastric and duodenal ulcers are the local expression of a general blood disease.

" Peptic " ulcers are only found in those parts of the intestinal canal in which the contents are acid. Bolton's experiments on the production of gastric ulcer showed that excess of hydrochloric acid delayed healing. In most cases of chronic gastric ulcer, as has been emphasized lately by Willcox, the total acidity is high; this is probably a factor in the initial development of the ulcer, but when the ulcer has become chronic this high acidity is not invariably found.

These considerations lead me to the belief that acute gastric ulcers are due to the autodigestion of areas of gastric mucous membrane, the resistance of which has been lowered as the result of toxic products acting directly on the gastric cells or giving rise to a swelling and erosion of lymphoid follicles. Chronic appendicitis is probably a frequent source of the septic infection. The lowered resistance of the gastric mucous membrane may possibly in some cases be produced by obstruction of small vessels either by emboli or by thrombosis.

The reason for the *chronicity* of ulcers is less clear, as is also the cause of their greater frequency in males. This latter may be related to the greater prevalence of disease of the appendix in the

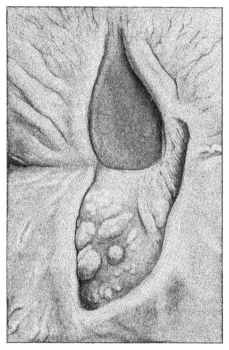

Fig. 373.—" Saddle-shaped " ulcer of lesser curvature, with pancreas exposed on the floor of its posterior portion.

(London Hospital Pathological Institute.)

male sex. Oral sepsis is present in most patients with chronic gastric ulcer; Mayo Robson believes that this is an important causal condition in a large number of cases. Few theories seem to fit in with the established fact that these ulcers heal after gastro-jejunostomy. The cause of non-healing may be continual irritation by abnormal gastric juice or by retention of food in the stomach owing to pyloric spasm.

Acute gastric ulcers are often multiple (according to Brinton, more than one ulcer is present in 21 per cent. of the cases), but chronic gastric and duodenal ulcers are usually single.

Site.—Ulcers of the stomach are usually situated on the lesser curvature towards the pylorus, and involve more often the posterior than the anterior wall. Those which are situated on the lesser curvature not infrequently involve both walls and constitute the so-called "saddle" ulcers (Fig. 373). The acute ulcers which perforate are most often situated on the anterior wall (Fig. 375).

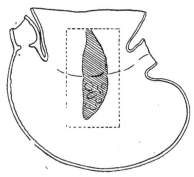

Fig. 374.—Diagram showing the situation of the ulcer in Fig. 373.

Morbid anatomy.— The acute ulcer sometimes called "round" is well defined and has a punched-out appearance. In shape it is conical, the deeper layers being affected to a less extent than the mucous membrane. The floor, usually formed of the muscular coat, is not covered with granulations, and post mortem no peritoneal affection is found. Microscopical examination reveals necrosis without any special infiltration with small lymphocyte - like cells or granulation tissue cells, and the mucous membrane is usually healthy right up to the margin of the ulcer.

In cases of acute ulcer leading to perforation, as seen at operation, the surrounding stomach wall may be œdematous, but this condition is absent post mortem, and is not marked if operation is performed within a short time after the perforation.

The edge of a chronic ulcer is often irregular, indurated and smooth, and the floor covered with scattered granulations. Satellite acute ulcers are sometimes present. The peritoneum covering it is thickened, and adhesions are often met with. When seen during life the peritoneum is rough and often red-speckled, and there is frequently a "sentinel" enlarged lymphatic gland between the layers of the neighbouring omentum. Adhesions to surrounding organs may take place, and in this way, with a continuance of the ulcerative process producing destruction of the stomach wall, the floor of the ulcer may be formed of pancreas or of liver. Blood-vessels may be laid bare, and the consequent weakening of their coats may lead to the formation of an aneurysm and to fatal hæmatemesis (Fig. 376).

Symptoms.—The most striking feature in connexion with the

symptoms of chronic gastric and chronic duodenal ulcers is their remission. In the former, severe attacks of pain and vomiting, lasting for a few days or weeks, intermit with periods of almost though rarely quite perfect digestive health; whilst in duodenal ulcer the patient may experience months of perfect health, before the onset of another attack.

Savariaud has stated that 20 per cent. of ulcers are latent; these are frequently on the lesser curvature. But this percentage is far too high; that gastric ulcers are common without the so-called classical symptoms is now well established, but few are really "latent." The classical symptoms are pain, vomiting, hæmatemesis. Pain is the most prominent feature, and is rarely absent. It is closely associated with the ingestion of food; it usually appears within an hour of a meal, there is always a definite latent period, and the pain persists until the stomach is emptied naturally or by vomiting. The pain is of a stabbing or burning character, situated in the epigastric region.

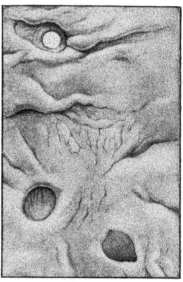

Fig. 375.—Multiple acute gastric ulcers, one of which has perforated. The stomach has been opened along its greater curvature. The ulcer which has perforated is on the anterior surface, and shows the typical characteristics of an acute ulcer.

(*London Hospital Pathological Institute.*)

On account of the frequent multiplicity of the lesions and complications, dogmatic statements are impossible regarding the relationship of the situation of the pain and tenderness, and the time at which it appears, to the situation of the ulcer. But it can be stated that in ulcers on the posterior surface and lesser curvature the pain is usually to the left of the middle line, and that the nearer the cardiac end of the stomach the lesion is situated the higher in the epigastric region is the site of the pain. This fact was first pointed out by Brinton, and stress has lately been laid on it by James Mackenzie. In pyloric ulcer the pain tends to appear later, and to be to the right of the middle line. In some cases of chronic ulcer situated on the lesser curve the pain appears late, and is definitely relieved by taking food.   The pain may be referred to the left dorsal region, and not infrequently, in an ulcer of the anterior surface, to the left shoulder.

The pain is often associated with tenderness, superficial and deep (*see* p. 303).   Superficial tenderness is uncommon, and is found in other gastric conditions ; it most often extends as a band around the body at the level of the 8th and 9th dorsal segments.   Deep tenderness in the epigastric region is usual, and is accompanied by rigidity of the rectus muscle ; in ulcers of the cardiac end it is most often met with over the upper part of the left rectus, in those of the pylorus over a similar part of the right rectus.

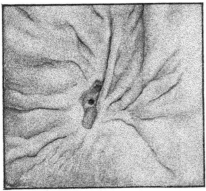

A patch of tenderness is sometimes present in the dorsal region to the left of the 9th and 10th dorsal spines.

In a large proportion of cases of chronic ulcer, free HCl and the total acidity of the gastric contents are increased slightly in amount, or only little altered from the normal ;

Fig. 376.—Portion of posterior wall of stomach, showing a chronic ulcer which had eroded the splenic artery.

(*London Hospital Museum.*)

but cases occur in which free HCl is diminished.

Vomiting is usual at some time during the course of the disease, and may be one of its most prominent features.   Its occurrence relieves the pain experienced from the ingestion of food.   The emesis may be self-induced, but this is more often the case when the ulcer is duodenal.   It must not, however, be forgotten that vomiting is infrequent in many cases of chronic ulcer.

Bleeding into the stomach takes place in the majority of cases of gastric ulcer.   Although it produces hæmatemesis in only about 50 per cent. of the cases, microscopical examination of the vomit or fæces will prove its existence.

Anæmia may be present in patients with acute and also with long-standing chronic ulcers.

Occasionally a definite **tumour** is felt, resembling that discovered in carcinoma of the stomach.   There is no *certain* means of differentiation, but examination of the stomach contents after a test meal may give valuable help (see p. 387).

Complications.—The following are the important complications: (1) Perforation, acute and chronic (p. 353); (2) hæmatemesis; (3) pyloric stenosis (see p. 327); (4) hour-glass stomach (see p. 321); (5) perigastritis (p. 358); (6) gastric fistula, internal and external (see p. 401); (7) carcinoma of stomach (see p. 378).

Diagnosis.—If a patient presents the symptoms of epigastric pain originating a short time after food, relieved by vomiting, and especially if he has hæmatemesis, he is suffering from a definite lesion of the mucous membrane of the stomach, in the form of either an erosion or an ulcer. It must, however, be remembered that, as shown by clinical observations and by the experiments of Bolton, lesions of the mucous membrane of the stomach occur in many diseases, and may present all the symptoms of ulcer. It should also be borne in mind that although the alimentary tract is divided for convenience of description into many parts, it is a whole, and that interference with the functions of any one section may cause trouble in the others.

When the symptoms occur in young women, considerable doubt should exist as to whether we are dealing with a case of true gastric ulcer. Young anæmic women often have pain after food, and vomit, with occasional hæmatemesis, yet their symptoms are certainly not in the majority of cases due to an ulcer, using the term in its usual significance.

There is a group in which hæmatemesis is a prominent symptom, called by Sir Bertrand Dawson " hæmorrhagic gastralgia," identical with that described by Hale White under the term " gastros taxis." These cases are not necessarily associated with anæmia, and although uncommon after 40, and most frequently met with in young women, may occur at any age and in the male sex. In some examined at operation and post mortem no ulcer has been found. But in many cases " erosions " have been present, seen during life, but escaping observation post mortem unless the stomach is examined with a lens. Hæmatemesis may be the first symptom (see p. 369).

Apart from these cases in which pain, vomiting, and hæmatemesis occur, there are others in which the symptoms are atypical, but which frequently prove to be due to chronic gastric ulcer. These diagnostic difficulties most often occur in women, but are not unknown in men. I have explored 11 such cases, in all of which symptoms had persisted for over three years. All had undergone systematic medical treatment. All were women; 4 had had hæmatemesis, all pain after food was relieved by vomiting. All were operated upon as cases of chronic gastric ulcer, although in 2 only did the operative findings come as a surprise. Their ages were 23, 24 (2), 25, 26, 34, 35, 37, 41, 47, 61, respectively. In none was a definite stomach lesion present, and in all the gall-bladder and appendix were healthy. No patient was the worse for exploration, and in the majority there was an improvement.

Even where the typical symptoms are present, particularly in women, the greatest care in examination must be taken. It must always be remembered that disease of the gall-bladder and of the colon or the appendix may cause "dyspepsia." The stomach symptoms associated with tabes, and with uræmia and diseases of the bladder and urethra, should be recognized, for gastro-jejunostomy has been performed on more than one patient suffering from these complaints. A careful study of the patient will ensure diagnosis of the last three groups, but no amount of careful study can at present prevent exploration in certain cases.

In the differential diagnosis there are six conditions requiring special study : (1) Gall-stones ; (2) gastric crises of tabes ; (3) duodenal ulcer ; (4) appendicitis ; (5) carcinoma ; (6) diseases of the colon.

Gall-stones.—It cannot be too often repeated that the "textbook symptoms" of cholelithiasis are late symptoms, and that a large number of patients with stones in the gall-bladder have no attacks of colic, but suffer from gastric symptoms, and are treated for "gastritis," "flatulent dyspepsia," or "gastric ulcer." It is no uncommon thing to find that a patient with gall-stones has been treated for acute gastritis or gastric ulcer, Kraus in 1884 described the early symptoms, and recently Moynihan and Mayo Robson have again laid stress upon them. These "inaugural symptoms" of gallstones are referred to the stomach ; the patient complains of pain or discomfort within an hour of taking food, relieved by belching or vomiting. There may be a feeling of chilliness after a meal, particularly in the evenings. In these cases there is not the same regularity in the occurrence of pain after meals as in gastric ulcer, and vomiting is more often associated with frequent retching, and does not so frequently relieve the pain. Careful investigation will usually enable a diagnosis to be made.

Tabes.—The gastric crises of tabes may cause difficulty in diagnosis, particularly when they occur early in the disease, before the appearance of pupil-changes or the loss of knee-jerks. In most cases, however, definite signs of tabes are present. The symptoms are usually attacks of epigastric pain, often with rigidity and hyperalgesia, accompanied by the vomiting of large quantities of fluid. It is a condition that should be considered in all anomalous stomach cases.

Appendicitis.—Cases have come under the care of most surgeons in which patients, after having been treated several years for "dyspepsia," develop an attack of acute appendicitis. In the early days of gastric surgery there is no doubt that cases of this nature were treated, without curative result, by gastro-jejunostomy. The symptoms may date from an acute attack of appendicitis, but as a rule no acute attack has been experienced, and there may have been no local symptoms pointing to appendicular disease. Until recently this condition has attracted little attention in this country, but papers on the subject have lately appeared from Moynihan, Paterson, and Soltau Fenwick; it was recognized some years ago by Ewald, and in America has been written about by Deaver, Ochsner, Murphy, and others. The symptoms may mimic either gastric or duodenal ulcer, but with care may in most cases be diagnosed from them. The chief complaint is of pain situated in the epigastrium, occurring in attacks, often due to exercise. Between the attacks there is often a continual gastric discomfort. The pain may come on shortly after food, or be delayed, and, as pointed out by Paterson, often radiates to the right iliac fossa. Vomiting is rarely present, but nausea is frequent.

During an attack, slight rigidity and deep tenderness may be present in the right iliac fossa, and the temperature is a little raised. Between the attacks, tenderness may be absent. Hæmatemesis may occur.

The symptoms have been attributed by W. J. Mayo and by Moynihan to pyloric spasm, by Soltau Fenwick and Paterson to hypersecretion of gastric juice. I believe the former to be the explanation in most cases of this nature. In a large number of the cases of "appendix dyspepsia" that have come under my care, free HCl has been absent and the total acidity low. It must be remembered, however, that disease of the appendix may give rise to "erosions" of the mucous membrane of the stomach, which may go on to chronic ulceration.

Careful attention to the history, confinement to bed, and examination during the attack should in most cases enable the surgeon to make the diagnosis.

Carcinoma.—The differential diagnosis between carcinoma and non-malignant gastric ulcer is discussed elsewhere (p. 386). It must first be remembered that in not a few cases carcinoma is directly implanted on chronic ulcer, and that in these cases there may be no symptoms or signs that the ulcer has become malignant; the usual history of chronic ulcer, extending over years, is obtained, with remissions of almost complete health, and the diagnosis of malignancy is only made at operation. The history of primary carcinoma is usually insidious, and includes the onset of gastric symptoms at middle age, a distaste for food, a gnawing pain, often not definitely relieved when the stomach is empty, and a steady downward progress. Vomiting is not so constant as in ulcer, and may be of the " coffee-grounds " type. The onset of symptoms of pyloric stenosis without previous history of gastric trouble usually means carcinoma.

Prognosis.—All modern observers are agreed that a chronic gastric ulcer carries with it a grave prognosis. It is well known that relapse after medical treatment and apparent cure is common.

The following figures illustrate the mortality and the chances of relapse under medical treatment. Taking hospital cases first, Mansell-Moullin has published the following figures: During the years 1897 to August, 1902, 500 patients whose cases were *diagnosed* as gastric ulcer were admitted into the London Hospital, of whom 402 were women, 98 men. Of these 18 per cent. died, 10 per cent. from peritonitis, 2 per cent. from hæmatemesis. These figures do not include death from remote complications such as pyloric stenosis, hour-glass stomach, perigastric adhesions, etc., but comprise many cases, particularly in women, of the so-called " medical " gastric ulcer.

The figures given by Habershon express more nearly the prognosis. Of 60 cases of chronic gastric ulcer in preoperative days 24 died, 11 of perforation, 7 of hæmorrhage, and 6 of exhaustion.

With regard to the liability to relapse in those cases treated medically, in Mansell-Moullin's statistics 42 per cent. had suffered before and been relieved by treatment. Greenhough and Joslin published the following results of medical treatment: Of 187 cases the initial mortality was 8 per cent. ; after five years, 115 patients could be traced, and of these 57 had had recurrence and 15 had died of gastric diseases. Paterson and Rhodes investigated the after-history of 147 patients who had been in the London Temperance Hospital under the care of Soltau Fenwick and Parkinson ; of these 72 could be traced, and 46 of them were not cured.

The results of the surgical treatment of chronic gastric ulcer and its complications are now becoming well known, and the operative mortality is falling. The following figures are instructive: Moynihan operated upon 334 cases with 21 deaths—6 per cent. ; Mayo Robson (excluding perforation) operated upon 400 cases with 12 deaths—3 per cent. ; and Mayo, 307, with a death-rate of 6·2 per cent.

We may conclude that the immediate mortality of the surgical treatment of chronic gastric ulcer, including perforation, is less than the immediate mortality of medical treatment; excluding perforation it is much less.

The final results are infinitely better. Large numbers of patients have now been traced after operation up to 17–18 years. Mayo Robson, Moynihan and Paterson (collected cases), Mayo, Rutherford Morrison, Busch, and others have published series of cases of definite chronic ulcers demonstrated at operation in which the patient was well when seen more than two years after the operation. Of these 80–90 per cent. were cured, another 5–10 per cent. were relieved, and the failures were less than 10 per cent.

Treatment.—The treatment of gastric ulcer is at first medical. Surgical treatment must not be considered, except in the case of perforation or certain cases of hæmatemesis, until all carious teeth have been attended to and the patient has been kept at rest in bed and subjected to medical treatment. If this fails to relieve, or relapse occurs, surgical treatment should be adopted as offering the patient almost certain relief with the prospect of cure in over 80 per cent. of cases at a very slight risk.

There is still some difference of opinion with regard to the actual surgical treatment of gastric ulcer. Two operations are performed —the direct, excision ; the indirect, gastro-jejunostomy—by which the condition of the stomach is influenced so as to allow the ulcer to heal.

Most surgeons are agreed that gastro-jejunostomy is the operation of choice in cases in which the ulcer is in the pyloric region of the stomach, but opinions are divided as to the treatment of ulcers situated on the lesser curvature, away from the pylorus. Moynihan and Mayo consider that ulcers in this situation should be treated directly by excision, as in their experience the results of treatment by gastro-enterostomy in such cases are not so good as in ulcers elsewhere. Rodman, however, on the grounds that carcinoma starts from chronic ulcer, and that hæmorrhage and perforation have followed gastro-jejunostomy successfully performed, advocates, even in pyloric ulcers, excision of the pylorus and lesser curvature with posterior gastro-jejunostomy, practically a partial gastrectomy. But it has to be proved that carcinoma develops in the scar of a healed ulcer, although Moynihan's cases are suggestive (*see* p. 352). Even after resection of the ulcer, relapse has occurred ; Mansell-Moullin, Robson, Sinclair White, Terrier, Deaver, and others have recorded such cases. Ulcers are also frequently multiple.

That an ulcer, although causing no obstruction, heals after gastro-jejunostomy is now established. I recorded a case in which the patient died of a cause other than gastric, twenty-eight months after I had performed gastro-jejunostomy for a large saddle-shaped ulcer on the lesser curvature, adherent to the pancreas. It had quite healed, and the scar was hardly visible. Sir Frederic Eve has recorded a case in which the ulcer was healed five weeks later. Similar cases have been described by others.

With regard to the after-effects, it has been urged that excision should be performed because perforation and hæmorrhage may occur before the ulcer is healed, or carcinoma may develop later. Isolated cases of perforation following gastro-jejunostomy for gastric ulcer have been published. More cases of hæmatemesis have been recorded, and fatal cases have been reported by Robson, Kocher, Mayo, etc., at periods when the patient was apparently well. In one patient who was under my care, one month after gastro-jejunostomy a sudden and fatal hæmorrhage occurred from an artery in the floor of a large ulcer adherent to the pancreas and spreading to the lesser curvature and anterior surface. It had originally been saddle-shaped, but its anterior part had healed after operation. As to *malignant disease*, cases have been recorded by Robson, Moynihan, Czerny, Deaver, and others in which a malignant tumour developed as long as three years and a half after gastro-jejunostomy had been performed. In two of my own cases—one of adherent ulcer on the lesser curvature, and the other of pyloric ulcer—malignant disease declared itself within twelve months. The first could not have been excised, the second could. Both these cases were instances of errors in diagnosis; the difficulties in distinguishing between the two conditions are notorious, and it is likely that in some of the recorded cases similar mistakes occurred. Perforation and hæmorrhage can be avoided by infolding the ulcer where possible, but the onset of malignant disease cannot be prevented. Against this are the records of many cases in which tumours thought to be malignant and irremovable at operation disappeared after gastro-jejunostomy. In one case under my care no tumour could be felt fourteen days later.

At the present time it may be said that **gastro-jejunostomy** is the operation of choice for chronic gastric ulcer, but it should be combined with infolding where possible, and, if there is any doubt as to malignancy, with excision of the ulcer or partial gastrectomy. The abdomen should be opened by an incision over the right rectus muscle dividing its anterior sheath. The muscle should then be pulled outwards and its posterior sheath and the peritoneum divided. After protecting the edges of the wound with gauze, the whole stomach and duodenum should be carefully examined in order to avoid such a catastrophe as performing gastro-jejunostomy to the pyloric pouch of an hour-glass stomach, an operation that has been invariably fatal. If no lesion is found on careful examination of both surfaces of the stomach, the posterior being inspected through an opening made in the transverse meso-colon, the cause of the trouble should be sought elsewhere—in the gall-bladder or appendix. Even when a lesion is found in the stomach these organs should always, if the patient's condition will permit, be examined, and any disease should be dealt with. The stomach should not be opened; if the lesion cannot be discovered by external examination it is not a chronic ulcer, and is unsuitable for surgical treatment. It cannot be too often insisted upon that gastro-jejunostomy must *never* be performed unless a definite lesion is present in the stomach; it must never be done for symptoms. A chronic ulcer will show definite signs of its presence on inspection or palpation. On inspection a rough, red-stippled area is usually seen, often somewhat puckered. If the ulcer be on the lesser curvature, an enlarged lymphatic gland is frequently present. In the diagnosis from carcinoma due weight must be placed on the history and on the chemical examination of the stomach contents. If the ulcer be malignant, induration is more marked, the peritoneum is often thickened and does not show the same rough red appearance, the lymphatic glands are enlarged and hard, and thickened lymphatics are frequently seen running from the growth to the glands.

The preferable operation is posterior gastro-jejunostomy (*see* p. 406), the opening in the stomach being vertical. When possible the ulcer should be excised or infolded in addition. If gastric adhesions render the posterior operation impossible, the anterior no-loop gastro-enterostomy should be done (*see* p. 408).

If there is any suspicion that the ulcer is malignant, a portion of its edge or an enlarged gland should be removed for rapid microscopical examination ; a gastro-jejunostomy suitable for use after partial gastrectomy should be performed, and the latter operation completed on receiving the pathologist's report.

After-treatment.—As soon as the patient has recovered from the anæsthetic he should be propped up in bed and remain in a sitting position. When any anæsthetic vomiting has ceased, feeding may be commenced. I am in the habit of ordering Benger's or Allenburys' food in preference to milk, but any form of bland diet may be given. Food should be increased cautiously ; many patients develop a ravenous appetite, but they should be cautioned against over-eating. It is wise to put the patient on alkalis ; a powder composed of equal parts of bismuth oxycarbonate, heavy magnesium carbonate, and sodium bicarbonate, in doses of ℥i three times a day, is useful.

It must be remembered that prolonged supervision is necessary after operation, which, though the most important, is only the first step in the treatment.

PERFORATION OF GASTRIC ULCER

Among the complications of gastric ulcer, perforation is the most serious, fully 95 per cent. of the cases thus complicated terminating fatally unless treated by operation. Various figures have been given stating the percentage of cases in which perforation occurs, but all such figures, based as they are upon a diagnosis of gastric ulcer made from symptoms, are useless.

The ulcer which perforates may be an acute one of a few hours' or days' duration, or a chronic one which has been in existence for many years. In many cases gastric symptoms suggestive of ulceration have been present for a considerable time. Thus, of 28 cases which have been under my care. in 16 symptoms had been present over two years, in 2 ten years, and in 1 thirteen years. In 1 case only were the symptoms of less than two months' duration (a week).

Perforation of a gastric ulcer occurs most often in young women; thus, of 132 cases treated at the London Hospital in ten years (1899-1908), 92 were women, of whom 55 were between the ages of 15 and 25. The age-incidence in men is higher; in the 40 males, only 6 occurred in this decennium, 14 between 25 and 35, 13 between 35 and 45. No satisfactory explanation can be given of this difference, for of the 107 cases of chronic gastric ulcer in women treated surgically during the same time only 12 occurred in this decennium, 43 between 25 and 35, and 27 between 35 and 45, corresponding well to the ages at which chronic ulcers are met with in men, viz. among 100, 24 between 25 and 35, 42 between 35 and 45.

Ulcers which perforate are usually situated on the anterior wall of the stomach, nearer the lesser than the greater curvature, and the pylorus than the cardia; no facts have been adduced to explain why ulcers in this situation are more common in young women. Among the 28 cases operated upon by myself the perforation was on the anterior wall in 25, but in several the ulcer was on the lesser curvature and saddle-shaped. Perforations may be multiple; Deaver and Ashurst state that in about 20 per cent. of cases two or more perforations have been found; but among my own cases there was 1 only in which two ulcers had perforated.

The immediate cause of the perforation is the separation of a slough or spread of the ulceration, but it may occur from over-distension of the stomach, or as the result of a sudden strain. As pointed out by Brinton, it is "often directly traceable to mechanical violence, such as coughing, sneezing, convulsion or constriction of the belly." Alexander Miles found that of 30 cases of perforated gastric ulcer treated by him, in 15 the perforation occurred while the patient was at rest; only 6 were engaged in such a way as to involve muscular strain.

The perforation may be acute, subacute, or chronic (the first is the more common; among my cases 2 were chronic and 3 subacute); it is usually rounded; it varies in size, but as a rule is not larger in diameter than a small pea.

The perforation is *acute* when the giving way of the ulcer allows the contents of the stomach to obtain access to the general peritoneal cavity. In a *subacute* perforation the stomach is empty, or extravasation is limited by adhesions to the abdominal wall, the under surface of the liver, or the omentum. In this type of case recovery without operation may take place if the patient be kept at rest and starved. A *chronic* perforation most often occurs when the ulcer is on the posterior wall. There may be no sudden onset of additional symptoms, and the diagnosis may be impossible until a subphrenic or a perigastric abscess forms.

Symptoms.—It has been stated that perforation may be the first sign of the presence of a gastric ulcer. In my experience this is unusual; in all the cases under my care symptoms had been present, in most for a considerable time, in one for a week only; in a few the symptoms have increased in severity for a short time preceding perforation. This is also the experience of Moynihan, who states: " The perforation of an ulcer of the stomach is a catastrophe which, in my experience, never comes unannounced."

The patient is suddenly seized with agonizing pain in the epigastric region; in some cases the pain shoots to the left shoulder. If seen shortly after perforation, shock is, as a rule, absent, and the pulse-rate is not increased; this should be borne in mind. Board-like rigidity and deep tenderness appear early, both signs being first present and most marked in the epigastric region. In a few cases this early rigidity may be absent, but tenderness is always present. Gradually the pulse-rate rises, collapse sets in, and the abdomen becomes distended, indicating that the most favourable time for operation has passed. The initial severe pain passes off usually in less than an hour.

Vomiting occurs shortly after the onset of the pain in about half the cases, but is usually not repeated, and is not frequent until peritonitis has developed. In many cases the temperature is subnormal directly after the perforation. Liver-dullness may be absent if much gas has escaped into the peritoneal cavity, but it is not a sign on which reliance can be placed. General subcutaneous emphysema has been noticed as a rare complication.

Cases have been recorded in which death occurred from the severe pain or shock of perforation. In a case which recently came under my notice, death took place two hours after perforation of an acute ulcer, in a girl of 19.

In subacute perforation there are often for several days premonitory symptoms of stabbing pain, or a feeling of aching or stiffness, but at the time of perforation the symptoms are less acute. Unless operated on, the condition usually leads to the formation of a perigastric abscess (see p. 373).

Diagnosis.—No difficulty arises in the majority of cases. The sudden onset of acute abdominal pain in a young woman who has had gastric symptoms previously should lead to the correct diagnosis. In men it is often difficult to decide before operation whether the ulcer is gastric or duodenal, but this is a matter of no importance. But cases occur in which no previous history of gastric trouble can be obtained. In many catastrophes in the upper abdomen no definite diagnosis can be made, but these are cases in which the correct treatment is operative—e.g. perforation of the gall-bladder, or acute pancreatitis.

Acute appendicitis may be simulated by a subacute perforation of the stomach, but with much less frequency than by perforation of duodenal ulcers.

Ruptured tubal pregnancy should also give rise to no difficulty in diagnosis if attention be paid to the history, the onset of the symptoms, and the appearance of the patient.

In acute intestinal obstruction there is the same sudden onset of agonizing pain, but vomiting is a constant feature and the localization of the pain is different.

Acute dilatation of the stomach and gastric volvulus should not be confused with perforation of the viscus.

Rare conditions that have misled are mesenteric thrombosis, ptomaine poisoning, abdominal crises in diabetes (Downes and O'Brien), gastric crises of tabes, and hæmorrhage into the ovary at about the time of menstruation (Waring).

Cases have occurred in which there has been a sudden onset of severe abdominal pain accompanied by rigidity in patients the subjects of gastric ulcer, in whom at operation no perforation was discovered, and other cases in which no cause was found for the symptoms. The phenomenon was called " pseudo-perforation " by Manges, who recorded a case of this nature.

Very rarely, as in the case recorded by Moore, another lesion is present; in this case perforated gastric ulcer was complicated by acute appendicitis.

Prognosis.—Death is inevitable in over 95 per cent. of the cases not treated by operation. The prognosis depends upon the time after perforation at which operation can be performed; if the patient is seen within the first twenty-four hours the death-rate should be not more than 10 per cent.

Sinclair Kirk has recorded 11 cases in which he operated, with recovery in all. In 8 cases the operation was done within 5 hours of perforation, in 1 at 7, in 1 at 10, and in 1 at 20 hours.

The death-rate at the present time in large numbers of cases is about 50 per cent. Thus, Gross and Gross collected the reports of 369 operations with a death-rate of nearly 51 per cent. The death-rate at St. Thomas's Hospital (Sargent) for the fifteen years up to 1904 was 55 per cent., at St. Bartholomew's between 1897 and 1905, 49 per cent. (69 cases). During the years 1899-1908 there were 132 cases of perforated gastric ulcers operated upon at the London Hospital, with a death-rate of 67 per cent.; but of this number less than 5 were within 12 hours of perforation.

During the last nine years I have operated upon 28 cases, with 16 recoveries; of these 10 were seen within 24 hours of perforation—at 4 (2 cases), 6, 9, 10, 11, 12 (2 cases), 18, 22 hours—and recovery took place in all; the remainder were over this period—from 26 hours to 3 weeks.

Treatment.—Abdominal section should be performed at once; no time should be wasted in waiting for " shock " to pass off, for this will be best relieved by immediate operation. It must be remembered that if the case is seen early there may be no shock.

The abdomen should be opened in the middle line. In many cases, as soon as the peritoneum is reached it is seen to be blown out in a bladder-like way by the air contained in the peritoneal cavity. The stomach should be quickly found. As a rule the perforation is easily discovered, as it is usually on the anterior wall. Unless the case be very recent, it will generally be surrounded by yellow lymph. If the ulcer is not seen on the anterior surface or in the duodenum, a wide opening should be made in the gastro-colic omentum and the posterior surface examined. If no ulcer is present, the gall-bladder and pancreas must be examined, and then the appendix and pelvic organs. The perforation should be infolded, chromic gut being used, and the area buried by a continuous stitch of silk. It is sometimes impossible to close the perforation in this way on account of the friability of the tissues immediately around the ulcer or the amount of induration present; in these cases the ulcer should be rapidly excised, or, if the condition of the patient will not permit, a piece of omentum may be brought up and stitched over the ulcer, or, if this is impossible, the perforation should be covered by iodoform gauze packing.

As perforation of two ulcers has occurred simultaneously in many recorded cases, search should always be made for other lesions.

Gastro-jejunostomy should be performed at the same time in all cases in which closure of the perforation produces pyloric contraction or any deformity of the stomach likely to interfere with its action, when more than one ulcer is present, or when the ulcer that has perforated is a chronic one. It is unnecessary in perforation of an acute ulcer on the anterior wall. The performance of this operation at the time of closure of the perforation will lead to a more rapid convalescence and the prevention of after-trouble.

Various opinions have been held with regard to the need for this step. W. J. Mayo found that only one out of 18 patients needed gastro-jejunostomy later, and Hale White states: "Judging from the results at Guy's Hospital, it appears that patients who survive an operation for perforated gastric ulcer do so well that gastro-enterostomy is unnecessary." But this has not been the experience of most observers. Paterson found 23 per cent. of patients relapse within a year of operation. Of the 16 patients upon whom I operated and who recovered, I performed gastro-jejunostomy at the time in 6, and excised the ulcer in 1; gastro-jejunostomy was necessary at a later date in 4.

After the perforation has been closed and gastro-jejunostomy performed, if this has been considered necessary, all extravasation should be gently wiped away and the abdomen closed without drainage, unless the extravasation has been considerable, when a tube, brought out on the loin, should be placed in the right or left kidney pouch according to whether the extravasation has been from an ulcer at the pyloric or the cardiac end. If the peritoneal soiling has been general, it will be well to drain suprapubically also.

After-treatment.—After operation the patient should be nursed in the propped-up position and, as soon as postanæsthetic vomiting has passed off, should be given small quantities of water. It is unnecessary to institute rectal feeding, for within thirty-six hours of operation the patient should be taking Benger's food, or albumin-water and glucose.

Careful attention must be paid to the mouth, to avoid parotitis.

As soon as discharge ceases the tube should be removed.

If general peritonitis is present, nothing should be given by the mouth until vomiting has ceased and the condition of the patient shows that feeding is safe. Continuous saline infusion is given per rectum. After from twenty-four to thirty-six hours, if the condition of the patient is satisfactory, water may be given by the mouth, and a start made on albumin-water and glucose, Benger's food, or milk and water, but if this causes increase in pulse-rate or vomiting it should not be persisted in. On no account should aperients be given, and the resumption of food should be gradual.

A continuing temperature with gradual loss of flesh should raise suspicion that a subphrenic abscess is present ; this should be sought (*see* p. 374), and treated in the usual way.

After the patient is free from danger, all carious teeth should be removed and alkalis given.

Ultimate prognosis.—If the ulcer which perforated is acute, situated on the anterior surface of the stomach and capable of being infolded, no further symptoms will develop in most cases. If, on the other hand, the ulcer is a chronic one, the infolding may be difficult and part of the ulcer may escape ; for example, if a saddle-shaped ulcer on the lesser curvature perforates on its anterior wall, this part may be infolded and healed, but the remainder of the ulcer is unaffected, and, unless excision or a simultaneous gastro-jejunostomy be done, symptoms will recur.

PERIGASTRITIS—GASTRIC ADHESIONS

Adhesions connecting the stomach to the abdominal wall or to other viscera are commonly due to gastric or duodenal ulcers, but may be due to diseases of other abdominal viscera, most commonly the gall-bladder.

Through the attachment of the great omentum to the stomach, this organ may be interfered with in disease of any part of the abdomen. In one patient upon whom I operated, gastric symptoms, which at one time had been thought to be due to gastric ulcer, were found to be caused by adhesions of the great omentum to the uterus at the site of removal of the left Fallopian tube.

Adhesions resulting from gastric or duodenal ulcers are most common to the pancreas and to the liver ; in 123 cases recorded by Fenwick they bound the stomach to the pancreas in 49, to the liver in 33, to the colon in 7, and to the liver and colon together in 4.

In the majority of cases, adhesions, whether due to extrinsic or intrinsic causes, give rise to no symptoms whatever. In the pyloric region, as the result of constriction or fixation of the pylorus at a higher level than normal, dilatation may result (*see* p. 327). Adhesion of the stomach to the anterior abdominal wall or constriction by adhesion may lead to hour-glass stomach. In such cases as these definite symptoms of stenosis will be present.

It is in the cases in which pain is the prominent feature that difficulties are most likely to occur. Pain arises most often when the adhesions are to the most movable portion of the stomach, the greater curvature. Hale White, speaking of this subject, says: "I am not sure, but I think they most often give rise to symptoms when they connect the stomach with the bowel."

The pain is often worse after food, but it may be absent for days and weeks, and in some cases bears no relation to meals. It is often worse on exertion, and the patient may complain that the pain is increased if she reaches above the head or stands quite erect. The long-continued pain may set up neurasthenic symptoms.

There may be distinct deep tenderness with muscular rigidity over the area occupied by the adhesions.

Diagnosis.—This must rest on the history of previous abdominal trouble such as might cause a local peritonitis.

Treatment.—If the adhesions have caused hour-glass stomach or gastric dilatation, the appropriate treatment for these conditions must be carried out. When pain is the chief complaint and is of sufficient severity to interfere with the patient's work, operation should be undertaken for the purpose of separating the adhesions, care being exercised to avoid overlooking any perforation of stomach which may have been closed by them. The adhesions should be cleanly divided, and both ends ligatured. If a large raw surface is left, the edge of the omentum may be used to cover it.

Attempts at preventing the re-formation of adhesions by covering the raw surface with Cargile membrane or by leaving saline solution in the abdominal cavity have not been very successful.

Symptoms may persist after the division of adhesions, particularly in women in whom neurasthenia has supervened.

DUODENAL ULCER

Ulcers resembling those occurring in the stomach, and probably caused in a similar way (*see* p. 340), are frequently found in the duodenum. They may be divided into the acute and the chronic.

Etiology.—As in the stomach, the *acute* ulcers may be found complicating many diseases, especially those in which sepsis is present. There is a close association between chronic appendicitis and duodenal ulcer; it is probable that the appendix is the source of the infection in many cases.

Burns.—Ulcers occurring in the duodenum complicating severe burns were described by Curling in 1842 (Fig. 377); and it is said they may also be present in the stomach, and in the intestine lower down. Usually single, they are met with most often in the first portion and begin as hæmorrhagic erosions. They are said to occur, as a rule, from seven to fourteen days after the burn, but they may be discovered earlier—in one case (Parfick) they were s e e n within eighteen. hours. T h e s e ulcers often lead to a fatal issue within a few days from hæmorrhage or perforation. They were more frequently met with by older writers. Thus, Fenwick, from the statistics of Holmes, Erichsen, Perry and Shaw, found this complication in 6·2 per cent. of all fatal cases of burns. These ulcers are now not often found after burns, and some authors deny that the two c o n d i t i o n s are associated. V a r i o u s explanations have been given of the development of these acute ulcers, but they are probably of toxæmic origin, and can thus be brought into line with other acute peptic ulcers (p. 342).

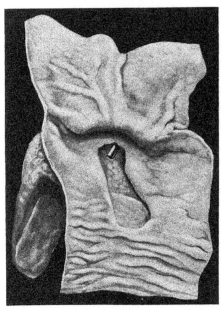

Fig. 377.—Duodenal ulcer following burns, from a girl 7 years of age, in whom death took place eight days later from hæmorrhage from the p a n c r e a t i c o - duodenal artery. (*Curling's case.*)

(*Royal College of Surgeons Museum.*)

Age.—Duodenal ulcers may be met with at any age. Cases have been recorded of the perforation of a duodenal ulcer in an infant of 21 hours, and of death from hæmorrhage from a duodenal ulcer in an infant 2 days old.

Among 273 cases collected by Collin, 16 were under a year. In these the ulcers were acute, usually complicating some septic disease and found post mortem.

Duodenal ulcer as seen clinically, the *chronic* ulcer, is a disease of adult life, the patient most often coming under surgical observation between the ages of 30 and 50. In many, however, symptoms were noticed much earlier in life; for instance, in one patient of 53 upon whom I operated, symptoms had been present for thirty-five years, and in another of 68 for forty-eight.

Sex.—All are agreed that men are more often affected than women.

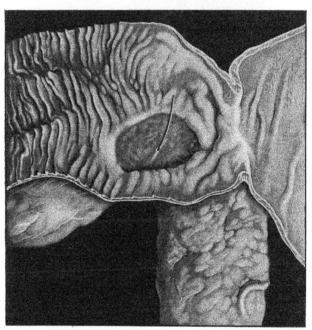

Fig. 378.—Chronic ulcer, situated on the posterior wall of the first part of the duodenum, which had eroded the pancreatico-duodenal artery. A bristle is in the artery; the body of the pancreas has been displaced downwards.

Of Mayo Robson's cases 86 per cent. were males, of the Mayos' 73 per cent., and of Moynihan's 73·6 per cent. Among my own cases operated up to December, 1911, 70 in number, 10 were in women. This may be connected with the greater frequency of diseases of the appendix in men. Mayo has observed that the first portion of the duodenum in men is nearly always ascending, and suggests that the alkaline reaction of the bile and pancreatic juice more readily neutralizes the acid chyme in the upper duodenum in women than in men.

Situation.—Ulcers occur most often in the supra-ampullary portion of the duodenum, over 95 per cent. being found within an inch of the pylorus. The ulcer is usually solitary, and situated on the upper and anterior wall ; next in order of frequency, on the posterior wall.   An ulcer in this latter situation is particularly liable to be associated with hæmorrhage, which may prove rapidly fatal from erosion of the pancreatico-duodenal artery

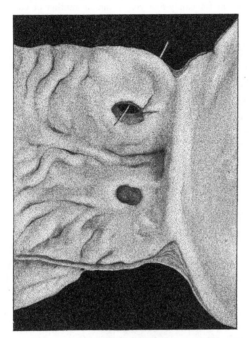

Fig. 379.—Chronic ulcer on the posterior wall, with acute perforated ulcer on the anterior surface.   Duodenum opened from below.

(London Hospital Pathological Institute.)

(Fig. 378).   Occasionally two ulcers are present on opposite sides of the intestine—contact ulcers (*see* Fig. 379).

The **morbid anatomy** of duodenal ulcer resembles that of gastric ulcer, with which it may coexist.

Symptoms.—A chronic duodenal ulcer may be latent until perforation occurs.   In the majority of patients, however, it gives rise to a definite train of symptoms.   In a few cases it cannot be distinguished from a gastric ulcer, and in still fewer the diagnosis of peptic ulcer is not made at all.

Thus we may conveniently make four groups :—
1. Those with typical symptoms.
2. Those with symptoms indistinguishable from gastric ulcer.
3. Those in which diagnosis is impossible.
4. Those presenting no symptoms till perforation.

The onset of the disease is usually insidious ; at first there is only a sense of uneasiness, or a feeling of distension. Pain is rarely absent, and is the most important symptom ; it appears about two hours after food, and lasts until the next meal, by which it is relieved—hence the name " hunger-pain," applied to it by Moynihan. A characteristic feature of the pain is that in many cases it wakens the patient about 1 or 2 a.m. It is epigastric and may pass round to the right side, is often relieved by pressure, and may be accompanied by eructation of gas or regurgitation of a little bitter fluid, followed by relief. Occasionally it is spasmodic, doubling the patient up and resembling biliary colic. It is sometimes noted that the period of relief from the pain is greater after the ingestion of solid than of liquid food. The appetite often remains good ; indeed, it may be better during the attack than at other times.

An important feature is the complete remission of symptoms, an attack lasting a few weeks being followed by a period of perfect health which may last for months. An attack is particularly prone to come on in the winter, and may result from cold, worry, or overwork.

Spontaneous vomiting is very unusual unless stenosis occurs ; but self-induced vomiting, rare in gastric ulcer, is noted in many cases of duodenal ulcer.

During the attack, rigidity of the upper segment of the right rectus muscle and deep tenderness may be present, but in many cases abdominal examination is negative.

Symptoms such as those described above are present in most cases in which an ulcer is situated in the first part of the duodenum.

It must be remembered, however, that the presence of post-prandial or nocturnal pain, relieved by a warm drink or by bicarbonate of soda, does not justify a certain diagnosis of duodenal ulcer ; occasionally, when the ulcer is situated on the lesser curvature of the stomach, pain is similarly relieved, but the symptoms are never perfectly typical. It is in this type of case that a duodenal ulcer may be diagnosed and a gastric one found ; the converse rarely or never. Disease of the gall-bladder or appendix may cause hunger-pain. It may, however, be laid down that recurrent attacks of hunger-pain are always due to a definite organic lesion, one that can be dealt with surgically.

Occasionally the ulcer is situated in the second part of the duodenum. In these cases the symptoms are often atypical, and jaundice may occur. I have recorded cases of this nature in which it was impossible to make a certain diagnosis between duodenal ulcer and gall-stones.

Complications.—Stenosis of the pylorus may result after many years; this sequel brought the patients under my care in 18 out of 70 cases of chronic ulcer.

Hæmorrhage.—It is impossible to estimate the frequency with which bleeding occurs. The blood may be vomited, but generally only appears in the fæces. Slight hæmorrhage, such as may be discovered by tests for " occult blood," is probable in most cases. Craven Moore found it in all the cases under his care. Severe hæmorrhage is a late and serious complication. The bleeding may come on without warning and cause sudden fainting, followed by the passage of a tarry motion, with or without the vomiting of blood. In other cases it may occur insidiously without the knowledge of the patient. The bleeding may be fatal, the source of the blood being the gastro-duodenal, superior pancreatico-duodenal, right gastro-epiploic, or pyloric arteries. In a few cases death has been sudden.

Jaundice may develop as the result of the cicatrization of ulcers of the second part, or of the spread of inflammation into the common bile-duct, but is a rare complication.

Pancreatitis may be present, due to a spread of the associated duodenal inflammation. In a large number of cases of chronic duodenal ulcer the Cammidge reaction may be obtained.

Diagnosis.—In about 85 per cent. of the cases the typical character of the recurring attacks of hunger-pain will render the diagnosis almost certain. Difficulty arises in those which do not conform to this type. It must not be considered that hunger-pain, or pain two or three hours after food relieved by taking food, is found only in association with duodenal ulcer, for it occasionally occurs also in cases of gastric ulcer. In cholelithiasis, attacks of pain two or three hours after food may cause duodenal ulcer to be thought of, but in these cases the pain is not relieved by a warm drink or soda bicarbonate, as in duodenal ulcer; moreover, in cholelithiasis retching and vomiting are common, whilst they are usually absent in duodenal ulcer.

In doubtful cases the fæces may be tested for traces of blood—" occult " hæmorrhage.

The examination of the gastric contents after a test meal is of great service in enabling a diagnosis to be made. Chronic duodenal ulcer uncomplicated by secondary gastric dilatation is associated with an excess of free HCl and the total acidity is high. In cholelithiasis this is unusual; in long-standing cases free HCl is usually absent and the total acidity is low.

Prognosis.—Chronic ulcer of the duodenum is a grave disease. Its mortality after non-operative treatment has not been worked out as in the case of gastric ulcer, for until recently it was only recognized when giving rise to late symptoms—hæmorrhage, perforation, or stenosis. It is, therefore, quite impossible to estimate its mortality accurately, but if hæmorrhage or perforation has occurred the death-rate is high.

On the other hand, operative treatment not only offers relief, but enables the ulcer to heal.

The results of operation are extremely good. Moynihan, between 1900 and 1909, operated upon 228 patients, with a death-rate of less than 2 per cent., and no death among the last 116 cases : 163 were traced, and of these 144 were cured (79 per cent.), 18 improved, and only 1 " no better." Similarly, good results have been recorded by all who have worked at the subject. In 70 patients with chronic ulcer upon whom I had operated up to December, 1911, there was 1 death—from " aspiration" broncho-pneumonia. All are improved, and all but one of those operated on over two years ago are quite well.

Treatment.—At the first attack the patient should have a thorough trial of medical treatment with rest in bed. It is impossible to estimate the prospect of success by this treatment, but it has failed to cure in many cases. Ambulatory treatment is certainly a failure ; I have recently operated upon 2 patients in whom perforation had occurred while under this treatment.

Operation should be carried out in all cases of duodenal ulcer in which thorough medical treatment has failed to cure. Although the condition was first treated by **gastro-enterostomy** by Codevilla in 1893, it is only of recent years that its correct treatment has been recognized owing, in great measure, to the work of Moynihan, the Mayos, and Mayo Robson.

The abdomen should be opened by displacing the right rectus muscle. The ulcer is usually found on the upper and anterior part of the first portion of the duodenum. The peritoneum over it presents a speckled reddish appearance, and a definite induration can be felt between the finger and thumb. When the ulcer is situated on the posterior portion of the duodenum, it may usually be felt through the anterior wall or by picking up the duodenum between finger and thumb. In many cases adhesions are present binding the duodenum to the gall-bladder or liver. In every case in which the condition of the patient permits, the gall-bladder and appendix should be examined, and surgically treated if necessary.

After examining the stomach for signs of ulcer, posterior no-loop gastro-jejunostomy should be carried out. That this is sufficient in most cases is shown not only by the long series recorded in which absolute relief of symptoms occurred, but by demonstration at a second operation performed for some other condition.

In one patient upon whom I operated the ulcer was demonstrated as healed during the course of an operation undertaken for another condition three years later. At the operation I had found " a large indurated mass on the anterior surface of the first part of the duodenum adherent to the liver." The surgeon who performed the second operation wrote: " The duodenum was quite free from induration and was loosely adherent to the liver. There was a greyish-white scar on its anterior surface ¾ in. from pylorus, which was, however, quite soft and no thicker than the neighbouring gut. The anastomosis was quite perfect, with the mesocolon merely adherent to the suture line." In another patient I opened the abdomen four years later for another condition, and found that the ulcer had healed. Similar cases have been recorded by Moynihan.

But death has occurred from hæmorrhage or perforation after a successful gastro-jejunostomy had been performed, and Moynihan has recorded a case in which, on opening the abdomen three years later for recurrence of symptoms, two recent ulcers were found close to the large scar of the old one. For these reasons the ulcer should be infolded if it is situated on the anterior surface ; if on the posterior, the duodenum should be obliterated by infolding the anterior wall.

The after-treatment should be similar to that carried out in chronic gastric ulcer.

Hæmorrhage must be looked upon as a serious symptom, and operation carried out as soon as the patient can stand it, usually within forty-eight hours. It will rarely be justifiable to operate during the course of the bleeding, but if the patient has had a severe hæmorrhage, and the bleeding recurs while he is absolutely at rest, operation without loss of time is indicated. The ulcer should be infolded, the gastro-duodenal artery ligatured, and gastro-jejunostomy done.

PERFORATION OF DUODENAL ULCER

It has been stated that perforation is a relatively more frequent accident in duodenal than in gastric ulcer, but this is impossible of direct proof, for we have no means of knowing the number of patients suffering from this lesion. The old figures (Chvostek, 42 per cent. ; Collin, 69 per cent.) certainly over-state the frequency, and were compiled before our present knowledge of the condition. It is more common than in chronic gastric ulcer, for chronic duodenal ulcer is most often situated on the anterior and upper wall of the duodenum. That it is a fatal termination and not infrequently occurs while the patient is under treatment is certain.

The perforation is more common on the anterior wall of the first part of the duodenum—90 per cent. of the cases. (Fig. 380.)

Symptoms.—A few years ago it was thought that duodenal ulcer was often latent, and that the first symptom was in many cases perforation. Now that the symptoms of duodenal ulcer are better known, it is recognized that in most cases symptoms have been present for years, and that the ulcer which has perforated is a chronic one.

Thus, in 14 out of 15 cases recorded by Mitchell, a history of previous "dyspepsia" was present, in the majority of the cases, typical of chronic ulcer. I have found the same in most of the cases of perforation in which I made careful inquiries; the last four occurred while the patient was under medical treatment.

The perforation may be acute, subacute, or chronic. It is much more frequently subacute than in gastric ulcer, and consequently the symptoms may not be so definite as those of a perforated gastric ulcer.

If the ulcer is situated close to the pylorus, and the opening is a large one, there is a sudden escape of gastric contents, causing severe epigastric pain, followed by abdominal rigidity, with the same absence of early severe shock as in perforation of a gastric ulcer. But if the

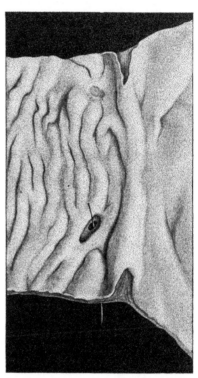

Fig. 380.—Perforation of an acute ulcer situated on the anterior wall of the first part of the duodenum. Small chronic ulcer on the posterior wall; stomach and duodenum opened from above.

(*London Hospital Pathological Institute.*)

perforation is a small one, or is situated at the junction of the first and second parts of the duodenum, or in the second part, the escaped fluid may track down into the right kidney pouch. Maynard Smith has experimentally investigated the course taken by fluids escaping from the duodenum, with results corresponding to those found clinically. The fluid in every case ran down and collected in the right kidney pouch, then passed down along the outer side of the ascending colon as far as the pelvis, and overflowed into this.

In these cases the symptoms are by no means typical, and, in the absence of a previous history pointing to duodenal ulcer, are very liable to be mistaken for appendicitis. It should be borne in mind that the two diseases may coexist, and that cases of simultaneous perforation of a duodenal ulcer and acute appendicitis are not unknown.

Thus, there are two types of perforation—those in which, from the immediate symptoms, the diagnosis of a perforated peptic ulcer is possible; and those in which the onset is more gradual, the symptoms that bring the patient under observation resembling those of appendicitis or subphrenic abscess. Fortunately the first is the larger group.

Diagnosis.—In the first group the diagnosis cannot be made from a perforated gastric ulcer except on the previous history. In the cases with subacute symptoms of perforation or with signs resembling those of appendicitis, only the greatest care in eliciting the previous history and the history of the onset of the lesion will enable the diagnosis to be made. In most cases this will be possible; the onset of "acute abdominal" symptoms in an adult male should always raise the suspicion that the duodenum is at fault.

Occasionally the perforation is retroperitoneal, with the gradual formation of a swelling in the right loin, usually associated with contraction of the psoas muscle. The abscess, as in a case recorded by Wagner, may simulate a psoas abscess due to spinal disease, and may point in the inguinal region. There is no absolutely sudden onset, but pain with a raised temperature. If the previous symptoms of ulcer have not been typical the diagnosis is not made until after the abscess has been opened and a duodenal fistula forms. These cases are rare; one successfully treated by operation has been recorded by Lawford Knaggs.

It might be supposed that if the abdomen has been opened on the diagnosis of a perforated peptic ulcer no further difficulty will arise, yet in one such case the discovery of fat necrosis at the root of the mesentery led me to abandon further search. In this case an ulcer of the second part of the duodenum had perforated and permitted the escape of pancreatic juice into the peritoneal cavity. A similar instance of fat necrosis associated with a perforated duodenal ulcer has been since recorded by H. M. Richter.

Treatment.—The abdomen should be opened through the right rectus muscle. As a rule the ulcer is at once seen. It should be infolded and gastro-jejunostomy performed if the condition of the patient admit. After examining for further perforations the right kidney pouch should be carefully sponged out and the abdomen closed. If necessary the right renal pouch is to be drained, and, in addition, if there has been extensive peritoneal soiling, a tube may be placed suprapubically. The after-treatment follows the lines laid down for cases of perforated gastric ulcer (p. 358).

Prognosis.—At the present time, owing chiefly to the less acute onset of many cases of perforation, the death-rate is higher than in similar perforations of the stomach.

Mayo Robson collected 155 cases, with a mortality of 66 per cent.; during 1899–1908, 42 cases were operated upon at the London Hospital, with a death-rate of 80 per cent.; up to December, 1911, I had operated upon 20 cases, with 9 recoveries.

A. B. Mitchell of Belfast has published a series of 16 consecutive operations for perforation, without a single death. Of these cases, 11 were operated upon within 12 hours of perforation, 6 within 5 hours, 1 each at $17\frac{1}{2}$, 18, 25, 36, and 49 hours after perforation. In my own cases, successful results attended operations done 4, 5, $6\frac{1}{2}$, 7, 12, 14, 17, 20, and 21 hours after perforation, whilst death followed those performed after 6 days, 5 days, 4 days, 3 days, 70 hours, 65 hours, 40 hours, 30 hours, 25 hours, 12 hours, and 6 hours respectively. In this last case I found fat necrosis and did not search for the duodenal perforation.

The death-rate in the first 29 cases recorded in 1899 (Pagenstecher) was nearly 86 per cent., and the mortality has been gradually falling. As knowledge of the early symptoms which accompany perforation becomes widely spread, earlier operation will render treatment more successful, and recognition of chronic duodenal ulcer will lead to the prevention of perforation by appropriate treatment.

HÆMATEMESIS

Hæmatemesis occurs in many diseases, in the majority of which there is a definite lesion of the stomach, but it may arise secondarily in cirrhosis of the liver or in Banti's disease.

In cirrhosis of the liver the bleeding usually takes place from a ruptured œsophageal varix. As shown by Preble, in over two-thirds of the cases the bleeding was the first symptom calling attention to the disease. In Banti's disease the history of anæmia and the presence of the enlarged spleen will lead to the correct diagnosis.

Cases of hæmatemesis fall into three groups: (1) Those in which the bleeding is the first obvious symptom of disease. (2) Hæmatemesis occurring after operation. (3) Hæmatemesis occurring in patients presenting the symptoms of chronic gastric or duodenal ulcer.

1. BLEEDING WITHOUT PREMONITORY SYMPTOMS

In this group the patients are usually young anæmic women. The hæmorrhage is the first symptom in 75 per cent. of the cases; in the remainder it may have been preceded for a few days or weeks by symptoms suggestive of gastric ulcer. The hæmorrhage is alarming and profuse, but is very rarely fatal. Tuffier has stated that the death-rate is only 1·7 per cent. when medically treated ; this corresponds with my experience.

Instances have been recorded in which at operation or at the post-mortem examination no ulcer could be discovered. Hale White collected 29 such examples of this condition, and suggested for it the name gastrostaxis.

It is difficult to examine the interior of the stomach satisfactorily during life, and recent acute ulcers or erosions are easily overlooked even post mortem unless the stomach be carefully examined with a lens. It is probable that there is a definite lesion of the mucous membrane in all the cases in this group.

Charles Miller has described swelling and necrosis of the lymphoid follicles in cases of this description in which the patient died from hæmorrhage or the operation for it. Fred. J. Smith has found small ulcers, hardly visible to the naked eye, leading directly into blood-vessels.

Treatment.—Operation should *never* be undertaken in these cases. The death-rate after operation is over 60 per cent., and the bleeding has recurred after all forms of treatment.

Absolute rest in bed should be insisted upon and a hypodermic of morphia given. High rectal injection of hot water from 112° to 120° F. (Tripier), repeated once or twice, may be useful. Nothing should be given by mouth for forty-eight hours, salines being given per rectum every six hours. At the end of forty-eight hours feeding may be carefully begun, small quantities of albumin-water being first given, and the quantity gradually increased if well taken, followed by Benger's food or milk-and-water.

2. Postoperative Hæmatemesis

Hæmorrhage from the stomach occurs occasionally after operation upon the abdomen, and in rare instances after operations upon other parts of the body. In most cases the operation has been for some septic condition. In these cases the general condition of the patient is bad and indicative of a severe toxæmia. In most instances the hæmatemesis occurs within twenty-four hours of the operation, although it may be delayed, particularly in such cases as appendicitis in which there is prolonged sepsis. As a rule the blood vomited is altered in colour, and the name " black vomit " has been given to it.

The death-rate of this condition is high. Purves estimated it at 69 per cent. This is in accordance with experience at the London Hospital.

Several theories have been put forward with regard to its causation : (1) That it is due to sepsis. (2) That it is " dependent on a reflex nervous influence " (Mayo Robson). (3) That it is due to injury to the omentum (v. Eiselsberg). (4) That it is due to the anæsthetic.

Sepsis, as first shown by Rodman, is the cause in most cases. It is now known that gastric erosions and gastric ulcers are relatively common complications of septic conditions. The hæmorrhage has the same origin as that in the first group, from definite lesions of the mucous membrane of the stomach.

Thus, during the years 1907-9, 19 acute ulcers—18 of stomach and 1 of duodénum—were found at the Pathological Institute of the London Hospital in patients who died shortly after operation. In none of these cases had hæmatemesis or melæna occurred. In 12 the operations had been undertaken for acute appendicitis, in 3 for acute intestinal obstruction, in 1 for infective gangrene of the leg, in 1 for papilloma of bladder in a patient with pyuria, and in 2 for disease of the gall-bladder. During the same period 8 patients died with postoperative hæmatemesis. In 3 cases it originated after operation for acute appendicitis, in 2 after operation upon the gall-bladder, and in 1 each after external urethrotomy, hysterectomy, and epithelioma of tongue. In the last two of these cases the hæmorrhage arose from a chronic gastric ulcer which had eroded the coronary artery, and a chronic duodenal ulcer with an erosion of the gastro-duodenal artery. Of the remainder, in 1 case erosions were found in the duodenum, in 2 cases an acute gastric ulcer was found, in 1 a bleeding erosion was discovered at operation, in 1 no cause could be found post mortem, in another no post-mortem was obtained.

Postoperative hæmatemesis is the result of septic gastritis in the majority of cases, but hæmatemesis may occur from a chronic ulcer which has been in existence for some time without giving rise to symptoms sufficiently severe to need treatment. Mansell-Moullin has recorded a case in which a young man aged 23 died from profuse hæmatemesis forty-eight hours after an exploratory incision made in the left iliac fossa for inoperable carcinoma ; at the post-mortem no cause was found in the stomach, but it is possible that an erosion was overlooked.

Treatment.—Patients in whom this condition arises are always desperately ill. If the vomit is black, frequent, and small in amount, gentle lavage with warm water, to which ʒi of bicarbonate of soda to the pint has been added, should be employed, and repeated if necessary. The toxæmia should be combated by continuous saline injection per rectum.

3. HÆMATEMESIS FROM A CHRONIC GASTRIC OR DUODENAL ULCER

This is a serious complication and leads not infrequently to a fatal result. Cecil Wall investigated the death-rate among the patients admitted into the London Hospital with hæmatemesis due to chronic gastric ulcer, and found that it was 12½ per cent. in men, 6½ per cent. in women. It is not yet sufficiently realized that death from this cause is common. The bleeding occurs usually from an artery of medium size, although it may take place as the result of ulceration into a vein. A small aneurysm often forms on an artery exposed in the floor of the ulcer, ruptures, and gives rise to profuse bleeding, the artery being unable to retract. The hæmatemesis may be acute and lead to death so rapidly that there is no time for surgical treatment; this was the result in 8 out of 54 fatal cases collected by Savariaud: in these cases it most often occurs from the splenic artery. Usually, however, the bleeding ceases spontaneously, only to recur later, with perhaps a fatal result. The coronary, pancreatico-duodenal, and right gastro-epiploic are the usual sources of the bleeding.

Treatment.—In this group, unlike the first, operation must be carried out in all cases. It must be undertaken as soon after the cessation of the first bleeding as the patient's condition will permit; this will usually be in thirty-six to forty-eight hours. During this time absolute rest and the avoidance of oral feeding are essential. If in spite of this treatment the bleeding continues or recurs, operation should be resorted to without delay. During the period of waiting after the first attack, a careful watch must be kept to see that bleeding is not continuing although no blood is being vomited.

In this group the blood is usually escaping from an artery; direct treatment of the bleeding-point is therefore necessary. It has been stated that gastro-jejunostomy is sufficient to arrest the bleeding; this is probably true when the blood is coming from a small vessel, but there is no way of telling the size of the vessel, and it is safer to treat the ulcer directly. That gastro-jejunostomy is not sufficient to arrest arterial hæmorrhage is seen in the cases in which fatal hæmatemesis from an artery in the floor of a chronic ulcer occurs some weeks after a successful gastro-jejunostomy. In a case under my care in which this happened, gastro-jejunostomy was performed in a patient with a large saddle-shaped ulcer of stomach which had perforated anteriorly and was firmly adherent to the pancreas posteriorly. The patient did extremely well until the day on which he was to leave hospital, a month after operation, when he had a fatal hæmatemesis. At the post-mortem examination the ulcer had healed anteriorly, but posteriorly the pancreas was exposed in the floor of the ulcer and a small aneurysm of the splenic artery had ruptured.

After opening the abdomen, the stomach should be carefully examined, and if an ulcer is seen on the lesser curvature it should, if possible, be infolded, after ligature of the vessel on either side of it, or excised. If this is impossible from its size or the presence of adhesions, or if the ulcer is situated on the posterior surface of the stomach and adherent to the pancreas, the stomach should be opened, the floor of the ulcer carefully examined, and any vessels which have ruptured tied on both sides. In one case I was able successfully to ligate on both sides of an opening in a large artery in the floor of an ulcer on the posterior wall. If the condition of the patient permits, gastro-jejunostomy should be done at the same time.

If the ulcer is duodenal, it should be infolded, and the gastro-duodenal artery tied; if on account of adhesions or ulceration the anterior wall cannot be satisfactorily infolded so as to press upon the affected vessel (usually the gastro-duodenal), the gut should be opened and the vessel ligated. Posterior gastro-jejunostomy should then be done.

If the stomach appears to be normal, no operation should be performed, but the abdomen closed.

PERIGASTRIC ABSCESS

This is usually due to the perforation of a chronic gastric ulcer, or to imperfect drainage of the abdominal cavity after operation for perforation.

When a perigastric abscess is the result of an ulcer on the anterior wall of the stomach, this viscus forms the lower boundary of the

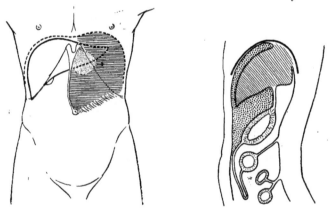

Fig. 381.—Diagrams to illustrate abscess in left anterior intraperitoneal fossa. (*Barnard.*)

abscess cavity, the gastro-hepatic omentum the posterior wall, and the liver the upper wall. Such an abscess may burst through the skin, or may open into the colon, causing a gastro-colic fistula, or may become subphrenic.

As a rule, ulcers which perforate chronically are situated on the posterior surface of the stomach, and a subphrenic abscess results (p. 572).

Subphrenic abscess (*see also* p. 572) is most commonly caused by perforation of a gastric or duodenal ulcer. Of 76 cases recorded by Barnard, it was due to this cause in 26, the ulcer being gastric in 21 and duodenal in 5 cases. The fossa affected is usually the left anterior intraperitoneal (Barnard). This fossa is bounded above by the diaphragm, below and to the right by the left lobe of the liver, on the left by the spleen, and below by adhesions of the omentum to the abdominal wall (Fig. 381). Signs of interference with the base of the left lung are usually present.

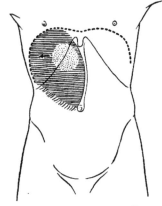

An abdominal swelling can be recognized occupying a triangular area limited by the costal margin on the outer side, and by a line convex to the right joining the umbilicus to the ensiform and the ensiform to the costal margin. Gas is usually present, giving rise to resonance at the upper part of the swelling (Fig. 381).

When the perforation is at the pylorus or in the duodenum the right anterior intraperitoneal space may be affected (Fig. 382). Of 27 abscesses of this type, 4 were the result of perforation of a gastric and 2 of the perforation of a duodenal ulcer.

Fig. 382.—Diagram to illustrate abscess in right anterior intraperitoneal fossa. (*Barnard.*)

This fossa is situated between the diaphragm above, the right lobe of the liver below, and the falciform ligament to the left.

The right posterior fossa (subhepatic fossa, right renal fossa) is rarely affected. Of 10 abscesses in this situation, 1 was due to a gastric and 1 to a duodenal ulcer.

Rarely the abscess involves the lesser sac (left posterior intraperitoneal, Barnard); of 3 cases of this nature it was due to perforated gastric ulcer in 2, but the lesser sac was not affected alone.

The abscess may burst spontaneously into a bronchus, into the pleura, with the formation of a pyopneumothorax, into the stomach or intestine, or, rarely, through the skin.

Treatment.—If the presence of pus beneath the diaphragm is suspected, careful exploration under an anæsthetic must be undertaken. An exploring syringe having a needle 3 in. long should be used. As recommended by Barnard, search should first be made in the scapular line, from the 10th space to the 6th. If no pus is found here, the spaces in the mid-axillary line should be similarly explored. When pus is found the rib below should be resected, the diaphragm fixed to the intercostal muscles with catgut stitches, and the abscess opened and drained.

Anterior abscesses should only be drained from the front when no pus is discovered by thorough posterior exploration.

BENIGN TUMOURS

Benign tumours of the stomach and duodenum are rare, and may be divided into three groups :—

1. Connective-tissue tumours.
2. Glandular tumours (adenomas).
3. Cysts.

1. CONNECTIVE-TISSUE TUMOURS

This group of tumours includes—i. Fibromas. ii. Fibro-myomas. iii. Lipomas.

i. FIBROMAS

These are rarely met with. They may occur as polypoid tumours in the pyloric region, single or multiple. (Fig. 383.)

They may be encapsuled in the gastric wall, as in the case reported

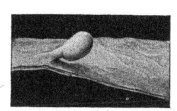 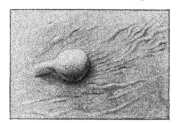

Fig. 383.—Fibroma of stomach.
(*London Hospital Museum.*)

by W. G. Spencer in which he successfully removed a fibroma weighing 7 oz. from the posterior wall of the stomach of a woman of 46.

According to Fenwick, no case hitherto recorded has been above suspicion of malignancy.

Treatment.—Pedunculated tumours should be removed by cutting through the pedicle and suturing the mucous membrane. When embedded in the gastric wall they should be enucleated or excised with the affected part of the stomach.

ii. MYOMAS AND FIBRO-MYOMAS

These constitute the commonest variety of simple tumour of the stomach ; 61 cases (Thomson of Galveston) have been published since the first was recorded by Morgagni in 1762.

Arising in the muscular tissue, usually along one of the curvatures, they are mostly single, and may project into the stomach or grow externally; the internal and external varieties are about equally common. Those that project into the cavity of the stomach rarely attain a size larger than a walnut; they frequently become ulcerated, and may cause hæmatemesis or pyloric obstruction. The external

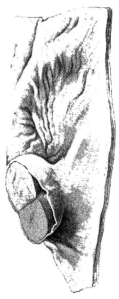

form may attain a large size and may contract adhesions to various organs. Herman has recorded the successful removal of a tumour of this nature. Similar tumours may arise in the duodenum.

The condition is met with in adult life. Fenwick states that it is more common in males, but of 27 of the 49 cases analysed by Deaver and Ashurst, in which the sex was stated, 16 were females.

On section the tumour is firm and of a whitish colour, and under the microscope is seen to be made up of bundles of unstriped muscle fibres mixed with strands of fibrous tissue concentrically arranged.

Myxomatous degeneration may occur, and cases have been recorded in which secondary growths were present in the liver and in the peritoneum. Cysts may originate from hæmorrhage. The tumour may contain angiomatous or adenomatous tissue.

Treatment. — When "internal," a myoma should be shelled out, or, if this be impossible, it should be excised together with the portion of gastric wall from which it springs. When external, its pedicle should be clamped and divided, and the stump covered with peritoneum after ligature of the necessary vessels.

Fig. 384.—Submucous encapsuled lipoma of stomach.

(*London Hospital Museum.*)

Twenty operations have been recorded for this condition, including 2 in which gastro-enterostomy was done on the supposition that the tumour was malignant.

iii. LIPOMAS

Fatty tumours may originate in subserous or submucous coats, usually the latter, and may in rare instances become pedunculated. They form lobulated tumours projecting into the stomach, covered usually by healthy mucous membrane (Fig. 384).

2. ADENOMAS

Under this heading are included both the solitary and the multiple pedunculated tumours. The latter are usually called polyadenomas or mucous polypi. (Fig. 385.)

Adenomas are usually found in the pyloric region, and constitute the commonest variety of gastric polypi. The tumour may reach the size of an apple, and may produce pyloric obstruction, as in the

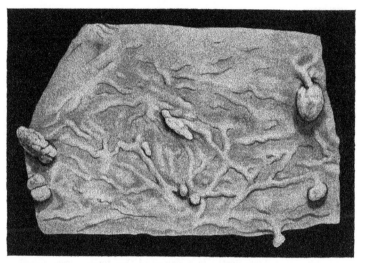

Fig. 385.—Mucous polypi.

(Royal College of Surgeons Museum.)

cases operated upon by Mayo Robson, Moynihan, and Sir William Bennett, or may cause fatal intussusception.

Multiple mucous polypi are more common in men than in women, are rare before the age of 40, and are generally found in conjunction with chronic gastritis. Rarely larger than cherries, they are evenly distributed over the stomach, and may extend into the duodenum. The greater part of each polypus is composed of mucous membrane in which the glands are dilated and tortuous, while frequently they are cystic.

Treatment follows the lines as laid down for pedunculated tumours elsewhere. Six cases have been recorded, in 5 of which recovery ensued.

3. CYSTS.

Cysts of the stomach are rare. They may occur in consequence of injury (traumatic cysts), or as the result of degeneration of tumours (degeneration cysts); while hydatid cysts may develop in the wall of the stomach, and in one instance, recorded in 1732, a dermoid cyst was said to be present. Retention cysts may arise from the obstruction of ducts in chronic gastritis, but they are devoid of clinical importance. Gastric cysts produce symptoms which resemble those of other benign tumours, but in addition they are liable to rupture or to become infected, causing a perigastric abscess or general peritonitis.

Symptoms of benign tumours.—In many cases benign tumours give rise to no symptoms unless they obstruct the pyloric or cardiac orifices; but if large and situated in the body of the stomach they may cause pain of a dragging character. Vomiting is unusual unless the tumour obstructs the pylorus. Hæmatemesis may arise in adenomas or in myomas, when the mucous membrane covering them has become ulcerated.

Diagnosis of benign tumours.—The possibility of a tumour being benign should be remembered, for unnecessarily severe operations have been performed—for example, partial gastrectomy for myoma.

MALIGNANT TUMOURS

CARCINOMA OF THE STOMACH

This is a disease of appalling frequency. It has been estimated to be the cause of death in over 4,000 people in England annually; during the years 1897-1904, 36,331 deaths were registered as due to gastric cancer. Dowd states that 9,000 deaths from cancer of the stomach were recorded in the United States in 1900. Virchow estimated that nearly 35 per cent. of all cancers that terminated fatally originated in the stomach. Häberlin, analysing the records of over 27,000 cases of carcinoma, found that 41 per cent. were connected with the stomach. In England and Wales it is the seat of disease in 22 per cent. of the fatal cases.

Etiology.—Carcinoma of the stomach may be met with at any age, but is most common between the ages of 40 and 70.

Thus, in 230 cases of carcinoma of the stomach admitted to the London Hospital between the years 1899-1908, in which the diagnosis was verified by operation or post-mortem examination, 196 occurred during this period, the greatest number being between 50 and 60. From a study of 2,604 post-mortems on patients who had died from gastric carcinoma, Fenwick found the age of death to be between 60 and 70 in 77 per cent. of the cases. It is rare under 20, according to Osler and McCrae 2·5 per cent., but among the London Hospital cases only 1 was below the age of 20. Six cases have been reported in children under 10, but of these only 2 can be definitely claimed as examples of carcinoma.

Sex.—Men are affected more frequently than women. Fenwick found that in 3,679 post-mortem examinations on cases of gastric cancer, 2,162—i.e. 60 per cent. of the subjects—were males.

Race.—Bainbridge has stated that the black races are almost immune, and cancer of the stomach is said to be practically unknown among the natives in Natal, Gambia, and West Africa.

Gastric ulcer.—It is held by all surgeons who have worked at the question that chronic gastric ulcer predisposes to the development of gastric carcinoma. Evidence of this has been gradually accumulating since its possibility was first discussed by Cruveilhier in 1839, and Rokitansky a year later. Dittrich, in 1848, described 6 cases in which carcinoma developed in the immediate vicinity of active or healed ulcers. The evidence of the relationship has of late been entirely surgical ; in fact, physicians generally have been somewhat sceptical with regard to it.

Osler and McCrae in 1900, in their work on " Cancer of the Stomach," found that in only 4 out of 150 cases was there a history of ulcer ; they say : " We may conclude, so far as the figures show anything, that the victims of chronic dyspepsia and the various forms of gastritis are not more prone to malignant disease than other individuals." The great development of gastric surgery since that date has led to other views. Among 87 patients with carcinoma of the stomach upon whom I operated up to December, 1911, there was in 31 a definite history pointing to chronic gastric ulcer, symptoms having been present for from five to twenty-eight years. Mayo Robson, in cases in which he operated, found a suggestive history in 59 per cent. ; Moynihan, in 60 per cent. Mumford and Stone traced 60 patients who had been treated at the Massachusetts General Hospital for " chronic indigestion," and subsequently died, no less than half with gastric cancer.

The most convincing evidence has been put forward by Wilson and MacCarty as the result of their examination of specimens removed by operation in the Mayos' clinic. In 71 per cent. (109 out of 153 cases) there was naked-eye and microscopical evidence that carcinoma had developed from pre-existing ulcers.

The facts that carcinoma and chronic gastric ulcer are both more common in men than in women, and that they have their usual seat in the same part of the stomach, are suggestive of a close relationship between them.

There can, in my opinion, be no doubt that gastric ulcer is a predisposing cause of cancer of the stomach in a large proportion of cases.

Pathology. — Carcinoma may start primarily in the stomach or affect it secondarily. The secondary variety is comparatively rare and of little surgical importance ; it occurred in 7 per cent. of the 265 post-mortem examinations of cancer of the stomach recorded by Fenwick, and Hale White states that it occurs in 6 to 7 per cent. of the cases. In the other published series the percentage has been as low as 1, which is in agreement with experience at the London Hospital.

Gastric Carcinoma arises most often as the result of *direct* extension from the pancreas, colon, or gall-bladder, or from the œsophagus. In this group must also be placed those cases, by no means uncommon, following carcinoma of the breast. It may be secondary to carcinoma of the upper alimentary tract (auto-inoculation). More rarely still does it arise as a metastasis.

Primary carcinoma of the stomach may be composed of spheroidal or cylindrical cells ; either may undergo colloid degeneration. If the fibrous stroma is abundant, the adjective " scirrhus " is applied ; if small in amount, the growth is known as a " medullary " or " encephaloid " carcinoma.

In *spheroidal-celled* carcinoma the cells resemble those of the gastric tubules ; this variety is more than twice as common as the *cylindrical* or columnar-celled (Perry and Shaw, Fenwick), and is the usual type of " malignant ulcer." It was found by Fenwick to be " hard " in 19 out of 41 cases. " Colloid " carcinoma—the result of a mucoid or colloid degeneration which, though usually affecting the cells, may affect the stroma as well—is found in about 7 per cent. of cases. Neither form has a special preference for any portion of the stomach, but the columnar-celled variety is most common in the pyloric region, where it usually springs as a soft red fungoid growth. Either form may infiltrate the whole organ ("leather-bottle" stomach), rendering it small in the spheroidal-celled variety, rarely diminishing its size in the columnar. (Fig. 386.)

Situation.—The older authorities were of opinion that 60 per cent. of all gastric cancers are situated at the pylorus. But modern observations show that the percentage is not so great as this ; Boas, in 125 cases, found the pylorus affected in 34 (27 per cent.), while in 87 cases upon which I have operated the growth was on the lesser curvature in 52. The cardiac end is affected in 9·8 per cent. (Fenwick).

Growths are occasionally multiple ; in most of the recorded cases they have been on opposed surfaces of the viscus.

Carcinoma commences in the deeper layers of the mucous membrane ; if at the edge of an ulcer, it is usually in that edge nearest the pylorus.

Method of spread.—This may be direct, in the stomach itself or to adjacent organs immediately or through adhesion ; or indirect, by lymphatics or by blood-vessels.

Cancer in the stomach tends to spread along the lesser curvature, and, as first pointed out by Rokitansky, rarely affects the duodenum. Although Brinton found the duodenum involved in 10 out of 125 cases, this high percentage has not been borne out by later observers ; thus, in 131 cases, Fenwick found this structure involved in 2 only. However, as the result of microscopic examination of 63 specimens removed by operation, Borrmann found the cut edge of the duodenum involved in 20. On the other hand, carcinoma of the cardiac end of the stomach frequently involves the œsophagus, and vice versa.

Growth extends in the submucosa early and widely ; while the induration marks the limit of infiltration of the mucous membrane, the growth extends in the submucosa for several centimetres beyond. The area of involvement of the serous and muscular coat is always less. Adjacent organs may be directly affected, most frequently the pancreas, then the liver and colon, rarely the spleen.

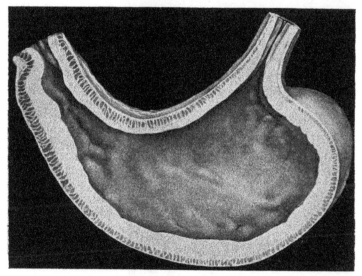

Fig. 386.—" Leather bottle " stomach.

(*Royal College of Surgeons Museum.*)

Adhesions are present in about 80 per cent. of cases at the time of death, and constitute an important method of spread.

Lymphatic spread.—The lymphatic system of the stomach has already been described (p. 300). In carcinoma of the pylorus and lesser curvature the lower coronary group of glands is first affected. Occasionally a lymphatic vessel runs past this group of glands and terminates directly in one of the upper coronary set ; this is well shown in Fig. 387, a photograph of a portion of the stomach which I removed. In carcinoma of this region the subpyloric glands are usually affected, and lymphatic vessels may run directly to the suprapancreatic glands and even to the biliary chain.

Hey Groves has recently called attention to the spread of carcinoma in the great omentum in advanced cases, and has shown that the growth may be disseminated by adhesion of the great omentum to neighbouring organs. Dobson and Jamieson have drawn attention to the tendency shown by the glands associated with the right gastro-epiploic artery to extend into the great omentum, but. there are no efferent vessels here that drain into glands other · than those of the gastro-epiploic, subpyloric, or splenic groups.

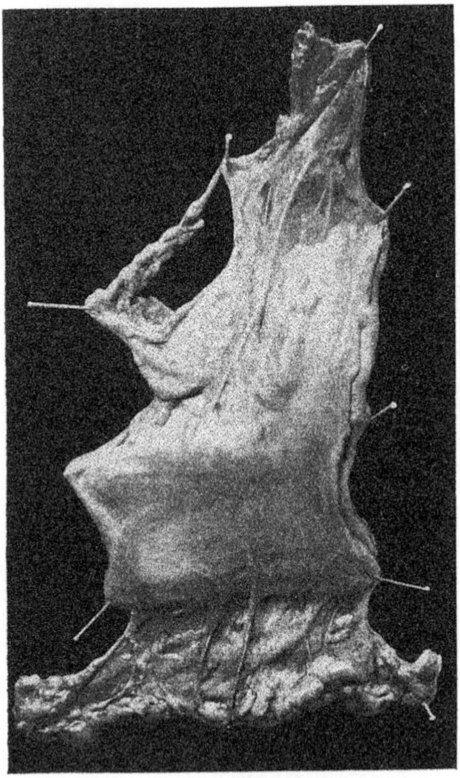

Lymphatic invasion is early and constant, and present in practically every case at the time of operation. Cunéo found the glands of the lesser curvature involved in 87 per cent. of cases examined, those of the greater curvature in 66 per cent. Lengemann, in the examination of 20 specimens removed by operation, found that the subpyloric group of glands was involved in 60 per cent. of cases, while Cunéo had found them to be affected in 2 per cent. only. Jamieson and Dobson support Lengemann's observations, which are in accord with my own experience.

Fig. 387.—Portion of stomach removed at operation, showing a lymphatic vessel containing growth that runs directly to one of the upper group of coronary glands.

(*Photograph taken from a case of the author's.*)

In a late stage of the disease the glands at the hilum of the liver, those around the cœliac axis, the superior mesenteric glands, the biliary glands, the mesocolic and the lumbar glands may be involved.

As the glands at the hilum of the liver merely receive vessels from the liver for transmission to the right suprapancreatic and biliary groups, and have no vessels directly connecting with any gland-group receiving lymphatics from the stomach, they must become infected in a retrograde manner or from a secondary growth in the liver.

Henoch, in 1863, first recorded enlargement of the left supraclavicular glands in gastric carcinoma. An enlargement of these glands is said to take place in 3 per cent. of cases. Involvement of the right group is a rare event.

Vascular infection.—This is usually through the veins of the portal system, and produces secondary growths in the liver. It is most common in carcinoma of the body of the stomach ; carcinoma of the pyloric end tends to affect the liver by direct spread. Rarely, the systemic veins disseminate the growth, either through direct invasion of the inferior vena cava, or via the thoracic duct or liver.

Summary.—Glandular invasion is early and almost invariable, while next in order of frequency secondary deposits are found in the liver, great omentum, and pancreas.

Symptoms.—These will vary with the situation of the growth. In carcinoma of the pylorus or cardiac orifice, symptoms of obstruction appear early ; but in carcinoma of the prepyloric portion the growth does not produce obstruction until late, and the symptoms are therefore less marked.

The cases can be divided, according to symptoms, into three groups : (1) Following previous gastric disease. (2) Occurring in previously healthy persons. (3) " Latent."

1. This will comprise at least 50 per cent. of the cases, and in many instances there will be the typical history of chronic gastric ulcer—attacks, at irregular intervals, of pain after food, relieved, it may be, by vomiting. It may be noticed that in the last attack the pain is not so readily relieved by rest or vomiting, becomes almost constant, assumes a gnawing character, and wakes the patient at night. There may also be a distaste for food, particularly meat, which was not present in the previous attacks. In some few cases no change in the character of the symptoms is noticed, but at the operation for supposed chronic gastric ulcer carcinoma is found. Occasionally the history is of a gastric illness, with symptoms of ulceration several years before, followed by apparently perfect recovery.

2. In this group the onset may be sudden, an acute hæmatemesis occurring in a previously healthy person, succeeded by a sense of gastric discomfort. In other cases the symptoms follow, according to the patient, an error in diet a short time before. But as a rule the onset is more gradual. As Brinton wrote : " An elderly person

. . . begins to suffer from a capricious appetite ' '; a distaste for food may be first noticed, perhaps a distaste for meat only. This was at one time considered an important diagnostic point, but in 87 cases in which I made inquiry it was only noted as the first symptom in 3, though it is usually present when the disease has advanced.

Pain is the most constant feature, and is present in 85 per cent. of the cases. It is not so sharp or so localized as in ulcer, is often not relieved when the stomach is empty, and is seldom relieved by rest.

Vomiting may be absent or infrequent when the growth is pre-pyloric, and does little to relieve the pain; it frequently occurs independently of food, is often offensive, and contains small quantities of blood. In growths causing pyloric obstruction, vomiting is often the first symptom. Careful examination of the vomit will show the presence of *blood* in practically every case. As a rule it is slight, and may only be revealed by the test for " occult " hæmorrhage; if greater in amount it may impart a " coffee-grounds " appearance to the vomit. Bleeding sufficient to cause hæmatemesis is unusual; Brinton estimated its frequency as 6 per cent. Fatal hæmorrhage occurs in not more than 1 per cent. of the cases.

When the growth is diffuse, involving the whole of the stomach ("leather-bottle " stomach), there is inability to take more than a certain amount of food without causing vomiting, and the amount that can be taken gradually diminishes.

A palpable *tumour* is present at some time during the course of over 70 per cent. of the cases; but it must be remembered that it is a late sign. It has been stated (Czerny, Rindfleisch) that the presence of a tumour means that the disease is inoperable. This is not so. Instances have been recorded, among others by Mayo Robson and Kocher, of patients alive and well six or seven years after partial gastrectomy for carcinoma, although a tumour had been palpable before operation. While the majority of tumours are felt in the umbilical region, a tumour due to carcinoma of the pylorus may be found in almost any part of the abdomen, while those due to growths of the lesser curvature and to "leather-bottle " stomach are seen in the epigastric and left hypochondriac regions.

Inspection of the abdomen will generally reveal the tumour moving on respiration. Tumours of the pylorus can be usually moved from side to side, and vary in the position they occupy according to the condition of the stomach. Many of these tumours receive transmitted pulsation from the aorta. Very rarely indeed the patient comes under observation because the tumour has been noticed and no other signs are present. Inflation of the stomach will sometimes aid the diagnosis in obscure cases.

In some cases, as first pointed out by Wickham Legg in 1880, metastases are seen at the umbilicus.

Anæmia, loss of weight, and change in gastric secretion are other symptoms to be found in all late cases.

Anæmia is present in all advanced cases; in a few the resemblance of the symptoms to those of pernicious anæmia has led to error of diagnosis and treatment, but examination of the blood will prevent this mistake. The blood-changes in carcinoma of the stomach are those of a secondary anæmia. The red corpuscles are rarely reduced lower than 3,000,000, the average of 59 cases recorded by Osler and McCrae being 3,712,186. There is a slight leucocytosis in most cases. It has been stated by Müller that digestive leucocytosis is absent in carcinoma of the stomach. Very little reliance can be placed on this test, for it is present in nearly half the cases examined (Osler and McCrae, Fenwick).

Progressive **loss of weight** may very rarely be the first sign of disease. Thus, in one patient under my care, a man of 57, progressive loss of weight, from 16 st. 3 lb. to 12 st. 6 lb., was noticed for twelve months before the onset of any gastric symptom.

Changes in **gastric secretion** are present in the late stages of the disease. Golding Bird, in 1843, pointed out that free HCl was absent in cases of cancer of the stomach. Among 495 cases published by various authors, free HCl was absent in 89 per cent. (Fenwick). It has been stated that free HCl is only present in those cases which originate from ulcer; it is certainly usually present in patients with a previous history of long-standing gastric trouble, and absent in those in whom the carcinoma develops without previous history of gastric disease. It is a test on which too much stress should not be laid, for it is a late sign and due to concomitant chronic gastritis. Hammerschlag, from the examination of mucosa removed from the stomach in cases of gastro-jejunostomy, found that when free HCl was absent the specific glandular elements had disappeared and been replaced by cylindrical epithelium.

Free HCl may be present throughout the whole course of the disease, and it may be absent from the gastric juice in patients with carcinoma of other organs (Mansell-Moullin, Moore, Palmer). This statement is disputed by Willcox, who has found free HCl present in the gastric contents of patients with carcinoma of organs even contiguous to the stomach. This is in agreement with my own experience. It has been stated (Seidelin) that free HCl is absent in 40 per cent. of people over the age of 50.

Fragments of growth, blood, sarcinæ, and the Oppler-Boas bacillus may be found on *microscopical examination of the vomit* (p. 311). Salomon has stated that the presence of nucleo-albumin and mucin.

tested by Esbach's reagent, in the washings of a fasting stomach is in favour of carcinoma. These are also late signs.

3. As already pointed out, malignant disease of the stomach may be *latent*, progressive loss of weight perhaps being the first sign of its presence. In other cases, ascites or a tumour due to secondary growth is first noticed.

Fenwick was able to collect from the records of the London Hospital, during the twenty years preceding 1902, 14 cases in which " the presence of ascites constituted the sole indication of cancer of the stomach." In at least half of these there was no evidence to connect the ascites with a malignant growth of the stomach.

Cases with ascites fall into two groups—(*a*) those in which the ascites is the first symptom seriously to attract the patient's attention, and (*b*) those in which, following indefinite abdominal symptoms, there is a sudden onset of acute pain and swelling. Four cases have been under my care ; in all the ascites had been preceded by vague abdominal symptoms of which no notice was taken, in 2 the onset of ascites was gradual, in 2 so acute that the diagnosis of a perforative lesion was made.

In cases in which metastases call attention to the disease the secondary growths are usually in the liver ; but a malignant ovarian tumour may be the first sign for which the patient comes under observation.

Perforation may be acute or subacute. Acute perforation takes place in about 3 per cent. of cases, but occasionally a subacute perforation with the formation of a perigastric abscess occurs. One example of each was present in 87 cases under my care.

Fistulæ may open externally or into the colon, rarely into the duodenum (*see* p. 402).

Thrombosis of veins may occur in the late stage. Trousseau wrote : " Should you, when in doubt as to the nature of an affection of the stomach, observe a vein becoming inflamed in the arm or leg, you may dispel your doubt and pronounce in a positive manner that there is a cancer."

Fever is present in nearly a third of the cases at some period during the course.

Jaundice is stated to occur in 13 per cent. of cases (Fenwick), and is usually due to extension of the growth to the head of the pancreas.

Diagnosis.—At the present time a *certain* diagnosis at the most favourable period for removal is impossible. All the signs which make for a positive diagnosis are late signs.

Help may be expected in the future from the use of the gastroscope, and it may be that examination of the blood will be of service.

Kelling, Crile, and others have attempted the early diagnosis by means of a hæmolytic test. Wideroe, Crile, and Paus found a positive reaction in over 60 per cent. of the cases. All the patients with malignant disease who failed to give a positive reaction had advanced disease. E. C. Hort has shown that the power of inhibiting tryptic digestion is much greater in the serum of patients suffering from carcinoma ; but as the antitryptic index is raised in many other diseases it is chiefly helpful from its negative side, although in Hort's cases the test was of no value in 6 out of 100. It is suggested that absence of a rise in the antitryptic index of the serum may be of value in the diagnosis of chronic gastric ulcer from carcinoma. Unfortunately, neither of these tests is sufficiently reliable to help materially with the diagnosis. It can only be laid down that surgical treatment should be considered in all cases in which digestive symptoms in an adult fail to respond to thorough meidcal treatment, or relapse, and that exploration should be undertaken in all cases in which the disease is due to some structural alteration in the stomach.

A careful examination of the gastric contents should be made. Absence of free HCl, diminution of the total acidity, as well as the presence of lactic acid and the Oppler-Boas bacillus, are signs suggestive of carcinoma.

In patients in whom carcinoma originates in a previously healthy stomach, free HCl is usually absent and the total acidity is low by the time they come under observation. Whether this obtains within a few weeks of the onset of the symptoms remains for further investigation.

When the malignant growth supervenes on a chronic gastric ulcer, free HCl is usually present in about normal amount, and the total acidity corresponds. These are the cases in which diagnostic help is so much needed ; no information of any value is given. Again, in cases of chronic gastritis of long duration and in certain cases of chronic ulcer and after severe hæmorrhage, free HCl may be absent.

It is evident that too much reliance must not be placed upon the result of gastric analysis, but, taken with other symptoms, it is particularly helpful in those cases in which gastric symptoms appear for the first time in adults.

The vomit and fæces should also be examined for occult blood.

All are agreed that exploration should be undertaken when any suspicion of cancer exists, without waiting for the diagnosis to be made certain.

When a tumour is present it must be diagnosed from tumour of the gall-bladder and colon ; if other means have failed, distension of the stomach with air will in most cases enable this to be done.

Even when the abdomen has been opened and the stomach exposed it may be impossible to make the diagnosis of malignancy without microscopical examination. It is in these cases that the result of a previous chemical examination of the gastric contents after a test meal may be invaluable. In recorded cases the condition has been diagnosed at the operation as carcinoma and treated by partial gastrectomy, yet subsequent microscopic examination has revealed chronic ulcer only, and a supposed palliative operation has led to complete disappearance of the tumour and proved to be curative. Points to be considered are the appearance and feel of the tumour, its method of spread, and affection of lymphatic glands. In carcinoma of the stomach the peritoneum is usually thickened and opaque, small outlying patches of the same nature are seen, and the lymphatics are often marked out. The shaggy, red-stippled appearance of the peritoneum, and the thickening with a depressed centre, seen in chronic gastric ulcer, are rarely present. On palpation, distinct irregular induration may be felt. If there is doubt a portion of the suspected growth should be removed and submitted to rapid microscopical examination. Even in this way it may be impossible to make a definite diagnosis.

Treatment.—The treatment of suspected carcinoma is surgical ; if the question that a growth is present is raised, valuable time should not be wasted. In the words of Hale White : " If symptoms of serious chronic indigestion first appear after the age of 40, organic disease of the stomach should be strongly suspected, and, if a comparatively short period of medical treatment does not effect a cure, it may be quite justifiable to open the abdomen." Were his advice carried into effect, many patients would be operated upon in the precancerous stage, the percentage of cases found suitable for radical treatment increased, and the ultimate results rendered more favourable than they are at present. The percentage of cases suitable for resection must vary in every clinic, and will become greater as time goes on. As an average the following may be given : In my series of 87 cases, 21 were treated by excision ; these figures almost correspond with those given by Poncet, Delore and Leriche (in 137 cases operated upon excision was performed in 40), and with those from the Breslau clinic given by Küttner (102 excisions in 366 cases of carcinoma).

Operation should be undertaken in all cases of suspected or proved carcinoma of the stomach, unless obviously inoperable by reason of secondary growths, the surgeon being prepared to do a partial or a complete gastrectomy.

The surgical treatment can be summed up shortly : the operation of choice is partial gastrectomy ; in certain cases total gastrectomy may be necessary. *Simple gastro-jejunostomy should only be performed when the growth is producing pyloric obstruction ; in other cases no good results.* If cardiac obstruction is present, gastrostomy may be done ; in certain cases jejunostomy may be advisable.

The incision should be made through the right rectus muscle or in the middle line, and the stomach examined. The question of malignancy must first be settled. If doubt exists, a portion of the ulcer or a gland is removed and examined microscopically while a gastro-jejunostomy suitable for use after partial gastrectomy is being performed. If a rapid microscopic examination cannot be obtained the abdomen should be closed, and a second operation undertaken at a later date if the section reveals malignancy or the progress of the case renders the diagnosis certain. If the suspected carcinoma is situated on the lesser curvature the absence of relief as the result of the gastro-jejunostomy will clinch the diagnosis.

If the growth is obviously malignant its operability must be settled. The decision depends upon the presence and degree of adhesions and infiltration of other structures, particularly the liver and pancreas, of massive glandular enlargements, and of secondary deposits in the peritoneum or at a distance. In every case a careful examination should be made before this question is decided. If from the presence of adhesions it is impossible to make out the nature of any tumour present, gastro-jejunostomy should be performed, and a further operation undertaken after the lapse of a fortnight. If the mass has been due to chronic ulcer, great improvement will have taken place ; in all probability the tumour will have almost completely disappeared, or, even if it be carcinomatous, the subsidence of the coincident inflammatory swelling will have made operation easier.

The death-rate of *simple exploration* without further interference is small ; Mayo Robson estimates it at from 3 to 5 per cent. Among 39 personal cases, 1 died the following day—a patient in whom the disease was very advanced and operation was undertaken to attempt to give some relief to the incessant vomiting, but his condition was so bad that even jejunostomy was thought inadvisable.

Occasionally after an exploratory operation a period of improvement sets in and all symptoms disappear, for a time raising a doubt as to the correctness of the diagnosis. Three such cases have been under my care.

A man of 48 who had had symptoms for eight weeks was explored in October, 1903, a large malignant growth on the lesser curvature being found. He left hospital a month later, feeling quite well. All symptoms were in abeyance for fourteen months ; they then returned, and he died in hospital in March, 1905, the diagnosis being confirmed at autopsy. A case has been recorded by Keen and Stewart in which symptoms were in abeyance for seventeen months after exploration.

When possible, partial gastrectomy should be carried out (p. 404). In a few cases it may be justifiable to excise at the same time a portion of the liver where the pylorus has become adherent to it, or where the growth has directly attacked it, or a portion of the transverse colon where this is involved.

Total gastrectomy is rarely necessary except in cases of diffuse growth—"leather-bottle" stomach.

With regard to the immediate mortality : Deaver and Ashurst collected 747 cases of *partial gastrectomy* with an immediate mortality of a little over 25 per cent.   This may be taken as about the average immediate mortality at the present time, although individual surgeons have obtained better results—thus, the Mayos' 226 cases with 12·4 per cent. deaths ; Maydl, 16 per cent. ; Mayo Robson, 13 per cent.

Of my 21 cases of partial gastrectomy 3 died as the result of operation ; 1, in whom I excised a wedge-shaped portion of the liver, two months later with a biliary fistula ; another died of shock within twenty-four hours. In the other case the wound was sutured hurriedly with through-and-through stitches on account of the patient's condition, but these gave way on the fourth day, and he died of broncho-pneumonia five days after the second anæsthetic.   Patients are alive without recurrence twenty-seven months, twenty-two months, twenty months, twelve months, eleven months, six months, and four months after operation.   Of those in whom recurrence took place, the earliest was at three months, the latest at thirty months.

In 127 cases analysed by Hey Groves in which the cause of death was given, peritonitis accounted for 78, shock 23, lung complications 20.

With improved methods of operating, the death-rate should certainly be no more than 15 per cent.

As to the after-results, cases have been recorded well fourteen years (Braun), thirteen years, twelve years (Lemoin), eleven and a half years (Maydl), eight years (Goldschwend), five years and ten months (Poncet) after operation.

The average duration of life after partial gastrectomy in cases in which recurrence takes place is about eighteen months.   The quality of the life is good, and death occurs less painfully.   Recurrence is rare after two years ; if life is prolonged beyond four years, there is a good prospect of cure.   From the collected statistics of Paterson, 15 per cent. of the number operated upon lived five years or more. In 140 resections of stomach for carcinoma recorded by Kocher (1910), 20 per cent. remained well for over four years.

At the present time it is safe to say that the general operative mortality is about 25 per cent. ; of the 75 per cent. who recover, 60 per cent. will succumb to the disease within three years, after a period of comparative comfort, and 15 will survive over five years and may possibly be cured.   These figures will show great improvement in the future.

The death-rate of total gastrectomy appears to be about 40 per cent.; in 27 cases collected by Paterson it was 36 per cent. The average duration of life in those in which recurrence took place was nineteen months; 17 per cent. were free from symptoms five years after operation; 1 was well at eight, and 1 at seven years after operation.

Gastro-jejunostomy should be performed for the relief of symptoms when pyloric obstruction is present. The death-rate in these cases is considerably higher than when the operation is performed for simple diseases.

Poncet, Delore and Leriche have recorded 87 cases with 33 per cent. death-rate; Kindl, 21 per cent.; Moynihan, 35 cases, 14 per cent. death-rate; Sherren, 27 cases, 5 deaths.

With regard to the duration of life: this cannot be predicted. The average appears to be about six months, but the operation must be done only in the cases stated. The longest duration in my cases was two years, with absolute comfort for twenty-two months; another lived fifteen months, with comfort for thirteen; a third nine months, with comfort for eight; whilst in the others death took place within six months; but the relief afforded by the operation in all made it worth doing. Unless the growth is causing pyloric obstruction, relief of symptoms is not obtained.

The radical treatment of carcinoma of the cardiac end of the stomach is at present in the experimental stage. The researches of Sauerbruch, Willy Meyer, Janeway and Green, Meltzer and Auer, Brauer, and others have raised hope that it may be possible to extend operative interference to this portion of the stomach. Three cases have been recorded in which operation was carried out, the growth being removed and œsophago-gastrostomy done (Wendel, Wiener, Janeway and Green): death occurred from secondary hæmorrhage in the first case, in the second from subphrenic abscess twelve days after operation; and the third died fifty-four hours later with an empyema.

Gastrostomy should be performed when it becomes impossible to take food. The immediate mortality is not high, and an interval of comfort of from three to six months, in some cases as long as eighteen, is given.

Jejunostomy is an operation rarely advisable for carcinoma of the stomach, though it may be performed to obtain relief from pain and vomiting. Patients seldom survive operation longer than a few weeks. The immediate mortality in 127 cases of jejunostomy collected by Billon was 29 per cent., and the majority of patients succumbed under two months; only one lived for a year.

CARCINOMA OF THE DUODENUM

Carcinoma of the duodenum is rare. Maydl and Schlesinger found that it represented 2 per cent. of the primary malignant growths of intestine. Fenwick states its comparative frequency as compared with carcinoma of the stomach as 1 to 20; but if anything this over-states the frequency.

It is more common in men than in women (Fenwick, 37 men, 14 women), and is most common between the ages of 40 and 50. It may originate in a chronic ulcer; according to Fenwick, at least 10 instances have been recorded. In 3 cases observed by Mayo, in one certainly and in another probably, it had its origin in this manner; the third case was too far advanced to enable any opinion to be given. In some cases it has been associated with gall-stones.

It most frequently arises in the second part of the duodenum. In 41 cases collected by Rolleston, 24 had their origin here, 8 in the first part; while in 51 collected by Fenwick, 29 were in the second part, 11 in the first, 7 in the third. It may be secondary to carcinoma of the pancreas, of the gall-bladder or bile-ducts.

The growth is usually cylindrical-celled, and has a constricting effect, like a similar growth elsewhere. When composed of spheroidal cells it forms a soft, flat mass or a deep fungating ulcer. Colloid degeneration may occur.

Symptoms.—These vary with the portion of the duodenum involved.

1. In the **supra-ampullary** variety the symptoms resemble pyloric carcinoma and may very rarely follow those of chronic ulcer. Diagnosis from pyloric carcinoma is impossible. A fixed or only slightly mobile tumour can usually be felt in the right hypochondrium.

2. Carcinoma in the **peri-ampullary** portion most often arises in the mucous membrane covering the biliary papilla. Usually, owing to the involvement of the papilla, jaundice is present (in 23 out of 25 of Mathieu's cases); it is often intermittent, thus differing from that due to carcinoma of the head of the pancreas or of the common bile-duct.

Painless jaundice is usually the first symptom, and is followed by gastric symptoms due to dilatation. The gall-bladder is usually distended, and occasionally a fixed tumour can be felt in the right hypochondrium near the middle line. (Plate 90.)

Not infrequently infection and suppurative cholangitis occurs.

3. In the **infra-ampullary** cases the stomach and duodenum are dilated, and the symptoms resemble those of pyloric obstruction, but with one important difference, viz. that the vomit always contains bile and pancreatic juice. The latter can be demonstrated by the digestion of fibrin after a few grains of sodium bicarbonate have been added to the filtered vomit. Intermittent attacks of intestinal obstruction are also common.

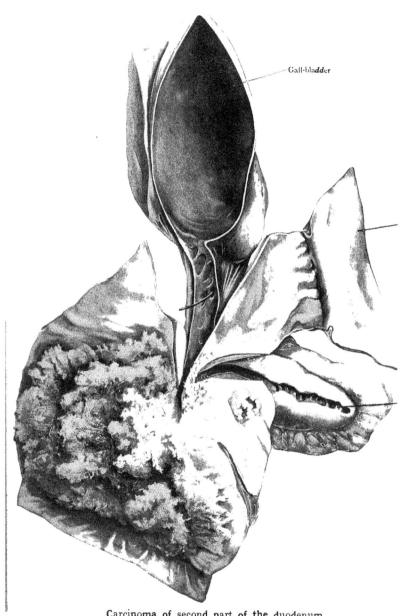

Gall-bladder

Carcinoma of second part of the duodenum.

(Pathological Institute, London Hospital.)

PLATE 90.

Prognosis.—The average duration of life is about seven months (Fenwick). Hæmorrhage, perforation, abscess, external or internal fistula, may complicate the course of the disease.

Treatment. — Palliative treatment is frequently all that is possible. In most cases this will consist in gastro-jejunostomy, but, when obstructive jaundice is present, relief may be obtained by chole-cystenterostomy. When the growth involves the first portion of the duodenum, removal, together with the adjacent portion of stomach, subpyloric and right gastro-epiploic glands, should be carried out. Carcinoma of the third part of the duodenum has been successfully removed by Syme. Hitherto, operations for malignant growth of the second portion of the duodenum have been palliative only, the growth being locally excised and the common bile-duct re-implanted. Cases have been recorded—by Körte, in which the patient was alive nearly four years after the operation; by Deaver, in which the patient was alive and well one year after operation; and by Czerny, Halsted, and W. J. Mayo, in which the patient died a few days after operation. Radical operation in this situation will always necessitate removal of a portion of the pancreas in addition to the duodenum. The duodenum and head of the pancreas were first removed by Codivilla in 1898, gastro-jejunostomy and cholecystenterostomy being performed, and the patient dying twenty-four days later.

Attention has again been directed to this possibility by the recent work of French surgeons. Desjardins, in 1907, and Sauvé, in 1908, published suggested methods of operation, which, however, had the same failing, that they were operations intended to be completed in one stage. As patients with obstructive jaundice stand prolonged operative procedures badly, Kausch, in 1909, devised and carried out successfully a two-stage operation which is an advance in the surgery of this region. At the first operation the gall-bladder was united to the jejunum and entero-anastomosis done below. At the second operation, performed after disappearance of the jaundice, a posterior gastro-enterostomy was made, the pylorus divided and closed, and the descending portion of duodenum removed. The common bile-duct was ligatured after as much as necessary had been removed, a portion of the head of the pancreas excised, and the lower duodenal end then drawn over the stump. The case was reported a month after operation.

SARCOMA OF THE STOMACH

Sarcoma of the stomach is a comparatively rare disease. It was first recorded by Sibley in 1816; Schlesinger, in 1897 was able to collect 35 cases; Howard, in 1902, 61 cases; Ziesche and Davidsohn, in 1900, 150 cases.

It may occur at any age, but is most common between the ages of 30 and 50. The sexes are equally affected, except in fibro-sarcoma, which is more common in women.

Fenwick estimated that sarcomas constitute from 3 to 8 per cent. of all tumours of the stomach.

The growth may be composed of round or spindle cells, and the intercellular substance may be very scanty, or it may be definitely fibrous. Myomatous, myxomatous, or angiomatous tissue may be found in any given case.

The round-celled sarcoma is the most common type (60 per cent.), spindle-celled the next (36 per cent.).

Four types can be recognized: (1) Round-celled sarcoma. (2) Spindle-celled sarcoma. (3) Lympho-sarcoma. (4) Secondary to sarcoma of retroperitoneal glands.

1. *Round-celled* sarcoma commences in the submucous tissue, and may be diffuse or may form a circumscribed tumour projecting into the lumen of the stomach. It occurs most commouly in the pyloric region and along the greater curvature, but rarely gives rise to pyloric obstruction. The whole organ may be affected. Metastases are commonly present.

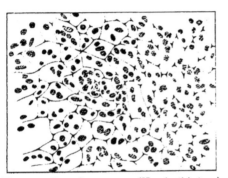

Fig. 388.—Lympho-sarcoma (Kundrath's type).

(*Salaman, Proc. of Path. Soc.*)

2. *Spindle-celled* sarcomas, fibro - sarcomas, myo-sarcomas or endotheliomas usually form circumscribed tumours springing from the greater curvature, and presenting a polypoid mass. They are all liable to myxomatous change and cyst-formation. They tend to project towards the serous coat, and may fill the greater part of the abdominal cavity.

3. *Lympho-sarcomas* are composed of lymphoid cells in a fibrillar meshwork (Kundrath, *see* Fig. 388). Originating in a lymph follicle of mucous membrane, or a lymphatic gland in the pharynx or any part of the intestinal tract, they may spread along the wall of these tubes and bring about dilatation of the lumen. In some cases polypoid submucous growths are present.

In the stomach they originate in the submucous tissue, and may spread throughout the intestinal tract, thus differing from round-celled sarcoma, which is confined to the stomach.

The growth, although commencing in the submucous tissue, infiltrates all the coats of the stomach and thus causes marked increase in thickness of the wall; in the case described by Salaman it measured at one place 1½ in. According to Salaman, 12 cases of this nature have been recorded. Some of these tumours have been described as lymphadenomas of stomach, a condition which, if it occurs at all, is very rare.

4. *Secondary to retroperitoneal glands.*—The intestinal tract is never, or rarely affected in true lymphadenoma. It is well known that, in lymphadenoma in other parts of the body, glands which for years have been clinically " lymphadenomatous " may coalesce and infiltrate

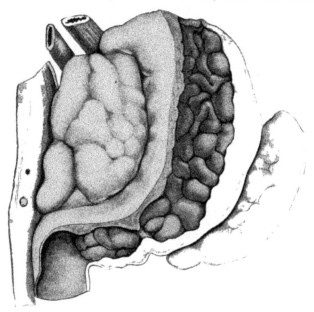

Fig. 389.—Secondary involvement of stomach in " lymph-adenoma."

(*Salaman, Proc. of Path. Soc.*)

the surrounding tissues. It is probable that the cases in which the stomach is involved secondarily to neighbouring glands are instances of this nature (Fig. 389). Many groups of glands and the tonsils are usually involved. Salaman collected 8 cases and suggested the name lymphadeno-sarcoma for these growths.

Symptoms.—The symptoms of round-celled sarcoma resemble those of carcinoma of the stomach. A tumour is present in about 30 per cent. of these cases. Hæmorrhage is rare. Secondary deposits in the skin are not uncommon.

Chemical examination of the gastric contents gives a result similar to that found in gastric carcinoma (p. 385).

In the spindle-celled variety gastric symptoms may be absent, but hæmatemesis was observed in half the cases. A tumour is nearly always present, smooth, painless, and mobile.

Prognosis.—The average duration of life is about fifteen months in round-celled sarcoma, twenty-eight months in spindle-celled. Death usually occurs from exhaustion. Perforation has taken place in 10 per cent. of the cases of round-celled sarcoma.

Treatment.—This is the same as for carcinoma. Ziesche and Davidsohn have collected records of 53 operations, in 32 of which resection was carried out, with a mortality of 25 per cent.

Partial gastrectomy on the lines of that carried out for carcinoma is necessary in all cases of diffuse growth. In the pedunculated form, removal of the growth with the portion of gastric wall from which it springs is all that is necessary.

Gastro-jejunostomy should be carried out when resection is impossible and pyloric obstruction is present.

SARCOMA OF THE DUODENUM

Primary sarcoma of the duodenum is extremely rare. As a rule it is round-celled and involves the whole duodenum. Obstruction is rarely produced, the lumen of the gut being usually increased.

TUBERCULOSIS, SYPHILIS, FISTULÆ, ETC.

TUBERCULOSIS OF THE STOMACH

Tuberculosis of the stomach is usually secondary to tuberculosis elsewhere, most often in the lung. It may occur as a primary lesion ; Barchasch states that 6 cases had been recorded up to 1907. Of 107 cases studied by Ricard and Chevrier, in 3 only was the stomach alone involved. It is more uncommon than tuberculous infection of the intestine ; thus, in over 3,000 autopsies on tuberculous subjects (Dürk, Simmonds, Letulle) the stomach was affected 13 times only, whereas intestinal infection is stated to occur in over 50 per cent. of post-mortems on tuberculous subjects.

Infection probably occurs through an erosion becoming infected by the tubercle bacillus.

Tuberculosis of the stomach presents two clinical types—(1) hypertrophic ; (2) ulcerative.

1. The hypertrophic variety usually affects the pyloric region, and, as in other parts of the alimentary canal, is frequently mistaken for carcinoma. This is the least usual form of disease, and shows itself by symptoms of stenosis.

2. A tuberculous ulcer usually occurs in the body of the stomach, frequently runs transversely to the axis of the viscus, and has all the characters of a tuberculous ulcer elsewhere.

The **symptoms** are variable. Perforation and hæmatemesis rarely occur. In one patient, a man of 34 who was under my care with a tuberculous ulcer of the anterior wall of the stomach, the symptoms were indefinite and consisted of epigastric pain and vomiting without definite relation to food. In addition to the tuberculous ulcer of stomach, tuberculous peritonitis was present. Exploration was followed by recovery, and the patient is in perfect health at the time of writing, four years after operation.

Prognosis depends upon the presence and condition of tubercle elsewhere in the body.

Treatment.—Operation should only be carried out to relieve pyloric obstruction, when gastro-jejunostomy should be performed. Otherwise the patient should be subjected to general treatment, as adopted for tuberculosis elsewhere.

SYPHILIS OF THE STOMACH

Tertiary syphilitic lesions may be found in the stomach, but they are rare, not more than 50 cases having been recorded. The disease starts in the submucous tissue, and may be diffuse or localized. Ulceration follows in both varieties; perforation may occur; a stricture may be produced at either orifice, more frequently at the pyloric; or a tumour may form, simulating carcinoma. Of 12 cases observed by Bird, 11 were situated in the pyloric region.

The disease is most common in men between the ages of 25 and 40. Fenwick states that pain and vomiting are more severe and hæmorrhage is less common than in simple ulcer.

Diagnosis.—There is no single symptom or combination of symptoms which will enable the diagnosis to be made from a chronic gastric ulcer or malignant growth. Its presence should be suspected when gastric symptoms occur in a syphilitic patient, and will be confirmed if, after resistance to the usual measures of treatment, they subside under mercury and iodides.

Partial gastrectomy has been performed (Tuffier, Bird) for what was considered to be carcinoma but proved to be a gummatous tumour. In nearly all the cases other abdominal manifestations of syphilis are present. Stress is laid upon peritoneal involvement and the occurrence of gummata in the liver. With regard to the former, Bird has frequently noted the presence of bluish striæ following the course of the lymphatics, or of opaque bluish-white patches on the peritoneal coat.

It must be remembered that gastric symptoms frequently arise in patients taking antisyphilitic remedies by the mouth, and that gastric syphilis is a late manifestation.

Treatment.—The usual antisyphilitic remedies should be given. If pyloric or cardiac stenosis is present, unaffected by drugs, gastro-jejunostomy or gastrotomy must be undertaken.

PLASTIC LINITIS (CIRRHOSIS OF STOMACH; FIBRO-MATOSIS OF STOMACH—Alexis Thomson)

This rare disease, first named cirrhosis of stomach by Andral in 1845, was accurately described by Brinton in 1859. It is characterized by a diffuse fibrous thickening usually starting at the pyloric region, chiefly involving the submucous coat, and diminishing the capacity of the stomach. Writers are by no means agreed that this condition is a clinical entity, but there seems to be no doubt that, although rare, such a condition exists. Definite cases have been recorded by Osler, Leith, Sheldon, and Jonnesco. It may be impossible, even after microscopical examination of the stomach or, in most cases, of the enlarged lymphatic glands, to say if the condition is simple (plastic linitis) or malignant (diffuse scirrhus carcinoma), for the section examined may show no sign of malignancy, but secondary deposits of carcinoma may be present in the liver; or the after-course only may render the diagnosis certain. I have had 4 cases under my care; in 3 the section of the stomach wall showed no sign of malignancy, but in one of these secondary growths were present in the liver, and in another the after-progress left no doubt that the growth was malignant.

The causation of the condition is obscure when those cases secondary to diffuse atrophic carcinoma are excluded.

It is a disease of adult life more common in men than in women. The stomach is of normal size or contracted; it may be freely mobile or fixed by adhesions; externally it presents a peculiar pearly-white appearance. On section it is found to be of diminished capacity, and all its coats stand out (*see* Fig. 386). The thickening chiefly affects the submucous coat, which is many times the normal thickness. The mucous membrane is not usually affected. The change is, as a rule, most marked in the pyloric region.

Symptoms.—As pointed out by Brinton, the condition may be found after death, no symptoms having been produced during life.

It is a disease of insidious onset, with pain and vomiting. The patient loses weight, and a tumour is usually found extending from under the left costal margin. Rarely, free fluid may be present in the peritoneal cavity. Free HCl is usually absent from the gastric contents after a test meal.

Diagnosis.—This should be suggested by a tumour under the left costal margin, if there is difficulty in inflating the stomach and the stomach will not hold more than a small quantity of fluid.

Treatment.—When possible, gastrectomy, complete or partial, should be done, for it is impossible to be certain whether the condition is simple or malignant. Moynihan has recorded a case which appeared clinically to be one of plastic linitis, for which he successfully performed total gastrectomy; microscopic examination later showed the growth to be malignant. Where this treatment is not feasible, gastro-jejunostomy should be performed if the condition of the stomach will permit. Sheldon has recorded a case well three and a half years, Deaver one well two and a half years after this operation. It may be necessary to perform jejunostomy.

PHLEGMONOUS GASTRITIS (SUBMUCOUS GASTRITIS; SUPPURATIVE LINITIS)

This is a rare condition of diffuse inflammation of the submucous layer of the stomach, occasionally going on to suppuration.

Since the recognition of the disease by P. Borel, in 1656, the number of recorded cases is under 100. The condition is more common in men than in women, and may occur at any age, but is most often seen between 20 and 40. In 25 per cent. of the cases there is a history of chronic alcoholism.

Etiology and pathology.—Phlegmonous gastritis is an infective cellulitic inflammation of the submucous tissue of the stomach, which may diffusely involve the whole stomach or be localized. The infecting micro-organism present is usually a streptococcus. In a case recorded by J. E. Adams a pure culture of pneumococcus was obtained. The organism may obtain entrance through an ulcer, simple or malignant, or a wound, accidental or operative. In some cases the origin of the infection cannot be discovered; in others it is associated with some acute infective disease, such as typhoid or puerperal fever; whilst cases have been recorded following the ingestion of infected food. There are, therefore, two groups—primary, in which the infection occurs through a lesion of the stomach wall; and secondary, complicating other diseases. J. E. Adams has recently suggested that the term primary should be applied only to those cases in which no naked-eye lesion of the gastric wall can be discovered; secondary, to those in which the infection spreads from an ulcer, simple or malignant, or from an operation wound. But as it is probable that in all, except those complicating disease elsewhere, the micro-organism gains entrance through the wall of the stomach, the term primary should not be limited to those in which the seat of entrance is visible to the naked eye.

The stomach-wall is increased in thickness, often to eight or nine times its normal size. The peritoneal coat in the early stage is unaltered, but in the later stage shows signs of inflammation. The mucous membrane is swollen and often hyperæmic and ecchymotic. The submucous coat is markedly thickened, yellowish-white in appearance, and soft, and occasionally presents tiny abscesses. Peritonitis is found in most of the cases. When the disease is circumscribed the pyloric end is most often affected, and a localized abscess may form.

A similar condition may occur in the duodenum. Ungermann has recently collected 6 cases of phlegmonous duodenitis, in 3 of which the disease was localized in the duodenum alone. The inflammation was most marked in the region of the biliary papilla.

Symptoms.—The onset is usually sudden, with severe epigastric pain, vomiting, and prostration. The pain is constant and accompanied at first by localized rigidity. The patient is obviously suffering from some acute septic condition; the pulse is feeble, the temperature is elevated, and the tongue is dry and furred. Later the signs of general peritonitis are added.

Prognosis.—No case of generalized phlegmonous gastritis has recovered. In a case of the localized variety, in which a definite abscess formed, recovery followed operation and evacuation of the abscess (Bovée); and in a similar case spontaneous recovery followed rupture of the abscess into the stomach, the pus being vomited.

Diagnosis.—This has so far never been made before operation; and when we consider that it has to be made from a perforative lesion of the stomach or duodenum and acute pancreatitis, it is unlikely that it will often be possible. The history of alcoholism, the frequent vomiting, and the profound general disturbance should cause the condition to be suspected.

In the localized form, after an acute onset the symptoms abate, and a swelling palpable through the abdominal wall may form. This may rupture into the peritoneal cavity, causing general peritonitis, or into the stomach; recovery has followed the latter accident.

Treatment.—In the diffuse variety, if exploration is undertaken before general peritonitis has supervened, multiple incisions down to the submucosa should be made after packing over the stomach area with gauze. In the localized form, incision and drainage should be carried out.

GASTRIC AND DUODENAL FISTULÆ

Fistulæ connected with either stomach or duodenum are rare. The fistula may be an "internal" one connecting the organ with another viscus, or an "external" one opening on the surface of the body. Of gastric fistulæ, the internal is the more common; a duodenal fistula is much rarer, and here the external fistula is more frequent than the internal.

GASTRIC FISTULÆ

On account of the development of gastric surgery these cases are rarer now than formerly; external gastric fistulæ are particularly uncommon.

External Fistulæ

Fall into two groups, the traumatic and the pathological, the latter being divided into primary, in which the causal disease originates in the stomach, and secondary, in which it begins in a neighbouring organ. Lieblein and Hilgenreiner based their article (*Deutsche Chirurgie*) in 1905 on 120 published cases. Formerly gastric ulcer was the most common cause; now it is rarely seen except in advanced malignant disease.

1. Traumatic.—Alexis St. Martin was the most celebrated example of this condition. Fistulæ rarely form nowadays as the result of injuries to the stomach, immediate operation saving the patient from this risk. Cases have been recorded in which a foreign body swallowed has perforated the stomach, caused a perigastric abscess which has opened externally, and thus led to a gastric fistula. A fistula occasionally follows operations upon the stomach and neighbouring organs; and cases have been recorded following operations upon pancreatic cysts, cholecysto-gastrostomy, gastro-enterostomy, and nephrectomy.

2. Pathological. (*a*) *Primary.*—In both simple and malignant ulcers of the stomach, fistula may be a secondary result of subacute perforation, a perigastric abscess forming, which is opened or bursts through the anterior abdominal wall. In a few cases the fistula may be the result of the direct involvement of the abdominal wall.

Cases have been recorded in which the stomach was contained in a strangulated ventral hernia, and a fistula followed operation.

(*b*) *Secondary.*—These are usually due to disease of the liver and gall-bladder; cases have also been recorded after operation upon hydatid cysts of liver, etc.

Symptoms.—The characteristic feature is the discharge of stomach contents from an opening, situated in most cases in the lower epigastric region, the umbilical region, or the left hypochondrium. If it is small, very little effect is produced on the general condition of the patient; if the discharge is great the patient wastes, and much discomfort is caused by irritation of the skin.

The diagnosis may have to be made from duodenal fistula; this is usually easy from the position of the external opening, and is facilitated by noting the characters of the discharge and the lapse of time between ingestion of food and its appearance at the opening. In a gastric fistula, food generally appears within a short time of

2 *a*

ingestion, while delay occurs in duodenal fistula and the discharge is often bile-stained.

Prognosis.—This depends upon the causation. Patients have lived as long as thirty-five years after the formation of the fistula. If the pylorus is unobstructed and the fistula not large, spontaneous healing will occur; thus, it takes place in most postoperative cases and in those following the perforation of ulcers on the anterior surface of the stomach.

Treatment.—Resort to operative treatment should not be hurried unless the escape of gastric contents is great. In these cases, after packing the external opening with gauze and thoroughly cleaning the skin in its neighbourhood, an elliptical incision should be made around it, the peritoneal cavity opened, the fistulous tract dissected down to the stomach, and the opening closed. If the fistulæ is due to malignant disease, or the condition of the patient will not permit of extensive operation, jejunostomy may be performed. Where the condition is not interfering with the general health, it may be left in the hope that it will eventually close.

Internal Fistulæ

These may be the result of injuries (usually operative), or of disease, primary or secondary. The communication is most frequently with the colon, more rarely with the gall-bladder, duodenum (Plate 91), lung, pancreas, urinary tract, or œsophagus.

Gastro-colic fistula is usually the result of carcinoma (65 out of 84 cases—Chavannaz), mostly of the stomach, much less frequently of the colon. It may result from simple ulcer, tuberculous disease of colon, perigastric abscess due to disease of neighbouring organs, or ulcer of the jejunum following gastro-jejunostomy.

The fistulous opening in the stomach is most common at the greater curvature near the pyloric end; that in the colon, in the middle of the transverse part.

Symptoms.—The condition may exist without giving rise to symptoms, but in the majority of cases they are definite and consist of fæcal vomiting and diarrhœa, the motions containing undigested food which in some cases appears soon after it has been taken. In many cases a similarity between motion and vomit has been noticed.

Diagnosis may be confirmed, if this is necessary, by distending the stomach or colon with air. No difficulty arises except in hysterical women.

Sir Frederick Treves recorded an example—a woman of 20 vomited formed fæces, and an enema of methylene blue a few minutes after it was given; at operation, all abdominal organs were normal. The patient had undergone two operations previously. Similar cases have been reported by others.

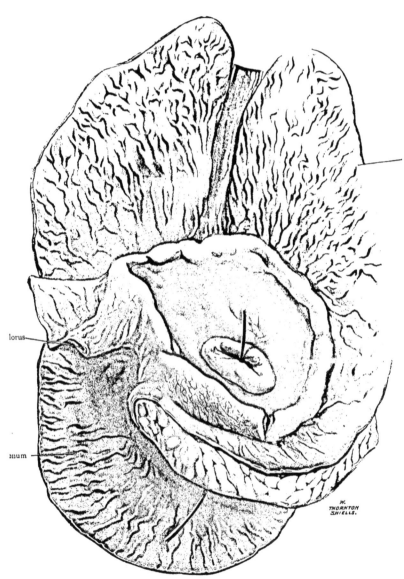

lorus

anum

W.
THORNTON
SHIELLS.

Gastro-duodenal fistula, the result of carcinoma of the stomach.
The probe passes from stomach to duodenum.

(*Pathological Institute, London Hospital.*)

PLATE 91.

No mistakes should occur if the existence of these cases is remembered, for they occur in well-nourished, hysterical women, whereas the patients with gastro-colic fistula are obviously ill.

Prognosis.—This is bad. Spontaneous closure is said to have occurred in two cases.

Treatment will depend upon the causation. If this is malignant growth, wide dissection followed by end-to-end suture of colon and partial gastrectomy (p. 404) should be performed if possible. If the growth is too far advanced to admit of this, short-circuiting operations should be done.

Other kinds of Internal Fistulæ

Fistulous communications between the gall-bladder and biliary passages and stomach or duodenum, although relatively rare, are, after the gastro-colic, the most common form of fistula. Cases have been recorded in which patients vomited gall-stones ; more often the fistulous communication is with the duodenum, and no symptoms result unless a stone passes into the intestines large enough to cause intestinal obstruction.

The symptoms of a stomach-gall-bladder fistula are usually bilious vomiting and, in some cases, dilatation of the stomach due to surrounding adhesions.

Treatment.—The gall-bladder should be separated from the stomach, and the opening into the latter closed. The gall-bladder should be drained or removed, according to its condition, and gastro-jejunostomy done if necessary.

DUODENAL FISTULÆ

These are rare. They may follow operation upon gall-bladder, duodenum, or kidney, particularly the first-named, the duodenum being torn, or injured by the pressure of a drainage-tube. When the duodenum has been mobilized for the purpose of removing a stone from the retroduodenal portion of the common duct, a fistula may result. Fistula is not an uncommon sequel to the perforation of a duodenal ulcer ; it may follow suture, the opening of a subdiaphragmatic abscess or of one due to retroperitoneal perforation ; the external opening is usually in the right hypochondrium, but in the case last mentioned may be in the loin or even in the inguinal region.

Internal fistulæ have been described, the duodenum communicating with stomach or colon. These are pathological curiosities. The only common form is that between duodenum and gall-bladder secondary to disease of the latter.

Prognosis.—In the cases following operation the fistula usually heals spontaneously. Recovery is recorded in one case only (Lawford Knaggs) following perforation of an ulcer.

Treatment.—The treatment is on the same lines as in external gastric fistulæ (p. 402). If spontaneous closure does not occur or delay is inadvisable, gastro-jejunostomy should be performed with simultaneous closure of the pylorus by infolding. This was carried out in Lawford Knaggs' case.

GASTRIC OPERATIONS

General considerations.—Care must be taken to render the upper part of the alimentary tract as sterile as possible ; the mouth must be attended to, and all septic teeth treated. For twenty-four hours before operation, nothing but sterile milk or Benger's food should be given. If examination gives evidence of gastric stasis, the stomach should be washed out an hour before operation ; if dilatation is great, lavage should be employed twice a day for several days before operation is undertaken.

When the abdomen has been opened, the whole of the stomach and duodenum must be carefully examined ; then the condition of other organs—particularly the gall-bladder and appendix—investigated.

After recovering from the effects of the anæsthetic the patient should be propped up in bed, and nursed as far as possible in this position. When lying down the dorsal position is unnecessary, and the patient may be turned from side to side as desired. Vomiting is unusual, and during the first twenty-four hours the patient should be allowed to drink as much water as he wishes. On the day following operation, milk, Benger's food, bread and milk, and tea can be given, and solid food usually by the second week. For the first week or ten days the patient is better in bed, but he may be allowed up about the tenth day. This rule may be broken without fear of evil consequences, if confinement to bed is inadvisable, unless the wound has been allowed to remain open for drainage. An action of the bowels should be obtained by enema the day following operation.

GASTRECTOMY

Gastrectomy may be described under two headings, partial and complete. The term *partial gastrectomy* should be restricted to a definite operation, i.e. removal of the pyloric portion of the stomach together with the whole of the lesser curvature and a varying portion of the greater curvature, never less than its pyloric half. When small portions of the stomach-wall are removed the operation should be called resection. In *complete gastrectomy* the whole of the stomach is removed, from the duodenum to the œsophagus.

Partial Gastrectomy

In this operation, when carried out (as it usually is) for malignant disease, in addition to the part of the stomach mentioned above, the primary lymphatic glands, the lesser omentum, and as much as possible of the great omentum must be removed, together with about an inch of the duodenum.

Closure of the gastric and duodenal cut ends and anastomosis by gastro-enterostomy (Billroth II.) is certainly preferable either to Billroth's original operation of pylorectomy combined with end-to-end junction (Billroth I., 1881), or to Kocher's modification in which he closed the cut end of the stomach and implanted the open duodenal end into the posterior gastric wall. If sufficient stomach is removed both of these methods are difficult and are liable to permit leakage.

After ligaturing and dividing the lesser omentum close to the liver, and the pyloric and gastro-duodenal arteries close to their origin from the hepatic, the operator divides the left gastro-epiploic artery between ligatures, and then inserts his hand into the lesser sac behind the stomach so as to free it, if necessary, from the pancreas, and to separate the anterior layers of the great omentum from the transverse mesocolon. Care is necessary at this stage to avoid the middle colic artery. Injury to this vessel has resulted in the death of the patient from gangrene and perforation of the transverse colon.

The duodenum is then divided between clamps at least an inch beyond the pylorus, and closed with through-and-through stitches of fine chromic gut, buried by a continuous silk stitch. All the fatty tissue and glands in the angle between the stomach and duodenum must be removed.

The coronary artery is then sought at its origin and divided, and all the tissue here removed down to the stomach. The stomach can then be pulled well over to the left. Posterior gastro-jejunostomy should be performed, the stomach removed between two clamps, and the cut end closed in a manner similar to that adopted for the duodenum. The right suprapancreatic glands lying along the hepatic artery should be then sought for and removed.

It may be necessary to excise the whole or a portion of the transverse colon with the stomach, either because it is invaded by the growth or because its blood-supply is endangered.

Hey Groves has suggested that operation in two stages would lower the death-rate. A two-stage operation should only be performed in pyloric carcinoma when the condition of the patient is bad, or when the diagnosis is uncertain. A preliminary gastro-jejunostomy is useless if the growth is not producing obstruction. In two cases of my own, after gastro-jejunostomy for early malignant growth of the pylorus, in which the condition of the patient did not justify a one-stage operation, the second stage was refused on account of the great improvement which had taken place, and both patients died within eighteen months.

Rodman's operation.—This is a variety of partial gastrectomy performed for indurated ulcer of the pyloric end of the stomach in cases in which the diagnosis from carcinoma is uncertain. Rodman excises the ulcer-bearing area in all cases of pyloric ulcer. His operation differs from that just described in that the whole of the lesser curvature, the duodenum, or glands need not be removed, but both duodenum and stomach should be closed and posterior gastro-jejunostomy performed.

COMPLETE GASTRECTOMY

The operation is begun as in partial gastrectomy, but the entire great omentum and then the gastro-splenic omentum are ligatured off. After division of the coronary artery the stomach can be pulled well out. It should not be removed yet, but a coil of jejunum brought up, clamped, and united to the extreme cardiac end of the stomach by stitches passing through serous and muscular coats. An opening is then made in both, and gradually enlarged as stitches are put in through all the coats of each viscus, the stomach in this way being removed. Finally, the operation is completed by the insertion of an anterior row of sero-muscular stitches; or the jejunum may be divided completely, its distal end anastomosed to the œsophagus, and its proximal into its distal portion.

GASTRO-ENTEROSTOMY

This operation consists in making an anastomosis between the stomach and the small intestine. The jejunum is usually chosen (gastro-jejunostomy), in a few cases the duodenum (gastro-duodenostomy).

GASTRO-JEJUNOSTOMY

This may be performed to the anterior or posterior surface of the stomach. The latter is the operation of choice. At first a loop was left between the anastomosis and the duodeno-jejunal junction, but this should never be done (see p. 413).

Posterior Gastro-Jejunostomy

After careful examination of the stomach, the transverse colon and omentum are withdrawn from the abdomen and an opening made in the transverse mesocolon, beginning close to the point at which it is in contact with the jejunum. The opening should then be enlarged, care being taken to avoid injury to vessels. The portion of stomach wall which is to be used for the anastomosis is drawn through this opening and clamped in a vertical direction from the lesser to the greater curvature. The duodeno-jejunal flexure is now carefully examined (the jejunum at its origin should always be seen) (p. 299). The jejunum is then stretched tightly from the duodeno-

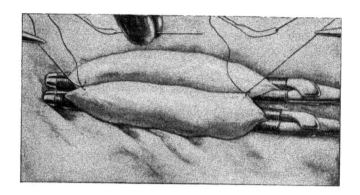

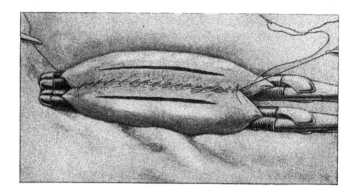

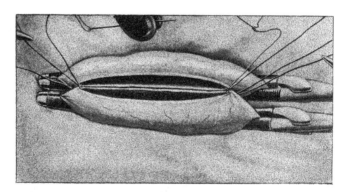

Fig. 390.—Gastro-jejunostomy by the four-stitch method.
(*See* text, *p.* 408.)

jejunal flexure and a second clamp applied, care being taken that the jejunum does not become twisted longitudinally. At least 3 in. of stomach and jejunum should be in the clamps. A strip of gauze should be placed between the clamps, the stomach and jejunum brought together, and the omentum, colon, and rest of the stomach returned to the abdomen. In performing the anastomosis four stitches are used, two of silk and two of chromic gut. The stomach and jejunum are first united by two silk stitches passing through serous and muscular coats at least 3 in. apart (Fig. 390). The thread at the patient's right is then taken, and a continuous sero-muscular stitch inserted from right to left. On reaching the left stitch it is tied off, and its end tied to the loose end of the left stitch. The viscera are opened, redundant mucous membrane is removed, and a chromic-gut stitch passed at each end of the opening through all the coats of the stomach and jejunum. The right-hand needle is then taken and a continuous stitch inserted, care being exercised to pass the needle through all the coats and to insert them sufficiently closely to stop all bleeding. This stitch is tied off in a way similar to that adopted for the silk. The left stitch of chromic gut is inserted continuously from left to right and tied off. After removal of the clamps the left silk stitch is taken, and the sero-muscular suture finished anteriorly.

The posterior surface of the anastomosis is inspected by pulling on the gauze, and finally the opening in the mesocolon is stitched to the stomach close to the line of anastomosis. Performed in this way the results are most satisfactory.

Various modifications have been suggested and used. Mayo unites the jejunum to the stomach in such a manner that it passes to the left. This has not proved so satisfactory in the hands of other surgeons as the vertical operation described above.

Anterior Gastro-Jejunostomy

This was the original operation performed by Wölfer in 1881. It should only be carried out when conditions render the posterior operation impossible. As usually performed it is a " loop " operation. A portion of the jejunum 18 to 24 in. from the duodeno-jejunal flexure is taken and brought up beneath and then in front of the transverse colon, and united to the anterior surface of the stomach. This loop is unnecessary and dangerous. Since 1904 I have always performed the anterior operation without a loop. This operation is, I believe, original, the nearest approach to it being the operation described by Brenner in 1891, in which the jejunum was brought to the stomach by the same route but a long loop was left. The duodeno-jejunal junction is found and an opening made in the transverse mesocolon and gastro-colic omentum immediately over it ; a portion of jejunum

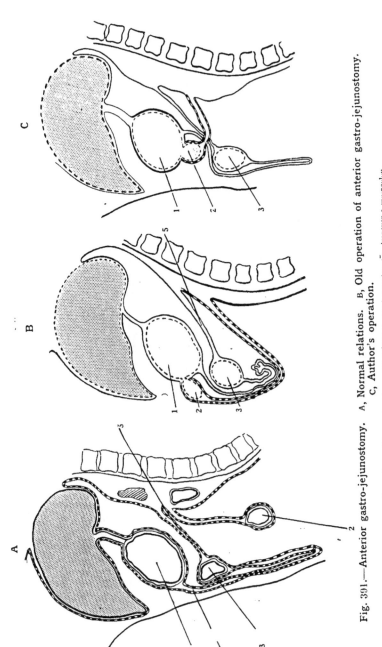

Fig. 391.—Anterior gastro-jejunostomy. A, Normal relations. B, Old operation of anterior gastro-jejunostomy. C, Author's operation.

1, Stomach ; 2, jejunum ; 3, transverse colon ; 4, great omentum ; 5, transverse mesocolon.

close to the duodeno-jejunal flexure is brought up through this and
united to the anterior surface of the stomach (Fig. 390).   At the
end of the operation the opening in the great omentum is stitched
around the stomach.

I have performed this operation now on 26 occasions, and have

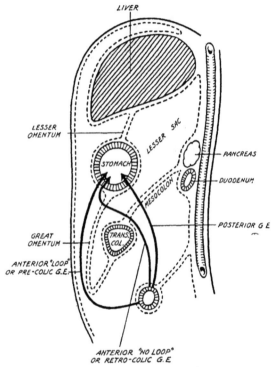

Fig. 392.—To illustrate the three methods of gastro-jejunostomy.

never had trouble, convalescence being as smooth as after the
posterior no-loop operation, with complete absence of any biliary
regurgitation.   The first patient upon whom I performed the operation, for a saddle-shaped chronic gastric ulcer, died of another
cause twenty-eight months later; the ulcer was healed, and the
anastomosis was described by the pathologist as posterior.

Gastro-Enterostomy in Y : Roux's Operation

In this modification of posterior gastro-jejunostomy the jejunum
is completely divided 10 or 12 in. below the duodeno-jejunal flexure,

its distal end implanted into the posterior surface of the stomach, and its proximal into the jejunum about 4 in. below its junction with the stomach.

The operation should not be performed if it is possible to do either of those just described. It is liable to be followed by ulcer of the jejunum (*see* p. 414).

Results of gastro-jejunostomy.—It is beyond dispute that the performance of gastro-jejunostomy is followed by the healing of

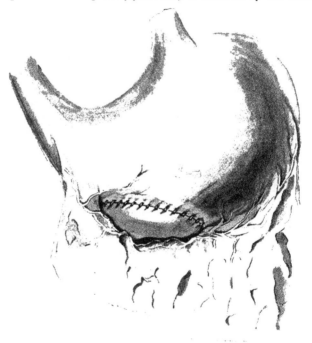

Fig. 393.—Anterior no-loop gastro-jejunostomy, completed except for suturing the opening in the great omentum around the anastomosis.

a chronic ulcer of the stomach or duodenum (*see* p. 351).   Much work has been done on the X-ray examination of the stomach after experimental gastro-jejunostomy on animals, with results that are widely divergent from those obtained in a similar examination on patients. Cannon and Blake, Kelling, and Delbet considered that nothing passed out by the anastomotic opening.   In one of Cannon and Blakes' experiments, in which an exceptionally large opening was found in the pyloric portion of the stomach, some of the food passed out by this channel. On the other hand, Pers of Copenhagen published in 1909 the results of X-ray examination of 40 patients upon whom he had performed gastro-jejunostomy, and found that in 38, irrespectively of the permeability of the pylorus, a bismuth meal passed only through the anastomosis, that in one case it passed through both anastomosis and pylorus, and that in one its course could not be ascertained. In 24 cases the food began to leave the stomach at once. This is in agreement with a case recorded by H. M. W. Gray, in which, after gastro-jejunostomy, pyloric obstruction not being present, food preferred to leave by the anastomotic opening.

Cases have been recorded in which, after gastro-jejunostomy carried out for the treatment of a duodenal fistula, food still passed through the pylorus and escaped at the fistula.

In comparing these results with those of animal experiments, and using them to aid in explaining the occurrences after gastro-jejunostomy for non-obstructive chronic ulcer, it must be remembered that in the one the stomach was healthy, in the other diseased. To settle the question a series of X-ray examinations is needed, taken immediately after operation and at intervals until the ulcer has healed. I believe, from the few cases I have examined with the screen, that after gastro-jejunostomy for chronic ulcer the food passes out by the anastomotic opening, owing to the presence of pyloric spasm, but that when the ulcer has healed this aperture may be no longer used, though by remaining as a safety-valve it prevents an ulcer from again becoming chronic.

Bolton's experiments have proved the importance of impaired motility in preventing the healing of ulcers.

After gastro-jejunostomy the total acidity of the gastric contents is lowered (Willcox, Paterson). This is due partly to the escape of bile or pancreatic juice into the stomach, and also in all probability, as pointed out by Paterson, to the earlier secretion of pancreatic juice and consequent earlier diminution of gastric secretion due to the presence of an acid fluid in the jejunum.

The beneficial effect of gastro-jejunostomy in allowing ulcers to heal is twofold. In the first place, by more rapid emptying of the stomach it prevents irritation of the ulcer; secondly, it leads to diminution of HCl. That the first is a factor is shown by the immediate relief given by operation : it is no uncommon thing to find a patient, a week after gastro-jejunostomy, able to eat solid food ; it is inconceivable that a large ulcer should be healed in a few days by diminution of gastric acidity only.

That the operation has no evil effects on nutrition is proved by the normal growth and development of children who have had gastro-jejunostomy done in infancy for infantile pyloric stenosis. It has been shown by the investigations of Paterson on the absorption of fat and of nitrogen from a mixed diet after gastro-jejunostomy, that the percentage absorbed, although very slightly below the average, is within the limits observed in healthy individuals.

Complications.—The following complications may occur after gastro-jejunostomy, the majority being due to faulty technique : (1) Hæmorrhage ; (2) regurgitant vomiting ; (3) peptic ulcer of jejunum ; (4) intestinal obstruction (internal hernia) ; (5) diarrhœa ; (6) contraction of opening.

1. Several cases have been recorded recently in which **severe hæmorrhage** has followed the operation of gastro-jejunostomy ; in one fatal case the source of the bleeding was discovered to be a vein in the gastric mucous membrane. This has led some to advocate the abandonment of the use of clamps during the operation, on the ground that they prevent the surgeon from seeing vessels that may be bleeding ; others advise that the clamps be loosened after the posterior row of stitches has been inserted. Hæmorrhage is due to faulty application of the inner suture, probably in that it fails to penetrate all the coats of the stomach at one spot ; this may easily occur if too much or too little mucous membrane is removed. It can be prevented by careful suturing.

The only instance of severe hæmatemesis that has occurred in my cases was some years ago, before I used clamps. Three hours after operation the patient vomited about a pint of blood, but no untoward result followed.

The hæmorrhage may in a few cases come from the ulcer itself ; this may be avoided by infolding the ulcer.

2. **Regurgitant vomiting** (vicious circle).—This is rarely met with after the modern no-loop operation. It is due in most cases to faulty technique. In the early days of gastro-jejunostomy it was a much-dreaded and very fatal complication.

Various theories were at one time put forward with regard to it. At first it was thought to be due to the presence of bile in the stomach, but this has been disproved both by animal experiment and as the result of operation. In a case of ruptured duodenum, Moynihan closed both ends and joined the jejunum to the stomach. All the bile and pancreatic juice had to pass through the stomach, but no vomiting ensued.

It is the result of intestinal obstruction, and is due, in most cases, to leaving a loop of jejunum between the flexure and the anastomosis. This becomes " bile-logged," and the fluid, unable to escape, passes backwards into the stomach. In other cases the weight of the loop may cause a kink at the anastomosis. In a few cases a kink may obstruct the efferent opening, or adhesions obstruct the jejunum beyond. As has been pointed out by Paul, Stanmore Bishop, and myself, regurgitant vomiting is liable to arise not only from faulty technique but also from operation upon unsuitable cases, particularly cases of atonic dyspepsia. The only two severe cases of regurgitant vomiting I have met with were in cases in which no lesion was demonstrated in the stomach; both recovered. These are cases which would not now be treated by operation.

Symptoms.—Vomiting after gastro-jejunostomy is uncommon; in most cases no vomiting at all takes place. When, from the presence of adhesions or from trouble in administering the anæsthetic, operation proves to be difficult, copious bilious vomiting may occur, but passes off within forty-eight hours; this I am in the habit of referring to as "paralytic." If it persists longer it is probably truly regurgitant. In the typical case vomiting does not develop for several days after operation. Bilious vomiting may first appear many weeks or months later, although it is unusual to see it after the third week.

In severe cases, large quantities of bile-stained fluid are vomited once or twice a day. The vomit gushes up with very little effort, and as a rule contains no food. Emaciation is rapid, and death occurs unless relief is given. These cases are rare with modern methods of operating.

In less severe cases, vomiting of a similar nature occurs at irregular intervals. In still slighter cases there is regurgitation of small quantities of bilious fluid. In the slight cases the patient may put on weight and obtain complete relief from the symptoms for which the operation was performed.

Treatment.—Lavage should be employed once or twice a day, and continued until the passage of the stomach-tube reveals no excess of fluid in the stomach. In the severe cases coming on soon after operation, if lavage does not speedily relieve, further operation must be undertaken. If a loop has been left, it is usually found distended. Entero-anastomosis between the afferent and efferent limbs should be performed, or the afferent limb divided and implanted into the efferent below the anastomosis (Roux's operation). It may happen that neither is possible, there being no loop; in these cases entero-enterostomy should be carried out by the method employed by Finney for gastro-duodenostomy (p. 418), or a communication made with the second part of the duodenum.

If the operation was performed for symptoms only, and no lesion of stomach found, the anastomosis should be excised and the continuity of intestine re-established.

3. **Peptic jejunal ulcer.**—Ulceration of the jejunum after gastro-

jejunostomy is an uncommon condition. It was first described by Braun in 1889 ; twenty years later, Paterson was able to publish the result of his investigation of 52 certain and 11 doubtful cases. Since that date, cases have been recorded by Battle, Lion and Moreau (2), Maylard, Rubritius, Florschutz ; and I have had two under my care.

The first, a male aged 47, had had a posterior gastro-jejunostomy with entero-anastomosis performed by another surgeon three years previously. Owing to the recurrence of symptoms, I explored and found a chronic ulcer in the jejunum immediately opposite to the opening in the stomach. In the other case I had performed posterior no-loop gastro-jejunostomy six months previously, in a man of 39, for chronic duodenal ulcer. He was suddenly seized with hæmatemesis. At the operation I found a typical round chronic ulcer on the anterior surface of the jejunum, an inch distal to the anastomosis. I excised the ulcer, and he has remained well.

It is impossible to estimate the frequency with which this complication occurs, but it is probably not more than 1 per cent.

The ulcer is usually solitary, and resembles in every respect that met with in the stomach or duodenum. It may be of the acute or the chronic type, and is usually situate in the efferent limb, within an inch of the anastomotic opening. Occasionally, ulceration may be present at the site of anastomosis, involving both stomach and duodenum ; to this type Paterson gave the name of gastro-jejunal. This latter type appears to be the direct result of operation in most cases, and is often associated with infection of an inner silk suture ; non-absorbable material should not be used for this stitch.

Jejunal ulcers have been met with most often in men, and have not been recorded after gastro-jejunostomy for carcinoma of the stomach ; but in one case, published by Einar Key, death occurred from the perforation of a jejunal ulcer, twenty days after partial gastrectomy with anterior gastro-jejunostomy had been performed for carcinoma of the stomach.

Ulcer has been met with after all forms of gastro-jejunostomy, anterior and posterior, with or without a loop, or entero-anastomosis and " en Y " (Roux's operation). It is undoubtedly met with most often after the Y-type of operation (including the loop operations in which entero-anastomosis has been performed), and after anterior loop operations. It is most uncommon after the posterior no-loop operation. Paterson stated, in 1909, that so far no instance had been recorded. Moynihan states that it may occur after the posterior no-loop method ; the case I have recorded bears this out.

Its frequency after the anterior operation is undoubted ; thus, Rubritius has recorded its occurrence in 3 out of 33 cases of anterior gastro-jejunostomy performed by him ; it did not occur among the 45 posterior operations. Mayo Robson observed it once among 30 anterior operations, but not once after 300 posterior operations; W. J. Mayo, not once in 715 operations.

The ulcer appears to be due to a continuance of the conditions that lead to the formation of the original gastric ulcer. (p. 341), the frequency of this complication after the Y and long-loop type of operations being due to their less efficient action in diminishing hyperacidity and to the action of the gastric juice on mucous membrane unused to it. Hyperacidity is frequently present (in 13 out of 18 cases, Paterson).

Those cases in which the ulceration occurs at the anastomotic margin are probably due to infection.

Symptoms.—These may arise at any time from a few days to years after the operation; the shortest recorded interval has been two days, and the longest eight years. In more than half the cases, symptoms appear within a year, in 75 per cent. within two years, of operation.

The cases fall into three groups—(i) those with acute symptoms of perforation or hæmorrhage; (ii) those with symptoms suggesting recurrence of the original trouble; (iii) those with perforation into the colon.

i. Perforation may occur within a few days of operation; as a rule it is about a year later, but it has taken place five years after operation. The patient in the interval has usually been quite free from symptoms. The ulcer may be either an acute or a chronic one. In two instances (Battle, Maylard) after anterior gastro-enterostomy, the patient suffered on two occasions from perforation of a jejunal ulcer. Operation in both patients on both occasions was successful.

The symptoms resemble those of perforated gastric ulcer, and the differential diagnosis is impossible.

ii. About two-thirds of all the recorded cases fall into this group. In some, particularly after the anterior operation, an abdominal tumour develops as the result of a subacute perforation and adhesions to the abdominal wall. The swelling is usually in the region of the upper left rectus muscle. Occasionally a jejunal fistula forms.

iii. In 8 recorded cases (Kaufmann, Czerny, Gosset, Herczel, Cackovic, Florschutz, Lion and Moreau 2), perforation took place into the transverse colon, and in 1 case (Kaufmann) there was a gastro-colic fistula with closure of the gastro-jejunostomy opening. In all the gastro-jejunostomy was posterior, in one (Lion and Moreau) Roux's operation was performed. The ulcer is usually chronic, and symptoms of pain and discomfort after food are followed by vomiting of fæcal material or of vomit with a fæcal odour. In many cases undigested food is passed soon after it is taken.

Treatment.—This should be preventive. The operation should be of the no-loop type and, if possible, posterior. If from the presence of adhesions this is impossible, then the anterior no-loop operation that I have described should be done (p. 408). The anastomotic opening should be large. The appendix should be removed if the condition of the patient permits. Treatment must not cease with the performance of gastro-enterostomy (p. 353).

When perforation has occurred, laparotomy with immediate suture must be carried out. This is the life-saving measure ; but the causes leading to the production of the ulcer may still be acting, for in several cases after the successful suture of a perforation another has occurred at a later date. The condition of the stomach and the size of the anastomotic opening are to be investigated ; if the latter is too small or has closed, the defect must be remedied if possible. The appendix should, if possible, be removed. During recovery, means should be taken to prevent hyperacidity ; and if the operation is found to have been faulty, rectification of this should be discussed. In the second group of causes, prolonged medical treatment should be tried. If this fails, operation should be performed, the anastomosis excised, and a fresh no-loop operation done or both limbs implanted into the stomach.

In the third group, the viscera should be separated, the opening in the colon closed, and a fresh gastro-jejunostomy performed.

4. Intestinal obstruction.—After posterior operations, internal hernia has occurred into the lesser sac (Moynihan, Hartmann, Ashurst). This is to be prevented by suturing the edge of the opening in the mesocolon to the stomach.

Strangulation has taken place beneath the loop formed in anterior gastro-jejunostomy, more rarely in posterior. Barker recorded a case following the latter in which nearly the whole of the small intestine had passed through, and had in addition become twisted on itself.

In anterior loop gastro-enterostomy the colon may be compressed.

5. Diarrhœa occasionally occurs after gastro-jejunostomy. It has been noticed most often in cases of carcinoma. Its causation is unknown. As a rule it soon passes off, but has been fatal. In one case which proved fatal, Kelling could discover no cause post mortem.

6. Contracture and closure of the opening is due to gastro-jejunal ulceration. It more often followed operation performed with the aid of Murphy's button, with its necessary ulceration of the margins of the opening. If healing by first intention takes place, closure will not occur. The inner layer of suture should be of absorbable material to avoid late infection.

Anterior versus posterior gastro-enterostomy.—The *posterior* gastro-jejunostomy is the operation of choice, for the following reasons : 1. It affords better drainage of the stomach, inasmuch as the posterior is also the inferior wall. 2. A higher part

2 b

of the jejunum can be used for anastomosis, and thus less of this important part of the intestine is looped up and thrown out of use. 3. There is no necessity for the formation of a loop with its attendant dangers of internal hernia and obstruction, and therefore symptoms of the so-called " vicious circle " or regurgitant vomiting. 4. There is less danger of the formation of a peptic ulcer.

If the *anterior* method be carried out without a loop in the way I have described the results are as good as in the posterior, but, as it is more difficult of employment and alters the anatomical relation of parts more, it should not be employed where the posterior operation is possible. (Fig. 393.)

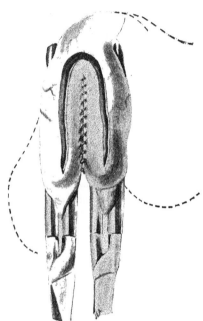

Fig. 394.—Finney's operation of gastro-duodenostomy.

GASTRO-DUODENOSTOMY

This operation is rarely employed, except as Finney's modification, which is explained by Fig. 394. It is useful in cases of fibrous stricture of the pylorus and certain cases of gastroptosis.

JEJUNOSTOMY

This should be done by Mayo Robson's method. A loop of jejunum is taken as high as possible, allowing sufficient length to reach the abdominal wall easily. The two arms of the loop are short-circuited by lateral anastomosis. An opening is made at the top of the loop, then a No. 12 catheter is inserted and passed for 3 in. into the distal limb of the loop, and the margin of the opening inverted by two purse-string sutures. The apex of the loop is fixed to the skin.

BIBLIOGRAPHY

Brinton, *Lectures on the Diseases of the Stomach*, 2nd edit. London, 1864.
Deaver, *J. B.*, and A. P. C. Ashurst, *Surgery of the Upper Abdomen*, vol. i. 1909.
Fenwick, W. Soltau, *Cancer and other Tumours of the Stomach* (1902); and *Ulcer of the Stomach and Duodenum and its Consequences* (1900).

BIBLIOGRAPHY 419

Habershon, S. H., *Diseases of the Stomach.* 1909.
Moynihan, B. G. A., *Duodenal Ulcer.* 1910.
Osler and McCrae, *Cancer of the Stomach.* 1900.
Paterson, Herbert J., *Gastric Surgery.* 1906.
Robson, A. W. M., and **B. G. A. Moynihan,** *Diseases of the Stomach and their Surgical Treatment,* 2nd edit. 1904.

ANATOMY AND PHYSIOLOGY

Barclay, A. E., *Proc. Roy. Soc. Med.,* Feb., 1909; *Brit. Med. Journ.,* 1910, ii. 537.
Cannon, *Amer. Journ. Phys.,* 1898, i. 359.
Dobson, J. F., and *J. K.* **Jamieson,** *Lancet,* 1907, i. 1061.
Gray, H. M. W., *Lancet,* 1908, ii. 224; 1910, ii. 1610. Also correspondence in numbers for Dec. 10, 17, 22, 31.
Hertz, A. F., *Brit. Med. Journ.,* 1908, i. 130; 1911, i. 477; *Quarterly Journ. Med.,* July, 1910.

CLINICAL EXAMINATION, ETC.

Head, H., *Brain,* 1893, xvi. 1; 1894, xvii. 339.
Head, Rivers, and Sherren, *Brain,* Nov., 1905.
Hertz, A. F., *The Sensibility of the Alimentary Canal.* 1911.
Hill, W., *Brit. Med. Journ.,* 1911, Oct. 28.
Lennander, *Mitt. a. d. Grenzgeb. d. Med. u. Chir.,* Bd. x., Hefte 1, 2; Bd. xv., Heft 5; Bd. xvi, Heft 1; *Deuts. Zeits. f. Chir.,* Nov., 1905.
Mackenzie, James, *Brit. Med. Journ.,* June 23, 30, 1906; *Symptoms and their Interpretation,* 1909.
Panton, P. N., and **H. L. Tidy,** "On the Analysis of Gastric Contents," *Quarterly Journ. Med.,* July, 1911, vol. iv., No. 16.
Sherren, James, *Clin. Journ.,* June 28, 1905.
Willcox, W. H., *Med. Soc. Trans.,* xxxi. 229; *Lancet,* 1910, i. 1119.

MALFORMATIONS

Barnard, H. L., contributions to *Abdominal Surgery,* edited by James Sherren, p. 144.
Clogg, H. S., *Lancet,* 1904, ii. 1770.
Keith, Arthur, *Brit. Med. Journ.,* 1910, i. 303.
Kuliga, *Beitr. z. path. Anat.,* 1903, xxxiii. 481.

INFANTILE STENOSIS

Burghard, F. F., *Trans. Clin. Soc.,* xl. 122.
Cautley and Dent, *Med.-Chir. Trans.,* 1903, lxxxvi. 471; *Brit. Med. Journ.,* 1906, ii. 939.
Hutchison, Robert, *Brit. Med. Journ.,* 1910, ii. 1021.
Nicoll, J. H., *Glasg. Med. Journ.,* 1906, lxv. 253.
Stiles, Harold, *Brit. Med. Journ.,* 1906, ii. 943; 1909, ii. 752.
Still, G. F., *Lancet,* March 11, 1905; *Common Disorders and Diseases of Childhood.*
Sutherland, G. A., *Trans. Clin. Soc.,* xl. 98.
Thomson, John, *Clinical Examination and Treatment of Sick Children.*
Voelcker, Arthur, *Trans. Clin. Soc.,* xl. 108.
Willcox, W. H., and **R. Miller,** *Lancet,* Dec. 14, 1907.

HOUR-GLASS STOMACH

Delamere et Dieulafé, *Bull. et Mém. de la Soc. Anat.,* Paris, 1906, viii. 467.
Downes, W. A., *Ann. of Surg.,* 1909, ii. 552, 646.
Moynihan, B. G. A., *Med.-Chir. Trans.,* lxxxvii. 143; *Brit. Med. Journ.,* 1904, i. 414.
Veyrassat, *Rev. de Chir.,* Aug., Sept., Dec., 1908, xxxviii. 269, 403, 761.
Wölfer, *Beitr. z. klin. Chir.,* 1895, xiii. 221.

ACUTE DILATATION OF THE STOMACH

Box, C. R., and Cuthbert Wallace, *Clin. Soc. Trans.*, 1898, xxxi. 241; *Lancet*, 1901, ii. 1259; 1911, ii. 214.
Laffer, Walter B., *Ann. of Surg.*, 1908, i. 390.
Nicholls, A. G., *Internat. Clin.*, 1908, iv. 80.
Thomson, H. Campbell, *Acute Dilatation of the Stomach.* 1902.

INJURIES OF THE STOMACH AND DUODENUM

Berry, J., and Paul L. Giuseppi, *Proc. Roy. Soc. Med.*, Surgical Section, Oct. 13, 1908, p. 41.
Forgue et Jeanbrau, *Rev. de Chir.*, 1903, xxviii. 285.
Meerwein, *Beitr. z. klin. Chir.*, 1907, liii. 496.

CHRONIC GASTRIC AND DUODENAL ULCER

Bolton, Charles, *Med. Soc. Trans.*, xxxi. 249; *Proc. Roy. Soc.*, 1904, lxxiv. 135; 1907, B lxxix. 53; 1910, B lxxxii. 233; *Brit. Med. Journ.*, 1910, i.1221, ii. 1963.
Dawson, Sir Bertrand, *Med. Soc. Trans.*, 1902, xxvi. 55; *Brit. Med. Journ.*, May 9, 1908; *Lancet*, 1911, i. 1124.
English, T. Crisp, *Med.-Chir. Trans.*, 1904, lxxxvii. 27.
Eve, Sir Frederic, *Lancet*, 1908, i. 1822.
Fenwick, W. Soltau, *Lancet*, 1910, i. 706.
Kindl, *Beitr. z. klin. Chir.*, Bd. lxiii., Heft 1.
Mayo, W. J., *Ann. of Surg.*, 1908, i. 885; 1911, ii. 313.
Miles, Alexander, *Edin. Med. Journ.*, 1906, pp. 106, 223.
Miller, Charles, *Arch. Path. Inst. London Hospital*, 1906, i. 39.
Moullin, C. Mansell-, *Lancet*, 1910, ii. 993; *Med.-Chir. Trans.*, xc. 275.
Moynihan, B. G. A., *Ann. of Surg.*, 1908, i. 873; *Brit. Med. Journ.*, 1910, i. 241; *Med.-Chir. Trans.*, 1906, lxxxiv. 471; *Proc. Roy. Soc. Med.*, Surgical Section, Dec. 14, 1909, p. 69; Jan. 11, 1910, p. 97 (discussion).
Paterson, H. J., *Lancet*, 1910, i. 708; 1911, i. 97.
Robson, A. W. Mayo, *Brit. Med. Journ.*, 1907, i. 248; *Med.-Chir. Trans.*, 1907, xc. 228, and discussion; *Med. Soc. Trans.*, 1902, xxvi. 72, and discussion.
Rodman, W. L., *Journ. Amer. Med. Assoc.*, 1908, i. 165.
Sherren, James, *Trans. Clin. Soc.*, 1907, xl. 156; *Med. Press*, April 7 and 14, 1909; *Lancet*, April 1, 1911; *Lond. Hosp. Gaz.*, Oct., 1911.
Smith, Maynard, *Lancet*, 1906, i. 895.
White, W. Hale, *Lancet*, 1906, ii. 1189; *Med.-Chir. Trans.*, xc. 215; *Lancet*, 1910, i. 1819.

CARCINOMA OF THE STOMACH

Braun, *Deuts. Zeits. f. Chir.*, 1907, lxxxvii. 275.
Goldschwend, *von Langenbecks Archiv*, Bd. lxxxviii., Heft 1.
Groves, E. W. Hey, *Brit. Med. Journ.*, 1910, i. 366.
Janeway and Green, *Ann. of Surg.*, 1910, ii. 67.
Kocher, *Mitt: a. d. Grenzgeb. d. Med. u. Chir.*, Bd. xx., Heft 5.
Mayo, W. J., *Journ. of Amer. Med. Assoc.*, 1910, liv. 608.
Moullin, C. Mansell-, *Lancet*, 1910, i. 415.
Moynihan, B. G. A., *Trans. Clin. Soc. Lond.*, 1906, xxxix. 84; *Brit. Med. Journ.*, 1906, i. 370; 1909, i. 830.
Paterson, H. J., *Brit. Med. Journ.*, 1910, ii. 953.
Poncet, Delore, et Leriche, *Gaz. des Hôp.*, 1909, 35.
Robson, A. W. Mayo, *Med.-Chir. Trans.*, 1907, xc. 232.
Sherren, James, *Clin. Journ.*, Oct. 19 and 26, 1910; *Brit. Med. Journ.*, June 24, 1911.
Wilson and MacCarty, *Amer. Journ. Med. Sci.*, Dec., 1909.

CARCINOMA OF THE DUODENUM

Coffey, R. C., *Ann. of Surg.*, 1909, ii. 1238.
Desjardins, *Rev. de Chir.*, June 10, 1907.

Kausch, *Zentralbl. f. Chir.*, 1909, p. 1351.
Mayo, W. J., *Ann. of Surg.*, 1907, ii. 890.
Rolleston, *Diseases of Intestine and Peritoneum* (Nothnagel, English translation), p. 440.
Sauvé, *Rev. de Chir.*, Feb. 10, 1908.
Wendel, *Arch. f. klin. Chir.*, 1907, lxxxiii. 635.

SARCOMA OF THE STOMACH
von Eiselsberg, *Arch. f. klin. Chir.*, 1897, xl. 599.
Howard, *Journ. of Amer. Med. Assoc.*, July, 1902.
Maylard, A. E., and J. Anderson, *Ann. of Surg.*, 1910, ii. 506.
Salaman, R. N., *Trans. Path. Soc. Lond.*, 1904, lv. part iii. 324.
Sherren, James, *Brit. Med. Journ.*, 1911, ii. 593.
Yates, *Ann. of Surg.*, 1906, ii. 599-639.

PLASTIC LINITIS
Jonnesco et Grossman,*Rev. de Chir.*, 1908, xxxvi. 18.
Leith, R. F., Allbutt's *System of Medicine*, 1907, iii. 437.
Lyle, H. H. M., *Ann. of Surg.*, 1911, ii. 625.
Thomson, Alexis, *Brit. Med. Journ.*, 1910, ii. 949.

GASTRO-JEJUNOSTOMY
Brenner, *Wien. klin. Woch.*, 1892, v. 375.
Moullin, C. Mansell-, *Brit. Med. Journ.*, 1910, ii. 955 ; *Lancet*, 1905, i. 65.
Moynihan, G. B. A., *Brit. Med. Journ.*, 1908, p. 1092.
Paterson, Herbert J., *Lancet*, 1907, ii. 815.
Pers, *Zentralbl. f. Chir.*, 1909, p. 1417.

JEJUNAL ULCER
Connell, *Surg. of Gyn. and Obstet.*, 1908, p. 139.
Lion et Moreau, *Rev. de Chir.*, xxix. 5.
Moynihan, G. B. A., *Universal Med. Rec.*, 1912, i. 11 ; *Surg., Gyn., and Obstet.*, June, 1907 ; *Ann. of Surg.*, 1908, i. 1051.
Paterson, H. J., *Ann. of Surg.*, 1909, ii. 367.
Robson, A. W. Mayo, *Med.-Chir. Trans.*, lxxxvii. 339.
Rubritius, H., *Beitr. z. klin. Chir.*, 1910, lxvii. 222.
van Roojen, *Arch. f. klin. Chir.*, 1910, xci. 380.

THE INTESTINES

By ALEXANDER MILES, M.D., F.R.C.S.Ed.

For the purposes of this article, the intestines may be taken to
include that portion of the alimentary canal which extends from the
termination of the duodenum at the duodeno-jejunal junction to the
lower end of the pelvic colon, where it becomes continuous with the
rectum. Although the duodenum belongs anatomically to the small
intestine, its surgical associations are with the stomach, and are
considered in the preceding article. The affections of the vermiform
appendix and of the rectum are also most conveniently described
elsewhere (pp. 537 and 658).

ANATOMY

The **small intestine**, arbitrarily divided into jejunum and
ileum, is about 20 ft. in length, and with the exception of the first
part of the jejunum and the terminal part of the ileum, which are
fairly constant in their position, the numerous coils enjoy a wide
range of mobility, and show considerable variation in their disposition.
As a rule, however, the jejunum, which includes the first 8 ft. of the
canal, lies towards the upper and left part of the cavity, below the
level of the stomach, while the ileum, about 12 ft. in length, lies in
the lower and right regions. Although there is no definite point of
transition between the two portions, in the living subject the jejunum
can usually be distinguished from the ileum by its greater width, its
thicker and more vascular walls, its brighter colour, and the more
prominent yellow lines formed by the lacteals. The valvulæ conni-
ventes are larger and more closely approximated in the jejunum,
while the Peyer's patches are larger and more numerous in the ileum.

The arcades formed by the mesenteric vessels become more numerous
as we pass down the intestine, while the vessels entering into their
formation become smaller (Monks).

The **mesentery** is a double fold of peritoneum which connects
the small intestine to the posterior abdominal wall along a line 6 or
7 in. in length, extending from the left side of the second lumbar

vertebra downwards to the right iliac fossa. Between its layers are conveyed the blood-vessels—intestinal branches of the superior mesenteric artery and vein; the lymphatics, which are connected with numerous (40–150) mesenteric glands; and the nerves of the superior mesenteric plexus, derived from the solar plexus. Some fibres from the vagus ultimately reach the intestine. The bowel itself is enclosed in the free border of the mesentery, which thus furnishes it with its serous covering.

The ileo-cæcal junction.—The opening between the small and the large intestine—the ileo-cæcal orifice—is guarded by the ileo-cæcal valve, composed of two crescentic segments enclosing a slit-like opening, which, when the cæcum is distended, is closed and prevents regurgitation of its contents into the small intestine. In all likelihood, the circular fibres of the lowest part of the ileum form, as in some animals, a true muscular sphincter. A short distance below the valve, the vermiform process opens into the cæcum.

The **large intestine** extends from the cæcum, which occupies the right iliac fossa, to the beginning of the rectum in the pelvic cavity. It is about 5½ ft. in length; its widest part is the cæcum, which, when distended, has a diameter of about 3 in., and from this it gradually narrows till, at the lower end of the pelvic colon, it is only about 1½ in. in diameter.

When the abdomen is opened, the normal colon can be distinguished from the small intestine by its sacculated appearance, by the presence of three longitudinal muscular bands running along its surface, and by the appendices epiploicæ which project from its serous covering. When the bowel is greatly distended, and is covered with inflammatory exudate, it may be difficult to distinguish large from small intestine.

While it may be said that normally·the colon arches round the small intestine, the coils of which lie within the concavity of its curve, those segments of the bowel that are completely enveloped by peritoneum or that have a mesentery are subject to great variations in their disposition. The cæcum, for example, instead of lying in the right iliac fossa, may be found in the right lumbar region, even as high as the under aspect of the liver, or it may hang down into the pelvic cavity. The transverse colon, which normally arches across the abdomen in the upper part of the umbilical region, frequently dips downwards as a U- or V-shaped loop, reaching sometimes to the pubes, and thus increasing the sharpness of the angles at the hepatic and splenic flexures. When distended with gas, it may rise in front of the stomach. The pelvic colon also varies considerably in length and position. It may form a short, horseshoe-shaped loop of not more than 6 or 8 in., or may be two or three times as long, and be thrown into several curves, assuming an S- or Ω-shape, in which case it is not always easy during an operation to recognize the direction in which a particular part is running, especially if the bowel is distended. Being provided with a well-developed mesentery, it enjoys a wide range of movement, and when distended it may reach any part of the abdominal cavity.

The ascending colon, the hepatic and splenic flexures, and the descending and iliac portions are more constant in their position, as they are not completely enveloped by peritoneum, and are to some extent fixed to the posterior abdominal wall by areolar tissue.

Blood supply.—The cæcum and appendix are supplied by the ileo-colic branch of the superior mesenteric artery, the ascending colon by the right colic, and the transverse by the middle colic branch · of the same trunk.

The descending colon receives its blood from the left colic, and the iliac and pelvic colons from the sigmoid arteries, branches of the inferior mesenteric. The veins correspond to the arteries.

Lymphatics.—The lymphatics, after leaving the bowel, pass in the mesocolon to different groups of glands lying along the course of the branches of the superior and inferior mesenteric arteries. Their arrangement has been studied by Jamieson and Dobson, and is shown in Fig. 395.

PHYSIOLOGY OF THE INTESTINE

The functions of the intestine are—(1) to carry on the digestive processes begun in the stomach ; (2) to provide for the absorption of the products of digestion ; and (3) to excrete the indigestible residue. For the fulfilment of these functions the intestine is endowed with secretory and motor activities, and in addition the secretions of the liver and pancreas are poured into its lumen. The various enzymes act on the proteins, carbohydrates, and fats of the food, and transform them into substances that are capable of being absorbed into the lacteals and blood capillaries of the villi. The intimate mixing of the food with the digestive juices, and the passage of the chyme along the alimentary canal, are effected by the movements of the intestinal wall. Derangements may occur in the secretory or in the motor activities, or in both.

One other factor has to be noted—the decomposition of food-stuffs by bacteria. This occurs normally in the intestine, and is probably essential for health. The processes consist in the fermentation of carbohydrates, putrefaction of proteins, and conversion of fats into lower fatty acids. Some evidence has been brought forward to prove that disturbance of digestion may be associated with changes in the characters of the intestinal bacteria.

The secretion of ferments is confined to the small intestine, the liver, and the pancreas, and in the small intestine most of the absorption takes place. At the lower end of the ileum, bacterial fermentation of carbohydrates begins. In the large intestine, only small quantities of the food-stuffs are absorbed, but water is absorbed

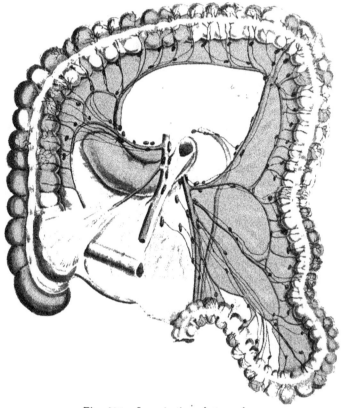

Fig. 395.—Lymphatics of the colon.

(From the Transactions of the Royal Society of Medicine. By courtesy of Mr. J. F. Dobson and Professor Jamieson. Reduced.)

readily. The fermentative and putrefactive processes reach their maximum in the cæcum and ascending colon, in which also digestion still goes on, ferments being present in the chyme which passes through the ileo-cæcal valve.

The secretory and absorptive function.—While derangements of the hepatic and pancreatic secretions have direct surgical bearings, the same cannot be said of changes in the *succus* *entericus.* We know, however, that if more than one-third, that is, a length of about 7 ft., of the small intestine is excised, digestion and absorption are decreased to such an extent as to lead to nutritional deficiency. Absorption is also much impaired in stenosis or paralysis of the bowel, as the result partly of venous stagnation in the wall, and partly of decomposition of the contents and consequent inflammatory changes. Decreased absorption in the colon is manifested chiefly by an excess of water in the fæces.

The effects of motor disturbances are more marked in surgical conditions, and for this reason the intestinal movements deserve mention in some detail.

MOVEMENTS OF THE SMALL INTESTINE

The small intestine exhibits several varieties of movement, the most important being *rhythmic segmentation movements* and *peristalsis*. These have been investigated in the excised gut, in anæsthetized animals with the peritoneal cavity opened, and in normal subjects by means of X-rays. The last method has been specially elaborated by Cannon, and his results have been confirmed in the human subject by Hertz. It consists in giving carbohydrate and protein food-substances in which a bismuth salt is suspended, and examining the shadows cast by the bismuth on the fluorescent screen.

Rhythmic segmentation.—Movements of rhythmic segmentation, which are the most frequent, are designed to mix the food with the intestinal secretions. While observations are being made through the fluorescent screen, one or more dark cord-like shadows are seen scattered over the field. These represent segments of the intestine which, for the time being, are at rest. If one of these shadows is watched, it will be observed that, following on this period of rest, it suddenly shows signs of activity, and definite nodes appear at regular intervals. The part of the intestine under observation is divided by the constrictions into " segments," which exist for a brief space of time. Then each segment is split into two " particles," and by the fusion of pairs of particles from adjoining segments, new segments are formed. Scarcely have they appeared than they in turn are halved, and a third series takes their place. The movements of segmentation occur at intervals of 7 to 10 seconds ; hence, within half an hour, each small mass of food will have been divided more than 200 times. By these rhythmic movements of segmentation, without changing its position in the intestine, the food is thoroughly mixed with the digestive juices, and brought into intimate contact with the absorptive folds of mucous membrane. In addition, the rhythmic contractions of the muscular wall pump blood from the submucous venous plexuses, and empty the lacteals.

Peristalsis.—When movements of segmentation have continued for some time, the food moves slowly for about 2 in. down the loop in which it lies. This is the movement of peristalsis, and it consists in a dilatation of the gut beyond the bolus, and a constriction on the proximal side of it (Bayliss and Starling). The waves travel at the rate of half an inch to an inch per minute after a meal, and four times as slowly during the fasting state. It is the incoordinated occurrence of constriction and relaxation that produces colic and admits of the possibility of intussusception.

The **other movements** of the small intestine are not yet clearly understood. Immediately after death, a swift wave may pass from the duodenum to the ileo-cæcal valve (Houkgeest), and possibly in its course it causes the multiple jejunal intussusceptions sometimes seen by the pathologist. The same movement may be produced during life by injecting a combination of drugs—ergot to stimulate the vagi, and calcium to inhibit the splanchnics (Meltzer and Auer). Shorter rushing waves may sometimes travel at a much higher rate than the peristaltic waves, and sweep the food without pause through several coils. Meltzer and Auer suggest that these may be an essential feature in purgation. Cannon has observed similar movements in the small intestine after administering an enema of soap and water. Physostigmin and ergot do not produce a true peristalsis, as, when they are introduced into the bowel or into the blood-stream, they cause violent local contractions, unaccompanied by any relaxation of the wall in front. These contractions are not transmitted along the bowel, and therefore are ineffectual in emptying it.

Antiperistalsis and vomiting of intestinal contents.—Although antiperistalsis has never been observed in the small intestine during the normal processes of digestion, the occurrence of continued vomiting of intestinal contents even after the stomach has been frequently washed out is a common clinical experience. Many attempts have been made to prove that " fæcal " vomiting is brought about merely by an exaggeration of a normal antiperistaltic movement, but the results are not conclusive. The first point to grasp is that the reflux of intestinal contents into the stomach occurs under two different conditions—one in which there is a mechanical obstruction to the onward passage of intestinal contents, and another in which there is paralysis of the intestinal wall.

In the first type, which is exemplified by strangulated hernia and malignant stenosis, intestinal movements are present in an exaggerated degree. Cannon experimentally produced a similar condition by tying a string round the gut in the upper part of the jejunum, and on watching the progress of a bismuth meal along the bowel he observed that the food passed out of the stomach normally, and was carried along the duodenum. When it reached the obstruction, powerful peristaltic waves followed each other in quick succession and hurled the contents against the barrier. As the intra-intestinal pressure rose, some of the fluid was squirted back through the narrowed lumen of the contracted portion by peristalsis. In this way, part of the contents might reach back to the pylorus, and so enter the stomach, without the occurrence of any antiperistaltic waves. In a second experiment, in which he stopped the progress of intestinal peristalsis by reversing one of the uppermost loops of the jejunum, antiperistaltic waves apparently occurred and carried the food back to the pylorus. Grützner administered enemata of saline solution in which were suspended starch grains, charcoal, lycopodium and other substances, and he recovered these particles from the stomach and small intestine. Such a result can only be explained by the occurrence of antiperistalsis.

When the intestine is paralysed, as in general peritonitis, it is difficult to conceive that one movement—that of antiperistalsis—should remain when the other movements are lost. In these cases, the "fæcal" vomiting is associated with distension of the bowel, the contents of which are decomposing and evolving gases that increase the pressure in the canal. This pressure may become so extreme that the bowel is kept from bursting only by the resistance of the abdominal wall. Hence, at any given point of the bowel, the contents will pass in the direction of least resistance. At the lower end of the ileum is the ileo-cæcal sphincter, which, we know, may be tightly contracted although no movements are occurring in the rest of the small intestine. If, as is probable, it is in the same condition in general peritonitis, then the accumulating gases and the copious secretion which they as irritants induce must gradually force their way upwards and finally reach the stomach, from which the gases are got rid of by frequent eructations and the liquids by vomiting.

The results following the administration of enemata in advanced general peritonitis favour the theory that the ileo-cæcal sphincter is strongly contracted. Once the colon has been cleared, the injected fluid is returned unaccompanied by any intestinal contents, although under normal conditions part of the enema reaches the small intestine and empties its lower coils.

In cases of strangulated hernia, the same explanation of "fæcal" vomiting is possible, because often it does not begin till all pain has ceased, and the distension of the intestine is extreme.

MOVEMENTS OF THE COLON

Antiperistalsis is the most frequent movement in the cæcum, and in the ascending and transverse colon. As soon as food enters the large intestine, a powerful contraction of the colon carries it some distance from the ileo-cæcal valve ; then antiperistaltic waves begin to pass rhythmically from the most advanced portion of the food, and travel backwards to the cæcum. These waves occur in " periods," during each of which they are small to begin with, gradually reach a maximum, and then die away. The period lasts for two to eight minutes in the cat, and periods recur at intervals of ten to thirty minutes, the bowel remaining at rest between them. In this way the food is thoroughly mixed and presented for absorption. As food accumulates, it reaches the neighbourhood of the splenic flexure, where the first " constriction ring " is usually seen. When the intra-intestinal pressure rises, as the food cannot force the ileo-cæcal sphincter, some of it may escape onwards through the ring. Though this explanation is the one commonly accepted, it is possible that the passage of the most advanced contents into the descending colon is brought about by waves of contractions behind them. Otherwise, the evacuation of the half-empty colon is difficult to explain. That contractions do pass from the cæcum along the whole length of the large intestine is proved by Hertz's observations on the act of defæcation in man.

In complete obstruction of the colon at some distance from its commencement, the antiperistaltic waves continue to drive the food backwards, and none of it can move onwards. As the pressure rises, the cæcum becomes dilated, and all the subjective symptoms may be referred to the right iliac fossa. In cancer of the pelvic colon, this sometimes leads to confusion in diagnosis.

Constriction rings.—With the increasing accumulation of food in the ascending and transverse colon, constrictions appear and separate the contents into a series of spherical masses. These increase in number, and gradually assume a position farther from the cæcum, so that they lie for the most part below the splenic flexure. In man, the first is about the middle of the transverse colon (Hertz). With the slow movement of the constriction rings, the contents are gradually pushed onwards along the descending and the pelvic colon. This movement corresponds with peristalsis in the small intestine, and each ring is associated with an area of dilatation in the gut below it.

Oscillating contractions of the walls of the sacculi have been observed in the excised colon (Elliott and Barclay-Smith). In all probability they assist in the churning of the contents.

In *defæcation* a strong contraction occurs to empty the distal colon. According to Hertz, who has actually observed the process in man by means of the fluorescent screen, the contraction starts at the cæcum, and proceeds along the whole length of the colon, driving the contents farther down. It is followed by similar waves, each of which empties the pelvic colon of part of its contents.

When *nutrient enemata* are administered, the contents lie at first in the descending and pelvic colon, and are then carried by anti-peristaltic waves towards the cæcum. Hence the function of anti-peristalsis is inherent in the colon throughout its whole length, although under normal conditions it is not called into action beyond the splenic flexure. The repeated passing of the waves mixes the contents of the enema with any digestive juices that may be present, and promotes absorption of the nutriment at least as far down as the splenic flexure ; beyond this there is little evidence of the absorption of anything except water. From Cannon's experiments on animals it seems likely that, if a bulky enema is administered, part of it reaches the lower ileum.

INNERVATION OF THE INTESTINE

The intestine can carry on its functions to a great extent independently of the central nervous system. In its walls lie two nerve-plexuses with ganglionic cells—Meissner's plexus in the submucosa, and Auerbach's plexus between the circular and longitudinal layers of muscle. Meissner's plexus is distributed to the mucous membrane, glands and villi, and is concerned with the secretory activities. Auerbach's plexus controls the movements of segmentation and peristalsis in the small intestine, and of antiperistalsis and the tonic constrictions in the colon. Hence these movements can be investigated in the excised gut, and they can be induced or inhibited by various mechanical and chemical stimuli. Thus, pinching of the gut, or the introduction of butyric or some other organic acid, stimulates peristalsis, and oxygen gas inhibits it. The best stimulus is a bolus introduced into the lumen, apparently because it produces a local distension of the bowel.

At the same time, the intestine is linked to, and its functions are under the influence of, the central nervous system. It is through these connexions that the emotions so commonly produce derangements of the alimentary functions. Cannon has shown in cats that excitement and anger stop segmentation and peristalsis in the small intestine, and antiperistalsis in the colon.

The small intestine is innervated by the vagi and the splanchnics. The latter are also distributed to the large intestine, and the fibres corresponding to those of the vagi are supplied by sacral nerve-roots through the pelvic visceral nerves. The extrinsic nerve supply gradually increases in activity, and the local mechanism decreases, from the ileo-cæcal valve to the anus. Thus, the strong contraction of the colon that produces defæcation is due to stimulation of the fibres of the sacral nerve roots.

The relationship between the three systems—local, sympathetic, and cerebro-spinal—is extremely complex, and is still imperfectly understood, but several facts have been experimentally established. Segmentation and peristalsis in the small intestine, and antiperistalsis and peristalsis in the colon, which are the result of a local reflex action effected through Auerbach's plexus, are inhibited by the splanchnic nerves, irritation of which, as in many acute abdominal inflammations, arrests the movements and produces constipation.

The vagi contain inhibitory and augmentor fibres for the small intestine. If they are cut and their distal ends stimulated, there may be temporary diminution or cessation of movements—that is, inhibition; but if the stimulation is repeated five or six times, inhibition is followed by augmentation of movements. After the vagi were cut, Cannon observed a definite weakness in peristaltic contractions, with, however, marked improvement in a few days; when both the vagi and the splanchnics were cut, the peristaltic contractions were practically normal in appearance, but the transit of food was slow.

The *ileo-cœcal valve* is also under nervous control. The existence of a definite sphincter muscle at the lower end of the ileum has been experimentally proved (Elliott). By impulses carried by the splanchnic nerves, it is kept in a condition of moderate tonic contraction, sufficient to prevent regurgitation of material from the cæcum. When these nerves are cut, free mingling of the contents of the small and large intestine takes place. It would also seem to be relaxed when large nutrient enemata are given, a special reflex perhaps called into play by the emptiness of the ileum. Stimulation of the splanchnic nerves, which stops intestinal movement, strongly contracts the ileocæcal valve. During the peristaltic movements of the lower ileum, the sphincter relaxes in front of each contraction and allows food to pass to the cæcum; when antiperistalsis begins in the colon, it closes and prevents regurgitation.

These considerations are of practical importance; for example, the early administration of fluids by the rectum, after an operation for removal of the appendix, may so increase the pressure within the cæcum as to burst the sutures with which the stump is invaginated, and this may lead to the formation of a fæcal fistula.

Sensibility of the Intestine and Peritoneum

In contrast to the parietal peritoneum, the normal intestine and the visceral peritoneum are insensitive to touch and pain. A loop of bowel may be pinched, incised, or even divided with the cautery without the patient feeling it, and advantage is often taken of this fact in carrying out the second stage of the operation of colostomy.

Interference with the blood supply of the intestine, irregular peristalsis, or the presence of irritants in the canal causes pain, but it is still uncertain whether such pain is referable to the bowel itself or to the parietes.

Ross first described visceral pain as being of two kinds—*splanchnic* and *somatic*, or, as it is now more frequently called, *referred* pain. Splanchnic pain is located by the brain in the viscus in which it originates, while somatic or referred pain is located in a definite area of the body wall. As an example of splanchnic pain may be cited the pain which is felt in the cæcum when that part of the gut is distended with flatus. In commencing appendicitis we have an example of referred pain, because, although the lesion is in the appendix, pain is felt in the vicinity of the umbilicus.

The existence of referred pain is now universally recognized, but there is an increasing number of clinicians, of whom Mackenzie was the pioneer, who dispute the existence of splanchnic pain. They believe that the viscera are not supplied with any nerve fibres that are capable, under either normal or abnormal conditions, of giving rise to sensations of pain. The evidence on this point is conflicting, but, if this view is correct, it is difficult to account for the fact that a patient can usually distinguish clearly between a superficial and a deep-seated pain in the abdomen.

Referred pain.—The accepted explanation of referred pain is that the intestine is supplied by splanchnic nerves, which are connected with cells in the spinal cord. When a lesion of the intestine exists, the splanchnic fibres supplying the diseased area are irritated and convey abnormal impulses to their spinal cells, which are thus stimulated to a condition of hypersensitiveness. These cells in turn irritate neighbouring sensory cells in the cornu, which send impulses along their axis cylinders to their peripheral distribution, and these impulses are interpreted by the brain as if they had originated at the periphery (Fig. 396).

The sensitive structures to which such stimuli may be referred are—(1) the skin and subcutaneous tissue, (2) the muscles of the parietes, and (3) the parietal peritoneum ; hence, referred pain may be manifested in any of these situations.

The most striking instances of referred pain are those in which the sensory nerves are distributed to a region remote from the diseased viscus ; for example, in affections of the bile passages, fibres of the phrenic nerve convey impulses to the 4th and 5th cervical segments. The sensory cells in these segments supply the skin over the deltoid ; hence, pain in disease of the bile passages is often referred to the region of the shoulder.

In affections of the alimentary canal, familiar examples of pain referred to the superficial structures are the pain of commencing appendicitis and of strangulation of small intestine, in each of which it is usually felt near the middle line in the vicinity of the umbilicus. In affections of the colon, the pain is usually referred to the hypogastrium.

Cutaneous hyperalgesia occurs in various abdominal inflammations, and its limits may be defined by stroking the surface if it is " superficial," or by pinching the skin if it is " deep."

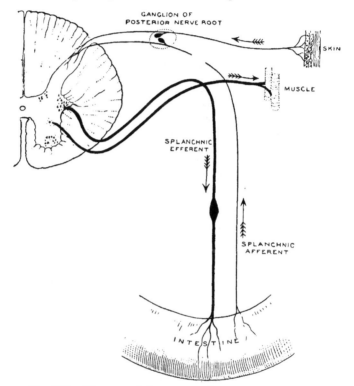

Fig. 396.—Diagram of the course of reflex pain (*see* text).

Muscular hyperalgesia may be present in intestinal disease, but it is difficult to differentiate from cutaneous hyperalgesia.

Muscular contraction and rigidity.—Motor cells in the cord may also be irritated by abnormal impulses conveyed by the splanchnic fibres (Fig. 396), and this irritation may manifest itself either by causing " muscular rigidity," or by disturbing the " abdominal reflex."

Muscular rigidity is the reflex which is best recognized and is a

2 c

symptom of great diagnostic value. The rigidity may extend widely and cause "boarding" of the whole anterior abdominal wall, or it may be localized to a small area. Unlike the muscles of the limbs, in which if part is stimulated the whole contracts, the muscles of the abdominal wall are capable of contracting in segments; hence, in limited intestinal lesions, a correspondingly small area of rigidity is present. The best examples of this are the rigid contraction of the upper portion of one or other rectus in cases of gastric or duodenal ulcer, and the "boarding" of the muscles of the right iliac fossa in localized appendicitis. The contraction may be so well defined as to simulate a definite tumour. In perforative conditions of the intestine, the rigidity involves the whole abdominal wall, being apparently due to reflexes set up by peritoneal irritation.

As a rule, in localized inflammatory conditions, the area of muscular contraction approximately overlies the inflamed viscus, but occasionally it is distant from it; for example, in some cases of pelvic appendicitis and of intussusception, the anal sphincter is in a state of spasm.

Clinically, this rigidity may be detected by noting that the respiratory movements of the abdominal wall are restricted or absent in the contracted area; and on palpation this region is firm and "boarded."

The reflex muscular contraction cannot be voluntarily inhibited, and the rigid segment is the last to relax during the induction of anæsthesia. In chronic conditions in which the rigidity is of long standing, and in exceptionally acute inflammatory affections, the contraction may not be overcome even when the anæsthetic is pushed to the utmost limit of safety, the fixation of the abdominal wall adding greatly to the difficulties of the operation.

In children who resist handling, it is more reliable to test the *abdominal reflex*. Any part of the muscle which is rigid does not twitch when the associated area of skin is stroked, as it is already in a state of contraction.

Vaso-motor reflexes.—It is a common clinical experience that if the abdominal wall is incised over an inflammatory lesion—for example, a gastric ulcer—the vessels may bleed more freely than normal. This is due to a vaso-motor reflex originating at the seat of the lesion and leading to dilatation of the blood-vessels.

Reflexes of peripheral origin.—The intestine may be affected reflexly by stimuli originating peripherally, its motor and secretory functions being disturbed in various directions. Thus, constipation or even complete obstruction, due to diminution or loss of peristalsis, may follow severe injuries, not only of the abdominal wall, but also of the chest, or even of the limbs.

Reflexes between different parts of the alimentary

canal.—Many of the clinical symptoms of disease in the intestine are to be explained by reflex influences exerted by one part of the tract on another, or even by one viscus on another. For example, vomiting of stomach contents is a symptom common to many lesions of the abdomen, apart from those of the stomach. Again, hyperchlorhydria may be induced by pathological changes in the vermiform appendix, which probably accounts for the condition spoken of as " appendicular dyspepsia."

Handling of one part of the intestine may inhibit the peristalsis in other parts, and lead to more or less complete stasis of intestinal contents. A striking example is the complete inhibition of gastric and intestinal movements which immediately follows a perforation or a bullet-wound of the stomach or intestine—a protective reflex which tends to prevent the escape of the bowel contents or their spread throughout the peritoneal cavity.

Cannon has shown in the cat that resection of a portion of the jejunum, with end-to-end suture, was followed by closure of the pyloric sphincter, which persisted for six hours—a period sufficiently long to admit of a protective plastic exudate forming at the seat of the anastomosis. When the resection was made low down in the ileum, the closure of the pylorus did not last so long, but the progress of the contents along the canal was retarded, a bismuth meal taking about seven hours to reach the seat of the anastomosis.

EXCRETORY FUNCTION OF THE INTESTINE

The fæces normally contain connective-tissue fibres, a small amount of muscle, traces of fat, fatty acids and soaps, remnants of starch, and inorganic crystals. Though many changes may take place in the constituents, probably the only one characteristic of disease of the small intestine is an increase in the starch granules.

The pigment of the fæces is urobilin. In health it is only found in the colon, but in obstructive conditions it may be present even in the jejunum. In the small intestine are found the bile pigments, bilirubin and biliverdin, which are transformed by the bacteria of the colon to urobilin. In purgation, however, the fæces may contain bile pigments.

With ordinary diet, the reaction of the stools is almost neutral. If the putrefaction of proteins is increased, as in intestinal tuberculosis and dysentery, it becomes alkaline ; and increased fermentation of carbohydrates produces acid stools.

The consistence of the fæces varies with the amounts of water, fat, mucus, and indigestible residue that they contain. Scybala are composed of food taken some days previously, and are formed in the sacculi of the colon.

The chief abnormal constituents of the fæces are mucus, blood, and pus. *Mucus* in more than a trace is present only in pathological conditions. If coloured yellow by bilirubin, it comes from the small intestine ; if white, it comes from the colon or rectum (Harley and Goodbody). In membranous colitis, greyish shreds or casts are passed at intervals. These may or may not contain many epithelial cells. According to Leathes, the casts are composed of chitin derived from carbohydrates. Fibrin is also sometimes present in the shreds.

Blood in the fæces may occur in streaks or clots visible to the naked eye. In intestinal ulceration the clots are frequently adherent to mucus. If tarry, or like coffee-grounds, the blood comes from the small intestine or upper colon ; no red corpuscles are recognizable microscopically, and the blood pigment is transformed to hæmatin. If from the pelvic colon, the blood is not so intimately mixed with the fæces. For traces of blood, the benzidin test is the most delicate.

Pus is demonstrated microscopically. The cells are less or more disintegrated according as the disease is in the pelvic colon or higher up. In malignant disease, pus and blood occur after ulceration of the growth.

BACTERIAL DECOMPOSITION

In the contents of the alimentary canal, great masses of bacteria are to be seen microscopically, and it is commonly found that pathogenetic organisms, such as the pneumococcus and the streptococcus, show a greatly decreased virulence. It is often difficult to cultivate the organisms found in the intestinal canal, though bacteria which have escaped into the peritoneal cavity through the injured intestine are very readily grown on artificial media.

The bacterial masses are first met with at the lower end of the ileum, though micro-organisms are present in smaller numbers higher up. They are abundant in the colon—so abundant that on an ordinary diet they constitute 33 per cent. of the dried fæces (Strassburger). According to Schütz, the difficulty of cultivation is due to the influence of a vibrio which rapidly devitalizes the bacteria. There is no doubt that the healthy intestinal wall also plays an important part in destroying abnormal bacteria and regulating bacterial growth. In health the bacterial flora is extremely constant, and abnormal varieties are soon destroyed. The normal bacteria may be decreased by diet, but experimental observation has shown that they are little influenced by the so-called intestinal antiseptics.

Varieties of bacteria.—The majority belong to the *Bacillus. coli* group. In some conditions, these may reach the blood stream, and they appear to produce mental unrest. They are excreted in large numbers by the kidneys, and their presence in the bladder sometimes produces cystitis. Other organisms are the *Bacillus lactis aerogenes* and the *Bacillus putrificus*, an anaerobe. The most important pathogenetic organisms are those of typhoid, dysentery, and cholera, but streptococci and staphylococci, the bacillus of anthrax, and the *Bacillus pyocyaneus* may also be found. Tubercle bacilli can frequently be demonstrated, even when intestinal tuberculosis is not present and no bacilli are to be found in the sputum, but great care must be taken to distinguish them from the smegma bacillus which abounds at the anal orifice.

METHODS OF EXAMINATION

In the examination of the abdomen, the usual clinical methods are systematically employed. The patient should be flat on the back, with the shoulders slightly raised on a pillow, and the knees flexed so that the soles of the feet are flat on the bed. He should be instructed to breathe through the open mouth.

By **inspection** the presence of localized or general distension may be recognized, especially in spare subjects with thin abdominal walls. If the distension is extreme, the skin appears smooth, shining, and stretched, and when it is due to ascites the umbilicus may project beyond the surface.

The movements of the abdominal walls with natural respiration, and while the patient takes a series of full breaths, should be noted. This is better appreciated by bringing the eye to the level of the abdomen and looking across it than by looking down upon it. Abdominal movements of peristalsis can sometimes be seen through the parietes; and in cases of intestinal obstruction, various patterns formed by the dilated coils of gut may be recognized. The presence of dilated veins in the abdominal wall is suggestive of some obstruction to the portal circulation or of pressure on the vena cava.

Palpation.—The student should acquire the habit of examining all the external hernial orifices as the first step in the palpation of the abdomen. This having been done, the abdomen must be examined systematically, the flat of the hand (not the finger-tips) being lightly placed on the skin, and the examination should be so arranged that any manipulation likely to cause pain is reserved to the last. After observing the respiratory movement in each segment of the abdominal wall, the muscular rigidity is tested, any localized area of " boarding " being specially noted.

The condition of the wall having been thus determined, the hand is again passed over the abdomen to investigate the contents, each individual viscus and segment of the bowel being in turn felt for. At first only a moderate degree of pressure should be exercised ; later, if this is tolerated, deeper pressure can be made. In this way, local or general distension of the bowel, enlargement of a viscus, such as the gall-bladder, the spleen, or the pancreas, or the presence of a tumour may be recognized. If a localized swelling is detected, its size, shape, consistence, mobility, and degree of tenderness should be determined, and an attempt made to ascertain whether it moves with respiration. In estimating the degree of tenderness, more reliable information is obtained by watching the facial expression of the patient than from his verbal statements. A swelling in the line of the bowel should be firmly pressed upon with the finger-tips to see if it is indented or " pitted " by the pressure—an indication that it is a fæcal mass.

In testing for fluctuation when ascites is suspected, an assistant should press with the ulnar side of his hand in the line of the linea alba to cut off vibrations of the parietes.

The lateral aspects of the abdomen should be examined with one hand placed behind in the loin and the other over the abdomen in front.

It is sometimes useful to examine the patient lying on the side or in the knee-elbow position.

Percussion.—The note elicited by percussion over the hollow viscera is tympanitic, the pitch varying with the quantity of gas present and its tension. The character of the note is influenced by the presence of fluid or fæces in the viscus. Under pathological conditions, it is not always easy to identify one part of the intestinal tract from another by percussion alone, but the employment of combined *percussion and auscultation* is sometimes helpful. The stethoscope is placed over the viscus under examination, and by percussing close to it the characteristic note of that viscus is recognized. Percussion is then made well beyond the limits of the viscus, and a different note is elicited. If the percussion is now continued towards the stethoscope, the original note is again recognized when the limit of the viscus is reached. Variations in pitch of the note over different viscera may be detected by scratching the surface instead of percussing.

When a moderate amount of free fluid is present in the peritoneal cavity, as in ascites, the most dependent parts yield a dull note on percussion while the higher parts are tympanitic, as the intestine is floated up by the fluid. By changing the attitude of the patient, the dull and tympanitic areas are found to alter. When the ascites is extreme, this test is less convincing.

If the intestine is paralysed and full of fluid, a dull note may be elicited in the flanks, and, on succussion, splashing may be detected.

In every case the suprapubic region should be percussed to define the upper limit of the bladder, and if it is found to be distended it should be emptied, by the catheter if necessary, before the examination is completed.

Auscultation does not yield much information in abdominal conditions. In obstruction of the bowel, bubbling or gurgling sounds —" stenosis noises "—may be heard ; in relaxed and dilated bowel, splashing sounds may be elicited on succussion.

A digital examination of the rectum and vagina should be made in every case in which symptoms are referable to the intestine. Distension of the lower bowel with air or water is of doubtful value as a diagnostic measure, and is not devoid of risk.

The **Röntgen rays** are of value in determining the presence and position of foreign bodies in the intestine. After administration of a *bismuth meal*—say, bread and milk with which 2 oz. of subcarbonate of bismuth have been thoroughly mixed—the passage of the food along the intestinal canal can be traced by periodic observations made through the fluorescent screen, or by taking a series of X-ray photographs. For the investigation of conditions in the colon, an emulsion of bismuth in olive oil may be introduced directly into the bowel. The results obtained by these measures, when employed for the localization of an obstruction in the bowel, require to be carefully interpreted, and they should not be allowed to outweigh those obtained by ordinary clinical methods.[1]

The **sigmoidoscope** is of great value in investigating the condition of the lower bowel as far as the pelvic colon. The long tubular speculum, which carries a metal filament lamp to illuminate the bowel and is provided with a bellows by which air can be pumped in to distend the gut, is passed with the patient in the knee-elbow position or in the 'left Sims' position. In the introduction of the instrument, care must be taken by altering its axis to round the curves without pressing on the wall of the gut.

MALFORMATIONS

Development.—In the early embryo, the *primitive alimentary canal* is represented by an incomplete tubular cavity lying beneath the notochord, and continuous with the yolk sac. As the embryo becomes folded in its growth, this tube is differentiated into the *fore-gut*, from which are developed the pharynx, œsophagus, stomach, and duodenum as far down as the opening of the common bile-duct, as well as the organs formed as outgrowths from these ; the *hind-gut*, from which the rectum and a variable portion of the descending colon are developed ; and the *mid-gut*, which gives origin to the remainder of the intestinal canal. At first, the mid-gut is continuous with the cavity of the yolk sac, but in time the communication becomes narrowed and constitutes the *vitelline duct*, a remnant of which sometimes persists in the form of a Meckel's diverticulum.

[1] *See also* Vol. I., p. 622.

As development proceeds, the primitive canal becomes greatly elongated, and the mid-gut is differentiated into the large and small intestines, the junction being indicated by an outgrowth which eventually forms the cæcum.

Concurrently with the elongation of the tube and the development of its mesentery, which carries the superior mesenteric artery, there is a rotation of the mid-gut, which brings the large intestine across the duodenum, and the cæcum to the right side just below the liver. From this position it gradually descends to the right iliac fossa. The small intestine goes on increasing in length, and is thrown into the complicated series of coils characteristic of the adult bowel.

CONGENITAL CONSTRICTIONS AND OCCLUSIONS

The *small intestine* may be narrowed or occluded in a variety of ways. At the junction of the fore- and mid-guts, for example, the canal may be interrupted by a septum, or by an annular constriction, probably due to faulty development of the embryonic buds in which the liver and pancreas arise (Bland-Sutton). A complete segment of the bowel—jejunum or terminal portion of ileum—may be absent, together with a U-shaped portion of the mesentery ; sometimes there are multiple defects. Among the other congenital lesions of the jejunum and ileum that have been met with are septa, localized strictures, and adhesions from fœtal peritonitis. The segment above the obstruction is dilated and elongated, that below is contracted.

Congenital defects in the *colon* are usually met with at the various flexures, where portions may be absent or septa may occlude the lumen.

DIVERTICULA

Congenital diverticula are occasionally met with in the region of the *duodenum*, and in a certain proportion of cases masses of pancreatic tissue are found at the fundus of the pouch.

In the *small intestine* acquired diverticula are not common. They are usually multiple, varying in size from a pea to a hen's egg, and are found on the mesenteric edge of the bowel, particularly towards the lower end of the ileum. They consist of pouches of mucous membrane protruded through the muscular coat along the line of the small vessels that enter and leave the submucous tissue, and they push themselves between the layers of the mesentery. These diverticula are probably due to increased intra-intestinal pressure and irregular tonic contraction of the bowel. A case has been recorded by Alexis Thomson in which a localized focus of tuberculosis weakened the wall and admitted of the formation of a diverticulum ; and another in which an accessory pancreas was present at the apex of the diverticulum. (Plate 92.)

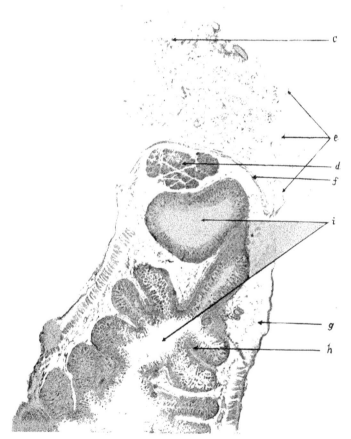

Complete longitudinal section of diverticulum with accessory
pancreas. × 5.

a, Extreme apex of diverticulum ; *b*, fat ; *c*, larger portion of accessory pancreas embedded in
extraperitoneal fat ; *d*, smaller portion of accessory pancreas ; *e*, blood-vessels ; *f*, longitudinal muscle fibres of coat of bowel ; *g*, circular-muscle fibres ; *h*, mucosa with villi and
solitary glands ; *i*, lumen of diverticulum.

(*By courtesy of Professor Alexis Thomson. Edin. Med. Journ., vol. xxiii., New Series.*)

PLATE 92.

Similar pressure diverticula are by no means uncommon in the *colon*, particularly in the pelvic colon and lower part of the descending colon. They are not confined to the line of the mesenteric attachment, but may form anywhere between the longitudinal muscular bands, and they sometimes pass into an appendix epiploica.

Usually multiple, they vary in size from a tiny saccule just admitting a probe, to an elongated pouch resembling at first sight a Meckel's diverticulum. Muscular tissue has been found in the

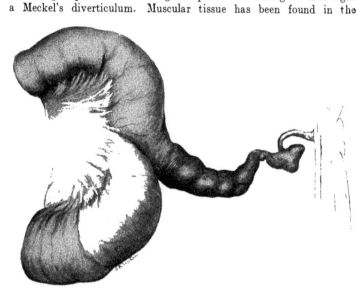

Fig. 397.—Meckel's diverticulum attached to abdominal wall.
(*Author's case.*)

wall of the pouch in some cases. They often contain concretions composed of inspissated fæcal matter, cholesterin, or calcium carbonate. The presence of such foreign bodies causes irritation of the mucous membrane—*diverticulitis* (p. 510)—and this may result in abscess formation and perforation, or may set up chronic pericolitis with the formation of an inflammatory cicatricial mass which may simulate malignant disease (p. 515). In some cases, the formation of an abscess has resulted in the production of fistulous communications with the bladder.

MECKEL'S DIVERTICULUM

Meckel's diverticulum is a congenital abnormality of the small intestine due to persistence of the intra-abdominal part of the vitelline duct, which, under normal conditions, should be obliterated during the sixth or seventh week of fœtal life. It usually springs from the convex free border of the ileum somewhere within 2 ft. of its termination at the ileo-cæcal valve.

Varieties.—As the process of obliteration may be arrested at any stage, this deformity manifests itself in many varieties. It has been estimated that a Meckel's diverticulum is present in 2 per cent. of human subjects, but in the vast majority of cases it is simply represented by a small thimble-like pouch which causes no trouble and gives rise to no inconvenience.

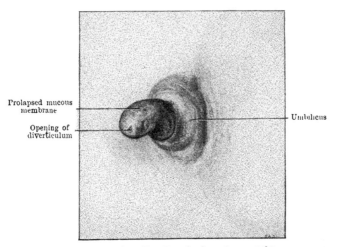

Prolapsed mucous membrane

Opening of diverticulum

Umbilicus

Fig. 398.—Patent Meckel's diverticulum in a child æt. 1 year.
(*Author's case.*)

It may persist as a patent canal, opening at the umbilicus at one end and into the ileum at the other, constituting one form of umbilical fistula. The mucous membrane is sometimes prolapsed, forming a reddish, conical projection at the umbilicus (Fig. 398), from which exudes a quantity of clear mucus, occasionally mixed with fæcal matter. Sometimes it forms a sinus, opening at the umbilicus but ending blindly a short distance inside the abdominal cavity. The most common form is a short tubular or saccular pouch of variable length (Fig. 399), with a well-formed mesentery, which passes in front of the ileum and has an artery running in its free border ; or the mesentery may be merely represented by a fibrous cord passing from the mesentery of the ileum to the tip of the diverticulum. In other cases it is narrowed down to a long, vermiform, or even filiform, process, which sometimes ends in a bulbous enlargement (Fig. 397).

On the other hand, it may become pear-shaped, or even spherical, and undergo considerable hypertrophic thickening, and, if it becomes occluded at each end, it forms a cystic tumour filled with mucus (Fig. 400).

The structure of the pervious portion of the diverticulum is similar to that of the lower ileum. A series of cases has recently been recorded in which masses of pancreatic t i s s u e were found embedded in the wall of the diverticulum, a condition which is probably to be explained by the fact that until the third week of development the mouth of the yolk sac extends up to the second part of the duodenum, where the pancreas has its origin.

The vascular cord of the diverticulum may be represented by an impervious fibrous band — *the terminal ligament*— which is attached to the anterior abdominal wall at, or some distance below, the umbilicus ˉ(Fig. 397). The end of a

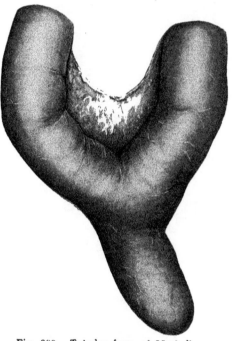

Fig. 399.—Tubular form of Meckel's diverticulum.

(Anatomical Museum, University of Edinburgh.)

free diverticulum or the terminal ligament may form new attachments to the mesentery of the ileum, to an adjacent coil of bowel, or to some other viscus, and form an arcade or ring through which a loop of bowel may pass and become strangulated (Fig. 401).

Complications.—1. Inflammation of a Meckel's diverticulum —diverticulitis—is attended with symptoms closely resembling those of appendicitis, a condition for which it is usually mistaken before the abdomen is opened.

2. In a considerable proportion of cases, the ileum is narrowed at, or more frequently just above, the level at which the diverticulum

arises. This narrowing may be due to defective development of the segment implicated, or to cicatricial contraction following ulceration of the gut at the opening of the pouch, or it may result from traction exerted on the gut by the diverticulum or its mesentery.

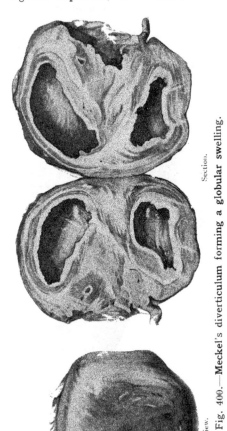

Section.

Surface view.

Fig. 400.—Meckel's diverticulum forming a globular swelling.

(By courtesy of Mr. J. W. Struthers. Edin. Med. Journ. vol. ii., 1911.)

3. **Intussusception** is sometimes originated by a Meckel's diverticulum becoming inverted and projecting into the lumen of the ileum, where it forms the apex of the intussusception.

4. **Volvulus** has been produced by the weight of a distended Meckel's diverticulum rotating the bowel on its mesenteric axis; or the diverticulum may itself be twisted on its long axis. The combination of volvulus and kinking is not uncommon.

5. By far the most common complication is **strangulation of the bowel** by the diverticulum acting as a band. When the diverticulum remains attached to the umbilicus and stretches across the abdomen (Fig. 397), a coil of bowel may be kinked over it, hanging like a towel over a rope. More frequently the free end, by forming new

attachments, has made a ring through which a loop of bowel slips (Fig. 401). When the apex remains free, and especially if it is long and ends in a rounded knob, a loop of bowel may be snared or noosed by it, and the knots thus formed may be most complicated.

The condition is most usually met with in young adult males, with no history of previous injury or peritonitis such as would give rise to the formation of a fibrous band. The obstructive symptoms are not always acute at the onset, as the diverticulum does not

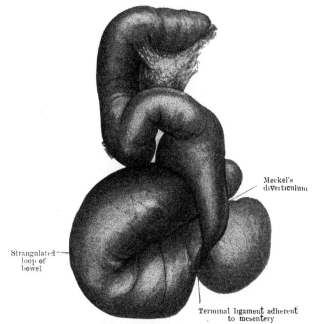

Fig. 401.—Meckel's diverticulum causing obstruction of the bowel by snaring a loop of small intestine.

(*Anatomical Museum, University of Edinburgh.*)

grasp the bowel tightly, but as it becomes œdematous and the constricted bowel distends they become more acute. Gangrene of the diverticulum soon supervenes, or perforation occurs, and peritonitis sets in early. There are no symptoms by which strangulation of the bowel by a Meckel's diverticulum can be distinguished from obstruction due to other forms of band.

6. A Meckel's diverticulum, either alone or together with the portion of ileum from which it springs, may form one of the contents of an inguinal hernia, less frequently of a femoral hernia (Littré's

hernia). Strangulation is a frequent complication of such hernias, but when the diverticulum alone is in the sac the symptoms are less acute than in strangulation of the ileum. Taxis is particularly dangerous, as the diverticulum is liable to rupture at its base ; and, owing to the poor blood supply, gangrene and perforation of the diverticulum rapidly occur.

The **clinical features** of these various complications differ but slightly from those of the same conditions arising from other causes, and the **treatment** is carried out on the same lines.

HIRSCHSPRUNG'S DISEASE OR "IDIOPATHIC DILATATION OF COLON"

The condition known as Hirschsprung's disease is usually met with in young children, and is characterized clinically by obstinate constipation dating from birth, and extreme distension and enlargement of the abdomen. The colon, in whole or in part, is greatly dilated and hypertrophied, without there being any organic obstruction distal to the dilated portion.

Morbid anatomy.—From a study of the recorded cases, it would appear that the anal canal and rectum are usually perfectly normal, the dilatation beginning in the lower part of the pelvic colon and affecting the whole of this segment of the bowel, so that it forms an enormous loop, sometimes as thick as a man's thigh, and extending up to the right costal margin. In most cases the dilatation affects the pelvic colon alone, but in some it extends to the iliac and descending portions of the colon. Less frequently the transverse colon is also enlarged, and still less frequently the ascending colon and cæcum. The small intestine invariably appears normal in size and structure.

The wall of the affected portion is greatly thickened, chiefly from enormous hypertrophy of the circular muscular coat. In cases of long standing there is considerable fibrous hyperplasia of the bowel wall—an evidence of "chronic interstitial colitis."

When scybalous masses are retained in the dilated bowel, numerous irregular ulcers of the mucosa, extending down to the circular muscular coat, are present. Perforation of such an ulcer has proved fatal. The dilated bowel contains great quantities of gas, a variable but usually small amount of semi-solid fæcal matter, and, occasionally, masses of hardened fæces.

On *microscopical examination* the mucosa shows some degree of leucocyte infiltration ; the muscularis mucosæ is slightly hypertrophied and shows interstitial fibrous changes ; and the submucous coat is more fibrous than normally, its blood-vessels are more numerous, and lymphocyte-like cells are collected round them in great numbers. The circular muscular coat shows an extreme degree of true muscular hypertrophy, being frequently four or five times its normal thickness. In old-standing cases the muscle may be replaced to some extent

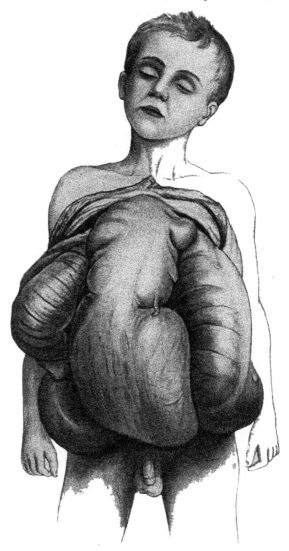

Fig. 402.—Case of Hirschsprung's disease.
(*From a photograph in the author's collection.*)

by dense connective-tissue fibres. The longitudinal muscular coat is also hypertrophied, but to a less extent than the circular coat. The serous coat shows some degree of fibrous thickening (D. P. D. Wilkie).

Etiology.—Great difference of opinion exists as to the determining cause of these changes in the colon, and it would appear that no one of the causative factors to which the condition has been assigned is sufficient to account for all the manifestations of the disease. It seems probable that a number of causes, some anatomical, others physiological, are at work. Such a combination as that suggested by Wilkie offers a rational and intelligible explanation of the sequence of events.

In the newly-born infant, the pelvic colon and its mesentery are relatively long and lax, and the mesocolon has an extensive attachment to the posterior abdominal wall, so that this segment of the bowel enjoys a wide range of mobility. At birth, the lower part of the large intestine, particularly the pelvic colon, is distended with meconium. If, from any cause, the muscular tone of the infant's bowel is below normal, it is easy to understand how this distension may proceed to such an extent as to render the bowel incapable of contracting on its contents and expelling them. The retained meconium soon undergoes bacterial decomposition, and fermentative gases are formed and add to the distension. From the combined weight of the contents and the gaseous distension, the mobile loop of the bowel may readily become bent or kinked, even to such an extent as to fold or press upon the upper end of the rectum and so occlude it, as by a valve. When the distension increases sufficiently, the pelvic colon rises into the abdomen and temporarily opens the valve, and some of the contents may escape.

In its efforts, only partly successful, to overcome the obstruction, the bowel wall becomes hypertrophied and thickened.

"The relation which the hypertrophy bears to the dilatation determines the fate of the case. When the hypertrophy fails to keep pace with the dilatation, we get early obstructive symptoms with distension, and frequently death from toxæmia in infancy or early childhood. When the hypertrophy is sufficient to compensate for the dilatation, the child may reach adult life, suffering only from a slightly swollen abdomen and a certain degree of constipation. Adult life being reached, compensation does not usually fail till the degenerative changes of old age begin to set in; then, from fibrous changes occurring in the hypertrophied wall, compensation fails, the bowel dilates further, and leads to the well-known symptoms" (Wilkie).

Clinical features.—The condition is much commoner in boys than in girls, and is usually met with during the first year of life, although its recognition may be delayed till later childhood, or even till adult life.

When the compensatory hypertrophy fails to overcome the distension, the symptoms appear in early infancy and tend to become acute. The most constant and characteristic symptom is obstinate constipation dating from birth, the bowels failing to move for several days at a time in spite of the free use of purgatives. Rectal injections usually afford temporary relief, but it is only by their constant repetition that the action of the bowels can be secured. The motions are, as a rule, small, soft, and very offensive, and some flatus may be passed. Occasionally small, hard scybalous masses are removed by an enema.

Flatulent distension is soon manifest, the abdomen becoming prominent, particularly in its upper part, and the lower ribs being raised and pushed outwards, so that the abdomen appears to be lengthened in contrast with the shortened thorax. The distended coils may form a pattern when a peristaltic wave passes along them, and loud borborygmi may be heard.

Sometimes the rectum is ballooned, sometimes it is contracted as if in a state of muscular spasm, but there is never any organic obstruction. Vomiting is not a constant symptom, and it almost never becomes fæcal.

. The pressure of the distended bowel upon the diaphragm interferes with respiration and with the heart's action. The patient becomes drowsy and listless, emaciates rapidly, and, unless relieved, dies of toxæmia or from the effects of perforation.

When the hypertrophy keeps pace with the dilatation, the symptoms are less urgent. Constipation may be as obstinate, but the abdominal distension is less marked, great quantities of flatus are passed, and there is seldom vomiting. The general nutrition is defective, and as the patient is constantly absorbing toxins from the colon, he becomes thin, sallow, and depressed. Sooner or later, however, compensation fails, and more acute symptoms of obstruction supervene, death resulting from toxæmia or from peritonitis following perforation.

Treatment.—In early cases in which there is reason to believe that the compensatory hypertrophy is efficient, medical measures designed to improve the muscular tone of the colon and to prevent fermentation of the contents are indicated. Such drugs as strychnine, belladonna, pituitary extract, and intestinal antiseptics may be administered. The frequent and systematic use of large high enemata is of great value, and it may be supplemented by abdominal massage and the use of electrical treatment.

When compensation is defective, or when medical measures have failed, recourse must be had to operative treatment, and this should be undertaken before the patient is suffering from toxæmia.

2 *d*

The appropriate operation can, as a rule, only be decided upon after the abdomen has been opened, and the actual state of affairs recognized.

When practicable, resection of the affected segment, with anastomosis of the bowel above and below, is the ideal operation, but as the dilatation often extends right down to the commencement of the rectum it is not always feasible. Entero-anastomosis, or short-circuiting of the bowel—the lower end of the ileum being anastomosed laterally with the pelvic colon—has in a few cases given relief.

Colostomy affords great relief in acute cases, and may tide the patient over till a more extensive operation can be undertaken. In many cases the relief afforded by a small colostomy opening acting as a safety-valve for the escape of flatus has added greatly to the comfort and safety of the patient.

Colopexy and coloplication have not yielded encouraging results.

ENTEROPTOSIS

(Glénard's Disease—Splanchnoptosis—Visceroptosis)

It is only necessary here to refer to the surgical aspects of this affection. A fuller description of its various manifestations will be found in works on Medicine.

Glénard, in 1885, first systematically described the condition, which consists in a sinking of the stomach, transverse colon, and right kidney to a lower level in the abdominal cavity than they normally occupy. Other viscera sometimes share in the prolapse.

Etiology.—The displacement is probably due to a combination of causes, by which the processes of peritoneum that naturally suspend the viscera become relaxed or stretched. Among the factors that bring this about may be mentioned weakness and atony of the muscles of the anterior abdominal wall resulting from repeated pregnancies, or following an exhausting illness; compression of the thorax and abdomen by tight corsets; excessive dragging on the suspensory ligaments by the weight of a dilated stomach, an overdistended colon, or a tumour; or the weight of an enlarged liver or spleen, pushing the organs down into the lower parts of the abdomen.

Clinical features.—Enteroptosis may exist to a marked degree without giving rise to any discomfort, and the severity of the symptoms is not proportionate to the degree of displacement of the viscera. As a rule, however, the patient complains of a constant sense of weight, and a dragging pain in the abdomen and loins, aggravated by exertion and relieved by lying down, and suffers from so-called "nervous dyspepsia," with pain and distension after taking food, flatulence, and hyperchlorhydria. There is usually obstinate constipation ; sometimes symptoms of mucous colitis develop. In many cases all the general symptoms of neurasthenia are present to a marked degree.

On examination of the abdomen, the epigastrium may be seen to be flattened, while the lower part of the abdomen is unduly prominent. By percussion, both borders of the stomach are found to be lower than normally, and the natural downward bend of the transverse colon is greatly exaggerated, sometimes to such an extent that the colon reaches the pubes. As the viscera change their position with the attitude assumed, the patient should be examined successively in the recumbent, the knee-elbow, and the erect position. The position of the stomach and colon may be demonstrated by X-ray examination after the introduction into the respective viscera of an emulsion of bismuth.

Treatment.—In mild cases, great benefit follows the Weir-Mitchell plan of treatment for the general neurasthenic condition ; and massage, electricity, and suitable exercises should be prescribed to improve the tone of the abdominal muscles.

The lower part of the abdomen should be supported by a suitable belt or bandage, applied while the patient is in the Trendelenburg position, and exerting pressure from below upwards.

In aggravated cases, or when these measures have failed, operative treatment may be considered, but when the neurasthenic element is prominent, even complete restoration of the viscera to their normal position often fails to relieve the symptoms.

Success has followed slinging up the stomach by "reefing" the lesser omentum. The stomach and transverse colon have been fixed to the abdominal wall, and other operations have been performed to restore individual viscera to their proper position. It is probable that when benefit follows the opening of the abdomen in these cases, it is largely due to the tightening up of the abdominal wall in suturing it, and special attention should always be directed to this part of the procedure.

Arbuthnot Lane recommends ileo-colostomy in severe and persistent cases, and, when pain is excessive, excision of the colon.

ABNORMAL ANUS

An opening deliberately made in the bowel to enable the intestinal contents to escape is spoken of as an *artificial anus*, and is to be distinguished from a *fœcal or intestinal fistula* which results from injury or disease.

ARTIFICIAL ANUS

The most common example of artificial anus is that made in the pelvic colon to empty the bowel when it is obstructed by malignant disease in the rectum (Fig. 403). Through a wound in the parietes a knuckle of the pelvic colon is brought out, and fixed by a glass rod passed through its mesentery. An opening is made on the convex aspect of the bowel, with the result that both the afferent and efferent tubes present on the surface, the mesenteric wall of the gut forming a septum or "spur" between them, which directs the flow out through the opening and prevents the contents reaching the distal or efferent tube.

As a rule, such an artificial anus is intended to be permanent, but similar openings are frequently made in this and other parts of the

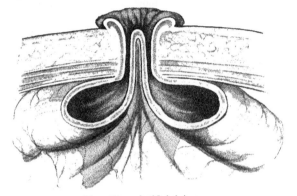

Fig. 403.—Artificial anus.

bowel as a temporary expedient, and when the necessity for the opening is past it should be closed.

The main difficulty in effecting the closure arises from the presence of the spur between the afferent and efferent loops. This may be destroyed by crushing it between the blades of a powerful clamp or "enterotome." The septum or spur is defined by passing a finger into each of the tubes of bowel, and, one blade of the enterotome being passed along each finger, the spur is crushed by closing the instrument. It is then supported by dressings and left in position till it causes necrosis of the spur and comes away, which usually happens in two to four days. The continuity of the bowel being thus restored, the external opening gradually closes.

A more certain and expeditious method is to separate the bowel from the abdominal wall by dissection, and invert the edges of the opening by sutures. The parietal wound is then closed. If it appears that the invagination of the opening in the bowel tends to narrow the lumen unduly, it is better to resect the segment implicated and establish a lateral anastomosis.

EXTERNAL INTESTINAL OR FÆCAL FISTULA

An external or fæcal fistula is an abnormal track leading from the lumen of the bowel to the surface of the skin, and giving exit to intestinal contents. As a rule, the opening in the bowel is a comparatively small one, and, so long as the lumen of the gut beyond is unobstructed, only a small proportion of the intestinal contents escapes to the surface.

Causes.—If the vitelline duct persists as a pervious tube when the umbilical cord separates after birth, a fistulous track is left in the form of a *patent Meckel's diverticulum* (Fig. 398). As a rule, only

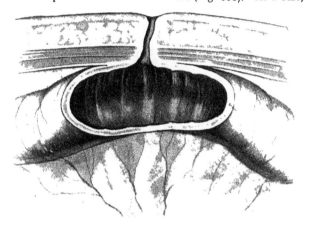

Fig. 404.—Fæcal fistula ; bowel adherent to parietal peritoneum.

a small quantity of clear mucus escapes from such an umbilical fistula, and the discharge may cease spontaneously, or after the lining membrane of the track has been destroyed by the actual cautery. If fæcal matter escapes, the abdomen should be opened and the diverticulum excised, the orifice of communication with the ileum being closed by suture.

A fistula may develop *after injury* of the bowel wall—for example, a contusion, a rupture, or a penetrating wound—or as a result of intestinal sutures having given way. If the bowel has become adherent to the parietal peritoneum before the fistula forms, the channel of communication is short (Fig. 404), and is often lined by the mucous membrane of the gut, which may even protrude from the opening. If, on the other hand, an abscess has developed in relation to the damaged portion of bowel, and has eventually worked its way to the surface, the fistulous track may be of considerable length, and is lined with granulation tissue, which yields a certain amount of pus (Fig. 405).

Fistulæ may also originate in *ulceration of the bowel*, such as some-times occurs in tuberculosis, in actinomycosis, and in malignant disease; or from *suppurative conditions* around it, notably in appendicitis with sloughing of the wall of the cæcum, and in perforation of the gut by foreign bodies. Sometimes the inflamed appendix becomes adherent to the parietes, and its lumen forms the track of the fistula —a condition of natural appendicostomy.

Clinical features.—An intestinal fistula may be met with anywhere on the abdominal wall, and it is not always easy to determine

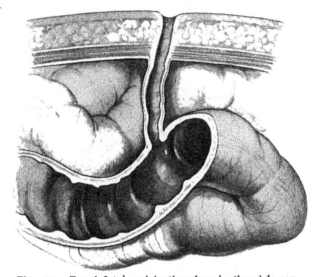

Fig. 405.—Fæcal fistula originating deep in the abdomen.

the part of the bowel with which it communicates. If the discharge is fluid, acid in reaction, and contains bile and undigested food, and if, further, it causes irritation and superficial ulceration of the skin, the opening probably leads into the upper part of the jejunum. This is rendered more probable if the patient emaciates rapidly and shows signs of starvation.

The discharge from a fistula opening into the lower part of the small intestine is usually neutral or alkaline in reaction, and is less irritating to the skin; bile and undigested food material cannot be distinctly recognized.

The discharge from a fistula in the colon is distinctly fæcal; in the cæcum it may be fluid and contain a considerable quantity of mucus; in the lower parts of the colon it is solid or semi-solid.

Treatment.—It is evident that if a fistula is associated with some irremovable disease of the bowel, such as carcinoma or tuberculosis, no attempt need be made to close it. If, on the other hand, it has resulted from some condition which has been overcome, such as an appendicular abscess, it should be dealt with.

It is to be borne in mind that those fistulæ that are lined with granulation tissue show a marked tendency to close spontaneously so long as the bowel beyond is unobstructed. If, after a reasonable time, this fails to take place, the patient should be confined to bed, the diet regulated so as to leave a minimum of residual material to pass through, and the granulation tissue gently scraped with a sharp spoon. If there is an abscess cavity in the track of the fistula, this should be opened up, and the wound packed lightly with iodoform worsted to induce it to heal from the bottom. Purgative medicines should be avoided, and the bowels emptied by enemata if necessary.

When the fistula is lined by mucous membrane, spontaneous closure seldom takes place, especially if there is a double loop of bowel with an intervening spur as in an artificial anus. It is then necessary to separate the bowel from the parietes by dissection, and to invaginate the aperture by sutures. If the opening is a large one and its closure by invagination unduly narrows the lumen, the segment of bowel implicated should be resected and a lateral anastomosis made.

Internal Intestinal Fistulæ

As a result of disease, particularly in malignant and tuberculous affections of the abdomen, fistulous communications are occasionally established between the intestine and other viscera. Sometimes an adventitious opening forms between two coils of bowel, but this is serious only if the upper opening is high in the jejunum and the lower one well down the bowel; in this case a long tract of the intestine is short-circuited, and is lost for purposes of absorption, with the result that the patient rapidly emaciates. The stools may contain unaltered bile and imperfectly digested food materials.

A communication is sometimes established between the stomach and the transverse colon as a result of malignant disease spreading from one of these organs to the other. Undigested food may appear in the stools, or fæcal matter may be vomited, with eructation of intestinal gases.

In malignant or tuberculous disease of the pelvic colon or rectum, and as a complication of chronic inflammatory diseases of the colon associated with diverticula, fistulæ may form with the bladder or urethra. This not only causes great discomfort, but is attended with considerable risk to life from the spread of infection to the kidneys.

Operative measures for the closure of such fistulæ are attended with some danger, and are only to be undertaken when the condition is endangering life and there is a reasonable prospect of curing the associated disease. The prospect of being able to cure the fistula is greatest when it has originated in a chronic inflammatory disease of the colon with diverticula, which is now known to be the commonest cause.

INJURIES

From the clinical point of view, it is convenient to divide injuries of the bowel into (1) those that are subcutaneous, and (2) open wounds —for example, gunshot injuries or stabs. It is by no means uncommon for the intestine and its associated processes of peritoneum to be damaged by external violence without any evidence of injury to the abdominal parietes, and the gravity of the patient's condition only becomes manifest when the effects of the injury declare themselves in the form of peritonitis, or by symptoms of internal hæmorrhage. These injuries are often associated with lesions of other viscera, such as rupture of the liver, spleen, or kidney, or intraperitoneal rupture of the bladder.

SUBCUTANEOUS INJURIES

Etiology.—For purposes of diagnosis, it is of great assistance to obtain an accurate description of the accident, as the lesion produced depends to a large extent upon the nature, intensity, and direction of the force applied.

Subcutaneous rupture of the intestine may be due to crushing, tearing, or bursting forms of violence.

Injuries produced by crushing.—The most common cause of subcutaneous injury to the bowel is the direct impact of a blunt object against the anterior abdominal wall ; for example, a kick from a horse, a blow with the fist, or a fall against a projecting object. The intestine, deprived for the moment of the protection of the abdominal muscles, which are taken unawares, is injured by being nipped between the impinging object and the bodies of the vertebræ. The centrally placed coils of small intestine—that is, those in the vicinity of the umbilicus—are most exposed to such forms of violence, particularly if the force is acting either directly backwards, or obliquely from without inwards. If the force acts in a direction away from the middle-line—downwards and outwards—the colon is more likely to be injured.

Injuries produced by tearing.—If the blow is a glancing one, acting from above, or if the body is squeezed, say, between buffers or by a wheel passing obliquely over it, the more movable segments of the bowel are driven before it, while the fixed portions, particularly the duodeno-jejunal junction, and less frequently the ileo-cæcal junction, the junction of the descending colon with the pelvic colon, or of the pelvic colon with the rectum, are liable to be torn across. Cases are recorded in which rupture of the small intestine has been produced by the impact of a bullet which grazed the abdominal wall without penetrating it. The mesentery may be torn from the bowel for a considerable distance, sometimes for several inches.

Injuries produced by bursting.—Only in rare cases is the bowel burst by increased intra-intestinal pressure induced by violence applied from without. This may occur if, for the moment, both ends of a coil of bowel distended with gas or food are occluded, and severe force is brought to bear on the full loop. It goes without saying that if the bowel is weakened by ulceration it is more liable to be ruptured by such a form of violence.

Morbid anatomy.—In the great majority of cases, the small intestine is the seat of rupture, and, as a rule, the bowel gives way only at one point. In about 10 per cent. of cases, however, it is torn at several points.

The wall of the intestine may be merely *contused*, blood being effused between its coats. If the effusion is in the mucous membrane, it may lead to hæmorrhage into the lumen, with blood-stained stools; or sloughing of the mucous membrane may ensue and lead to the formation of an ulcer. The lowering of the vitality of the bowel may admit of organisms traversing the walls and setting up localized peritonitis some days after the accident.

If only one or other of the coats is torn through—*incomplete rupture*—the immediate escape of the intestinal contents is prevented, but peritonitis may subsequently result, either from necrosis of the damaged portion or from the passage of organisms through it.

When all the coats are. torn through—*complete rupture*—the contents usually escape at once into the general peritoneal cavity, and set up septic peritonitis; but if the tear is small and the bowel is empty at the time, the mucous membrane may protrude and plug it, and adhesions form with the omentum or with adjacent coils and so prevent leakage. The circular muscles contract and so help to occlude the rupture, and it is possible that the portion of the bowel above the lesion is paralysed, and so does not send its contents on into the damaged segment. The presence of peritonitis, therefore, does not necessarily connote complete rupture of the bowel, nor does its absence necessarily indicate that the bowel has not been torn.

The colon is very seldom ruptured by direct violence. Berry and Giuseppi have collected 132 cases from the records of London hospitals during 15 years (1892-1907). As in the small intestine, the lesion may be a complete tear or a small perforation, and the devitalized bowel may subsequently give way at one or more points.

Cases are recorded in which those portions of the colon with an incomplete mesentery have ruptured into the retroperitoneal tissues, giving rise to localized suppuration, and in some instances to surgical emphysema from the escape of intestinal gases. The colon has been ruptured by large enemata given for the relief of constipation, and by foreign bodies entering the rectum.

Clinical features.—In many cases it is evident from the general appearance of the patient that he has sustained a grave abdominal injury, while in others, with equally severe lesions, there is nothing to cause anxiety. The three symptoms most constantly present, which strongly suggest perforation of the bowel, are pain, vomiting, and muscular rigidity.

The **pain** is usually severe and persistent, and is more or less diffused over the belly, but it is most intense at the site of the visceral lesion. Tenderness on palpation also is usually most marked over the rupture.

Vomiting often comes on at the time of the injury, continues after the stomach has emptied itself of food, and is attended by nausea. The presence of blood in the vomit indicates that the stomach or duodenum is the seat of the injury. If the vomit is bilious, the small intestine is probably injured. With the onset of peritonitis, the vomiting assumes the characteristic gulping character.

Muscular rigidity is the most valuable and characteristic sign, especially when accompanied by tenderness. The fixation of the abdominal walls, and the restricted action of the diaphragm, render the respiration almost entirely thoracic.

At first the abdomen is retracted to the extent of being scaphoid, but later it becomes prominent, either from paralytic distension of the bowel, or from the escape of gas into the peritoneal cavity. The early onset of tympanites is very significant of a rupture of the bowel.

Shock is sometimes so severe as to prove fatal within a few minutes; in other cases it is slight and evanescent. As a rule, all the classical symptoms of shock are present, but in quite a number of cases the patient has shown none, and has continued to work for some hours and been able to walk home or to the hospital before he began to feel ill. In these cases, the first sign of the injury is the onset of peritonitis.

Dullness in the flank may be due to empty, contracted bowel, or to extravasated blood, but it is not a reliable symptom, as the rigidity of the abdominal muscles may prevent its recognition. If the dullness changes with the position of the patient, it is usually due to fluid blood or urine in the peritoneal cavity. The dullness from fluid blood is usually most marked above the pubes.

The diminution of the area of liver dullness from the escape of gas into the peritoneal cavity is of no value, and this symptom should be ignored in forming a diagnosis, as it may be due to gaseous distension of the colon displacing the liver. Emphysema of the subperitoneal tissue is rare, except in cases of rupture at the duodeno-jejunal junction, or of the colon behind the peritoneum.

In the early stages the pulse has the character associated with shock, and, in the later stages, that associated with peritonitis. A rapid rise in the pulse-rate, especially if associated with a rise of temperature to 103° or 104° F., is usually of bad omen, as is also persistence of rapid, superficial breathing.

Inability to pass faeces or flatus is usually present, but the patient often empties the lower bowel soon after the accident, and if the motion contains blood, an injury to the bowel is strongly suggested.

Even after a careful analysis of all the symptoms it is often impossible to be certain whether or not the bowel has been ruptured, and it is seldom possible to localize the seat of the lesion when present.

Treatment.—When the nature of the accident and the symptoms presented by the patient render it probable that the intestine has been damaged, an exploratory operation should be performed, even although there is no conclusive evidence of visceral injury. Experience has shown that in many of these cases it is only when signs of peritonitis develop that a positive diagnosis can be made, and that operations carried out then are comparatively seldom successful. The best results have followed operations performed between seven and twelve hours after the accident, in the interval between the passing off of the initial shock and the onset of peritonitis.

The abdomen is opened over the seat of injury if this can be determined, and the lesion in the bowel or blood-vessels sought for and dealt with. If a single tear is found, it is closed by Lembert sutures inserted at right angles to the long axis of the gut. More extensive lesions necessitate resection of portions of the bowel, with lateral anastomosis. The peritoneum is then cleansed, and the abdomen closed, with or without drainage as may be found necessary.

OPEN WOUNDS

STAB WOUNDS

The presence of a penetrating wound of the abdominal wall always raises the presumption of a punctured or incised wound of the intestine. If the puncture in the bowel is a small one, the contraction of the muscular coat may close it, or the mucous membrane may protrude and prevent the escape of intestinal contents.

Nothing can be learnt by exploring the external wound with the probe, and this procedure is dangerous in that it may introduce infective material deeper into the tissues, or may determine an escape of intestinal contents by opening up a puncture which has been closed by natural means, or sealed off by fibrinous exudate.

The **clinical features** are similar to those of subcutaneous rupture (p. 458), and the external wound indicates the site of the injured loop of bowel, which is almost invariably immediately beneath the wound in the parietes.

The escape of gas or fæces, or the protrusion of the damaged loop of bowel through the external wound, removes all doubt as to the diagnosis, but in the absence of these signs it is often extremely difficult to decide whether the bowel has been injured or not. If the nature of the accident, the length and character of the weapon, and the position of the external wound render it probable that the bowel has been injured, an exploratory operation should always be performed at once. The existing wound is opened up and purified, the underlying coils of bowel examined, and any lesions found dealt with. If the puncture is small and single, it may be closed by a Lembert suture, introduced at right angles to the long axis of the bowel; if more extensive, it may be necessary to resect a portion of the gut and establish a lateral anastomosis. A considerable length of the bowel should be examined, as there may be more than one wound. The peritoneum is cleansed and the parietal wound closed, suitable provision being made for drainage. For the first few days the patient should be kept in the Fowler position.

Gunshot Wounds

The experience of military surgeons in warfare goes to show that injuries of the intestine produced by modern small-bore bullets are much less serious than were those due to the older and larger missiles. The puncture in the bowel made by a high-velocity conical bullet is extremely minute, and the mucous membrane protrudes and closes the aperture; and, as the peristalsis is immediately arrested by the shock, time is given for plastic lymph to be effused and adhesions to form between adjacent coils of intestine, or with a tag of omentum, before intestinal contents pass along the damaged segment, and thus leakage is prevented. This is the more likely to occur as the patient has often been fasting for some hours before being wounded.

The patient should, as far as possible, be left undisturbed for some hours after being wounded, in order that the formation of plastic lymph may not be interfered with. On no account should the wound be probed. In the South African War about one-third of the cases of injury of the small intestine, and about two-thirds of the cases of injury of the colon, recovered without operation. Operative interference should not be delayed if there is evidence of infection of the peritoneum or of severe internal hæmorrhage.

Pistol-shot wounds and wounds by sporting guns are more common in civil practice, and in their clinical aspects they resemble the injuries produced by pointed instruments rather than gunshot wounds. The intestinal injury is a contused and lacerated wound, and often, from the scattering of small shot, or from the close range at which the weapon was discharged, several coils of bowel are damaged.

The point of entrance of the bullet may be extremely minute. In one case operated upon by me, it was only discovered on opening up the folds of the umbilical cicatrix.

There may be considerable hæmorrhage into the peritoneal cavity from injury to a vessel in the abdominal wall, such as the deep epigastric, or from injury to the mesenteric vessels.

The **treatment** of gunshot or pistol-shot wounds consists in opening up the wound of entrance, and examining the whole length of the bowel. Each puncture is closed, and any contused area of bowel invaginated by a purse-string suture to prevent the risk of subsequent necrosis and leakage. It is not necessary to search for the bullet, which is usually embedded in bone or muscular tissue, where it does no harm.

INJURIES OF THE MESENTERY

The mesentery may be ruptured by violence inflicted on the anterior abdominal wall, or by penetrating wounds. Many of the fatal cases of gunshot wound of the abdomen occurring in warfare are due to injuries of the mesenteric and omental blood-vessels. As a rule other viscera are also implicated.

Profuse hæmorrhage usually takes place into the peritoneal cavity, with a rapidly fatal result. Sometimes the blood is effused between the leaves of the mesentery and forms a localized hæmatoma. In a case of this kind operated upon by me, a cake-like mass of clotted blood, about the size of the palm of the hand and nearly an inch thick, was found in the mesentery of a boy aged 13, about sixty hours after he had sustained a blow in the umbilical region. The clot was turned out, and the boy recovered.

The damage to the vessels may so interfere with the vascularity of the bowel that gangrene of the loop implicated ensues, and leads to a fatal result from peritonitis.

The symptoms resemble those of contusion or rupture of the bowel, but the signs of internal hæmorrhage are superadded.

The only **treatment** is to open the abdomen and secure the vessels. The tear in the mesentery should be closed, lest it form an aperture through which the bowel may subsequently pass and be strangulated.

FOREIGN BODIES IN THE INTESTINE

The great majority of foreign bodies that have been swallowed and have successfully passed the pylorus, safely traverse the remaining segments of the alimentary canal and are passed by the rectum. The facility with which large and irregular objects pass along the intestinal canal is remarkable.

In its passage along the bowel, a foreign body may become encrusted with fæcal matter and phosphates, and, while this may add to the bulk of the object, it at the same time renders its passage safer by rounding off sharp angles or filling up crevices and hooks, as, for example, in the case of a small tooth-plate. Some metallic objects undergo a certain degree of solution, while organic bodies, such as bones, may be partly digested.

Clinical features.—The passage of a foreign body along the intestine is seldom attended with any symptoms beyond slight colicky pain and occasional vomiting. The time taken for an insoluble body to traverse the bowel varies from forty-eight hours to two or three weeks. Irregular bodies are sometimes temporarily arrested and cause localized irritation of the mucous membrane with symptoms of enteritis, in the form of fever, severe griping pain and tenderness, distension, and diarrhœa, with pus and blood in the stools.

As the most common site of arrest is in the lower part of the ileum, at the ileo-cæcal valve, or in the cæcum, the local symptoms are generally referred to the right iliac fossa. If the body is long detained, localized peritonitis may ensue with muscular rigidity of the abdominal wall over the site of arrest. Foreign bodies may be permanently arrested at the narrowest part of the gut—that is, the ileo-cæcal region—or by a stricture of the bowel, the most common cause of which is malignant disease of the colon. In a few recorded cases, a foreign body has been arrested in a hernia, or in a pouch or diverticulum of the bowel.

Only in very rare cases does a foreign body arrested in a normal portion of the bowel cause obstruction, but when the lumen is narrowed by disease and becomes occluded by an object, such as a fruit-stone, a piece of bone, or a gall-stone, acute symptoms may supervene. The more serious effects of permanent arrest are due to septic complications following enteritis and ulceration, and ending in perforation. Cases have been recorded in which localized peritonitis has led to abscess formation, and the foreign body has passed into the abscess and escaped through the abdominal wall. In other cases the object has found its way into the bladder or other viscus.

Treatment.—To facilitate the passage of a foreign body along the intestine, the patient should be fed on such foods as porridge, pease-brose, or vegetables, which leave a considerable residue. In the ease of such bodies as tooth-plates, small lockets, or other objects with hooks or projections, it has been found useful to mix with the food a moderate quantity of chopped-up string, which, by the churning action of the stomach, is wound round the projections and prevents them catching on the mucous membrane. In the great majority of cases, there is no call to operate, unless serious symptoms develop. If a skiagram is taken to locate the foreign body and operation is decided upon, this should be done at once, as the body may change its position if there is any delay.

INTESTINAL OBSTRUCTION [1]

The term "intestinal obstruction" is a purely clinical one, and implies an interference with the passage of the bowel contents along the canal. The extent of the arrest varies widely, from a slight difficulty in obtaining a regular evacuation to sudden and complete arrest of the passage of fæces and flatus.

The primary cause of the obstruction is usually mechanical, and several different mechanisms may be responsible. For example, the lumen may be gradually narrowed by cicatricial contraction, resulting in a variable degree of stenosis or stricture ; the bowel may be blocked by a tumour of the wall gradually filling it up ; or one segment of bowel may be invaginated into another, as in intussusception. When due to such causes the obstruction is incomplete but progressive. Again, a loop of bowel may be twisted on its mesenteric axis, as in volvulus ; or be snared by a fibrous band, the margins of an aperture in the mesentery, or the neck of a hernial sac. Under these conditions, not only is the lumen immediately occluded, and the obstruction at once rendered complete, but the blood-vessels of the segment implicated are also occluded, and the nerve supply interfered with, so that the vitality of the bowel is endangered. To this condition, the term " strangulation " is applied.

Whatever the mechanical cause may be, sooner or later the nerve mechanism governing the peristaltic action of the bowel is interfered with, and a paralytic factor comes into play, adding to the difficulty the bowel has in emptying itself.

In certain forms of obstruction, notably that associated with generalized peritonitis, the cause is inherent in the bowel itself, consisting in a loss of muscular contractility—*paralytic obstruction.*

It is convenient to classify cases of obstruction of the bowel under the headings—(1) Acute or Sudden Obstruction ; (2) Chronic or Gradual Obstruction ; and (3) Chronic Obstruction becoming Acute.

[1] I desire here to express my indebtedness to the writings of the late H. L. Barnard.

1. Acute or Sudden Obstruction

Acute obstruction is always a serious condition, and is attended by a group of symptoms of which the most obvious are abdominal pain, persistent vomiting, distension with complete cessation of the passage of intestinal contents, and a greater or less degree of shock. The earliest of these symptoms—pain, vomiting, and shock—are not peculiar to obstruction, but are common to all acute abdominal affections, and are probably attributable to a profound impression made upon the sensory nerves of the abdomen rather than to the mere interference with the transmission of the bowel contents.

After the obstruction has lasted for some time, the patient passes into a condition of collapse and the general circulation is profoundly affected, the heart's action becoming weak and rapid as a result of the absorption of toxic material from the stagnating contents of the bowel above the seat of the block. At this stage, the relief of the obstruction may not suffice to save the life of the patient, as the amount of poisonous material absorbed may be so great as to prove fatal. It is evident, therefore, that, once a diagnosis of obstruction has been made, operative treatment should be undertaken at the earliest possible moment, to prevent the patient absorbing a fatal dose of toxins, and that no operation is complete that does not ensure a speedy evacuation of the segment above the block so that no further absorption may take place.

Pathology and morbid anatomy.—The most severe forms of acute obstruction are those due to sudden and complete occlusion of the bowel, as when a loop is impacted in a hernial aperture, or is snared by a band, or rotated on its mesentery, because not only is the passage of flatus and fæces completely arrested, but the vessels supplying the strangulated segment are occluded and the nerve supply interfered with.

The immediate effect of the strangulation is to excite a violent peristalsis, which results in forcing on the contents of *the segment below the obstruction,* so that this portion is emptied and passes into a condition of spasm. When seen a few hours after obstruction has begun, it is pale, contracted, and empty; and when handled, it feels firm. It is neither collapsed nor paralysed.

The segment above the obstruction rapidly becomes distended with intestinal fluids and gases. The fluids consist of liquid fæces, an excessive secretion of the glands of the alimentary canal, inflammatory exudate, and blood. When the disturbance of the circulation is so great as to interfere with absorption of gas from the intestine, the distension is added to by accumulation of flatus and by bacterial decomposition of the intestinal contents. At first, the walls are thin and pale, but in the course of a few hours they become deeply congested and œdematous, and the mucous membrane may show hæmorrhages and superficial erosions.

Distension is greatest when the small intestine is obstructed, because secretion of a considerable amount of fluid is reflexly stimulated. The distension gradually spreads upwards and may reach the duodenum or even the stomach. When the pelvic colon is the seat of the obstruction, the distension is less, because the higher reaches of the colon continue to absorb fluid.

In course of time, the surface epithelium of the mucous membrane is shed, and organisms pass through the wall and reach the peritoneal cavity, giving rise to peritonitis. Minute, sharply circumscribed ulcers may form as a result of necrosis of the mucous membrane, and these may lead to perforation (Kocher). Sometimes there are multiple pin-point perforations scattered over a segment of bowel.

The *strangulated* coil becomes deeply congested from interference with its venous return. At first, unless the strangulation is very tight, the arteries are not occluded, and they continue to force blood into the veins, with the result that the congestion is increased. The bowel becomes deep purple in colour, tense and œdematous, and blood-stained serum exudes into the lumen and the peritoneal cavity.

If the strangulation is so acute as to occlude the arteries at once, the affected segment is pale, grey or green, and flaccid, and it becomes gangrenous within a few hours. The occluded segment is distended with gas, which is probably carbonic dioxide that cannot be absorbed by the veins, and the distension may be enormous—for example, in volvulus of the pelvic colon. The tension of the strangulated coil is, as a rule, much greater than that of the distended bowel above the obstruction. The strangulated loop soon loses its power of preventing organisms passing through its wall, and in this way early infection of the peritoneum may take place. Sooner or later gangrene ensues from thrombosis of the vessels, and perforations of various sizes occur, leading to peritonitis.

Clinical features.—The clinical features of acute obstruction vary considerably according to the cause, but certain symptoms are common to all cases, whatever the cause, and these may be considered here.

It is to be borne in mind that obstruction itself is not the essential or all-important cause of the symptoms. The initial symptoms are evidence of " peritonism," or shock inflicted through the peritoneum ; the next to follow are due to interference with the onflow of the intestinal contents ; those of the later stages are signs of the absorption of toxins from the stagnating contents or from peritonitis.

As a rule, the onset is sudden, the patient having had no previous discomfort or feeling of illness, and it is seldom possible to attribute

2 e

the condition to any exciting cause. The first symptom is intense abdominal pain, which is usually so severe as to double the patient up, or cause him to writhe in agony on the floor. When the small intestine is implicated, the pain is continuous, and is referred to the region of the umbilicus. The higher up in the intestine the strangulation occurs, the tighter the constriction, and the greater the extent of bowel implicated the more severe is the pain. When the obstruction is in the more fixed parts of the bowel, such as the duodeno-jejunal junction, the ileo-cæcal junction, or the colon, the pain is usually correctly located in the affected segment.

After a time, when the nerves of the strangulated segment become exhausted, or when perforation occurs and the tension in the loop is relieved by the escape of gas and fluid, this initial pain may be temporarily alleviated.

Sooner or later, however, severe griping pain is experienced from the excessive peristaltic efforts of the bowel to force its contents along the tube. As the muscular coats become exhausted, this pain to some extent abates, and the relief may be contributed to by the poisoning of the nerve mechanism with toxins derived from the stagnating contents. The paralysis thus induced may prevent the bowel from emptying itself even if the obstruction is removed. Up to this point, the pain is not increased, and may even be relieved, by pressure, and there is no marked rigidity of the abdominal muscles.

Unless the obstruction is relieved, organisms pass through the wall of the gut and set up peritonitis, and this is associated with a characteristic stabbing pain, which is increased by pressure, and attended by rigidity of the abdominal muscles. In cases of extreme toxæmia, the abdominal muscles may relax and the tenderness disappear—symptoms of grave omen.

Vomiting almost always commences within a few hours of the onset of the pain. This early vomiting is a reflex symptom due to interference with the sympathetic nervous system, and is, as a rule, proportionate to the severity of the pain. It is attended with nausea, retching, and eructation, and affords no relief to the patient's suffering. It occurs independently of the taking of food, and is continuous and persistent. The vomited matter consists at first of the stomach contents ; later, it contains a large admixture of bile, which appears to be excreted in excessive quantities, and is permitted to enter the stomach by the relaxation of the pylorus induced by the alkalinity of the bile (Pavlov). As time goes on, the character of the vomiting changes, and assumes the characteristic regurgitant or gushing type, in which mouthfuls of dark-brown or yellowish fluid are brought up without retching or effort. The fluid has a highly offensive odour resembling that of fæces, but is not really fæcal in character. The

odour is due to bacterial decomposition of the intestinal fluids accumulated above the obstruction, and may be as marked in cases in which
the obstruction is high up in the jejunum as in obstruction of the
large intestine.   In fact, regurgitant vomiting occurs earlier and is
more severe the nearer the obstruction is to the stomach, and it is
often entirely absent when the colon is the seat of the obstruction.

The third symptom characteristic of the onset of acute obstruction
is **shock**, which is usually well marked within a few hours, and is at
first due to the profound impression made upon the sympathetic and
other nerve fibres distributed in the abdomen.   Later, the patient
passes into a condition of **collapse**, which is aggravated by the loss of
fluid from persistent vomiting and sweating, and by intoxication from
absorption of toxins formed in the decomposing contents of the bowel
above the obstruction.   The face is pale, the eyes are sunken, the pulse
is rapid, feeble, and thready, the respiration shallow and sighing, and
the temperature persistently subnormal.   The skin is covered with
a cold, clammy sweat.   The hands, the feet, and the tips of the nose
and ears become cold, blue, and shrivelled, and there is persistent,
insatiable thirst.   The patient often suffers greatly from cramps,
especially in the calf muscles.   He usually remains conscious ; indeed,
is often abnormally alert, even to the very end, and fails to realize
the gravity of his condition.

Frequently a motion is passed just after the onset of pain and
vomiting, the lower bowel being emptied by spasmodic contraction
of the segment below the obstruction.   Thereafter there is **complete
arrest of the passage of fæces and flatus,** and the patient has
no desire to defæcate, except in those cases in which the bowel is
strangulated low down, when there may be tenesmus.   Enemata
are often retained, and if returned the fluid flows away without force
and unaccompanied by fæces or flatus.

The presence of **indican in the urine** is fairly common in cases
of acute obstruction, but it is not characteristic of this condition, as
it may be a symptom of other acute affections.   It is due to bacterial
decomposition of proteins, resulting in the formation of indol in the
small intestine, which is excreted by the kidney as indican.   This
symptom is most marked in obstruction of the small intestine, and
is generally not present till the second or third day.

An examination of the abdomen in the early stages, as a rule,
gives little information.   The belly is usually flat, flaccid, and not
tender.   Later, it is more prominent, and when peritonitis begins
it becomes rigid.

Tympanites occurs to a greater or less extent in all forms of
acute obstruction, but is most marked in obstruction of the large
intestine, particularly in volvulus of the pelvic colon.   Distension

of a single loop of bowel is of no value in localizing the seat of the obstruction.

In primary acute obstruction, peristaltic waves are seldom visible, unless the patient is extremely emaciated. In the acute phase of a gradually increasing obstruction, they are often prominent and of diagnostic value.

Except in cases of intussusception, or of obstruction by foreign bodies or fæcal concretions, a localized tumour can rarely be palpated in the abdomen.

Differential diagnosis.—The initial symptoms of acute intestinal obstruction so closely resemble those of other acute abdominal conditions that it may be extremely difficult to distinguish between them. Among the possibilities that have to be considered at this stage are : (1) Acute appendicitis, (2) perforation of a gastric or duodenal ulcer, (3) rupture of a pyosalpinx or extra-uterine gestation, (4) rotation of the pedicle of an ovarian or uterine tumour, (5) acute pancreatitis, (6) embolism or thrombosis of the mesenteric vessels, (7) various forms of colic—biliary, renal, or intestinal.

By the time the symptoms characteristic of interference with the passage of the intestinal contents come to predominate, it is usually possible to exclude most of these conditions, and the question left for decision is the cause of the obstruction. A consideration of all the available clinical data may enable a correct opinion to be formed in many cases, but in others it is impossible to do more than make an intelligent guess as to the cause of the symptoms.

In the infant, the most likely causes are : (1) Strangulated external hernia, (2) intussusception, (3) one or other form of retroperitoneal hernia, (4) congenital abnormalities of the rectum or intestine. In the child over two years of age, the possibilities are: (1) Strangulated external hernia, (2) intussusception, (3) strangulation by Meckel's diverticulum, (4) strangulation by bands or adhesions, particularly if there is a history of tuberculous peritonitis, appendicitis, injury, or a previous operation ; (5) retroperitoneal hernia. In the adult, (1) strangulated external hernia, (2) volvulus, (3) strangulation by bands or through apertures, (4) retroperitoneal hernia, (5) impaction of a gall-stone or a fæcal concretion, and (6) pressure of tumours external to the bowel, are among the primary causes of acute obstruction. It is possible that a gradual narrowing of the bowel by cicatricial contraction or by the growth of a malignant tumour may culminate in complete obstruction without any premonitory signs of stenosis. In the aged, acute obstruction is usually due to (1) sudden blockage of the narrowed lumen in malignant disease of the colon, (2) strangulated external hernia, (3) intussusception, or (4) fæcal accumulation.

Diagnosis of the site of the obstruction.—The clinical distinctions between obstruction in the small intestine and in the colon are by no means well-marked. It may be said generally that the onset of obstruction in the small intestine is more acute, the initial shock is greater, the pain more intense, and the vomiting more copious and persistent than when the colon is blocked. The illness tends to run a more rapid course, and the vomiting becomes stercoraceous sooner.

Tympanites is more marked when the colon is the seat of the obstruction, and the dilated colon may be recognizable. The patterns formed by the distended bowel, the evidence afforded by percussion, and the situation of pain, are of no constant value in fixing the seat of obstruction.

Treatment.—Only when the patient's sufferings are extreme, and there is good reason to believe they may be due to some form of colic, should opium be administered in suspected cases of obstruction. If a single moderate dose of morphia, combined with atropine, fails to relieve the pain, no more should be given; and if a definite diagnosis cannot be arrived at, arrangements should be made for an immediate exploratory operation. Meanwhile, a turpentine enema should be administered, the patient lying on his left side with the pelvis raised. Nothing should be given by the mouth, except occasional sips of warm water. The use of ice is to be avoided.

Exploratory laparotomy.—Before the anæsthetic is administered the stomach should be washed out, and if the patient is unable to empty the bladder a catheter should be passed. The abdomen is opened below the umbilicus through the inner edge of one or other rectus. The incision should only be large enough to admit two or three fingers, and the cavity should be explored systematically. The cæcum is first examined, and if it is found distended, the colon should be traced down. If it is empty, the obstruction is probably in the small intestine. If a portion of empty and contracted small intestine is discovered, it should be traced upwards till it meets distended bowel at the seat of the lesion. If nothing but distended bowel can be found it is probably safest to secure the lowest loop that can be reached, and make a temporary artificial anus in it; when the bowel has been emptied and the patient tided over the dangerous period, a second operation may be done to discover and deal with the cause of the obstruction. Every endeavour should be made to prevent coils of distended bowel escaping from the peritoneal cavity, as experience shows that this greatly diminishes the patient's chance of recovery, even when the cause of the obstruction is found and removed.

When the cause of the obstruction is readily accessible and has been removed, if the bowel above is greatly distended it may be emptied, as suggested by Moynihan, by opening it, and passing a straight glass tube over which long stretches of the gut may be pulled.

The methods of dealing with the various lesions which cause obstruction will be referred to later.

2. Chronic or Gradual Obstruction

The freedom with which the bowel contents pass along the tube may be gradually interfered with in a variety of circumstances. In the great majority of cases, the interference occurs in the colon, and is due to mechanical causes, such as the growth of a tumour in the bowel wall slowly encroaching upon the lumen and narrowing it, the cicatricial contraction of inflammatory adhesions constricting, kinking, or binding down the bowel, or the pressure of an extrinsic tumour interfering with the peristaltic action of the gut or narrowing its lumen.

In these circumstances, either there is no disturbance of the vascular and nervous mechanism of the affected portion of bowel, or this is a factor of secondary importance and one which only comes into play late in the progress of the disease.

Sooner or later, if left alone, the interference with the function of the bowel becomes so great that symptoms of acute obstruction supervene, and in many cases the crisis comes on suddenly from some superadded complication. This phase will be considered separately, later (P. 474), as the clinical procedure is different.

Pathology and morbid anatomy.—Gradual obstruction is seen in its most typical form in malignant disease of the colon, in which, without completely occluding it, the growth gradually narrows the lumen of the bowel, either by filling it up or by cicatricial contraction, or by a combination of these processes.

In those portions of the bowel—the small intestine and the higher parts of the colon—in which the fæces are usually fluid, a very considerable degree of narrowing may exist without appreciable interference with the onflow, and there are no secondary structural changes in the bowel of any importance, or only a moderate degree of dilatation. When the narrowing has progressed sufficiently to interfere with the onward passage of the contents, the segment *above the seat of the obstruction* becomes distended, its walls, particularly the muscular coat, are hypertrophied as a result of prolonged and repeated attempts to force the passage, and the tube becomes elongated and tortuous.

Hypertrophy is most marked in the small intestine, the circular muscular fibres increasing in size and number so that the wall becomes thicker and firmer than normal (Fig. 431).

In the colon, dilatation is more prominent than hypertrophy, and in some conditions may reach extreme limits, the diameter of the bowel being as much as a foot (Fig. 402).

The mucous membrane is irritated by the products of decomposition in the stagnating contents, and is in a condition of chronic catarrh. Ulceration supervenes either as a result of the action of toxins on the inflamed and stretched mucous membrane—the "distension ulcers" of Kocher—or from the pressure of hard fæcal masses in the lower colon—so-called *stercoral ulcers* (Fig. 425). The ulceration may extend through the bowel and lead to peritonitis, or suppuration in the retroperitoneal tissue.

So long as the vascular mechanism of the bowel is intact, gases do not collect in the dilated portion, as they are absorbed into the circulation, or pass through the narrowed lumen into the bowel beyond.

The segment *below the obstruction* is pale and contracted, and, as a rule, empty, although in some cases the fæcal matter that escapes past the obstruction collects in the lower segment and may form a considerable mass there, and the bowel may even be moderately distended with gas.

Effects on the mesentery.—As it gradually becomes more and more distended, the bowel may force its way between the layers of its mesentery, so that this structure is appreciably shortened. Then the affected segment of bowel becomes abnormally fixed, and this may interfere with such operations as colostomy by rendering it difficult to bring the pelvic colon to the surface. If the stretching process continues, the peritoneum covering the bowel may split in the long axis of the gut—"striation of the mesentery."

Clinical features.—The symptoms of chronic obstruction come on insidiously and, from the way in which they are produced, the progress of the malady is often irregular and intermittent. There are periods, sometimes lasting for days or even weeks, during which the patient has little difficulty with the bowels, followed by others in which a satisfactory evacuation is only obtained by taking strong purgatives or with the aid of enemata.

The early symptoms—a feeling of discomfort or a moderate degree of pain and occasional attacks of vomiting, particularly after taking food, and a more or less constant feeling of uneasiness in the abdomen—are usually attributed by the patient to dyspepsia. There is great complaint of flatulence, which the patient has difficulty in getting to pass downwards. Either these symptoms are neglected, or treatment is directed towards the stomach. Morning diarrhœa—that is, passage of a fluid stool immediately on getting up—is a common and characteristic symptom of cancerous obstruction of the lower colon.

As time goes on, the patient finds a difficulty in securing a regular and satisfactory evacuation of the bowels, and succeeds in doing so only by taking purgatives, the dose and frequency of which require to be increased without, however, being followed by a corresponding result. Eventually, the medicine has no effect on the bowels, and only induces attacks of severe griping pain, which may be accompanied by vomiting, and are often relieved by making pressure on the abdomen or by rubbing it. Sometimes the pain is increased by pressure. When the obstruction is in the colon, the patient is often able to locate it very accurately by the point at which the pain reaches the maximum during a spasm of colic.

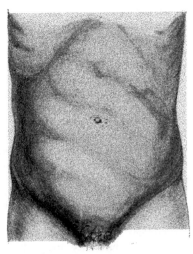

Fig. 406.—Dilated coils of small intestine forming "ladder" or "organ-pipe pattern," from a case of chronic tuberculous peritonitis with adhesions.

(From Treves's " Intestinal Obstruction.")

There is often a history of attacks of diarrhœa in which a small quantity of fæcal matter mixed with a considerable amount of mucus is passed, and these attacks are attended with great straining and are not followed by any feeling of relief. They are due to catarrhal inflammation of the mucous membrane set up by the fæcal masses retained above the seat of obstruction. As a rule, these attacks of spurious "diarrhœa" alternate with periods of marked constipation—a combination of circumstances which is very characteristic of chronic obstruction of the colon.

Gradually the bowel above the obstruction is distended and hypertrophied, the abdomen becomes more prominent, and visible peristaltic waves may be observed to pass along the gut from time to time. Visible peristalsis is perhaps the most certain clinical indication of chronic obstruction.

On rectal examination, it is frequently found that, after passing through the anal canal, the finger enters a wide open space, the walls of which it is difficult to reach. When touched, the mucous membrane is smooth, the rugæ having disappeared, and the rectum appears to be unduly fixed. This condition, known as " ballooning of the rectum," is due to paralysis of the gut, and is most frequently met with in cases of stenosis of the descending and pelvic portions of the colon.

When the small intestine is chronically distended, the contracting coils stand out as a series of tubular prominences running across the abdomen, suggesting the appearance of the rungs of a ladder, or a set of organ pipes—"ladder" or "organ-pipe pattern" (Fig. 406). When the distension affects principally the large intestine, the different parts of the colon may be recognized to be distended, but they seldom exhibit peristaltic waves so distinctly as does the small intestine (Fig. 407).

These waves of peristalsis are accompanied by attacks of colicky pain, and often by loud rumbling or gurgling sounds, spoken of as "stenosis noises" or "borborygmi," and on palpation the contracting loop of bowel is felt to become firm and rigid.

Gradually the symptoms become more severe and continuous. The digestion is seriously disturbed, the tongue and mouth become coated, the breath has an offensive fæcal odour, and the patient is poisoned by toxins absorbed from the stagnant and decomposing contents of the gut. Symptoms of collapse are present only when there is a marked degree of toxæmia.

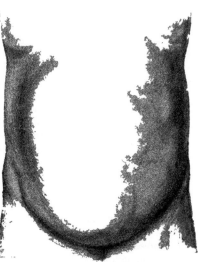

Fig. 407.—Dilatation of pelvic colon above a stricture.

(From Treves's "Intestinal Obstruction.")

Finally, death results, either from the toxæmia and exhaustion induced by it, or from the sudden occurrence of perforation and peritonitis.

Diagnosis.—There is never any difficulty in recognizing that the patient is suffering from chronic obstruction, but it may not be easy to form an opinion as to the cause. A careful analysis of all the clinical features, including the history, usually throws some light on the question. The following are among the possible causes : **In the child :** (1) Adhesions associated with tuberculous or other forms of peritonitis, (2) tuberculous disease of the bowel or mesenteric glands followed by cicatricial stenosis, (3) chronic forms of intussusception, (4) Hirschsprung's disease. **In the adult :** (1) Peritoneal adhesions, (2) cicatricial strictures, (3) malignant disease, (4) ileo-cæcal tuberculosis ; (5) fibromatosis of the colon, (6) actinomycosis, (7) primary chronic intussusception, (8) pressure of extrinsic tumours. **In the aged :** (1) Malignant disease, (2) chronic intussusception, (3) fæcal concretions, (4) fæcal accumulation.

The **treatment** of chronic obstruction depends upon the lesion causing it, and will be described later.

3. CHRONIC OBSTRUCTION TERMINATING ACUTELY

One of the most common terminations of gradually increasing stenosis of the bowel is the onset of symptoms of acute obstruction brought about by sudden occlusion of the narrowed lumen. This may be due to a hard fæcal mass, a gall-stone, or a foreign body blocking the aperture, or to congestion of the mucous membrane following the taking of a strong purgative. In other cases, it results from kinking or torsion of the affected segment brought about by rapid distension with gases, or by a sudden change of position. In advanced cases, the bowel may be exhausted by its attempts to overcome the obstruction, and become relaxed or even paralysed.

The changes in the bowel present a combination due to the gradual obstruction with the superadded effects of complete occlusion in the form of increased vascular engorgement and gaseous distension.

Unless relieved by operation, the condition usually terminates fatally, either by exhaustion induced by pain and vomiting, and interference with the action of the lungs and heart due to the distended bowel pressing upon the diaphragm, or by peritonitis set up by organisms passing through the wall of the gut or from perforation.

RETROPERITONEAL HERNIA

In the early embryo, the intestinal canal consists of an almost straight tube attached to the middle line of the body by a fold of peritoneum—the primitive mesentery. As the different segments of the alimentary canal and the associated glands are differentiated and assume the dimensions and position of the fully developed organs, this mesentery undergoes a corresponding series of changes, certain parts becoming elongated, while others become shortened and fixed. Without going into details, it may be said that, as a result of these and other changes, various peritoneal folds with intervening fossæ are developed on the posterior abdominal wall, particularly in relation to the flexures of the intestinal canal. The surgical significance of these fossæ lies in the fact that they may assume such dimensions as to form potential sacs into which a loop of bowel may pass and become strangulated.

The situations in which such retroperitoneal hernias may occur are (1) at the termination of the duodenum; (2) in the vicinity of the cæcum and appendix; (3) in the mesentery of the pelvic colon. Hernia into the foramen of Winslow, and diaphragmatic hernia, although not strictly retroperitoneal, are for convenience included in this section.

DUODENAL HERNIA

Numerous fossæ have been described in relation with the duodeno-jejunal junction. The most important for our present purpose is the *paraduodenal fossa*, which is situated on the left side of the ascending portion of the duodenum. Its left border is formed by the inferior mesenteric vein and its right by the duodeno-jejunal flexure. Its orifice looks downwards and to the right, its blind extremity being directed upwards and to the left. Into this fossa, the *left* form of duodenal hernia passes, and as it increases in size it extends down behind the transverse and descending colon.

The next most important is the *mesenterico-parietal fossa*. This lies in the mesentery of the jejunum, immediately below the duodenum and behind the superior mesenteric artery, which forms its anterior boundary. Its orifice looks to the left, and its base downwards and to the right, and into it the *right* form of duodenal hernia passes, extending down behind the transverse and ascending colon.

Clinical features.—Duodenal hernia has been met with at all ages; some of the recorded cases have occurred in infants. Its presence is never suspected unless strangulation has occurred, and even then, in the vast majority of cases, the cause of the obstruction has only been discovered on opening the abdomen.

The symptoms that may suggest the presence of a duodenal hernia are long-continued dyspepsia and irregularity of the bowels with colicky pains, and the presence of a circumscribed globular swelling, resembling a movable cyst, except that it is resonant on percussion and yields intestinal sounds on auscultation. Owing to the compression of the inferior mesenteric vein at the neck of the fossa, the patient usually suffers from piles, which bleed freely.

When *strangulation* ensues, all the symptoms of acute obstruction are present, and as it is usually the first part of the jejunum that is implicated, profound shock and persistent vomiting are prominent symptoms.

Treatment.—When, on opening the abdomen in a case of obstruction, the cause is found to be a strangulated duodenal hernia, the bowel must be withdrawn from the fossa without dividing the neck of the sac, in which runs the inferior mesenteric vein or the superior mesenteric artery. An attempt should be made to close the opening into the fossa by suturing its margins, and so prevent recurrence of the hernia.

PERICÆCAL HERNIA

Several fossæ are present in the vicinity of the ileo-cæcal junction, the most important from the surgical point of view being the *ileo-appendicular*, which lies between the ileo-appendicular or "bloodless" fold of Treves and the mesentery of the vermiform appendix; and the *retrocolic*, lying behind the cæcum and the lower part of the ascending colon.

The existence of a hernia into one or other of these pouches is never recognized unless strangulation occurs, and then the symptoms are those of acute obstruction. Usually, the hernia can readily be withdrawn from the sac, and the obliteration of the pouch is facilitated by removal of the appendix.

Hernia of the vermiform appendix alone into a fossa is not uncommon, and, if the appendix becomes strangulated, symptoms of acute appendicitis develop.

INTERSIGMOID HERNIA

This extremely rare form of hernia passes into the intersigmoid fossa, which is formed by the layers of the mesentery of the pelvic colon over the bifurcation of the common iliac artery and near the inner margin of the psoas muscle. The sigmoid vessels run in the fold of peritoneum which forms its anterior margin.

HERNIA INTO THE FORAMEN OF WINSLOW

Hernia through the foramen of Winslow is very rare, and is only possible when the foramen is exceptionally large, owing to some congenital abnormality.

When strangulation occurs, the usual signs of acute obstruction are present, the pain being intense and situated in the epigastrium, and a swelling, which is dull on light percussion but gives a resonant note on deeper percussion, can usually be made out. It is a curious fact that there is no evidence of pressure on the hepatic vessels or bile-duct, which run in the margin of the foramen.

The **treatment** consists in opening the abdomen and withdrawing the strangulated coil. As the structures in the margins of the foramen forbid division of the constricting agent, if reduction cannot be effected by traction the lesser sac of the peritoneum must be opened through the gastro-hepatic or gastro-colic omentum, and the distended bowel withdrawn and emptied. After the opening in the bowel is sutured, it is returned to the lesser sac and withdrawn through the foramen.

DIAPHRAGMATIC HERNIA

This term is applied to any protrusion of the abdominal contents through the diaphragm, although in nearly 90 per cent. of cases there is no peritoneal sac, and the condition is rather one of prolapse than of true hernia.

Morbid anatomy.—The protrusion may take place (1) through one or other of the natural openings in the diaphragm, particularly that for the œsophagus; (2) through a congenital deficiency in the muscle; (3) through a tear produced by indirect violence or muscular effort; or (4) through a direct wound of the muscle.

The condition is usually met with on the left side, where the diaphragm lacks the support of the liver. The size of the opening varies from a mere slit in the tendinous portion of the diaphragm to a complete absence of one half of the muscle.

As a rule the viscera are prolapsed into the left pleural cavity, and the organs most frequently implicated are the stomach, the colon, and the small intestine. The liver, pancreas, spleen, and left kidney have also been found in such hernias.

The majority of cases of congenital diaphragmatic hernia have been met with on post-mortem examination of still-born children, or of infants who have only survived a few days. Others have been found at the autopsy of adults who have never manifested any clinical signs of such a condition. In cases of traumatic origin, signs may develop soon after the injury, or not till long after.

Clinical features.—The condition has very seldom been accurately diagnosed during life. As the stomach is almost always present in the hernia, gastric discomfort constitutes the chief complaint, and the patient may be conscious that the food lodges in the region of the chest, where it produces a fixed pain.

On examination, an unnatural depression in the epigastric and left hypochondriac regions may be noted, with a corresponding fullness in the lower thoracic region. The thoracic signs are similar to those of pneumothorax, but are detectable chiefly in the lower part of the chest, and distinct intestinal gurgling may sometimes be heard on auscultation. The heart may be displaced and its action interfered with, causing palpitation, attacks of dyspnœa and oppression in the chest, with inability to lie on the left side.

These symptoms are influenced by the taking of food or fluid and sometimes by exertion, and the rapid variations in the physical signs help to differentiate this condition from pneumothorax.

Information may be obtained by taking an X-ray photograph after administering a bismuth meal, or following an injection of bismuth emulsion into the colon.

When the hernia is suddenly produced, there is intense dyspnœa and cyanosis, with severe præcordial pain and oppression, and the condition may rapidly prove fatal from shock or from compression of the lung.

Strangulation is associated with all the signs of acute obstruction. It may be determined in an old-standing hernia by some sudden and violent muscular effort, or by a crush of the body. In traumatic cases, the bowel may become strangulated at the moment it passes through the rent in the diaphragm.

Treatment.—In *recent traumatic cases*, an attempt should always be made to replace the prolapsed viscera in the peritoneal cavity. The rent in the diaphragm must be closed by suture, and to effect this it may be necessary to enlarge the wound and even to resect portions of one or more ribs.

When *strangulation* has occurred and the hernia is discovered on opening the abdomen, before any attempt is made to reduce it the pleural cavity should be opened by a U- or T-shaped incision, with resection of ribs, to avoid the risk of pulling a gangrenous or perforated loop of bowel into the peritoneal cavity, to enable the pleural cavity to be purified and drained, and to facilitate the subsequent closure of the opening in the diaphragm.

To avoid the risks of pneumothorax incident to free opening of the pleural cavity, such operations should, if possible, be done under altered atmospheric pressure.

PERITONEAL ADHESIONS

All varieties of inflammation of the peritoneum are liable to be followed by the formation of adhesions between adjacent serous surfaces. In certain circumstances—for example, after surgical operations on the bowel, as a sequel to drainage of the peritoneal cavity in cases of gastric or intestinal ulcers, cholecystitis, or disease of the mesenteric glands—the adhesions are confined to the vicinity of the irritant, and may only persist as long as the irritation lasts, serving a protective purpose and being absorbed when they are no longer required. On the other hand, as a sequel to such conditions as generalized septic or tuberculous peritonitis, the adhesions may involve the whole of the peritoneal membrane, matting the intestines into an inextricable mass, and fixing the viscera to one another and to the parietal peritoneum.

Between these extremes all degrees are met with, and the adhesions may take the form of broad thin sheets of fibrous tissue stretching between adjacent coils of bowel (Fig. 408), or narrow strands fixing one short loop to another, or they may be moulded into long cord-like bands passing from one part of the abdominal cavity to another.

The effect of adhesions on the function of the bowel bears no direct relation to their extent or disposition, and it is remarkable how little disturbance may result even when the whole intestine is matted into what appears to be a solid mass. When adhesions do give rise to symptoms, these may take the form of repeated attacks of colicky pain with vomiting, a moderately acute obstruction, or a gradually increasing interference with the passage of the intestinal contents.

Obstruction due to peritoneal adhesions.—The more acute form of obstruction is usually due to *kinking, bending,* or *twisting* of a short segment of bowel, which is suddenly dragged upon by an adhesion attached to its border so that the lumen is occluded. The traction may be due to distension of the coil by gas, or to some change in position. As this mechanism does not involve any serious interference with the blood supply of the affected coil, the symptoms are less acute than when the bowel is strangulated, for example, by a band. The cause of this form of obstruction is seldom diagnosed before the abdomen is opened, but the history of previous peritonitis or trauma should suggest the possibility of peritoneal adhesions.

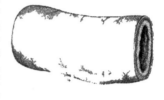

Limited adhesions may be separated and steps taken to prevent their re-formation by smearing the raw surfaces with sterilized vaseline oil.

The more gradual form of obstruction is due to *fixation* of a loop of bowel; to *localized constriction* by adhesions which encircle a segment; to *cicatricial contraction* of the mesentery; or to widespread adhesions *matting* a number of coils into a confused mass, as is frequently seen in cases of tuberculous peritonitis, or of disease of the mesenteric glands. The chronic symptoms—vague abdominal discomfort, colicky pains with occasional attacks of vomiting, gradually

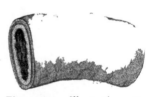

Fig. 408. — Illustrating the formation of a fibrous band between two coils of small intestine.

(*Museum, Royal College of Surgeons, Edinburgh.*)

increasing difficulty in securing a regular action of the bowels, and progressive distension—often culminate in acute obstruction.

This form of obstruction may usually be diagnosed from the history of previous disease in the glands or peritoneum, from the gradual progress of the symptoms, and in many cases from the detection of a localized swelling in the abdomen or on rectal examination.

If the adhesions cannot be separated and resection of the affected segments is impracticable, an anastomosis should be established between the bowel above and below the obstruction. If this is not possible at the timé, a temporary opening must be made in the bowel above the obstruction, and a more radical operation performed when the patient is in a better condition to stand it. The results of these operations have been very satisfactory, especially in cases due to tuberculosis.

STRANGULATION BY BANDS AND THROUGH ABNORMAL APERTURES

Strangulation by bands.—This is a common cause of acute obstruction. The constricting agent may be a solitary fibrous band

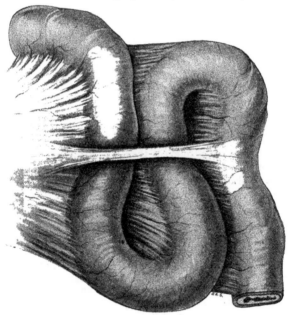

Fig. 409.—Obstruction of loop of small intestine by a band.
(Semi-diagrammatic.)

passing across the peritoneal cavity, a portion of the great omèntum that has formed abnormal attachments, a Meckel's diverticulum, or some misplaced and abnormally attached anatomical structure, such as the vermiform appendix or the Fallopian tube.

1. *Solitary peritoneal bands* result from the moulding and stretching of plastic exudate between two inflamed peritoneal surfaces. They are, therefore, most commonly found in the vicinity of the vermiform appendix (Fig. 411) and female pelvic organs, near hernial apertures,

or in relation with localized foci of tuberculosis either in the bowel or the mesenteric glands. Not infrequently a hand forms at the site of a previous operation.

As a rule, one end of the band is attached to the mesentery and the other to the parietal peritoneum, to another part of the mesentery, or to one of the viscera (Fig. 411). Occasionally one extremity becomes separated, and floats free among the viscera.

Bands vary in length from a fraction of an inch to several inches, and in thickness from a mere thread to a cord as thick as the finger. As a rule, they are round and cord-like, but sometimes they are flattened like a ribbon.

2. *Omental bands.* —The free edge of the great omentum not infrequently forms attachments with some part that has been the seat of inflammation, such as the region of the vermiform appendix, the Fallopian tube, tuberculous mesenteric glands, or a

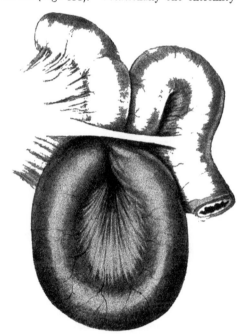

Fig. 410.—Obstruction of small intestine by a band, with volvulus of the strangulated loop. (Semi-diagrammatic.)

loop of intestine which has been injured or is the seat of ulceration ; and in course of time the adherent portion becomes so stretched and moulded as to constitute a band. Bands formed in this way are usually broader and stronger than peritoneal bands, and the fact that one end is always attached to the transverse colon, which is movable and yielding, explains why strangulation by an omental band is generally less acute than that caused by a fibrous cord.

There is often more than one omental band—a fact which must be borne in mind in cases of obstruction, lest the whole of the constricting agent be not divided.

2 f

3. A *Meckel's diverticulum* may cause obstruction by acting as a band (Fig. 401, p. 445).

4. *Bands formed by anatomical structures abnormally attached.*— Among anatomical structures which may act as bands and so cause obstruction may be mentioned the *vermiform appendix,* which may become attached to the right ovary, to the uterus, to an adjacent portion of mesentery (Fig. 412), or to the anterior abdominal wall.

The *Fallopian tube* (Plate 93), or even an enlarged *appendix epiploica,* may act in a similar manner.

I have operated on one case in which the *pedicle of a fibroid* of the uterus ensnared a coil of small intestine and caused obstruction, and on another in which the *pedicle of an ovarian cyst* was the cause of obstruction.

Strangulation through abnormal apertures.— In the majority of cases of obstruction due to this cause, the small intestine is

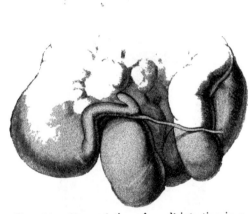

Fig. 411.—Strangulation of small intestine in a child by a cord-like band stretching between the vermiform appendix and a coil of small intestine.

(Author's case.)

prolapsed through an abnormal aperture in the mesentery of the lower ileum. Such apertures may be congenital, but are usually the result of a previous injury, the mesentery having been torn by a kick or crush of the abdomen, or divided in the course of an operation and not united again. In course of time the edges of the rent become smooth, rounded, and unyielding, and a ring or slit is formed into which a knuckle of bowel may at any time slip. Similar apertures may be met with in the great omentum, and less frequently in the mesentery of the transverse and descending colon. Slits are sometimes formed by stretched adhesions resulting from peritonitis, particularly in relation to the female pelvic organs.

Clinical features.—The symptoms are usually those of the most acute forms of intestinal obstruction (p. 465). Examination of the abdomen seldom reveals any localizing signs, and rectal examination is likewise negative. It is not uncommon, however, for a considerable quantity of blood to be passed by the rectum, and in children this may suggest the possibility of intussusception. A history that

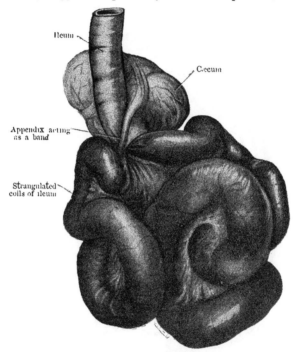

Ileum

Cæcum

Appendix acting as a band

Strangulated coils of ileum

Fig. 412.—Portion of small intestine strangulated by vermiform appendix acting as a band.

(*Anatomical Museum, University of Edinburgh.*)

the patient has previously suffered from some form of peritonitis, especially tuberculous, should suggest the presence of a band.

Treatment.—In the great majority of cases, it is impossible to arrive at a positive diagnosis as to the cause of the obstruction before the abdomen is opened. The escape of blood-stained fluid on opening the peritoneal cavity is strongly suggestive of the presence of a band or of volvulus. Any loop of contracted intestine that can be found should be traced upwards until the seat of obstruction is reached. If a band is discovered. it should, if possible, be divided between forceps and the secured ends removed.

When the bowel is prolapsed through an aperture, it is usually necessary to divide the constricting ring before it can be released, and in doing so care must be taken not to interfere unduly with the vessels of the mesentery lest the blood supply to the intestine be diminished. The opening should be closed by sutures to prevent recurrence of the protrusion. If the strangulated loop is gangrenous,

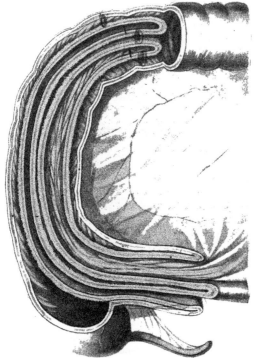

Fig. 413.—Diagram of intussusception.
(*Modified from R. C. Coffey.*)

t should be resected; but if the patient cannot stand this at the time, it must be brought to the surface, opened, and drained, the resection being postponed until the conditions are more favourable.

INTUSSUSCEPTION

Intussusception may be defined as the invagination of one part of the intestine into the lumen of the immediately adjoining part. In the great majority of cases it is the upper segment of bowel that passes into the lower.

The condition is most frequently met with in young children, and in them gives rise to one form of acute obstruction. When it occurs as a primary affection in the adult, the symptoms are usually those of a gradual or intermittent obstruction, which, however, may culminate in an acute and complete attack.

A typical intussusception forms a firm, rigid, sausage-like swelling, which, on account of the traction on the mesentery, usually assumes a semilunar or horseshoe shape. It is composed of three concentrically arranged tubes of bowel, which are differentiated from without inwards, as follows : (1) the *receiving tube* or *sheath ;* (2) the *returning tube ;* and (3) the *entering tube*. The entering and returning tubes together form the *intussusceptum*, and the receiving tube is the *intussuscipiens*.

The most advanced part of the intussusceptum, where the entering and returning layers join, is known as the *apex*, and is usually the starting-point of the invagination ; and the part at which the returning and receiving layers are continuous, and where the mesentery enters, is spoken of as the *neck*. In the space between the entering and returning layers, on the concave side of the intussusception, the mesentery is tightly packed (Fig. 413).

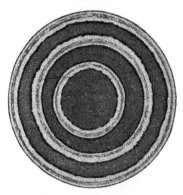

Fig. 414.—Cross-section of intussusception.

In vertical section, the mass consists of six layers, three on each side of the central canal ; and on transverse section, of three concentric rings, so arranged that mucous surfaces are in contact with mucous surfaces, and serous with serous (Fig. 414).

Multiple intussusceptions.—If the sheath is abnormally loose it may become folded on itself, forming a *double intussusception* (Fig. 416). In rare cases it is twice folded—*triple intussusception*.

According to the segment of bowel implicated, three types of intussusception are recognized : the *entero-colic*, in which the small intestine is invaginated into the colon ; the *colic*, in which the one part of the colon passes into the adjacent part ; and the *enteric*, in which one part of the small intestine is invaginated into another part.

Acute Intussusception in the Child

As the great majority of cases of intussusception occur in children and involve the ileo-cæcal region, giving rise to a form of acute

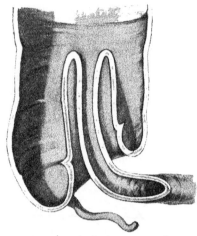

Fig. 415.—Single intussusception.

obstruction, it is convenient for clinical purposes to describe the condition in terms of this variety.

Three different forms are met with: (1) The *ileo-cæcal*, in which the ileo-cæcal valve forms the apex of the intussusception — this is the commonest form; (2) the *ileo-colic*, in which the invagination begins in the last few inches of the ileum (Fig. 417); and (3) the *cæcal*, in which the inverted cæcum forms the apex.

It is not always easy, however, in the course of an operation to distinguish these varieties of intussusception from one another.

Etiology.—The subjects of intussusception are usually lusty children in apparently perfect health, but it is generally possible to elicit a history of some recent slight disturbance of the bowels in the form of constipation or diarrhœa, in which the peristaltic function of the gut has been deranged, and it is probably to irregular muscular contraction that the commencement of the invagination is due. A portion of inflamed or swollen mucous membrane is pushed or pulled towards the lumen of the segment of gut just beyond, and acts as an irritant, setting up a reflex similar to that by which a bolus of food is passed along the bowel. The presence of a polypus,

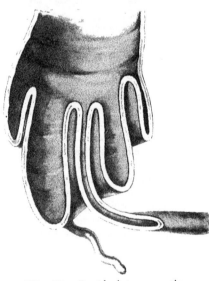

Fig. 416.—Double intussusception.

or of an inverted Meckel's diverticulum or vermiform appendix, renders such an explanation of the commencement of the invagination even more easily understood (Fig. 418). The apex of the intussusception, the first part to be invaginated, for all practical purposes remains constant, and, as it soon becomes congested and œdematous, it is impossible for more of the entering layer to roll

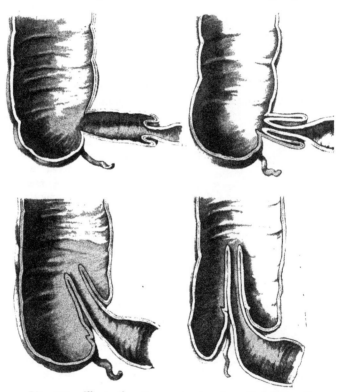

Fig. 417.—Illustrating the mechanism by which ileo-colic intussusceptions are formed.

(*Modified after P. C. L. Fitzwilliams*)

over and become part of the returning layer. The result is that the peristaltic efforts of the gut to force on the apex drag the sheath over the intussusceptum, so that the returning layer is gradually lengthened and the sheath creeps up the invaginated portion. An intussusception, therefore, increases at the expense of the sheath.

The frequency with which the intussusception originates in the ileo-cæcal region is to be explained by the anatomical and physiological arrangements of this part of the bowel, the last few inches of the ileum acting as a detrusor muscle to pass the intestinal contents through the ileo-colic sphincter, and being studded over with numerous Peyer's patches, which are liable to become inflamed and swollen. The greater size of the lumen of the colon as compared with the ileum, and the length and looseness of the meso-colon of the infant, also favour the folding of the receiving layer over the intussusceptum.

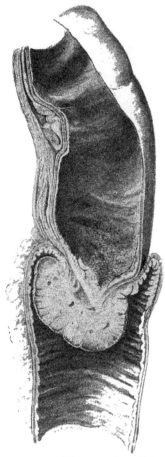

Fig. 418.—Adenoma of small in-testine causing intussusception.

(*Museum, Royal College of Surgeons, Edinburgh.*)

Morbid anatomy.—As the intussusceptum increases in length, the mesentery is dragged in between the entering and returning tubes, and the tension exerted through the mesentery causes the intussuscep-tion to become curved with its concavity towards the mesenteric attachment. At the same time, the whole intussusception is drawn back towards the promontory of the sa-crum where the mesentery is at-tached, and swings round in the direction of the hands of a watch till it may reach the left iliac fossa. In this process the mesentery is compressed, twisted, and stretched to such an extent that the vascular supply of the bowel is interfered with. At first the venous return is impeded, leading to engorgement and swelling of the invaginated bowel. As the congestion increases, blood is extravasated into the coats of the bowel, and an excess of mucus mixed with blood oozes from the mucous surfaces and is passed by the rectum.

The effects of the congestion are most marked in the returning tube, and towards the apex of the intussusception, which may become swollen into a knob, and this, together with adhesions formed between the apposed serous surfaces, renders the intussusception irreducible. The laxity of the outer wall of the cæcum admits of its slipping farther down than the rest of the intussusceptum, so that it may even be in advance of the true apex, and after reduction a characteristic "dimple" remains for a time on the lower and outer part of the cæcal wall (Fig. 419).

In time the swelling of the implicated bowel and the contraction of the sheath in its attempts to expel the intussusceptum occlude the lumen and lead to complete obstruction.

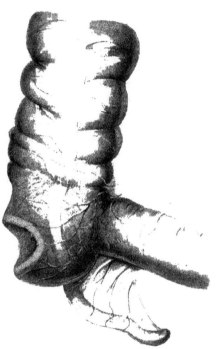

The interference with the nutrition of the bowel is followed by bacterial invasion of the coats, which may determine gangrene or lead to peritonitis.

The gangrene affeets first and chiefly the returning tube, then the entering tube, but it rarely implicates the sheath. In a certain number of cases the whole intussusceptum has undergone necrosis and been separated as a blackish-green tubular slough, varying in length from a few inches to several feet, and recovery

Fig. 419.—To illustrate the dimple in the wall of the cæcum after reduction of an intussusception.

(After D. C. L. Fitzwilliams.)

has in very rare instances followed the expulsion of such a slough.

Clinical features.—Intussusception is the most common cause of acute obstruction in children, and the clinical picture is usually so characteristic as to leave little doubt regarding the diagnosis. Nearly 75 per cent. of the cases occur during the first year of life, and about 70 per cent. are in boys. The subjects of this condition are, as a rule, fine lusty infants, and are in apparently perfect health when attacked.

The illness begins with an attack of severe intestinal colic, which causes the child to scream out and draw up his knees. The face is pale and manifests severe suffering; the eyes are bright and widely opened, as in fear. Soon after the onset of the pain, the child usually empties the stomach by vomiting, but the vomiting is not severe or persistent, and even in advanced cases it seldom becomes fæcal. The lower bowel is often emptied also, the motion being a normal one. This is followed by persistent tenesmus, a considerable quantity of mucus tinged with blood being expelled at frequent intervals. After a time, the symptoms abate, but they soon recur. In the intervals the patient may be unnaturally quiet and listless, but otherwise appears quite well. In most cases a general anæsthetic should be administered to admit of a satisfactory examination of the abdomen and rectum.

When the abdomen is examined it is often observed that the right iliac fossa is abnormally empty, and a firm, sausage-shaped swelling, curved with its concavity towards the umbilicus, can be felt in the line of the transverse or of the descending colon. The swelling may be recognized to harden and become more definite during the spasms of pain. There is seldom distension of the abdomen during the first two or three days.

The abdominal muscles are not rigid, and, so long as the swelling is not pressed upon, the child does not resent examination of the abdomen.

If the intussusception has reached the pelvic colon, as it does in about 25 per cent. of cases, it may be recognized on rectal examination as a soft, conical mass with a central slit-like depression resembling the os uteri, and the examining finger may be stained with bloody mucus like red-currant jelly. The sphincters are usually relaxed, but may be in a state of spasm. The intussusception seldom protrudes from the anus in acute cases.

As time goes on, the intervals between the attacks of colic are shorter, the pain becomes continuous, with occasional exacerbations, and the tenesmus is constant.

The child becomes exhausted, the facial appearance alters, dark rings appear round the eyes, and the abdomen becomes distended. If infection of the peritoneum takes place, the abdomen is tender and rigid, and other signs of peritonitis develop.

Differential diagnosis.—The only condition that may be mistaken for intussusception in infants is acute colitis, which is comparatively common at this age. The more gradual onset of the illness and the presence of bile in the matter passed from the rectum suggest a diagnosis of colitis; in intussusception the onset is sudden and the obstruction of the bowel prevents bile reaching the rectum.

Treatment.—Statistics show that every hour of delay in

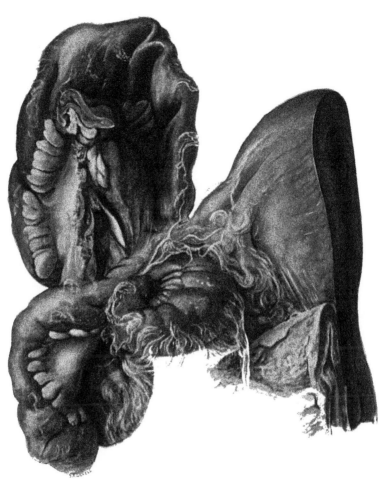

Strangulation of a loop of small intestine.

(*Museum, Royal College of Surgeons, Edinburgh.*)

PLATE 93.

operating diminishes the prospect of recovery. An incision is made over the most prominent part of the swelling, which is usually either in the line of the ascending colon, or in the vicinity of the umbilicus. The opening should be large enough to admit of ready access to the invaginated segment of bowel, so that it may be brought to the surface with as little handling as possible. In carrying out reduction of the invagination, the tumour should be straightened out as far as possible, after which pressure is made on the intussusceptum by compressing the sheath just beyond the apex. On no account should the entering loop be pulled upon, as this involves considerable risk of tearing the bowel. As a rule, in early cases reduction is easily effected in this way; but the last part may be difficult to reduce on account of the apex having become œdematous, in which case, to diminish the œdema, it should be gently squeezed for a few minutes through a pad of moist gauze. When the invagination has lasted for some considerable time, reduction may be prevented by adhesions between the apposed serous surfaces of the entering and returning tubes, or by swelling of the mesentery.

After reduction has been effected, the whole length of bowel implicated should be examined for evidence of threatening gangrene or of damage to the peritoneal coat. If there is any doubt as to the viability of the gut, it should be brought out and an artificial anus established.

To diminish the risk of recurrence, a longitudinal tuck or fold may be made in the mesentery of the ileum, or the mesentery may be stitched to the ascending mesocolon.

If it is impossible to effect complete reduction, or if, when reduced, the bowel is found to be gangrenous, the affected segment must be excised. By a continuous suture, the sheath and the intussusceptum are united at the neck of the intussusception; the sheath is then incised longitudinally, and the intussusceptum removed; and the operation is completed by closing the opening in the sheath, or by stitching its edges to the parietal peritoneum, and so forming an artificial anus.

If the sheath is gangrenous, the whole of the segment of bowel implicated must be resected.

The mortality after all forms of resection, whether with or without the formation of an artificial anus, is very high.

Chronic Intussusception in the Child

This is usually of the ileo-cæcal variety, and the condition may run a very slow course, associated with attacks of colicky pain, irregularity of the bowels, and the passage of blood in the stools. Visible peristalsis can sometimes be observed, particularly after a meal, and in some cases a tumour can be recognized on palpation. This tumour may change its position from time to time, and sometimes it reaches the rectum and is protruded from the anus, in which case it may be mistaken for a prolapse or a polypus.

The condition is treated on the same lines as acute intussusception

ACUTE INTUSSUSCEPTION IN THE ADULT

In the adult, intussusception is a rare cause of acute obstruction not more than 12 per cent. of all intussusceptions occurring in patients over 10 years of age.

Generally speaking, it may be said that the etiology is the same as in children, but more frequently some definite morbid condition of the bowel wall is present, such as an ulcerated polypus, a malignant tumour, or a diseased condition of the mucous membrane, which determines the invagination.

There is, therefore, usually a long history of gastro-intestinal disturbance, which culminates in acute obstruction. The intussusception may be of the entero-colic or of the enteric variety.

The clinical features are less characteristic than in the child, and the differential diagnosis from other causes of obstruction more difficult. On the whole, the symptoms are less acute than in children.

CHRONIC PRIMARY INTUSSUSCEPTION IN THE ADULT

Apart from cases in which chronic intussusception is due to tumour, ulceration, or tuberculosis of the bowel wall, a number of cases have been recorded in which the invagination was the primary condition leading to gradual obstruction of the bowel. Goodall of Boston has made a study of the literature of this subject, based upon 122 recorded cases.

Morbid anatomy.—The intussusception is usually of the entero-colic variety, the enteric and colic forms being comparatively rare. As a rule, there are numerous adhesions between the different layers, which render reduction impossible, but in some cases, in spite of the fact that the condition has lasted for weeks or even months, there have been remarkably few adhesions.

The lumen of the gut may be narrowed to the size of the little finger or even to that of a goose-quill, and sometimes a false opening forms which admits of the intestinal contents passing on.

Ulceration of the mucous membrane of the coils implicated is common, and the sheath frequently becomes perforated at several points, so that portions of the invaginated bowel project through it (Plate 94).

Clinical features.—The condition is usually met with in persons between 20 and 40 years of age, and appears to be twice as common in men as in women.

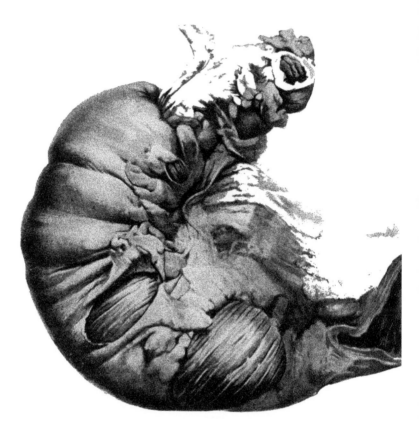

Chronic primary intussusception in an old man.

(*Author's case.*)

PLATE 94.

The symptoms may come on gradually in the form of gastro-intestinal disturbance with occasional attacks during which there is a threatening of obstruction, which, however, passes off in some hours. This state of affairs may last over a period of months or even years, and the illness runs a very obscure course.

The most constant symptom is the occurrence of repeated attacks of abdominal colic coming in paroxysms, and lasting for a period which may vary from a few minutes to some hours. It is characteristic of the pain that at the end of the attack it disappears suddenly, and the patient is at once quite comfortable again. This is especially the ease in the earlier stages, and it is attributed to the bowel becoming disinvaginated and to the sudden relief of congestion. In the later stages when adhesions have formed, the relief comes more gradually. At first the attacks recur every two or three days, but as time goes on the intervals become shorter, and there is more or less constant discomfort, with periodic exacerbations which are frequently determined by the taking of purgatives or unsuitable food, or by exertion.

Vomiting is seldom absent during an attack of pain, and may occur between attacks; recovery has followed an attack in which the vomiting was distinctly stercoraceous.

Constipation is not a constant symptom; in fact, there is often diarrhœa, the bowels moving three or four times a day, the motions being watery and offensive, and containing much mucus and often some blood. Tenesmus is a common symptom.

The patient gradually becomes exhausted from pain, is anxious and depressed, and soon shows signs of anæmia. Emaciation may be so extreme as to suggest malignant disease.

On examining the abdomen, distended coils of intestine can be recognized during an attack. In the entero-colic variety there is often a localized flattening of the right iliac fossa, while the rest of the abdomen is prominent.

In the majority of cases a localized, sausage-shaped tumour can be made out. It is usually ill defined towards its ends. It may be firm and elastic, or soft and doughy from fæcal accumulation. It is characteristic that the tumour varies in shape and size from time to time, and may even temporarily disappear. In some of the recorded cases the tumour only appeared during an attack of pain, and vanished with a gurgling sound when the pain ceased.

Symptoms of acute obstruction eventually supervene, or perforation occurs and gives rise to peritonitis. In a few cases spontaneous separation of the intussusceptum has taken place, but this has been followed by stenosis.

Differential diagnosis.—The majority of cases have hitherto been diagnosed only on opening the abdomen, or on post-mortem examination. The conditions for which it is most liable to be mis-taken are cancer of the bowel, ileo-cæcal tuberculosis, colitis, and recurrent appendicitis.

Treatment.—The only treatment is to open the abdomen and deal with the invagination. Hitherto the results obtained by resection have been satisfactory.

VOLVULUS

The term " volvulus " is applied to a condition in which a segment of bowel is twisted on its mesenteric axis. It is one of the most fatal of all forms of obstruction.

VOLVULUS OF THE PELVIC COLON

The pelvic colon is the segment of bowel implicated in about 75 per cent. of cases.

Etiology.—This portion of the colon, which approximates in shape to the letter Ω, is rendered liable to be twisted by the fact that its mesentery is comparatively narrow in proportion to the length of the bowel so that the two ends of the loop are approximated. The loop varies in length from about 8 in. to 2 ft., and the longer the loop in proportion to the width of its mesentery, the greater is the liability to volvulus.

The secondary changes in the mesocolon which further predispose to volvulus are—(1) *elongation*, such as may result, for example, from chronic constipation—the overloaded bowel by its weight hanging down into the pelvis and dragging upon the mesentery ; (2) *narrowing* of the base of attachment to the sacrum, resulting in closer approxi-mation of the two ends of the Ω-loop, produced, for instance, by inflammatory adhesions, by changes occurring in infected lymph-glands, or as a result of chronic inflammatory or ulcerative conditions in the bowel itself ; (3) *fixation* of the parietal attachment, as a result of thickening or adhesions due to inflammatory changes, forming an axis around which the bowel readily rotates.

The actual twisting is usually brought about by irregular peristalsis, induced, for example, by overloading of the pelvic colon in chronic constipation, or by efforts on the part of the bowel to expel a hardened mass of fæces, or by an excessive accumulation of flatus. The mere weight of an overloaded sigmoid may cause it to fall into the pelvis and twist its base. A violent straining effort, such as making a heavy lift, a sudden alteration in the intra-abdominal pressure, or even a change in the attitude of the patient may induce rotation.

As a rule, the upper part of the sigmoid rotates downwards and forwards, so that the rectum lies behind the twisted loop (Fig. 420). Less commonly, it passes backwards, and the rectum lies in front

(Fig. 421). The extent of the rotation varies from a half-twist—180°—to two or even three complete turns.

Morbid anatomy.—The gravity of the condition depends upon the tightness of the constriction at the base of the mesentery. If the twist does not implicate the blood-vessels in such a way as to occlude them, the symptoms are those of incarceration or incomplete obstruction ; but if the veins are occluded and the return of blood from the implicated segment is interfered with, symptoms of complete obstruction ensue. The twisted loop becomes intensely congested and œdematous, and assumes a dark purple colour. Hæmorrhages occur into the tissues, and serum, mixed with blood, escapes into the lumen of the gut and into the peritoneal cavity. The fluid found on opening the abdomen is of a brownish chocolate colour—a point of some diagnostic importance.

The twisted loop rapidly becomes enormously dilated, sometimes to such an extent that it nearly fills the abdominal cavity, pressing the small intestine backwards and towards the right. The diaphragm may be so pressed upon that the action of the heart and lungs is seriously impeded. The gas with which the bowel is distended is probably chiefly carbonic acid gas, which is not absorbed from the gut owing to the occlusion of the veins. Gases of putrefaction are also present, but the rapidity with which distension occurs makes it unlikely that they are the chief cause.

The dilatation of the sigmoid may be so great that the longitudinal striæ are not recognizable, and the peritoneal covering may split and gangrene of the gut take place. Under these conditions organisms soon pass through the wall of the bowel and, reaching the peritoneal surface, set up peritonitis, which speedily becomes generalized. Although patches of gangrene often form in the distended bowel, perforation, when it occurs, is usually above the twist.

Clinical features.—Volvulus of the pelvic colon is most frequently met with in adults in the prime of life, and is four times commoner in men than in women. There is generally a history of constipation. The symptoms usually come on suddenly, and the illness rapidly assumes the characters of acute and complete obstruction. There is sharp pain, with exacerbations of a colicky character. It is generally referred to the region of the umbilicus, and radiates along the colon to the left iliac fossa and to the lumbar region and back. In a comparatively short time definite tenderness can be detected in the left iliac fossa, a symptom which indicates the onset of peritonitis. There is frequently severe tenesmus, but nothing is passed by the bowel. Vomiting is seldom an early or a prominent symptom, as the seat of the lesion is low down in the large intestine, but hiccup and eructation of gas are in many cases persistent. The initial shock is not so severe as in most of the other forms of acute obstruction.

The most striking and characteristic local sign is the early and extreme degree of distension of the abdomen. Within a few hours the left side of the belly becomes prominent and yields a uniform drummy note on percussion, the colon becomes so dilated that it fills the abdomen, and the other viscera are pushed aside and cannot be located by percussion. The diaphragm may be displaced up as

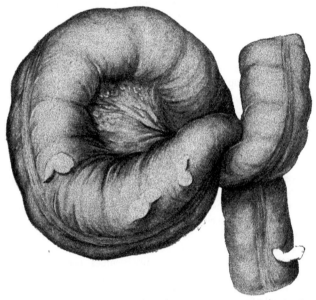

Fig. 420.—Volvulus of pelvic colon downwards and forwards.
(Semi-diagrammatic.)

far as the level of the third rib, with the result that the circulation and the respiration are seriously interfered with. Visible peristalsis is exceptional, as the bowel above the twisted loop is so pressed upon that it is incapable of contracting.

If unrelieved, the condition usually proves fatal in two or three days from peritonitis due to infection through the congested loop, or to perforation of the gut above the twist.

Only in rare cases is the obstruction *incomplete*. In these, the onset is less acute, and fæces and flatus may be passed in small quantities, or diarrhœa even may be present. In such cases, untwisting of the bowel may occur, with relief of the symptoms, but the condition is liable to recur from time to time if the pelvic colon becomes over-loaded.

Treatment.—When there is reason to suspect the presence of a volvulus within a few hours of the onset of obstructive symptoms, with the patient in the knee-elbow position a long rectal tube may be passed into the colon to withdraw gas and fluid.   If this is not imme-diately successful, it need not be repeated, and no time should be lost in opening the abdomen.   The incision should be large enough to

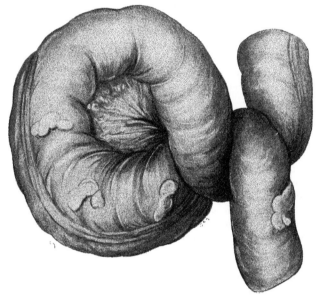

Fig. 421.—Volvulus of pelvic colon backwards.
(Semi-diagrammatic.)

admit of free access to the distended coil, and even of its being brought out of the abdomen.   After the abdomen has been opened, it may be possible, with one hand inside, to guide a rectal tube past the twist and so empty the distended loop of gas and fluid fæces.   If successful, this greatly simplifies the further manipulations ; if it fails, the loop must be opened and the twist undone.

If the gut is viable, the opening may be closed and the loop returned to the abdomen after any adhesions that may be present have been dealt with.   It is probably safer, however, to utilize the opening as an artificial anus till the patient has got over the immediate effects of the obstruction.

2 g

Primary resection is indicated only when the twisted loop is gangrenous, and then the divided ends of the bowel should be brought to the surface and drained, a lateral anastomosis being established later.

When the volvulus cannot be untwisted, an artificial anus should be established in the distended bowel above, and a tube inserted into the twisted loop to drain it. If the patient survives, the affected segment of gut is subsequently resected, and the continuity of the canal re-established by end-to-end suture or lateral anastomosis.

Attempts have been made to prevent recurrence of volvulus by stitching the pelvic colon to the parietal peritoneum or to the iliac fossa, but these have not proved successful. More satisfactory results have been attained by shortening the mesentery of the pelvic colon by a series of sutures introduced parallel to the bowel, care being taken not to interfere with the blood supply or to kink the bowel. If recurrence takes place, as it frequently does, the pelvic colon should be excised.

OTHER FORMS OF VOLVULUS

The other portions of the intestine that may be the seat of volvulus are—(1) the *ileo-cæcal junction,* and (2) the *small intestine.* So long as the mesenteric arrangements of these parts are normal, volvulus cannot take place; but if the mesentery is abnormally long, or its base of attachment narrowed or rendered rigid, then volvulus may occur.

Volvulus of the ileo-cæcal junction.—The twist may be limited to the cæcum, or may also involve the ascending colon, the last part of the ileum, or both. The conditions of occurrence are the same as in volvulus of the pelvic colon, and the circumstances which determine it similar.

The condition is less acute than when the pelvic colon is twisted. Vomiting is present, although not severe. The distension is not so extreme, and the distended cæcum may be recognizable in the right loin and iliac fossa, or in the left hypochondrium, as a defined resonant swelling about the size of a child's head. The difficulty of undoing the twist is greater than in volvulus of the pelvic colon.

Volvulus of the small intestine is rare. There are usually adhesions, which fix the gut and form an axis of rotation.

It may affect only one loop, or the entire ileum may be rotated. The rotation is usually in the direction of the hands of a watch, and amounts to one complete turn or more.

The symptoms vary in severity with the extent of bowel involved, and the tightness of the strangulation. The twisted segment may form a tangible mass in the middle of the abdomen. Vomiting is always an early and severe symptom.

The **treatment** of these forms of volvulus is carried out on the same lines as that of volvulus of the pelvic colon.

OBSTRUCTION DUE TO IMPACTION OF A GALL-STONE

The term " gall-stone ileus," or " gall-stone obstruction," is applied to a rare condition in which a large gall-stone has found its way into the intestinal canal and become impacted there. The gall-stone, which has formed in the gall-bladder and has reached such dimensions that it cannot pass along the bile-ducts, sets up irritation which leads to localized peritonitis around the gall-bladder and duodenum. The adjacent parts of these viscera become adherent, and the pressure of the gall-stone leads to the formation of a fistulous opening into the first or second part of the duodenum. It is in this way that the majority of large gall-stones enter the bowel, but cases have been recorded in which the stone had so dilated the cystic and common bile-ducts that these formed a continuous cavity from which it passed directly into the gut.

In rare cases, the stone ulcerates its way directly into the large intestine and is passed with the fæces without giving rise to obstructive symptoms.

If the stone is less than 1 in. in diameter, it usually passes safely along the intestinal canal, but if of larger dimensions it is liable to be arrested, and the larger the stone the higher up is impaction likely to take place. In the great majority of cases, impaction occurs in the lower part of the ileum. The occlusion of the bowel is due in part to the size of the stone, and in part to spasm of the circular muscular fibres induced by the irritation caused by the presence of a rough foreign body. If the lumen of the bowel is narrowed by cicatricial contraction or malignant disease, a comparatively small gall-stone may determine symptoms of acute obstruction if impacted in the orifice.

Clinical features.—The condition is most frequently met with in fat women between 55 and 65 years of age. There is usually the history that the patient has suffered for years from more or less constant, dull epigastric pain, with occasional exacerbations which have been attributed to dyspepsia. Only in a small proportion of cases is there a history of typical attacks of biliary colic associated with jaundice, doubtless because the stones that eventually cause obstruction are single, and do not engage in the common bile-duct or cause obstruction of its lumen. More recently the pain has been more severe and diffuse, as a result of the localized peritonitis and ulceration, associated with the formation of the fistulous tract by which the stone escapes into the bowel. At first, the stone projects into the duodenum and causes irritation, which gives rise to localized pain in the right hypochondrium and persistent vomiting. As the stone is passing along the small intestine, the pain is referred to the umbilicus.

When it becomes impacted, vomiting is the most prominent symptom. It is continuous and profuse, and at first the vomited material may be tinged with blood from the fistulous track; later, it is bile-stained, and it very soon becomes stercoraceous. The quantity of fluid vomited far exceeds that taken by the mouth.

Shock and collapse are less marked symptoms and are more delayed than in the case of most other forms of acute obstruction, presumably because the vascular and nervous mechanisms of the intestine are not interfered with. Arrest of the passage of fæces and flatus is not a constant symptom at the beginning of the illness. As the displacement of the stone from the duodenum is often brought about by the taking of a strong purge, the bowels may act several times after the onset of the pain and vomiting, and this is apt to be misleading in diagnosis. After the stone becomes firmly impacted, however, constipation is complete. Tenderness and rigidity of the abdomen are not marked, and distension is usually slight and not easily recognized owing to the obesity of the patient. It is sometimes possible to palpate the stone through the parietes or from the rectum while the patient is under an anæsthetic.

The **diagnosis** is always a matter of great difficulty, and is seldom made with certainty before the abdomen is opened, doubtless because the possibility of this cause for the symptoms is often overlooked. The late H. L. Barnard, who had an extensive experience of this condition, laid great stress upon the unusual character of the grouping of the symptoms as an aid in diagnosis.

Treatment.—As in other forms of acute obstruction, the only rational treatment is to remove the stone by operation, and the high mortality in this form of obstruction is chiefly due to delay in operating, although in addition the age and obesity of the patients render them unfavourable subjects for operation.

If this cause is suspected, the abdomen should be opened to one or other side of the middle line below the umbilicus, and the lower part of the cavity explored. As a rule, the cause of the obstruction is speedily discovered, as the stone is usually impacted low down in the ileum. If not, the ileo-cæcal junction should be found and the intestine traced upwards from it. When distended bowel predominates, the first presenting coil should be traced towards the right until the stone is reached. The occluded loop is then withdrawn from the wound and packed off with gauze, and opened in the long axis of the gut. The bowel is opened at some distance above the seat of impaction. The stone having been removed and the distended bowel emptied, the opening is closed by a Czerny-Lembert suture inserted at right angles to the long axis of the bowel. In some cases it has been necessary to resect the loop of bowel implicated.

If operation is impracticable, or is refused, belladonna and opium may be given to relieve the symptoms.

A **chronic form** of gall-stone obstruction has been described, in which the patient suffers from intermittent attacks of colicky pain with temporary incomplete obstruction, due to blocking of different parts of the gut as the stone passes along. Such attacks may occur at intervals of days or weeks, and any one of them may become acute.

ENTEROLITHS, INTESTINAL CALCULI, OR FÆCAL CONCRETIONS AND ACCUMULATIONS

Solid masses composed of phosphates of lime and magnesia, or triple phosphates, sometimes mixed with carbonate of lime, ammonia,

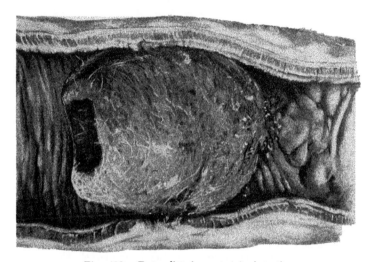

Fig. 422.—Enterolith impacted in intestine.

(From a photograph lent by Dr. T. Machardy.)

or soda, frequently form in the intestinal canal, particularly under conditions in which there is a long-continued catarrh of the bowel. Such enteroliths are often of stony hardness, but they seldom attain great dimensions. A similar form, composed chiefly of insoluble drugs, such as magnesia, salol, bismuth, or chalk, which the patient has been taking medicinally over a long period, is sometimes met with. A third variety, not so hard as the others, is composed chiefly of the indigestible residue of certain vegetable foods, notably oatmeal.

When such an adventitious object is arrested for a time in the lumen of the bowel or in a cul-de-sac in its wall, it gives rise to a degree of chronic enteritis, and the inflammatory products resulting from the irritation of the mucous membrane favour the adhesion of fæcal particles and lead to a gradual increase in the size of the concretion.

While these different concretions vary in composition, they have this in common, that they usually form on a nucleus of some organic substance, such as a fruit-stone, a mass of hairs, or a gall-stone.

ENTEROLITHS

Clinical features.—It is exceedingly rare for an enterolith to give rise to acute obstruction unless it is suddenly displaced from a diverticulum and becomes impacted in the lumen of the gut, and then the symptoms are similar to those of gall-stone ileus (p. 499).

While a concretion is in process of formation *in the ileum*, it may give rise to symptoms associated with enteritis—recurring attacks of colicky pain, vomiting, and diarrhœa, usually coming on two or three hours after a meal, and if ulceration of the mucous membrane has occurred, the motions may be stained with blood.. As it increases in size, it causes repeated mild obstructive attacks, attended with constipation and a moderate degree of distension, sometimes with visible peristalsis and severe vomiting. A palpable swelling, which is tender on pressure, may be recognizable in the lower part of the abdomen.

When the calculus forms *in the colon*, the prominent symptoms are severe coho with tenesmus, and the passage of watery stools containing mucus, pus, and sometimes blood. As the most common site is in the cæcum, the concretion may reach a considerable size, and can be felt as a rounded hard movable mass in the right iliac fossa, which is tender on pressure. A calculus situated in the colon seldom gives rise to acute obstructive symptoms.

The **treatment** consists in opening the abdomen, usually in the right iliac fossa, removing the concretion, and closing the bowel.

It is more than doubtful if, as has been alleged, an accumulation of intestinal worms ever causes obstruction of the bowels, the so-called *ileus verminosus*.

FÆCAL ACCUMULATIONS

We are here concerned only with that degree of habitual constipation which leads to an accumulation in the rectum and colon of fæcal masses, which become impacted in the bowel and may eventually cause complete obstruction. Considering the frequency of obstinate constipation, it is remarkable how seldom the bowel becomes obstructed by accumulated fæces.

As a rule, the clinical picture is one of gradually increasing obstruction, and it is probable that it is only when some additional factor, such as kinking or rotation of the overloaded pelvic colon, is super added that acute symptoms supervene. In some cases the onset of complete obstruction is precipitated by the taking of a violent purgative.

Morbid anatomy.—The masses that block the bowel may be single or multiple, and they vary in consistence from a putty-like substance to a body of stony hardness. They usually form in the pelvic colon, but may eventually fill the rectum, and extend into the ascending and transverse portions of the colon.

By their weight they may drag upon the pelvic colon so that it sinks down into the pelvis, and, by pressing upon the rectum, adds to the difficulty of emptying the bowel. The traction on the meso-colon causes it to elongate, and, by narrowing its base of attachment, predisposes to volvulus, which, if it occurs, sets up symptoms of acute obstruction. If the transverse colon is overloaded, it similarly is dragged down and forms a U- or V-shaped loop, which may reach the level of the pubes.

The pressure of the hardened masses on the mucous membrane leads to ulceration—*stercoral ulcers*—the mucosa becoming eroded in patches (p. 521).

Clinical features.—The condition is most commonly seen in elderly women who have for years suffered from constipation. As the bowel becomes loaded, there is a constant feeling of abdominal discomfort, the digestive functions are disturbed, there are flatulence and an unpleasant taste in the mouth, and the breath has an offensive odour. The skin may assume a dirty-greyish colour, giving the patient a swarthy appearance, and the pigment is sometimes deposited in patches. The patient suffers from painful tenesmus, due to the excessive efforts of the bowel to expel its contents, and when ulceration is present there are occasional attacks of spurious diarrhœa with the passage of sanious, muco-purulent discharge. The absorption of toxins is associated with a certain degree of febrile disturbance ; the patient emaciates, and becomes dull and lethargic, or even mentally depressed and melancholic.

On examination, a swelling can be felt in the line of the colon, which is usually distended. There is tenderness on making firm pressure over it, and the fæcal mass may pit on pressure.

On rectal examination, hard scybalæ, or a soft pultaceous mass, can sometimes be felt.

When acute obstruction supervenes there is intense colicky pain, and great distension of the intestines, which may displace the other abdominal and pelvic viscera and may even interfere with the action of the heart and respiration. Vomiting is a common symptom, but it is seldom urgent, and is rarely fæcal. The patient becomes collapsed, and, unless relief is obtained, the condition proves fatal, in the same way as in other forms of complete obstruction.

Treatment.—Before the onset of acute obstructive symptoms, to soften the scybalous masses and to lubricate the passage, several ounces of warm olive oil should be introduced into the bowel by means of a soft tube and funnel, and after an interval a large turpentine enema is administered.

It is often necessary to break down the hardened masses mechanically, and this is best done under an anæsthetic. The patient is placed in the lithotomy position, the anal sphincter is stretched, and with the gloved hand the scybalous masses are broken down, and then washed out. If there is evidence of stercoral ulceration, great care must be taken that the bowel be not perforated in this procedure.

When symptoms of acute obstruction are present, the abdomen must be opened and an artificial anus established. After the upper bowel has been emptied, the fæcal accumulation may be softened and removed by injections made through the artificial opening as well as by the anus.

Surgical treatment of habitual constipation.—Apart from those cases in which habitual constipation culminates in a fæcal obstruction of the bowel, attempts have been made to relieve the patient of the discomfort and ill-health induced by the chronic condition of the colon by surgical measures. The separation of adhesions between the colon and the parietes or adjacent viscera, which interfere mechanically with the peristaltic action of the bowel, is often followed by marked improvement. Mansell-Moullin has suggested and practised ileo-colostomy with some degree of success, but this operation is not always feasible, and has not proved very satisfactory.

Complete excision of the colon has been advocated by Arbuthnot Lane, the ileum being connected with the rectum, either by end-to-end suture or by lateral anastomosis.

In a certain number of cases it has been found that habitual constipation has been due to an hypertrophied condition of the rectal valves of Houston, and that removal of these thickened folds of mucous membrane by means of the knife or cautery has effected a cure of the condition.

POSTOPERATIVE OBSTRUCTION

This term is here used in relation to that form of acute obstruction which is an immediate and direct result of operation, and is mainly due to paralysis of the intestine. Obstruction due to strangulation by bands or to other mechanical effects of peritoneal adhesions resulting from a previous operation is described elsewhere (pp. 478, 480).

After abdominal operations, the bowel may become distended with gas, which the patient is unable to expel, either on account of a spasm of the anal sphincters or because of pain in the abdominal wound when he strains. As the flatus accumulates, the bowel is gradually stretched, and its muscular coat loses its tone and becomes paralysed. Paralysis of the bowel with symptoms of complete obstruction sometimes follows prolonged operations in which there has been excessive handling of the gut or forcible retraction of the edges of the wound. It is most liable to ensue if a large amount of bowel has had to be withdrawn from the abdominal cavity and the exposed coils have not been kept moist and warm.

In cases of localized sepsis—for example, appendicitis with abscess formation—there is often difficulty in securing an action of the bowels for some days after the operation. This may be due to paralysis of the loops of bowel in the vicinity of the abscess, or to adjacent coils being glued together by plastic lymph to such an extent that the peristaltic waves are arrested by the adhesions. Sometimes the obstruction is accounted for by too tight packing with gauze, or the pressure of a rigid drainage-tube on the bowel.

The most common and most serious cause of postoperative obstruction is general peritonitis, which may be due to spread of the disease for which the operation was performed, or to infection introduced at the operation. Occasionally, embolism or thrombosis of the mesenteric vessels causes paralytic obstruction.

Clinical features.—The most prominent symptoms are gradually increasing distension of the abdomen and a progressive rise in the pulse-rate. Sooner or later, mouthfuls of brown, fetid fluid regurgitate from the stomach almost continuously without retching or effort. In some cases, the fluid collects in the stomach for some hours and is ejected in large quantities, the emptying of the stomach giving great relief for a time. Occasionally no vomiting occurs till just before death, when a large quantity of brown, foul-smelling material, often mixed with blood, is brought up. The temperature usually remains persistently subnormal. Abdominal pain and colic are seldom complained of, and there is often an entire absence of muscular rigidity. The extremities soon become cold, blue, and clammy, although the rest of the body may maintain its warmth. The features are drawn and pinched, but the eyes are often bright and clear, and, although the patient looks extremely ill, he may express himself as feeling quite comfortable, and he usually fails to realize the gravity of his condition. It is seldom possible to distinguish between the paralytic and the mechanical forms.

Acute dilatation of the stomach or gastro-mesenteric ileus may closely simulate postoperative obstruction.

Treatment.—In the early stages of abdominal distension the introduction of a flatus tube into the rectum, or the administration of a turpentine or glycerine enema with Epsom salts, is usually sufficient to relieve the discomfort. If these measures fail, a hypodermic injection of $\frac{1}{30}$ gr. of eserin, combined with $\frac{1}{120}$ gr. of atropin, often stimulates the peristalsis. Pituitary extract sometimes acts in the same way.

If the abdominal wound has been packed or drained, it should be dressed, and the gauze or tube removed.

Great relief often follows washing out the stomach. Purgatives must not be given by the mouth, as they only increase the amount of fluid matter in the paralysed intestine, and large enemata should be avoided, as they are liable to be retained.

If the symptoms become worse, the wound should be reopened, and, if no definite cause for the obstruction be found, or if it cannot be removed, an artificial anus must be formed to drain the bowel. It may be necessary to open the intestine at several places.

EMBOLISM AND THROMBOSIS OF THE MESENTERIC BLOOD-VESSELS

The clinical picture in these conditions is one of acute intestinal obstruction of the paralytic type, and a diagnosis is seldom made before the abdomen is opened.

The pathological appearances and the clinical symptoms are much the same whether the obstruction is in the mesenteric artery or in the vein. The severity of the affection varies with the site and extent of the vascular interference, but even when only a limited area of bowel has its blood-vessels interfered with the condition is a grave one.

The patient is usually a man between 30 and 60 years of age, who suffers from infective endocarditis, mitral stenosis, or cirrhosis of the liver. Without warning, the general symptoms of acute intestinal obstruction suddenly develop, but there is often diarrhœa. the patient passing considerable quantities of blood, but getting no relief from movement of the bowels. There is likewise blood in the vomit.

If the abdomen is opened, it is found to contain a considerable quantity of dark, blood-stained fluid ; and the affected segment of intestine—varying from a few inches to the whole length of the small intestine and even part of the colon—is found of a dark chocolate colour, firm, swollen, and œdematous. When the condition has lasted for some time, the bowel shows signs of gangrene, and there is more or less generalized peritonitis.

The condition usually proves fatal in a few hours, and little benefit has followed excision of the affected portion of bowel.

ENTEROSPASM

The term "enterospasm" has been applied to a condition in which, as a result of spasmodic contraction of the circular fibres of a limited segment of the bowel, symptoms suggestive of acute intestinal obstruction develop.

Clinical features.—The condition is chiefly met with in neurotic women, between 20 and 50 years of age, who have suffered from chronic colitis with diarrhœa and blood-stained stools, or who have recently undergone a pelvic operation. Without obvious cause, the patient is seized with severe abdominal pain attended with vomiting, distension of the abdomen, and complete arrest of the passage of fæces and flatus. The attack may last for a few hours or for several days, and then pass off as suddenly as it began, and after the bowels have acted, the patient again feels perfectly well.

During the attack, a firm, sausage-shaped swelling can sometimes be made out in the position of the contracted gut, which is usually the pelvic colon.

In its less severe forms, in which there are merely repeated short, sharp attacks of colicky pain, with moderate flatulent distension, lasting for an hour or two, and then passing off completely, the condition is suggestive of recurrent appendicitis, renal or biliary colic.

It is characteristic of the affection that full doses of belladonna and hyoscyamus rapidly relieve the spasms, and the symptoms disappear. Opium acts in the same way, but should only be given for diagnostic purposes when there is reasonable certainty that no organic cause of obstruction exists.

Etiology.—The true nature of these attacks has only been recognized within recent years as a result of laparotomy having been performed for the relief of what was believed to be an organic obstruction. A careful search for the cause of the obstruction has only revealed a firm contraction of a portion of the bowel—usually the pelvic colon—varying in length from one to several inches. Above the contracted segment, which is pale, firm, and rigid, the bowel is distended with gas and fæces, and below, it is contracted and empty. In some cases the spasm has relaxed and come on again while the bowel was actually under observation.

In view of the almost constant history of chronic colitis with blood in the stools, it is probable that the spasm is set up by some local lesion of the mucous membrane, such as an ulcer.

Treatment.—It must be emphasized that enterospasm giving rise to symptoms so severe as to suggest acute obstruction is rare, and that treatment directed towards relief of spasm alone is seldom justified, and is only to be adopted when the various causes of organic obstruction can be definitely excluded. If any doubt remains, an exploratory laparotomy should be performed.

The use of morphia and other opiates should be avoided in view of the neurotic temperament of most of these patients, and if one full dose fails to give relief, the diagnosis of enterospasm has almost certainly been wrong.

Belladonna, hyoscyamus, and similar drugs relieve the spasms in true enterospasm, and their use may be supplemented by hot baths. Any coexisting inflammatory affection of the colon must, of course, be treated.

INFLAMMATORY AFFECTIONS

CHRONIC COLITIS

The term " chronic colitis " is, for convenience, applied to a condition in which the patient complains of recurring attacks of severe colicky pain, associated with the passage of an excessive amount of mucus in the stools, without there being any gross pathological lesion to account for the symptoms.

It cannot be too strongly emphasized that a diagnosis of " chronic colitis " should never be made until all the other affections of the bowel that may give rise to a similar train of symptoms have been excluded. These include malignant disease (p. 527), tuberculosis either of the hypertrophic or of the ulcerative type (p. 510), fibromatosis of the colon (p. 515), chronic appendicitis (p. 552), and localized peritonitis, or abscess in the vicinity of the colon.

Clinical features.—The severity of the symptoms varies in different cases, and even in the same patient at different times, and the disease tends to run a protracted course.

In the less severe form, which is the form usually met with in men who show no signs of neurasthenia, and are in other respects healthy, the patient complains of persistent abdominal discomfort, not amounting to pain, particularly after meals. The appetite is poor, and there is a tendency to constipation with flatulent distension. There are, however, occasional attacks of looseness of the bowels with pain and tenesmus, the motions consisting largely of mucus. The patient loses flesh rapidly, and often becomes markedly depressed or even melancholic. The local symptoms may be referred to the right iliac fossa, and it is then difficult to distinguish this condition from chronic appendicitis, with which indeed it is often associated, but whether as cause or effect it is impossible to say.

The more severe and typical form is most frequently met with in middle-aged women belonging to the upper classes, of a markedly neurotic temperament and in a poor state of health. It is common to find some uterine displacement or evidence of other pelvic disease in such subjects. The patient suffers from chronic dyspepsia with hyperacidity, and is habitually constipated, but has periodic attacks of severe colicky pain, attended with sickness and vomiting, and culminating in a spurious diarrhœa with the passage of large quantities of mucus intimately mixed with some pale fæculent matter, containing less than the normal amount of bile. The mucus is sometimes clear like white of egg or boiled sago, sometimes in flaky shreds, and sometimes it takes the form of fibrinous casts of the bowel, which may be several inches long. If broken up into strips, these casts are apt to be mistaken by the patient for intestinal worms. There is usually a moderate amount of blood in the motions, and occasionally intestinal sand is present. Sometimes the patient loses a considerable quantity of blood—*hæmorrhagic colitis.*

During an attack, tenderness can usually be located on making pressure over the colon, and the bowel may be felt to contract under the fingers, forming a firm, elongated, sausage-shaped swelling. There is an absence of muscular rigidity. On examining the pelvic colon with the sigmoidoscope, the mucous membrane may be found to be inflamed or ulcerated, and is covered with patches of shreddy mucus.

These acute attacks may recur every few weeks or months, but in the intervals the patient, as a rule, does not regain strength, and often becomes extremely emaciated. The absorption of toxins affects the nervous system, and aggravates the neurasthenic tendencies of the patient, who eventually passes into a condition of chronic invalidism.

Treatment.—Medical and dietetic treatment should always have a fair trial before recourse is had to operative measures. To relieve the acute symptoms during one of the paroxysmal attacks a hypodermic injection of morphia with atropine should be given to relax the spasm of the colon; then, the patient being placed in the knee-elbow position and directed to retain the enema as long as possible, about a pint of warm olive oil is slowly injected into the colon; after an hour or two, the colon is washed out with saline solution.

To correct the irritability of the colon, the patient must be put on a carefully selected diet. According to von Noorden—and my experience agrees with his—the diet should be a full one, and should consist of such things as fruit, vegetables, brown bread, and a moderate amount of butcher's meat, which leave a considerable indigestible residue. To prevent constipation and to render the fæces soft, a liberal allowance of fatty food should be given in the form of cream, butter, cod-liver oil emulsion, or petroleum preparations.

The local treatment consists in injecting from 6 to 8 oz. of warm olive oil into the colon every night. This is to be retained till morning, when the bowel is washed out with saline solution. The inflammation of the mucous membrane may be allayed by injections of one or other of the albuminous silver preparations, such as protargol or argyrol ($\frac{1}{2}$ to 1 per cent.).

Purgatives should be avoided if possible. If they cannot be dispensed with entirely, a small dose of castor oil should be taken regularly every four or five days till the tendency to constipation has been overcome.

When such measures are ineffectual, operative interference is necessary. The best results have followed appendicostomy, the appendix being brought out in the right iliac fossa and used as a means of irrigating the colon. Several pints of warm saline solution are injected into the colon through the artificial opening two, three or four times a day. As a rule, no antiseptic need be added, but benefit is sometimes derived from the silver salts. The irrigation must be kept up for several months, and the opening then allowed to close, which it usually does soon after the use of the injections is discontinued. During the treatment, the patient is able to continue his work and is seldom incommoded by the fistulous opening.

This procedure should be tried before recourse is had to right inguinal colostomy or ileo-sigmoidostomy.

PERICOLITIS

DIVERTICULITIS

Changes similar to those which occur in the vicinity of the cæcum as a result of appendicitis are frequently met with around other parts of the colon. These are most common in relation to the pelvic colon, and are generally due to infective processes originating in acquired diverticula—so-called *diverticulitis*.

The formation of a concretion in a diverticulum may be followed by ulceration or suppuration, and if the infective process spreads to the peritoneum, a localized abscess may form or a general peritonitis be set up.

Similar results may follow ulceration of the colon apart from the presence of a diverticulum—for example, a stercoral, tuberculous, or malignant ulcer, or an ulcer resulting from an injury produced by a foreign body, such as a fish or game bone.

The pathological processes, the clinical features, and the general principles of treatment are the same as those of allied conditions resulting from appendicitis.

TUBERCULOSIS OF THE INTESTINE

Tuberculosis affects the intestine in two distinct ways : (1) in the form of multiple ulcers, and (2) by the formation of localized tumour-like masses.

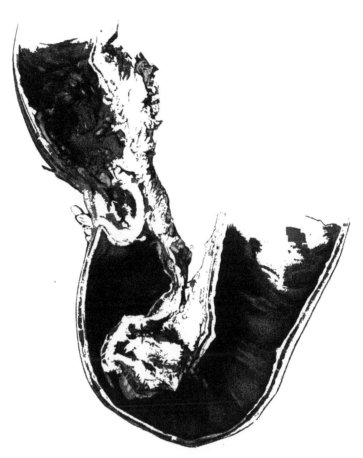

Tuberculosis of intestine, leading to multiple strictures.

(Museum, Royal College of Surgeons, Edinburgh.)

PLATE 95.

1. TUBERCULOUS ULCERATION

The ulcerative form is most frequently met with in young subjects who suffer from pulmonary phthisis or from some other tuberculous condition. Its chief surgical interest lies in the fact that the cicatricial contraction which accompanies the healing of such ulcers leads to stenosis of the bowel.

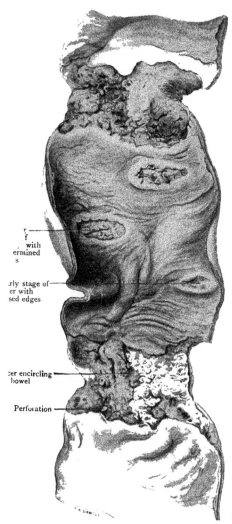

r f
, with ermined s

rly stage of er with sed edges

er encircling bowel

Perforation

The lower end of the ileum is the most common seat of the disease, the infection taking place from bacilli that have been swallowed in the sputum, or taken in with milk or other food, and have become implanted in the Peyer's patches and solitary glands. As the foci break down and caseate, they form small, irregularly oval ulcers in the mucous membrane, the edges of which are elevated (Fig. 423) and often indurated. Such ulcers tend to spread circularly round the gut, and, as they heal at one part while spreading at another, the contraction of the cicatricial tissue leads to stenosis of the bowel—one form of *tuberculous stricture* (Plates 95, 96). There may be several strictures scattered over a considerable length of intestine, the intervening segments being dilated and sacculated in a characteristic manner.

Neighbouring saccules

Fig. 423.—Tuberculous ulceration of the intestine.

(*Museum, Royal College of Surgeons, Edinburgh.*)

are liable to become adherent to one another or to the parietes, and this still further interferes with the passage of the intestinal contents. The peritoneal covering of the bowel is frequently scattered over with miliary tubercles, and the associated mesenteric glands are often enlarged and caseous.

The usual symptoms associated with gradual stenosis of the bowel are present—recurrent attacks of abdominal pain, gradually increasing distension of the abdomen, with visible peristalsis and gurgling intestinal sounds. One or more tumour-like masses may be felt through the abdominal wall or per rectum.

The nature of the lesion can usually be recognized from the other evidence of tuberculosis, by the von Pirquet test, or by discovering tubercle bacilli in the fæces ; but the diagnosis is sometimes only made after opening the abdomen.

The **treatment** consists in resecting the affected segment of gut when this is practicable, or in short-circuiting the bowel.

The **other complications** that may follow on tuberculous ulceration of the intestine are perforations (Fig. 423) with septic peritonitis (but this is rare owing to the thickening of the peritoneal coat and the formation of adhesions outside the affected segment of bowel); the development of a cold abscess, which, on bursting, may establish a fistula with an adjacent hollow viscus or with the surface ; and general tuberculous peritonitis. In so far as these conditions are amenable to surgical treatment, they are dealt with on the same lines as when they arise from other causes.

2. Ileo-Cæcal Tuberculosis

The hyperplastic or hypertrophic form of intestinal tuberculosis is almost always confined to the cæcum, although it may extend for some distance in the ascending colon, and frequently in the terminal part of the ileum. Occasionally the proximal part of the appendix is implicated.

Morbid anatomy.—This affection differs from other manifestations of tuberculosis in that the lesion is not a destructive one, but is attended with great increase in the bulk of the cæcum. The disease begins in the submucous or subperitoneal layers, and spreads to other coats of the bowel, which become diffusely infiltrated with small round cells among which are clumps of giant cells and calcareous deposits, and the wall is increased in thickness and rendered rigid by a deposit of plastic fibrous tissue. The condition tends to spread by the formation of fresh zones of hyperplasia in the distended bowel above the level of the primary focus (F. M. Caird). The thickened cæcum is usually included in a mass of fibro-adipose tissue of inflammatory origin.

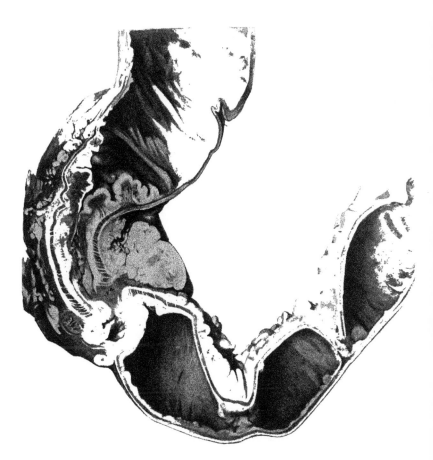

Ileo-cæcal tuberculosis.

(Author's case.)

PLATE 96.

Contraction of the mesocolon drags the cæcum upwards so that it may lie near the liver, and the ileum joins it at an obtuse angle. The glands in the mesentery may be enlarged, and form a solid mass which presses upon the gut (Fig. 424).

The cavity is diminished in size, and the lumen of the bowel may be narrowed down to a track no larger than a goose-quill. The ileo-

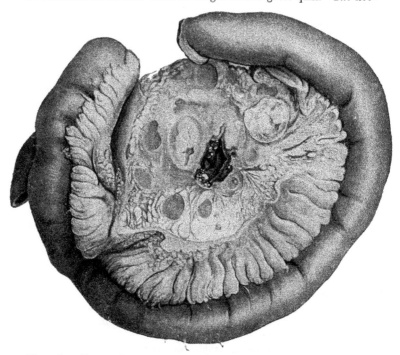

Fig. 424.—Tuberculous mesenteric glands forming a solid mass which pressed upon the bowel and caused obstruction.

(*Museum, Royal College of Surgeons, Edinburgh.*)

cæcal valve is shrivelled up and often cannot be recognized (Plates 95, 96).

The mucous membrane may be ulcerated or may present numerous villous processes projecting like polypi from its surface. These vegetations, which spring from the submucous tissue, have the structure of ordinary intestinal adenomas, and they vary in size from a mere thread to a hazel-nut.

Clinical features.—The condition is usually met with in patients between 20 and 40 years of age, who show slight, if any,

2 *h*

evidence of pulmonary disease. It may, however, occur at the extremes of life. It is insidious in its onset, and for many months may merely be associated with some loss of appetite and symptoms of indigestion, slight occasional discomfort in the right iliac fossa, and the passage of blood and mucus. As time goes on, the patient loses strength and emaciates, and he suffers from frequent attacks of griping pain, coming on usually two or three hours after meals, and from alternating constipation and diarrhœa. In some cases there is frequent vomiting, which affords the patient relief. There may be localized distension of the bowel, with loud borborygmi and visible peristalsis, the intestine presenting a characteristic ladder pattern (Fig. 406, p. 472).

Sooner or later, a palpable swelling can be detected in the right loin, the lower border being fairly well defined, while above it shades away in the colon. It is slightly mobile and tender, and yields an impaired note on percussion.

The illness may culminate in an attack of acute obstruction. Abscesses may form, and, if they rupture externally, may cause persistent sinuses, or a fæcal fistula. Generalized tuberculous peritonitis is a rare sequel.

Diagnosis.—Compared with cancer, with which it is most liable to be confused, the progress of the disease is slow, and there is a characteristic intermission in the symptoms, which may last for one or two years before becoming urgent. In some cases tuberculosis and cancer have coexisted. The differential diagnosis from chronic lesions resulting from appendicitis is seldom difficult. It is impossible to distinguish clinically between ileo-cæcal tuberculosis and fibromatosis of the colon affecting the cæcal region.

Treatment.—The treatment consists in excising the cæcum, and establishing a lateral anastomosis on the same lines as for cancer, and the results of this operation, whether performed in one or in two stages, have proved very satisfactory.

If this is found to be impossible, an anastomosis may be effected between the small intestine and the colon well beyond the limits of the disease.

ACTINOMYCOSIS

The cæcum is by far the most common seat of actinomycosis in the intestine, but the pelvic colon also is sometimes attacked.

The infection takes place from the mucous membrane and spreads through the various coats to the peritoneum, and thence to the abdominal wall, leading to the formation of abscesses and sinuses. In the mucous membrane lining the sinuses, or in the pus that escapes from them, the ray fungus may be found.

Before the disease infiltrates the parietes, the affected segment of bowel becomes greatly thickened and adherent to adjacent structures, the whole constituting a firm, ill-defined, diffuse mass, which simulates malignant disease or tuberculosis.

The **treatment** consists in opening up the sinuses and removing the infected tissues with the sharp spoon and scissors, but the difficulty of eradicating the whole disease renders this line of treatment unsatisfactory. Equally good results have been claimed for treatment by large doses of potassium iodide or of copper sulphate. Irrigation of the sinuses with a 1 per cent. solution of copper sulphate has proved beneficial (Bevan). Injections of iodipin are also of value.

FIBROMATOSIS OF THE COLON

Under this name may be described a condition frequently met with in the colon which in its clinical aspects and on naked-eye examination is almost indistinguishable from carcinoma or the hyperplastic form of intestinal tuberculosis.

In the majority of cases hitherto reported the nature of the condition has only been recognized after the growth had been removed in the belief that it was a malignant tumour, or on post-mortem examination. The microscopic appearances, however, show that the mass is inflammatory in character, and presents none of the signs of malignant disease.

It is highly probable that many of the cases which are recorded of malignant disease of the bowel having disappeared after colostomy or short-circuiting operations performed for obstruction were of this nature.

Morbid anatomy.—Any part of the colon may be involved, but the condition is most common in the pelvic colon and rectum. The affected segment of bowel, varying in length from one to several inches, is converted into a firm, rigid tube. The peritoneal coat is thick, rough and granular, and may show signs of adhesive inflammation. Beneath the serous coat is a uniform layer of dense fibro-adipose tissue, sometimes half an inch in thickness. The muscular coat may show some degree of atrophy, or may be unaltered in appearance.

More striking changes are seen in the submucous layer, which is greatly thickened by an overgrowth of dense fibrous tissue. This tends to contract, and in so doing drags upon the mucous membrane, which forms a series of irregular folds with deep recesses between them ; these are sometimes spoken of as " false diverticula."

The mucous surface may thus assume a festooned or cauliflower-like appearance, simulating that of multiple adenomas or papillomas. Ulcers form in the recesses of the thickened mucosa and burrow under the surface, making long, undermined tracts with overhanging flaps of mucous membrane. The ulceration may extend through all the coats of the bowel and lead to perforation. In some cases, the mucous membrane is unaltered in appearance, and no false diverticula are present.

The lumen of the bowel is usually considerably narrowed, sometimes to such an extent as to give rise to symptoms of obstruction.

On microscopical examination, the wall of the bowel is infiltrated with chronic inflammatory tissue, and there is an overgrowth of the mucous glands with aggregations of lymphoid cells between them. The epithelial cells of the glands may show proliferation, but they do not extend beyond their basement membranes, and have none of the appearances of carcinoma.

Etiology.—These changes resemble those met with in other organs as a result of chronic irritative conditions, and in all probability are due to infection taking place through some lesion of the mucosa— for example, an abrasion caused by a foreign body, a small ulcer, or the lodgment of a fæcal concretion in an acquired diverticulum, or in one of the deeper recesses of the mucosa. Cases are recorded in which the infection appeared to originate in other organs, such as the uterus and Fallopian tubes, with which the colon had formed adhesions.

Clinical features.—This condition is most frequently found in patients over 40 years of age, but it occurs also in younger subjects. The history of the illness is very like that of malignant disease of the colon. There is generally habitual constipation, with periodic attacks of diarrhœa, usually induced by the taking of a strong purgative, the motions often containing blood and mucus. The patient complains of persistent abdominal pain, and there is a progressive failure of health. When the disease extends into the rectum, a digital examination reveals a soft condition of the mucous membrane, which has been compared to thick velvet or moss, and considerable narrowing of the lumen. With the sigmoidoscope the excessive rugosity and thickening of the mucosa can be seen.

On examination, the pelvic colon is felt to stand out as a firm, sausage-shaped swelling, which is tender on pressure.

A positive diagnosis is seldom possible without an exploratory operation.

Treatment.—The only satisfactory treatment is to remove the affected segment of bowel. If there are symptoms of obstruction, or if the patient is not in a condition for such an operation, colostomy should be performed to empty the bowel, and the major operation undertaken at a later date. When the mass is considered irremovable, short-circuiting should be performed if it is practicable. In a considerable number of cases, these palliative operations have been followed by diminution or even disappearance of the swelling.

ULCERATION OF THE INTESTINE

It is important to distinguish between those cases in which ulceration is an accompaniment or complication of such diseases of the bowel as tuberculosis, malignant disease, and chronic obstruction from entero-liths or fæcal accumulation, and those in which it is due to some specific cause, such as typhoid, dysentery, or infection with particular organisms. In the former group, the symptoms due to the ulcer are superadded to, and cannot be distinguished from, those of the primary lesion, the treatment of which covers the treatment of the ulcer. In the latter group, the ulceration itself calls for treatment, or may lead to complications which bring the disease within the province of the surgeon.

PEPTIC ULCERS FOLLOWING GASTRO-ENTEROSTOMY [1]

In a small proportion of cases of gastro-enterostomy, performed for non-malignant affections of the stomach, ulceration occurs at the site of the anastomosis—*gastro-jejunal ulcer ;* or in the jejunum a short distance from the opening—*jejunal ulcer.*

The chief cause of the gastro-jejunal ulcer seems to be the hyper-acidity of the stomach contents, although Wilkie has shown experi-mentally that this alone is not sufficient to produce ulceration in intact mucous membranes. The other factors are the presence of a hæmatoma, or the formation of granulation tissue at the site of the anastomosis, which usually persists for about a week after the operation, the irritation caused by unabsorbable sutures in the granulating area, and the passage of solid food over the raw surface during the healing process.

The jejunal ulcer is probably due to the action of the acid contents of the stomach on the mucosa of the jejunum, which, under normal conditions, is exposed to an alkaline medium.

The fact that peptic ulcers almost never occur after gastro-enterostomy performed for cancer of the stomach, in which there is a deficiency of acid in the contents, supports the view that hyper-acidity is an important factor in their causation in non-malignant cases.

The prevention of these ulcers would seem to depend on securing rapid union of the apposed mucous surfaces by accurate suturing with an absorbable material such as catgut, on diminishing the acidity of the stomach contents or securing their neutralization by the bile and pancreatic secretions, and on careful dieting to diminish mechanical irritation of the healing surfaces. The posterior no-loop operation of gastro-enterostomy has seldom been followed by ulceration.

The ulcer, which is usually single, is small and rounded, and

[1] *See* also *ante,* p. 414.

has the same appearances as the peptic ulcer of the stomach or duodenum (p. 344).

The presence of a peptic ulcer should be suspected when symptoms similar to those for which the gastro-enterostomy was performed recur after the operation. This may happen within a few days, or not for many months. In some cases perforation has been the first evidence of the presence of an ulcer.

Treatment.—If medical measures fail, and if the hyperacidity persists, it may be necessary to enlarge the gastro-enterostomy opening, if this has contracted or is not sufficiently large, or to perform a gastro-enterostomy by the **Y**-method, implanting the proximal limb of the **Y** into the stomach, so that the bile and pancreatic secretions are mixed with the gastric juice before it reaches the jejunum (H. J. Paterson).

TYPHOID PERFORATION

It has been estimated that perforation of an ulcer occurs in about $2\frac{1}{2}$ to 3 per cent. of cases of typhoid fever. This complication usually arises during the second or third week of the fever, in patients who are under treatment for a severe attack, but it may be delayed until the patient is in the convalescent stage, or it may even occur in mild and "ambulant" cases and be the first manifestation of the disease.

The ulcer which perforates is usually situated in the lower end of the ileum, within 2 or 3 ft. of the ileo-cæcal junction. Occasionally more than one ulcer perforates.

The opening may be no larger than a pin's head, and is only discovered when some flaky lymph is removed from the serous covering of the bowel. When sloughing of the wall of the gut has taken place, the opening may be of considerable size. It is usually on the convex side of the bowel, where the blood supply is least.

Clinical features.—Perforation is most frequently met with in young adult males, but it may occur at all ages, and in both sexes. In patients who are seriously ill with general symptoms of typhoid fever the diagnosis of perforation is often extremely difficult, but if there are reasonable grounds for suspecting that the bowel has given way, an exploratory incision should at once be made. Experience abundantly proves that success largely depends on the shortness of the interval between the occurrence of perforation and the operation for its closure.

The symptoms that suggest perforation are the sudden onset of acute pain referred to the umbilicus or to the right lower half of the abdomen, with tenderness on pressure, and muscular rigidity, most marked in the right lower quadrant of the abdomen. There is nausea and vomiting, and other symptoms of acute infective peritonitis soon supervene.

Treatment.—The abdomen is opened in the middle line below the umbilicus, or in the right semilunar line, and if the patient's condition forbids the administration of a general anæsthetic, the operation can be done under local anæsthesia. The cæcum is first identified and examined, and then the lower coils of the ileum. The perforation may only be revealed by removing adherent flakes of lymph, and, when it is found, it is closed by Lembert sutures and sealed by an omental graft.

As multiple perforations are not uncommon, a thorough search should be made, and any suspicious area should be invaginated with a purse-string suture, and covered with an omental graft.

When there is a patch of gangrene on the bowel, and the patient cannot tolerate immediate resection, the affected loop should be brought to the surface, and an artificial anus established.

Cases have been recorded in which a second perforation occurred after the patient had recovered from an operation, and a second laparotomy was called for.

Dysenteric Ulceration

For a description of dysentery, the reader is referred to works on Medicine. Suffice it here to say that in the course of the disease extensive ulceration frequently occurs in the colon, particularly in the pelvic and descending portions. The typical dysenteric ulcer begins as a small yellow or grey erosion at the opening of one of the glands of the mucosa, and gradually spreads in the submucous layer, undermining the mucosa and eating into the muscular coat. The affected segment of bowel is studded over with such ulcers, which as they spread coalesce and may eventually cover a large area. The irritation causes the peritoneal coat to swell and form adhesions with surrounding structures, particularly with the omentum, which serves to prevent a generalized infection of the peritoneal cavity when perforation occurs, as it frequently does. Localized suppuration in the subperitoneal or in the extraperitoneal tissue is not uncommon. Abscess of the liver is also a frequent complication. The contraction which occurs in the healing of these extensive ulcers often leads to considerable stenosis of the bowel—*dysenteric stricture.*

Treatment.—When the disease does not yield to medical measures, surgical interference is indicated to secure rest for the colon, and to admit of the direct application of remedial agents to the inflamed and ulcerated mucous membrane. This is best effected by performing appendicostomy. The fluids most frequently employed for irrigation are saline solution and weak solutions of the albuminous silver salts, such as protargol or argyrol, from 4 to 8 pints being used three times a day.

If it is necessary to divert the fæces from the colon entirely, an artificial anus is made in the first part of the ascending colon, and through this irrigation can be carried out. The artificial anus is closed when the disease has been overcome.

When it is possible to implant the lower end of the divided ileum into the pelvic colon (ileo-sigmoidostomy) beyond the ulcerated area, this operation is preferable to the formation of an artificial anus.

ULCERATIVE COLITIS

Under this term are included certain forms of ulceration of the colon which cannot be ascribed to any specific organism or irritant, although they are closely allied to dysenteric ulceration.

The ulcers, which may be met with at various stages, vary greatly in size, some being no larger than a pea, while others destroy large tracts of the mucosa. The edges are raised and irregular, the base is covered with feeble granulations to which shreds of tenacious mucus adhere, and the surrounding mucous membrane is inflamed and red. The mucosa between the ulcers is œdematous and raised, so that it may assume the appearance of a series of polypi. The destructive process gradually spreads through the coats of the bowel, and may end in perforation, and set up a localized pericolitis or peritonitis. If a large artery is involved, copious hæmorrhage may result. Abscess of the liver is a rare complication of this type of ulceration—a point in which it differs from the dysenteric form.

Clinical features.—The disease is commonest in early adult life and affects the sexes equally. The outstanding symptom is diarrhœa attended with abdominal pain and tenderness along the line of the colon.

The bowels move very frequently, sometimes every two or three hours ; there is seldom tenesmus unless the rectum also is implicated. The motions are watery and contain only a small proportion of fæculent matter, but a great quantity of mucus, some pus, and often blood. The dejections are very offensive.

As the food passes through the bowel quickly and is imperfectly digested, the patient emaciates rapidly. The disease is a very intractable one, and is attended with a high mortality.

By the use of the sigmoidoscope, the ulcers in the pelvic colon may be seen.

Some cases run a less acute course, the symptoms disappearing and recurring at intervals.

Treatment.—General dietetic and medicinal treatment, carried out on the same lines as for other forms of inflammation and ulceration of the colon, should be tried in the first instance. The use of a bacillus coli vaccine has proved beneficial (Hale White). If these measures are not speedily followed by improvement, appendicostomy should be performed to enable the colon to be irrigated with saline solution or solutions of the silver salts. When the lesions are confined to the lower part of the colon, local applications may be employed with the aid of the sigmoidoscope.

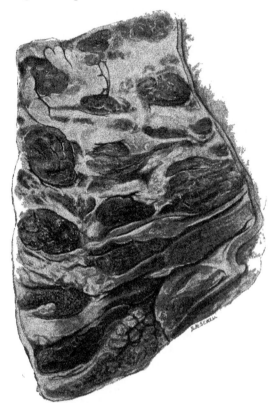

Fig. 425.—Stercoral ulcers of colon.

(*Museum, Royal College of Surgeons, Edinburgh.*)

STERCORAL ULCERS

The pressure of a hardened mass of fæces or an enterolith on the mucous membrane may give rise to ulceration—*stercoral ulcers*—the mucosa being eroded in patches (Fig. 425).

Such ulcers are most frequently met with in the rectum, the pelvic colon, and the cæcum, and they exude a blood-stained, muco-purulent discharge, which escapes with some fluid fæcal matter, giving rise to what is often misleadingly described by the patient as diarrhœa. Absorption of toxins takes place from the eroded surfaces, causing a variable degree of auto-intoxication. The ulcerative process may spread to the muscular and serous coats, and give rise to pericolitis and localized abscess, or perforation may occur and set up peritonitis.

STRICTURE OR STENOSIS

Narrowing of the lumen of the bowel is an incidental accompaniment of nearly all morbid conditions affecting the intestine, and on this factor many of the most troublesome symptoms and some of the most serious risks ultimately depend. In such diseases as carcinoma, the hypertrophic form of tuberculosis, actinomycosis, and fibromatosis of the colon, progressive organic stenosis is an almost constant result, but as this does not constitute the essential feature of these affections, it seems unnecessary and undesirable to differentiate and describe as separate conditions malignant, tuberculous, and other forms of stricture. The symptoms referable to the stenosis are more properly included with the other clinical features of each disease.

Stenosis resulting from the contraction of cicatricial tissue in or around the wall of the gut, however, requires special mention.

Cicatricial Stricture or Stenosis

The formation of cicatricial tissue in the wall of the bowel during the repair of destructive lesions is attended with a variable amount of narrowing of the lumen, but the stenosis rarely proceeds to such an extent as to cause complete obstruction.

The interference with the passage of the intestinal contents, however, is liable to be aggravated from time to time as a result of temporary congestion of the mucous membrane, or spasm of the circular muscular fibres. If to this is added a kinking or torsion of the affected loop, the lumen may be entirely occluded and acute symptoms suddenly supervene.

The most common cause of cicatricial stenosis is the healing of a tuberculous ulcer (p. 511). Syphilitic, typhoid, or dysenteric ulceration rarely gives rise to a sufficient degree of cicatricial contraction to cause symptoms of stenosis, and narrowing of the bowel seldom follows the reduction of an intussusception.

The two forms that call for special mention here are those that result from direct injury of the bowel, and from the effects of a temporary strangulation, as in hernia.

Traumatic stricture.—It occasionally happens that the process of repair in a portion of bowel which has been contused or ruptured by external violence, such as a kick or a blow, subsequently results in narrowing of the tube. Similarly, the cicatrix produced after closing a perforation of the gut by a purse-string or Lembert suture, or that resulting after resection or lateral anastomosis, may undergo such contraction as to lead to stenosis. This appears to be more common when mechanical means, such as a Murphy's button or a bone-bobbin, have been employed.

The symptoms of stenosis usually ensue from one to four months after the accident, but I had one case in which more than a year elapsed before acute obstruction followed the invagination of a number of punctures of the small intestine produced by an iron spike.

The affected segment of bowel has usually formed adhesions with the omentum, the parietal peritoneum, or adjacent coils of intestine, which favour the occurrence of kinking or bending, and so increase the liability to obstruction.

Stricture after strangulated hernia.—This is a comparatively rare sequel of strangulated hernia, and it almost always affects the small intestine.

It may follow reduction by taxis or by operation. The stricture forms at the site of the constriction groove ; sometimes there is narrowing at each end of the strangulated loop. As a rule, it is annular and so limited as to give the appearance of a string tied round the bowel ; occasionally an inch or more of the bowel is stenosed. In a case of strangulated obturator hernia operated on by me, in which the constriction groove was invaginated by a double Lembert suture, a diaphragm formed which in the course of four months had completely occluded the bowel (Fig. 426). Perforation occurred above this diaphragm. Recovery followed resection of the affected segment with lateral anastomosis.

Clinical features of cicatricial stricture.—The symptoms are those common to all forms of increasing stenosis of the bowel (p. 471). The history of a previous injury or operation, of a strangulated hernia reduced by taxis or otherwise, or of tuberculous disease of the bowel suggests this possibility.

In the small intestine and upper colon, where the contents of the bowel are normally liquid, a very considerable degree of narrowing may be present before signs of obstruction manifest themselves, while in the lower colon, where the contents are solid, a moderate degree of stenosis will cause symptoms.

Marked variability in the severity of the symptoms, due to periodic attacks of congestion or spasm, is suggestive of cicatricial stenosis.

It is often impossible to arrive at an accurate diagnosis until the abdomen is opened.

Treatment.—Before the onset of acute obstruction, the ideal method of treatment is resection of the affected loop of bowel, with closure of the divided ends, and restoration of the continuity of the canal by lateral anastomosis. If this is impracticable, the stenosed segment may be excluded by short-circuiting the bowel. The degree of narrowing is seldom so slight as to warrant a simple enteroplasty.

When symptoms of acute obstruction are present, a temporary

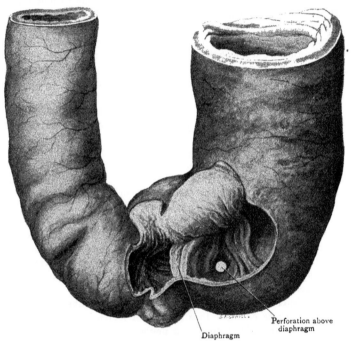

Perforation above diaphragm

Diaphragm

Fig. 426.—Stenosis of small intestine due to formation of a diaphragm at the seat of suture after strangulated hernia.

(*Author's case.*)

artificial anus should be established, and, after the bowel has been emptied, the stenosed portion may be dealt with by excision or short-circuiting according to circumstances.

TUMOURS

TUMOURS OF THE SMALL INTESTINE

The small intestine is seldom the seat of new growths, either innocent or malignant.

Innocent Tumours

Of the innocent tumours met with, perhaps the most common are **adenomas,** which arise in Lieberkühn's follicles and form pedunculated growths projecting into the lumen of the bowel. They may be solitary, or may be found scattered throughout the whole length of the intestine. They show less tendency to become malignant than similar tumours situated in the colon.

Fibromas and **lipomas** usually arise in the submucosa, and, becoming pedunculated, project into the bowel. They are almost always met with in the lower part of the ileum.[1]

Myomas originate in the muscular coat, and also tend to become pedunculated.

Angiomas are so rare that their occurrence has been denied.

Innocent tumours of the small intestine seldom give rise to trouble, unless they increase to such a size as to obstruct the lumen of the gut, or by dragging upon the wall of the bowel induce an intussusception. In either case, the symptoms are those of intestinal obstruction, and the presence of the tumour is only discovered after opening the abdomen.

Malignant Tumours

Malignant tumours are much less common in the small intestine than in the colon.

Carcinoma.[2]—Not more than 5 per cent. of carcinomas of the bowel affect the small intestine, and of these the great majority are found in the lower part of the ileum. The tumour is almost always of the columnar-celled variety, and tends to grow round the bowel, gradually narrowing the lumen. As the contents of the small intestine are fluid, the constriction of the bowel may progress till the lumen is reduced to the size of a crow-quill before signs of obstruction develop.

The exposed surface of the growth may ulcerate, and the changes characteristic of gradually increasing obstruction are evident in the bowel above and below the tumour. Secondary deposits are occasionally found in other parts of the bowel, but these seldom give rise to obstruction.

Clinical features.—The symptoms of cancer of the small intestine are less characteristic than those of cancer of the colon. Vomiting and pain are more severe and persistent, and the pain often follows the taking of food. The distended coils are centrally placed, and tend to assume a "ladder pattern," and strong, rapid peristaltic waves may be seen passing along them from time to time. Unless, however, a palpable swelling can be recognized, it is seldom possible to affirm more than that some form of stenosis is present.

[1] *See* Vol. I., p. 379.   [2] *See* Vol. I., p. 550.

Treatment.—When a positive diagnosis is impossible, and the symptoms of stenosis are progressive, the abdomen should be opened, and the cause sought for. If it is found to be a malignant growth of the small intestine, the affected segment should be excised, and a lateral anastomosis established.

Sarcoma.[1]—Sarcoma, although rare in the small intestine, is less infrequent there than in the colon.

The growth arises in the submucosa, and may project towards the lumen as a pedunculated tumour of the spindle-celled or round-celled variety, and may infiltrate the coats of the bowel, forming a localized thickening which encircles the tube, without, however, narrowing it. Indeed, the lumen is sometimes widened at first. In course of time the growth may encroach upon the lumen and cause stenosis, but this is a late development, as is also involvement of the serous coat.

Multiple growths sometimes occur. The lymphatics of the mesentery and omentum are soon infected, and metastasis to the liver and kidney occurs early.

Clinical features.—The disease is one of early life, sometimes occurring in infants. The symptoms are usually vague and are constitutional rather than local—progressive emaciation, loss of appetite, and great weakness. Eventually there may be irregularity of the bowels, with alternating constipation and diarrhoea, and vague abdominal pains. Sooner or later a palpable tumour is recognizable, and this rapidly increases in size.

The treatment is carried out on the same lines as for carcinoma, but if excision is to be successful it must be performed early.

TUMOURS OF THE COLON

INNOCENT TUMOURS

The same varieties of innocent tumours are met with in the colon as in the small intestine (p. 525), and they present very much the same appearances and give rise to the same symptoms.

The only form that requires special mention is the **multiple adenomas,**[2] first described by Virchow in 1863. These tumours may be present in enormous numbers, some small, flat, and sessile, others pedunculated and reaching the size of a cherry or even of a walnut. They are most numerous in the pelvic and descending portions of the colon, and as a rule extend into the rectum.

While originally composed of true adenomatous tissue with a covering of columnar epithelium derived from the mucous membrane, they show a marked tendency to become malignant, particularly when

---

[1] *See* Vol. I., p. 505.   [2] *See* Vol. I., p. 437.

they ulcerate, as they frequently do in the lower parts of the bowel, where they are subjected to irritation by hard fæces.

These growths are to be clearly distinguished from the polypoid condition of the mucous membrane frequently met with in cases of ileo-cæcal tuberculosis, stricture of the bowel, and fibromatosis of the colon.

Clinical features.—The most characteristic feature is severe and intractable diarrhœa, frequently attended with painful tenesmus. The stools contain a great quantity of mucus, which is often mixed with blood. There is constant pain in the abdomen and tenderness on pressure along the line of the colon, and the patient becomes anæmic and rapidly emaciates. The tumours may be felt on digital examination of the rectum, or they may be seen with the aid of the sigmoidoscope.

Treatment.—The only treatment that holds out any hope of complete or permanent relief is excision of the whole colon, but as the growths frequently invade the rectum also, this is not always practicable. The risk of the operation in suitable cases is compensated for by the prospect of getting rid of a condition which is likely sooner or later to assume malignant characters.

No extensive operation should be undertaken to remove the growths found in the rectum until it has been determined that the colon is free of them, as no benefit follows this procedure. Nor does colostomy with irrigation of the colon afford such relief as to compensate for the discomfort of the artificial anus.

MALIGNANT TUMOURS

Carcinoma.[1]—If we exclude the rectum, it may be said that 95 per cent. of cases of carcinoma of the intestine are met with in the colon. The tumour in the colon is nearly always the primary lesion, growths of metastatic origin being rare. I have met with one case in which cancer of the colon supervened in a patient whose breast I had removed for scirrhous carcinoma some years previously. Cases have been recorded in which more than one tumour was present in the bowel, probably as a result of direct infection by implantation, but cancers of different varieties may also be present in the same case.

As compared with cancer in other parts of the body, carcinoma of the colon is, on the whole, less malignant, the growth of the tumour being slower, the invasion of lymphatics taking place later, and metastasis occurring only at a late stage in the disease. It is not on this account, however, less serious, as the effect of the tumour in occluding the lumen of the gut and leading to obstruction of the bowels renders it a condition of great gravity.

[1] *See* Vol. I., p. 551.

Morbid anatomy.—The commonest variety is the columnar epithelioma, or adeno-carcinoma, originating in the glands of Lieberkühn. The tumour may form a cauliflower-like growth which projects

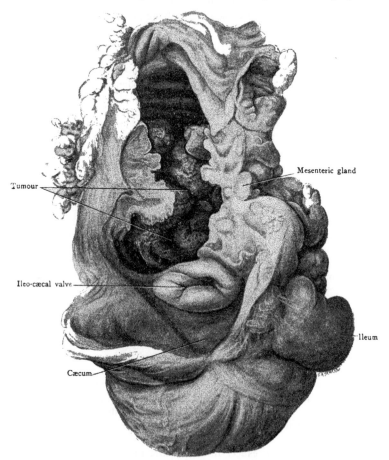

Tumour

Mesenteric gland

Ileo-cæcal valve

Ileum

Cæcum

Fig. 427.—Cancer of ascending colon filling lumen of bowel.

(*Museum, Royal College of Surgeons, Edinburgh.*)

into the lumen of the bowel, and soon ulcerates on the surface (Figs. 427, 428); or it may assume the scirrhous type, slowly encircling the bowel, and producing an annular stricture, sometimes so limited in extent as to give the appearance of a string tied tightly round the bowel (Fig. 429). In this form the lumen of the bowel may be almost completely occluded before the growth ulcerates. Colloid or encephaloid degeneration may occur in either form.

On mesial longitudinal section, the lumen of the bowel is found contracted, it may be to the size of a crow-quill, by a well-defined ridge or ring representing the oldest, central portion of the growth, while above and below this the cancer extends in the mucous membrane for about an inch in each direction (Fig. 430). The bowel above is distended, and its wall undergoes a moderate amount of hypertrophy. The mucous membrane is in a condition of catarrh and may become ulcerated.

The disease slowly spreads to the glands of the mesocolon, and also to the retroperitoneal glands, and when

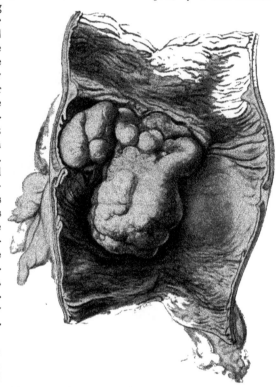

Fig. 428.—Cancer of colon forming cauliflower-like growth projecting into lumen of bowel.

(*Museum, Royal College of Surgeons, Edinburgh.*)

secondary deposits occur they almost always appear first in the liver. Secondary growths are not infrequent in the omentum, mesenteries, and peritoneum, and I have met with one case in which both ovaries were also the seat of secondary deposits. These are usually attended with a considerable amount of ascites. Spread by continuity to adjacent viscera, such as the stomach, the bladder, the female pelvic organs, and to neighbouring coils of small intestine, is not uncommon.

2 *i*

Cicatricial contraction of the mesocolon may fix the tumour and bind it to the parietes, and this in turn may lead to kinking or bending of the bowel and cause obstruction.

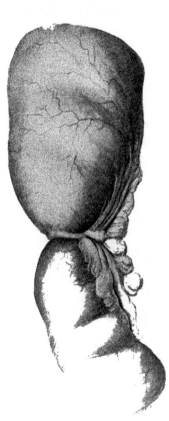 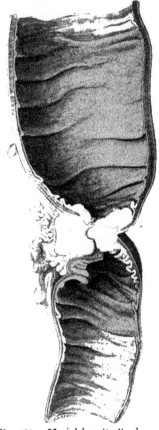

Fig. 429.—Annular stricture of bowel due to scirrhous cancer.

(This and the next figure are from specimens in the Museum of the Royal College of Surgeons, Edinburgh.)

Fig. 430.—Mesial longitudinal section of same specimen as Fig. 429, to show occlusion of lumen by scirrhous cancer. Note hypertrophy of muscular coat above stricture.

Cancer of the cæcum is liable to implicate the parietes, and in the retroperitoneal tissue cellulitis and abscess formation may occur, giving rise to symptoms which simulate appendicitis. The bursting of an abscess on the surface may establish a fæcal fistula.

Sites.—The pelvic colon is the most common seat of carcinoma, and next in order of frequency come the cæcum and the ascending colon, the transverse colon and splenic flexure, and lastly the hepatic flexure and descending colon.

Carcinoma of the pelvic colon sometimes originates in the cicatrix of a stercoral ulcer.

Clinical features. *Before the onset of complete obstruction.*—The extent to which the colon may be narrowed by a malignant stricture, without giving rise to any symptoms, is often remarkable, and in many cases attention is first directed to the condition by the onset of the symptoms of acute obstruction.

When the tumour manifests itself in its early stages, the symptoms are usually those of irritation of the bowel, and are common to many other conditions than cancer. It may be noticed that the patient is losing strength, is depressed and listless, and complains of vague abdominal discomfort, rarely amounting to pain. Loss of weight is not a prominent feature in the early stages; in fact, the patient may even be putting on weight. There is a gradually increasing difficulty in keeping the bowels regular, necessitating the frequent use of purgatives. The constipation gradually becomes more pronounced, and the medicines that previously procured a motion merely induce attacks of colicky pain and flatulent distension. Soon the patient begins to suffer from recurrent attacks of spurious diarrhœa, passing a small quantity of fæces, with a good deal of mucus and some flatus. This does not give him relief, and is usually followed by a further period of constipation. The sequence of alternating constipation and diarrhœa is very characteristic of cancer of the colon, and should always lead to a systematic examination of the abdomen. On examination, the stools are found to contain a small quantity of blood, sometimes only detectable by the microscope, or by the guaiac or the benzidine test. There is seldom a large hæmorrhage from the bowel. No importance is to be attached to the shape of the motions, unless the cancer actually implicates the anal canal.

Vomiting is seldom a constant or prominent symptom; when it occurs, it is usually in relation with the taking of food.

It is not always possible to detect a localized swelling in the abdomen, as, even when of considerable size, the growth may be obscured by the thickness of the abdominal wall, or by flatulent distension. When situated in the splenic or hepatic flexure it lies under cover of the ribs. When palpable, the tumour, although solid to the feel, is usually resonant on percussion, and it is not always tender. Frequently the swelling that is felt is due to an accumulation of fæces above a stricture, in which case it is comparatively soft and pits on pleasure. In other instances it is due to the omentum or an adjacent coil of bowel having become adherent to the tumour.

On examining the rectum, it is often observed that the external sphincter is tightly contracted, the anal canal unduly short, and the rectal cavity blown up with gas, so that the finger can scarcely reach its walls, a condition which is known as "ballooning of the rectum." This is most frequently observed when the stricture is in the pelvic colon, but is not a characteristic sign of cancer.

When ascites is present, there are usually advanced secondary deposits in the peritoneum, or in the liver.

As time goes on, the patient suffers greatly from recurring attacks of colic, during which visible coils of intestine may stand out and be felt to harden as a wave of peristalsis passes over them. There is increasing distension, and rumbling sounds are heard in the abdomen. The constipation becomes more marked, and, in spite of the taking of purgatives or enemata, the bowels may fail to act for days or even weeks, without acute symptoms of complete obstruction coming on.

When acute obstruction has supervened.—As a rule, acute symptoms appear suddenly in a patient who has for some time shown signs of gradually increasing stenosis. In a considerable proportion of cases, however, the compensation has been so efficient that the muscular hypertrophy has been able to overcome the obstruction, and it is only when a severe strain is suddenly thrown upon the musculature of the dilated bowel—for example by the taking of a strong purgative, or by a foreign body or a hardened fæcal mass becoming impacted in the stricture—that the compensation fails and signs of acute obstruction manifest themselves. The usual symptoms of acute obstruction are present, and there may be nothing, apart from the previous history, to indicate either the cause or the seat of the obstruction. The whole colon above the stricture usually becomes greatly dilated, the dilatation supervening rapidly, and being so marked that, when the abdomen is opened, the longitudinal striæ cannot be recognized, and the peritoneal coat often splits with the removal of the support of the abdominal wall. The distended bowel forces its way between the layers of the mesentery, which may become so much shortened as to anchor the gut. Patches of gangrene may form on the dilated bowel and perforation occur, leading to peritonitis, which adds to the distension. Sometimes the cæcum alone is acutely distended, the other parts of the colon above the obstruction showing only moderate dilatation. This is probably due to the ileo-cæcal valve remaining competent and to violent anti-peristalsis forcing gas and fluid fæces back to the cæcum.

When the colon is full and bulges into the flanks, it yields a dull note on percussion, and an apparent sense of fluctuation with distinct splashing may be detected on succussion.

If peritonitis is present, there is muscular rigidity and fixation, and if perforation has occurred the whole abdomen is uniformly blown up and yields a high-pitched, drummy note.

Pain is not always referred to the position of the obstruction ; when peritonitis is present it is generally referred to the seat of infection.

Vomiting is a late symptom, and, although it may be persistent, it seldom becomes stercoraceous. Hiccup is often very intractable. The patient may linger on for some days in this condition, but ultimately succumbs to toxæmia or to exhaustion from the persistent vomiting and loss of fluid.

Cancer of the cæcum (Fig. 431).—A palpable tumour is more frequently to be made out when the cancer affects the cæcum, and flatulent distension and exaggerated peristalsis of the lower coils of the ileum are often detectable. The pain frequently bears a distinct relation to the taking of food.

Cancer of the transverse colon.—When a tumour is palpable, it is centrally placed, and is usually freely movable. It may be of considerable size, as it is not uncommon for the omentum to be rolled up and incorporated in the growth, or for the lesser omentum and even the stomach to be invaded. The distension is most evident in the right flank.

Cancer of the splenic flexure.—As the growth is under cover of the ribs, it cannot be palpated. The distension affects the transverse colon, and the cæcum is sometimes very greatly distended. Peristalsis is usually too feeble to be recognized. Pain is often worst before defæcation.

Cancer of the descending and pelvic colon.—There is usually a palpable tumour in the left iliac fossa, which may be fixed by contraction of the mesocolon, but in some cases is so movable that it can be pushed towards the middle of the abdomen or even to the right side. The tumour can sometimes be felt on bimanual examination, or it may be seen with the sigmoidoscope, or its position can be recognized by X-ray examination after injecting an emulsion of bismuth into the bowel. The whole length of the colon is distended, the cæcum often being blown up to an enormous extent, and in rare cases the distension involves also the small intestine, producing a characteristic "ladder pattern." It is in cancer of the pelvic colon that ballooning of the rectum is most frequently present. Constipation is more marked than in cancer higher up, but it alternates, or may even be associated with persistent and painful tenesmus and the passage of mucus.

Complications.—In addition to complete obstruction of the bowels, which is sooner or later an almost inevitable sequel to malignant disease of the colon, various other complications may arise. The growth may, for example, form attachments with an adjacent portion of the alimentary canal, and gradually invade it, with the result that an *internal fistula* is established. So long as two adjacent coils become

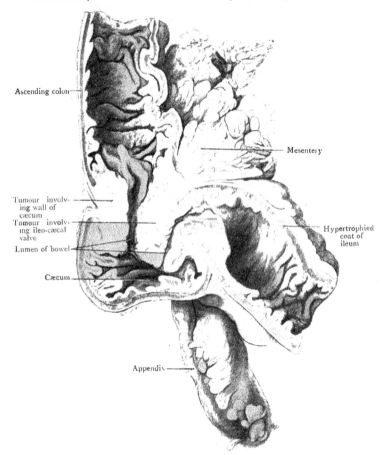

Ascending colon

Mesentery

Tumour involving wall of cæcum

Tumour involving ileo-cæcal valve

Lumen of bowel

Hypertrophied coat of ileum

Cæcum

Appendix

Fig. 431.—Cancer of the cæcum.

(*Author's case.*)

connected, the effects of the formation of such a fistula are not necessarily serious, but when portions of the canal widely separated from one another become fused, the short-circuiting may seriously interfere with the nutrition of the patient—for example, when the stomach is invaded by a growth of the transverse colon. It has happened that a fistulous communication between the intestine above and that beyond the cancer has temporarily relieved an obstruction. Fistulæ may also form between the colon and the bladder. I have observed two cases in which flatus was passed with the urine ; in one this continued for about a fortnight, and then ceased, and did not recur during the fifteen months the patient survived; post-mortem the opening was found occluded by cicatricial tissue apparently due to peritonitic adhesions. Similar fistulæ may also form with the urethra, the vagina, or the skin.

Intussusception is occasionally induced, and *kinking* of the bowel may occur and lead to acute obstruction.

Differential diagnosis.—In the absence of acute obstructive symptoms, the diagnosis of cancer of the colon does not present great difficulty. It is to be borne in mind that in the colon cancer occurs at an earlier age than in most other situations. Many of the patients appear to be in good general health, and show no sign of what is spoken of as a cancerous cachexia. This cachectic condition only ensues in the terminal stages of the disease when the diagnosis is no longer in doubt. The conditions that have to be borne in mind when the symptoms are referred to the region of the cæcum are ileo-cæcal tuberculosis, enterolith, and inflammatory swellings originating in the appendix ; in the region of the ascending colon and hepatic flexure, affections of the right kidney, the liver and gall-bladder, the stomach and pylorus, and the omentum ; in the splenic flexure and descending colon, affections of the left kidney and spleen ; in the pelvic colon, diseases of the uterine appendages, fibromatosis of the colon, and fæcal accumulation.

When symptoms of acute obstruction are present, apart from the history, there is nothing characteristic of cancerous stricture, and all other causes of obstruction have to be considered. It is often impossible to arrive at a diagnosis without opening the abdomen.

Treatment.—As the disease remains for a considerable time confined to the bowel and is slow to implicate the mesenteric glands, a radical operation, if undertaken before there is much distension of the bowel above the stricture and before obstructive symptoms have appeared, affords a considerable prospect of permanent cure. The radical operation consists in removing the affected segment, as well as several inches of the bowel above and below it, together with the lymphatic vessels draining the bowel, the glands into which these lymphatics open, and the connective tissue in which they lie. The continuity of the tube is re-established either by end-to-end suture or by lateral anastomosis. With the patient in the Trendelenburg position, an incision is made which will give free access to the tumour. To enable the ends to be brought together without tension, it is advisable to "mobilize" the segment to be dealt with, by dividing the reflection of the peritoneum on to the parietes and stripping it towards the middle line.

In the great majority of cases, the patient is already suffering from obstructive symptoms before the question of operation is raised, and the bowel is more or less distended above the stricture. When acute obstructive symptoms are present, it is seldom possible to locate the tumour, and the abdomen is best opened to the right of the middle line below the level of the umbilicus. Under these conditions, the resection should always be done by the "two-stage" method, the obstruction being relieved by opening and draining the distended bowel, and the growth removed at a later date. If it is possible at the first operation to bring the tumour out to the surface, this should be done, as it greatly facilitates the second stage of removal.

The second stage should be carried through as soon as the bowel has been completely emptied and the patient has sufficiently recovered from the effects of the obstruction and the primary operation. This is usually in from three to seven days.

If, after relieving the obstruction, it is found to be impossible to resect the growth, the patient may be saved the discomfort of a permanent artificial anus and his life may be prolonged by entero-anastomosis, the bowel above and below the stricture being united.

Sarcoma of the colon.—Sarcoma of the colon is a rare disease, and is usually met with in the cæcum. It occurs in young subjects as a diffuse infiltration of the coats of the bowel, converting it into a rigid tube. The mucous membrane as a rule is tightly stretched over the tumour, which tends to grow towards the lumen of the bowel. Obstruction is not a common manifestation of the disease. As a rule, the disease is characterized by a general weakness, loss of flesh, and the development of a rapidly growing abdominal swelling.

If the disease is diagnosed early, the affected segment of bowel should be removed on the same lines as for carcinoma, and experience has shown that the results of early operation are on the whole satisfactory.

BIBLIOGRAPHY

Barnard, H. L., *Contributions to Abdominal Surgery.* 1910.
Berry and Giuseppi, *Proc. Roy. Soc. Med.*, Nov., 1908.
Caird, F. M., *Scot. Med. and Surg. Journ.*, 1904, xiv.
Goodall, Harry W., *Boston Med. and Surg. Journ.*, April, 1910.
Hartmann, *Rev. de Chir.*, Feb., 1907.
Keith, Arthur, *Brit. Med. Journ.*, Feb. 5, 1910.
Miles, Alexander, *Edin. Med. Journ.*, 1910, i.
Paterson, H. J., *Proc. Roy. Soc. Med.*, June, 1909.
Pavlov, *The Work of the Digestive Glands*, 2nd Edit. 1910.
Proc. Roy. Soc. Med., 1909, pp. 59–99, Discussion in Med. Sec. on Ulcerative Colitis.
Thomson, Alexis, *Edin. Med. Journ.*, April, 1908.
Wilkie, D. P. D., *Edin. Med. Journ.*, 1909, ii., and Oct., 1910.

THE APPENDIX

By PERCY SARGENT, M.A., M.B., B.C.CANTAB.,
F.R.C.S.ENG.

Anatomy and physiology.—The appendix is a blind tubular diverticulum springing from the inner and posterior aspect of the cæcum at a point about 2 in. from the ileo-cæcal valve. In the fœtus and in the infant it forms the apex of the cæcum, and when this condition persists in adult life the cæcum is said to be of the fœtal type. The sacculations of the adult cæcum which displace the appendix from its apical position are of secondary formation. The appendix attains its maximum development in young adult life, and after middle age it is said slowly to atrophy. In old age it may be found represented by a mere fibrous cord.

Length.—The average length of the appendix is between 3 and 4 in., varying from $\frac{1}{2}$ in. or even less up to as much as 9 in. (R. Berry). Whilst its average diameter is about $\frac{1}{4}$ in., its lumen, unless occupied by pathological material, is very narrow. The cæcal orifice is sometimes marked by a feebly developed valve-like fold of mucous membrane (Gerlach's valve).

Position.—The appendix occupies no constant anatomical position, the variations in this respect being due to its free mobility. The situations in which it is most frequently found are (1) to the inner side of the cæcum, pointing upwards and leftwards towards the spleen (38 per cent., H. P. Hawkins); (2) pointing upwards behind the cæcum, where it often occupies and is concealed in, the retrocolic fossa (26 per cent.); and (3) hanging over the pelvic brim (17 per cent.). It will be readily understood that the position in which the appendix happens to lie when it becomes acutely inflamed or perforated will determine the situation of a resulting abscess or the direction of spread of a diffuse peritonitis.

Surface marking.—McBurney's point is situated upon a line drawn from the anterior superior iliac spine to the umbilicus (spino-umbilical line) and about 2 in. internally to the iliac spine. This does not represent the situation of the appendix, but is said to be, as a rule, the point of greatest tenderness in appendicitis. Munro's point is the spot at which the spino-umbilical line crosses the outer border of the rectus muscle or linea semilunaris. According to A. Keith, the ileo-cæcal valve is the part of the intestine which most often lies directly beneath Munro's point, so that the appendicular orifice will usually be found about an inch below and to the outer side of Munro's point.

Structure.—The coats of the appendix consist of (1) a mucous membrane, containing innumerable Lieberkühn's glands, and resting upon a very faintly marked muscularis mucosæ; (2) a submucous layer, extremely rich in lymphoid tissue; (3) a muscular layer, comprising inner circular and outer longitudinal strata corresponding with the muscular layers of the cæcum, but differing in the fact that the outer layer is disposed uniformly over the surface instead of being grouped into distinct bands; and (4) a peritoneal coat, separated from the muscle by a small amount of subserous connective tissue. The peritoneal covering is complete, except just along the line of attachment of the mesentery where the vessels enter and leave the organ. The meso-appendix connects the little process to the mesentery of the termination of the ileum, springing from its inferior aspect, and is often so short as to render the appendix tortuous; it is sometimes heavily loaded with fat.

Blood-vessels.—The appendix is supplied by a branch of the ileo-cæcal artery, the termination of the superior mesenteric, which passes down behind the termination of the ileum, and enters the meso-appendix, to be distributed to the organ by a series of circularly-disposed branches. The veins are arranged in a similar manner, and are radicles of the portal system.

Lymphatics.—The lymphatics are collected into four or five trunks which pass with the appendicular artery between the layers of the meso-appendix and travel behind the termination of the ileum to end in the ileo-cæcal glands—a group of some five or six glands situated between the layers of the mesentery of the small intestine in the upper ileo-cæcal angle (Poirier and Cunéo).

Peritoneal relations.—The clinical significance of the various positions in which the appendix may be found will be readily understood when considered in connexion with the peritoneal watersheds (p. 559). In addition to the meso-appendix, there is a second peritoneal fold, occasionally well marked, which passes from the anterior aspect of the termination of the ileum to the front of the appendicular mesentery. This is the ileo-cæcal fold (the so-called " bloodless fold "), which bounds the ileo-cæcal fossa. The appendix is frequently lodged in the retrocæcal fossa, a peritoneal pouch which may be demonstrated by drawing the caput coli upwards.

Physiology.—The appendix is a vestigial structure whose functions, if any, are of little moment. Experience has amply proved that its removal is followed by no demonstrable alteration in the economy. It has been variously credited with the provision of some secretion which prevents fæcal hardening in the cæcum ; with being concerned in the digestion of vegetable material ; with providing a fluid which stimulates peristaltic activity in the cæcum ; and, on account of the large quantity of lymphoid tissue which it contains, with having to do with the disposal of bacteria. W. Macewen believes that the appendix possesses definite and important functions. He regards it as a sort of culture-tube from which, in response to the stimulus provided by the passage of the intestinal contents over its orifice, bacteria in a proper state of activity are from time to time discharged into the cæcum, where they assist in the disintegration of undigested food-stuffs.

Misplacement of the appendix.—The various positions occupied by an appendix lying in the right iliac region can scarcely be termed abnormalities, as there is no " normal " position with which to compare them. The organ is, however, sometimes found in situations so remote from its usual position as to constitute misplacements, and such variations are due either to (a) arrest in the development and descent of the cæcum, or (b) the presence of abnormally long and voluminous mesenteries.

(a) **Misplacement due to arrest of development.**—During the development of the colon the cæcum passes from the left hypochondrium across the upper part of the abdomen to the under surface of the liver, and then downwards until it reaches its final adult position in the right iliac fossa. Arrest of development may cause the appendix to occupy any position upon this line of descent ; consequently it has been found near the spleen, in the epigastrium, beneath the liver, and at various points in the right loin between the liver and the right iliac fossa.

(b) **Mesenteric abnormalities.**—A long mesocolon, such as that which predisposes to the production of a volvulus of the cæcum, is not infrequently responsible for abnormal positions of the appendix, especially when combined with elongation of the meso-appendix. Thus the appendix may be entirely in the pelvis, where it may be adherent to the uterus, broad ligament, or bladder ; it may lie entirely upon the left side of the body, and be found in the left loin or left iliac fossa ; or it may occupy any position amongst the intestinal coils. A long meso-appendix, apart from any abnormality of the mesocolon, may allow of abnormal positions being assumed by the appendix through its tip becoming adherent to other viscera and being pulled upon by them. Thus the tip of a long appendix with a long mesentery, having become adherent to the pelvic colon, may be drawn upon so that it stretches across the abdomen and lies partly upon the left iliac fossa. Similarly it may become pulled upon, elongated, and displaced by any coil of small intestine to which it may have become adherent.

Just as mesenteric abnormalities permit of the appendix being found in many abnormal positions within the abdomen, so they also allow of its appearance in hernial sacs, and the organ has often been found in right-sided femoral and inguinal hernias; less often in umbilical and in left-sided femoral and inguinal hernias. It may be found either alone or in company with other viscera.

In the rare instances of transposition of viscera, the cæcum and appendix are found in the left iliac fossa, but with their relations to one another and to other viscera otherwise unaltered.

APPENDICITIS

Etiology.—Appendicitis is a disease essentially dependent upon bacterial activity, which may be brought about or contributed to by a number of subsidiary causes.

Bacteriology.—The great majority of cases of appendicitis are caused by the Bacillus coli (*see* Peritonitis, p. 565). Other organisms have from time to time been found in or around an inflamed appendix, such as the Pneumococcus (J. Eyre), the pathogenetic staphylococci (Tavel and Lanz), the Streptococcus pyogenes (Cushing), certain anaerobes (Veillon and Zuber), and the Bacillus pyocyaneus (Dudgeon and Sargent); and whilst it must be admitted that any of these organisms may be occasional causes of the disease, yet there is no doubt that the colon bacillus is by far the most frequent causal agent (Dudgeon and Sargent).

Accessory causes.—*Age* is a most important factor in the incidence of appendicitis, and its greater frequency in young adult life is probably related to the maximum development of the lymphoid tissue which is noted at that period. The disease is rare in infancy and becomes increasingly frequent between the ages of 10 and 20, when the maximum is reached; from 20 to 30 the age-incidence falls but little; whilst from 30 to 40 the diminution is considerable; after 40 it becomes less and less frequent, until in old age it is as rare as in infancy.

Sex can scarcely be cited as a cause, for there is no obvious reason, anatomical or pathological, why the disease should occur more often in one sex than in the other. Yet it is a fact that all large series of cases show a distinct preponderance of males, the proportion of males to females being variously estimated as lying between 2 to 1 and 3 to 1.

Heredity.—There is some reason for thinking that the tendency to appendicitis runs in families. If this is so it may perhaps be ascribed to similarity of anatomical conformation favouring the disease, to

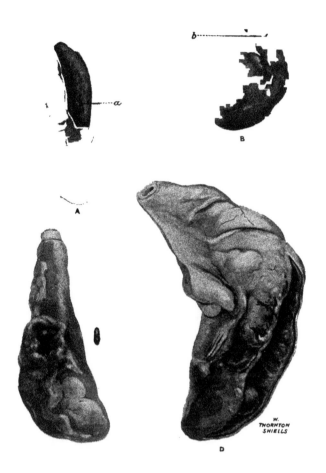

A. Appendix distended by a large concretion. The serous and muscular coats have been cut away to show the mucosa stretched over the concretion, and ulcerated at *a*. (*Specimen* 1107E, *St. Thomas's Hospital Museum.*)

B. Acutely inflamed appendix from a boy aged 7, removed fifteen hours after the onset. At *b* the wall consists of the serous coat only; the mucosa is gangrenous. The patient recovered.

C. Perforated appendix, with concretion, from a woman aged 35, removed forty-eight hours after the onset. The patient recovered.

D. Gangrenous appendix, with concretion, from a fatal case. (*Specimen* 1107E A, *St. Thomas's Hospital Museum.*)

PLATE 97.

similar lack of resistance to B. coli infection, or to similar habits of diet in members of the same family.

Dietetic errors and *chronic constipation* undoubtedly influence the incidence of the disease. Conversely, it seems probable that chronic disease of the appendix is a factor in the production of various intestinal disorders, so that the diseased appendix becomes a link in a vicious circle.

Injury has been credited with being a factor in the causation of appendicitis, since a certain number of patients give a history either of some abrupt and unaccustomed strain or of a direct abdominal injury (6·6 per cent., von Neumann). Byrom Robinson has suggested that the injury caused by the constant action of the underlying psoas muscle may be responsible for some cases.

· *Foreign bodies and concretions.*—Pins, bristles, hairs, grains of corn, fruit-seeds, and other foreign bodies have been found in inflamed appendices, but their occurrence is so uncommon as to constitute a curiosity. Fæcal concretions, on the other hand, are found in about 25 per cent. of cases.

Parasites.—Threadworms are not infrequently found in appendices removed at operation. In 200 post-mortem examinations of children, G. F. Still found the oxyuris in the appendix 25 times.

Inflammation of adjacent structures, such as an ovarian cyst, may involve the appendix secondarily; on the other hand, these structures may be secondarily infected from a diseased appendix. The coexistence of pelvic disease with appendicitis is well known.

Many other factors have, on slender grounds for the most part, been cited as causes of appendicitis, such as exposure to cold, rheumatism, and influenza. These need but passing notice.

Appendices in abnormal situations are very prone to become the seat of disease, as for example in hernias. In a similar manner the appendix utilized in the operation of appendicostomy is very liable to become inflamed and gangrenous. When this happens it is possible to watch the course of a case of appendicitis in the abdominal wall, and uncomplicated by peritoneal involvement.

Morbid anatomy (Plate 97).—Inflammatory changes in the appendix may be of any degree, from those of a superficial catarrh up to total gangrene. In the mildest cases the mucous membrane is swollen and reddened, with but slight infiltration of the more external layers, and with little or no periappendicular effusion. An increase of secretion occurs which, if the appendix be patent, escapes into the cæcum, and the inflammation subsides, leaving little trace behind. Repeated attacks of such a catarrhal inflammation leave the appendix thickened, firm to the touch, and often adherent to surrounding structures; its lumen is narrowed, and the lining membrane is swollen and mottled in appearance. In some instances the lumen is wholly or partly obliterated (Fig. 432).

If the secretion in a catarrhal appendicitis is unable to escape freely into the cæcum, several results may occur, depending partly upon the completeness of the obstruction, but chiefly upon the degree of bacterial activity within the organ.

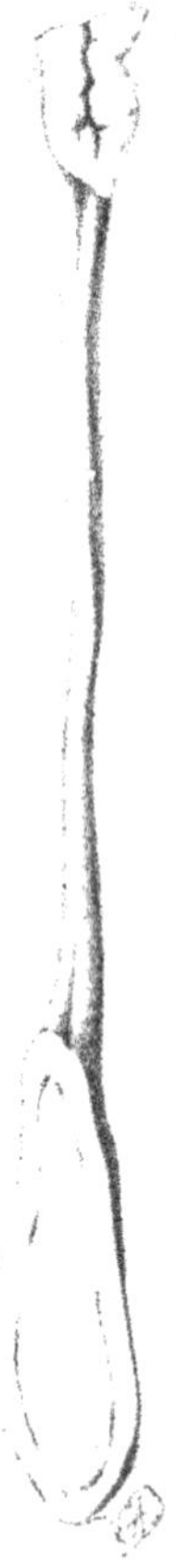

With complete obstruction and mild bacterial activity a cyst may result, containing clear or turbid fluid, and occasionally attaining a large size (Fig. 433). The fluid may prove to be sterile.

With only partial obstruction a concretion may be formed consisting of a mass of inspissated mucus and fæcal matter. These concretions frequently present, on section, a laminated appearance, as though added to from time to time by the deposition of fresh layers (Fig. 434). In appearance they often resemble a cherry-stone or a date-stone; and it is this resemblance which has given rise to the popular notions as to the danger of swallowing such objects. -Occasionally a concretion attains a large size and resembles a gall-stone. Once a concretion has formed and is unable to escape into the cæcum, it becomes a source not only of discomfort but also of danger to its possessor, inducing repeated attacks of inflammation, and threatening ulceration and perforation. If a concretion is able to escape into the cæcum, or to be shifted to a different spot in the appendix, the ulcerated surface against which it lay becomes cicatrized, and a stricture results.

When the bacterial activity is great the inflammatory changes are of a more pronounced nature, and a more advanced series of changes takes place. The inflammation involves the whole thickness of the appendicular wall, and the bacteria are able to pass into the subserous tissue and finally to infect the peritoneum. The most virulent forms of peritonitis can occur from the migration of bacteria through the wall of an inflamed but unperforated appendix. Bacterial invasion of the peritoneal cavity may take place in other ways also—(1) thrombosis of the appendicular vessels followed by gangrene of the organ *en masse ;* (2) localized gangrene from vascular disturbance, or from pressure over a concretion, leading to rupture or perforation of the appendix

Fig. 432.—An appendix, 4½ in. long, with bulbous end; the greater part of it has been converted into a cord-like structure. (*St. Thomas's Hospital Museum.*)

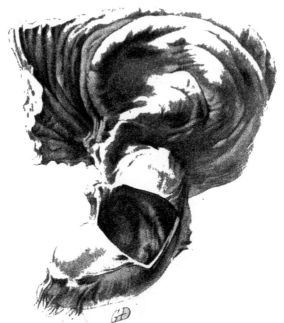

Fig. 433.—An appendix which has been converted into a cyst.
(*Specimen* 1098, *St. Thomas's Hospital Museum.*)

at the gangrenous spot (Fig. 435); (3) ulceration over a concretion, or deep ulceration independent of the presence of a concretion, followed
by rupture of the appendix at that spot. A
foreign body sometimes, but rarely, acts in the
same manner as a concretion, and a sharp-
pointed foreign body such as a pin may perforate the appendix mechanically (Fig. 436).

When those processes which entail the passage
of bacteria through the appendicular wall take
place slowly and gradually, the natural defensive powers of the peritoneum are called into
play (*see* under Peritonitis, p. 562). Around an
inflamed appendix there is always a little turbid
peritoneal exudate, rich in phagocytes, which is
capable of dealing with the bacteria coming from
the appendix, provided that an overwhelming
amount of virulent material be not suddenly

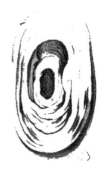

Fig. 434.—Section
of a large appendi-
cular concretion,
showing the lami-
nation.

(*Specimen* 1002,
*St. Thomas's Hospital
Museum.*)

discharged into the peritoneal cavity. This constitutes the first and chief line of resistance. The second protective process lies in the formation of adhesions, so that when the perforation does occur it is not into the general cavity but into a localized portion of it (Fig. 437). In this manner the effect of the bacterial invasion of the peritoneal cavity, whether with or without gross perforation of the appendix, is the production of a localized abscess.

When these protective agencies, either from want of time or from lack of resistance on the part of the individual, fail to limit the infection, a diffuse, spreading peritonitis results.

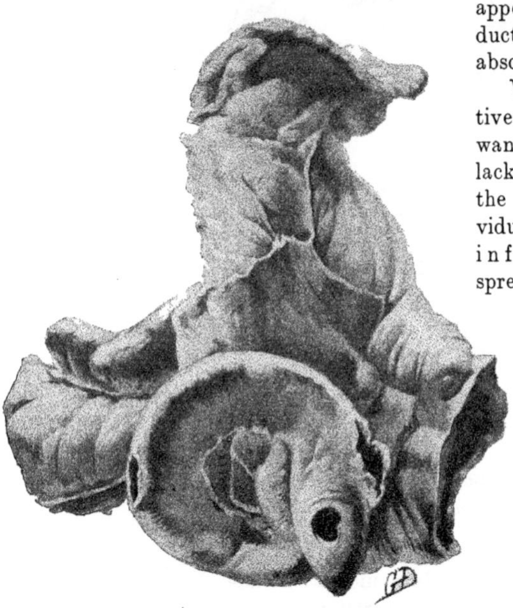

A. ACUTE FORMS OF APPENDICITIS

Clinical features.— The various morbid conditions of the appendix indicated above bear but little relation to the clinical course of the disease. A

Fig. 435.—A gangrenous perforated appendix, from a fatal case.

(*Specimen* 1103, *St. Thomas's Hospital Museum.*)

rapidly fatal diffuse peritonitis may spread from an appendix which to the naked eye appears only reddened and swollen, but unperforated, or a gangrenous perforated appendix may be found in a completely localized abscess cavity. Nor is there any means of recognizing clinically the presence of constrictions, adhesions, or concretions, with the possible exception of the latter, which have sometimes been demonstrated by means of the X-rays. It is not possible, therefore, to make clinical subdivisions to correspond with the various pathological conditions enumerated above.

Appendicitis presents itself in many different degrees of severity, all of which pass by gentle gradations into one another. Nevertheless, certain common types of the acute disease may be recognized, so that the clinical course may conveniently be described under three headings :—

— 1. Acute or subacute attacks, without perforation or gangrene, and associated with a mild and local peritonitis in the immediate neighbourhood of the appendix.

— 2. Acute attacks associated with ulceration, perforation, or gangrene, resulting in the formation of a localized abscess around the appendix.

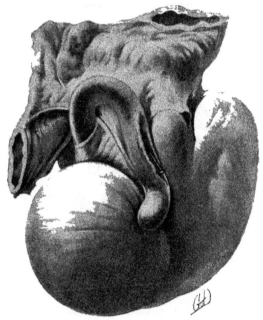

Fig. 436.—Perforation of the appendix by a pin.

(Specimen 1098B, *St. Thomas's Hospital Museum.)*

— 3. Acute attacks associated with the passage of virulent bacteria from the inflamed appendix into the peritoneal cavity, either with or without gross perforation or gangrene, and resulting in a diffuse, spreading peritonitis.

For the sake of brevity these may respectively be termed—(1) acute appendicitis, (2) appendicitis with local abscess, and (3) appendicitis with diffuse peritonitis.

1. ACUTE APPENDICITIS

Symptoms.—The attack may be sudden and unexpected, or it may be preceded by certain symptoms which are termed prodromal.

2 *j*

Amongst these may be mentioned an indefinite feeling of malaise, indigestion, constipation, diarrhœa, and vague abdominal discomfort.

Whether preceded by prodromal symptoms or not, the attack begins with an acute pain in the abdomen, often quite sudden in its onset, which at first cannot be localized and may be referred to the epigastrium or to the umbilicus. The pain is rapidly followed by nausea and vomiting, and this is very soon succeeded by a rise of temperature, occasionally with an initial rigor, accompanied by the usual constitutional symptoms of toxic fever. The bowels may act once or twice after the onset, but then constipation usually becomes a prominent feature. Exceptionally the bowels act naturally throughout, and some of the severer cases are attended with diarrhœa.

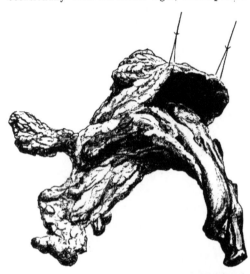

Fig. 437.—From a case of acute appendicitis of three days' duration in a youth aged 17. The distal end had perforated into an omental pocket.

Examination shortly after the onset shows the abdomen to be rigid, motionless, and uniformly tender; these signs soon become localized to the right iliac region, and the spot of most acute tenderness is commonly found to correspond with McBurney's point. The abdomen is usually a little distended, and may be markedly so ; the distension may be limited to the lower half of the abdomen, and even to the right iliac region. Very soon an indefinite swelling can be felt in the right iliac fossa, which in two or three days becomes palpable as a more or less definite mass. Muscular rigidity often causes a localized swelling which may readily be mistaken for a subjacent inflammatory tumour. In some cases symptoms referable to the bladder are present, namely, pain, frequency of micturition, or retention of urine. Rectal pain and tenesmus may also be experienced. In these instances examination per rectum usually reveals the presence of a tender inflammatory mass in the right side of the pelvis.

Meanwhile the temperature is raised, ranging from 100° to 103° or
104°; the pulse-rate is correspondingly accelerated, the tongue is
furred, and the appetite lost.   These symptoms last from about three
to ten days according to the severity of the attack.

2. APPENDICITIS WITH LOCAL ABSCESS

The **symptoms** at first are the same as those described above,
except that they are usually more severe, though this is not necessarily
the ease.   The probability of abscess formation increases in proportion as the symptoms of fever and the local signs persist beyond the
customary time for an ordinary attack to last.   The presence of a tumour
in the right iliac fossa which increases in size and definition, especially
when diarrhœa replaces the initial constipation, or the existence of a
tender pelvic mass together with vesical symptoms at a time when an
ordinary attack would naturally be clearing up, indicates the formation
of an abscess.   The patient prefers to lie with the right thigh drawn
up, full extension being painful.

Leucocytosis is regarded by some as of value in the diagnosis of
abscess; but, like the elevation of temperature, it is to be taken as
an indication of absorption and reaction rather than of the actual
presence of pus, for a large completely walled-off abscess may exist
without either leucocytosis or fever.

In a neglected case the skin of the abdominal wall may become
œdematous and reddened, and it may even be possible to detect fluctuation; but this is a sign which is rarely present, and should never
be expected.   If untreated the pus may make its way to the surface,
but it is much more likely to rupture into the general peritoneal cavity,
the bowel, vagina, or bladder; or it may track upwards to the subphrenic region and rupture into the pleura or respiratory passages.

3. APPENDICITIS WITH DIFFUSE PERITONITIS

The rupture or perforation of a diseased appendix, giving rise to
a diffuse peritonitis, may be abrupt and unexpected.

A patient, apparently in perfect health, may be suddenly seized
with violent abdominal pain and vomiting, and rapidly evince the
symptoms of profound collapse.   Often there are premonitory symptoms of a more or less definite character pointing to appendicitis, but
in most cases the onset of the peritonitis is sudden or at least rapid.
In some instances the actual moment of perforation is indicated
by sudden relief of the pain due to distension of an acutely inflamed
appendix; in others the peritonitis spreads swiftly, but more insidiously, from an imperfectly shut-off collection of pus around the appendix; in others, again, the rupture of a localized abscess provides the
starting-point of a diffuse peritonitis.

The symptoms of this form of acute appendicitis are therefore those of diffuse peritonitis (*see* p. 567), either of sudden and unexpected onset, added to those of a pre-existing acute appendicitis, with or without periappendicular abscess.

Diagnosis of acute forms of appendicitis.—The diagnosis of an ordinary attack of acute appendicitis presents little difficulty, nor, as a rule, do the history, symptoms, and physical signs of the cases complicated by gross peritoneal infection leave much room for doubt as to the nature of the illness. In the less acute cases the difficulty is greater, particularly as there is a growing tendency to ascribe, often on slender evidence, vague abdominal symptoms of all kinds to pathological conditions of the appendix.

The diagnosis embraces two distinct considerations, namely, the discrimination of appendicitis from other conditions, and the recognition of the stage and severity of the appendicitis.

1. **Acute appendicitis may be simulated by—**

(*a*) *Pelvic causes.*—Salpingitis, pyosalpinx, ruptured tubal pregnancy, and inflammation or the twisting of the pedicle of a small ovarian cyst, are to be eliminated by the history, together with a careful bimanual examination of the pelvis. At the same time, the possibility of associated pelvic and appendicular disease must not be overlooked.

(*b*) *Renal causes.*—Movable kidney with Dietl's crises, renal calculus, and ureteral calculus, all may give rise to symptoms resembling acute or subacute appendicitis. The character and position of the pain, the absence of fever and of constipation, the examination of the urine, and X-ray investigation should serve to eliminate these sources of error.

(*c*) *Hepatic causes*, such as cholecystitis and cholelithiasis, can generally be distinguished by the position of the tenderness, a history or the presence of jaundice, and the radiation of the pain to the shoulder. Disease of a subhepatic appendix may simulate affections of the gall-bladder very closely, and, on the other hand, a large, tender, low-lying gall-bladder has been mistaken for an appendix abscess.

(*d*) *Gastric and duodenal ulcer* are to be excluded by inquiry into the relation of pain to ingestion of food, and the absence of epigastric tenderness, melæna, hæmatemesis, and gastric dilatation.

(*e*) *The onset of pneumonia and of pleurisy* occasionally mimics appendicitis by causing acute abdominal pain and rigidity. A careful examination of the chest should prevent error in such cases.

2. **Diagnosis of the severity and degree of the appendicitis.**—At the onset there is no means of telling whether the attack is one which will run a mild course and subside spontaneously, or

whether it will proceed to abscess formation or the involvement of the peritoneum in a diffuse, spreading inflammation. The acuteness of the onset is but a poor indication of the probable course of events, because an apparently mild attack may go on to the formation of an abscess, or may, from perforation or gangrene, at any moment present the most urgent symptoms of spreading peritonitis.

When the patient has not been seen from the commencement of the attack, and the course has been so atypical that the disease could not be recognized until two or three days have elapsed, the diagnosis of the degree and severity of the appendicitis becomes a matter of some difficulty. In watching a case of this kind so that surgical treatment may be adopted at the right moment, it is of the utmost importance to avoid the administration of morphia or opium, since these drugs may completely obscure symptoms of great gravity. The presence of a definite tumour, felt either through the abdominal wall or per rectum, which is increasing in size, or at least not diminishing, after several days of illness, together with continued fever and high leuco-cytosis, especially if accompanied by diarrhœa, indicates the formation of an abscess. At this stage spontaneous relief may occur from the discharge of pus into the bowel. This would be indicated by the passage of pus and blood per rectum, followed by a fall of temperature and an amelioration of the febrile symptoms. On the other hand, the pus may approach the surface, when the abscess will be felt as a definite rounded tumour. As localization becomes more complete, toxic absorption diminishes, so that even without evacuation of the pus the febrile symptoms in such cases subside, and the presence of a large abscess, full of the most evil-smelling pus, is not incompatible with a normal temperature and a clean tongue.

The symptoms which indicate a spreading peritonitis are an accelerating pulse-rate and a subnormal temperature, vomiting, "facies Hippocratica," and increasing abdominal distension and rigidity. Hiccup is a symptom of grave import.

Treatment.—Many slight attacks of acute appendicitis subside spontaneously, but, inasmuch as there is no means of distinguishing these cases at the onset, the decision to postpone operation carries with it a grave responsibility. With cases running a mild course, which are not seen or are not diagnosed for several days, and in which operation is strongly opposed by the patient or his friends, non-operative treatment may be adopted, for the details of which reference must be made to the textbooks of Medicine. The main points in the treatment are complete rest in bed until all pain and tenderness have disappeared, a restricted diet, a regular action of the bowels secured by enemata and mild aperients, fomentations to the abdomen, and the avoidance of opium.

Surgical treatment of acute appendicitis.—The best time for operation is during the first twenty-four hours of the attack, and the earlier the better. The advantages are obvious, for not only is the mortality in this stage no greater than that of "interval" appendicectomy, but the patient is saved from the risks of diffuse peritonitis and abscess formation, the attack is cut short, and the abdominal wall is not weakened by the use of drainage tubes.

Cases not seen or not recognized until the third, fourth, or fifth day of illness present greater difficulty. The attack may then be about to subside ; a small localized periappendicular abscess may have opened into the bowel ; or the appendix may be deeply situated amongst adhesions and surrounded by a small localized collection of pus, the disturbance of which might possibly prove to be the starting-point of a diffuse peritonitis. The difficulty of decision may be increased by the previous administration of opium ; this may be completely masking symptoms which, in the absence of this disturbing factor, would indicate immediate operation, such as vomiting, increasing distension and rigidity, and an accelerating pulse-rate.

The operation for acute appendicitis within the first few hours of the onset differs in no essential respect from that of an interval appendicectomy, provided that perforation and gangrene have not taken place. When these gross changes have occurred, as they occasionally do even at so early a stage, the operation must be completed in the manner described under the next heading.

Treatment of acute appendicitis with diffuse peritonitis. —Immediate operation is the only course to be adopted, for the delay of even two or three hours may turn the scale between recovery and death. The operation embraces two essentials, namely, the removal of the appendix and the treatment of the peritoneum. These, together with the after-treatment, are described under Peritonitis (p. 569).

The mere opening and draining of the abdomen in the right iliac fossa without removal of the appendix has been recommended in the belief that in desperate cases the immediate danger is thus best tided over. Statistics show this view to be erroneous. During the years 1894 to 1903, 38 cases were so treated at St. Thomas's Hospital, with a mortality of 97·3 per cent. Contrasted with this result, the operation of removal of the appendix, combined with some attempt to cleanse the peritoneum during the same period, showed a mortality of 81·2 per cent. These cases were almost all subjected to general lavage of the peritoneal cavity, a procedure which is now recognized to have been wrong, and which doubtless contributed towards that exceedingly high mortality. Since the adoption of strictly local treatment of the peritoneum, generally by dry swabbing, the death-rate has fallen in the striking manner indicated in the chart (Fig. 438). The figures given here are not those of selected cases of spreading peritonitis in an early stage, but they embrace all the cases admitted to hospital with diffuse peritonitis, however desperate, which were subjected to operation.

Treatment of appendicitis with local abscess.—An appendix abscess must, like an abscess anywhere else, be opened as soon as a diagnosis has been arrived at. Delay involves greater risks than immediate action, the possible results being rupture of the abscess into the general peritoneal cavity, into the bowel, or into the bladder; the formation of a subphrenic abscess; retroperitoneal cellulitis; and the formation of dense adhesions which may later give rise to intestinal obstruction and other troubles.

The incision is most conveniently p l a c e d over the spot at which the pus is judged to be closest to the surface and should take the form of a muscle-splitting operation. For the m a j o r i t y, either McBurney's "gridiron"

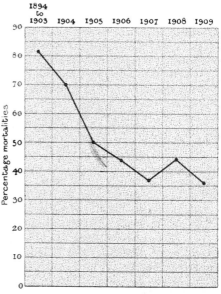

Fig. 438.—Diagram of mortality percentages in operation for removal of the appendix.

opening, or an opening which separates the fibres of the right rectus muscle below the umbilicus, is best; abscesses situated far back in the loin may be reached through a "split-muscle" opening similar to that of McBurney; and occasionally it is advisable to open the abscess by an incision through the posterior vaginal fornix. In a neglected case the abdominal wall may be oedematous, and the skin may even be reddened over a pointing abscess, so that the pus can be reached by little more than a skin incision. In others the parietal peritoneum forms part of the abscess wall, so that the pus can be readily evacuated without opening the general peritoneal cavity. In most cases, however, the peritoneal cavity is opened into as soon as the parietal peritoneum is incised. When this happens the general cavity must be carefully packed off with gauze strips and the abscess gently opened into with the finger. As soon as the pus has ceased to flow, one or more large rubber tubes are inserted into the abscess cavity, and the wound is sutured around them. The gauze strips which were used to shut off the peritoneal cavity may with advantage be left *in situ* for two or three days.

The question of immediate removal of the appendix is one that has received considerable attention, and upon which different surgeons hold different views.

According to the St. Thomas's Hospital statistics, the mortality is practically the same whether the appendix is removed at once or not.

Clearly, when the appendix is readily felt in the abscess cavity, and can easily be removed without much disturbance, the operation should be completed in one stage, because the illness is thereby shortened, and the patient is saved the necessity of a subsequent operation. But if the appendix is not found at once, it is probable that the patient's interests are best served by making no deliberate search for it, but leaving its removal to be effected at a second operation some weeks later. The mortality of cases of appendix abscess is about 15 per cent.

That the appendix ought to be removed subsequently is now almost universally admitted. There is no evidence to support the old belief that an attack of appendicitis which ends in suppuration is curative, and that no further trouble is likely to occur. All the available evidence points in the opposite direction. Recurrent attacks of acute appendicitis and recurrent abscesses are common, and even acute attacks, with diffuse and fatal peritonitis, are occasionally encountered. The St. Thomas's Hospital series contains detailed descriptions of 49 appendices removed at periods varying from two to twelve months after recovery from an abscess. In no single instance was the appendix obliterated; 44·9 per cent. showed well-marked constrictions, 27·5 per cent. the healed scars of previous perforation, 16·3 per cent. contained one or more concretions, 10·2 per cent. were cystic and contained pus, 14·2 per cent. were large and greatly thickened, 20·4 per cent. were free from adhesions, 6·1 per cent. were " catarrhal " or " practically normal," and 4·1 per cent. contained unhealed ulcers. The conclusion arrived at from a critical study of the 1,075 cases in this series was, that of the subjects of appendix abscess in whom the appendix is not removed, a minimum of 10 per cent. will suffer from further serious trouble.

B. CHRONIC AND RELAPSING APPENDICITIS

The term " relapsing appendicitis " is used to describe those cases in which there are recurring attacks of an acute or chronic character. Each individual attack comes into its own particular category, and is more often of a subacute or chronic nature.

Chronic appendicitis includes cases in which a pathological condition of the appendix gives rise to a variety of more or less vague abdominal symptoms. "Appendicular colic" may conveniently be included in this class. By it is meant an attack of abdominal pain, more or less severe, with or without vomiting, unaccompanied by fever, lasting but a few minutes or hours, and having a great tendency to recur at intervals. Such attacks are ascribed to temporary kinking and distension of the appendix, to obstruction of its lumen by stricture, or to attempts to extrude a concretion. Exactly how such attacks are caused, how far they are related to definite structural changes in the appendix, and what is their relation to appendicitis, are matters of speculation. Naturally, a diagnosis of appendicular colic would be made only with the greatest caution, and after the most careful exclusion of other causes of similar abdominal pain, such as renal colic.

A large number of different symptoms are ascribed to chronic disease of the appendix. Among these may be mentioned—

1. More or less persistent abdominal discomfort, increased by exertion or constipation, and not necessarily referred to the right iliac region.

2. Attacks of "appendicular colic."

3. Chronic constipation and anæmia.

4. Chronic diarrhœa and some forms of colitis.

5. Chronic "dyspepsia," and even hæmatemesis, melæna, and "hunger pain."

The **diagnosis** of chronic appendicitis ought never to be made hastily and without due consideration of the many other conditions which may give rise to similar symptoms. Affections of the ovary and Fallopian tube must be eliminated by careful bimanual pelvic examination; renal and ureteral calculus by the X-rays and the examination of the urine, but remembering that concretions in the appendix have sometimes been demonstrated by the X-rays. Nephroptosis often causes considerable difficulty, and the coexistence of a movable kidney and a diseased appendix may necessitate diagnosis by exploratory laparotomy, followed by both appendicectomy and nephropexy. Chronic disease of the appendix may give rise to many of the symptoms of gall-stones, cholecystitis, and duodenal ulcer, so that in difficult cases the diagnosis has to be made by exploratory operation.

When a palpable tumour is present in the region of the appendix, and more or less vague abdominal symptoms are complained of, the probability of the case being one of chronic appendicitis is great, yet several other conditions can give rise to identical symptoms and signs. Amongst these the chief are tuberculosis, actinomycosis, and carcinoma of the cæcum, chronic cæcal intussusception, tuberculous peritonitis, tuberculous mesenteric glands, and sarcoma of the ventral aspect of the ilium. The differential diagnosis of these conditions is not always possible without an abdominal exploration.

Appendicectomy.—The removal of the appendix in the quiet period is an operation which is practically devoid of danger to life, and, if properly performed, is without risk of subsequent weakness of the abdominal wall. No special preparation is needed beyond the customary emptying of the bowels by enema on the morning of the operation, and the shaving and thorough cleansing of the skin at and around the site of the operation.

The method of entering the abdominal cavity is a matter of great importance. Formerly the incision was made either directly through the muscles, or through the semilunar line ; both these methods have rightly been abandoned by nearly all surgeons at the present day, as almost inevitably being followed by a postoperative ventral hernia.

The method of splitting the right rectus muscle in the direction of its fibres has been referred to in dealing with acute appendicitis ; there it possesses certain advantages which do not necessarily hold good in the case of an interval operation for appendicectomy.

There are two chief methods, namely, the "*gridiron*" *incision* of McBurney, and the *temporary displacement of the rectus muscle* devised by W. H. Battle. In the former the skin incision crosses the spino-umbilical line at a point $1\frac{1}{2}$ in. from the antero-superior iliac spine, and is made to divide the aponeurosis of the external oblique in the same direction and for the same distance. Retractors are employed to spread the skin and aponeurosis apart as widely as possible, and the fascia covering the internal oblique is divided at right angles to the first incision. The knife is then laid aside, and by blunt dissection the internal oblique and transversalis abdominis muscles are split in the direction of their fibres, which at this point is as nearly as possible identical. The transversalis fascia is thus exposed, and, together with the peritoneum, is divided in a direction parallel with the skin incision. Battle's incision crosses the spino-umbilical line at right angles near its middle, and exposes the anterior layer of the rectus sheath, which is then divided a little internally to the skin incision and in the same direction. The outer border of the rectus muscle is now freed and drawn inwards with a retractor. The posterior layer of the rectus sheath, together with the underlying peritoneum, is next divided either vertically or transversely, care being taken to avoid division of the motor nerves to the rectus, which are readily identified as soon as the muscle has been drawn aside.

Both these incisions are useful, and are followed by no weakness of the abdominal wall, but Battle's has this advantage over McBurney's, namely, that it can be extended upwards and downwards if the exigencies of any particular case require a larger abdominal opening, whereas the additional room which can be obtained in McBurney's incision by firm retraction is very small. Since it is never possible to be sure beforehand whether the identification and separation of the appendix will be easy or difficult, Battle's incision is the more generally useful.

Whichever abdominal incision is adopted, the first care of the surgeon on opening the peritoneum is to ascertain the position of the appendix. As a rule, the cæcum first comes into view, and then it is an easy matter to find the appendix by following downwards the anterior muscle-band of the cæcum. Any adhesions which may be present are next carefully separated, and the appendix is brought out of the wound and isolated from the peritoneal cavity with strips of gauze. The mesoappendix having been ligatured and divided, the little process is ready for amputation. Innumerable details of technique have been devised, most of which are perfectly satisfactory. Probably the two methods most frequently adopted in this country are Barker's " cuff " method and Kocher's " clamp " method. In the former the peritoneum is divided about a quarter of an inch from the base of the appendix, and turned back towards the cæcum. The rest of the appendix is ligatured and cut away, the stump being touched with a drop of pure carbolic acid. The little cuff of peritoneum is then used to cover in the stump. In the latter method a strong crushing clamp is applied to the base of the appendix close to the cæcum. This instrument divides the inner coats, which retract in either direction, leaving a flat band of crushed peritoneum which can be divided without opening the lumen of the appendix at all. This band is ligatured and divided, and the tiny stump is invaginated into the cæcal wall with a single purse-string suture. When the appendix is inflamed and swollen, the clamp method is unsatisfactory, as the instrument is often found to shear the appendix across.

RARE DISEASES OF THE APPENDIX

Diseases of the appendix other than those due to pyogenetic bacteria are rare, and still more rarely do they cause symptoms independently of secondary infection. It is usually a superadded acute inflammation which directs attention to the appendix, and, as a rule, the tumour or other rare condition is discovered accidentally when the appendix is removed.

TUMOURS

Although very rare, primary appendicular tumours are probably sometimes overlooked, owing to their small size and freedom from recognizable symptoms or to involvement in the necrosis of the appendix.

Innocent tumours are mere pathological curiosities. Up to 1906 Rolleston and Lawrence Jones found 42 undoubted records of primary malignant growth starting in the appendix, of which 37 were carcinoma, 3 endothelioma, and 2 sarcoma. The size varied from that of a pea to that of a marble, and in nearly half the cases the growth was situated in the distal third of the appendix. Metastatic growths are recorded as having been present in only 12 per cent. The average age of the patients was—for the carcinomas 30·6 years, for the endotheliomas 30·3 years, and for the sarcomas 39 years, the average being thus lower than that for carcinoma in other parts of the intestinal tract by 17 years.

The commonest type is represented by a small, white, firm growth consisting of polyhedral or spheroidal cells showing an alveolar arrangement, and often exhibiting vacuolation. The commoner type of carcinoma of the appendix differs, therefore, from the common type of carcinoma of the alimentary canal elsewhere in being spheroidal-celled instead of columnar-celled. These spheroidal-celled growths are also comparatively benign in their clinical character. In no case was a diagnosis made before operation, and the reasons which led to the operation were either symptoms of acute, chronic, or recurrent appendicitis, symptoms referable to the female pelvic organs, or persistent fistula following abscess in the right iliac fossa.

Secondary involvement of the appendix in malignant growths of the cæcum and other parts is less uncommon. In a series of 3,770 autopsies mentioned by Kelly, there was not a single example of primary tumour of the appendix, but there were 11 cases in which the organ was secondarily involved in malignant growth—10 times by carcinoma, and once by sarcoma.

TUBERCULOSIS

While the appendix is not infrequently involved secondarily in tuberculous disease arising in the ileo-cæcal region, or from a tuberculous ovary or Fallopian tube, it is rarely the primary seat of the disease; even then it gives rise to no symptoms by which it can be recognized clinically.

In 2,000 autopsies upon patients who had died of tuberculosis, Fenwick and Dodwell found 17 cases in which the intestinal ulceration was limited to the appendix.

ACTINOMYCOSIS

Abdominal actinomycosis is most often found in the cæcal region, and in several reported cases there is no doubt that the appendix was the seat of the primary disease. The streptothrix has been demonstrated in the appendix, and more than once in company with a grain of corn. The pathology of the disease differs in no essential respect from that of actinomycosis elsewhere. (For Ileo-Cæcal Actinomycosis *see* Vol. I., p. 876.)

INTUSSUSCEPTION, HERNIAS, INTESTINAL OBSTRUCTION

The appendix is almost necessarily involved in **intussusceptions** of the cæcal, ileo-cæcal, and ileo-colic varieties, and is prone to have its vascularity gravely. interfered with thereby. On reducing such an intussusception, it is sometimes advisable to amputate the appendix, even though the little extra time required may add to the patient's danger.

Primary intussusception or inversion of the appendix itself is rare, but Battle and Corner have succeeded in collecting 17 cases from the literature. It is suggested that in the attempt to extrude a concretion the mucous membrane becomes prolapsed into the cæcum, and that this is followed by inversion of the cæcum and then of the ascending colon, so that a complicated form of intussusception is produced.

Involvement in **hernias** has been already alluded to (p. 540). According to Kelly, the appendix is present in from 1 to 2 per cent. of all hernias. A large proportion of the cases occurs in infants, when the appendix can sometimes be felt in the hernia as a rounded cord. It is commonly adherent, at any rate in the cases which are operated upon, and in congenital inguinal hernia has been found adherent to the testis. In hernial sacs the appendix has been found strangulated, inflamed, and perforated; and in this connexion an interesting point has been noted by Battle and Corner, namely, that when strangulated in a hernia the appendix is more often found alone than in company with other viscera.

Intestinal obstruction is sometimes produced by the incarceration of a coil of intestine beneath a band formed by the adherent appendix.

BIBLIOGRAPHY

Battle and **Corner,** *Surgery of the Diseases of the Appendix.* London, 1904.
Cushing, Harvey, *Johns Hopkins Hosp. Repts.*, 1904, vol. viii.
Dudgeon and **Sargent,** *Bacteriology of Peritonitis.* London, 1905.
Fenwick and **Dodwell,** *Lancet,* 1894.
Hawkins, H. P., *Diseases of the Vermiform Appendix.* London, 1895.
Macewen, Sir W., *Lancet,* Oct. 8. 1904.
Poirier and **Cunéo,** *The Lymphatics.* London, 1903.
Robinson, Byrom, quoted by Battle and Corner.
Rolleston and **Lawrence Jones,** *Med.-Chir. Trans., London,* lxxxix. 125.
Sargent, Percy, *Lancet,* Sept., 1905.
Still, G. F., *Brit. Med. Journ.,* April 15, 1899.
Tavel and **Lanz,** *Rev. de Chir.,* Paris, 1904.
Veillon and **Zuber,** *Arch. de Méd. Expér.,* July, 1898.
Wallace and **Sargent,** *St. Thomas's Hosp. Repts.,* 1904.

THE PERITONEUM

By PERCY SARGENT, M.A., M.B., B.C.Cantab., F.R.C.S.Eng.

Anatomy and physiology.—The peritoneum is a thin, smooth, elastic membrane consisting of a layer of flattened endothelial cells resting upon a layer of subendothelial connective tissue. This membrane lines the walls of the abdominal cavity (parietal layer), and covers with a varying degree of completeness the abdominal and pelvic viscera (visceral layer). Its superficial area is stated to equal that of the skin. Outside the peritoneal membrane proper is the subperitoneal connective tissue, which, in certain situations, is heavily loaded with fat.

The so-called peritoneal cavity is only a potential space. for its smooth opposing surfaces are everywhere in contact, being separated in health only by a minimal amount of lubricating fluid. It is only by artificial or accidental separation of these opposing surfaces that a cavity is produced.

In the male the peritoneum forms a completely closed sac ; in the female the interior of the Fallopian tube communicates directly with the interior of the potential peritoneal cavity through a minute orifice—the ostium abdominale.

Peritoneal compartments and pouches.—Anatomists divide the peritoneal sac into two main compartments, the greater and the lesser, communicating with one another by a narrow passage, the walls of which are normally in contact with one another. This is the foramen of Winslow, which is situated at the right side of the first lumbar vertebra close to the neck of the gall-bladder. The greater sac is further subdivided, from clinical considerations, into certain areas into which fluids tend to gravitate ; these very readily become shut off into more or less definite compartments by the agglutination of neighbouring areas of peritoneum.

With the body supine, the lumbar spine presents a well-marked forward projection with a deep fossa on either side. A similar projection is afforded by the pelvic brim and the superjacent psoas muscles. To these projections, which play so important a part in directing the course of fluid effusions, C. R. Box has given the name of *abdominal watersheds* (Figs. 439 and 440).

There are thus three large wells into which fluids tend to gravitate, namely, the pelvic cavity and the right and left lumbar regions. But the course which effused fluid takes is further influenced by the arrangement of certain peritoneal folds and of the fixed portions of

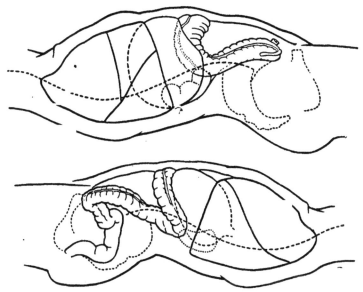

Figs. 439 and 440.—Diagrams to show the "peritoneal watersheds."
(*C. R. Box.*) (*See* text.)

the intestine. "Thus the transverse mesocolon and great omentum, passing across the belly cavity, mark off an upper from a lower territory, which communicate with one another only in the lumbar regions. This partition is more complete on the left than the right side, especially when the phrenicocolic fold of peritoneum, which passes from the left end of the transverse colon to the diaphragm below the spleen, is well marked. A similar fold is sometimes present on the right side." (C. R. Box.)

Above this transverse mesocolic shelf, and on the right slope of the vertebral watershed, lie the pylorus, the commencement of the duodenum, the gall-bladder, and the right lobe of the liver; in a similar position on the left side lie the stomach and spleen. Effusions resulting from the perforation or inflammation of these structures will consequently be directed, in the one case towards the right kidney, and in the other towards the spleen.

Near the summit of the pelvic ridge on the right side the appendix often lies, so that a purulent effusion resulting from a diseased appendix, if it does not gravitate towards the pelvic cavity, is directed upwards alongside the colon towards the right renal or subhepatic pouch. From the arrangement both of the watersheds and of the peritoneal folds, together with the anatomical disposition of the viscera which are most frequently the source of intraperitoneal effusion, namely the appendix, pylorus, duodenum, and bile passages, it will be seen that the right renal pouch is a region of great clinical importance. The boundaries of this pouch are: " above and in front, the right lobe of the liver and its ligaments; below, the hepatic flexure of the colon and its attachment to the posterior abdominal wall; internally, the peritoneum covering the descending duodenum and the lumbar spine, and stretching forwards to the foramen of Winslow; externally, the parietal peritoneum of the lumbar region."

The subphrenic region is also of special importance. A subphrenic abscess on the left side lies between the spleen, stomach, and left lobe of the liver on the one hand, and the diaphragm on the other, being separated by the diaphragm, from the lower border of the lung, the pleural cavity, and the chest wall; below, it is limited by the phrenico-colic fold, and to the right by the falciform ligament. Similarly, a right-sided subphrenic abscess, lying between the right dome of the diaphragm and the liver, may be limited leftwards by the falciform ligament.

There are, in addition, certain smaller pouches which may become the seat of internal hernias, the chief of which are the paraduodenal, superior duodenal, and inferior duodenal fossæ at the left side of the 2nd lumbar vertebræ; the retrocolic, ileo-cæcal, and ileo-colic fossæ in the right iliac fossa; and the fossa intersigmoidea close to the left sacro-iliac joint, marking the position at which the ureter crosses the external iliac artery. None of these fossæ is of constant occurrence.

Lymphatics.—There is no direct communication between the peritoneal cavity and the lymphatic system, though fluids and solid particles are readily removed from the peritoneal cavity into the lymphatics. There are no " stomata " between the endothelial cells, nor, over the greater part of the peritoneal membrane, are there any subendothelial lymphatic spaces. The diaphragmatic peritoneum, however, presents a vast number of pits or wells, penetrating between the tendon bundles, which are microscopic diverticula of the peritoneum, and, like it, are lined in their whole extent by endothelial cells.

The peritoneal cavity is very intimately related with the subpleural diaphragmatic lymphatics, which present, according to MacCalium, a network of branching lymphatic trunks, whose efferent vessels pass to the mediastinal and abdominal lymphatic glands. From these lymphatic vessels diverticula or pouches pass downwards through the muscular and tendinous tissue of the diaphragm, where they come into the most intimate relation with the peritoneum, being only separated from it by a delicate basement membrane.

Nerves.—Ramström has shown by dissection the ramifications of the lower intercostal nerves in the serous covering of the abdominal wall. Whilst the parietal peritoneum is said to be sensitive, the visceral portion is devoid of sensation both in health and in disease (Cushing and Lennander). The nerves are derived from the same source whence arises the cutaneous and muscular supply of the abdominal wall, namely, the last seven thoracic trunks; this fact accounts for the reflex muscular rigidity and the superficial tenderness in peritonitis.

Functions of the peritoneum.—In health the peritoneum serves to permit the intestinal and other intra-abdominal movements to take place painlessly and with a minimal amount of friction. Its various folds attach the viscera to one another and to the parietes, and also serve to carry the blood-vessels and other structures from the abdominal wall to the viscera.

The great omentum has special functions. In addition to that of protection, fat storage, and the part which, in injury and disease, if is able to play in sealing an accidental opening in the bowel or in the abdominal wall, it takes a special share in the disposal of bacteria and other solid substances which may find their way into the peritoneal cavity (H. E. Durham; Dudgeon and Ross).

The absorptive powers of the peritoneum are very great, and both fluids and solid particles such as bacteria are removed from the peritoneal cavity with great readiness and rapidity. The fluids are mainly taken up by the lymphatics, but may also, when under pressure, pass directly into the blood-vessels; the solid particles are removed by the lymphatics alone, provided that the membrane is intact. This lymphatic absorption occurs only over the diaphragm and omentum, and the removal of solid particles takes place chiefly by phagocytosis, the particles being carried first into the pits described above, and thence into the subperitoneal lymphatic vessels and spaces (Muscatello).

The experiments of Buxton and Torrey and others have shown that inert particles and bacteria also find their way into the lymphatics without the aid of phagocytosis; and Muscatello thinks that the passage of the phagocytes leaves minute apertures through which particles can afterwards be drawn by the suction action of the diaphragm and its lymphatic currents.

Absorption from the peritoneal cavity is normally aided by the pressure of the continual respiratory movements of the abdominal

2 k

walls, the suction action of the diaphragm, and the peristaltic movements of the intestines. In disease other factors come into play, some hindering and others assisting absorption.

Amongst the chief additional factors which assist absorption are— (1) phagocytosis, (2) increased intra-abdominal pressure, (3) endothelial exfoliation.

Those which diminish absorption are—(1) diminution of respiratory movements, (2) diminution of peristalsis, (3) fibrinous deposition upon the peritoneal surface, (4) agglutination of intestinal coils and omentum, (5) lowering of intra-abdominal pressure by laparotomy, (6) toxæmic fall in blood pressure.

Defences of the peritoneum against bacterial infection.— The introduction of foreign matter, whether sterile or not, is the signal for the appearance in the peritoneal cavity of an effusion of fluid rich in leucocytes, their number varying with the nature of the foreign matter. Any lesion of a peritoneum-covered organ, such as the strangulation of a coil of intestine, inflammation of the appendix, or the twisting of the pedicle of an ovarian cyst, is rapidly followed by the appearance in the fluid of a white staphylococcus of extremely low pathogenetic properties (Dudgeon and Sargent) ; with its appearance the exudate becomes rich in leucocytes, and it is upon the phagocytic action of these white cells, assisted by the body fluids, that the removal of the pathogenetic organisms chiefly depends. If this defensive reaction has time to become well marked before any large quantity of infective material has gained access to the peritoneal cavity, the peritonitis which has started at the point of entrance of the infection may be stopped from becoming diffused over a fatally large area, either by complete absorption or by loculation of the effusion. This shutting-off process is brought about by the gluing together of adjacent peritoneal areas with a plastic exudate, and is assisted by the diminution of respiratory and peristaltic movements. The fibrinous deposit upon the peritoneal surface also serves to limit the absorption of toxins into the subendothelial blood-vessels, and to entangle and hold harmless a certain amount of the foreign matter until such time as it can be gradually and safely removed by phagocytosis. (Plate 98.)

INJURIES OF THE PERITONEUM

1. WOUNDS AND CONTUSIONS

The peritoneum is rarely injured, either in open wounds or contusions, sufficiently to cause clinical symptoms apart from comitant damage to the abdominal viscera. The visceral injury at overshadows that of the peritoneum ; later the resulting peritonitis becomes the predominant feature. Contusions of, and hæmorrhage

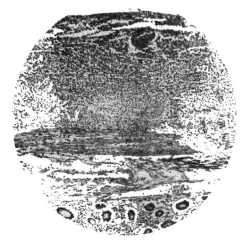

Fig. 1.—Section of intestine from a case of peritonitis of sixteen hours' duration. showing inflammatory deposit which becomes less as the mucous coat is approached. (" B " eyepiece ; ⅔ obj.)

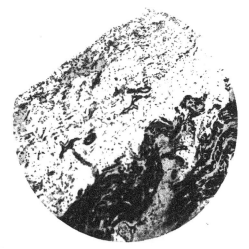

Fig. 2.—Section of diaphragm, showing organization of fibrinous deposit in a case of chronic septic peritonitis. (" B " eyepiece ; ⅔ obj.)

PLATE 98.

into, the mesentery may, in the absence of other intra-abdominal injury, cause serious symptoms, and even lead to an abdominal exploration. Laceration of the mesentery or omentum alone is responsible for a certain number of cases of intraperitoneal hæmorrhage.

Clean wounds of the peritoneum heal with great readiness; infected wounds also heal readily if the virulence and number of the bacteria introduced are not beyond the very considerable defensive powers of the peritoneum. It is, indeed, this property of rapid healing which permits of anastomotic operations being safely performed upon the stomach and intestines. The omentum plays an important part in abdominal injuries. It may become rolled around and isolate infective material, and may even prevent leakage from a perforated organ by becoming adherent to and sealing the opening. It also possesses the special property of dealing with bacteria by phagocytosis upon its surface, of which mention has already been made.

2. INTRAPERITONEAL HÆMORRHAGE

Traumatic intraperitoneal hæmorrhage may take place from torn or incised mesenteric or omental vessels without any visceral injury. The results which follow such hæmorrhage vary with the quantity of blood effused, and may be summarized as follows : (a) Death from loss of blood alone; (b) diffuse peritonitis; (c) formation of a localized hæmatocele, which may suppurate later and so produce one of the varieties of localized intraperitoneal abscess; (d) partial absorption, with the formation of persistent adhesions; (e) complete absorption.

Peritonitis, either diffuse or localized, results from the effusion of blood into the peritoneal cavity, quite apart from infection at the time of the injury. Any effusion of blood into the peritoneal cavity which is sufficient in amount to be capable of diagnosis ought to be operated upon. The abdomen must be opened, the bleeding-point secured, the blood and clot washed away with sterile normal saline solution, and the abdomen closed without drainage.

3. RETROPERITONEAL HÆMORRHAGE

In abdominal contusions, especially when associated with fracture of the pelvis, blood sometimes escapes into the retroperitoneal cellular tissues in such quantity as to cause severe symptoms of hæmorrhage. The case is then usually looked upon as one of intraperitoneal hæmorrhage, nor are there any definite signs by which the two conditions may be distinguished with certainty, even when a more or less localized swelling can be felt. The diagnosis has therefore to be made by exploratory laparotomy. When a diffuse retroperitoneal hæmorrhage is found the wound should be closed without drainage, for the blood will be absorbed spontaneously. Even a large perinephric swelling may be so absorbed, though incision may be required for secondary suppuration of the hæmatoma.

DISEASES OF THE PERITONEUM

I. INFLAMMATORY

A. ACUTE DIFFUSE PERITONITIS

Definition.—A spreading inflammation of the peritoneum which is unlimited by adhesions. To this form the term "general peritonitis" is sometimes applied, but it is best abandoned as incorrectly implying that the whole peritoneal surface is involved.

The cause of such peritoneal inflammation is in all cases bacterial infection. A spreading inflammation can be caused by injection into the peritoneal cavity of sterile irritating fluids, and to these experimental forms the terms "aseptic" and "chemical" peritonitis were formerly applied. In the same way it was long thought that peritonitis resulting from hæmorrhage into the unopened peritoneal cavity could cause a "chemical" peritonitis, and the same expression was also formerly applied to the peritonitis which occurs in the early stages of intestinal obstruction. Bacteriological examination of the peritoneal surface, especially that covering the great omentum, as well as of the exudate, has thrown grave doubt upon the existence of a non-bacterial peritonitis.

According to Dudgeon and Sargent, the *Staphylococcus albus* appears to have a distinct and definite part to play in peritonitis. It makes its appearance early in inflammatory affections of the peritoneum, from whatever cause they may arise, and can be isolated from the exudate and from the surface of the bowel or omentum. It is found in the sacs of strangulated hernias and in the clot from an intraperitoneal hæmorrhage, as well as in the early stages of inflammation or strangulation of the abdominal viscera. It is probably protective in function, determining the appearance of a fluid exudate rich in phagocytes, which do not degenerate in its presence, and having also to do with the formation of adhesions.

Just as the resistance of the peritoneum to infection can be artificially raised by the preliminary injection of various sterile fluids, notably nucleic acid (von Mikulicz), so the injection of a culture of this white staphylococcus into the peritoneal cavity of an animal is able to protect it against an otherwise fatal dose of the colon bacillus (Dudgeon and Sargent).

Many different organisms are found to cause peritonitis in man, the most important by far being the colon bacillus. These organisms vary greatly in pathogenicity as regards the peritoneum. The most virulent is the *Streptococcus pyogenes*, and next to that the *Bacillus pyocyaneus*. The colon bacillus is sometimes extremely virulent, the differences in behaviour being due to the particular strain present, and to the patient's powers of resistance. The course of a case of peritonitis depends upon many factors, the chief of which are the nature and virulence of the infecting organism, the dosage, the suddenness with which the peritoneum is invaded, and the power of resistance of the individual patient.

Infection may reach the peritoneum by many different channels :—

    (a) From the exterior of the body, either through an accidental or an operation wound or along the Fallopian tube.

    (b) From some part of the alimentary canal.

    (c) From disease of an adjacent organ other than the alimentary canal, such as the gall-bladder or the pancreas.

    (d) From an adjacent pathological structure such as a retroperitoneal abscess or an inflamed ovarian cyst.

    (e) From the blood-stream (hæmic infection).

The following are the most common forms of acute diffuse peritonitis :—

1. COLON BACILLUS PERITONITIS

The great majority of these cases originate from disease of the vermiform appendix. Perforation of that organ is a frequent though not a necessary starting-point, for the colon bacillus can infect the peritoneum through an acutely inflamed or gangrenous though unperforated appendix ; it may spread from an imperfectly localized collection of pus around a diseased appendix ; or it may result from the rupture of an appendix abscess. Other causes of colon bacillus peritonitis are—penetrating wounds, contusions or lacerations of the intestine ; intestinal obstruction of any kind ; perforation of any form of ulcer, simple or malignant, of the intestine ; acute inflammation, gangrene, or perforation of the gall-bladder ; acute pancreatitis ; suppuration and rupture of an ovarian cyst ; and inflammation, gangrene, or perforation of a Meckel's diverticulum.

The exudate in these cases is usually large in amount ; that in the immediate neighbourhood of the causative lesion is turbid, and may be, but is not necessarily, of an offensive odour, whilst in more remote parts of the peritoneal cavity it is less turbid and odourless. Coverslip preparations from this odourless exudate usually show innumerable leucocytes and cocci ; in the exudate nearer the focus of infection are seen cocci, bacilli, and phagocytes, many of which are degenerated. As the peritonitis spreads, bacilli are found in the exudate farther and farther from the focus of infection ; the intestinal coils become progressively more reddened, distended, and agglutinated; and flakes of fibrin are found both floating in the exudate and adherent to the inflamed peritoneum.

2. ACUTE STREPTOCOCCAL PERITONITIS

The *Streptococcus pyogenes* may reach the peritoneum by direct infection through accidental or even operation wounds, in puerperal sepsis, and by the blood-stream in septicæmia. Possibly also it may in some cases come from disease of the alimentary canal or from an infected ovarian cyst. It also occurs as a terminal event in some cases of cutaneous erysipelas. It is the most rapidly fatal variety of peritonitis, in part perhaps because it takes the form, when originating from the uterus, of a rapidly spreading subserous cellulitis (Murphy) : in part certainly because the intraperitoneal phagocytosis appears powerless against this form of infection.

There are no distinctive appearances by which streptococcal peritonitis can be recognized at operation. As a rule, the exudate is large in amount, odourless, and only slightly turbid ; intestinal distension is not great, and agglutination of coils is absent; fibrinous flakes are scanty or absent. Cover-slip preparations show chains of cocci, together with large numbers of polynuclear cells, apparently in a healthy state, but non-phagocytic as regards the streptococci. There is little doubt that the terminal event in most of these cases is a streptococcal septicæmia.

3. ACUTE PNEUMOCOCCAL PERITONITIS

Whilst this form of peritonitis is more commonly secondary to some pre-existing pneumococcal lesion elsewhere, it does occur as a primary affection. When *primary*, the pneumococcus may reach the peritoneum through the blood, and possibly more directly from the bowel ; it has been known to extend from a pyometra along the Fallopian tube (Dudgeon and Sargent). When *secondary*, the infection may come from a neighbouring pneumococcal affection, such as pleuritis ; or the peritonitis may be septicæmic in origin, the peritoneum being then infected through the blood-stream from some focus at a distance, such as an otitis media. The pneumococcus is said to have been found in the exudate in a certain number of cases of gastric perforation. The exudate in pneumococcal peritonitis is usually large in amount and greenish in colour, contains a quantity of fibrinous flakes, and is quite odourless. There are, however, no definite clinical signs by which it can be recognized, the only certain method being the bacteriological examination of the exudate. It may be suspected at operation if the exudate shows the above-mentioned characteristics, whilst no definite lesion can be found to account for the peritonitis, especially when the patient is a child.

4. ACUTE GONOCOCCAL PERITONITIS

Acute diffused gonococcal peritonitis is occasionally met with The organism reaches the peritoneum either through the open mouth of a Fallopian tube, or by leakage from or rupture of a pyosalpinx. It does not readily affect the peritoneum, and when it does so is apt to produce a form of peritonitis which, although sometimes of sudden or acute onset, usually runs a mild and favourable course, and is unaccompanied by intestinal distension. The exudate is scanty, usually clear or only very slightly turbid, and distinctly viscid. Cover-slip preparations occasionally show intracellular diplococci.

5. OTHER FORMS OF ACUTE PERITONITIS

The organisms more rarely found in acute diffuse peritonitis are *B. pyocyaneus*, *Staphylococcus pyogenes aureus* and other forms of pyogenetic staphylococci, and *B. typhosus*. The last-named may reach the peritoneum from a suppurating mesenteric gland (Körte), and perhaps from the intestine without perforation. The peritonitis resulting from perforation of a typhoid ulcer is a mixed infection, the colon bacillus predominating.

Veillon and Zuber have described certain anaerobic organisms as occurring in peritonitis, as also have Tavel and Lanz. Dudgeon and Sargent only once found an anaerobic organism, namely, the *B. aerogenes capsulatus*, and consider that anaerobes do not play an important part in peritonitis.

Symptoms of acute diffuse peritonitis.—The clinical history and symptoms of the disease or injury which has allowed the infection to reach the peritoneum are dealt with elsewhere. In the later stages the peritoneal symptoms so overshadow those of the original lesion that in the majority of cases its nature can only be ascertained by the operation which the peritonitis makes imperative.

The onset is often sudden, or at least rapid, and is accompanied by *abdominal pain*. At first diffuse, the pain may, after a short time, become sufficiently localized to be of diagnostic value ; later, again, it becomes generalized over the whole abdomen.

Vomiting is a symptom which is rarely absent. It is persistent, and accompanied by nausea and straining, differing in these respects from the vomiting of intestinal obstruction. The vomitus is commonly green in colour, and does not become fæculent. The occurrence of " black vomit " is one of the most serious symptoms in a bad case of peritonitis. *Constipation* is present from the outset, and becomes more marked with the progressive paralysis of the intestine. The tongue, at first furred and moist, soon becomes dry and brown.

The *temperature* affords little information. At the onset it may be subnormal from the shock of a perforation or strangulation ; on the other hand, it is often raised at first, and sometimes the onset is marked by a rigor. As the peritonitis spreads, the temperature falls to and below the normal.

The *pulse-rate* is of much greater importance. Rapid at the onset, it may become slowed as the initial shock passes off, only to. rise again steadily and progressively with the spread of the peritonitis. At the same time it becomes feeble and "thready." One of the most reliable indications of a spreading peritonitis is the coexistence of a rising pulse-rate and a falling temperature.

The *facies* is important. The patient quickly assumes a characteristic appearance, the face being pale, drawn, and anxious-looking, whilst dark rings appear round the sunken eyes. The *mental condition* is clear, and in fatal cases the patient is only too conscious of his condition until the end.

Examination of the abdomen by inspection, palpation, and percussion should be thoroughly and systematically carried out. The abdomen is *rigid* and often extremely *tender*, and the abdominal *respiratory movements are diminished.* In the early stages this rigidity and the diminution of respiratory movements may be so localized as to afford valuable evidence as to the situation of the starting-point of the peritonitis. Later, the whole abdomen becomes rigid and motionless. As the disease progresses, the abdomen, which may at first have been flat, or even sunken, becomes progressively *distended* from intestinal paralysis, and the distension may become so great as seriously to interfere with respiration. The presence of free fluid may sometimes be ascertained by the somewhat fallacious sign of *shifting dullness* in the flanks.

In peritonitis from intestinal perforation there may, in addition, be evidence of *free gas* in the peritoneal cavity. This is shown by diminution or absence of the normal area of liver dullness, especially when it occurs in a flat abdomen. Intestinal distension may simulate this sign very closely.

In old persons many of the above-mentioned symptoms may be absent. The abdomen is sometimes observed to be both soft and mobile, even in the presence of an acute spreading peritonitis. Similarly, both rigidity and immobility are often absent in postoperative peritonitis.

Nearly all these symptoms and signs may be modified or abolished by the administration of opium. A patient under its influence may look comparatively well, vomiting may be absent, the pulse may be only slightly accelerated, the abdomen may be soft and moving with respiration, and examination may not be resented.

Diagnosis.—Acute peritonitis has to be diagnosed from intestinal obstruction, the clinical features of which are detailed at p. 465. In addition to establishing the fact that diffuse peritonitis is present, an attempt must be made to ascertain the starting-point of the peritoneal infection.

Treatment.—The presence of acute diffuse peritonitis urgently demands operation, every hour that passes between onset and operation rendering the prognosis increasingly grave. Whilst preparations are being made for the operation the patient should not be allowed to lie flat upon the back, but should be propped up in bed almost in a sitting posture (Fowler's position, Fig. 466, p. 639); if he has to be transferred to hospital a similar posture should be adopted on the journey. Opium should not be given, not only on account of its tendency to diminish intestinal movements and add to the paralytic distension of the bowel, but also because it inhibits intraperitoneal phagocytosis (Dudgeon and Ross).

The operation consists of two essential parts, namely, the removal of the focus of infection, and the treatment of the peritoneum.

1. **Removal of the focus of infection.**—If before operation a decision has been arrived at as to the source of the infection, the abdomen should be opened as nearly as possible over that point. When the source of infection is uncertain, the most generally useful incision is that which separates the fibres of the right rectus muscle just below the umbilicus, as this allows the appendix region to be explored at once, and also gives easy access to the pelvic organs. The methods of dealing with any particular lesion that may be found are discussed elsewhere under various headings, such as Removal of the Appendix (P. 554), Suture of a Ruptured Gastric Ulcer (p. 357), Removal of Suppurating Tubes (p. 1054), and so on.

2. **Method of dealing with the peritoneum.**—The error of attempting to cleanse the peritoneum by heroic methods of lavage has been amply demonstrated both by clinical results and on pathological grounds. No amount of washing will rid the peritoneum of infective material, while the disturbance occasioned by such manipulations tends to spread infection beyond the area already involved, destroys the phagocytes which alone can effectively deal with the micro-organisms, injures the delicate peritoneal endothelium, so rendering hæmic absorption more easy, and increases the shock of the operation. Once the focus of infection has been removed, the less that is done to the peritoneum the better, and all manipulations ought to be of the gentlest possible character. Any collection of pus which may lie in the immediate neighbourhood of the starting-point of the infection, and any pools of fluid that may have collected in the pelvis or lumbar regions, may be gently mopped up with dry sterilized gauze. On no account should flakes of " lymph " be peeled off the bowel.

This done,.a drainage tube of large calibre may be inserted down to the site of the lesion, either through the original wound or through some new opening—in the loin, for example—which may be considered more suitable for drainage. Gauze strips are sometimes used for this purpose, but they do not act well as drains, and their removal is attended by considerable pain. The "cigarette" drain, which consists of a piece of "green protective" or rubber tissue wrapped round a loosely arranged roll of gauze in the form of a cigarette, is sometimes used, but is not so effective as a tube. A good plan is to pass a narrow strip of gauze down the rubber tube ; this can easily be changed, and serves the purpose of preventing the tube from becoming blocked by coagulated blood and pus.

Sometimes lavage of the peritoneal cavity is advisable, as in those cases of ruptured gastric or duodenal ulcer in which the peritoneal cavity is flooded with acrid gastric contents and solid particles of food, and in certain cases of intraperitoneal hæmorrhage when it is desirable to wash away large quantities of blood and clot. In such instances the interference with intraperitoneal phagocytosis is of less moment than the desirability of ridding the peritoneum of foreign matter. Drainage is not always necessary. It is not required in intraperitoneal hæmorrhage, in peritonitis from an inflamed cyst, in gonorrhœal peritonitis, or in the great majority of cases of ruptured gastric ulcer. These are all instances of peritonitis in which the infection is of a mild type. In colon bacillus infections, on the other hand, represented by the vast majority of cases of peritonitis of intestinal origin, it is usually advisable to leave a drain down to the original site of the infection.

After-treatment.—Posture is important. The Fowler position is now widely adopted, the patient being propped up almost in a sitting position, with the object of preventing the gravitation of fluid upwards towards the diaphragm (Fig. 466, p. 639). If this position be used, careful watch should be kept for any collection of pus in the pelvis.

When the patient has been put back into bed, every effort must be directed towards combating shock. The various means of dealing with this condition are explained in Vol. I., p. 330.

It is of the utmost importance to get the bowels opened freely as soon as possible ; a dose of calomel may be followed by repeated doses of magnesium sulphate until a free action is obtained, and enemata containing turpentine are often useful. Subcutaneous injection of pituitary extract ($\mathrm{m}$xv of a 20 per cent. solution) appears to be useful in stimulating peristaltic action. In this connexion it should be remembered that the administration of opium is to be avoided.

The continuous administration of saline solution per rectum by Murphy's method has many advocates, and good results are obtained by its use. A pliable tube of soft metal, provided with many openings, is inserted in the rectum, and connected with a reservoir containing normal saline solution maintained at a temperature of 105° to 110° F. The reservoir is raised from one to two feet above the level of the buttocks, and the fluid allowed to run slowly in. By this means some twelve or more pints of fluid can be absorbed in a day. Care must be taken to keep the quantity within reasonable limits, lest the lungs become waterlogged.

If drainage-tubes have been used, they should not be allowed to remain in place for more than three or four days. By that time they will have done all that can be done by drainage, and longer retention may be followed by a troublesome sinus and an unnecessary weakening of the abdominal wall.

Vomiting may be controlled by small repeated doses of tincture of iodine or of cocaine ; sometimes gastric lavage may be advantageously employed.

The use, in cases of *B. coli* peritonitis, of a multivalent anti-coli serum has yielded promising results, and may be given a trial.

Complications of acute diffuse peritonitis.—Most of the fatal cases terminate by septic intoxication, and many from a general septicæmia. When, with the removal of the focus of infection, and the placing of the peritoneum under the best conditions for dealing with the remaining infection, death from these causes has been averted, the chief complications to be looked for are the following :—

1. **Intestinal obstruction.**—Paralytic distension is very common, and, unless peristaltic action is quickly restored, death from septic absorption will soon occur. But, apart from this paralytic form of obstruction, mechanical obstruction may occur from adhesions and kinking of the bowel. This is shown by inability to get the bowels open in spite of the presence of peristalsis, by increasing distension, and by renewed vomiting which sooner or later becomes fæculent in type. A further operation (enterostomy or enterolysis) may possibly succeed, but the outlook in such cases is extremely grave.

2. **Cellulitis and gangrene** of the abdominal wall around the wound are occasional, but very uncommon, complications.

3. **Residual abscesses.**—After the subsidence of a diffuse peritonitis a localized collection of pus may appear anywhere within the peritoneal cavity. The commonest variety is the subphrenic abscess (*see* p. 572) ; whilst after the use of the Fowler position, without efficient drainage of the pelvis, a pelvic accumulation of pus may occur.

4. **Pneumonia and empyema.**—These complications sometimes occur within the first week or fortnight after the operation for diffuse peritonitis.

B. LOCALIZED INTRAPERITONEAL SUPPURATION

Localized collections of pus within the peritoneal cavity may result from a large number of different causes. The commonest variety is the localized appendix abscess; others are due to disease of the female pelvic organs, to slow leakage from a gastric or duodenal ulcer, to inflammatory processes around a cancerous growth of the intestine, and to disease of the gall-bladder, bile-ducts, or pancreas; others are those already described as "residual" abscesses, which may occur in any part of the peritoneal cavity after the subsidence of a diffuse peritonitis; whilst others, again, are due to the chronic forms of tuberculous or pneumococcal peritonitis, to be described later. Suppurative epiploitis constitutes still another variety of localized abscess.

The situations in which such abscesses tend to form have already been indicated in describing the anatomy of the peritoneal compartments; but it not infrequently happens that adhesions alter the course of a tracking collection of pus, and that perforation of the peritoneum forming the abscess wall may allow the pus to escape into the retroperitoneal tissue, so as to form an abscess in situations uninfluenced by the anatomical disposition of the peritoneum.

In addition to the symptoms of the disease from which the abscess originated, those presented by a localized intraperitoneal abscess are abdominal pain and tenderness, together with toxæmia. The course may be very slow and the diagnosis difficult. In the simpler cases a firm and definite intra-abdominal tumour may be felt; others have to be diagnosed by the general symptoms, added to those of pressure effects upon neighbouring structures such as the base of the lung.

One variety of localized abscess must be considered separately, namely, subphrenic or subdiaphragmatic abscess.

Subphrenic Abscess

Definition.—A collection of pus beneath the diaphragm, lying on the right side between the liver and diaphragm, and on the left between the diaphragm and the stomach and spleen. The term is often used to include abscesses situated in the right kidney well, when the pus is really subhepatic rather than subphrenic.

Causation.—The possible causes of subphrenic abscess are very numerous, for almost any intra-abdominal lesion may give rise to it, whilst occasionally the spread is in the reverse direction, suppuration above the diaphragm giving rise to infection below. The most common causes are perforation of an ulcer of the stomach or duodenum, suppurative conditions of the liver and its ducts, and appendicitis. Renal, pancreatic, and traumatic suppurations are occasional causes,

Pathology.—The bacteriology of subphrenic abscess is as varied as that of peritonitis. Pus spreading from the primary focus may find itself at once in the subphrenic region, or it may reach this region from a distance, traversing intraperitoneally the anatomical routes already considered, or paths determined by adhesions, or spreading in the retroperitoneal tissue of the posterior abdominal wall. Perforation of the diaphragm is said to be more likely to occur in the last-named class of case. In a certain number of cases (about 15 per cent.) the cavity of a subphrenic abscess contains gas, which may be present either as the result of bacterial activity within the abscess, or may have gained admission by direct continuity from the alimentary canal, or even from the air-passages.

Symptoms and diagnosis.—The onset may be very acute and present most of the features of an abdominal "catastrophe"; it may be subacute, with pain in the upper part of the abdomen, fever, and possibly a rigor, and pain in the shoulder is common. Pain and tenderness over the lower ribs, and limitation of the respiratory movements, together with cough, slight expectoration, and irregular fever, following upon a history of gastric ulcer, an operation for suppurative appendicitis, or other recognizable cause of subphrenic suppuration, would make up a clinical picture of such a case. The onset may, on the other hand, be so slow and insidious, and present so few localizing symptoms and physical signs, as to make the diagnosis a matter of the greatest difficulty.

As the symptoms and causes vary within such wide limits, so also do the physical signs. Broadly speaking, the physical signs are those of a limited collection of fluid at the base of the lung. In a well-marked case there may be an area of dullness sharply marked off from the resonance of the lung above, together with loss of breath sounds and diminution or loss of vocal fremitus and resonance. When the abscess contains gas there may be on percussion a characteristic series of changes from the dull area below, through a tympanitic area, up to the normal pulmonary resonance. Alteration of the position of the patient may cause alteration of the position of the resonant area as the gas and pus adjust themselves to the new position.

The lower lobe of the lung may be so compressed as to present a zone of tubular breathing and impaired resonance above the level of absolute dullness. If the collection is a large one, the liver may be pushed downwards so as to be easily palpable below the costal margin; the heart may be displaced upwards. A screen examination with the X-rays sometimes proves most valuable by indicating the level and degree of mobility of the diaphragm.

The diagnosis is often complicated by the presence of clear or purulent fluid in the pleural cavity above the subphrenic collection. The diaphragm is sometimes perforated, so that the subphrenic and pleural collections of pus communicate with one another.

Exploratory puncture with an aspirating needle cannot be too severely condemned. The procedure is far more dangerous than an exploratory operation, and a negative result is valueless.

Treatment.—The abscess must be opened as soon as its presence has been determined. The actual site of the opening will be indicated by the situation of the pus, as shown by percussion, position of tenderness, palpation, and X - ray examination. Occasionally such an abscess, if coming forward, can be reached by an incision through the anterior abdominal wall below the costal margin, and posteriorly situated collections have been reached by an incision below the costal margin behind, though in doing this there is risk of accidentally wounding and infecting the pleura.

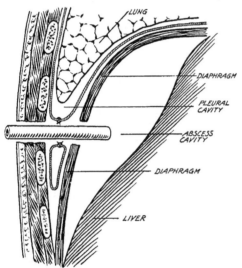

Fig. 441.—Diagram showing structures traversed in opening a subphrenic abscess.

The method adapted to the majority of cases is that of deliberately traversing the pleural cavity and diaphragm. The structures which have to be traversed are shown diagrammatically in Fig. 441. If the patient is very ill the operation can be done under local anæsthesia.

The operation, briefly, consists in resecting portions of two or three ribs over the site of the abscess, opening the pleural cavity, suturing the diaphragm to the costal pleura, so as to shut off the pleural cavity, incising the diaphragm, and inserting a drainage-tube. Some surgeons prefer to perform this operation in two stages, the first stage being directed to shutting off the pleural cavity, and the second to opening the abscess. The danger of infecting the pleura in the one-stage operation has been exaggerated, and there is little to be said in favour of the two-stage procedure. In some cases an empyema is present in addition to the subphrenic abscess; when this is so, doubt may arise as to whether there is also pus beneath the diaphragm ; the operator would then be content to drain the empyema and to await events.

Prognosis.—Rare instances have occurred of spontaneous termination either by absorption or evacuation of the pus. With such reported exceptions the condition, if unrelieved by operation, terminates fatally, sometimes after a very prolonged period of illness. Extension or rupture of the abscess may take place into the pleural cavity, the pericardium, the bronchi, or the general peritoneal cavity, and the patient dies from these complications or from prolonged suppuration and septic poisoning. Early operation, on 'the other hand, offers a fairly good prospect of recovery, and the mortality of such cases may be placed at between 30 and 40 per cent.

There is a tendency to the formation of fresh loculi of pus even after the primary collection has been evacuated, and in the event of the temperature not subsiding, fresh efforts should be made to find such collections.

C. CHRONIC FORMS OF PERITONITIS

1. CHRONIC SEPTIC PERITONITIS

Localized intraperitoneal abscess has already been considered (p. 572). A form of peritonitis intermediate between these cases and those of acute diffuse peritonitis can sometimes be recognized, coming on after the subsidence of an acute diffuse peritonitis, and characterized clinically by irregular fever, diarrhœa, and progressive emaciation ; from time to time collections of pus large enough to be recognized and opened make their appearance. Post mortem there is a general matting together of the abdominal contents, in the midst of which are found loculi of pus of various sizes, which often communicate with one another by narrow fistulous tracks, and an extreme thickening of the peritoneum from fibrinous deposit more or less organized (Plate 98, Fig. 2). In such cases the pyogenetic staphylococci, the colon bacillus, and the *Bacillus pyocyaneus* have been found.

2. CHRONIC GONOCOCCAL PERITONITIS

The gonococcus, whilst only an occasional cause of acute diffuse peritonitis, frequently produces a chronic form of peritonitis which, from its almost invariable starting-point in the Fallopian tubes, chiefly concerns the pelvic peritoneum. The resulting peritonitis is slow and insidious in its course, produces few or no symptoms apart from those of the initial lesions, and leads to the formation of adhesions which may mat together the pelvic viscera and may cause intestinal obstruction.

3. Chronic Pneumococcal Peritonitis

Like the gonococcus, the pneumococcus may produce either an acute and diffuse, or a localized and chronic peritonitis. The chronic form closely resembles tuberculous peritonitis, both in its clinical course and in its local effects upon the peritoneum, and the two diseases can scarcely be distinguished except by a bacteriological examination. The diagnosis may have to rest upon the discovery of some recognizable pneumococcal or tuberculous lesión elsewhere.

D. TUBERCULOUS PERITONITIS

The forms in which peritoneal tuberculosis occurs are—

1. The miliary form, in which the peritoneum is affected merely as part of a general miliary tuberculosis. This form is of no surgical interest.

2. A form in which the peritoneal affection is either primary or—being secondary, as is more common—constitutes the predominant feature of the case.

The infection reaches the peritoneum either through the blood-stream from some focus at a distance, such as the lung; or more directly from a neighbouring focus, such as intestinal ulceration, a tuberculous mesenteric gland, or a tuberculous Fallopian tube.

Clinically the disease appears in two chief varieties, which, however, merge into one another, namely, the *ascitic* and the *adhesive*. In the former the exudation is the chief clinical feature, the peritoneum being studded with tuberculous nodules of varying sizes ; in the latter the intestines and omentum are matted together in an inextricable mass, in the midst of which are collections of broken-down caseous material of various sizes. Such collections are liable to become secondarily infected with pyogenetic organisms from the intestine, and to form acute or subacute intraperitoneal abscesses. With one or more of these abscesses the intestine may communicate by fistulous tracks, and such abscesses becoming adherent to and perforating the abdominal wall, or being opened surgically, may produce intractable fæcal fistulæ. The umbilicus is a common site for such a fistula to arise spontaneously.

Symptoms.—Tuberculous peritonitis is chiefly a disease of childhood and young adult life, though it is sometimes met with in older patients. It runs a slow course, and is characterized principally by progressive emaciation which may be accompanied by irregular slight fever. Attacks of pain and vomiting occur at intervals, but, unless proceeding from a definite intestinal obstruction, they are not severe. In some cases diarrhœa is a marked feature. Secondary infection of intraperitoneal abscesses may cause more acute symptoms and may necessitate incision.

Examination of the abdomen reveals, in the ascitic variety, the physical signs of free fluid within the abdomen. The distension may become very marked, so that the belly wall appears tense and shiny, with dilated veins upon its surface and a prominent umbilicus ; respiratory and cardiac embarrassment may thus be caused. The fluid may find its way into a patent funicular process, and, unless there is something to call attention to the abdomen, such a case may easily be mistaken for one of simple congenital hydrocele.

In the adhesive variety it is often possible to feel nodules or irregular masses of various sizes scattered throughout the abdomen.

Diagnosis.—A characteristic case presents little difficulty, though it may be closely mimicked by the chronic form of pneumococcal peritonitis.

On the other hand, tuberculous peritonitis may assume forms in which the diagnosis is a matter of the greatest difficulty and may have to be decided by exploratory laparotomy. Thus, *malignant disease of the peritoneum*, especially when accompanied by the presence of palpable masses and of ascites, may be quite indistinguishable from tuberculous peritonitis except by surgical exploration. An encysted collection of fluid in tuberculous peritonitis may readily be mistaken for an *ovarian cyst*, or for a *local intraperitoneal abscess due to some other cause*.

In a case with acute onset, accompanied by fever and diarrhœa, the diagnosis from *enteric fever* may be most difficult. The greater irregularity of the fever, especially when observed over a period of several weeks, together with the absence of rash, of splenic enlargement, and of bronchitis, and the negative Widal reaction, would serve to distinguish tuberculous peritonitis. Some assistance may be gained from Calmette's or von Pirquet's tuberculin test.

Treatment.—Treatment by medical means, hygienic and dietetic, such as is suitable for tuberculosis in general, may be followed by good results. Tuberculin may also be tried in suitable cases. The tapping of a large ascitic collection may afford relief, but does not give such good results as laparotomy, and is by no means free from the risk of puncturing adherent intestine.

Treatment by surgical means is often indicated, and is frequently followed by results sufficiently good to be justly denominated cures. It is chiefly in the ascitic form that operation holds out such favourable prospects. The operation is of the simplest character, and consists in making a small incision, some two or three inches long, through one or other rectus abdominis muscle in the direction of its fibres. The fluid is allowed to escape, and the little wound is closed and dressed with collodion. No advantage appears to attach to the flushing or mopping-out of the peritoneal cavity, still less to the introduction of antiseptics. Occasionally a definite tuberculous focus of origin can be removed at the same time, such as a Fallopian tube or a lymphatic

2 *l*

gland. The coexistence of phthisis or other tuberculous focus, unless of an advanced character, is no contra-indication to operation.

Other operative measures are called for in certain cases, as for the relief of intestinal obstruction, or the opening of localized infected abscesses. When fistulæ are present, no surgical procedure is likely to be of any benefit.

Prognosis.—The immediate result of operation in the ascitic form, and in dealing with encysted collections of exudate, is strikingly beneficial, whilst the operative risk is very small. Rorsch's series of collected cases showed an operation mortality of 5·6 per cent., 70 per cent. of immediate cures, and 14·8 per cent. of cures of two or more years' duration.

II. TUMOURS

The peritoneum is often involved secondarily by malignant growths, but is rarely the seat of a primary tumour. It is said to be sometimes the seat of a primary endothelioma and of colloid carcinoma. Other neoplasms, described as peritoneal tumours, such as lipomas, are in reality connective-tissue tumours of the retroperitoneal tissues.

Carcinoma and sarcoma of the gastro-intestinal tract, uterus, ovaries, and biliary passages often involve the peritoneum, the affection taking the form of nodules of growth of various sizes everywhere studding the serous membrane, and involving in particular the omentum, which tends to become rolled up into cake-like masses, especially in the upper part of the abdomen. The growth may consist of hard nodules, but is sometimes of gelatinous consistency.

Effusion of fluid into the peritoneal cavity is the rule, the fluid being clear or straw-coloured and often blood-stained.

The symptoms of such peritoneal involvement by malignant growth are usually overshadowed by those of the primary tumour. Sometimes, however, the primary growth is small and so situated as to produce no symptoms, in which case those of the peritoneal involvement will predominate. The existence of ascites, together with the presence of nodules or large masses palpable on abdominal examination, in a patient of or beyond middle age, would point to the possibility of intraperitoneal carcinomatosis. Similar cases of sarcomatosis occur in children and young people, and such a condition may be very difficult to distinguish from tuberculous peritonitis (*see* above).

The treatment can only be symptomatic.

HYDATID CYSTS

These cysts sometimes arise primarily in the omentum. Multiple hydatid cysts occasionally result from rupture into the peritoneal cavity of a primary cyst in the liver or elsewhere.

MESENTERIC CYSTS

Apart from hydatids, the origin of mesenteric cysts is obscure. They are usually unilocular, contain clear or milky fluid, and may attain a very large size. Possibly traumatism accounts for a certain number of the cases, though it is more likely that the injury merely calls attention to a cyst which had previously caused no symptoms.

The presence of a freely movable painless tumour is usually all that the clinical picture presents, though indefinite pain or intestinal disturbance may call attention to the disease. The diagnosis is usually only made with any certainty by exploratory operation.

Treatment.—Removal by means of an incision through the overlying mesenteric peritoneum, with due regard to the position of the intestinal blood-vessels, is the most satisfactory method. When the cyst cannot be so shelled out without risk of damage to the blood supply of the overlying or adjacent intestine, it may be brought up to the abdominal wound and opened, the lips of the incision in the cyst being sutured to the abdominal wall and a tube or gauze drain inserted.

III. ASCITES

Any non-inflammatory collection of serous fluid in the peritoneal cavity is called ascites. It is the result of such circulatory disturbances as arise from cardiac or pulmonary disease ; from portal obstruction of hepatic origin, such as cirrhosis ; or from renal disease. It is therefore not a disease of the peritoneum, but a secondary transudation of fluid into the peritoneal cavity symptomatic of disease elsewhere. Its symptoms and treatment will therefore be found dealt with in the various articles devoted to those causes.

For chylous ascites, *see* under Lymphatic System, Vol. III., p. 84.

BIBLIOGRAPHY

Box, C. R., *Lancet,* March 26, 1910.
Box and **Eccles,** *Clinical Applied Anatomy.* London, 1906.
Buxton and **Torrey,** *Journ. of Med. Research,* xiv. 5.
Durham, H. E., *Med.-Chir. Trans.,* London, lxxx. 191.
Dudgeon and **Sargent,** *Bacteriology of Peritonitis.* London, 1905.
Gohn, A., *Wien. klin. Woch.,* 1904, xvii. 207.
Lennander, *Mittheil. Grenz.,* 1902.
MacCallum, *Johns Hopkins Hosp. Bull.,* 1903, xiv.
von Mikulicz, Cavendish Lecture, 1904.
Muscatello, *Virchows Arch.,* cxlii.
Ramström, Inaug. Dissert., Wiesbaden.
Veillon et **Zuber,** *Arch. de Méd. Expér.,* July, 1898.

HERNIA

BY LAWRIE McGAVIN, F.R.C.S.ENG.

Structure of a hernia.—With certain exceptions a hernia consists of (1) a sac, (2) its coverings, and (3) its contents.

In some hernias, to be described later, the sac is partially or wholly absent, and in some, although present, it may be devoid of contents from time to time.

The hernial sac consists of peritoneum, and is either present at birth, or is formed subsequently as the result of pathological changes in the abdominal wall. It is usually described as having a neck, a body, and a fundus.

The *neck* is that part which occupies the aperture through which the hernia escaped. It is commonly narrow, being constricted by the surrounding tissues, and when unoccupied is flattened from before backwards. Occasionally, however, it is the widest part of the sac. In its earliest condition, the peritoneum of the neck resembles that from which it springs; it is quite free from the surrounding structures, and is lined by normal glistening endothelium. In children it is very thin, and in all inguinal or femoral hernias the posterior wall is thinner than the anterior.

The *body* is usually wider than the neck, and is at first unilocular. Subsequently it may enlarge to remarkable dimensions and become altered in character. A sac may exist which has never been occupied by contents, in which case it rarely attains to great size and may retain the original character of the parietal peritoneum.

The *fundus*, or extreme end, is usually, though not always, the oldest part of the sac. Since the iliac peritoneum is more readily dragged down than the parietal, there is in inguinal and femoral hernias a tendency for the original point of protrusion to lag behind; the fundus may thus be formed from the peritoneum which was derived from the iliac fossa.

Formation of hernial sacs.—Hernial sacs may have their origin as—

1. **Preformed (congenital) sacs.**—The opinion is becoming more general that many sacs, hitherto looked upon as acquired,

are in reality congenital diverticula. This, as pointed out by Hamilton Russell, is especially the ease with femoral hernias, and probably applies to the inguinal variety as well.

The sacs of *undoubtedly* congenital origin are those which occur (*a*) into the patent vaginal process in the male, (*b*) into the patent canal of Nuck in the female, (*c*) at the patent umbilical ring in the infant. These are considered later.

2. **Distension diverticula (acquired sacs).**—These occur as the result of muscular weakness at certain sites in the abdominal wall, assisted by forced expiratory efforts which repeatedly raise the intra-abdominal pressure. They are commonly thicker in the wall and more adherent at the neck than the sacs of congenital origin, and are often wide-mouthed from the first, especially when they are of the variety met with in direct hernia; they are frequently multilocular, and are rarely empty.

3. **Traction diverticula.**—For the formation of a sac by the constant drag of a tumour attached to some portion of the peritoneal surface, the action of gravity is necessary; and for this reason such sacs are rarely seen in any position other than the pelvic floor. Sacs are, however, formed in the inguinal region by the dragging of tumours of the cord or testis, or by the weight of large hydroceles. Lipomas of the spermatic cord are often found at the fundus of a sac, suggesting the possibility that the sac has arisen first by traction and then by distension.

4. **Downward displacement of the peritoneum.**—This method of formation is rare; it is usually seen in cases of hernia associated with general enteroptosis (Glénard's disease); and results in the presence of a complete sac only at the *commencement* of the trouble, for in time the iliac peritoneum slips down, and what was the posterior wall of the sac becomes first the fundus and then the anterior wall, the posterior wall now being deficient, and its place being taken by the down-slipping cæcum on the right side, or the sigmoid on the left; a partial sac is thus eventually formed (Fig. 457). Such sacs are more often met with in direct than in oblique inguinal hernias.

The congenital sac.—Prior to birth, two well-recognized processes of peritoneum exist, which should be obliterated when the infant is born. These are (1) the umbilical process, and (2) the funiculo-vaginal process of the testis in the male, or the canal of Nuck in the female.

The first rarely persists long; containing at birth a small coil of ileum in connexion with Meckel's diverticulum, it commonly closes within a few days. Remaining unobliterated, however, it forms the sac of a " congenital umbilical hernia."

The second is more important. In both sexes the inguinal canal is occupied shortly before birth by a tubular process of peritoneum, which passes into the scrotum of the male, forming the processus vaginalis of the testis, and in the female into the labium majus, forming the canal of Nuck. The latter should be, and usually is, entirely obliterated; exceptionally it remains patent and forms the sac of a " congenital hernia of the canal of Nuck." The former should be obliterated as far as the testis, the remainder forming the tunica vaginalis of that organ. If the

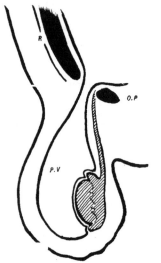
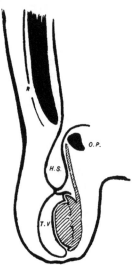

Fig. 442.—Sac of hernia into processus vaginalis.

P.V., Processus vaginalis; O.P., pubes; R., rectus muscle.

Fig. 443.—Sac of hernia into funicular process.

H.S., Hernial sac; T.V., tunica vaginalis; O.P., pubes; R., rectus muscle.

process remains patent in its whole length and at any time contains viscera, the sac thus formed is that of a " congenital hernia of the vaginal process " (Fig. 442). If the process is obliterated at the upper pole of the testis but in free communication with the peritoneal cavity above this point, the sac is that of a " congenital hernia of the funicular process " (Fig. 443). Two other forms of congenital sac are met with, and are known as "infantile " and " encysted infantile." In the first, there is what looks like an acquired sac immediately behind, and bulging into, the sac of a congenital hernia of the vaginal process or funicular process (Fig. 444). In the second, the neck of the vaginal process would seem to have been obliterated only at the internal abdominal ring, by a septum which, having been stretched and forced downwards, has formed a second sac dependent *within the lumen of the first* (Fig. 445). A better term for the first of these sacs would be "retrofunicular," and for the second "intrafunicular." It is doubtful if the second sac in the first of these forms is really of congenital origin.

The congenital sac differs but slightly from the acquired sac in its general appearance; it is, however, usually narrower at the

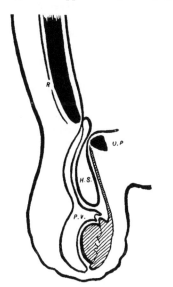 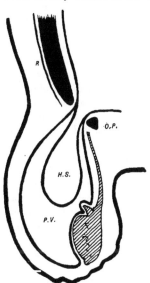

Fig. 444.—Sac of infantile
hernia; common variety.

P.V., Processus vaginalis; H.S, hernial
sac; O.P, pubes; R., rectus muscle.

Fig. 445.—Sac of encysted
infantile hernia.

P.V., Processus vaginalis; H.S, hernial
sac; O.P., pubes; R., rectus muscle.

neck, less adherent to its surroundings, and freer from thickening and cicatrization of its walls; it is frequently empty or contains only fluid.

Contents of hernial sacs.—In a reducible hernia the contents may vary, but in an irreducible one they are usually constant. The commonest content is the *omentum*, owing to its weight, length, mobility, and lobulated character, which facilitate its engagement in the hernial orifices. Occasionally its free margin becomes adherent to the posterior edge of the aperture, and a part above is invaginated into the sac so as to form an omental lining or "omental sac"; the recognition of this condition is important during operation, owing to the danger of including a contained knuckle of gut when ligating the omentum.

Next in frequency is the *bowel* itself. The part most commonly involved in inguinal and femoral hernias, especially on the right side, is the lower part of the ileum ; on the left side, the ilio-pelvic colon is often found. Very rarely the intestinal canal of one side will trespass into a sac of the opposite side. Thus, sigmoid is at times found on the right side (Eccles, Kelly, Griffiths), and appendix, cæcum, and ascending colon have been found in a sac on the left (Owen Richards). Such cases are of extreme rarity, and suggest either general enteroptosis, elongation of the mesocolon, or transposition of viscera.

The presence of the *vermiform appendix* in right-sided sacs has been frequently noted, at times in a state of acute inflammation. I have met with such a condition in 4 per cent. of cases.

A *Meckel's diverticulum* may be met with in inguinal sacs, and may be mistaken, when much atrophied, for an adhesion band ; the discovery of its true nature is thus a matter of some importance.

The *ovary and Fallopian tube* are met with occasionally in inguinal and even femoral sacs, the tube being often adherent at its fimbriated extremity. I have also found a small pedunculated fibro-myoma of the uterus in an inguinal sac.

Although the *bladder* is more commonly found in the extra-peritoneal varieties of hernia, a process of it may present in the sac of an inguinal or a femoral hernia.

The sac of an umbilical hernia rarely contains anything except omentum, transverse colon, and mesocolon ; it may, however, contain small intestine or a Meckel's diverticulum.

Fluid may be found in hernial sacs, and, unless due to ascites, points to some local irritation of the sac or its contents. Thus, it is seen constantly in strangulation, or where strangulation has undergone spontaneous resolution ; it may also be associated with injury to the sac, with pressure by a badly fitted truss, or, at times, with localized tuberculous or malignant disease of the sac or its contents.

Loose bodies may be found in hernial sacs, usually in the form of calcareous or fibro-cartilaginous masses varying in size from a pea to a horse-bean ; these are usually detached appendices epiploicæ which have undergone secondary histological change.

Diagnosis of hernial contents.—The presence of bowel is usually determined from the elastic character of the tumour, the gurgling of fluid and gas when it is handled, the resonance to percussion, the occurrence of visible peristalsis, and the plastic sensation due to the presence of fæces.

Recurrent attacks of pain and tenderness in a sac, especially if accompanied by pyrexia and vomiting, but in the absence of definite signs of strangulation, should suggest the presence of an inflamed appendix. Its presence may at times be diagnosed by palpation, from the peculiar shape of the organ, and from the tenderness on pressure being referred to McBurney's point, or to the umbilicus.

Omentum in the sac gives rise to a spongy, lobulated mass of ill-defined outline, usually irreducible, dull to percussion throughout the length of the inguinal canal, although in the scrotum there may be areas of resonance which are due to bowel. It lacks the tenseness and rounded character of hydrocele, and the plastic character of fæces.

The presence of an ovary is generally indicated by tenderness and enlargement of the hernia coincident with each menstrual period, irregularity of these periods, some displacement of the uterus to the side of the hernia, and absence of the ovary of that side when a bimanual examination is made. In either femoral or inguinal hernia its characteristic shape and sensation on pressure may be elicited in the quiescent period.

Hernias which contain cæcum, colon, or sigmoid are usually very large with wide necks, contain fæces from time to time, and are often associated with constipation and incarceration.

It is not always possible to be certain of the presence of the bladder in the sac of a hernia, since only a small part of its wall may be involved, but it should be suspected in all cases of direct inguinal and in femoral hernia accompanied by urinary symptoms, whether in the way of frequency, pain, strangury, or unexplained cystitis; and in cases where an overfull bladder is associated repeatedly with an increase, and micturition with a decrease, in the size of the hernia. In femoral hernia the bladder should never be forgotten, whether symptoms are present or not, since it is frequently found at operation without any external evidence. Where doubt exists, it may be cleared up by the passage of a sound per urethram, after the bladder has been emptied; it may thus be possible, especially in the female, to direct the beak of the sound into the diverticulum in the sac, and so avoid an accident during operation.

Coverings of the sac.—These naturally depend on the variety of hernia in question, and will be discussed as each variety is considered.

Secondary changes in the sac.—Although at first a simple protrusion of almost unaltered peritoneum, the sac does not long remain in this condition; it is influenced especially by pressure and irritation from without, and by the character and weight of its contents. At first it is thin, avascular, usually unilocular, and easily reducible into the abdomen; but with the constantly increasing weight of its contents it becomes stretched, and tends to grow in length rather than in width, provided no pressure is brought to bear upon it from without.

1. Thickening of the walls.—This increase in size demands an increase in nutrition; the sac soon becomes adherent to the surrounding structures, develops new vessels on its outer surface, and becomes very much thicker; in hernias of large dimensions and long standing the walls may measure as much as an eighth to a quarter of an inch in thickness, and assume the consistence of the pericardium. These changes are chiefly seen in irreducible omental hernias, where the omentum has become widely adherent to the sac wall, which thus receives a blood supply from within as well as from without. Thickening is also favoured by the chronic congestion produced by the pressure of an ill-fitting truss upon the veins about the neck of the sac.

2. Thickening below the neck.—The changes above mentioned are frequently most marked just below the neck of the sac, especially if a truss has been worn, this part becoming densely adherent to the tissues about it and often developing into an almost fibro-cartilaginous ring, while the true neck and the structures composing the inguinal or femoral canal become thinned out and matted together owing to the pressure of the truss. In such cases the omentum in the sac is usually adherent to the entire circumference of the neck.

3. Cartilaginous and calcareous degeneration.—These are only met with in hernial sacs of large dimensions and long standing. The areas of degeneration are usually discrete, and seldom involve the entire sac wall.

4. Obliteration of the neck.—Occasionally a sac containing fluid is seen in which the original communication with the abdominal cavity has been cut off. The cause is to be sought in some antecedent inflammation at the neck of the sac by which the passage has been sealed. The pressure of a truss on a strand of unreduced omentum may be the cause; occasionally the obliteration appears to be spontaneous, no truss having been worn. Such a fortunate result is only possible in sacs having very narrow necks; the condition is termed " hydrocele of a hernial sac."

5. Cysts in hernial sacs.—In certain cases a hernial sac will be found to include one or more cysts containing fluid, giving the impression of a second sac within the first. These cysts will be found to have no connexion with the abdominal cavity or the tunica vaginalis. They are developed in or between the sac walls and its coverings. They are commonly due to lymphatic dilatation or to subserous effusions resulting from irritation or injury, and have no pathological importance.

6. **Acute inflammation.**—This is rarely seen except in the sacs of very large irreducible hernias ; it is of the nature of a localized peritonitis, is predisposed to by direct injury, and usually results in resolution with the formation of extensive adhesions between the sac and its contents. At times it may give rise to strangulation of these contents, or may progress to complete sloughing or gangrene. It is especially prone to occur in the victims of Bright's disease, in whom the prognosis is consequently very unfavourable.

7. **Loculation.**—Although due at times to congenital abnormality, the formation of secondary loculi in hernial sacs is also seen as the result of inflammation about the inguinal and femoral regions, and is an almost constant feature of umbilical hernias of any size. It is especially prone to occur in recurrent hernias of rapid formation. The presence of omentum densely adherent to the sac wall below the neck may compel the wall above the adhesion to bulge laterally through the separated fibres of its coverings. Thus the original sac may have one or more secondary loculi, opening usually near the neck, and often as large as, or even larger than, the parent sac.

8. **Localized disease.**—Although extremely rare, cases have been reported of the presence of disease apparently confined to hernial sacs. I have met with three such cases : in two elderly men, masses in the fundi of the sacs proved on section to be spheroidal-celled carcinomas ; in the third, a middle-aged man, an apparently localized tuberculous mass was found.

Secondary changes in the coverings.—In some cases the coverings, owing to very rapid increase in the size of the hernia, become extremely thin, their fibres being widely separated and atrophic, the common condition in umbilical hernia ; on the other hand, those which develop slowly and steadily frequently undergo marked hypertrophy, the muscular coverings especially appearing as a definite thick layer. In such cases the blood supply is markedly increased, and large vessels are seen ramifying over the surface of the sac, while the coverings are matted together and often densely adherent.

Occasionally, in very large umbilical and ventral hernias, whose coverings are atrophic, the skin at the most dependent part becomes œdematous and inflamed, and a slough appears, or what is more common, a recurrent superficial ulcer. Such changes are due to interference with the blood supply and to the influence of gravity.

Secondary changes in the contents.—As regards the omentum, the most noteworthy changes are the remarkable and often rapid increase which takes place in its volume when it remains permanently in the sac, and its proneness to become adherent to its surroundings. This increase is independent of any general increase

in obesity of the patient, and depends chiefly on interference with
the venous return from the omentum, since the most marked examples
are met with where this organ is adherent to the neck of the sac ; at
the same time it is not entirely due to œdema, distension of vessels,
nor to intrusion of fresh omentum, but in part arises from actual
hypertrophy.

Adhesions in hernial sacs may concern—

1. *The sac only.*—Fibrous bands, the result of old inflammation,
   are at times found passing from one side to the other;
   these may subsequently become stretched-and form " bridles,"
   just as they do in the abdominal cavity.   Their only
   surgical importance is that they predispose to strangulation, and, especially if they cross the neck, are apt to
   ensnare a loop of bowel when reduction is attempted, thus
   giving rise to one of the varieties of " reduction *en masse* "
   (p. 644). They may occur simply as elevated cicatricial bands
   on the inner surface.   Again, an actual septum may be produced by these adhesions, the sac being thus divided into
   an upper and a lower compartment, the latter of which,
   filling with fluid, becomes a hydrocele of the sac.

2. *The sac wall and the contents.*—When adhesions occur between
   these two they commonly result from inflammation of the
   omentum.   Bowel is rarely found adherent to the sac unless
   affected by inflammation arising in the omentum, or unless
   itself diseased.   Thus a loop of bowel containing tuberculous
   ulcers, an appendix when inflamed, or a portion of large
   bowel inflamed as the result of stercoral ulceration, may
   acquire adhesions to the sac at any point.   Similarly the
   ovary and Fallopian tube may become adherent to the wall.

3. *The contents alone.*—Rarely, adhesions occur in the sac without
   affecting its walls.   The contents may be so bound together
   as to prevent reduction, the cause being, as before, the
   presence of inflamed omentum, etc.

The **intestine**, when long retained in a sac by adhesions, frequently
undergoes marked hypertrophy. In certain cases, owing to some
constriction at the neck of the sac, not sufficient to cause actual
strangulation, it may become permanently narrowed at one or more
points by a ring-like atrophy of the muscular wall and subsequent
fibrosis at these points.

In umbilical and ventral hernias the bowel may become adherent
to the thinned-out cutaneo-peritoneal sac, and may then be affected
by the sloughing above mentioned, a fæcal or intestinal fistula resulting.

Occasionally an **appendix** or an **ovary** occupying a hernial sac
undergoes an attack of acute inflammation, and if the presence of

these organs has not been diagnosed, the case may be treated simply as one of inflamed sac, with the result that an abscess forms, and in the one case a fæcal fistula, and in the other sloughing of the ovary and its tube, is the result.

Etiology of hernia.—It has been customary hitherto to divide all hernias into two classes, viz. (1) those dependent on some arrest in the development of the abdominal wall at or previous to birth, and therefore known as *congenital ;* and (2) those which, owing to weakening of the abdominal wall at its most vulnerable points by subsequent strains and injuries, originate in later life, and are known therefore as *acquired*. Much doubt has been thrown on the accuracy of the latter term by Hamilton Russell, whose theory is dealt with later (p. 590).

Whether a hernia be congenital or acquired, certain factors are essential to its formation—(1) a weak spot in the abdominal wall, and (2) an increase in the intra-abdominal pressure.

1. Weak spots in the abdominal wall.—Inasmuch as fibrous tissue lacks the power of resistance to strain and of recovery after stretching possessed by muscle, all areas in the abdominal wall that depend for their strength upon either aponeuroses or cicatrices are to be considered as weak spots.

If the entire abdominal wall were guarded by muscular tissue alone, hernia would probably be comparatively rare. The naturally weak points of the abdominal wall are as follows : The inguinal canal ; the femoral canal ; the umbilicus ; the median line of the abdomen ; the lumbar (Petit's) triangle ; the obturator foramen ; the sciatic notch ; the intermuscular spaces in the levator ani ; and the costo-xiphoid interspace.

2. Increase of intra-abdominal pressure.—This is probably only a potent factor—(i) When it is *quickly developed*, as in rapid ascites or in general obesity. (ii) When it is *sudden, powerful, or intermittent,* as in heavy manual labour, in the playing of wind instruments, in coughing or screaming, in repeated pregnancies in weakly women, or in the straining necessitated by phimosis, stricture, constipation, etc. (iii) *When gradual pressure is suddenly relieved and followed by intermittent increase,* e.g. when large old-standing pelvic tumours are removed in asthmatic or bronchitic patients. Gradual increase alone has probably but little influence.

Defæcation and hernia.—Although the squatting position during defæcation is both natural and anatomically and physiologically correct, most modern conveniences demand a sedentary posture, in which the groins are undefended, the abdominal muscles lack a *point d'appui,* and consequently the effort required is a serious tax on the weak spots. If the effort to support the abdomen on the thighs is

made in the sedentary form of convenience, it can only be done by
lowering the head to the level of the knees, a dangerous position for
old people when making any expulsive effort. Both for young and
old the sedentary posture is a bad one and favours the occurrence
of hernia at the groins.

Congenital theory of hernia.—The production of a hernial
sac in later life by alterations in pressure alone has been questioned
from time to time, and especially by Hamilton Russell, who believes that "acquired oblique inguinal hernia in the young subject
has probably no existence in fact." He maintains that, with the
possible exception of some cases of direct inguinal hernia, all hernias,
whether inguinal or femoral (and probably ischiatic and obturator
as well), are the result of the presence of congenitally formed sacs,
and are *not* acquired. The grounds on which the belief is founded
are (1) the results of post-mortem examinations ; (2) the examination of sacs removed by operation ; (3) the results of operations in
which simple removal of the sac constituted the entire procedure ;
(4) the accidental discovery during operation of preformed peritoneal
diverticula which had never been occupied by a hernia. I have
found, in a woman of 47, both inguinal and both femoral canals patent
and occupied by such diverticula, none of which had ever contained
a hernia.[1] (5) The *sudden* descent of hernias in adults into sacs having
the anatomical characters of acquired, but the histological characters
of congenital, sacs ; (6) the curious disposition of certain femoral
sacs along the branches of the femoral artery ; (7) the association of
hernial sacs with other congenital anomalies, such as hypospadias,
ectopia vesicæ, congenital dislocation of the hip, and talipes. Russell
believes that inguinal sacs are simply diverticula from the original
processus vaginalis, while the sacs found in cases of femoral hernia,
etc., are prolongations of the peritoneal lining of the abdomen, which
are drawn out along the course of the branches of the femoral artery
during the development of the embryonic limb-buds.

There is much to be said for the congenital theory of hernia, with
which I am myself in sympathy, but space does not permit of a full
discussion of this subject.

Clinical characters of hernia.—The contents of hernias, of whatever variety, are in nearly every case, in their earliest
stages, capable of being returned into the abdominal cavity by slight
pressure, and often disappear spontaneously on the patient lying down.
Such hernias are known by the term *reducible*. Even the sac in rare
cases, especially in children, can for a period be reduced, but later,
becoming adherent to its surroundings, it remains *in situ*, the contents

---

[1] Since this was written the patient has developed an inguinal hernia of the
right side.

only going back. When the contents can no longer be returned, the term *irreducible* is applied to the hernia.

Causes of irreducibility.—(*a*) Adhesions of the contents to the sac. (*b*) The matting together of the contents. (*c*) Lack of room inside the abdomen for the contents of very large and long-standing hernias. (*d*) The presence of secondary diverticula at the neck of the sac, the contents passing into these rather than into the abdomen (*see* Interstitial Hernia, p. 610). (*e*) The presence of any tumour in the sac, whether of the contents or of the sac itself. (*f*) The presence of enlarged inguinal or femoral glands. (*g*) Increase of intra-abdominal pressure, whether voluntary on account of tenderness during manipulation, or from the presence of tumours, ascites, etc., in the abdomen. (*h*) The presence of fæcal masses, undigested food, foreign bodies, gall-stones, etc., in the bowel contained in the sac. Such a condition is termed *incarceration ;* when due to impaction of fæces it is obviously only probable in the large intestine. (*i*) Inflammation or œdema of the sac or its contents. (*j*) Tumours of the inguinal canal or of the cord ; these are commonly either fibromas, lipomas, or hydroceles.

Strangulation.—Occasionally the contents of a hernia become strangulated—i.e. not only are these contents irreducible, but the blood circulation and the passage of flatus and fæces through them is interfered with to such an extent as to result in gangrene, sloughing, and perforation if the condition is not relieved by natural or artificial means.

Incarceration can only take place when the sac contains bowel, whereas strangulation may affect any of the contents of the sac.

Characters of incarcerated hernia.—More commonly seen in elderly men or in women who are subject to chronic constipation, incarceration is almost confined to the umbilical and inguino-scrotal forms of hernia. On examining the hernia, it will be found to be globular in outline, heavy, often devoid of tenderness and pain, and having the consistence of half-dried putty, so that its form can be moulded by the fingers. It is, of course, dull to percussion.

It is clear that if no fæcal matter can pass the site of hernia, a time will very soon arrive when, the whole of the large bowel becoming full, the small intestine must begin to regurgitate its contents into the stomach. Such a condition is less serious than actual strangulation only because in it there is no arrest of circulation.

Frequently, incarceration may persist for a considerable time, the obstruction being partial in character and partaking of the nature of obstinate constipation ; on the other hand, it may lead to strangulation from the continued increase of pressure of the fæcal contents. The premonitory signs of this are the presence or increase of umbilical pain, tenderness in the hernia, distension of the abdomen, and the presence of peristaltic waves. Such signs are an indication for early operation.

ANATOMICAL VARIETIES OF HERNIA

Of the weak spots of the abdominal wall at which hernias may appear, the *inguinal canal* is by far the most frequently involved; here two varieties of hernia are met with, viz. *oblique* and *direct*.

Oblique inguinal hernia (Fig. 446).—This form of hernia makes its exit at the internal abdominal ring, and, passing along

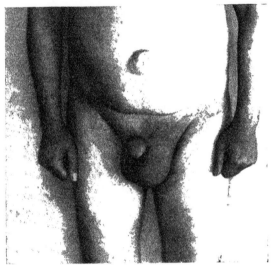

Fig. 446.—Oblique inguinal hernia becoming inguino-scrotal; also early umbilical hernia.

the spermatic cord in the male, or the round ligament of the uterus in the female, leaves the canal at the external abdominal ring, and enters, in the former case the scrotum (Fig. 447), and in the latter the labium majus. The neck of the sac thus has the deep epigastric artery as *its immediate internal relation*.

An oblique inguinal hernia is invariably clothed by certain struc-tures known as its " coverings "; these are best described in order of dissection, thus : (1) skin ; (2) superficial fascia ; (3) aponeurosis of the external oblique muscle and its arciform or intercolumnar fibres, commonly called the " external spermatic fascia " ; (4) cremasteric fascia, which is simply the stretched fibres of the cremaster muscle ; (5) " internal spermatic fascia " or infundibuliform fascia, a finger-like process of the transversalis fascia ; and (6) the extraperitoneal fascia which overlies the peritoneum. These coverings, with the exception of the cremaster, which is often hypertrophied in old-standing cases, are not, as a rule, easily demonstrable, being usually fused together.

In large hernias which have existed for many years, the internal ring often becomes so much distended that its inner edge is shifted inwards ; similarly, when the hernia is of the scrotal variety the outer edge of the external ring becomes displaced outwards, so that in time the two rings are found to be superimposed, and several fingers, or even the whole hand, may be passed into the abdomen, the oblique character of the hernia being then apparently lost. The relative position of the deep epigastric artery, however, will always show the true nature of the hernia ; the position of the structures of the spermatic cord will also help to distinguish it, for, although in large hernias they may be much separated by pressure, they will still lie *deep to the sac*.

Associated with the hernia there is often a marked weakening of the whole inguinal region, permitting of much bulging when the patient stands up or strains, and this is especially common where the hernia is bilateral. It may be due, in elderly subjects with large hernias, to the presence of the hernia itself, but in young subjects it is often congenital, and will be found to be caused by a high origin of the internal oblique muscle and a defect in its development.

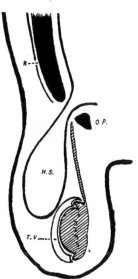

Fig. 447.—Sac of ordinary inguinal hernia.

H S., Hernial sac; T.V., tunica vaginalis; O.P., pubes; R, rectus muscle.

The progress of an inguinal hernia may be comparatively slow till it reaches the external abdominal ring, from which time the force of gravity favours its descent, and it rapidly enlarges, becoming "inguino-scrotal" (Fig. 446) or "inguino-labial" according to the sex of the patient. Where, however, the sac is that which has been described as "congenital vaginal" or "congenital funicular," the development of the hernia is in some cases actually immediate, the swelling appearing suddenly on some unusual expiratory effort.

On arriving at the scrotum, many of these hernias, especially in elderly subjects, attain an enormous size, and cause great discomfort owing to their weight and to the fact that the penis is frequently

2 *m*

retracted into the mass so as to disappear out of sight, micturition being thus rendered difficult. (Fig. 448.) Such hernias are usually quite irreducible, frequently become incarcerated, but are seldom strangulated, owing to the width of the neck of the sac. The skin over such scrotal hernias is frequently eczematous, excoriated, or even sloughy, owing to the dribbling of urine during micturition.

Direct inguinal hernia.— In this variety the hernia, in place of making its exit by the internal abdominal ring, leaves the abdomen *internally to the deep epigastric artery.* It thus enters the in-

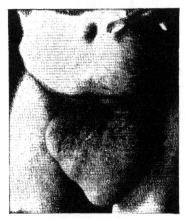

Fig. 448.—Scrotal hernia; cured by double-filigree method.

(*Author's case.*)

guinal canal through its posterior wall, carrying the stretched fibres of the conjoined tendon of the internal oblique and transversalis muscles with it. It then takes the same course as the oblique variety, passing into the scrotum or labium through the external abdominal ring. It is probably the only variety of hernia which can truly be said to be acquired, and even in some cases it, too, is possibly congenital in origin. The coverings of direct hernia are exactly similar to those of oblique, except that the cremasteric fascia of the latter is replaced by the conjoined tendon in the former, and that the term " infundibuliform " is not usually applied to the transversalis fascia here. The sac lies *posteriorly* to the spermatic cord, which it often separates widely by pressure.

The following characters of direct hernia differentiate it from oblique hernia : (1) It occurs at a later period of life. (2) It is slower in its development, less frequently becomes scrotal, and more often rises towards the pubic region. (3) The neck of the sac is wide, and the hernia is often a mere bulging. (4) It is much less liable to strangulation, and is as a rule reducible. (5) It more often contains small bowel, and not infrequently a portion of the bladder. (6) It much more frequently results in a very large gap in the abdominal wall, and consequently more cases require filigree-implantation for their cure. (7) It is more commonly bilateral. (8) From the first, one or more fingers may be passed directly back into the abdomen, whereas this can only be done in the case of oblique hernia of long standing and large dimensions, and rarely even then owing to irreducibility. (9) In thin subjects it is at times possible, with the finger in the ring, to feel the pulsation of the deep epigastric artery along the outer edge of the neck of the sac.

Symptoms and diagnosis of inguinal hernia.—In most cases subjective symptoms are entirely absent, and the patient is unaware of anything amiss until a swelling is accidentally found, or attention is directed to it by a medical man. Occasionally there is a feeling of dragging in the loin of that side, or actual shooting pain caused by the stretching of the fascial planes; this may be accompanied by nausea or actual retching, a small piece of omentum or a knuckle of bowel being nipped during sudden flexion of the thigh. There is also a sense of weakness and insecurity in the groin on coughing, which, even in patients ignorant of the presence or nature of a hernia, prompts them to support it by manual pressure. At times the presence of a varicocele at an unusual period of life may call attention to the trouble, or the patient may complain of gurgling in the region of the groin when making any expiratory effort.

When the hernia has reached the length of producing an obvious swelling in the groin and is reducible, the diagnosis is simple; thus, the reduction, on applying pressure, is rapid, and often accompanied by a gurgling sound if bowel be present; if the tips of the fingers be placed over the external abdominal ring, and the patient be directed to cough, a distinct impulse will be felt, which will be still more obvious if the little finger be passed gently into the ring by invaginating before its tip the skin of the scrotum. By careful palpation the swelling will be found to lie *above the level of Poupart's ligament*, and, if it has reached the external abdominal ring, *internally to the spine of the pubes*. The empty sac may also be felt as a thickening in the course of the cord.

Where the hernia is confined to the inguinal canal (i.e. a " bubonocele ") and is *irreducible*, there is more difficulty; it is then necessary to differentiate between hernia and the following inguinal swellings :—

(a) *Encysted hydrocele of the spermatic cord, or canal of Nuck.*—This is firm, elastic, usually of small size, dull to percussion, fixed in position, and not usually tender. Using a small frontal-sinus transillumination lamp, it will be found to be translucent; the intestine in infants, however, is also translucent.

(b) *Retained testis.*—Testes retained in the inguinal canal are practically always mobile; they retain their characteristic sensation of tenderness to pressure, and are nearly always in association with an unobliterated processus vaginalis.

(c) A *lipoma of the spermatic cord* is softer, more lobulated, and quite devoid of tenderness.

(d) A *fibroma of the inguinal canal* begins at the *inner end* of the canal, arising as a rule from the sheath of the rectus abdominis muscle, and is very fixed and hard ; it is painless, of slow growth, and of rare occurrence.

(e) *Glandular swellings* may be recognized by their marked lobulation, association with other such swellings, rapid increase in size, and tendency to break down, and by the rarity with which single glands are affected here.

(f) For the differentiation from *femoral hernia, see* p. 598.

When the hernia is scrotal, the diagnosis is again easy except in some cases of old-standing hydrocele of the vaginal process, in which reduction of the fluid is accomplished only gradually, and the walls are too thick to allow of translucency. The following points will help : The mass is dull to percussion ; this means either fluid, omentum, or incarceration. Fluid gives a smooth, tense, heavy tumour, which in this case will reduce very slowly, and as slowly return, and which will often give a characteristic " thrill " to one hand when flicked smartly by the finger of the other. Omentum is rarely reducible in large hernias, is always lobulated, and seldom tense. Incarceration produces constitutional disturbance, and has the characters already described (*see* p. 591).

At times it may be difficult to diagnose the presence of a hydrocele of the tunica vaginalis when in association with an irreducible omental scrotal hernia, if both are of long standing. There is, however, generally a slight constriction to be felt between the two, but the question is not one of much practical importance. Such a case is shown in Fig. 459.

From hydrocele of a hernial sac, or from a large vaginal hydrocele, a hernia may be diagnosed by the fact that in the former conditions the swelling is localized to the lower two-thirds of the scrotum, is tense, elastic, heavy, painless, dull to percussion, devoid of tenderness, often translucent, and by the cord being distinctly felt for a space between the upper end of the swelling and the external abdominal ring.

Femoral hernia.—All structures which leave the abdomen to pass into the limbs or abdominal wall carry with them for a short space an investment from the transversalis fascia which lines the abdomen, and which is gradually lost on their surface. In the case of the femoral vessels this investment, known as the " crural or femoral sheath," is well marked, and is constituted by a downward prolongation of the transversalis fascia in front and the iliacus fascia behind. It forms a funnel-shaped passage which is subdivided into three compartments by two fascial partitions. The outer of these contains the femoral artery, the middle contains the femoral vein, and the inner, which is known as the femoral or crural canal, is unoccupied save for a lymphatic gland and a small plug of extraperitoneal fat. It is along this inner canal that the contents of a femoral or crural hernia descend. Its mouth is known as the " crural ring."

The anterior wall of the canal formed by transversalis fascia is covered by the falciform "ligament," derived from the iliac portion of the fascia lata, whilst behind the posterior wall (formed of iliacus fascia) passes the pubic portion of the fascia lata. The outer wall is the septum between the canal and the femoral vein, whilst to the inner side of the inner wall lies Gimbernat's ligament above and the pectineus muscle below (internally and posteriorly). Overlying the lower end of the canal is the saphenous "opening" in the fascia lata of the thigh ; this is closed by the cribriform fascia, which transmits some lymphatics and veins. The "crural ring" is closed by a thick mass of areolar and often fatty tissue, the septum crurale. The immediate relations of this ring are as follows :—

Internally : Gimbernat's ligament, the little, sharp-edged, triangular band of fascia which fills in the pubic angle between the inner end of Poupart's ligament and the horizontal ramus of the pubes. *Externally :* The femoral vein. *Anteriorly :* Poupart's ligament. *Posteriorly :* The horizontal ramus of the pubes.

In the course of its descent, a femoral hernia, leaving the abdomen through the crural ring, passes down to the bottom of the crural canal, and, taking the line of least resistance, passes forwards through the saphenous "opening" and appears as a swelling in the groin. In its passage, therefore, it acquires the following coverings, which are given in order of dissection, viz. (*a*) skin ; (*b*) superficial fascia ; (*c*) cribriform fascia ; (*d*) crural sheath ; (*e*) septum crurale ; (*f*) extraperitoneal fascia ; (*g*) sac of the hernia.

If Hamilton Russell's theory be accepted, the sac of a femoral hernia is always of congenital origin, and may occupy one of three positions ; this is due to the fact that the peritoneal process from which it is formed is, in the course of the growth of the limb-bud in the embryo, drawn out from the abdomen along the line of the vessels proceeding from the femoral artery. Thus at times the sac will be found passing inwards along the course of the external pudic, upwards along that of the superficial epigastric, or outwards following the superficial circumflex iliac artery. A compromise between the latter two positions is the more common, the sac passing out of the saphenous opening and then turning upwards and outwards to a position between the two latter vessels. At times more than one sac may be present ; this is said to be one of the chief causes of the recurrence of femoral hernia after operation, one of the sacs being overlooked at the time.

As regards frequency, femoral hernia is much more common in

women than in men, in the proportion of 6 to 1 ; it is, however, less common in women than inguinal hernia, and is usually met with at a rather more advanced age. The presence of a femoral hernia, owing to the depth of its origin, the receding angle of the groin, and the fact that it is rarely of large size, is frequently overlooked, and in stout patients its diagnosis is not always an easy matter. Its characteristic features are these : It is nearly always irreducible from the first ; the neck is always very narrow ; omentum is its usual content, bowel being rarely found in it except when strangulation reveals its presence ; owing to the narrowness of the neck, strangulation is frequent and severe, the chief element of danger being found in the presence of the resistant, knife-like edge of Gimbernat's ligament, which tends to cut into the surface of the distended bowel.

Diagnosis of femoral hernia. — 1. The resemblance of a femoral to an *inguinal hernia* may at times be very close on casual inspection ; the distinction, however, depends on the relationship of the neck of the sac to the spine of the pubis. On careful palpation, the spine will be found to lie externally to and below the neck of an inguinal, and above and internally to that of a femoral sac ; but, as the latter frequently passes upwards and overlies the inner third of Poupart's ligament and becomes to some extent fixed there, careful examination is at times required to differentiate these hernias. The femoral variety is most closely simulated by the inguinal bubonocele, but in the latter case reduction is effected by pressure directed backwards and outwards, whereas in the former the direction of pressure must be downwards ; very commonly the hernia is not capable of reduction at all. Again, an irreducible bubonocele cannot be moved in any direction, while a femoral hernia is often capable of being pushed downwards or laterally. On attempting to pull a femoral hernia upwards over Poupart's ligament, it will be found to have a firm anchorage at the saphenous opening, and the neck of the sac will be distinctly felt if the tips of the fingers are placed just over the opening and moved to and fro across it like the teeth of a saw. I have seen an irregular form of inguinal hernia following an attempt at radical cure, in which the sac descended *beneath* Poupart's ligament into the thigh, appearing at the saphenous opening ; such a condition can hardly be diagnosed from femoral hernia.

2. *Enlarged femoral glands* are generally distinguished by being (a) firmer and more lobulated ; (b) often discrete ; (c) commonly bilateral and in association with other glandular enlargements ; (d) if not bilateral, often dependent upon inflammatory conditions of the lower extremity ; (e) not accompanied by dragging sensations in the groin or loin ; (f) often movable in *any* direction, or, if fixed, lacking the definite " neck " above-mentioned ; (g) prone to a rapid enlarge-

ment, which is accompanied by signs of softening. At the same time they may coexist with a hernia, and in stout patients are often impossible to differentiate from that condition.

3. *Saphena varix* is easily distinguished by its cystic character, and by the fact that it can be readily emptied by pressure, and by compression of the vein below, the swelling refilling at once on the release of pressure even when the patient is in the supine position (when fluctuation can often be felt between vein and swelling). It is, further, almost always part of a general varicosity of the saphena vein.

4. *Aneurysm of the femoral artery* exhibits the characteristic expansile pulsation which can be arrested by pressure on the external iliac artery, when the swelling will be, in part at least, reduced without gurgling. It is, like saphena varix, cystic in character, and the swelling reappears on the release of pressure. The stethoscope will reveal the usual bruit of an aneurysm. It is important to recognize the *expansile* character of the impulse here, since tumours overlying the vessel (e.g. an omental hernia, or a mass of glands) may receive transmitted pulsation from it.

5. A *psoas abscess*, when presenting beneath Poupart's ligament, produces a swelling which, although appearing externally to the vessels, occupies much the same position and gives the same impulse on coughing as a femoral hernia. It lacks, however, the "neck," is cystic in character, is commonly associated with some tenderness or kyphosis of the lumbar spine, may be accompanied by wasting, and fluctuation can often be made out between the femoral swelling and that in the iliac fossa.

The most important points to remember with regard to femoral hernia are—(1) Its liability to early strangulation. (2) The danger of early ulceration of bowel when strangulated. (3) The close relationship to the bladder on the inner (a diverticulum from the latter often projecting into the sac), and to the femoral vein on the outer side. (4) The possible presence of the aberrant branch of the obturator artery, which may pass along the inner aspect of the neck of the sac, and be in danger of division during the operation of kelotomy (*see* Strangulated Hernia, p. 649).

The contents of a femoral are, for all practical purposes, the same as those of an inguinal hernia, except that large intestine is less frequently, and the urinary bladder more frequently, met with.[1]

Umbilical hernia.—Except when congenital in origin, this

---

[1] Brunner's and Maydl's statistics would seem to show a greater frequency of the bladder in *inguinal* hernias; the bladder is more often seen as a simple bulging in inguinal hernia, but as a true diverticulum projecting into the sac it is commoner in femoral hernia.

form of hernia is rarely seen before middle life, and is much commoner after than before 40. Like femoral hernia, it is almost confined
to the female sex, and especially to women who have borne many
children and have become obese.

Six points especially characterize umbilical hernia : (1) Its markedly
progressive tendency. Unlike the forms already mentioned, there is
almost no limit to the size which it may attain, and sacs are occasionally met with containing more than half the intestinal contents of the
abdomen. (2) The tendency to
widespread loculation of the
sac. (3) The extensive and
rapid formation of adhesions,
leading to (4) early irreducibility. (5) The proneness to,
and dangerous na-
ture of, strangula-
tion here. (6) The
difficulty of accom-
plishing a radical
cure.

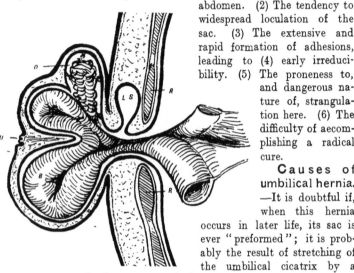

Fig. 449.—Umbilical hernia, showing
sacculation in superficial fascia
(transverse section).

L.S., Lateral sacculus ; B., bowel ; O., omentum ;
R., rectus muscle ; U., umbilicus.

Causes of
umbilical hernia.
—It is doubtful if,
when this hernia
occurs in later life, its sac is
ever " preformed " ; it is probably the result of stretching of
the umbilical cicatrix by a
gradual increase of intra-
abdominal pressure, or by the
long-continued intermittent increase of such pressure. Thus
it is most commonly seen as
the result of (a) repeated pregnancy ; (b) general obesity in women
about the menopause ; (c) accumulation of ascitic fluid ; (d) the
repeated strain thrown on the abdominal wall by the constant
coughing of chronic bronchitis and emphysema.

Clinical features of umbilical hernia.—At first there may be
nothing seen externally, and the patient's attention may be drawn
to the trouble owing to dragging pain at the umbilicus, often accompanied by nausea and flatulent distension of the abdomen. There may
be tenderness in the umbilical region, and frequently the symptoms are increased by the act of lying down, the explanation being
that if the omentum happens to be adherent at this point and the

stomach full, the supine position results in a falling back of the latter and a dragging upon the former. Where such a "blind hernia" is present, it may in a very stout patient become strangulated without the external evidence of a swelling to assist the diagnosis. Owing to the thickness and the loose character of the subcutaneous and extraperitoneal fat layers, the expansion of the hernial contents causes the sac to bulge in various directions along the lines of least resistance into either or both of these layers (but especially into the former). The result is that in small hernias the swelling is hidden in the fat, while in large ones there is produced a two-storied and complicated arrangement of secondary sac-culi, radiating from the central passage which represents the original sac (Fig. 449). If, then, the hernia commences by the protrusion of a lateral sacculus into the extraperi-toneal, or into the deep portion of the subcutaneous layer, a "blind hernia" is produced (Fig. 450).

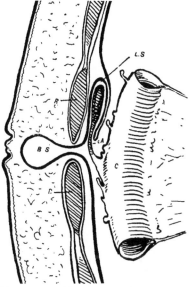

Fig. 450.—"Blind hernia" of umbilicus; appendix epiploica occupying lateral sacculus (transverse section).

B.S., "Blind" sac; L.S., lateral sacculus; A., appendix epiploica; C., colon; R., rectus muscle.

More commonly there will be noticed at the umbilicus a slight protrusion which transmits an impulse on coughing. In the early stages, at least, it can always be easily reduced, and the sharp edges of the ring can then be felt.

. At a later period these hernias may assume gigantic proportions, spreading out on either side on the abdomen in an ill-defined and lobulated mass, or projecting directly forwards, with a tendency, by their own weight, to sink down and overhang the pubes (Fig. 451).

At an early stage the sac becomes adherent to the coverings—peritoneum, aponeuroses, and skin being welded into one layer; later, as distension increases, these coverings become thinned out, so that the intestinal movements may be observed through them. At the same time, extensive adhesions are formed between the contents themselves (the omentum being chiefly involved) and the sac walls. In very large pendulous hernias the skin at the most dependent part is often reddened, chronically inflamed and œdematous, and sometimes shows desquamation or ulceration; whilst a broad band of intertrigo

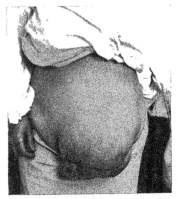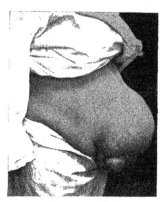

Fig. 451.—Large umbilical hernia, before operation.
(*Same case* as in Fig. 452.)

Front and side views.

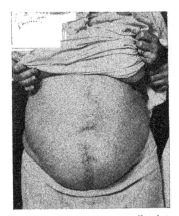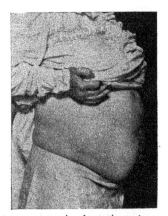

Fig. 452.—Large umbilical hernia cured by implantation of filigree measuring 9 in. × 5 in. (*Author's case.*)

Front and side views.

appears at the lower edge of the hernial neck. Cases are reported of fæcal fistulæ resulting from such ulceration opening into bowel in the sac.

The contents of these hernias are usually omentum and transverse colon, but small intestine is common, and stomach may be encountered. Reduction is seldom possible in long-standing cases, owing to the sacculation already mentioned, and when strangulation occurs the prognosis is bad owing to the obesity of the patient and the pulmonary complications frequently associated with it.

The discomfort induced by a large umbilical hernia may be very great; apart from the constant drag on the abdominal contents, the weight to be supported, the interference with clothing, and the unsightliness of the patient's figure, there is constant liability to attacks of colic, nausea, constipation, or actual incarceration of the hernia. Little can be done to relieve these troubles except by operation, and the risk of this is, in very stout patients, considerable.

Congenital umbilical hernia.—It is customary to apply this term to hernia at the navel in infants and young children when it occurs in the first few months of life. Two forms of it are described. In one there is intestine present in the umbilical cord at birth, *retraction not yet having taken place*. Here the umbilicus is represented by a circular gap, the spread-out membranes of the cord covering the loop of intestine, and fusing with the skin at the margins of the gap. In such a case, these avascular amniotic membranes may become gangrenous or may rupture, leaving a factitious ectopia of the viscera; in most cases of this kind death results from septic peritonitis. If the membranes retain their integrity sufficiently long to permit of the retraction of the bowel, the aperture may close, but, the cicatrix being weak, a hernia may develop at the site of closure at a later date. In the other form of this hernia there is complete retraction of the bowel at the time of birth, but the sound *closure of the aperture is delayed*. In such cases there will be a bulging of the degenerate skin at the umbilicus on any expiratory effort, and subsequently from lack of treatment, or from improper treatment, a large hernia may develop. To this variety the term "infantile" may be applied.

Although these hernias, when correctly treated, rarely give rise to serious trouble during infancy or adolescence, they do at times become strangulated. In any case, the cicatrix of a "delayed closure" is never so perfect as that of the normal umbilicus; a small peritoneal dimple, which must be regarded as a predisposing factor in the umbilical hernia of later life, frequently remains to mark the site on the visceral surface of the parietes.

Ventral hernia.—This may be spontaneous or acquired, the latter being very much the commoner. Apart from umbilical hernia, which is only a special form of ventral hernia, protrusions of viscera may occur in the middle line above that point (median epigastric hernia), or below it (median hypogastric hernia), or may occupy the entire length of the linea alba (complete median hernia). They may also occur at other points in the abdominal wall, but in this case they are invariably traumatic and are known as "lateral ventral hernias."

Spontaneous hernia (median) is rarely seen except in association with large umbilical hernias, where it is usually an extension *downwards* of the rupture, the lower segment of the umbilical ring having given way and the recti muscles having become separated. Above the umbilicus it is more often separate, and is sufficiently rare to suggest the possibility of a congenital origin ; and this is supported by the fact that it is not usually seen in stout patients, and is not, therefore, the direct result of distension. It is perhaps less rare in men than in women.

The presence of subperitoneal lipomas has been noted in many instances, and is found to be a causative factor in some cases of ventral hernia, more especially of the median epigastric variety. Insinuating themselves into some slight deficiency in the transversalis fascia, or the fascia of the posterior sheath of the rectus muscle, these small tumours gradually expand the cavity which they have invaded, and by their traction at times draw after them the process of peritoneum to which they are attached. Thus a true hernial sac is formed. These hernias are also found occasionally in the linea semilunaris, and many femoral hernias probably owe their origin to the presence of the lipomatous material in the crural canal.

Complete median hernia results from wide separation of the recti muscles, and is more frequently seen in thin women who have borne many children than in those who are markedly obese ; it is also seen in elderly men of feeble muscular development who have been subjected to hard manual labour. Although rarely sufficiently marked to require operative interference, it is none the less in the nature of a hernia, and may result in considerable weakness and bodily discomfort. It extends usually from the ensiform cartilage to the pubes, the actual extent being easily ascertained by making the patient raise the head and shoulders from the supine position without the support of the hands. The hernia will at once show as an elevated ridge along the linea alba, the actual gap being felt by passing the ulnar edge of the hand into it. .

It is probable that this condition originates in a congenital wideness of the linea alba, and is only aggravated by subsequent exertion, as many young subjects are met with who exhibit wide separation without actual hernia. Adhesions, irreducibility, and strangulation are never met with in this form of hernia, although they occur in the epigastric variety.

Hernia through scar tissue.—Space does not permit of a discussion of the pathology of these hernias, but the following points should be noted :—

1. Hernia never occurs through the *muscular wall* of the abdomen except as the result of its conversion at some point into scar tissue.

2. This may occur as the result of suppuration or ulceration, transverse division of the muscular fibres with subsequent stretched union, destruction by disease, or extensive division of the nerves supplying the muscles.

3. The whole thickness of the abdominal wall being converted into scar tissue, there is no true sac ; all the layers are welded together and the contents are invariably adherent, often densely so.

4. Owing to the alteration in structure of the muscle fibres, and to the fact that only by the primary union of healthy muscle can such a hernia be prevented from recurring, these hernias are particularly difficult to cure, and often necessitate extensive and difficult plastic operations.

5. Where approximation of the above nature cannot be accomplished, recurrence can only be prevented by converting the distensible cicatrix into material which cannot stretch (*see* Bartlett's Method, p. 629).

6. The period requisite for the formation of a fully organized cicatrix produced by a primary union is probably not less than forty to sixty days.

Such a hernia may follow the cicatricial weakening of any part of the abdominal wall either by accident, by disease, or by inadequacy of suturing of operative wounds—whether due to faulty technique or to the character of the operation, as in drainage of abscesses or of the gall-bladder.

However produced, traumatic ventral hernia is, like umbilical hernia, constantly progressive, crippling to the patient, and difficult to repair ; it is not amenable, as a rule, to any form of truss or belt. In spite of the extensive adhesions found in the sac, possibly because of them, strangulation is seldom seen, the excursions of the contents being very limited.

Lumbar hernia.—A hernia appearing through the lateral aspect of the abdomen—that is, between the iliac crest and the last rib—is known as lumbar. It is by no means common, and much doubt exists as to the etiology of those cases which are not definitely traumatic. In some cases it is apparently congenital, depending on defects in the musculature, or on absence of the last rib ; in others it follows the development of abscesses arising in the muscular wall or in connexion with caries of the twelfth rib ; the commonest form, however, is that which follows stretching of the scar resulting from operations upon the kidneys, especially where prolonged drainage has been employed. The congenital form may appear in two different situations, viz. (a) behind the posterior axillary line and just beneath the last rib, and (b) anteriorly to that line and immediately above the crest of the ilium. The upper of these hernial sites is the less common of the two; it is the position frequently occupied by a lumbar abscess, and from this it must be diagnosed, since both hernia and abscess are elastic, reducible to some extent, and give an impulse on coughing.

The lower hernial site is that which is known as " Petit's triangle " ; it is bounded below by the crest of the ilium, in front by the posterior margin of the external oblique muscle, and behind by the anterior margin of the latissimus dorsi muscle. The hernia is rarely more than a slight bulging, and only when there is a distinct deficiency in the extent of origin of these muscles can the triangle be said to exist. Where hernia follows operations upon the kidneys the bulging will occupy the whole space between the ilium and the last rib. Owing to the transverse division of the muscle fibres in these operations, the difficulty of approximation, and the frequent necessity for drainage, this hernia, when it occurs, is extensive and very disabling.

Of whatever variety, lumbar hernia rarely contains anything but omentum and ascending or descending colon; the sac resembles that of other ventral hernias, being ultimately incorporated with the integuments. Operative treatment is only called for in cases of hernia of large dimensions following operations on the loins, and may then present considerable difficulty.

The following four varieties of hernia are of sufficient rarity to merit being considered as pathological curiosities.

1. Obturator hernia.—The protrusion in this case occurs through the small obturator canal, the insignificant aperture existing at the upper and anterior part of the obturator foramen for the passage of the obturator vessels and nerve. Always of great rarity, it is commoner in women than in men, and owes its importance to its danger and the difficulty of its diagnosis. The hernial contents, which are most frequently intestinal (less commonly the colon and pelvic organs), in their passage through the canal have the obturator nerve external to and above them, and, arriving outside the pelvis, are covered by the pectineus muscle. The hernia may never go beyond this point, and is very liable to immediate strangulation on its first escape. It may, however, pass on downwards, forwards, and inwards, and arrive at the space between the adductor longus and the femoral vessels. Here it may at times be felt as a rounded swelling rather deeply situated, and may be confounded with a femoral hernia ; but it is always less mobile, has no palpable neck, and occupies a position rather more internal than the latter.

The diagnosis of obturator hernia is always difficult, so much so that it is not infrequently only made in the post-mortem room. Strangulation is usually the first symptom, and in the absence of any swelling at any of the hernial rings the condition may be found at an exploratory laparotomy; but the relation of the hernia to the obturator nerve, which it often compresses, may give rise to pain referred to the hip- or knee-joints, or along the inner side of the thigh and knee, or even the calf. Localized tenderness internal to the femoral vessels in the presence of signs of obstruction should suggest the possibility of this condition. It should not be forgotten that in this hernia especially, as in the two following varieties, a portion of the lateral aspect of the bowel only may be involved (Richter's hernia), and therefore the signs of obstruction may not be complete, flatus passing, and even fæces at times.

2, 3. **Gluteal and sciatic hernia.**—In the region of the buttock there are three apertures through which a hernia may escape from the pelvis, viz. (1) the great sacro-sciatic notch, above the pyriformis muscle; (2) the same, below that muscle (these two hernias are known as gluteal); and (3) the lesser sacro-sciatic notch, when the hernia is known as sciatic. All of these hernias are of very rare occurrence, and, like obturator hernia, are usually only met with when strangulated. But they *may* be recognized whilst still simply irreducible, or even in rare cases reducible; and in such cases the swelling which is felt in the gluteal region or, in the case of the sciatic hernia, just at or below the gluteal fold, must be differentiated from that produced by a subfascial lipoma, a chronic abscess in connexion with the hip- or the sacro-iliac joint, an aneurysm of the gluteal or sciatic vessels, or cysts or other tumours of this region.

Pressure of the hernia on the sciatic nerve may cause local tenderness or deep-seated pain down the back of the thigh, and thus suggest sciatica; or in the case of the gluteal hernia there may be pain referred to the hip-joint. Owing to the thickness of the coverings an impulse on coughing is rarely felt, and for the same reason absence of pulsation does not entirely obscure the possibility of aneurysm. In aneurysm, however, throbbing pain may be present, and, although this might suggest an acute abscess, the absence of constitutional symptoms and the duration of the tumour without rapid increase in size would negative the diagnosis. Lipomas are commonly devoid of pain or tenderness, and are of such size as to render a mistake improbable, at least as regards hernia. Cold abscesses not in connexion with joints or bone disease are also painless and definitely fluctuating; otherwise they are only part of a condition giving rise to definite symptoms. The following points should be remembered :—

(1) All gluteal swellings of doubtful origin should be exposed by open incision.

(2) Puncture by exploring needles should be avoided owing to the possibility of aneurysm or hernia.

(3) The possibility of the existence of these rare hernias should never be forgotten in obscure cases of intestinal obstruction.

(4) Strangulation is usually tight and the mortality high, therefore no time should be lost in clearing up the diagnosis.

These hernias may contain any of the organs commonly found in inguinal or femoral sacs, and are less frequently seen in children than in adults ; and the sexes appear to be equally affected.

4. Perineal hernia.—This is rare. Protrusions are seen (a) to one side or other of the perineum in the male, or in either labium in the female ; (b) in the ischio-rectal fossæ, or (c) through the lateral vaginal wall.

Passing between the fibres of the levator ani muscle, these hernias invariably carry before them a covering of the peritoneum and the pelvic fascia. They are of commoner occurrence in the female—owing probably to the greater width of the pelvis, the presence of the vagina, and the great strain imposed upon the pelvic floor by childbirth—and are especially prone to

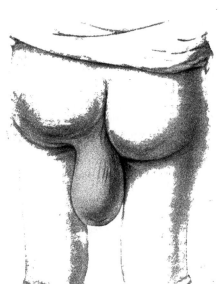

Fig. 453.—Subperitoneal fibroma simulating perineal hernia.

(From 'Annals of Surgery.')

occur after rupture of the perineum. Lacerated wounds may originate them, and of these I have met with two cases, one following a deep wound from a broken chamber utensil, and the other a fall on a wooden paling.

The diagnosis is not always easy, since these hernias are frequently closely simulated by pedunculated subperitoneal fibromas (Figs. 453 and 454). Such tumours are commonly, as in my case, easily reducible, soft, elastic, associated with a definite ring to be felt in the pelvic floor, and give a marked impulse on coughing. These fibromas may, indeed, by their weight and traction originate a perineal hernia. Perineal hernia has been seen following trans-sacral excision of the rectum. A cold abscess of the ischio-rectal fossa, originating in disease of the tuber ischii, the ilium, or even the spine, may also simulate this condition.

As, however, perineal hernias almost always contain intestine, the resonance on percussion and the gurgling on reduction should indicate the diagnosis. Bowel has been opened on one occasion in mistake

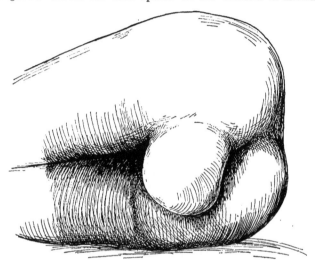

Fig. 454.—Perineal myxo-fibroma simulating hernia.

(*Author's case.*)

for an abscess, and excised in another in mistake for a polypoid vaginal tumour. As the bladder may easily be contained in a perineal hernia, the question should be determined by the use of a sound, the beak being turned downwards into the sac, while it is palpated from without. Frequency of micturition, desire accompanied by inability to perform the act, or the presence of constantly turbid urine should suggest the possibility of the presence of the bladder. When appearing in the vagina these hernias suggest at first sight the occurrence of a cyst or an abscess of the vaginal wall, until they are found to be reducible.

These hernias rarely, if ever, become strangulated, but are very diffi-cult to cure, and are very crippling, from the feeling of insecurity which characterizes them.

Interstitial hernia.—In certain cases of inguinal hernia, espe-cially those of the oblique variety, there is an irregularity of the sac,

2 *n*

which consists in the development of lateral diverticula in, or even of a complete congenital displacement of the whole sac into, the planes of the abdominal wall. Such hernias are known as interstitial or interparietal, and are in more than half the cases in association with maldevelopment or arrested descent of the testis (Fig. 455). The following are the varieties most commonly met with, in the order of frequency :—

1. Patent processus vaginalis in scrotum, with lateral diverticulum lying between—
    (a) Peritoneum and transversalis fascia (properitoneal).
    (b) Internal oblique muscle and external oblique aponeurosis.
    (c) Transversalis fascia and muscle.
    (d) Peritoneum and iliacus fascia (retroperitoneal).
2. Processus vaginalis absent from scrotum and sac found lying between—
    (a) External oblique aponeurosis and skin.
    (b) Peritoneum and iliacus fascia.

Many variations of the above may be met with, and at times more than one diverticulum may be present.

It is quite obvious that these hernias are all dependent upon some congenital abnormality. Their chief importance lies in the possibility of the lateral sac being overlooked in the performance of a radical operation ; in the chance of reduction being effected from one diverticulum into another ; and in the occurrence of strangulation in these diverticula. The intimate union of the transversalis with the internal oblique muscle renders the occurrence of a diverticulum between these muscles very rare, although such cases have been recorded. Interstitial hernia has been attributed to forcible and oft-repeated clumsy efforts at reduction ; this is a mistaken theory. Such attempts could only lead, where no diverticulum is present, to displacement of the *whole* sac, or rupture of its neck. These cases come under the heading of " Reduction *en masse* " (p. 645), and are not true interstitial hernias. The danger of strangulation in interstitial hernias is considerable, and only occasionally is their presence diagnosed before operation. Some bulging of the abdominal wall above and outside the internal abdominal ring may be noticed, or it may be possible to feel the diverticulum fill up, on reduction being effected from the scrotum ; this latter being then kept empty, the diverticulum may be detected by gurgling, or sudden emptying, on reduction of its contents being effected.

The abnormalities which have been noted in association with these hernias are—(1) Retention, maldevelopment, and ectopia of the testis. (2) Absence of the cremaster muscle. (3) Superimposition of the abdominal rings. (4) Partial obliteration of the external abdominal ring.

Umbilical hernia is so constantly associated with diverticulation of the sac that it cannot be considered as an irregular hernia, nor as interstitial, although the diverticula are at times found both between the peritoneum and the posterior sheath of the rectus muscle, and between the anterior sheath and the superficial fascia.

Traumatic interstitial hernia.—This is the result of ruptures or pathological lesions of the abdominal wall in which only the deeper layers have been affected; it is consequently a very rare condition. It has been seen following rupture of a section of the rectus muscle. Such a case occurred in my own practice; the bowel was found between the muscle and its anterior sheath, the rupture having taken place between the two lower lineæ transversæ on the left side. Deep-seated gummata or chronic abscesses which have resolved under treatment may result in the formation of such a hernia. However they are produced, they can remain interstitial only for a time; in course of years the coverings become thinned out, fused together, and amalgam-ated with the sac, and their interstitial character is thus to a great extent lost.

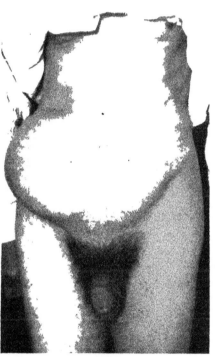

Fig. 455.—Interstitial hernia and retained testis.

(*Author's case.*)

The diagnosis is not usually difficult; an elastic, hyper-resonant swelling, exhibiting intestinal gurgling, in the substance of the abdominal wall can hardly be mistaken for anything else than hernia. If the sac contains only omentum the case is not so obvious, for, impulse being probably absent owing to adhesions, the lobulation and doughiness of the mass might suggest a lipoma or other form of tumour.

Partial enterocele (Richter's hernia).—Occasionally a portion only of the lateral wall of the bowel may protrude through a hernial ring, or through some adventitious opening (Fig. 456). The ileum is the part most commonly affected, and though the site of the hernia may be very various, the condition is most often seen at the femoral ring. A rare form of hernia, it is said to be more frequent in women than in men, and in adults than in children. The hernia is always small in size, being rarely larger than a marble, and the ring, wherever it may be, is always narrow ; thus strangulation is commonly the first evidence of the trouble. Its chief importance lies in the fact that the strangulation fails to give rise to two of its cardinal signs, viz. complete obstruction and fæcal vomiting. The entire lumen of the bowel not being involved in the ring, flatus and fæces may continue to pass from time to time, and consequently fæcal vomiting may be absent. Therefore gangrene of the constricted portion may easily supervene before a diagnosis is reached. Reduction is rarely possible, and even when it is accomplished by operation, the constricted neck, which is on the antimesenteric aspect of the bowel, may be permanently altered by the development of cicatricial tissue in its wall, with the result that the herniated portion remains as a permanent diverticulum.

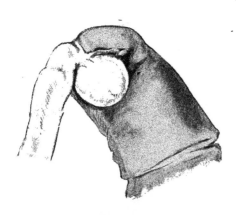

Fig. 456.—Richter's hernia.

(From Gould and Warren's " International Text-Book of Surgery.")

The hernia is rarely diagnosed ; the mortality is consequently high (60–65 per cent.), even when operation is undertaken. In some cases, however, gangrene has supervened and a spontaneous recovery has resulted, leaving the patient with a fæcal fistula into the scrotum, or at the groin or umbilicus.

Hernia of Meckel's diverticulum (Littré's hernia).— Although only differing from the last-mentioned variety in its embryonic origin, this hernia must be mentioned separately, since the lateral diverticulum is in this case the cause of the hernia and not the result.

Meckel's diverticulum, the unobliterated remains of the vitellointestinal duct, when present, springs from the antimesenteric aspect of the ileum, usually within 3 ft. of the ileo-cæcal valve, and is generally attached by a terminal narrow band to the umbilical site. Strictly speaking, therefore, it should be associated with umbilical hernia. Since, however, it may be found in the sacs of other hernias, it is given a special place, and the term has been loosely applied to any hernia in which the diverticulum is involved. The diverticulum varies from a mere prominence on the surface of the bowel to a tube 3 to 5 in. in length, with, at times, a diameter almost as great as the bowel from which it springs. Its strangulation therefore produces symptoms and results exactly similar to those of Richter's hernia, with the exception that when the diverticulum is well developed the operative treatment is simplified and the mortality is lessened.

Hernia in the absence of a sac. — Although it is hardly accurate to say that a hernia may occur without a sac, certain protrusions of viscera do occur uncovered, or only partially covered, by parietal peritoneum. In these cases a sac either has disappeared by an alteration in the position of the hernia, or can be found lying to one side of the main mass of the protrusion. Such instances are to be found in hernias of the cæcum, sigmoid, and bladder.

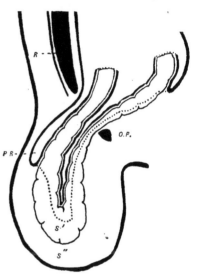

Fig. 457.—Extraperitoneal hernia of sigmoid.

o.p , Pubes ; R., rectus muscle ; p.r., peritoneal reflection ; s.', sigmoid colon ; s.'', scrotum.

Hernias of the cæcum and sigmoid frequently differ in no respect from other inguinal hernias, and these organs are of moderately common occurrence in large hernial sacs. But at times, especially in general enteroptosis (Glénard's disease), the cæcum and sigmoid descend from the iliac fossæ by a process of slipping of the iliac peritoneum (*hernie en glissade*), leaving the abdomen either as a direct or, much less commonly, as an indirect hernia. At first a sac is present, but later, as the hernia enlarges, the peritoneum of which it was composed assumes a more and more anterior position, the bowel coming down from behind it. Ultimately only a partial sac is to be found in front and high up, the bowel itself forming the posterior and inferior wall of the sac (Fig. 457). Some of these cases, supposed to be congenital, are conjecturally attributed to overaction of the gubernaculum testis, but elongation of the mesentery and enteroptosis furnishes a better explanation.

Hernia of the bladder.—The bladder is occasionally met with projecting into the sacs of inguinal or femoral hernias ; at other times it is seen, especially in the direct form of inguinal hernia in elderly subjects, with prostatic obstruction or pulmonary diatheses, and in the perineal and pudendal hernias, presenting as a bulging fleshy mass quite uncovered by peritoneum. In such cases great care must be exercised not to mistake it for a thick-walled sac. The presence of loose muscular fibres running in various directions and of large veins on its surface should be noticed, and any doubt as to its character cleared up by the passage of a rigid bougie, the beak of the instrument being turned into the protrusion. The nature of the hernia may be suspected when, in such patients, a history is obtained of the swelling being more marked before, and less prominent after, micturition. The chief characteristics of hernias which lack a peritoneal sac are those of irreducibility and liability to incarceration ; this applies especially to hernias of the cæcum and sigmoid.

TREATMENT OF HERNIA IN GENERAL

The following points must be considered, bearing in mind that only two methods are available, viz. palliative and operative, and that only the latter is *curative*.

Age. Infancy. — Hernia has occasionally been cured spontaneously in quite young children. In most cases it is *not* cured, for, although apparently so, it frequently reappears in early adult life. The difficulty of treating young children by palliative means is considerable, for the following reasons : (1) Their restlessness and irritability and constant crying tend to force the rings open and shift the truss. (2) Their skins are tender, and in the poorer classes are easily excoriated by the accumulation of dirt and sweat beneath the truss. (3) Constant increase in size demands a relay of fresh trusses. (4) The tissues are so delicate that the perpetual pressure of a truss probably does more harm than good. (5) The ignorance of the mothers in the poorer classes, and the question of expense, result in the treatment being improperly and intermittently applied.

The objections to operation during infancy are the possibility of spontaneous cure, the delicacy and weakness of the tissues, and the danger of fatality or of sepsis.

In **young adults** a hernia can only be cured by operation. The surgeon's decision will be influenced by the following factors :—

1. The well-known progressive tendency of hernia.

2. The influence of hard manual labour on the one hand, and of sedentary occupation on the other ; both of which conditions favour the growth of a hernia.

3. The constant danger of strangulation.

4. The influence now exerted by the Employers' Liability Act, which makes it very difficult for any man who is ruptured to obtain employment.

5. The greater prospect of permanent cure the earlier the operation is undertaken. The longer the hernia has been in existence the less this prospect can be entertained, at least so far as the ordinary methods of operating are concerned.

In old age.—At the age of 50 and over, hernias tend to become very large and the tissues much degenerated, and, although operation is still capable of curing many of these patients, the risk to life and the difficulties of the operation are greater, while the ordinary form of operation is useless, recurrence being the general rule. In such cases the use of my double-filigree operation (p. 622) is strongly advisable.

PALLIATIVE TREATMENT OF HERNIA

This consists essentially in (a) the reduction of the hernia, and (b) the application of some form of truss to prevent its re-descent.

In the earlier stages of hernia the saccular contents return to the abdomen, by their own weight, on the patient lying down. Later on, for reasons already given, there is some delay in the process, and manual pressure is required to effect the reduction ; even this may at first fail, and the return may only be accomplished after some hours of recumbency, with or without the use of the ice-bag and the Trendelenburg position, both of which tend to empty the vessels of the omentum and reduce the size of the swelling.

Reduction by manipulation.—The patient is placed in the recumbent position, the thighs are flexed upon the abdomen to relax the abdominal muscles, and, in the case of inguinal and femoral hernia, are rotated inwards to relax the fascia of the thigh and the neck of the sac. The latter is then grasped by the hand in such a way as to straighten out the body of the sac, while with the other hand pressure is evenly applied to the fundus, gently but firmly, in such a manner as to favour the return first of that portion of the contents occupying the neck, following which the contents of the fundus will usually slip back easily. In the case of omentum alone, the sudden flaccidity of the sac will indicate the completion of the process, while in that of bowel the characteristic gurgle of air and fluid will be both felt and heard at the moment of reduction.

Gentleness is most essential in these manipulations, since roughness or clumsy force, if the hernia is difficult of reduction, can only result in pain to the patient ; in bruising and inflammation of the sac and its contents, thus producing early irreducibility ; and possibly even in rupture of the sac, " reduction *en masse*," and strangulation. On no account should force replace patience and skill.

At times a hernia may be irreducible simply from the fact that any attempt at reduction is resisted by the patient, owing to griping pains, the abdominal muscles being involuntarily contracted at each attempt ; this difficulty may be overcome by making the patient keep the mouth wide open and instructing him to breathe deeply and not to hold his breath. This failing, a general anæsthetic or, preferably, spinal analgesia may be employed, the muscular relaxation provided by this latter method being very marked.

The direction of pressure during reduction will vary with the position of the sac. In umbilical hernia it should be directly backwards, but these hernias are so commonly irreducible at an early date that, when they do not reduce spontaneously, little success is to be expected from manipulations. The direction in inguinal hernia should be upwards and outwards towards the iliac spine. In femoral hernia it will depend much on the direction of the fundus of the sac. This reduction is always more difficult to effect owing to the tendency of the sac to turn upwards to Poupart's ligament, the narrowness of the canal, and the sharp edges of the saphenous opening and Gimbernat's ligament, besides which the sac cannot be lifted in the hand as in the case of inguinal hernia. In most cases the pressure must be in a downward and inward direction.

The dangers of using undue force are dealt with under " Reduction *en masse* " (p. 645).

Treatment by truss.—The disadvantages of trusses are as follows :—

1. They do not *cure* any hernia (a very small proportion in quite young infants possibly excepted).

2. They are inconvenient and often uncomfortable.

3. They are costly for poor patients, who, as a rule, soon wear them out.

4. They are frequently badly fitted or not fitted at all.

5. In a few years the hernia, growing larger, overcomes the truss.

6. Their pressure tends to thin out and mat together the underlying tissues, rendering any future operation much more difficult and the chances of cure much more remote.

7. In young children a constant change of truss is necessary, to ensure accuracy of fit at different ages.

8. Although useless and dangerous in irreducible hernias, they are often applied to these by ignorant patients.

If used, the truss must fulfil the following conditions : it must fit the patient ; be neither too strong nor too weak in the spring ; be of a pattern intended for the variety of hernia under treatment ; and only be applied in the recumbent position *after* the hernia has been reduced

For a description of the numerous forms of truss the reader is referred to the surgical instrument-makers' catalogues. · The most popular variety is the circular spring truss ; a modification of this with a prolonged perineal pad, known as the "rat-tail" truss, is sometimes more efficient for large inguino-scrotal hernias. The "Moc-main" truss gives more with the movements of the body, but is readily damaged.

· For inguinal hernias in children the best forms are the india-rubber horseshoe-shaped truss and the woollen-skein truss. The former is the better, but is expensive, for new ones must be bought as the child grows, and the rubber deteriorates on the moist skin of a young child and may cause irritation. The skein is applied as follows : A thick skein of undyed berlin wool is passed round the waist from behind forwards ; the end on the side of the hernia is threaded through its fellow and drawn taut, so that the crossing lies immediately over the inguinal canal. With the child in the recumbent position the hernia is reduced, a cotton-wool pad placed beneath the crossing, and the free end of the skein carried back through the perineum and fixed to the girdle portion just to the outer side of the sacro-iliac joint. The skein should not be removed in the bath, but replaced by a dry one afterwards.

For umbilical hernia in an infant a binder over a pad is sufficient ; no pad small enough to enter the umbilical ring must be used. Nothing is better than a leaden disc covered with lint or cotton-wool and sewn to the binder.

Indications for use of a truss.—Unless there is some definite contra-indication to operation, the surgeon will do well to advise a radical cure at any age. Trusses may, however, be advisable in infants under 18 months of age, in patients refusing operation or out of reach of surgical assistance, in those in whom any surgical interference is contra-indicated, e.g. in the victims of hæmophilia, diabetes, or nephritis, and sometimes in very old people. The *characters of a well-fitting truss* should be as follows : (1) The spring should lie closely to the pelvis without undue pressure at any point. (2) It should control the hernia when the patient, standing with legs wide apart and thighs everted, and stooping so as to rest his hands on his knees, exerts his full expiratory force. (3) The pad should be soft and elastic, and rather flat. (4) The pad should fall not on the external abdominal ring, but on the whole length of the inguinal canal.

OPERATIVE TREATMENT

The principles governing a true radical cure are—(1) complete removal of the sac; (2) closure of the hernial aperture; and (3) the production of an unstretchable cicatrix.

In some cases the first of these will suffice, but in most cases all three are required, and in a few the last is the most essential.

Indications for operation.—Some form of operation is especially indicated in—(1) patients between the ages of 18 months and 65 years; (2) all wage-earning workmen (in view of the Employers' Liability Act); (3) married women, or women about to marry; (4) patients going out of reach of surgical help; (5) where the hernia is irreducible; (6) where there have been signs of strangulation; (7) where there is a gradual increase in size; (8) where the hernia is associated with an undescended testis; (9) where a truss, having been worn, no longer controls the hernia.

As regards *contra-indications*, it may be said that since the introduction of filigree implantation these have been greatly reduced in number. It is open to question whether the operation is desirable in patients over the age of 65, and the physical condition of the patient must be the determining factor here. In hernias of such gigantic size that the return of the abdominal contents presents a serious risk of paralytic ileus, operation should not be attempted without serious consideration. In cases of hæmophilia, diabetes, albuminuria of pathological origin, and severe anæmia, operation is definitely contra-indicated.

Chief factors tending to a successful result.—Although many minor points must be considered, the success of a hernial operation largely depends on observance of the following conditions :—

1. **Complete obliteration of the sac and its diverticula.** —This is considered by some surgeons to be the chief essential of the operation, and in quite young children it is so to a great extent, but it cannot be admitted in the case of adults. In them the long-continued presence of the hernial contents has widened and stretched the ring, and converted much of the sound muscular tissue into fibrous material. Further, the presence of lateral sacculi, especially in femoral hernia, must be remembered, since, if overlooked, the reappearance of the hernia may be accounted as a recurrence when it is only an evidence of faulty technique.

2. **Avoidance of tension in suturing.**—Neglect of this precaution will result in the rapid cutting out of the deep sutures, the recession of the muscles covering the gap, and the formation of an excess of fibrous cicatrix.

3. **Perfect dryness of the wound.**—The result of oozing of

blood, serum, and liquid fat into an operation wound is, in the first place, to furnish a nidus for bacterial growth, which is especially favoured in the vicinity of the groins and genitals ; secondly, it separates the layers of the abdominal wall near the wound ; and, thirdly, it increases the amount of fibrous tissue by organization of the exudate, and thus tends ultimately to atrophy of the muscular layers involved in it.

4. **Sufficiently prolonged convalescence.**—Few things tend so greatly to vitiate the result of hernial operations as an undue curtailment of convalescence. Young cicatrices are easily stretched long after the occurrence of primary union. The present-day custom of discharging hospital patients at the end of fourteen to twenty-one days is a directly predisposing cause of recurrence.

OPERATIVE TREATMENT OF INGUINAL HERNIA

The operation may be divided into two essential parts, viz. (a) the obliteration of the sac, and (b) the closure of the canal. In *Bassini's* operation, the one usually adopted, the sac is emptied and removed, the open neck being closed either by transfixion and ligature or, if wide, by suturing ; this method secures good results and is advised. *Barker* recommended ligature and removal of the sac, the stump being afterwards carried upwards by the two ends of the ligature passed through the abdominal wall and tied together there. *Macewen* puckered up the sac like a venetian blind by a purse-string suture from below upwards, and fixed it as a pad over the internal abdominal ring. In *Kocher's* first operation the fundus was passed through the muscles above the internal ring, from within outwards, the sac drawn after it and then turned downwards and fixed to the anterior surface of the external oblique aponeurosis. Later, Kocher invaginated the sac into the abdomen like an inverted glove-finger, and, bringing it out through peritoneum and muscles, fixed it as above.

To close the inguinal canal, two methods may be mentioned— (1) *Halsted's*, in which the inguinal canal is obliterated by suturing all the layers of the abdominal wall *behind* the cord, which therefore is made to run subcutaneously to the scrotum ; (2) *Bassini's*, in which, after removal of the sac, the conjoint tendon is stitched to Poupart's ligament behind the cord, and the gap in the external oblique closed in front of it, so as to maintain the valvular action of the canal.

Choice of anæsthetic.—The best results are obtained with spinal analgesia, which procures a maximum of muscular relaxation, avoids postoperative vomiting, and minimizes oozing and congestion. (*See* Vol. I., p. 688.)

Bassini's operation (Fig. 458).—This operation may be divided into three stages—(1) isolation, ligature, and removal of the sac ; (2) closure of the inguinal canal ; and (3) completion of the operation.

1. The incision extends from a point just external to the pubic spine outwards, parallel to and slightly above Poupart's ligament, for a distance of 4 in. or more. In the case of a scrotal hernia it may be necessary to extend it downwards over the outer aspect of the scrotum, but this should be avoided, if possible, for three reasons : firstly, for fear of sepsis ; secondly, on account of the troublesome oozing following division of the hernial coverings here ; and thirdly, because of the difficulty of bandaging the scrotum.

The aponeurosis is next split from the external abdominal ring

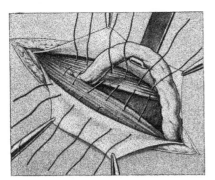

outwards, and the edges held widely apart by flat retractors—*not* by pressure forceps, which tend to tear the edges and make it difficult to cover a thick cord or implant a filigree. The spermatic cord is raised from its bed, and the sac sought. If three fingers are passed beneath the cord, and the coverings are divided in its length by a light touch of the knife and then peeled upwards and downwards with the point of a pair of dissect-

Fig. 458.—Bassini's method of closing inguinal canal.

(*From "Annals of Surgery."*)

ing forceps, there will be no difficulty in recognizing the transverse white fold which marks the fundus of the sac.

Then, avoiding injury of the cord-like vas, the sac is stripped from the surrounding tissues as high as its origin from the parietal peritoneum, and the fundus, held up by three pairs of pressure forceps, is opened. A finger is introduced, the sac is explored, any adherent omentum being detached, and the bowel reduced ; lateral sacculi must be dissected out and removed with the sac. The finger being still kept in the latter, to prevent the escape of contents, the neck is transfixed by a needle carrying a ligature, and is firmly tied off as close to the abdominal wall as possible. The sac is then removed at a short distance from the ligature.

The dangers to be avoided at this stage are as follows : (*a*) Puncture of the bladder, where this organ lies close to the neck of the sac. (*b*) Transfixion of the bowel from omitting to guard it with the finger. (*c*) Tying-in a loop of bowel or piece of omentum which has protruded at the last moment on removal of the finger. (d) Slipping of a ligature placed upon a thick-walled and vascular sac. (e) Tying-in or dividing a loop of the vas deferens close to the deep surface of the neck of the sac.

2. With the finger or the handle of a scalpel the peritoneum is peeled back from the deep aspect of Poupart's ligament so as to display its shining white fibres, and the conjoined tendon is similarly peeled back from the overlying aponeurosis of the external oblique as far as possible. At this point the question will arise as to the necessity of reinforcing the inguinal canal by the method described on p. 622; where the patient is young, the musculature good, and the hernia not of unusual size nor recurrent, this will not be necessary. The cord is held out of the way, and five or more stout chromicized, iodized catgut sutures inserted through a half-inch grip of the conjoined tendon and through the upturned edge of Poupart's ligament, from the pubic spine to the internal abdominal ring. The wound is flushed out with normal saline and thoroughly dried, and the sutures are then tied *just sufficiently tightly to approximate the structures included*, and so to remake the posterior wall of the inguinal canal.

Care must be taken—(a) to avoid puncturing the deep epigastric vessels; (b) to take up a good thickness of the conjoined tendon in the sutures; (c) not to tie these sutures to the extent of strangulation; (d) to avoid mattress-sutures, which of necessity cause strangulation of tissue; (e) to take up only the deep fibres of Poupart's ligament, and *not* the free cut edge of the oblique aponeurosis.

3. The cord is replaced in position, and the wound in the aponeurosis closed, the edges being caught up in the manner of a Lembert's suture, which prevents the tendency to split, sufficient room being left for the escape of the cord from the canal without undue constriction. Finally, in stout patients the superficial fascia may be approximated by one or two sutures so as to obliterate any " dead. space," and the skin incision is closed by interrupted silkworm-gut sutures, or preferably by Michel's clip-sutures. The dressings and bandages applied, in order to avoid any strain being brought upon the sutures the patient's knee and hip should be flexed and kept in this position during his removal to bed, when at some distance from the scene of operation; this is best done by passing a figure-of-eight bandage round the leg and thigh, and fixing the limb to that of the sound side in a position of *adduction and internal rotation*.

Operative Treatment of Large Scrotal Hernia

Few large scrotal hernias can be cured by any method which relies upon the patient's tissues alone. The musculature is no longer firm and resilient, and frequently the inguinal region external to the internal abdominal ring is· weak and bulging. In very ·large scrotal hernias the sac, especially the body and fundus, is thick, vascular, and adherent, and the attempt to strip this out of the scrotum results in much troublesome oozing of blood and fat, which not only distends the cavity of the scrotum but also invades the layers of the coverings of the sac, making it impossible to evacuate the clot. It is thus often unwise to attempt the removal of such a sac; it is better simply to detach it sufficiently at the neck to enable it to be ligated and divided here; thus the risk of a scrotal hæmatoma is avoided at the cost of a comparatively slight increase in the size of the scrotum. This increase may be considerably reduced by the use of a large-sized Keetley's suspender, worn for some weeks after the operation.

If the scrotum is very long and flabby, a section of it may be removed, but no attempt should be made to cut away the thick coverings of the sac, since much time must be lost in catching and tying divided vessels.

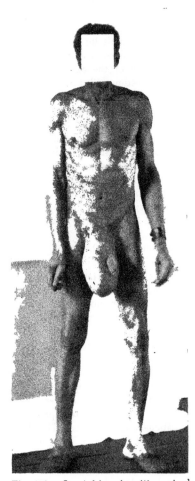

Fig. 459.—Scrotal hernia with vaginal hydrocele, cured by filigree implantation. (*Author's case.*)

Double-filigree operation: author's method. Principles involved.[1]—" It was with the idea of bringing *all* cases of hernia, especially those of great size and those of recurrence, within the scope of

---

[1] This passage is extracted from the *Brit. Med. Journ.*, Aug. 14, 1909, where fuller details will be found.

operative treatment, of doing away entirely with the truss, and of establishing a method of treatment which should honestly deserve the term 'radical cure,' that I devised, in 1905, the method which is known as the 'double-filigree method,' and which has been used since that time with the best results. The principles which underlie it are, simply, the removal of the sac, the approximation of the conjoined tendon to Poupart's ligament, and the rendering absolutely unstretchable of the whole operative cicatrix by the introduction of a scaffolding of silver wire known as 'filigree.' When a filigree of silver wire such as will presently be described is introduced into the tissues of the inguinal canal, presuming that it is perfectly aseptic, the first effect is that of local irritation of the parts in contact with it; this results in the exudation of lymph, which rapidly organizes about the filigree, and in a very short time new vessels and young fibrous tissue are produced, and grow around, among,

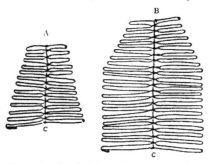

Fig. 460.—Pubic (A) and iliac (B) sections of author's filigree for inguinal hernia. (c) Midrib.

and between the wires of the filigree to such an extent that ere long a solid plaque is formed that once and for all converts the inguinal canal into a sound, resistant area which will neither stretch nor bulge, the muscles, peritoneum, and aponeurosis being welded together by the filigree, which acts much as the backbone of a sole does upon the tissues which it supports, with this difference, that the ends of the filigree wires, being in the form of a loop, are capable of acting as retaining sutures, whereas the bones of the sole only act as a scaffolding for support."

Method of constructing filigrees.—These are made in two sections (Fig. 460), a pubic (A) and an iliac (B). The former measures $1\frac{1}{2}$ in. in length (the normal length of the inguinal canal), $\frac{3}{4}$ in. in width at the narrow end, and $1\frac{1}{2}$ in. at the wide end. All filigrees being constructed on the principle of eight loops to the inch, there will be thirteen loops on either side of the pubic section.

The iliac section is constructed in such a way that its inner third corresponds in shape and size to the outer two-thirds of the pubic section. Its outer end must meet the requirements of the case, being trapezoid, square, or, what is more usual, oblong, and of a total length of 2½ to 3 in., as may be found necessary. The wire must be of unalloyed silver, and of the same gauge for all filigrees, viz. No. 28 standard wire gauge.

A board of soft wood or cork is taken, and on it is placed and fixed by pins a sheet of white paper; upon this the plan of the filigrees to be made is drawn out accurately. Stout pins are then inserted vertically, as in Fig. 461, and an odd one, the "anchor" pin (Fig. 461, A), is placed to the left of the wider end of the plan from which to start, the wire being given a turn or so round it. The wire now runs from the end pin on one side to the second from the end of the other, and so on from side to side, a pin being missed each time, and the wire being carried round the outer side of the pins. Having reached the last pin on one side, it is carried across to that of the other, and so begins to travel back to the pin from which it started, when the anchor pin (A) is removed, and the ends of the wire are neatly twisted together round the outer side of the first pin of the row and cut off short.

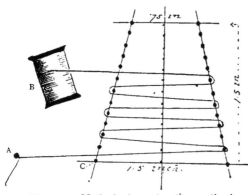

Fig. 461.—Method of constructing author's filigree.

It will now be seen that the crossing of the wires falls evenly down the centre of the filigree, and the mid-rib (Fig. 460, c) is attached. This is done by taking a separate short strand of wire and fixing it to the centre of the strand at the wide end; from this point it is carried along the centre of the filigree, a turn being made round each point of crossing of the wires, at which points it is firmly pinched by a pair of dissecting forceps to fix it in position. On reaching the opposite end of the filigree the mid-rib is finished off by being attached to the last strand in the same manner as that by which it was fixed to the first. The surplus being cut off short and the pins removed, the filigree is complete. A little practice is required to produce the most perfect work, as the pull of the wire must be kept equal at all points and breakages avoided, since joins are not only clumsy but difficult to effect.

Method of implantation.—The filigrees should be placed in ether for five minutes to remove all grease from them, and should be left in the sterilizer *in the centre of the most actively boiling area* till the moment of implantation, when they are lifted straight from the sterilizer into the wound.

The operation is at first conducted exactly as in performing an ordinary Bassini's closure, except that the aponeurosis should be split to a point rather farther out, and the peritoneum must be more freely separated from the posterior surface of the conjoined tendon, as must the latter be from the aponeurosis overlying it. From this point the steps are as follows : The sac having been isolated and dealt with, the cord is held out of the way, and the first two of the sutures which are to approximate the conjoined tendon to Poupart's ligament are inserted, and their ends are caught by pressure forceps. These sutures being held aside by the assistant, the pubic section of the filigree is placed upon the peritoneum, its narrow end being close to the pubic spine, and its wide end at the inner margin of the internal abdominal ring. If the peritoneum is very loose and inclined to sag, a fine suture may be used to unite it to the filigree ; as a rule, however, this is unnecessary, and all that is required is to bring the conjoined tendon into close apposition with Poupart's ligament *over the filigree* by the two sutures already inserted, and then to insert as many more as may be deemed necessary, care being

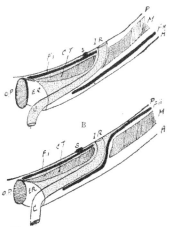

Fig. 462.—Positions of filigree sections in inguinal canal.

A, In ordinary cases ; B, where there is excessive weakness of inguinal region.

taken to keep the bed in which it lies as dry as possible. In cases in which the muscular wall of the abdomen external to the internal ring is sound and strong, the cord is placed in position, and the iliac section of the filigree is taken from the sterilizer and placed beneath the aponeurosis in such a way that its inner end lies over the internal abdominal ring and upon the cord for a space of $\frac{3}{4}$ in., the outer end being carried outwards and laid upon the surface of the internal oblique muscle, one or two sutures holding it in place (Fig. 462, A). If the above-mentioned weakness is present, the muscular wall is divided from the ring outwards towards the iliac spine for about an inch, and is separated from the peritoneum by the handle of a scalpel ; upon this peritoneum the outer end of the iliac section is laid, being lightly sutured in place, and the muscles are brought together again over it (Fig. 462, B), the inner end

2 o

lying as already described. Finally, the aponeurosis is sutured in place, and the wound closed by means of Michel's clips, which are removed on the fifth day.

It will be seen that the cord comes to be " sandwiched " between two layers of filigree in the canal, the natural relations of which are hardly altered; and further that the area outside the internal abdominal ring is fortified by a filigree which may be made of any size that is deemed necessary.

Granted a primary union of the wound, the hernial gap will be found to become as impermeable and as unstretchable as a pad of leather. There will be neither pain nor discomfort afterwards; there is not the least fear of interference with the cord or with the functions of the testis; the necessity for any form of truss is done away with permanently, and the operation thus offers the patient a radical cure in the truest sense of the word.

OPERATIVE TREATMENT OF FEMORAL HERNIA

The skin incision in this case is a vertical one over the site of the saphenous opening, and extends from $\frac{1}{2}$ in. above the inner point of trisection of Poupart's ligament downwards for a distance of 4 in. A network of veins will be met with, formed from the superficial epigastric and circumflex iliac, and the superficial - external pudic vessels; these must be divided between ligatures. The sac will usually be found without difficulty, lying in the superficial fascia and directed towards the centre of Poupart's ligament, the neck being long and narrow, and curving round the falciform process of the fascia lata to reach the parietal peritoneum.

The neck should be entirely freed from its surroundings as high as possible, and treated exactly as described under inguinal hernia, the first four of the precautionary points there mentioned being again borne in mind.

The necessity of using some means for closing the femoral canal has been much debated by surgeons, and the following methods may be mentioned here :—

1. Three or four catgut sutures (*not* mattress sutures) may be passed deeply through the substance of the pectineus muscle, and then through the falciform process and lower edge of Poupart's ligament, so that, when tied, these two structures are closely approximated, and the saphenous opening is partially obliterated. This method does not, however, close the upper end of the femoral canal, and involves the exercise of considerable tension if the saphenous opening is to be even narrowed; for this reason the sutures probably cut out early and do more harm than good.

2. An attempt has been made to cover the gap by turning up a flap

of the pectineus muscle and fascia, and suturing it to Poupart's ligament. The only effect of this has been to damage the. pectineus muscle, and, since the transplanted flap undergoes fibroid degeneration, no good results from it.

3. An attempt has also been made to suture Poupart's ligament to the horizontal ramus of the pubes, by passing deep sutures round the ramus or through the periosteum covering it.

4. With a similar object an endeavour has been made to unite these two structures by the use of steel staples driven through the ligament into the bone. The method fails owing to the rarefying osteitis which shortly loosens the grip of the staples, and is moreover dangerous, since the points of the loosened staples are apt to wound the bladder and femoral vessels.

5. The femoral canal has been plugged with decalcified bone or with a graft of bone raised from the ramus of the pubes.

6. I have attempted to close the crural ring by means of a "spider-web" filigree introduced from behind Poupart's ligament (Fig. 465). The incision was made above and parallel to the ligament. The operation was difficult, and it is as yet too early to judge of its merits.

These operations are founded on an erroneous belief that femoral hernia has a special tendency to recur. Such recurrences as are seen are frequently due, as Hamilton Russell has pointed out, to incomplete removal of the sac, or to the overlooking of lateral diverticula, which are especially common in this form of hernia. If it is thought necessary, owing to the unusual length of a femoral canal, to treat the sac in any special way, the best method is probably that of Kocher, which has already been described.

In young subjects nothing more is necessary than to remove the sac *completely* after ligature, and close the wound by suture or clips; but care must be taken to leave no lateral sacculus overlooked.

The difficulty of closing the femoral canal is an anatomical one. The outer wall of the canal being formed of the flaccid femoral vein, complete closure without compression or obliteration of this vein is practically impossible, and any method of closing the saphenous opening, whether by silver filigree or simple suture of its margins, still leaves the femoral canal unguarded, and causes compression of the long saphenous vein.

If it is intended to utilize the first method of narrowing the canal, care must be taken in passing the sutures to guard the femoral vein from puncture as the point of the needle passes beneath Poupart's ligament, and to avoid passing the point so deeply that the peritoneum is in danger of being wounded.

In some cases, especially of strangulated femoral hernia, it is advantageous also to expose the neck of the sac from above Poupart's ligament, so gaining access to the entrance to the canal.

Operative Treatment of Umbilical Hernia

The points to be aimed at are complete removal of the sac and the closure of the abdomen *in separate layers*.

The incision is made in the middle line of the abdomen above and below the hernia, the actual prominence being enclosed by an ellipse between these incisions. Where there is a deep layer of superficial fascia, the skin incision must be long enough to give free access to the hernia. The abdomen is opened above the level of the hernia and a finger is introduced to search for adhesions. These are separated, and the incision is then carried through the whole thickness of the abdominal wall along one side of the tumour, and the sac everted and emptied of its contents. Any degenerate omentum is ligated and removed, care being taken to see that all vessels in the stump are fully secured. The sac, including its cutaneous covering, is then removed close to the neck of the hernia. If the gap is very wide it is often well to avoid too free a removal of the peritoneal sac, lest difficulty be found in closing the abdomen without the exercise of tension. The bowels are now retained by a large gauze pad placed within the abdomen, and the peritoneum is closed by a continuous suture, the pad being removed before closure. The margins of the rectus sheath are laid open above and below the gap, and the edges of the posterior layers approximated like those of the peritoneum. The rectus muscles are brought out of their sheaths, and their edges united by interrupted sutures which should include a considerable thickness of the muscle on either side, without the least constriction. If approximation can only be effected by the exercise of tension, either the muscles must be more freely brought out, or the case must be treated by filigree implantation (*see* p. 629).

In freeing the muscles it is necessary to detach them from the lineæ transversæ which bind them to their sheaths. This is easily done, but, as these lineæ transversæ carry large vessels, care must be taken to arrest all bleeding before proceeding to unite the muscles. Only round-bodied curved needles should be used here, since bayonet-edged or Hagedorn's needles are liable to divide muscular branches of the vessels, and so give rise to bleeding and cause loss of time. The anterior layers of the rectus sheaths are now united by a continuous suture ; one or two interrupted sutures are inserted to hold the superficial fascia together and obliterate dead spaces, and finally the skin incision is closed by Michel's clips. A firm binder should be applied for the first twenty-four hours, and the patient should be placed in the semi-recumbent position.

Where the hernia has attained to rather larger dimensions, various attempts have been made to strengthen the abdominal wall by the overlapping of its aponeurosis; but in view of the brilliant results achieved by Bartlett's method (*see* below), and of the great tendency of all umbilical and ventral hernias to recur, the wisdom of these operations is doubtful, since, in the event of recurrence after their performance, the accomplishment of Bartlett's method is rendered much more difficult. The best of these overlapping operations is that of William Mayo. The incisions are transverse and elliptical, and are carried down to the neck of the sac, after which the aponeurotic surfaces are cleared for a distance around this point. The sac, its coverings, and its omental contents, are removed by a circular incision without dissection. A transverse incision is made through the abdominal aponeurosis (posterior rectus sheath) for an inch or less on either side, and the peritoneum is separated from the upper of the two flaps thus made. Sutures are now passed through the aponeurotic layer of the upper flap, about 3 in. from its free margin from without inwards, then through the free margin of the lower flap, and back again through the upper flap from within outwards, and are sufficiently drawn upon to approximate the peritoneal edges, which are closed by a continuous suture. This done, the sutures are so tightened that the lower aponeurotic flap is drawn into the space between the upper flap and the peritoneum, where it is fixed. The free margin of the upper flap is then sutured to the surface of the aponeurosis below, and the skin incision finally closed.

The operation is not suitable for very large hernias, and the separation of the peritoneum is frequently difficult owing to old adhesions.

Bartlett's method of filigree implantation: author's modification.—For hernias which have grown so large that any prospect of cure by ordinary means is out of the question, this method is the only one which can be relied upon. It is simple and extremely effective, but often necessitates a very extensive and tedious operation.

The filigree which I use (Fig. 463) is a modification of Willard Bartlett's original pattern in that it is barrel-shaped in outline, and has two side ribs as well as a mid-rib. It is made in precisely the same manner as the filigrees for inguinal hernia (p. 624), except as regards shape and size. The method is in all respects that of Bartlett, except that the filigree is implanted between the rectus muscle and the posterior layer of its sheath, instead of upon the peritoneum.

The operation is conducted in precisely the same manner as already detailed for small hernias, except that the incision must be very much more extensive, often indeed from the ensiform cartilage to the pubes

(Fig. 452). The rectus sheath must be very freely opened on either side, and a complete separation of both muscles effected from both anterior and posterior layers. As soon as the edges of the peritoneum, together with those of the posterior layers,[1] are united, all oozing is arrested, and the edges of the recti muscles being widely retracted, the filigree is lifted straight from the sterilizer and at once introduced into the wound, being laid upon the posterior layer of the sheath of the muscle. There is no need to suture it in place, since, being of the exact width of the sheath, it cannot get out of place. The recti muscles are now approximated as far as possible over it, and the anterior layer of the sheath is also closed by a continuous suture. No drainage is used, and the wound is closed by the clips from end to end.

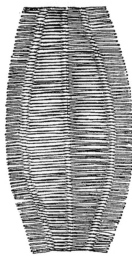

Fig. 463.—Author's modification of Bartlett's abdominal filigree.

Before operation is undertaken, the size of the filigree to be used must be determined. The vertical length of the hernial gap should be measured, and the filigree made at least one-third longer than this measurement; the width remains constant—$4\frac{1}{2}$ to 5 in.

When successfully implanted, these filigrees do away entirely with the necessity for any kind of belt or truss after convalescence. The patient may wear an abdominal binder for a month from the date of the operation, when consolidation will be complete. No inconvenience or discomfort is felt subsequently, nor does the method interfere with pregnancy.

OPERATIVE TREATMENT OF VENTRAL HERNIA

What has been said of umbilical applies equally well to ventral hernia. These gaps are from the first so large as to preclude any operation by the superimposition of flaps, and the tendency to recurrence is so great that only a few are cured by direct approximation of the abdominal wall in tiers. It is, therefore, best to treat them by filigree implantation from the first.

Since they are commonly the result of trauma or of operative interference, they present greater difficulties than simple umbilical

---

[1] Unless these are taken together the peritoneum will be much torn by the sutures.

hernias owing to the nature of the cicatrix and adhesions ; this is especially so where there has been extensive suppuration, or where abdominal drainage has been employed.

The majority are situated between the umbilicus and the pubes (Fig. 464), and consequently there is a deficiency of the posterior sheath of the rectus in the lower half of this area. The filigree must therefore lie on the posterior sheath in its upper, and on the peritoneum in its lower half, and should come well down below the crest of the pubes.

Appendicular and other lateral hernias.—Whenever drainage of an appendicular abscess, or reposition after cæcostomy or colostomy, has been performed, a ventral hernia is to be expected ; and, owing to the disposition of the muscular layers here, recurrence is almost certain to follow any attempt to cure such a hernia by simple approximation of such layers. The situation is not one which lends itself to the application of belts or trusses, and the discomfort of this variety of hernia is greater in proportion than that of any other form of ventral hernia, since the sac always contains the cæcum and ileo-cæcal valve or the sigmoid, which structures are usually adherent to its walls.

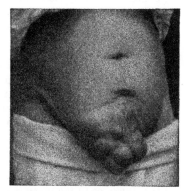

Fig. 464.—Ventral hernia following laparotomy, cured by implantation of 9-in. filigree. (*Author's case.*)

For this reason also much of the peritoneum may be sacrificed in detaching these adhesions. In a case of mine[1] it was impossible to close the gap in the peritoneum, an area of 3 by 1½ in. remaining to be closed. The omentum being too short to suture into the gap, the cæcum and ileum were united together and sewn to the edges of the peritoneal gap in order that a filigree measuring 9 by 5 in. might be implanted. The case was successful, and the patient has since married and has borne a child. The filigree in such cases as these is introduced as follows :—

The skin cicatrix having been excised by an elliptical incision running obliquely from the loin to the pubes, the abdomen is opened at the upper end and the adhesions determined as above detailed. The peritoneum is separated as widely as possible from the abdominal muscles external to the incision, and the rectus sheath is opened extensively along its outer edge. The muscle is then freed from the

[1] *Lancet,* Nov. 23, 1907.

sheath above and from the peritoneum below the semilunar fold of Douglas. When the oozing is arrested and the edges of the peritoneum are approximated, the filigree is introduced so that its inner loops rest on the posterior sheath of the rectus muscle above, and on the peritoneum below, while its outer loops lie on the peritoneum only and are deep to the abdominal muscles. The rectus is then brought well out of its sheath and is sutured to the transversalis and internal oblique muscles over the filigree, while the anterior layer of the sheath is united to the external oblique aponeurosis. The skin incision is finally closed in the usual way.

When implanting a filigree in a case in which the abscess has been drained without the removal of the appendix, it is essential, for obvious reasons, to effect this removal at the time of implantation. Bartlett himself goes so far as to implant a filigree in cases in which suppuration is actually present, knowing that granulation will occur through the filigree ; thus he avoids a second operation. To this, however, I am opposed, for the following reasons :—

1. The cases in which an appendix can be safely removed from a suppurating cavity are comparatively few.

2. The implantation requires the more extensive opening up of muscular layers, involving a fresh area of infection.

3. Cases are at times seen of secondary sinuses after the removal of a gangrenous appendix, owing either to the infection of the ligature of the stump, or to the presence of small portions of concretion overlooked at the operation.

4. The presence of a filigree in a suppurating area renders the process of healing much more prolonged.

5. There is always the chance of damage occurring to the filigree, or of its becoming displaced in the repeated dressings necessary during healing.

6. In the process of healing, the filigree is apt to be pushed out by the granulations to a more superficial position than that which it should properly occupy.

It is better surgery to allow the cavity to close, and then at a subsequent date to implant a filigree under aseptic conditions.

Operative Treatment of Lumbar Hernia

When occurring at Petit's triangle, hernia may often be cured by simple approximation of the muscles ; but if the gap be wide, it must also be submitted to filigree implantation. When the hernia appears in the upper region of the loin this is the only sound method of treatment, especially when it is the result of an operation on the kidney. Here the muscles have been divided transversely, much of their nerve supply has been damaged, and extensive fibrosis and atrophy have occurred. The filigree may be placed upon or deep to the transversalis fascia, the latter being the simpler method. The operation is by no means so simple as in the case of the abdomen, owing to the narrowness and depth of the costo-iliac space and the unyielding nature of the fascia. The filigree should measure about 4 to 5 in. in length and 3 to 4 in. in width, and should be of the same shape as the abdominal filigree.

OPERATIVE TREATMENT OF GLUTEAL AND SCIATIC HERNIA

These hernias may occasionally be operated upon when not stran-

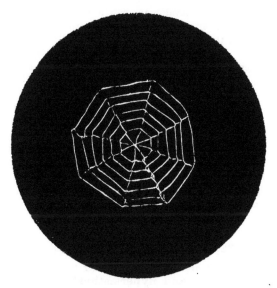

Fig. 465.—Author's spider-web filigree for use in perineal and femoral hernia.

gulated. The incision and dissection are in all respects the same as for ligature of the respective arteries, the essential point being to obtain very free access to the parts. The difficulties are chiefly those of depth, the presence of the network of vessels, and the difficulty of effecting reduction. In dividing the constriction, care must be taken of the vessels and nerves in the vicinity, and, as these are numerous and their courses not always regular, it is wiser to depend on clear exposure of the parts than to be guided by any anatomical rule. In case of failure, abdominal section should be performed as for obturator hernia (*see* p. 650).

Operative Treatment of Perineal Hernia

The majority of perineal hernias should be attacked by the combined abdomino-perineal route. They are extremely difficult to deal with, and so variable in their character that no definite rule can be laid down for their operative treatment. The difficulties to be overcome are the reposition and retention in place of the pelvic organs, especially the bladder, which at times occupies the sac; and the depth of the hernial ring both from within and from without. The Trendelenburg position is, of course, essential, and there are no sound structures to assist in closing the gap. My spider-web filigree (Fig. 465) may be used, being implanted either beneath the peritoneum from within, or beneath the levator ani muscle from without, as may be found easiest. In either case it should lie between the peritoneum and the muscle, the sac having been invaginated and tied off within the abdomen. In women this may necessitate the separation of the broad ligament from the pelvic floor, but that is of little consequence, since it can easily be sutured in place again. Where the hernia is found to contain the ovary, broad ligament, uterus, and bladder, it will be advisable to complete the operation by performing a ventro-fixation of the uterus, and possibly removal of the ovary and tube of the affected side at the same time.

The greatest care must be taken to ascertain the presence or absence of the bladder in these cases, since any injury to it in so deep a wound is difficult to repair. On one occasion a pudendal hernia appearing in the labium majus was mistaken for a vaginal polypus, and, being ligatured and removed, was found to contain a length of intestine and a mass of omentum (Graser, *see* Bibliography).

POSTOPERATIVE COMPLICATIONS OF HERNIA

These fortunately are few. The following have been noted:—

1. **Chronic pain and hyperæsthesia of the cicatrix.** —This is probably due to the inclusion of some of the cutaneous nerves in the ligatures and sutures. If severe and genuine (many of these patients are malingerers or neurotic youths), the cicatrix may be undercut with a tenotomy knife where the condition is one of hyperæsthesia; but where chronic pain is complained of it is better to open up the old wound down to the aponeurosis, or even to the conjoined tendon, and divide high up any nerves found in the course of dissection. Where pain is complained of only in wet or cold weather, the condition is not to be benefited by operation.

2. **Formation of a hæmatoma.**—This may occur in the course of the inguinal canal or in the scrotum. It is not uncommon after extensive stripping away of large adherent sacs in scrotal hernias.

Unless very extensive or causing a distinct rise of temperature, these hæmatomas should not be opened, especially when in the scrotum; it is almost impossible to evacuate all the clot from this region, since, besides occupying the cavity of the scrotum, it has extensively invaded the layers of the hernial coverings, from which it cannot be dislodged. It is better to use the ice-bag for the first twenty-four hours, and hot fomentations or simply pressure after this. Unless very large, these swellings nearly always subside in time. When suppuration occurs they must be freely opened, but in such cases the hernia commonly recurs.

3. **Atrophy of the testis.**—This is due either to (*a*) damage to the vas deferens by cutting or crushing; (*b*) damage to the spermatic artery; or (*c*) compression of the spermatic cord by too tight suturing of the canal. When atrophy is established there is no remedy.

4. **Formation of a varicocele.**—This is also due to tight suturing, and is, indeed, often a stage in the previous condition. When suturing is complete, the external abdominal ring should with difficulty admit the tip of the little finger.

5. **Torsion of the testis.**—As the result of twisting the organ round in the process of removing a patent processus vaginalis, especially in cases of retained testis, this accident may occur, the testis being finally left in the scrotum with the digital fossa, as it should be, on the outside, but with a complete twist of the cord above it. Such an accident may give rise to pain, swelling of the scrotum, vomiting, distension of the abdomen, and constipation; the case may thus resemble one of intestinal obstruction. The accident can only be the outcome of carelessness.

6. **Persistent vomiting.**—The importance of this lies in its effect on the result of the operation. Its cause may be (*a*) the anæsthetic; (*b*) intestinal obstruction; (*c*) torsion of the testis; (*d*) general peritonitis; or (*e*) paralytic ileus.

The danger of forcible and prolonged vomiting is that it strains or ruptures the sutures, tears the conjoined tendon, stretches the young cicatrix of the union, and causes fresh oozing into the tissues, all of which effects tend to produce recurrence. Since the introduction of spinal analgesia into my practice there has been only one case of prolonged vomiting (viz. five hours); this was in a woman, and was not violent. The use of spinal analgesia is a strong factor in the prevention of recurrence.

7. **Intestinal obstruction.**—This may result from the tying-in of a loop of bowel in the neck of the sac, or from the production of a volvulus, or the forcing of a loop of bowel through a rent in the omentum or mesentery by a rough attempt to return large masses of hernial contents. The prophylaxis is obvious; the treatment, immediate laparotomy.

8. **Fæcal or urinary fistulæ.**—These are the outcome of direct injury to the bowel or bladder, from transfixion by sutures or inclusion in ligatures ; or, in the case of the bowel, they are due to subsequent sloughing at the site of constriction when a strangulated loop has been released and returned to the abdomen.

Either of these conditions may improve spontaneously after a time, or may require an operation to effect a cure. In the case of the bladder, a catheter should be tied in and the cavity washed out twice a day without forcible distension ; the patient should be given such drugs as urotropine in 10-gr. doses ; acid sodium phosphate ℥ss, salol 10 gr., etc., in such vehicles as infusion of buchu, pareira, barley-water, etc.

When the bowel has been damaged, much will depend on the level of the injury. If it be in the upper regions of the jejunum, emaciation will ensue rapidly ; whereas fistula of the colon produces little change in the nutrition.

9. **Suppuration.**—Owing to the situation of inguinal and femoral operations, asepsis is more difficult to ensure than in the case of ventral or umbilical hernia. But in all cases the greatest care must be taken to avoid infection of the wound, since suppuration is almost certain to be followed by recurrence. Absorbent and unabsorbable sutures like silk and linen thread should be avoided, since they often give rise to sinuses of prolonged duration. The safest material is probably catgut soaked in ether and then treated by Moskowitz's iodine method, or some of the specially prepared brands in sealed tubes ; these latter are, however, very costly. Where deep suppuration occurs, nothing is gained by waiting except where a filigree has been implanted ; the wound should be reopened, all sutures removed, the wound swabbed out with pure carbolic or lysol, and lightly packed with gauze. After healing, any recurrence must be treated by filigree implantation.

Suppuration following filigree implantation.—In the case of inguinal hernia it is wiser not to remove the filigree at once—many cases heal soundly with constant washing out; but there is certainly a tendency for the iliac section to shift its position upwards, when the hernia may recur beneath it. In such a case I have been able successfully to close the gap by the implantation of a fresh iliac section after the wound had healed, without removing that which had shifted.

In the case of umbilical and ventral filigrees there is little chance of displacement, since they are held in position by the outer margins of the rectus sheath. Thorough syringing of the wound, which should be opened at the lower end, will overcome the difficulty, peroxide of hydrogen being used in a 5-to-8-volume solution. The ultimate result is simply to render the abdominal wall firmer than ever, owing to the greater amount of cicatricial tissue produced around the filigree.

Care should be taken not to disturb the wires of the filigree by the introduction of probes, etc., for the presence of loose wires in the sinus is the surest means of preventing healing.

10. **Retention of urine.**—In all operations on the groins or perineum this is liable to occur from time to time ; it would appear to be less frequent where the operation is performed under spinal analgesia. In any case, it is a temporary complication of no great importance, and is readily overcome by the use of a catheter.

11. **Orchitis and epididymitis.**—This is seen in a certain proportion of inguinal hernias. It usually comes on within the first four or five days after operation, and may last for a week or ten days, gradually subsiding on the application of hot fomentations, or the use of glycerine and belladonna ; the patient's bowels should be kept freely open, and the testes should be kept raised upon a pad of soft wool supported on a band of strapping passed across the thighs. The prognosis is good, suppuration being rare, and little damage resulting to the testes. The trouble is probably due to rough handling of the vas and to congestion of the pampiniform plexus of veins.

12. **Paralytic ileus.**—This is by far the most serious complication of hernial operations, and is rarely met with except in the case of prolonged manipulation of the bowels in dealing with unusually large hernias, especially umbilical ones in plethoric subjects. The symptoms are those of gradually oncoming intestinal obstruction, and unless the bowels can be induced to move, the case is likely to terminate rapidly. If distension occurs and cannot be relieved by the rectal tube and turpentine enemata, time should not be wasted in the administration of drugs, but the abdomen should be opened and the cæcum or distal end of the ileum brought out of the wound, and a Paul's tube inserted, after which strychnine, sulphate of magnesium, croton oil, etc., may be given. Eserine salicylate and pituitrin are also of value, and may be given hypodermically. Where vomiting has actually set in, the prognosis is very grave ; and where the vomit is fæcal the case is, as a rule, hopeless.

In extreme cases, where the manipulation gives reason to fear the possibility of ileus, prevention is better than cure, and the cæcum should be opened at the time of operation, a Paul's tube being inserted and the bowels evacuated at once.[1] Such drastic treatment must, of course, be reserved for the most exceptional cases.

Recurrence of hernia after operation.—Although less commonly seen than formerly, recurrence is still far from rare, and may be met with as the result of—

1. Suppuration, which accounts for about 60 per cent. of all cases.

---

[1] On this subject the reader is referred to a valuable article by Victor Bonney (*see* Bibliography).

2. Badly chosen cases and unsuitable methods. Thus, even Bassini's method is incapable of dealing with large hernias, especially in men over 40, and in the presence of atrophied abdominal walls. Operations done under general anæsthesia on patients the subjects of asthma or bronchitis are likely to result in failure. Simple approximation of the abdominal layers in umbilical or ventral hernias of any size is generally quite useless.

3. Tightly tied sutures—especially if "mattress sutures" are used, since strangulation of the tissues is produced and the sutures cut out too soon. The forcible dragging down of the conjoined tendon is apt to produce a separation of the muscular fibres above the level of the inguinal canal. The practice of dragging up the neck of the sac by sutures passed through the abdominal wall and then tied produces a cicatrix and therefore a weak spot in the muscle, and this may easily be the starting point of a recurrence. In my opinion the practice is unsound and should be abandoned.

4. Unduly short convalescence: this should *never be less* than three weeks in bed, and one week on a couch or chair.

5. Postoperative vomiting : this is best avoided by the use of spinal analgesia.

6. The overlooking of lateral sacculi in a hernia : this, however, is rather a failure to cure than a recurrence.

7. Omission to relax the tension on the sutures after operation, by flexion of the knee and hip.

8. Constipation, which induces straining, especially when the patient has to use a bed-pan. The bowels should be kept loose and the semi-recumbent (Fowler) position permitted during the act.

9. Distension due to flatulence : this applies especially to abdominal hernia.

10. Allowing the patient to come round from the anæsthetic before application of the bandages. A sudden spasm of vomiting is often enough to rupture the deep sutures and undo the whole of the work.

After-treatment of hernial operations.—Firm bandaging should be the rule after operation, a soft, thick pad of wool being placed over the part to prevent any oozing. On his return to bed the patient's hips and knees should be semiflexed, and kept in this position by means of a rest or pillow for a period of a fortnight in cases of inguinal and femoral hernia when any plastic closure has been attempted.

For some time after the bandages are discarded, while the cicatrix is still young, the rings should be supported by the pressure of the hand during defæcation, coughing, or other expulsive effort. *On no account should any form of truss be applied.*

In young children, care must be taken to prevent the soiling of the dressings with urine or fæces, by frequent inspection of the bandages and immediate redressing where necessary. With very young and restless children it may even be advisable to apply some form of retentive apparatus, such as a vertical suspension as for fractured femur, or a Thomas's hip splint slightly bent to a suitable shape and fixed by plaster bandages.

Elderly subjects should be treated either with a bed-rest or a double inclined plane, the latter being very much the better (Fig. 466). In this position the flatulent distension often occurring after operations on umbilical and ventral hernias is more easily dealt with. The treatment may be assisted by the retention *in situ* of the rectal tube, and the administration of enemata of turpentine, asafœtida, etc., and of

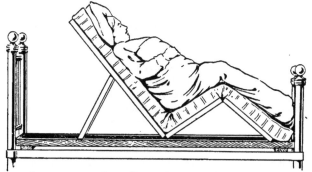

Fig. 466.—Double inclined plane (Fowler's position).
(From "Annals of Surgery.")

carminatives by the mouth. Calomel given in grain doses every hour up to 5–8 gr., or tincture of nux vomica ♏vi–x every three hours, will often help where there is no vomiting.

Unless the patient complains of discomfort, the binder applied after operation should not be loosened for twenty-four hours; a tight binder is a great safeguard to the sutures after a general anæsthetic, but it may be a source of danger to the patient's respiration if distension is marked.

STRANGULATED HERNIA

Strangulation—that is, the constriction of a viscus, usually the bowel, in such a manner as to cause arrest of its circulation as well as of its natural function—is one of the commonest of surgical emergencies. It may occur at any time in the life-history of a hernia, and is not infrequently the first evidence of the presence of hernia. It is met with in all the forms of hernia already mentioned, as well as in certain others known as " internal hernias," since they are confined to the abdominal cavity; in these latter strangulation is the rule, and they are rarely seen except in this condition.

The effects of strangulation vary according to the age and condition of the patient, the portion of the bowel involved, and the tightness of the constriction. Thus, although if unrelieved, either spontaneously or by operation, the inevitable result is death, this result is much more rapid when the patient is old and feeble or excessively plethoric, and the constriction tight and high up in the intestinal canal. In such cases the fatal result may ensue in the course of three or four days, whereas in less unfavourable cases seven to ten days may elapse. The cause of death is commonly exhaustion, peritonitis, or septic pneumonia.

Cardinal symptoms of strangulation.—These are essentially those of intestinal obstruction, viz. (1) vomiting; (2) absolute constipation both as to flatus and fæces; (3) gradual distension of the abdomen; and (4) the appearance of an irreducible swelling in the neighbourhood of one or other of the hernial sites.

1. **Vomiting.**—At first this may be mere effortless regurgitation of the gastric contents, preceded by a sense of overfullness of the stomach, possibly in spite of the fact that no food has been taken. In the course of a few hours the vomiting becomes worse and is accompanied by active retching, bitter greenish-yellow bile-stained fluid being ejected in mouthfuls. As time goes on, the vomiting progresses, undiminished by drugs, and large quantities of foul-smelling brown liquid are brought up, having a distinctly fæculent odour. Ultimately, if the condition is unrelieved and the patient lives sufficiently long, the actual contents of the large bowel may be vomited; this, however, is rare.

2. **Constipation.**—This may not at first be complete, some of the contents of the rectum below the constriction being voided; but it very soon becomes absolute, neither fæces nor flatus passing the anus. An occasional exception to this is met with in the case of Richter's hernia (p. 612), especially when low down in the ileum, slight action of the bowels and little vomiting being present throughout. The diagnosis is thus rendered very difficult.

3. **Distension of the abdomen.**—When increasing rapidly, and especially when supervening on rigidity of the parietes, this is a sign of great importance. It may be due to gas within the bowel or free in the peritoneal cavity. The diagnosis is not always easy. Stress is laid by some writers on the absence of liver dullness, but the sign is very deceptive, the bowel at times being able to insinuate itself between the liver and the abdominal wall, thus giving rise to the belief that there is free gas in the peritoneal cavity. However, taken in conjunction with other signs of abdominal disaster, such as sweating, collapse, rapid pulse, and marked abdominal facies, it is of value. The rapidity

of the onset of distension must be considered in the diagnosis of its cause. Thus a gradual, slow development is the rule in strangulation, whereas rapid and acute increase suggests perforation of the bowel.

Distension may occur even when omentum only is strangulated, the paralysis which originates it being due to reflex inhibition of the splanchnic nerves.

4. Appearance of a swelling.—The above signs, in association with a swelling at the umbilicus, groin, saphenous opening, or other hernial site (especially when the swelling is irreducible or has recently become so, is tender on manipulation, and transmits no expansile impulse on coughing), presents a picture the significance of which should be obvious. The swelling is always tender, and the pain is referred to the umbilical region.

For the rest, the condition of the patient is as follows : The tongue is thickly coated, at first with dirty white fur, later becoming dry and brown, and sordes form on the lips. The patient's face assumes the sunken, anxious appearance known as "facies Hippocratica," his voice becomes feeble and conversation is carried on in whispered gasps, articulation being indistinct owing to dryness of the tongue. The breath becomes horribly foul, the pulse rapid and running, the temperature often subnormal ; gradually exhaustion sets in, and the patient dies in a comatose, asthenic condition. At times death is due to inhalation of fæculent vomit and subsequent gangrene of the lung or septic pneumonia ; or, the bowel becoming gangrenous, general septic peritonitis terminates the case.

Varieties of strangulated hernia.—All the forms of hernia may undergo strangulation, but that most frequently affected *in proportion* is the femoral variety, although inguinal strangulation is the more often met with. Umbilical is less frequent, but more serious, since it occurs in obese and elderly women of plethoric habit. Ventral hernia rarely becomes strangulated, owing to the wide neck of the sac ; whereas obturator, sciatic, and gluteal hernias are rarely seen except in the condition of strangulation, which generally occurs on their first appearance.

Retrograde strangulation.—This is a rare variety, first described by Maydl, in which the contents of the sac remain normal, but in which a part of such contents having retraced its steps and passed into the abdomen again, becomes there strangulated. It has been described affecting bowel, omentum, the appendix, and Fallopian tube. (Sultan, *see* Bibliography).

Causes of strangulation.—A hernia which has been spontaneously reducible for years may become strangulated as the result of—

1. **Some excessive exertion,** such as the lifting of a heavy

2 *p*

weight, defæcation, vomiting, coughing, etc., the immediate effect being the forcing of a fresh mass of omentum or a coil of bowel into the sac, the neck of which is too narrow for it ; or the production of a volvulus of bowel already in the sac.

2. **Some violence applied from without,** such as foolhardy and clumsy attempts at the reduction of an irreducible hernia ; the result being its conversion into one of the forms of "reduction *en masse*," the setting up of an inflammatory œdema of the sac or its contents ; or the forcing of the bowel through a rent in the omentum.

3. **Simple rapid increase,** from overgrowth of fat, of the omental contents of the sac.

4. **Sudden distension of the bowel** in the sac from acute enteritis.

5. **Gradual increase** in the bulk of an incarcerating mass in the bowel.

6. **The growth of a tumour** in the sac.

Of the above causes, the first is by far the commonest.

Pathology of strangulation. — The process may be divided into three stages, between which there is no real dividing line, but which are easily recognizable at operation and are important as a guide to treatment and prognosis. The first stage is that of congestion from venous engorgement, the bowel being cyanosed and the omentum dark and covered by large loops of over-filled veins. As the result of this, œdema of the contents shortly occurs, and the pressure within the sac is increased. Soon the engorgement becomes so great that fluid accumulates in the sac, and this is frequently turbid or blood-stained. The sac is now tense, and the bowel becomes deep-purple in colour, and blood may be effused into its lumen.

The second stage is marked by the loss by the bowel of its smooth, glistening appearance, by its blackish-grey colour, and by its wet-wash-leather consistence. The fluid now becomes distinctly fæculent in odour.

The third stage is that of actual gangrene of the bowel, or of ulceration and perforation at the site of constriction.

In the case of Richter's hernia, where only the lateral wall of the bowel is involved, it is clear that perforation may take place without the signs already described as characterizing strangulation being present.

Results of untreated strangulation.—The prognosis is usually fatal ; at times, however, recovery takes place as the result of the formation of a fæcal fistula on the surface of the body.

Strangulated inguinal hernia.—Inguinal hernia becomes strangulated more frequently in males than in females, owing probably to the nature of their work ; the immediate cause is usually the descent of a fresh mass of omentum, and it is more commonly the latter which is strangulated. The constricting agent is to be found either in the rigid pillars of the external abdominal ring, or in the fibrous band which commonly surrounds the neck of the sac. Only occasionally is the hernia strangulated on its first appearance. Owing to the wider nature of the ring and canal here, the symptoms take rather longer to establish themselves than in the case of femoral hernia.

These hernias are usually scrotal, and on examination the scrotum will be found to be distended, hard, tender, dull to percussion, or, when bowel is present, with resonance diminished owing to the presence of fluid in the sac. No expansile impulse is felt on making the patient cough. Any attempt at reduction is resisted owing to the pain, and the patient lies with the thigh of the affected side drawn up and inverted in an endeavour to relax the tension. In many cases there is rigidity of the abdominal muscles on the affected side, and retention of urine is not uncommon. Pain may be complained of in the testis and loin owing to pressure on the constituents of the cord, and in time cramping pain referred to the umbilicus is felt. In the case of women, the ovary may be contained in the sac, in which case pain is referred to the " bottom of the back " (sacralgia) as well as to the umbilicus, and may be aggravated by raising the cervix uteri per vaginam. The appendix in a strangulated hernia gives rise to no sign by which its presence can be recognized.

Strangulated femoral hernia. — As compared with inguinal, this strangulation is more serious in that (1) being less outwardly obvious, it is more liable to be overlooked ; (2) being transmitted through a narrower canal, it is more acute in its onset ; and (3) with the sharp edge of Gimbernat's ligament always in close contact with it, ulceration is more prone to occur early.

It is seen especially in women (since in them femoral hernia is commoner) at all ages, but chiefly between the ages of 30 and 50. The tumour produced is usually quite a small one, and if of recent occurrence may easily be mistaken for an enlarged gland ; there is, however, no periglandular thickening, in spite of the tenderness, the mass is spherical rather than lobulated, and not adherent to the skin, and unless the sac is inflamed there is no redness over it, such as usually denotes femoral adenitis.

The cause of strangulation is similar to that in inguinal hernia, but the constricting agent is always the knife-edge of Gimbernat's ligament. This structure is so prominent that reduction, either spontaneous or intentional, is almost impossible and is seldom seen. For this reason, too, any prolonged effort at taxis is more dangerous than in inguinal hernia ; " reduction *en masse* " is less, while rupture of the bowel is more likely to occur as a result.

Strangulated umbilical hernia.—This condition is almost confined to women of the age of 40 to 60, especially those who are markedly obese, of plethoric habit, and frequently the subjects of chronic asthma and bronchitis. For these reasons umbilical strangulation is very dangerous, and its mortality high. Reduction can very rarely be effected owing to the size of the mass, its omental adhesions, the tightness of the constriction, and the numerous lateral sacculi present. The constricting agent is in this case the neck of the sac itself, and this is often of almost cartilaginous consistence. The especially dangerous nature of the strangulation is further due to the following factors :—

1. The depth and extent of the wound necessary for its relief.

2. The jejunum as well as the transverse colon and omentum being at times involved, the shock is proportionately greater than when the lower end of the ileum is in question.

3. The size of the mass to be exposed and returned ; many feet of bowel being frequently involved.

4. The fact that such patients are bad subjects for any kind of operation, more especially those which involve resection, anastomosis, or drainage of the intestine.

5. If jejunostomy is required, rapid emaciation is likely to result.

6. The amount of handling necessary to replace these large hernias in an abdomen already full of tensely distended bowel frequently leads to the occurrence of paralytic ileus.

Case for case, strangulated umbilical hernia is attended by a worse prognosis than any other form of external strangulation, and therefore admits of less delay in its relief ; next to it comes femoral, and lastly inguinal strangulation.

TREATMENT OF STRANGULATED HERNIA

The only sound and safe method when strangulation of any variety of hernia has been diagnosed is immediate operation.

Employment of taxis.—When a case of apparent strangulation comes under consideration, the question will arise as to the justifiability of taxis for its reduction. In only a few cases, however, is it possible, and in fewer still is it safe ; it should only be used as a last resource, as where a patient obstinately refuses any operation. If it can ever be said to be justified, it can only be where the trouble is of but a few hours' duration ; in a hernia hitherto easily reducible ; where there is absence of pain and tenderness ; and even then it should be of the gentlest kind, and should neither be prolonged nor repeated.

Dangers of forcible taxis.—1. " Reduction *en masse* " (Figs. 467 to 474). The following remarks apply especially to *inguinal* hernia.

When a hernia which is irreducible or strangulated is subjected to forcible manipulation with a view to its reduction, certain displacements of the sac or of its contents may result; these displacements, known as " reduction *en masse*," may be thus enumerated :—

(1) The whole sac with its unreduced contents may be displaced upwards—(i) subcutaneously between the skin and the abdominal wall ; (ii) interstitially between the internal and external oblique muscles (Fig. 467), or between the transversalis muscle and the peritoneum (properitoneal) (Fig. 468) ; (iii) behind the iliac peritoneum, cæcum, or sigmoid (retroperitoneal).

(2) The sac may be ruptured circularly at the neck and *the contents* forced into any of the above positions, the body and fundus remaining behind (Fig. 469).

(3) The sac may be ruptured laterally and the contents forced through the rent either interstitially as above, or simply into the scrotum (Fig. 470).

(4) The contents may be forced from the main sac to a lateral diverticulum (Fig. 471).

(5) The contents may be forced through a rent in the omentum and the whole reduced into the abdomen, the sac remaining behind (Fig. 472).

(6) The bowel may be reduced across an adhesion at the neck of the sac (Fig. 474).

2. The bowel may be torn across at the neck of the sac (Fig. 473), general peritonitis rapidly terminating the case.

3. Short of rupture, serious hæmorrhage may be produced in the sac ; or such bruising may take place that gangrene rapidly supervenes.

" Reduction *en masse* " is thus a very serious condition, since it suggests for the moment that reduction has been correctly performed, although an irreducible hernia may have been converted into a strangulated one, while a strangulated hernia may be allowed to persist. When suspected, the only possible treatment is immediate laparotomy. The possibility of the occurrence of " reduction *en masse* " should be thought of where a very sudden reduction effected under considerable pressure is accompanied by sharp pain, and is followed by persistence of the signs of strangulation, or by those of general peritonitis. The mortality of operation in such cases is, of course, very high.

In very early cases it may be possible to assist taxis by placing the patient in the Trendelenburg position, and applying an ice-bag for some time before the attempt is made ; or by the use of ether applied drop by drop to the swelling. These methods may reduce the volume of gases in the intestine and diminish the congestion to some extent, but on the other hand there is the danger of producing thrombosis in the constricted vessels. In any case, time is thus lost.

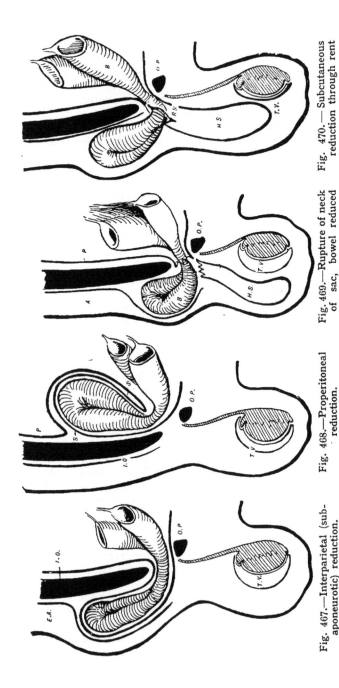

Fig. 467.—Interparietal (sub-aponeurotic) reduction.

E.A., External oblique aponeurosis ; I.O., internal oblique muscle ; O.P., pubes ; T.V., tunica vaginalis.

Fig. 468.—Properitoneal reduction.

P., Peritoneum ; S., sac in peritoneal position ; I.O., conjoined internal oblique and transversalis muscles ; O.P., pubes ; T.V., tunica vaginalis.

Fig. 469.—Rupture of neck of sac, bowel reduced interparietally.

A., Aponeurosis ; B., bowel ; H.S., hernial sac ; P., peritoneum ; O.P., pubes ; T.V., tunica vaginalis.

Fig. 470.— Subcutaneous reduction through rent in sac.

H.S., Hernial sac ; T.V., tunica vaginalis ; O.P., pubes ; B., bowel ; R.S., rent in sac.

REDUCTION "EN MASSE."

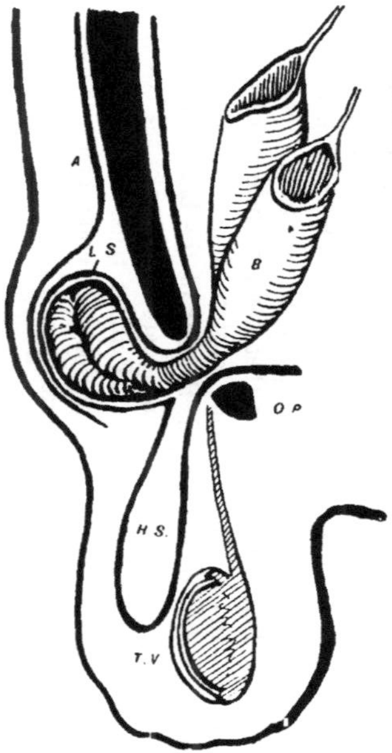

Fig. 471.—Reduction into lateral sacculus.

L.S., Lateral sacculus ; H.S., hernial sac ; A., aponeurosis ; B., bowel ; T.V., tunica vaginalis.

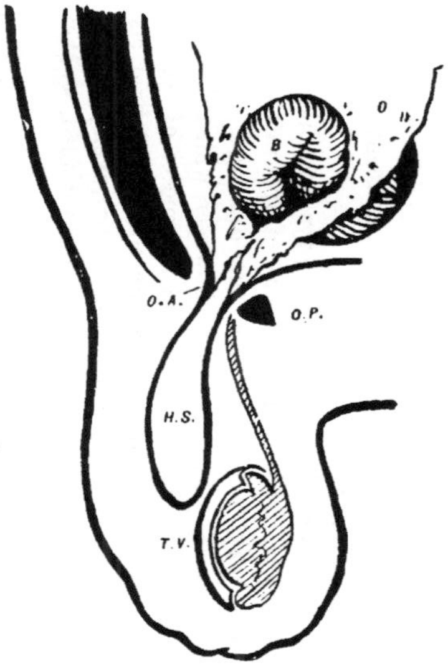

Fig. 472.—Reduction through rent in omentum.

H.S., Hernial sac ; O.P., pubes ; T.V., tunica vaginalis ; O., omentum ; O.A., omental adhesion ; B., bowel.

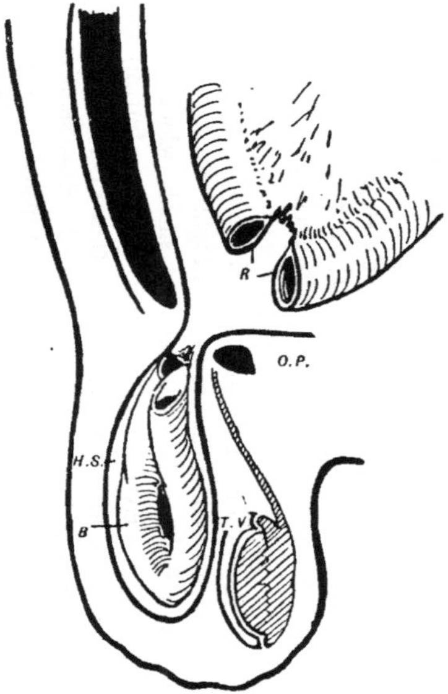

Fig. 473.—Rupture of bowel at neck of sac.

H.S., Hernial sac ; B., bowel ; R., point of rupture ; O.P., pubes ; T.V., tunica vaginalis.

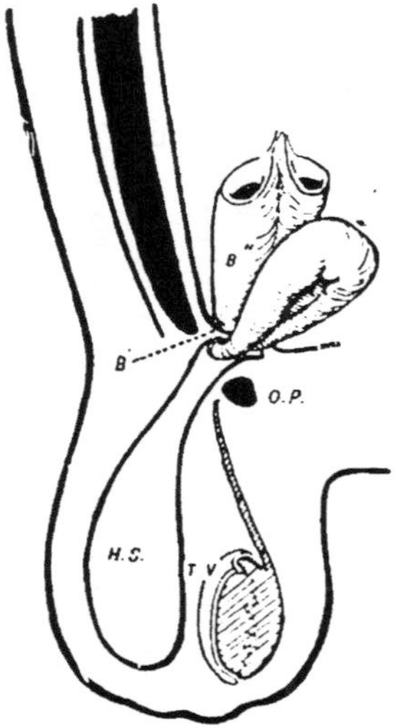

Fig. 474.— Reduction across an adhesion at neck of sac.

A', Adhesion band ; B', bowel ; O.P., pubes ; H.S., hernial sac ; T.V., tunica vaginalis.

REDUCTION "EN MASSE."

A better method is to submit the patient to spinal analgesia, or to chloroform anæsthesia, proceeding at once to operation if taxis fails.

OPERATIVE TREATMENT OF STRANGULATED HERNIA

Precautions.—The following precautions must be observed prior to operation :—

1. The preliminary cleansing is best done by swabbing with acetone, followed by painting with iodine (*see* Vol. I., p. 266), *without* the previous use of soap and water.

2. In every case where possible the patient's stomach should be washed out. This is especially necessary where a general anæsthetic is to be employed, the danger of inhalation of fæculent vomit being considerable. Septic pneumonia following, or even asphxyia during operation may be the result of neglecting this precaution. In any case the material, if retained in the stomach, is highly toxic.

3. Every precaution must be taken against shock, which is often marked in these cases. Extract of pituitary gland (pituitrin) may be given hypodermically an hour before operation or on the table ; while during the operation two or three pints of dextrose solution (2½ per cent.), in normal saline, may be intravenously infused. The body must be kept warm.

4. Rapidity of operation should be aimed at, and no attempt made to complete the operation by radical cure at the moment if the patient is showing signs of exhaustion.

5. Since the condition of the bowel is always an unknown quantity, nothing should be overlooked in the way of apparatus, when it is obtainable, which may be required for the drainage, resection, or anastomosis of the bowel. In emergencies, however, wide rubber tubing may take the place of a Paul's tube ; and flat pieces of wood, their ends surrounded by rubber bands, make excellent intestinal clamps.

6. Neither purgatives nor enemata should be given ; the former are dangerous and useless, and the latter, being retained, as they are sure to be, will probably be voided on the table.

Kelotomy.—The incision should in all cases be a wide one ; much time may be lost in attempting to operate through a cramped space. All structures are divided down to the sac itself, from which they should be separated, provided the patient's condition does not compel haste. The fundus of the sac is then caught up in three pairs of pressure forceps, and is opened. This must be done carefully with the edge (not the point) of the scalpel, the flat of the blade lying on the surface of the sac ; unless this is done, there is danger of the bowel being carried by the sudden rush of fluid under tension in the sac, or by the sudden expansion of flatus, against the point of the knife, and so being injured. The escaping fluid should be caught on a pad and its colour and smell noted. If it be turbid, blood-stained, or fæculent, care should be observed in handling the bowel, since such signs point to ulceration at the point of constriction ; no attempt should be made as yet to draw down the bowel for inspection, in view of this possibility. The sac is opened to the neck, and the colour and surface of the bowel or of the omentum must be noted. The bowel must now be released by division of the constriction, the method depending on the variety of hernia.

In inguinal hernia.—If the hernia is an oblique one, a Cooper's hernia director is passed along between the bowel and the neck of the sac, so that its groove faces the anterior superior spine ; the hernia knife is passed along it on the flat, and the back of the knife being turned into the groove, the two instruments are pushed along together, their handles more or less widely separated according to the depth of incision required. In this way the neck of the sac is divided *upwards and outwards* so as to avoid the deep epigastric vessels which lie along its inner side. If the hernia is a direct one, the incision must be made *upwards and inwards,* the director being passed along the inner aspect of the bowel. In spite of the width of the director, bowel will at times tend to overlap its edges, especially in wide-necked sacs with much bowel ; the greatest care must be taken in these cases not to injure the latter.

In femoral hernia.—Here the structure to be divided is Gimbernat's ligament, which lies just internally to the neck of the sac. In doing this the occasional peculiar origin of the obturator artery from the deep epigastric must be remembered. This vessel should arise from the anterior branch of the internal iliac artery, giving off, just before it enters the foramen, the little pubic branch which anastomoses with the pubic branch of the deep epigastric. Occasionally this branch may be so large, and the obturator itself so small, that the latter may be said to arise from the deep epigastric. In this case the vessel will be found to occupy one of three positions : (*a*) It may lie at some distance internally to the sac ; (*b*) it may cross the posterior aspect of Gimbernat's ligament ; or (*c*) it may closely follow its external margin, hugging the neck of the sac. In the last position it would almost certainly be divided in the act of incising the constriction. Statistics as to the frequency of this accident do not help to prevent its occurrence ; the constriction *must* be divided, and if by chance the accident should happen, three courses are open to the surgeon : (*a*) The bowel being returned, an effort may be made to catch the vessel in the wound—a very difficult matter owing to the narrowness and depth of the latter. (*b*) The deep epigastric may be tied ; this may fail owing to the free collateral circulation here. (*c*) The tying of the deep epigastric may be supplemented by ligature of the external iliac artery. Fortunately the accident is of rare occurrence; it may to some extent be avoided by using a hernia knife with a slightly blunted edge, since the tense ligament is more readily cut than the lax vessel. The director should be passed with the groove facing the pubic spine, and the incision made directly inwards, no more being done than is necessary to free the bowel.

In umbilical hernia.—The incision may be made upwards or downwards, usually without danger; the director is rarely necessary, since the constriction, being due to the fibres of the linea alba, can be divided from without; if there is still a constriction due to the neck of the sac, this too can be dealt with from without.

Operative treatment of obturator hernia.—For reasons already given (*see* p. 606), this hernia is rarely submitted to operation except when strangulated. The skin incision should be made vertically downwards and inwards from a point 1 in. external to the pubic spine, for a distance of 5 or 6 in. This will lie along the inner edge of the femoral vein. The femoral vessels are retracted outwards and a separation is effected between the adductor longus and pectineus muscles. The bulging of the hernial sac either through the obturator canal or through the muscle fibres should now be seen. If access to the parts is difficult, the fibres of the pectineus muscle may be divided, care being taken to avoid its nerve which lies behind it. If an attempt to reduce the hernia fails, a hernia director is passed along the neck of the sac *above or below*, and the hernia knife passed along it so as to divide the constriction either upwards or downwards, the vessels usually lying anteriorly or posteriorly to the neck of the sac. Failing success in reduction by this method, the abdomen should be opened to the hernial side of the middle line, and reduction effected by gentle traction from within, the greatest care being taken not to rupture the bowel, nor to allow of the escape of foul-smelling or blood-stained fluid into the abdominal cavity. The sac is then transfixed, tied, and removed, and the wound is closed.

Gluteal and sciatic hernias can be released by a downward incision, but in these cases the irregularity of the vascular anastomosis may be considerable, and the best rule is that of free access to the parts by a wide incision, the division being effected by careful dissection.

Is the bowel recoverable?—As soon as the constriction has been divided, the state of the bowel must be ascertained. It should be gently withdrawn from the wound, remembering always that the release must be sufficiently free to permit of this being done without the least force; for if at this moment a tear should occur at the constriction, the bowel above being tensely filled with liquid fæces and flatus, the lower abdomen is immediately flooded and the patient's doom is sealed.

Bowel may be classified as "safe," "doubtful," or "dangerous." It is **"safe"** when—(1) there is no lymph on its surface; (2) it has not lost its gloss; (3) œdema and bogginess are absent; (4) there is neither ecchymosis nor constriction-slough at or near the neck; (5) it gradually returns to its normal colour on being released; (6) the mesentery is not discoloured by blood extravasation; (7) the fluid in the sac is clear and free from odour.

It is **"doubtful"** if—(1) there is much delay in the return of colour on being released; (2) it has lost its gloss; (3) the fluid is blood-stained.

It is **"dangerous"** when—(1) it is black and boggy; (2) the constriction remains clearly outlined on the surface; (3) the fluid is foul and blood-stained.

"*Safe*" intestine may be returned to the abdomen after being gently washed with normal saline at a temperature of 110° F.; after which, if the patient's condition is good, the usual radical operation may be performed. Otherwise, the wound is closed and a pad applied to prevent the return of the hernia; the radical operation being deferred till later.

"*Doubtful*" or "*dangerous*" bowel.—Two courses are open to the surgeon here. He may either resect the strangulated portion, reuniting the cut ends by some form of intestinal anastomosis, or, fixing the loop in the wound, he may open it and introduce a Paul's tube. The choice of method will depend chiefly on the condition of the patient. Resection is the ideal method and should be done even where the bowel is "doubtful," but the decision to attempt it must be influenced also by (1) the length of bowel to be resected; (2) the portion of the bowel involved; (3) the character of the strangulation; (4) the experience of the operator; (5) the availability of skilled assistance; and (6) the patient's surroundings, as regards light, cleanliness, and materials for so serious an operation. Roughly speaking, resection is indicated (a) where the patient is not over 60, is not exhausted by vomiting, and cardiac and pulmonary disease are absent; (b) where the small intestine is involved; (c) where the amount of bowel involved is not so great as to preclude the possibility of success;[1] (d) where the operation is done by one skilled in surgical technique and rapid operating; and (e) where it can be done under spinal analgesia. Strangulated omentum should *always* be resected.

Formation of a fæcal or intestinal fistula.—This

[1] A length of anything over 3 feet must be looked upon as serious, although as much as 11 feet has been successfully removed. Spinal analgesia has greatly lessened the danger of resection; thus, in the Seamen's Hospital, Gwynne Williams has successfully resected 7 feet of small intestine under its influence in a patient of over 60, without increase of shock, although the strangulation was a double one.

is the only safe treatment where the patient is old, feeble, and exhausted by pain and vomiting, and where the mass is too great for resection and anastomosis. It should also be done, as a rule, in strangulation of the large bowel, in preference to primary resection, which has a higher mortality than in the case of the small bowel, because (1) the blood supply is less extensive and more longitudinal, and therefore union is more difficult to secure ; (2) the contents are more solid and therefore more irritating ; (3) the arrangement of the musculature is less adapted to anastomosis ; and (4) flatus accumulates with greater rapidity here.

It should not, however, be done when there is reason to suppose that the strangulation is high, for although life *can* be saved by artificial feeding through the jejunum for a considerable period, as proved by me in conjunction with Bruce · Clarke, it is extremely difficult, and would not succeed in all cases alike.

Points regarding the methods of operating.—When resection and anastomosis is proposed in the case of inguinal or femoral hernia, it is better that the operation should be done *in situ* than that the abdomen should be opened and the damaged bowel withdrawn through the abdominal wound for the purpose. When a perforation exists there is danger of soiling the peritoneum ; while even when none is present, the manipulation necessary to reduce the damaged bowel, especially when wrapped in gauze as a precautionary measure, is likely to result in a tear and in extravasation of the contents. In performing the anastomosis the hernial aperture must be enlarged, the bowel must be well drawn through the ring from the abdomen, thoroughly cleansed, and reduced. Where foul fluid is present, a light gauze wick or a " cigarette " drain should be placed in the wound for twenty-four hours.

The surgeon may be faced with the difficulty of dealing with a section of intestine which is gangrenous, or at least " dangerous," at two or more points.[1] He must rapidly determine on one of three courses : he must either (*a*) perform two or more separate resections ; (*b*) resect the whole length of bowel involved ; or (*c*) bring the whole length outside the abdomen and make an intestinal fistula or an artificial anus. Each case must be judged on its merits, and the following points will help in the decision :—

1. A large section may be resected and an anastomosis performed more rapidly than two short sections ; thus a prolonged operation is avoided.

2. When, however, the section to be removed is very long (6 to 8 ft.) the shock may be equally great ; in even longer sections it may be much greater than from the resection of two separate sections.

[1] This was so in Williams's case, referred to on p. 651 (footnote).

3. When the gangrenous portions are situated one in the small and the other in the large bowel, the former may be resected and the latter converted into an artificial anus for the time being, when the patient cannot stand two resections.

4. Extensive resections are attended by a mortality which is largely in inverse ratio to the skill and rapidity of the operator. For this reason, in unpractised hands, the emergency is best met by the third method, viz. exclusion of the affected loop and the formation of an intestinal fistula.

For this purpose, the sound bowel having been brought down to

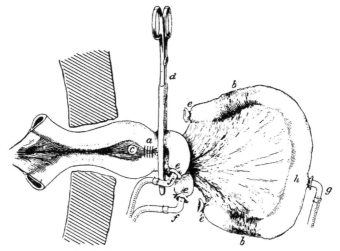

Fig. 475.—Exclusion of gangrenous bowel and formation of intestinal fistula.

a, Sutures joining loops ; *b, b*, gangrenous sections ; *c*, rod supporting bowel ; *d*, bowel clamp : *e, e, e, e*, ligatures on bowel ; *f, f*, Paul's tubes in cut ends; *g*, Paul's tube in excluded loop ; *h*, site of incision in loop.

the ring, the entering and returning coils are connected side by side by one or two interrupted sutures (Fig. 475, *a*) some distance from the gangrenous portions (*b*), and are supported by a short length of rubber-covered glass rod (*c*) passed beneath the union. A clamp (*d*) is applied just distally to the union, and a ligature (*e*) is placed round each portion of the bowel about 1½ in. beyond the clamp. Finally, the bowel is divided between the clamp and the ligatures ; a Paul's tube (*f*) is introduced into each cut end, being fixed by a purse-string suture, and the clamp is removed. An incision should be made into the loop at the point (*h*), and, if necessary, a third Paul's tube (*g*) introduced to prevent it from becoming distended with gas and fluid. The fistula may be rapidly made in this way, and the loop with its mesentery may be removed on recovery of the patient at the end of three or four days; the anastomosis may be deferred till later unless the fistula is high up in the bowel, when it should be done at the earliest possible date. It may even be done at the time of the first operation; in this case a lateral anastomosis by means of a Murphy's or a Jaboulay's button is the method indicated.

Where the case is so urgent as to demand it, the loop must be secured to the skin incision and the Paul's tube inserted without the above elaboration. The making of an intestinal fistula *in situ* in the case of femoral hernia is attended by certain difficulties: the proximity of the femoral and saphenous veins renders the femoral canal a bad site for the discharge of fæces; moreover, the canal is often too long and narrow to allow of satisfactory evacuation of the bowel, or its reduction from within by laparotomy, when swathed in gauze. In such a case, where the patient is able to stand it, the abdomen may be opened above the pubes; the gangrenous loop and its mesentery are surrounded by a double ligature and divided between, the mass being cut away. The cut ends are then washed, swabbed over with pure carbolic acid, washed again, and seized with a clamp and drawn through the wound into the abdomen, the remaining bowels being kept out of the way as far as possible; finally, the ends are brought out of the abdominal wound, and are treated by anastomosis, or with Paul's tubes, in the manner above described.

After-treatment of strangulated hernia.—The indications are—to combat shock, support the patient's strength, and provide against complications.

In a quite uncomplicated case nothing more is, as a rule, necessary than to secure sleep and provide fluid diet. The bowels should be moved at first only by enemata, and after forty-eight hours by calomel given in grain doses every hour up to 5-8 gr., this being assisted when needful by a dose of salts, or Apenta or other mineral water. Strychnine hypodermically or nux vomica by the mouth will lessen the chances of paralytic ileus; by some, pituitary extract or eserine salicylate given hypodermically is thought to be also of use.

Where there has been severe strangulation with fæculent vomit, infusion with normal saline or, better still, dextrose saline intravenously (2·5 per cent.) or per rectum (8 per cent.), should be practised. Two or three pints may be given intravenously; but, per rectum the continuous method should be used, the solution being introduced at the rate of half a pint an hour, till the blood pressure is sufficiently raised. The addition of adrenalin solution, 1 drachm to the pint, will often help considerably in the intravenous method.

If not done before operation, the stomach should be washed out as soon as the patient's condition admits of it, and salol in 5-grain doses administered. The semi-recumbent position (Fig. 466, p. 639) should be adopted, and the expectoration of fæculent sputum encouraged by the use of ammonium carbonate in 5-grain doses, or other suitable drug.

When resection and anastomosis has been performed, it is in the highest degree important to prevent any distension of the bowel ; this is best accomplished by the use of the soft rectal tube passed high and retained *in situ*, or by the occasional use of enemata of turpentine or asafœtida.

The feeding of these patients is not, as a rule, difficult. Where no damage to the bowel has occurred it may be carried out on ordinary lines. When resection and anastomosis has been done, nothing but fluids should be given for at least forty-eight hours. Albumin water, beef-juice, egg-flip, white wine whey, Brand's jelly, veal or chicken jelly, junket, calf's-foot jelly, etc., may be given ; dextrose solution per rectum is in itself a food, and has a very high calorific value. On the fourth day, if the patient is progressing well, Benger's food, pounded fish or chicken, etc., may be given in small quantities frequently. Full diet should not be allowed for a fortnight from the time of operation.

Opium and morphia are best avoided ; they mask symptoms and cause constipation. Pain must be relieved, if possible, by aspirin in 10-grain doses, and sleep provided by such drugs as veronal 5 gr., chloralamide 30 gr., or trional 20 gr. When the case has ended in the establishment of an intestinal fistula, the bowels may be cleared out at once, and feeding started as soon as the stomach has been cleansed and the sickness has ceased.

In the event of recovery the Paul's tube will become detached in about three days, and the question will then arise as to the reconstitution of the bowel. This, unless the stoma is high in the canal (jejunum), should not be attempted before the strength is recovered, since there is a danger of union failing owing to weakness and anæmia. In the higher regions the attempt must be made at the earliest possible date by simple suture without detachment of the skin union ; failing this, detachment should be done, and the lips of the bowel wound should be inverted by two rows of Lembert's sutures. Where this fails, or where there is a marked " spur," resection and anastomosis affords the only chance of arresting the rapid emaciation which occurs. The abdominal wound should not be closed in these cases, as the tissues are obviously infected ; it should be allowed to close by granulation, any subsequent hernia being cured by filigree-implantation.

After-complications of kelotomy for strangulated hernia.—1. Septic broncho-pneumonia is not infrequent when fæcal vomiting has occurred. The prognosis is grave, especially in elderly subjects, and the case may progress to abscess and gangrene of the lung.

2. General peritonitis may result from subsequent sloughing or perforation of the returned bowel. The only possible treatment is immediate laparotomy and cleansing of the abdomen, the bowel being brought into the wound as already described, and the abdomen drained through both loins and above the pubes. The prognosis is usually fatal, recovery, when it occurs, depending on the interval which has elapsed, the amount of extravasation, and the strength of the patient.

3. Paralytic ileus may supervene on release of the strangulation, or may be actually present when the case is first seen, the vomiting, distension, and inability to pass flatus persisting. No time should be lost in opening the cæcum or lower end of the ileum. Owing to the vomiting, drugs can seldom be given by the mouth, and, if the ileus is absolute, little can be done. When the strangulation has been seen late in the case this danger is to be feared ; it is well to open the abdomen by a small incision above the umbilicus, and, drawing out a loop of the jejunum, to inject into it 3 or 4 drachms of magnesium sulphate with 10 minims of tincture of nux vomica, closing the puncture by a fine purse-string suture. Puncture of the coils of intestine by means of a trocar and cannula is a tedious process, and seldom succeeds. The prognosis is commonly fatal, and prophylaxis is better than attempts at cure. Eserine or pituitrin hypodermically will help.

4. Stenosis may occur at the site of constriction, or when anastomosis has been performed, especially when a Murphy's button has been used. In a case of my own, stenosis followed simple reduction four months after operation in another hospital, and resulted in adhesion to the abdominal wall, ulceration above the constriction, and a fæcal abscess of the abdominal wall. This necessitated excision of the cæcum, appendix, and ten inches of ileum, and, on recovery, the cure of the resulting hernia by implantation of a large abdominal filigree.

Symptoms of dyspepsia, distension, anorexia, and constipation should suggest the possibility of this complication, especially where the bowel has been slow in recovering its vitality at the original operation.

Prognosis in strangulated hernia.—The probabilities of recovery in an uncomplicated case depend on the duration and character of the vomiting, the age of the patient, and his general condition. Up to the time of the vomit becoming fæculent the patient is well within the period of grace ; when this point has been passed and the odour of the vomit shows the presence of jejunal contents, the prognosis must be considered grave, especially if the vomit is copious, frequent, and forcible ; when the vomit is actually fæcal the time of grace has passed, and, as Handley has pointed out, this sign must be looked upon as a *præsagium mortis.*

The older the patient, the worse the prognosis, since in these cases exhaustion sets in rapidly, and the inability to expectorate the foul sputum and mucus from the larynx is very distressing.

When, in a strangulated hernia of some standing, and in which vomiting has been active the vomiting suddenly ceases, the patient going into collapse or, as sometimes happens, saying *he feels better*, a grave suspicion should be entertained of rupture or perforation of the bowel.

Elderly subjects are more affected by the shock of a tight constriction than are young adults, and the exhaustion produced by the vomitless retching of a high jejunal strangulation is in them more profound than when the vomit is in quantity and possibly even fæculent.

In cases complicated by gangrene, perforation, and peritonitis, or in which resection has been performed, it is obvious that the gravity of the prognosis will be proportionate to the duration and height of the strangulation, the period elapsing between perforation and operation, and the length of the section of bowel removed.

BIBLIOGRAPHY

Bartlett, Willard, *Journ. of Amer. Med. Assoc.*, 1903, i. 47.
Bonney, Victor, *Arch. of Middx. Hosp.*, Nov., 1910, p. 27.
Clarke, Bruce, *Lancet*, 1907, i. 8.
Graser, von Bergmann's *System of Surgery*, iv. 622.
McGavin, Lawrie, *Trans. Clin. Soc.*, 1907, p. 134 ; *Trans. Roy. Soc. Med.*, Clin. Sec., 1909, ii. 156 ; *Lancet*, 1907, ii. 1445 ; *Brit. Med. Journ.*, 1907, ii. 1395 ; Aug. 14, 1911.
Mayo, William, *Ann. of Surg.*, 1901, ii. 276 ; *Journ. of Amer. Med. Assoc.*, July, 1903.
Richards, Owen, *Lancet*, 1899, ii. 1386.
Russell, Hamilton, *Lancet*, 1899, ii. 1353 ; 1902, i. 1519 ; 1904, i. 707.
Sultan, *Saunders' Hand-Atlas*, "Hernia," p. 106.

THE RECTUM AND ANAL CANAL

By H. S. CLOGG, M.S.Lond., F.R.C.S.Eng.

Anatomy.—The **rectum** commences in front of the 3rd (sometimes the 2nd) sacral vertebra, and ends by passing through the pelvic diaphragm, about 1½ in. below and in front of the tip of the coccyx, opposite the lower part of the prostate in the male, and the lower fourth of the vagina in the female. It lies entirely within the pelvic cavity, and measures about 6 in. in the adult. Its relations are seen

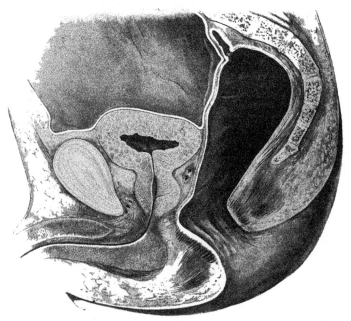

Fig. 476.—Male pelvis in vertical median section, showing the rectum and anal canal in section, their anterior and posterior relations, and the recto-vesical reflexion of the peritoneum.

in Figs. 476, 477, and 478. Narrowest above, it frequently shows a distinct constriction at its junction with the pelvic colon, and here a physiological sphincter exists, for the rectum is a passage, and not a reservoir, for fæces. Just above its termination a dilatation known as the *ampulla* is present.

The upper part, except a narrow strip of posterior surface, is covered with peritoneum. The serous membrane gradually leaves the sides, and finally the anterior wall; the level of reflexion varies slightly, but is commonly about 3 in. from the anal margin; in the child it is relatively lower than in the adult. The peritoneum is intimately attached to the bowel above, but more loosely below.

The *longitudinal muscle fibres* are principally collected into an anterior and a posterior bundle, which are relatively shorter than the rectum itself; hence when distended the bowel shows lateral inflexions of its walls. The *circular muscle fibres* form a complete investment. The thick, vascular *mucosa* presents numerous folds in the empty gut. Lymphoid nodules are found in the mucosa and submucosa; Lieberkühn's follicles are abundant; the surface epithelium is columnar.

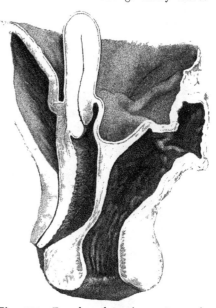

Fig. 477.—Female pelvic viscera in vertical section, showing the relation of the rectum to the vagina and the recto-vaginal reflexion of the peritoneum.

The *rectal valves* (*valves of Houston*, Fig. 479) are circular, crescentic, or spiral folds, best seen in the distended gut, and composed of all the tissues of the bowel wall, except perhaps some of the outer longitudinal muscle fibres. They correspond in position to the lateral inflexions of the wall, and have a similar origin. There are commonly one well-marked right valve and two less definite left ones, the former being immediately above the peritoneal reflexion and the latter equidistant above and below it.

The anal canal is an antero-posterior slit-like passage, about 1 in. long, leading downwards and backwards to the anal orifice, and forming an angle of 90° with the rectum (Fig. 476). On each side is the ischio-rectal fossa; in front the membranous urethra and its enclosing muscles in the male, and in the female the perineal body, separating it from the vagina; behind is a mass of muscular and connective tissue—the ano-coccygeal body. The

longitudinal muscle fibres of the rectum are prolonged as a thin investment
to the canal. and the levator ani also encloses it.   The circular muscle fibres
are considerably thickened, and constitute the *internal sphincter*.   This is
about 1 in. in vertical extent, and is easily detected on digital examination.
Being merely a thickening of circular muscle fibres, it should have a similar
action, and should, therefore, empty the bowel (Cunningham).   Clinical
experience, however, teaches that
whereas the external sphincter may
be cut with impunity, division of
both sphincters may cause fæcal
incontinence.

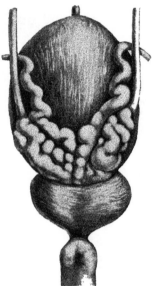

Fig. 478.—Base of the bladder,
vesiculæ seminales, vasa deferentia, ureters, prostate,
membranous urethra, and
bulb of the corpus spongiosum, to show the structures
in relation anteriorly to the
male rectum and anal canal.

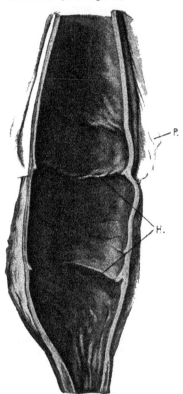

Fig. 479.—The rectum opened
anteriorly.

P., Peritoneum of the anterior and lateral walls of
the rectum. and the lower limit anteriorly ; H., the
valves of Houston, one of which is immediately
above the peritoneal reflexion.

The anal canal shows eight or nine vertical folds composed of mucous
membrane and muscularis mucosæ—the *columns of Morgagni* (Fig. 480).
These are permanent, not effaced by distension, well marked in the fœtus,
and constant throughout life.   Occasionally they are ill marked, rarely
they are absent.   The columns are broader below, and gradually taper above.
Their bases (anal ends) are connected by a circumferential irregular " zig-zag "

line a little above the anus, thought by some to indicate the line of fusion of the hind-gut and proctodæum (p. 666). The intervening depressions—the *rectal sinuses of Morgagni*—end abruptly below and are guarded by the miniature *anal valves* (the intercolumnar portions of the " zig-zag " line). The sinuses and valves vary in development, and are better marked posteriorly. The appearance below the " zig-zag " line is whitish, resembling modified skin, whilst above it resembles modified mucous membrane. Squamous epithelium lines the lower part of the canal, and extends to the bases of the columns, columnar epithelium extending to the sinuses. The transformation of epithelium is a gradual one. Sometimes minute tiny pits or depressions

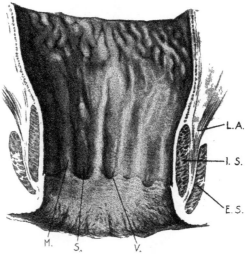

Fig. 480.—The lower rectum and anal canal, incised longitudinally and held widely open.

ᴇ.ꜱ., External sphincter muscle ; ɪ.ꜱ., internal sphincter muscle : ʟ.ᴀ., levator ani muscle ᴍ., columns of Morgagni ; ꜱ., sinus of Morgagni ; ᴠ., anal valve.

are seen on the mucosa of the lower rectum and anal canal. It has been stated that infective diseases may originate in these depressions.

Muscles and fasciæ.—The *external sphincter* is a subcutaneous muscle, about 1 in. in breadth, encircling the anus, attached posteriorly to the coccyx, and anteriorly to the central point of the perineum. It is superficial to the internal sphincter muscle, the sulcus between the two being readily detected on digital examination of the anal canal. It overlies the fat of the ischio-rectal fossa. It is supplied by the inferior hæmorrhoidal and perineal branch of the 4th sacral nerves.

The *levator ani* and the *coccygeus* form the pelvic floor or diaphragm ; they are enclosed in sheaths derived from the pelvic fascia, and with their fascial prolongations help to support the bowel.

The *levator ani* is attached to the back of the os pubis in front and the ischial spine posteriorly, and between these two points to the pelvic fascia, near its " white line." The fibres pass downwards and backwards—the anterior ones being almost horizontal and the posterior ones nearly vertical—to be inserted into the central point of the perineum and into the wall of the anal canal, blending with the external sphincter, while behind the anus the two muscles meet in a median raphe between the anus and the coccyx. and the most posterior fibres are attached to the lower sacral and coccygeal vertebræ (Fig. 481). The upper surface is separated by the pelvic fascia from the prostate, or vagina, and the rectum ; the inferior surface, covered by the anal fascia, bounds the ischio-rectal fossa. It is supplied by the

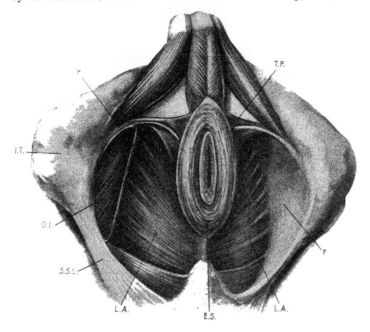

Fig. 481.—The ischio-rectal fossæ. The attachment of the external sphincter muscle to the coccyx has been removed.

I.T., Ischial tuberosity ; S.S.L., great sacro-sciatic ligament ; T.P., transverse perineal muscle ; E S., external sphincter muscle ; L.A., levator ani muscle ; F. (on the right side), the fascia covering the obturator internus muscle ; F. (on the left side), the cut edge of the fascia which has been removed. showing O.I., the obturator internus muscle.

perineal branch of the pudic nerve, and by the 3rd and 4th sacral nerves on its pelvic aspect.

The fibres of the levatores ani passing from the back of the os pubis to meet behind the anus will, when contracted, firmly grip the anal canal, reducing it to an antero-posterior slit. These fibres of the levatores, therefore, form a sphincter to the anal canal, and can often be detected by digital examination per rectum.

The *coccygeus* is attached to the ischial spine, the adjacent pelvic fascia and the side of the coccyx. It is in contact anteriorly with the levator ani.

and posteriorly with the lesser sacro-sciatic ligament. It is supplied on its pelvic surface by the 3rd and 4th sacral nerves.

The *extraperitoneal tissue* in the pelvis, almost devoid of fat, extends along the rectum as far as the anal canal. It supports the bowel, and conveys the vessels to the rectum.

The *pelvic fascia* lines the pelvis and supplies sheaths for the muscles and supports for the pelvic viscera. Lining the levator ani on its pelvic aspect is a strong fibrous layer, which at the insertion of the muscle is attached to the deep layer of the triangular ligament, the bowel wall, and behind this is continuous with the layer of the opposite side above the raphe of insertion of the levatores ani muscles, and is prolonged posteriorly over the coccygeus muscle. The rectum receives from this layer a sheath which gradually thins below and becomes lost where the anal canal commences.

Ischio-rectal fossa (Fig. 481).—This fossa, occupied by fat, is bounded externally by the pelvic fascia covering the obturator internus muscle ; internally by the anal fascia clothing the levator ani and coccygeus muscles ; anteriorly by the junction of the anal fascia and deep layer of the triangular ligament : posteriorly by the sacro-sciatic ligament and gluteus maximus muscle. The fossa is overlapped posteriorly by the gluteus maximus, and internally by the external sphincter ; between these two the subcutaneous is continuous with the ischio-rectal fat. The depth of the fossa varies, but in an average adult measures about 2½ in. The pudic vessels and nerve run in a fascial tunnel in the outer wall of the fossa, and the inferior hæmorrhoidal vessels and nerve cross the fat in the fossa.

Arteries.—The *superior hæmorrhoidal*, a continuation of the inferior mesenteric trunk, supplies the muscular and mucous coats in the upper part, and the mucosa only in the lower inch or so, one terminal vessel being found in each column of Morgagni. The *middle hæmorrhoidals*, one on each side, from the internal iliac arteries, supply the muscular walls of the lower rectum and the mucosa of the upper anal canal. The *inferior hæmorrhoidals*, two or three on each side, from the pudic vessels, supply the muscles principally, but branches also pass to the mucosa through the interval between the two sphincter muscles or in the immediate neighbourhood. The *middle sacral* gives one or two small branches to the muscular wall, some of which may penetrate to the mucosa.

A plexus, the *hæmorrhoidal plexus*, is formed in the submucous tissue by the anastomosis of the branches of all these arteries.

Veins.—The veins are valveless. In each column of Morgagni is found a plexiform arrangement of veins, some of which may show dilatations. Leaving the upper end of each column are one or more veins which, after passing a variable distance in the submucosa, perforate the muscular wall and join the superior hæmorrhoidal vessels. When in the submucosa the veins freely communicate with one another, forming the *internal venous hæmorrhoidal plexus*.

In the perianal skin are a number of radially arranged veins, communicating with one another by a circular vein. These connect above with the radicles of the superior hæmorrhoidal veins in the columns of Morgagni. The veins of the anal margin and the anal canal chiefly contribute to the formation of the inferior hæmorrhoidal veins. Veins accompanying the middle hæmorrhoidal arteries are also present. On the outer surface of the rectal wall is a rich venous plexus contributed to by all the veins which pass out from the mucosa through the bowel wall, and hence all the hæmorrhoidal veins are brought freely into communication with one another. A free anastomosis is established, therefore, between the portal and the systemic venous circulations.

Lymphatics.—These, playing such an important part in cancer, are best considered in connexion with that disease (p. 717).

Anamnesis and examination.—Methodical inquiry should be made into the history of *pain, hæmorrhage, discharge, frequency of bowel action, the shape and size of the motions*, and the presence of any *swelling* at or near the anal margin.

Pain, as distinguished from mere discomfort, is often absent in rectal diseases until some complication arises, but is usually present in lesions of the anal canal. Pain from mobility of the coccyx and pain referred from diseases of the urinary or genital tract must be differentiated from that of rectal origin. *Hæmorrhage* of rectal origin is bright red, but bright-red blood occasionally arises from diseases higher in the alimentary tract. *Discharge* from the anal margin is constant, whereas from the rectum it is only voided in response to the desire for defæcation. The normal *frequency of bowel action* should be ascertained, and any departure from this noted. Constipation causes some diseases, results from others. In proctitis and ulceration a characteristic spurious diarrhœa occurs; urgent calls to stool, frequently repeated, especially in the early morning, expel little but flatus, mucus, and perhaps blood; the motions may or may not be fæcal-stained, or may even contain some fæces. After expulsion of all secretion from the inflamed surface several hours of comparative comfort may ensue. The *shape of the motion* is determined by the last orifice through which it passes, i.e. the anus; therefore narrowing of the lumen of the bowel does not alter the shape of the motion unless the anal sphincteric power is destroyed. Hypertrophy of the sphincter and abnormal, spasmodic action, which occur in some diseases of the anal margin, may flatten the motion or give it a tapering extremity. In stricture of the bowel, simple or malignant, the typical motion consists of small isolated fragments.

Though a carefully obtained history will often suggest the correct diagnosis, visual examination of the perineum is always, and digital examination of the rectum usually, necessary. For the latter, the well-lubricated finger should be inserted very gently and slowly, pressure being made away from any painful condition of the anal margin. The diagnosis of many rectal and anal diseases is possible without further examination, but visual inspection of the interior of the bowel is sometimes necessary. A *duckbill speculum* permits efficient inspection of the anal canal and lower rectum; for the upper rectum the sigmoidoscope is necessary.

The *sigmoidoscope* (Fig. 482) consists essentially of a metal cylindrical tube fitted with an obturator to facilitate its introduction, and graduated on its exterior to indicate the distance passed into the bowel. When the obturator is withdrawn a long rod carrying a light at its distal end is introduced into the tube. The proximal end of the rod fits into the tube by a metal collar carrying the electric terminals, and closed by a glass window fitted in a metal rim. A small hand-bellows attached to the proximal end of the tube permits inflation of the rectum during examination.

The instrument, warmed and well lubricated, may be introduced with or without anæsthesia. In nervous patients, or those with painful affections, an anæsthetic is necessary. The bowels must be previously thoroughly emptied by aperients and enemata. If blood, discharge, or fæces obscure the view, they may be removed by cotton-wool pledgets on the applicator.

The introduction of the sigmoidoscope, and the interpretation of the picture seen, require practice. Houston's valves may offer some impediment to its passage, but this is easily overcome by a little manipulation; their appearance is too characteristic to cause confusion with a pathological condition. A little practice is required to facilitate the passage of the instrument along the sacro-coccygeal curve. Any stricture, simple or malignant, or any tumour pressing upon the bowel will naturally cause some impediment to the passage of the tube. The correct interpretation of the appearance observed requires experience, and implies sigmoidoscopic familiarity with the normal rectum.

The sigmoidoscope affords invaluable diagnostic aid in rectal lesions situated beyond the reach of the finger. It is invaluable also in the diagnosis of ulcer-

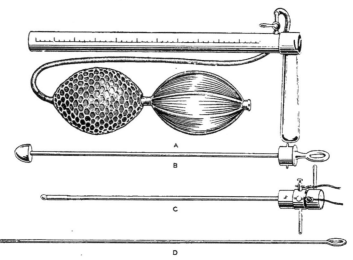

Fig. 482.—The sigmoidoscope.

A, The metal graduated tube with hand-bellows attached; B, the obturator; C, the rod carrying the light at the distal end and the terminals at the proximal end; D, the applicator.

ations, high-lying polypi, and malignant disease of the upper rectum. When it is used in cases of ulceration great care must be exercised to avoid perforation of the diseased bowel wall.

MALFORMATIONS

It is impossible in the very early human embryo to differentiate the allantois and the hind-gut. but as the hind-end of the embryo grows, the body-stalk, originally attached at the hind-end, becomes more ventral, as also does the termination of the allantois, so that a U-shaped bend, the *hind-gut*, is formed in the dorsal part of the tube. At this stage, therefore, there is a common chamber, the *cloaca*, into which open the hind-gut and the allantois. The opening of the hind-gut into the cloaca disappears early. As the hind-end of the embryo grows backwards, the dorsal part grows more rapidly than the ventral, and carries with it the hind-gut beyond the allantois, the *postallantoic* gut, a new formation entirely separated from the cloaca, but without an external opening at this stage. At the site of the future perineum, ventral to the termination of the postallantoic gut, the epiblast becomes thickened, constituting the *anal plug*. This thickening soon breaks down, and the *anal pit* or *proctodæum* is formed. The proctodæum meets the termination of the postallantoic gut towards its ventral surface, the two being separated by a thin membrane, which later disappears. The very short portion of the postallantoic gut dorsal and posterior to its fusion with the proctodæum disappears.

The cloaca forms no part of the rectum, but early becomes separated from it. The cloaca, receiving the openings of the genital ducts, becomes, in the male, the trigone of the bladder and the urethra to just below the openings of the genital ducts, that is, to just beyond the verumontanum. In the female, the Müllerian ducts open into the cloaca between the allantois anteriorly, and the original aperture of the hind-gut posteriorly. Later, the ducts migrate to the posterior part of the body, and their communications with the cloaca become lost. The vagina is for a great part of fœtal life a solid structure and not a canal, but later the Müllerian ducts tunnel a passage through this to the hind-end of the embryo. The cloaca becomes the trigone of the bladder, the urethra, and the space between the labia minora.

Thus the rectum and anal canal consist of three developmental portions— (1) the hind-gut, (2) the postallantoic gut, and (3) the proctodæum. The posterior limit of the body cavity serves to mark the junction of the hind-gut and the postallantoic gut. This point in the fully developed body is at the reflexion of the peritoneum from the rectum to the bladder or the vagina. The posterior limit of the postallantoic gut is the level of the anal sinuses. The proctodæum forms the anal canal below this level.[1]

Keith explains the abnormalities by comparative anatomy and physiology. " Above all," he says, " the process of impregnation has to be kept in mind, for it was by the evolution of the penis that the rectum attained an opening on the perineum." The cloaca of the frog is represented in the mammal by the trigone of the bladder and the urethra ; it is a passage that conveys the urine, genital products, and fæces to their destination. The fæces have no lodgment there. The rectum opens higher up than the urinary and genital ducts. Rarely in the human subject does the rectum open into the trigone of the bladder, and this exactly reproduces the amphibian form. In the tortoise and turtle the rectal orifice has moved along the dorsal wall of the cloaca nearer the tail than the genital and urinary ducts, i.e. exactly in the position where the abnormal rectum commonly ends in the human subject, in the urethra just beyond the verumontanum. The termination of the rectum as a fibrous cord on the base of the prostate represents a stage of arrest in passing from the amphibian to the tortoise form. In the tortoise and turtle the cloaca is becoming modified for sexual purposes, and is less capable of serving as a fæcal passage, and hence its orifice has moved nearer to the perineum. In Monotremes the sexual modifications are carried further, the rectum opening into that part of the cloaca derived from the ingrowth of ectoderm, the endodermal cloaca becoming the urino-genital sinus. During the evolution of the higher vertebrates the anus has migrated from an intracloacal to an extracloacal or perineal position. The various forms of malformation represent arrested stages of migration.

According to Keith, both the external and internal sphincter muscles are

---

[1] This description follows that which is given by F. Wood-Jones, and is the only one which will satisfactorily explain the various malformations.

developed from the proctodæum, which would, therefore, form the anal canal as far as the upper limit of the columns of Morgagni. Wood-Jones, however, considers that the anal sinuses limit the perineal invagination. Whether the sphincter muscles are developed in the absence of the proctodæum appears not to have been determined. In two cases where the rectum ended blindly at the base of the prostate and the proctodæal invagination was not developed, but the site of the anus merely marked by a little cutaneous eminence. I found a few muscle fibres in the position and having the course of the external sphincter. There was certainly no development of the internal sphincter. If the external sphincter were developed in such cases, operation might be undertaken with some prospect of success ; but if it were not developed, however brilliant the first results of the operation might appear, there could be no possibility of control.

Malformations are conveniently classified according to Wood-Jones's account of the development as follows :—

1. PERSISTENCE OF THE ORIGINAL COMMUNICATION WITH THE CLOACA

i. *Males.*—The common abnormality is the ending of the rectum in the urethra at the lower end of the verumontanum, immediately

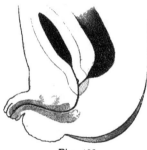 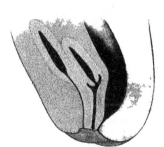

<table>
<tr><td align="center">Fig. 483.</td><td align="center">Fig. 484.</td></tr>
</table>

Fig. 483.—Rectum opening into the urethra immediately below the uterus masculinus, represented by a slight depression in the floor of the urethra.
Fig. 484.—Rectum opening into the navicular fossa of the vulval cleft.

beyond the openings of the uterus masculinus and the vasa deferentia (Fig. 483). The opening is too small to allow the passage of fæces ; it seems to be provided with a sphincter. The opening has been seen in the trigone of the bladder (amphibian form), at the internal meatus, and at the apex of the prostate.

Cases are also recorded in which the rectum opened into the frænum of the prepuce, the under surface of the penis, the raphe of the scrotum or the perineum. According to Keith, " it occasionally happens that not only is the perineal orifice of the cloaca carried forwards on the outgrowing penis, but the rectal orifice is also transplanted with it."

One specimen in the Royal College of Surgeons Museum is unique (Keith) in that the rectum has two openings—(a) the proctodæum has grown in and opened into the rectum, forming an anus in the usual position, and (b) the cloacal orifice has been prolonged forwards, and opens into the median raphe of the scrotum near the root of the penis.

ii. *Females.*—The commonest abnormality is where the rectum opens into the navicular fossa of the vulval cleft (Fig. 484), that is, in a position corresponding to the abnormal opening in the male subject. Some reports state that a sphincter exists at the opening.

The rectum has been seen opening into the vagina. Such cases, according to Keith's observations, are associated with a divided vagina, the arrested rectum probably preventing the fusion of the Müllerian ducts to form the vagina. In a few cases the vulva and clitoris are

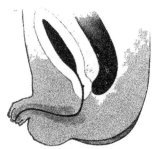 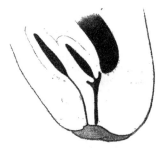

Fig. 485. — Rectum ending blindly at the back of the prostate gland.   Fig. 486.—Rectum ending blindly at the upper level of the posterior fornix of the vagina.

prolonged to form a urethra, and the rectum has been seen opening in the floor of this urethra immediately below the orifice.

2. Non-Development or Imperfect Development of the Postallantoic Gut

i. The postallantoic gut may be practically non-existent, the rectum ending blindly at the base of the prostate (Fig. 485) or at the upper level of the vagina (Fig. 486). A fibrous cord may attach the termination of the rectum to these viscera (Figs. 487 and 488).

ii. The postallantoic gut may grow backwards imperfectly, becoming separated from the prostate or the vagina (Fig. 489). It may end as a fibrous cord attached either to the proctodæal invagination (Fig. 490), or, if this be not developed, to the site of the normal anus.

3. Non-Development or Ill-Development of the Proctodæum

The proctodæum and the postallantoic gut may themselves be well formed, but the original membrane separating them may partially

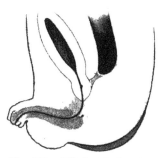

Fig. 487.—Blind end of rectum attached to the prostate by a fibrous cord.

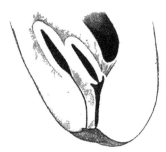

Fig. 488.—Blind end of rectum attached by a fibrous cord to the posterior vaginal vault.

or completely persist; in the former case a fibrous stricture, in the latter an absolute barrier, results (Fig. 491).

The proctodæum may be very feebly developed, or there may be

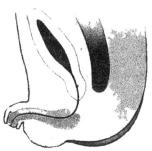

Fig. 489.—Postallantoic gut separated from the prostate and ending blindly at some distance from the peri-neum; there is no develop-ment of the proctodæum.

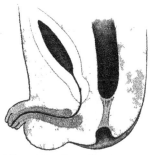

Fig. 490.—Postallantoic gut attached to the proctodæum by a fibrous cord; both the postallantoic gut and the proctodæum are imperfectly developed.

no depression at all. In some cases there is nothing to mark the site of the normal anus; in others there is an eminence at this site.

The condition of development of the proctodæum is no measure of· the degree of development of the rectum. Usually, when the rectum ends in the vulva the proctodæum is absent. When the rectum ends in the prostatic urethra the proctodæum, as a rule, is absent or imperfectly developed. Generally speaking, the nearer the rectum is to the perineum the better developed is the proctodæum, but to this there are many exceptions. Conversely, if a well-developed proctodæum be present, it does not always follow that the rectum is well developed.

The **symptoms** depend upon the type of deformity present. When a narrowing at the junction of the postallantoic gut and procto-

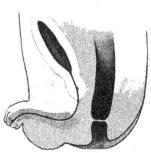

Fig. 491.—Postallantoic gut and proctodæum fully developed, but the two cavities separated by a thin membrane.

dæum only is present, the severity of obstruction will depend upon the tightness of the stricture. The stricture may be very slight, and symptoms may be practically absent ; on the other hand, obstinate constipation and abdominal distension may be present. Symptoms may be delayed for some time after birth in this variety.

When there is no outlet for the meconium, abdominal distension and vomiting will be present soon after birth. Rapid wasting occurs, and, if the condition be not relieved within a few days, death ensues.

When the rectum opens into the vulva the opening is often sufficient to allow the passage of meconium. Adult age has been reached with this deformity, sometimes with very little inconvenience, except constipation or recurrent attacks of subacute intestinal obstruction relieved by aperients.

When the rectum opens into the urethra the outlook is far less favourable, for the opening is rarely large enough to transmit the fæces, and symptoms of intestinal obstruction in various degrees are soon evident. In a few cases, however, life has been prolonged for three or four years, but rarely longer.

Treatment.—This may be considered with reference to **(1)** those cases in which the intestinal canal ends blindly and there is no outlet for its contents, and (2) those in which there is an outlet in an abnormal situation.

1. Immediate relief is necessary, failing which death will occur within a few days. The deformity is often overlooked through carelessness for the first day or so of the infant's life, and recognized only when symptoms of intestinal obstruction appear. When relief has

been given by the simplest method, a considerable proportion of the infants will die, even when operation is undertaken early.

i. *The deformity consists of a membrane of varying thickness between the proctodæum and the rectum.*—The proctodæum is well developed, and a marked bulging of the rectum into it will be felt when the infant strains. All that is necessary is to incise the membrane and remove as much of it as possible. Some degree of congenital narrowing of the lumen of the bowel may be present at the site of attachment of the membrane to the bowel wall. This must be overcome by the frequent passage of a finger or the bougie.

ii. *The proctodæum may or may not be developed, and there is no evidence to show the degree of development of the rectum.* —Two methods of procedure are possible—(a) immediate colostomy, and some weeks or months later the establishment of an anus in a normal position, or (b) an immediate attempt to form an anus in the normal position by a perineal dissection. In deciding between these alternatives it must be remembered that the degree of development of the proctodæum is not proportional to that of the development of the rectum, which, with a well-developed proctodæum, may be found as high as the base of the prostate or the vagina ; that the only permissible method of forming the anus in the perineum is freely to separate the rectum from its connexions, and draw it to the anal margin, or the skin of the future anus, without tension—a dissection which, if the rectum ends high, will be very difficult to execute in an infant two or three days old suffering from intestinal obstruction, and will very probably be fatal ; that the mere exposure and opening of the rectum, allowing the contents to escape through the track thus made, will only be followed by irremediable stricture, which of itself will sooner or later prove fatal ; that the most rapid method of giving relief should be chosen ; and that the immediate results of colostomy are superior to those of a primary perineal anus. As a general rule, therefore, it is best to perform colostomy. This should be done through as small an incision as possible in the left iliac region. The excoriation of the skin which will occur around the opening, may, with care, be kept well under control, and is probably no worse than that which occurs in the perineum when an anus is made there.

Later, at a time which will vary with the condition of the child's health, an attempt is made to form a perineal anus. It may be necessary, if the postallantoic gut be absent, to remove the coccyx. Any muscle fibres should be carefully preserved. The rectum must be separated from its surroundings (which will often mean a free opening of the peritoneal cavity), and so mobilized that it may be sutured to the skin of the perineum without tension. Later the colostomy is closed. This operation, if the rectum is low in the perineum and the proctodæum (with the sphincters) is developed, may give a good result. If, on the other hand, the rectum lies high, the operation will be severe and the prognosis grave. When recovery ensues, three accidents may befall the anus : (*a*) A stricture may occur ; this will not happen if the bowel, which has been brought well down, and sutured to the skin, does not later recede. A stricture has probably always resulted in those cases where the bowel has been blindly opened at some depth in the perineum, and a fistulous track established between the bowel and the perineum. This is not an anus. (*b*) There may be deficient sphincteric control of the new anus. If the proctodæum is developed, and care has been taken to preserve the sphincters, then control may be obtained ; but in the absence of development of the proctodæum the internal sphincter is absent, and probably the external, if developed at all, is very poor, and there will be no control. (*c*) In some cases prolapse of the mucous membrane has occurred. This is likely to happen when there is no sphincteric closure of the anus.

2. The treatment of this group may differ with the sex of the patient and with the severity of symptoms. In the female the opening in the vulval cleft is frequently of sufficient size to allow the escape of the intestinal contents, it is provided with a sphincter, and the proctodæum is very frequently absent. It would therefore seem best to leave things alone. Transplanting the anus from the vulva to the perineum would merely substitute an anus in the normal position without control for the one in the abnormal position with control. If, however, the aperture is too small, an anus should be made in the normal site.

In the male the condition is different, for the aperture is nearly always too small, and some relief from obstruction is required. If this is not necessary in early infancy it will become so later. In such cases the urgency of symptoms and age of the child will decide whether a primary colostomy or a perineal dissection should be performed.

HÆMORRHOIDS, OR PILES

This term includes a variety of conditions dependent primarily, in the majority of cases, upon a varicosity of the veins of the lower rectum and anal canal.

Etiology.—The condition is most common in middle life, and affects both sexes equally. Although not unknown, it is very rare in childhood ; indeed, an instance of congenital piles is recorded. It appears to be certain that there is an hereditary predisposition.

Mechanical congestion of the rectal veins is the exciting cause, and habitual constipation one of the most important etiological factors. During normal defæcation temporary dilatation of the valveless lower rectal and anal veins is encouraged by (1) the passage of fæces through the rectum exerting pressure in a direction reverse to that of the blood-flow in the ascending veins; (2) the contraction of the muscular walls of the bowel tending to constrict the apertures through which the veins pass; (3) the raising of the blood pressure in both the portal and caval systems during forced expiratory efforts, and (4) the loss of support to the veins due to relaxation of the sphincters and levatores ani. In habitual constipation, fæces are more or less constantly retained in the rectum, and, becoming unduly solid from absorption of water, cause constant pressure on the ascending veins. The contraction of the rectal wall is increased in force, and expulsive expiratory efforts are prolonged. Ultimately, the repeated and severe venous distension so induced terminates in permanent varicosity.

Other forms of mechanical venous obstruction, acting alone or in combination with constipation, are sometimes responsible for piles. The condition may be associated with local pressure by the gravid uterus or pelvic tumours, with the general back pressure of cardiac and pulmonary diseases, and with the portal obstruction of hepatic cirrhosis, or of hepatic congestion in those who habitually eat and drink to excess.

In some cases local irritation seems to produce or to aggravate hæmorrhoids; thus, etiological association has been claimed with worms in children, and with fissures, ulcerations, and fistulæ, and even with diarrhœa; while the mechanical results of rectal accumulations of fæces may be aided by their irritant effects.

Classification.—Anatomically, piles are divided into *external* and *internal*. In the former the tumour is covered with skin, and in the latter with mucous membrane. This is also a useful clinical classification, since the symptoms, complications, and treatment differ.

External Piles

Several different conditions are included, some only of which satisfy the definition.

1. *Dilatation of the Anal Veins*

The veins surrounding the anal margin are dilated, and during straining form a distinct swelling; when straining ceases the veins subside, leaving the skin loose. The condition is always associated with constipation, and is frequently accompanied by internal piles.

The **symptoms** are merely a feeling of fullness and uneasiness after defæcation. Spasmodic contraction of the sphincter may occur, and in time the muscle may become hypertrophied.

Treatment should be directed to inducing regular action of the bowels. In some cases where the sphincter is markedly hypertrophied its division may give relief.

2 *r*

2. The Thrombotic Pile

This term does not always indicate the true pathology. It implies the formation of a thrombus in one of the anal veins. This may occur in a few cases, but more commonly the prime condition is a rupture of a vein. The usual history is that more or less suddenly, and generally during some straining effort, there appears at the anal margin a swelling which consists of extravasated blood, fluid, tense and cystic at first, but later clotted and more firm. Should the swelling be a primary intravenous thrombosis, it is comparatively smaller and not cystic. Although generally single, occasionally more than one swelling may form. The tumour is tender and painful, especially during defæcation, which is therefore postponed as long as possible. Walking aggravates the pain, and sitting may be impossible.

The terminations are : (1) *Resolution.* This may occur if the swelling is small, and irritation and constipation are prevented. Some three or four weeks are required before the blood is completely absorbed. (2) *Suppuration.* The clot becomes infected with pyogenetic organisms, and an anal abscess results (p. 684). (3) The clot is *incompletely absorbed*, being transformed into fibrous tissue. A variety of cutaneous pile is thus formed (*see* below). (4) Rarely the skin gives way, the clot is extruded, and a natural cure results.

The **treatment** is at first symptomatic. Daily easy action of the bowels should be ensured by a mild aperient. Pain should be relieved by the application of lead lotion, or sometimes hot moist applications are more gratifying. No further treatment is required in most cases. Should, however, the swelling show no sign of diminishing in a few days, the overlying skin should be anæsthetized with eucaine, and incised in a direction radiating from the anal margin. The clot should be expressed, and the cavity allowed to heal from the bottom.

The condition is liable to recur, therefore straining efforts and constipation are to be avoided.

3. Cutaneous Piles or Redundant Folds of Perianal Skin

In appearance the folds are an exaggeration of those normally present around the anal margin. In structure there is an increase of connective tissue ; there is also in some cases a dilatation of the anal veins, but this is by no means constant.

Etiology.—As indicated above, the cutaneous pile may arise from the thrombotic one, either by the organization of the clot or by increase in the surrounding tissues due to the irritation caused by it. In other cases constipation is the prime factor. Excoriation of the skin of the anal margin by the passage of hard fæcal masses leads to a mild infection, and therefore to some œdema of the normal rugæ; the recurrence of this process induces chronic inflammatory tissue change, and therefore the formation of redundant folds. Should the perianal veins be also dilated, these will tend to increase the size of the folds. The enlargement of the perianal folds hinders the proper cleansing of the skin after defæcation, and therefore predisposes to additional excoriation of the skin in the crevices, from which a further infection or even a true fissure may arise. Hence the condition, when once established, is always liable to become aggravated.

Symptoms.—A mere redundancy of the perianal folds gives rise to few symptoms. The repeated attacks of inflammation are accompanied by pain, especially during defæcation, and hence the patient refrains from the act as long as possible. Difficulty in thoroughly cleansing the parts after defæcation may cause pruritus ani (p. 727), and the frequent rubbing to relieve this symptom will aggravate the condition.

Treatment.—The first care is to treat efficiently the constipation. After defæcation the anus should be thoroughly cleansed with water, dried, and then washed with oil. A soothing ointment or powder—e.g. bismuth or zinc combined with starch—should be applied. Should this fail to relieve, operative measures are indicated. A general anæsthetic is necessary. About two-thirds of the redundant fold is removed, leaving sufficient of the base to allow the sides to fall together. Each cutaneous pile may be thus removed without fear of stricture. As in all operations in this region, complete bodily rest should be enforced until the wound has healed, otherwise troublesome fissures or ulcerations may develop.

4. The True External Pile

In this condition there is a tumour (rarely more than one) at the anal margin. It is composed of dilated veins and hypertrophied connective tissue, the result of repeated irritation. Thrombosis may occur in the veins.

In the absence of acute inflammation, **symptoms** are slight, and are similar to those of the foregoing variety. When inflammation is present, acute pain and spasmodic contractions of the external sphincter render the condition very distressing. Not infrequently a fissure may develop at the base of the pile.

The **treatment** in all cases is removal. Sufficient of the skin covering the base of each tumour should be retained to allow the sides to fall together so that undue contraction may be avoided.

INTERNAL PILES

These consist primarily of a dilatation of the radicles of the superior hæmorrhoidal vein, and secorlarily of connective-tissue increase in

the columns of Morgagni; in the early stage internal piles are merely.
enlargements of these columns (Fig. 492), and appear as longitudinal.
sessile folds of mucous membrane. Later they increase and become more
globular, or rarely pedunculated. Entering the upper level of the.
tumour is an artery, the terminal branch of the superior hæmorrhoidal
artery. Occasionally, several arteries enter the pile, the latter being
then so vascular as to deserve the name arterial pile. Sometimes, as
the result of periphlebitis, the blood in the dilated veins coagulates,
and organization of the clot may occur, with the result that the pile
is reduced to a small fibrous mass.

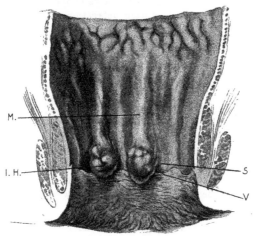

Fig. 492.—Lower rectum and anal canal opened vertically,
and the edges held widely apart.   From a preparation.

M., column of Morgagni; s., sinus of Morgagni; v., anal valve; I.H., internal hæmorrhoids, in
the early stage, showing the pile to be an enlargement of the column of Morgagni.

Symptoms.—Some discomfort and a feeling of incomplete emptying of the bowel may be experienced, but true pain is not present
unless some complication occurs. *Bleeding* is the common symptom.
At first it happens only during defæcation, either at every act, or
it may be at intervals of days, weeks, or months. Later, hæmorrhage
may occur at other times, e.g. during active exercise. The amount
of blood lost varies between a few drops only at the end of defæcation
and a continuous loss sufficient to induce grave anæmia in a few weeks.
The source of the blood is an abrasion on the mucosa.

As internal hæmorrhoids increase in size they tend to *prolapse*
through the anus. This protrusion differs from that of a pedunculated
growth which is thrust bodily through the orifice. The pile, being

sessile, when extruded is accompanied by an eversion of the skin of the anal canal, giving rise to the erroneous belief that external piles are also present. When the anal canal reverts to the normal, external piles, if present, will be seen. Internal piles project at first only during defæcation, retreating when the act ceases, but frequent recurrence of the prolapse relaxes the sphincteric tone, and protrusion may occur during any expiratory effort, sudden exertion, or even walking. The mucous membrane of a pile frequently extruded may become inflamed and secrete a mucoid discharge which may cause pruritus ani (p. 727). Superficial ulceration or even suppuration may occur. On the other hand, a pile prolapsed may become so tightly gripped by the sphincter muscles that it is only with difficulty reduced. If allowed to remain prolapsed, it will rapidly swell from interference with its vascular circulation, acute infection is liable to occur, and this may be followed by ulceration, or gangrene of the whole or part of the pile. If gangrene occur the extruded mass may separate and a cure result, but such a sequel should only be permitted in exceptional cases.

The **diagnosis** of internal piles should be easy if a proper examination be made by means of a speculum and reflected light. If pain be excessive, probably some complication is present, e.g. a fissure or suppuration. Careful examination easily demonstrates that the protruded mass consists of the mucosa of the anal canal, and that it is not derived from a point higher in the bowel as is a polyp or an intussusception ; moreover the pedicle of a polyp is readily felt on digital examination. Intussusception in the rectum probably does not occur in the absence of a tumour.

Treatment.—Palliative measures are indicated at first in many cases. They may suffice where bleeding is trivial, protrusion slight or absent, and the prime cause of the piles, e.g. gestation or a pelvic tumour, has been removed. In old age associated with arterial degeneration, bleeding from internal piles may be regarded as favourable, tending to deplete the circulation. In more than one such case, where piles have been removed, cerebral hæmorrhage has followed. In cases of chronic cardiac or pulmonary disease, or portal obstruction, operative treatment is contra-indicated. In portal obstruction, hæmorrhage relieving the portal circulation tends to prevent ascites and hæmatemesis.

The first care must be to keep the bowels regular by the systematic and judicious administration of aperients. There is no one aperient which can be vaunted ; several may have to be tried before the one which suits the patient is found ; saline purgatives are generally inadvisable. Undue hardness of the motion must be prevented by the injection into the bowel of warm olive oil. The diet must be regulated, and especially in those who habitually eat and drink excessively.

Alcohol is better avoided. Regular exercise should be taken. Under such treatment many cases are immensely relieved, as regards both bleeding and protrusion. Should bleeding still continue, an astringent application should be employed, e.g. an injection of a solution of sulphate of iron or adrenalin, a powder such as dried sulphate of iron, bismuth, or zinc, a suppository containing gallic or tannic acid, or an ointment, of which the principal ingredient may be one of the foregoing, or hamamelis.

Operative treatment should be advised when palliative measures have failed. It is indicated when bleeding is continuous, when prolapse is frequent, when there is a persistent discharge causing pruritus ani, when fissure is present, or when inflammation, sloughing or gangrene has occurred.

There are four methods of operation—(1) the clamp and cautery, (2) the ligature, (3) the excision of individual piles, and (4) the

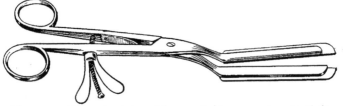

Fig. 493.—Clamp for internal hæmorrhoids preparatory to their cauterization.

removal of a complete ring of mucosa, the so-called " pile-bearing area " (Whitehead's operation).

1. Clamp and cautery.—It is claimed for this operation that the after-pain is less than when other methods are employed, the convalescence is shortened, and there is no tendency to a contraction of the anal canal. Practical experience shows that, provided the cautery is used at a *dull*-red heat, reactionary hæmorrhage is not more frequent after this than after the other methods. The method is better not employed when external piles requiring removal are also present. It is strongly indicated where the piles are acutely inflamed, sloughing or gangrenous, for no foreign body is left in the wound.

After dilatation of the sphincters, each pile is grasped at its base by a special clamp (Fig. 493), and then seared off by the knife of a Paquelin cautery. The clamp is gradually relaxed, and if any bleeding is seen the clamp should be tightened and the stump again cauterized ; this is repeated until all bleeding has ceased.

2. Ligature.—This is the method which has most advocates. It may be employed in any case, but is especially indicated where

inflammation is absent and the number of piles is limited. It should be reserved for those cases in which the piles are not more than four or five in number, and form definite tumour masses, with healthy mucosa between them. On the other hand, where practically the whole mucosa is the seat of hæmorrhoidal changes, and where prolapse is great, Whitehead's operation will give a better result.

To perform the ligature operation the sphincters are thoroughly stretched and the piles allowed to protrude. Each pile is seized in ring-forceps. A curved incision is made through the cutaneous ring formed by the everted anal canal about midway between its outer margin and the muco-cutaneous junction corresponding to the base of

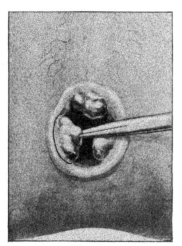 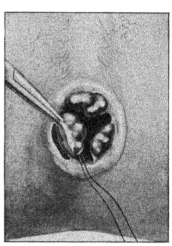

| Fig. 494. | Fig. 495. |

The operation for removal of an internal pile. (*See text.*)

the pile, the ends of the incision terminating in the mucous membrane at the sides of the pile (Fig. 494). The incision is deepened through the subcutaneous tissue to the external sphincter muscle, which is recognized and avoided (Fig. 495). By continuing the dissection up the anal canal a pedicle containing the vessels of the pile is formed. This is transfixed, ligatured tightly, and the pile cut away not too closely to the ligature, for fear the latter should slip from the stump. The stump will separate, with the ligature, in about ten days' time.

3. **Excision of each individual hæmorrhoid** is a modification of the ligature operation. The pile is seized longitudinally by a long narrow clamp, and its upper pole, including the main vessels, is transfixed and ligatured just above the end of the clamp. The projecting

hæmorrhoid is cut off, the edges of the mucous membrane sutured with the long ends of the ligature, and the clamp removed.

4. **Whitehead's operation** is performed as follows: An incision is made circumferentially through the skin of the anal canal immediately outside the muco-cutaneous junction (Fig. 496). The incision is deepened until the external sphincter muscle is exposed (Fig. 497). The mucous membrane in its entirety is dissected off the underlying structures until healthy mucosa above is reached (Fig. 498). The diseased mucosa is removed, and the healthy cut edge is sutured to the skin of the anal margin (Fig. 499).

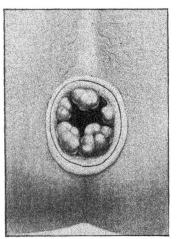
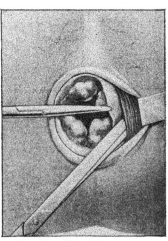

Fig. 496.   Fig. 497.

First and second stages of Whitehead's operation. (*See text.*)

After-treatment.—Shortly after the operation a hypodermic injection of morphia is given. The bowels are confined for four days. If the bowel has been thoroughly emptied before operation, there will be no difficulty in this; should it be thought desirable, a catechu and opium mixture may be given for the purpose. On the night of the third day an aperient is administered, and in order to soften the motion, and so to lessen pain, some warm oil is injected into the rectum. Just before the bowels act some cocaine ointment may be applied to the wound. The wound must be kept scrupulously clean, and particular attention paid to it after defæcation.

The **complications** that may arise after the operation are—

(a) *Hæmorrhage.*—This occurs either from the slipping of a ligature or from an unoccluded vessel. It is evidenced by the general signs of loss of blood, and the saturated condition of the dressing. It must be remembered that considerable hæmorrhage may occur into the rectum before appearing outside. It is unusual, and is probably not more frequent after one method of operation than another. The treatment must be prompt. The patient is anæsthetized, the rectum irrigated to remove all clots, and examination made for the bleeding-point. If this can be found, it should be ligatured. In all probability bleeding will have ceased, and all that can be done is to pass a tube, to which a petticoat of lint has been tied, into the rectum, and to pack gauze between the tube and the petticoat to prevent a recurrence.

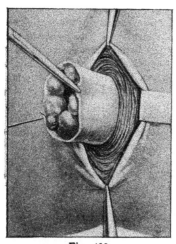 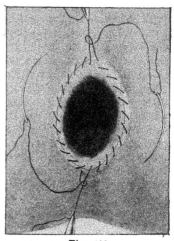

Fig. 498.   Fig. 499.

Third and fourth stages of Whitehead's operation. (*See text.*)

(b) *Infection.*—Severe sepsis rarely occurs, but occasionally, especially when the operation is undertaken for inflamed or sloughing piles, some septic infection may ensue and lead to troublesome ulceration, which will increase the tendency to stricture. Specific infections, e.g. tetanus and pyæmia, have been known to occur, but they are extremely rare.

(c) *Œdematous tags of skin* at the anal margin are frequently present within a few days of the operation. These are due either to an inflammatory disturbance or to interference with the venous circulation. They occur alike after the ligature and the Whitehead operation. In the great majority of cases, if the operation has been properly performed, they subside under the application of astringent lotions. In a few cases, however, they may have to be removed under local anæsthesia.

(*d*) Temporary *loss of control* is naturally present after forcible stretching of the sphincter muscle, but in the majority of cases is partially recovered from within a few hours. Removal of the sensitive area of the mucous membrane is partially responsible for loss of control ; hence the time for return of control is longer after the Whitehead than after the ligature or the clamp-and-cautery method of operating. But recovery after the Whitehead method is usually complete in a fortnight, and practically always in three weeks. When the sphincter has been stretched by piles for months or years before operation, and again forcibly at operation, re-establishment of muscular power is slower. In such cases the sphincters should not be stretched more than is absolutely necessary.

(*e*) *Stricture.*—This never follows the clamp-and-cautery method or the excision of individual piles. It may follow the ligature or the Whitehead operation. In the latter, union by first intention practically never occurs, but, the stitches giving way about the fourth or fifth day, the mucosa retracts for a variable distance. The tendency to stricture is proportionate to the degree of retraction of the mucosa. In the ligature operation healthy mucosa is left between the raw surfaces, and from this epithelium will be regenerated. Hence the tendency to stricture is greater after the Whitehead than after the ligature operation. After either operation an examination should be made during the third or fourth weeks, and any contraction will then be evident. By frequent digital stretching when the fibrous tissue is still young, a stricture of sufficient degree to cause symptoms may usually be entirely prevented.

Hæmorrhoids occasionally recur, or, more strictly speaking, fresh piles form. This is, however, most unusual if all have been properly removed, and if sufficient care be taken to avoid the causes which are held responsible for the production of piles. Naturally, recurrence would be comparatively more frequent after the clamp-and-cautery, the excision of the individual pile and the ligature methods of operating than after the Whitehead operation. But it is stated that it may occur even after the excision of the " pile-bearing area."

ANAL FISSURE

Definition.—An elongated narrow ulcer in the long axis of the anal canal within the sphere of influence of the external sphincter muscle.

Etiology and pathology.—Anal fissure occurs most frequently in adult life ; it is rare in childhood and uncommon in old age. Chronic constipation is the usual predisposing cause ; in it the sphincters tend to become hypertrophied and indurated, the anal canal to lose elasticity and dilatability ; the hard scybalous mass actually tears the skin of the anal orifice. Healing is prevented by the stretching due to defæcation and by the activity of the external sphincter muscle. A fissure is usually, though not always, single ; multiple fissures suggest syphilis, but this is not invariable. A fissure is somewhat pear-shaped or triangular in form, broader below than above, situated between the normal rugæ of the anal orifice, and of varying length and depth. Often the upper extremity is at the lower margin of, or even overlies, the internal sphincter muscle, and the lower extremity is at the lower margin of the external sphincter muscle. At first it is quite superficial, but later its base may be formed by the muscles. In a minority of cases there is an œdematous tag of skin, the so-called " sentinel pile," at the lower end of the fissure and partly obscuring it. This may occasionally be an anal valve, torn down during defæcation, but more often is one of the normal rugæ, œdematous through infection from the fissure.

Fissure may rarely result from partial detachment during defæcation of a polypus originating low in the rectum, or from laceration during the passage of a foreign body. It may also follow direct infection due to imperfect cleansing of the crevices between the circumanal rugæ.

Symptoms.—Pain of a characteristic and often pathognomonic type is the one symptom. It occurs during defæcation, and lasts for a variable time after. It is often most intense, incapacitating the patient for an hour or more. It is of a tearing character, and radiates from the anus to the perineum, thighs, and back. Its severity causes voluntary abstention from defæcation, with consequences disastrous to the fissure. Sometimes pain is not so severe, but passes off as soon as the bowels are relieved. The degree of pain appears to vary with the depth of the fissure. The skin of the anal canal is richly supplied with sensory nerves, some of which are probably exposed, as points of exquisite tenderness may be found by passing a probe over the surface of the fissure. The passage of fæces over the raw, sensitive surface is responsible for the pain during defæcation, and the spasm of the sphincter muscle for its persistence. Hæmorrhage during defæcation may occur ; this is usually a mere drop, but occasionally is more extensive. A little pus is secreted from the fissure, and may cause pruritus ani (p. 727). The spasmodic contractions of the sphincter muscle during defæcation may render the motions somewhat flattened or tapering in shape.

The examination must be conducted with all gentleness. On separating the circumanal folds a fissure will be readily seen. A digital examination is usually necessary to determine the presence or absence of coexisting disease.

Treatment.—Palliative measures should first be tried, and will often greatly relieve a recent and superficial fissure. Constipation must be effectually treated, and the motion rendered as soft as possible by the injection of oil into the bowel. For pain, a cocaine ointment may be applied. To promote healing, a stimulating ointment or powder, e.g. calomel or resin, should be used. If these measures fail to cure in three or four weeks, operation should be earnestly advised, for this painful disease causes rapid loss of flesh and great depression.

The object of **operative** treatment is to secure temporary paralysis of the external sphincter muscle by its division. If the fissure is recent and not associated with other conditions requiring operation, local anæsthesia may be employed, but whenever possible a general anæsthetic should be given to ensure more thorough treatment. In the former case the base of the fissure is infiltrated with eucaine and adrenalin, and divided, together with the superficial fibres of the external sphincter muscle. The "sentinel pile," if present, must be removed, otherwise healing will not follow. If general anæsthesia be adopted, the sphincters are dilated, and the anal margin everted with the finger inside, so as to bring the fissure into full view. An incision is then made through the fissure and the whole external sphincter muscle, and prolonged on to the skin for ½ in. The wound must be carefully cleansed after defæcation, and made to heal from the bottom. One division only of the sphincter is necessary to secure the healing of multiple fissures. Permanent loss of control never follows the operation.

ABSCESS

Suppuration originating in disease of the rectum and anal canal occurs in definite anatomical situations. The following varieties of abscess may be distinguished, viz. (I) subcutaneous, (2) ischio-rectal, (3) submucous, (4) pelvi-rectal, and (5) labial. (Fig. 500.)

1. Subcutaneous Abscess

This is situated in the subcutaneous tissue at or near the anal margin. It originates from infection of either a sebaceous follicle (the follicular abscess), a fissure, or an external pile. The follicular abscess is usually single, but may be multiple if more than one follicle be infected. It is situated close to, but not at the anal margin, and has no tendency to burrow towards the anal canal; hence a fistula does not follow. The diagnosis is obvious, and the treatment by a free radial incision is simple.

An abscess originating in a fissure, or in a thrombotic or inflamed external pile, is situated at the anal margin, and tends to burrow towards and open into the anal canal as well as on the surface of the skin at a variable distance from the anal margin. A complete subcutaneous fistula, therefore, frequently results. This tendency to open into the anal canal should be anticipated in the treatment, which consists in freely opening the abscess into the anal canal by a radial incision. The incision is entirely superficial to the external sphincter muscle.

2. ISCHIO-RECTAL ABSCESS

The ill-nourished condition of the fat of the ischio-rectal fossa predisposes it to infection. The infection may arise from any inflammatory process in the lower part of the bowel, and it extends to the fossa via the weak point in the bowel wall, i.e. the interval between the two sphincter muscles.

Etiology.—An inflamed internal pile, an ulcer in one of the sinuses of Morgagni, the upper extremity of an anal fissure, or ulceration following operations, may all cause an ischio-rectal abscess. But frequently none of these lesions is found, and in all probability bacteria can escape through the bowel wall without any recognizable lesion of the latter. A little accumulation of fæcal material in one of the sinuses of Morgagni may excite some inflammation from which the fossa may be infected. Rarely a foreign body has been known to perforate the bowel wall, and has been found in the pus of the abscess. The bacterium causing the suppuration is either the Bacillus coli, or the common pyogenetic coccus alone or in association with the former.

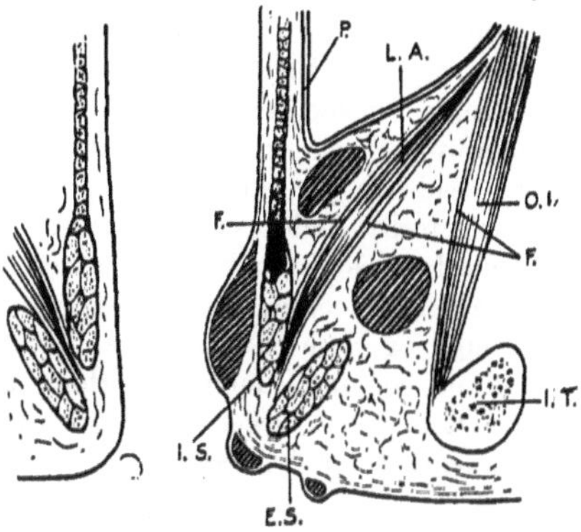

Fig. 500.—Imaginary section, in the coronal plane, of the rectum, anal canal, and perirectal tissues, illustrating the various positions of abscesses.

I.T., Ischial tuberosity ; E.S., external sphincter muscle ; I.S., internal sphincter muscle ; L.A., levator ani muscle ; O.I., obturator internus muscle ; F., fascia covering the obturator internus and levatores ani muscles ; P., peritoneum. The shaded areas represent abscesses, which are thus seen in the submucous tissue, at the anal margin, under the skin a little distance from the anal margin, in the ischio-rectal fossa, and between the levator ani muscle and the peritoneum, the potential pelvi-rectal space.

Suppuration tends to spread (1) towards the skin over the fossa ; (2) towards the bowel, usually between the two sphincters, or occasionally through the fibres of the external or internal sphincter, the site of pointing or rupture being determined often by that of the origin of the infection ; (3) less commonly between the levator ani and the ano-coccygeal ligament posteriorly, to the fossa of the opposite side ; (4) very rarely through the levator ani to the pelvi-rectal space ; (5) uncommonly to the anterior part of the perineum or labium majus.

The **symptoms** are those attending acute suppuration. A fullness

,in the fossa may be appreciated both externally and internally. If allowed to progress, redness and œdema of the skin, and eventually fluctuation, will appear.

Treatment.—An acute inflammatory mass in the ischio-rectal fossa should be incised at once, even before the presence of pus is .certain. Early operation will materially shorten convalescence and ,perhaps prevent the subsequent formation of a fistula.

Under anæsthesia a curved incision is made, parallel to the anal margin over the most prominent part of the swelling, and extended anteriorly and posteriorly beyond the limits of the swelling. A second incision is made at right angles to this outwards, well beyond the limits of the induration. The finger is inserted into the cavity, and all septa broken down. Free opening is necessary to prevent the burrowing of pus, which so constantly results from any smaller incision and leads to persistent sinus or fistula. The abscess usually heals satisfactorily under such treatment, but a sinus may persist, or a fistula form, and require further treatment. At the time of evacuating the abscess a communication with the rectum may be present, usually through or close to the space between the two sphincters. Should this be so, or if merely a thin stratum of mucosa separate the abscess from the bowel cavity, the case should be treated as fistula or cutaneous sinus (p. 689).

3. Submucous Abscess

An abscess in the submucosa of the lower rectum shows a marked tendency to track towards the anal margin and open there, but also burrows to some extent laterally in the bowel wall. Usually this abscess bursts of its own accord, but if seen before this occurs it should be opened at its lower margin. Healing is generally rapid, but occasionally a submucous track persists and should be freely laid open in the longitudinal direction, care being taken to check all hæmorrhage, which may be free from one of the terminal branches of the superior hæmorrhoidal artery.

4. Pelvi-Rectal Abscess

This abscess is a suppurative cellulitis of the connective tissue between the levator ani muscle and the peritoneum. This tissue is continuous with that between the layers of the pelvic mesocolon and the broad ligament, and also with that surrounding the prostate and the neck of the bladder. Disease of the latter organs, rather than of the rectum, is more frequently responsible for a pelvi-rectal abscess. But occasionally ulceration of the rectum, malignant disease, or perforation by a foreign body may cause an infection of the connective tissue surrounding the bowel above the levator ani.

The ultra-acute pelvi-rectal infection frequently terminates in acute peritonitis or gangrenous cellulitis. The more subacute or chronic cases present the symptoms of pelvic cellulitis ; unless rectal disease is known to exist, the cause may be entirely overlooked. Rectal examination may demonstrate a unilateral fullness above the level of the internal sphincter muscle. Pus may escape into the bowel with relief of symptoms, but drainage will probably be imperfect and the abscess reaccumulate. Sometimes the pus may track through the levator ani, or posteriorly through the median raphe, to the ischio-rectal fossa, and eventually reach the surface through one or more openings. In other cases the pus may track to the iliac or lumbar regions, or even through the sacro-sciatic foramen to the buttock.

Treatment is a difficult matter, and depends to some extent upon the cause. Any etiological rectal disease must be appropriately treated. Incisions into the abscess cavity must be free, and may be necessary in the perineum or the iliac region, or both. When a pelvi-rectal abscess has burst into the ischio-rectal fossa, it is to be opened as already explained, and the aperture through the levator ani enlarged with forceps and freely drained.

5. LABIAL ABSCESS

This abscess is generally confined to the labium majus. It arises from disease of the anterior part of the lower rectum or anal canal. It is incised in a manner similar to that adopted for the ischio-rectal abscess.

FISTULA AND SINUS

A fistula is a suppurating track opening both on to the cutaneous surface and into the lumen of the bowel. A sinus, on the other hand, has only one opening, which may either be on to the cutaneous surface, the *cutaneous sinus,* or into the lumen of the bowel, the *rectal sinus.* Both the sinus and the fistula, when of rectal origin, are practically always preceded by one or other variety of perirectal abscess. Rarely will a foreign body, such as a fish-bone, perforate the rectal wall without the formation of any definite abscess, causing at first a rectal sinus and later a fistula.

FISTULA

A fistula may be superficial, intermuscular, or supramuscular, according to its position in the bowel wall (Fig. 501).

Superficial fistula.—The track is superficial to the external sphincter, or may pass between the superficial fibres of the muscle. It results from a subcutaneous abscess opening both on to the surface and into the anal canal at the anal margin. The internal orifice of the fistula may be seen at the base of a fissure, or as a small ulcer at the anal margin. The external orifice is near the anus, and the track is seldom more than 1½ in. in length. Since the fistula is so superficial, the discharge so slight, and the inner opening not really into the lumen of the bowel but at the anal margin, and free from the entry of fæces, there is no tendency to the purulent accumulations and burrowing of the pus which so frequently occur in the deeper fistulæ. The external opening is, therefore, practically always single. The fistula may be situated anywhere around the anus, but is very frequently located posteriorly. The track may pursue a straight or slightly curved course.

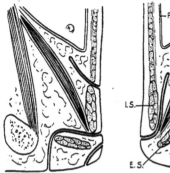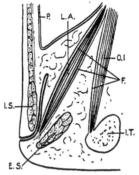

The symptoms of a superficial fistula are slight. Pain is acute before the abscess is emptied, but as there is no tendency to burrowing, it is practically absent when the fistulous track is established. The discharge is comparatively little. The internal orifice is easily detected, and the fistula readily permits the

Fig. 501.—Section similar to that in Fig. 500, illustrating the positions of sinuses and fistulæ.

On the left side are the superficial and intermuscular fistulæ, and the internal sinus opening into the bowel above the internal sphincter muscle. On the right is the internal sinus extending into the pelvi-rectal space and opening into the bowel between the sphincter muscles and above the levator ani muscle. For lettering, *see* Fig. 500.

passage of a probe. The walls of a superficial fistula have been known to become completely epithelialized from the margins of the orifices.

The **treatment** consists in laying the track completely open and allowing the wound to granulate. When the track passes between the superficial fibres of the external sphincter, this muscle must be completely divided at right angles to the direction of its fibres, in order to secure rest.

The **intermuscular fistula** results from an ischio-rectal abscess. Spontaneous rupture of an ischio-rectal abscess will almost certainly lead to imperfect drainage, and the pus tends to burrow in various directions, and not infrequently towards the bowel. But even when drainage is timely and efficient a fistula may form; for the abscess originates from and may be in close proximity to a lesion, e.g. an ulcer, in the bowel, and, in fact, may communicate with the interior of the bowel from the beginning, or the diseased bowel wall may be readily perforated at a later date. The internal opening of the fistula is between the internal and external sphincter muscles, or in the immediate vicinity, the track passing through the fibres of one or other muscle. The reasons for this fact are that the disease which, originally caused the abscess is situated in this region of the bowel; the sloping internal boundary of the abscess (the levator ani and its fascia) passes to the bowel between the sphincter muscles, and will direct the pus to this space; the main branches of the inferior hæmorrhoidal vessels enter the bowel here, and may influence the direction in which suppuration extends. The internal opening is generally single. When two internal openings are present there are either two distinct fistulæ, or the second opening is higher and at the upper extremity of a submucous track, an offshoot of the original abscess. The opening is frequently situated posteriorly just to one side of the mid-line. This is probably explained either by the better development of the sinuses of Morgagni posteriorly, the original infection being, therefore, more likely to arise from this part of the bowel, or by the greater interval between the sphincters posteriorly permitting pus to track there more readily.

The external opening of the fistula is at first single. Imperfect drainage and burrowing of pus frequently lead to secondary abscesses, which open spontaneously, and hence multiple external openings are by no means uncommon. They may be situated in the skin over any part of the ischio-rectal fossa, or at some distance from this, in the buttocks or the perineum. An ischio-rectal abscess may track from one fossa to the other. The external openings of a fistula may therefore be on opposite sides of the anus. The name "horseshoe-shaped" fistula has been given to this variety. When the internal orifice has its common posterior position the fistulous track is curved or tortuous. When, however, the internal orifice is situated laterally the external orifice is generally immediately opposite, and the fistula is short and direct.

The **symptoms** of an intermuscular fistula are various. If untreated, secondary abscesses form sooner or later, and are attended by the symptoms of pent-up pus. Flatus, and rarely fæces, may escape from a fistula. On examination, the external orifices are readily detected. The internal orifice may generally be felt or seen, but sometimes it cannot, and then without the aid of an anæsthetic the diagnosis between a fistula and a cutaneous sinus is impossible. The track of an old-standing fistula may be felt as an indurated cord in the tissues. The passage of a probe is often impeded by the tortuosity of the fistula, and is unnecessary before operation.

Treatment.—Operation is the only satisfactory treatment of an
2 *s*

intermuscular fistula, and in the absence of any special contra-indication should be earnestly advised. It consists essentially in slitting up the original fistulous track and all secondary sinuses leading from it. In order to do this the internal orifice *must be found.* If the probe can be passed along the whole length of the fistulous track, all structures superficial to it are divided, including the external sphincter muscle. If a probe cannot be passed right through, it should be introduced either from the cutaneous surface or the internal orifice as far as possible, the sinus slit up, and the other aperture carefully sought and enlarged. It is imperative that no artificial opening be made into the bowel and then enlarged on the supposition that it is the fistula. The original communication with the bowel must in all cases be found, and this opened up, otherwise the fistula obviously will not heal. When the main track has been thus treated, all secondary offshoots must be freely enlarged, and ample drainage provided for them. A submucous track, not infrequently present, should also be freely slit up. The external sphincter muscle should only be divided in one place, and transversely to the direction of its fibres. If this rule be followed, incontinence of fæces will not result. All overhanging edges of skin and mucous membrane must be removed. The wound must be carefully dressed to ensure healing from the bottom.

Should operation be refused or inadvisable, scrupulous cleanliness must be enforced, and stimulating lotions e.g. silver nitrate, copper sulphate, Friar's balsam, tincture of iodine, injected along the track.

A **supramuscular fistula** tracks through the bowel wall above the internal sphincter muscle, and arises from rectal ulceration, pelvi-rectal abscesses, or very rarely from the burrowing of an ischio-rectal abscess through the levator ani muscle with secondary rupture into the bowel. The orifices vary greatly in position ; not infrequently they are multiple internally. Suppuration may extend right around the bowel in the pelvi-rectal space, both anteriorly and posteriorly, reaching the surface through many points. The course and direction of these fistulæ and their symptomatology are so indefinite that no concise account of them can be given.

The **treatment** is largely that of the original disease ; thus, malignant disease frequently demands a palliative colostomy. Ulceration and stricture are discussed later (pp. 698, 704). For the fistula itself the only certain plan is to lay the track freely open and pack lightly with gauze. In some cases it is possible to excise the whole lining membrane of the split fistula, to close the opening into the bowel, and then to close the track, at any rate in its deeper part, by a series of buried catgut sutures, special care being taken to reconstitute the divided internal sphincter.

But as splitting of the whole track involves division of both sphincters it entails grave risk of fæcal incontinence; therefore less drastic measures may be tried first. The external part of the fistula may be laid open, and the rest syringed periodically with stimulating lotions, such as silver nitrate or tincture of iodine. This will sometimes be successful. Division of both sphincters should be reserved for fistulæ causing severe trouble, and should only be done with the patient's full knowledge of the possible consequences.

For the treatment of tuberculous fistulæ, *see* p. 695.

SINUS

The **cutaneous sinus** results from an ischio-rectal abscess, or occasionally from a pelvi-rectal abscess, reaching the surface through the levator ani and ischio-rectal fossa. The imperfect drainage of the sinus, the constant movements to which it is subjected, and its frequent extension to the sphere of influence of the sphincter muscles, are factors which tend to prevent healing.

The differentiation between a cutaneous sinus and a fistula is often difficult, and requires patience and manipulative skill. Inability to pass a probe through the sinus into the bowel does not necessarily mean that no communication exists. The passage of fæces or flatus through the track, or the discovery of an internal opening, establishes the diagnosis of fistula.

The **treatment** of a cutaneous sinus is very similar to that of a fistula. It must be freely opened up, and will then often be found to track towards the bowel, being only separated from it by a thin layer of tissue. The track generally passes towards the interval between the sphincters. When it is certain that there is no aperture of communication with the bowel, one should be made by passing the probe through the thinnest portion between the sphincters, thus converting the sinus into a fistula; as such it is then treated. Should, however, the track pass in connexion with the bowel above the level of the internal sphincter muscle, this treatment should not be advised, for it would mean division of the internal sphincter, and in all probability incontinence of fæces would result. In such cases the sinuses may be enlarged, free drainage provided, and some stimulating lotion injected from time to time. The whole sinus wall may sometimes be excised.

In the **rectal sinus** the aperture of communication with the bowel may be situated between the two sphincter muscles, or in close proximity, or less frequently above the level of the internal sphincter muscle. The rectal sinus results from the rupture of an ischio-rectal or a pelvi-rectal abscess into the bowel. Drainage is nearly always inefficient; the orifice into the bowel frequently becomes temporarily occluded, and pus reaccumulates. The **symptoms** are those of recurring attacks of perirectal suppuration with periodical discharges of pus from the bowel. On examination an induration may be felt in the ischio-rectal fossa, more evident at times than at others. With a speculum the internal orifice may be seen, and pus observed to issue from it.

Cure cannot be expected without operation, since the drainage from the abscess into the bowel is always inefficient.

Treatment.—(a) *When the internal orifice is between the sphincter muscles* a probe should, if possible, be passed through the orifice, directed towards the surface, and its end exposed by incising the tissues superficial to it. Or, if the swelling is palpable, it may be incised from the surface. In either case the sinus is converted into a fistula and treated as such. (b) *When the orifice is above the internal sphincter muscle* the operation performed as above would necessarily divide the muscle, and incontinence of fæces would probably result. A rectal sinus above the internal sphincter nearly always arises from some ulceration of the bowel, and this must be treated. The abscess should be incised from the surface, efficient drainage provided, and the track through the bowel wall treated as for a fistula in this region (p. 690).

Complicated Fistulæ

Under this heading are included some of the rarer forms of rectal fistulæ. Two varieties may be considered : (1) the fistula communicating with some adjacent viscus—the bladder, the urethra, or the vagina ; and (2) the fistula dependent originally upon some chronic bone disease.

1. (a) **Recto-vesical fistula.**—This may be caused by rectal ulceration spreading to the bladder, by a pelvi-rectal abscess opening both into the bowel and the bladder, or more rarely by injuries, such as bullet wounds or buffer crushes.

The typical **symptoms** of a recto-vesical fistula are those caused by the escape of the contents of one viscus into the other. Urine may pass into the rectum or fæces into the bladder, and theoretically it would seem that both may occur. Practically, however, a valve-like action develops, and the current is only in one direction. Severe cystitis and the presence of fæces in the bladder cause extreme suffering and painful micturition. Excoriation of the skin of the anal region may occur from the constant passage over it of urine.

The **treatment** varies with the cause of the fistula. If this is due to malignant disease, and fæces are entering the bladder, a palliative colostomy is indicated, though the less distressing symptoms of urine escaping into the bowel will not, of course, be relieved. Cystostomy may be necessary in some cases where micturition is extremely painful. When the fistula is narrow and of inflammatory origin, success has attended cauterization through a long rectal speculum, with or without a preliminary posterior proctotomy. When this fails, or when the orifice is large, cure can only be obtained by perineal dissection, separating the rectum from the prostate and bladder, paring the edges and suturing them. The operation is severe and difficult, and often attended with failure.

(*b*) **Recto-urethral fistula** usually results from urethral disease (e.g. a stricture), and very rarely from penetrating wounds. The symptoms are those of the original urethral disease and the passage of urine into the bowel during micturition. The treatment is, in the first place, that of the original disease. A stricture should be dilated and the urine drawn off by catheter. This simple measure may be successful. If it fail, the fistula should be exposed by a dissection from the perineum, and the apertures closed with sutures.

(*c*) **Recto-vaginal fistula** may be due to any form of perirectal suppuration which opens both into the bowel and the vagina, to injuries during parturition, to tuberculous or syphilitic infection of either the bowel or the vagina or both, and also to cancer originating in either viscus. The symptoms peculiar to a recto-vaginal fistula are the passage of flatus and fæces from the bowel to the vagina. The treatment of the fistula obviously depends upon the cause. If due to malignant ulceration the disease in all probability will be too extensive for removal, and a palliative colostomy is indicated. Syphilitic and tuberculous disease must be appropriately treated before any attempt is made to close the fistula. When the aperture is of small size, cauterization may effect a cure. In other cases the edges of the fistula may be pared and sutured either from the vagina or from the rectum as seems most accessible. In yet others the fistula may be exposed by a perineal dissection, the edges of the openings pared, and approximated by sutures.

2. **Fistula dependent upon bone disease.**—Abscesses arising from bone disease occasionally open into the rectum. A psoas abscess which enters the pelvis by perforating the sheath of the muscle, an abscess originating from the sacrum or ischium, or perhaps more frequently an abscess due to coccygeal caries, are examples of those which may communicate with the rectum. The diagnosis is usually easy from the history of the case and the physical examination. Radiography may, when necessary, aid the diagnosis of bone disease. The treatment of these fistulæ is that of the original bone disease.

INFLAMMATION—PROCTITIS

Much remains to be learnt about the bacteriology of proctitis, and the classification adopted is clinical rather than pathological. For clinical purposes proctitis may be considered under the heads of Simple Catarrhal Proctitis, Gangrenous Proctitis, Proctitis due to Specific Organisms, and Ulcerations.

Acute catarrhal proctitis may be caused by injury, by the irritation of scybalous masses, violent purgatives, or thread-worms, or it may be a part of a generalized colitis.

The **symptoms** are rectal tenesmus and the passage of muco-pus tinged with blood. The mucosa is very swollen and vasculàr. The frequent straining at defæcation renders the swollen mucosa liable to prolapse. Reflex urinary symptoms are frequently present.

The course and terminations are various. Some cases resolve in a few days, others become chronic, and occasionally ulceration follows.

Chronic catarrhal proctitis is usually a sequel of the acute form, and the symptoms are similar but modified in degree. The rectal mucosa is swollen, pale and œdematous, and covered with tenacious muco-pus. Cell proliferation in the submucous tissue leads to considerable thickening of the rectal wall. Superficial ulceration may be present.

Treatment.—In the acute form, rest in bed, a diet which leaves the least residue, and regulation of the bowels with mild aperients are essential. Occasional hot hip-baths give relief. When the disease has become chronic similar treatment is necessary, and the rectum should be irrigated with some astringent lotion through a double-channelled catheter, or, better, a direct application of silver nitrate or iodine should be made to the diseased mucosa.

DIFFUSE SEPTIC AND GANGRENOUS PROCTITIS

This is, nowadays, a very rare condition. Formerly it was seen after operations upon the rectum, and was apparently infectious. The infective process involved the rectum and the perirectal tissues, and was not infrequently fatal. If recovery took place, it only did so after prolonged suppuration and sloughing, leaving the tissues permanently damaged, e.g. by strictures of the bowel and destruction of the sphincter muscles.

PROCTITIS DUE TO SPECIFIC ORGANISMS

Gonorrhœal proctitis is rare. It occurs more frequently in the female by direct infection from the vagina ; in the male it results from unnatural coitus. The symptoms are those of catarrhal proctitis. The diagnosis is founded upon the bacteriological examination. The treatment is similar in the acute stage to that of catarrhal proctitis. When the disease has become chronic, douches of protargol, chinosol, or some mercurial lotion should be employed, or a direct application of one of these substances should be made to the diseased mucosa.

Diphtheria very rarely attacks the rectum and anal canal. Occasionally it has been seen in association with the disease in the throat, and it is said that the lesions in the perineum have preceded those in the more common situations. It is also stated that diphtheria has followed an operation in this region. The signs, diagnosis, and treatment are similar to those of the disease in the usual situations.

Tuberculosis is not uncommon, and is usually secondary to pulmonary disease. It is stated, however, that the lesion may be primary, the bacilli entering with the food. Imperfect gastric digestion may permit the passage of undestroyed bacilli, which may lodge in the anal sinuses and there cause single or multiple tuberculous ulcers. The ulcer is small and shows no tendency to spread widely over the surface of the bowel, though it is very apt to perforate to the perirectal tissues. Usually the first indication of the disease is a slowly forming ischio-rectal abscess, which differs from the acute abscess already described in its slower development and less severe symptoms. The abscess tends to burrow in the fossa, eventually making its way to the surface and discharging through one or more openings which show the undermined edges and bluish discoloration of the surrounding skin, and the prominent pale granulations characteristic of tuberculous sinuses.

Clinically the tuberculous fistula may generally be differentiated by the following points : The buttocks are thin and the ischio-rectal fossa feebly developed ; the perineal hair is abundant, long and silky ; the abscess preceding the fistula forms insidiously, the external orifice is more or less characteristic of a tuberculous sinus, the discharge is thin and watery, and the internal opening is often easily felt and seen, being sometimes so large as to admit the finger-tip. It can only be certainly diagnosed by finding the tubercle bacillus in the discharge, or by the microscopy of the granulation tissue lining the sinus.

For treatment the subjects of tuberculous fistula may be divided into three classes :

(a) *Fistula associated with advanced pulmonary tuberculosis.*—As little should be done as is consistent with relief of symptoms. If the abscess has not burst externally, but a rectal sinus is present, considerable pain may be caused by the passage of fæces into and the accumulation of pus in the cavity. Under local anæsthesia external drainage should be provided. No active interference should be considered if free drainage is already established.

(b) *Fistula associated with chronic tuberculosis.*—In the majority of these cases an attempt may be made to cure the fistula, and with considerable prospect of success.

(c) *Fistula not associated with pulmonary tuberculosis.*—In these cases there is a liability to the later development of pulmonary tuberculosis. Every endeavour should be made to cure the fistula. All the tracks should be slit up and their walls scraped, or in some cases the whole track may be dissected out. The communication with the bowel should be laid open as in the simple fistula. The wound may be partially closed by sutures, and primary union in part may be anticipated.

Of greater rarity than the above is the variety in which *the tubercles are deposited irregularly in the mucous or submucous tissues of the bowel wall* (Fig. 502). These degenerate, and finally *ulceration* ensues. The tuberculous ulcer may be seen on any part of the rectal wall. At first it is superficial with thin undermined edges, and on its floor may perhaps be seen caseating areas. The surrounding mucosa becomes much swollen, and probably shows yellowish areas of caseating tuberele. Adjacent ulcers will coalesce until a considerable part of the rectal wall is involved; indeed, in some advanced cases almost the entire rectum may be invaded. The ulceration may spread to the

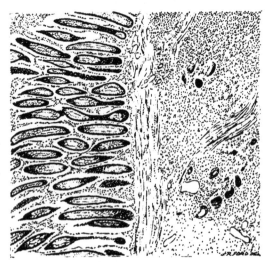

Fig. 502.—Section, taken near the edge of the ulcer, from a case of extensive tuberculous ulceration of the rectum, showing the submucous tuberculous infiltration.

anal canal and destroy the sphincters. The depth of a tuberculous ulcer is very variable. If it is allowed to progress the muscular wall may become eroded, the peritoneum involved, or suppuration may occur in the pelvi-rectal space or in the ischio-rectal fossa.

The symptoms are those of ulceration of the rectum, described at p. 698. The condition has to be diagnosed from chronic septic ulceration, syphilis, and malignant disease. In a great majority of cases pulmonary tuberculosis is present. Diagnosis is only established by the examination of the granulation tissue or the discovery of the tubercle bacillus in the scrapings of the ulcer. The latter is generally an easy matter in this form of ulceration. The course of the disease varies

Since pulmonary tuberculosis is usually present, the rectal ulceration tends to progress even when treated. In a few cases, under treatment the disease runs a more chronic course ; fibrosis occurs, and in part the ulceration may heal.

Although tuberculous disease is often given as a rare cause of rectal stricture, the evidence is by no means conclusive that the healing of a deep tuberculous ulcer ever progresses sufficiently to narrow the lumen materially.

The treatment of tuberculous ulceration of the rectum depends upon the severity of the pulmonary affection and the extent of the ulceration. In advanced pulmonary disease very little can be done, except by astringent injections, to relieve the distress caused by the constant discharge. If the pulmonary affection permits of any operative procedure, and the ulcer is of only moderate size, it may be excised. If larger, the ulcer should be thoroughly scraped and the raw surface cauterized, or smeared with pure carbolic acid, and dusted with iodoform powder. This may have to be repeated should the ulceration spread, or a fresh ulcer arise. When the disease is extensive the only method of cure is by complete excision of the rectum. This, in the great majority of cases, is not permissible on account of the pulmonary affection. Perirectal suppuration must be treated as already described.

A third variety of tuberculous disease occurs in which *the inflammation is limited to the skin of the anal canal and the immediate perianal region*. Excluding the cutaneous affection which occurs around the orifices of tuberculous fistulæ, tuberculosis of the anal skin is very rare. When occurring the disease is very chronic, involves the anal canal, but does not tend to spread to the mucosa. The appearance resembles that of hypertrophic lupus. The bacilli are difficult of detection in this lesion, but the microscopic structure of the granuloma is characteristic. The affected area of skin should be completely removed.

Syphilis.—Various syphilitic lesions occur in the rectum and anal canal. The primary chancre has been observed rarely at the anal margin, and even on the rectal mucosa. In the secondary period moist papules and condylomata occur at the anal margin, and may extend into the anal canal; multiple fissures similar to those in the lips and tongue occur at the anal margin, and mucous tubercles have been seen on the rectal mucosa. In the tertiary period, multiple localized gummata and diffuse gummatous infiltration may occur in the submucosa and spread deeply into the muscular walls, but they are decidedly rare. Ulceration may follow, and the coalescence of several large ulcers may cause wide and irregular tissue destruction. A gummatous ulcer has been known to invade neighbouring parts, e.g. the bladder and vagina, and fistulæ may occur between these viscera.

Although it has been customary to assign to tertiary syphilis a prominent place in the etiology of chronic rectal ulceration, probably it is
but seldom an effective cause.

There is a decidedly rare form of diffuse gummatous infiltration,
called by Fournier the " ano-rectal syphiloma." Commencing in the
submucous tissue, it involves a considerable part of the rectal wall,
with or without implication of the anal canal. Ulceration may or
may not occur. The bowel wall is converted into a rigid and much
thickened tube, which later becomes diminished in size by fibrous
contraction. It appears to be analogous to the diffuse syphilitic
deposit which occurs in other viscera, e.g. the liver and testicles. Antisyphilitic treatment in the early stage gives good results, but later,
when fibrosis has occurred, is of little value.

Chancroids (*see* Vol. I., p. 834) occur on the skin in the
vicinity of the anus. They are much more common in the female,
and arise by direct infection from the vulval discharge. The sores are
multiple, and in appearance, prognosis and treatment are similar to
those occurring on the genitals. Occasionally, the ulcerating chancroid
may, without doubt, extend into the rectum. According to some, this
is one cause of chronic ulceration of the rectum, but it must be a
decidedly rare one.

Dysentery.—Many different forms of rectal ulceration have
been ascribed to dysentery, but the term should be reserved for cases
caused by the organisms of tropical dysentery. The rectum may be
involved in true dysentery, but probably only in association with
disease in the colon. The ulcerations are then superficial, and in their
healing give rise to but little contraction. It is stated, however, that
occasionally a stricture productive of symptoms may follow.

Actinomycosis may very rarely occur in the perianal skin and
in the anal canal.

ULCERATION

Septic ulceration of rectal sinuses.—When well developed, the sinuses peculiarly lend themselves to the lodgment of fæcal
material, which may cause abrasions and open the path for septic
infection. Though occasionally two or more may be present, the ulcer
is usually single, situated dorsally, and may be as large as a three-
penny piece. Symptoms may be absent ; but sometimes pain radiating
around the perineum and down the thighs is present without any
relation to defæcation ; it differs from that of a fissure, since the ulcer
is above the level of the external sphincter muscle. Sometimes there
are traces of blood and pus in the motions, and pruritus ani may
be present. Discovery of an ulcer in a sinus, concealed by a swollen
valve, may be difficult without anæsthesia ; hence a faulty diagnosis of

rectal neuralgia has been made in some cases. An ulcer in the sinus may cause infection in the ischio-rectal fossa, and possibly may rarely be the starting-point of chronic diffuse ulceration.

Ulceration caused by injuries.—Accidental wounds of the rectum are rare, but may initiate chronic diffuse ulceration. Ulceration has followed injury with the stem of an enema tube, and also wounds made for the removal of hæmorrhoids, etc. ; this postoperative danger is enhanced if the patient be feeble and resume the upright posture before the wound has healed. Some authorities consider that erosions of the mucosa by hard scybalous masses may be a possible starting-point of a progressive ulceration. Portions of the rectal wall may be so severely damaged by the passage of the fœtal head during labour that an infective gangrene may ensue. In such cases large portions of the mucosa or even the deeper parts of the bowel wall may slough. This latter cause is held by some to be a cause of chronic septic ulceration, and in this way it is sought to explain the greater frequency of ulceration in the female sex.

Follicular ulceration is rare. Numerous ulcers, more or less circular, and with sharply cut edges, involve the whole thickness of the mucosa, and may be associated with a similar condition throughout almost the entire colon. In some cases the condition seems to have a relationship to chronic renal disease. It probably plays no part in the etiology of chronic rectal ulceration.

Chronic diffuse ulceration.—Excluding tuberculous disease, where the diagnosis is made upon bacteriological or pathological grounds, most cases of chronic diffuse ulceration are of obscure origin. Whatever be the prime cause, the common organisms of suppuration, viz. streptococci, staphylococci, and the Bacillus coli, are in great part responsible for the spread and chronicity of the ulceration. Hence it is that some put forward syphilis as a primary cause, others maintain that chancroid is more often responsible than syphilis, some think that gonorrhœa may be the initial lesion, and others maintain with very good reason that some form of injury, particularly injury to the rectal wall during labour, is the most important cause. It is certain that women are more often affected than men, and a reference to these causes will show how much more frequently the female sex is predisposed.

Symptoms of chronic diffuse ulceration.—Whatever the cause, the symptoms are characteristic. The accumulation of the discharges in the lower bowel creates a frequent reflex desire to defæcate. Since the lower bowel contains scarcely any fæcal material, little but flatus, mucus, pus, and perhaps blood, is passed. This frequency of defæcation is particularly present in the early morning immediately the patient assumes the upright position, or at any other time during the day after resting for a while. The remainder of the day the patient may spend in comparative comfort. But as the ulceration progresses and the discharges become more copious the desire to go to stool will be felt more and more frequently during the day, until it may be that a call must be answered every hour. The quantity of pus and blood passed will vary considerably, depending upon the extent and depth of the ulceration. Pain is not a marked feature in the early stages, but later some pain in the perineum, in the back, or radiating down the thighs is very common. Reflex urinary symptoms may be present.

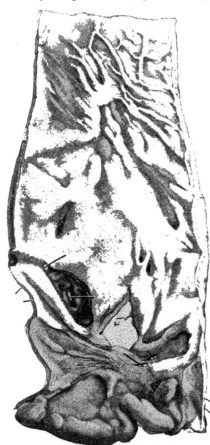

Fig. 503.—Extensive ulceration of the rectum, reaching from the anus (which is surrounded with piles) to some 6 inches above. The walls of the bowel are considerably thickened, and several perforations are seen. The cause was supposed to be syphilis.

A progressive loss of weight and strength due to the continual discharges, the loss of appetite and insufficiency of food, and the unhealthy life which has to be led by these sufferers, will certainly be present sooner or later. In a considerable number of cases some narrowing of the lumen of the bowel will occur, and the symptoms of chronic intestinal obstruction add to the suffering and malnutrition of the patients. Perirectal suppuration is common. Distant foci of inflammation, particularly involving the joints, not infrequently occur, as they may in any infective disease.

The ulceration in some cases extends to the pelvic colon, and over this viscus pain may be experienced and tenderness elicited. The pelvic and iliac colons may be felt as thickened cylinders. Plastic peritonitis is commonly present, and localized suppuration or diffuse peritonitis may occur either from perforation of an ulcer or migration of the bacteria through the unhealthy bowel wall.

On examination with the sigmoidoscope the diagnosis is easy, but the cause of the ulceration often remains undetermined. The sigmoidoscope may fail to demonstrate the upper limit of the disease, either because its passage is prevented by a stricture or because its length is insufficient. In such cases the extent of bowel involvement can only be decided by abdominal exploration.

Treatment of ulceration of the rectum and anal canal. — This depends to a slight extent upon the cause, but far more upon the situation and extent, of the ulceration. If it be due to a specific organism, the recognized treatment of this, either by drugs or by vaccines, is indicated. Such cases

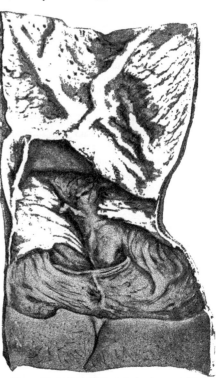

Fig. 504.—Extensive ulceration of the rectum, of unknown origin.

form a small minority, for when cases are first seen the ulceration has become chronic, and is in great part dependent upon the common pyogenetic bacteria ; the infection is a mixed one, and vaccines are probably useless. In all cases absolute rest in bed is essential; the diet should be very light and calculated to leave the smallest possible residue, and the bowels should be carefully regulated by aperients to prevent accumulation of fæcal material in the rectum.

When the ulceration involves the anal canal only, or at the most the lower rectum, the sphincters are to be stretched under anæsthesia, and some application made direct to the ulcerated surface. Nitric acid, carbolic acid, or other strong caustic may be applied. Or the ulcer may be curetted and covered with some antiseptic powder, such as iodoform. Hot hip-baths and enemata containing some antiseptic, such as perchloride of mercury, or chinosol, should be given daily. The application of the caustic may have to be repeated. Such treatment may succeed in early cases where ulceration is of very limited extent.

When, however, the ulceration is higher in the bowel, but still of limited extent, similar treatment may be employed, but is very often attended with complete failure. In fact, rectal ulceration which is at all extensive and long continued is very rarely cured by enemata or direct applications.

Zinc cataphoresis.—The principle of this treatment, according to Ironside Bruce, "is that zinc sulphate is broken up by the galvanic current, the zinc ions travel towards the negative pole, and are thus driven into the tissues surrounding the positive pole. The SO_4 so liberated combines with the metallic zinc of the positive pole to form again zinc sulphate. The method of application is exceedingly simple. The necessary apparatus is as follows : A zinc rod, 6 in. in length, with suitable connexion at the end for the purpose of attaching it to the positive pole of a galvanic supply ; a large indifferent electrode to connect the negative pole. The zinc rod is covered with four layers of lint, which is saturated with a 4 per cent. solution of zinc sulphate (in distilled water). The negative electrode is soaked in plain water to ensure a good contact. The patient being suitably placed, lying on the side, with the aid of a little vaseline as a lubricant the positive pole is introduced in the rectum to a distance well above the ulcerated area. The indifferent electrode is placed over the sacrum or on the abdomen ; to this is attached the negative pole of the source of the galvanic current, the positive pole being attached to the zinc rod. It is necessary to have a milliamperemeter in circuit. All connexions having been made secure, the circuit is completed, and the resistance cut out until the meter stands at 20 ma. In one or two minutes the amount of current will increase to 25–30 ma., and it is kept at this figure for ten minutes. Such an application is made once every two weeks. This method is quite sufficient where the ulceration is confined to the lower portion of the bowel, but where the disease extends higher up, slightly more complicated apparatus is necessary."

This treatment, although of comparatively recent date, seems worthy of a thorough trial. Should it fail, operative measures have to be considered.

Excision of the diseased bowel would seem to be the ideal method of treatment. Superficial ulcers of comparatively small size may be excised and the margins of the mucosa sutured. If the ulceration is superficial and involves only the anal canal, or at most the lower inch of the rectum, it may be possible to excise the diseased mucosa—Whitehead's operation (p. 680). This operation has, however, a very limited sphere of practicability, as ulceration in this region generally responds to more simple methods of treatment. It must be insisted that all the diseased mucosa should be removed and healthy mucosa sutured to the skin of the anal margin, or success cannot be anticipated.

When ulceration involves the higher bowel and extends more deeply, the rectum in whole or in part may be excised by a method similar to that for excision of a cancerous rectum, save that the perirectal tissues need not be removed (p. 721). Should the ulceration extend to the pelvic colon (as determined by laparotomy), excision is still possible by the combined abdomino-perineal operation (p. 723). Excision is only practicable when the whole diseased area can be removed, the sphincter muscle and its nerve supply preserved, and healthy bowel sutured to healthy bowel or to the skin of the anal margin without undue tension. It is contra-indicated when perirectal suppuration, sinuses, and fistulæ are present. At all times it is a serious operation, and one not to be lightly undertaken. Its severity is increased in the enfeebled subjects of chronic ulceration, and the difficulties of the operation are magnified by the perirectal infiltration which is often present.

Colostomy is merely a palliative operation, whose object, by diverting the passage of fæces, is to give entire rest to the diseased bowel. It is the only procedure in many cases where perirectal suppuration, sinuses, and fistulæ are present. Where excision is impossible, either from the general condition of the patient or upon anatomical grounds, and where simpler forms of treatment have failed to alleviate symptoms, colostomy is indicated. There will naturally be considerable aversion on the part of the patient to the operation, but his condition is often enormously improved by it, and his life rendered more tolerable. Following the operation, energetic treatment locally must be persevered with. The bowel must be thoroughly cleansed, and this may be more effectually done through the colostomy opening than from the anus. Should the ulceration heal, certainly some degree of stricture will result. If this can be effectually treated (p. 705) it may be possible to close the colostomy opening. More often the colostomy must remain permanently, for, when the ulceration has been so extensive as to warrant colostomy, in the healing process the bowel becomes so deformed that the satisfactory treatment of the stricture is impossible, and its covering is so delicate that ulceration is liable to recur upon the slightest provocation.

STRICTURE

The lumen of the rectum may be narrowed by extrinsic causes, e.g. enlargements of the prostate, pelvic cellulitis, uterine tumours, or hydatid cysts of the pelvis, which are all described in their appropriate places. A stricture implies that the narrowing is produced by some abnormality or pathological change in the bowel wall itself.

A stricture may be (1) *congenital* (p. 669); (2) *spasmodic ;* (3) the result of *inflammatory changes in the bowel wall.* Congenital stricture is not very common. Although the condition is congenital in origin, symptoms may not occur until later life. The stricture is situated in the anal canal or at its junction with the rectum. Spasmodic stricture is extremely rare. Inflammatory changes in the bowel wall may narrow the lumen in one of two ways—(a) by a diffuse mucous, submucous, and muscular infiltration, such as may occur in the localized gummata, the diffuse ano-rectal syphiloma (p. 698), and to some extent in diffuse tuberculosis of the bowel (p. 696); (b) much more commonly by the fibrous contraction which necessarily results from the healing of any deep and extensive ulceration (p. 699). Diffuse inflammatory infiltration and fibroid contraction may occur together.

The **pathological appearances** depend upon the cause. Congenital strictures are felt by the finger as a tight ring ; postoperative strictures in the anal canal are felt as a fibrous ring surrounding the lumen of the bowel ; in such cases there is no deep infiltration of the bowel walls. Where fibrous contraction results from the healing of rectal ulceration the degree and extent of the stricture will vary enormously. In the majority of cases which come under observation active ulceration is still present. The stricture is usually within reach of the examining finger, but occasionally it is higher, and may be at the junction of the rectum and the pelvic colon. It is sometimes annular, surrounding the lumen as a fibrous ring ; in other cases the contraction takes place on one side only, with the result that the wall is puckered up at this site ; again, in others a considerable extent of the bowel is involved in the contraction. Polypoid masses of infiltrated mucous and submucous tissue may be seen projecting into the rectum. Hæmorrhoids frequently accompany a stricture, and are probably caused by the pressure upon the hæmorrhoidal veins. The bowel above the stricture becomes hypertrophied and dilated. Fæcal masses retained above a stricture will cause ulceration, or aggravate that already existing.

Symptoms.—Most commonly the symptoms of stricture are slowly engrafted upon those of ulceration. The passage of fæces becomes increasingly difficult : they are retained above the stricture for a variable time, and then expelled piecemeal, so that the motion consists of small, hard, isolated fragments.   There are periods of days together when no motion may be passed.   If the stricture is low down, near the anal margin, e.g. the congenital stricture, or that following operations upon the anal canal, the motion may sometimes be flat-tened or ribbon-shaped.   This is unusual (p. 664).   Since ulceration is so commonly present, the passage of blood, pus, and mucus is more or less constant.   Even if ulceration be absent, the irritation of fæces retained above the stricture will excite a catarrh of the bowel, shown by the passage of mucus, and perhaps blood.   The patients complain of diarrhœa—the spurious diarrhœa of proctitis or ulceration.   Sooner or later, symptoms of intestinal obstruction appear—i.e. flatulent dis-tension, probably aggravated by food; unpleasant rumblings of wind in the bowels, accompanied by colicky peristaltic pains ; and an increasing demand for purgatives to obtain an action of the bowels.   Later, if the stricture be allowed to progress, the compensation of the colon, taxed to its utmost, fails : distension progresses, and the obstruction terminates acutely or subacutely (p. 719).   The colon, filled with the contents of the small bowel and its own secretion and gases, is distended so greatly that its circulation is impeded, and infection of its walls results.   Local infective necrosis of its wall may occur, and acute perforative peritonitis follow.   The perforation will usually be low in the pelvic colon, where distension is greatest and bacterial life most rampant, but it may be, as in any case of colonic obstruction, in the cæcum.

The **diagnosis** is readily made by digital and, if necessary, by careful sigmoidoscopic examination.   Occasionally difficulty may arise in differentiating the simple from the malignant stricture.   In simple fibrous contraction there cannot be doubt, but where there is narrowing of the bowel associated with irregular polypoid masses projecting into its lumen the similarity to cancer is sometimes very great.   In the simple disease there will be a long history of ulceration of the bowel, probably commencing at an age when malignant disease is unusual. The polypoid masses have not the characteristically hard and irregular surface of a carcinoma.   If doubt exists, a portion of the edge of the thickening should be submitted to microscopy.

The **treatment** varies with the site and extent of the stricture, and with the presence or absence of ulceration.

Dilatation.—Strictures situated in the anal canal, e.g. the con-genital form and those following operations upon the anal canal, may be treated satisfactorily by dilatation with Hegar's dilators.   Before dilatation, if the stricture is very firm, it may be advisable to incise it at four points situated at the extremities of two diameters at right angles to one another.   Dilatation will have to be maintained for some time, perhaps during the rest of life.   Simple strictures of the

2 t

lower rectum, say the last inch, may, in the absence of ulceration, be treated in the same manner. Dilatation of a stricture higher in the rectum is often a difficult matter, but in the absence of ulceration a soft rubber dilator may be passed through the sigmoidoscope tube : a stiff metal instrument is dangerous, since it may readily perforate the bowel wall and cause perirectal inflammation.

Complete proctotomy.—The bowel and tissues posteriorly are divided completely from a level above the stricture in the median line, the knife emerging at the tip of the coccyx. Strictures associated with ulceration may be treated in this manner. Good drainage is secured, threatened obstruction overcome, and ulceration given a chance to heal. The after-treatment of this septic wound requires unremitting care, and during the healing contraction will occur, and constant dilatation will be required. Probably several weeks or even months will elapse before healing is complete. Incontinence of fæces is present at first, but is generally recovered from when healing is complete.

Excision.—In strictures of the anal canal which do not respond to dilatation, Whitehead's operation may be performed. This may be a simple operation in congenital stricture, but in postoperative strictures the scar tissue may be dense, adherent to deeper parts, and difficult to dissect. The method probably has a very limited practicability, as most of these strictures can be readily dilated.

In higher-lying strictures the affected bowel may be excised. The principles involved are similar to those of excision of an ulcerated rectum (p. 702). The excision of these strictures is a severe and difficult operation, and must never be lightly undertaken. It should be reserved, in suitable subjects, for high-lying undilatable or ulcerated strictures. In some measure, excision may be looked upon as an alternative to complete proctotomy. If successful, its advantages are the shortened convalescence and the restoration of the lumen of the bowel. It is, however, a much more severe and formidable operation.

Colostomy may be necessary to relieve urgent obstruction. It is indicated in the majority of cases which are complicated with perirectal suppuration, sinuses, and fistulæ. Patients enfeebled by prolonged ulceration are often best treated by colostomy, for they are in no condition to stand the severe operation of excision, or the prolonged suppuration after complete proctotomy. By care after the operation, the ulceration may heal. It may then be feasible to dilate the stricture or possibly to excise it. Later the colostomy may perhaps be closed (p. 703).

PROLAPSE

Prolapse may be defined as a protrusion through the anal orifice of parts normally situated within. It may be *partial* (Fig. 505), when rectal mucosa alone protrudes, or *complete* (Fig. 506), when all the coats of the bowel project.

Etiology.—The condition may occur at any age, but is peculiarly frequent at the extremes of life, babies and young children furnishing a large proportion of cases.

Normally during defæcation a narrow ring of mucosa protrudes from the anus, and recedes immediately after the completion of the act; if recession does not immediately occur, prolapse may be said to be present. Any swelling of this ring of mucosa, inflammatory or otherwise, predisposes to prolapse. Such swelling, in babies and young children, may be due to the irritation of worms, but probably this

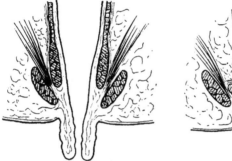 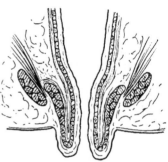

Fig. 505.—Partial prolapse, only the mucosa involved.

Fig. 506.—Complete prolapse, the whole thickness of the bowel wall protruded.

cause has been much exaggerated. In diarrhœa the mucosa may be swollen, straining is severe and prolonged, and a child suffering from this affection is often allowed to remain seated on the chamber for an indefinite period, thus favouring prolapse. The straining due to phimosis or to vesical calculus is often held responsible, but careful inquiry shows that this alone plays very little, if any, part in the etiology. In adults similar causes may be prevalent, but much more commonly the predisposing cause is a hæmorrhoidal swelling of the mucosa (p. 676). In elderly subjects hæmorrhoids may be present, but at this age the straining and local venous engorgement due to urinary trouble, such as urethral obstruction from enlargement of the prostate, are often responsible.

Once partial prolapse is established, it tends to be progressive, unless promptly and efficiently treated. The sphincters become stretched and partly lose tone, thus favouring the increase of the protrusion.

Complete prolapse usually results from a neglected partial prolapse, and generally evolves gradually, but occasionally the prolapse may be complete and well developed from the beginning.

The conditions essential for complete prolapse are—(1) stretching and eventually relaxation of the supporting tissues of the rectum —the pelvic fascia, and the fat of the ischio-rectal fossæ ; (2) a long mesentery to the pelvic colon ; (3) relaxation of the sphincter muscles.

Complete prolapse is practically never found in a healthy fat baby, but only in the wasted baby with loss of perirectal fat. It is especially seen in association with severe diarrhœa, or with some specific fevers, e.g. measles and whooping-cough ; the severe cough in these diseases excites the formation of the prolapse. The relatively straighter course of the child's pelvis predisposes to the condition, especially if defæcation is permitted in the sitting posture, in which the rectum is practically a straight tube.

In adults complete prolapse is more common in women who have borne children, due, no doubt, to a laceration of some of the supporting tissues of the rectum during labour.

In elderly subjects a partial protrusion is liable to become complete, for at this age the absorption of fatty tissues supporting the rectum is probable, and the sphincters easily lose tone.

At any age a polypus may cause prolapse, partial or complete. Such a protrusion is more of the nature of an intussusception than a true prolapse, the part bearing the tumour becoming invaginated into the lower rectum. Intussusceptions of the rectum probably do not occur in the absence of a tumour.

Clinical manifestations.—The appearances are quite distinctive. Projecting from the anus is a more or less cylindrical mass covered with mucosa, and varying from a mere ring of mucosa in the partial, to a thick cylinder of bowel, 5 or 6 in. long, in the complete variety. In the smaller protrusions the cylinder is more or less straight, but in the larger it is slightly curved. The mucosa may have a normal appearance if not subjected to irritation, and if it be only loosely grasped by the sphincter ; but when irritated or tightly gripped, it becomes of a dark-red or even purple colour. In cases which have been allowed to protrude for some time, abrasions of the mucosa may occur, and in some ulceration or acute infective gangrene may supervene. In others considerable thickening of the prolapsed part from inflammatory infiltration into the mucous and submucous tissues will occur. The mucosa in the larger protrusions is seen to be arranged in parallel and concentric folds, and the orifice is not infrequently more or less occluded by one of these folds.

In complete prolapse the peritoneum covering the anterior surface of the rectum will be drawn down, and in large protrusions it must pass through the anal orifice with the bowel. A hernial sac is thus constituted which may or may not contain an abdominal viscus. In a few cases the hernial contents have been known to protrude at the anal orifice in front of the prolapsed bowel, which is displaced posteriorly and its orifice directed backwards. The contents are naturally, in the great majority of cases, small intestine, but the ovaries and bladder have been found. Occasionally, adhesions may form, rendering the contents irreducible. Attempts at reduction in such cases have sometimes resulted in rupture of the rectum and protrusion of the herniated gut through the rent.

Diagnosis.—The only protrusions from the anus which may be mistaken for prolapse are the simple polypus (very rarely a malignant neoplasm), hæmorrhoids, and an intussusception. A polypus is easily recognized by its pedicle, alongside which the finger can be passed into the bowel. Hæmorrhoids form a series of tumours surrounding the anal orifice. An intussusception may at times cause a little difficulty. In a pure prolapse the mucosa is continuous with the skin at the anal margin ; or at times, the anal canal not being everted, there is a very shallow recess at the base of the prolapse, whereas in an intussusception there is a distinct sulcus into which the finger may be passed freely all around.

Treatment.—Any prolapse should be immediately replaced. In order to do this the child should be laid across the knee, or the adult upon the left side, and the prolapse well oiled and firmly grasped with the hand. Gentle pressure in the majority of cases will succeed in reduction. The part protruded last is the apex, and this must be returned first. If reduction be not done immediately, inflammatory changes and those resulting from the grip of the sphincters may produce serious consequences, and render replacement very difficult or impossible.

Recurrence must be prevented by removal of the cause. Thus, in children, diarrhœa and the feeble wasted condition must receive treatment, and, above all, the child must not pass the motions in the sitting posture, but must assume the squatting position on a low pan ; in this position the lower sacrum and coccyx are bent and the rectum is more supported than in the sitting posture. In children this line of treatment will usually cure the disease, but in a very small minority, in spite of all care, the prolapse will recur, demanding some form of operative treatment. In adults similar lines of treatment should be instituted in the first place, but in the majority of these no cure will result, and further treatment is indicated.

Numerous pessaries have been invented to prevent prolapse, but all are unsatisfactory, and should only be employed when there are special contra-indications to operation.

Many and varied operative procedures have been performed for prolapse of the rectum, among which the following may be mentioned :—

1. **Searing the mucous membrane with the actual cautery.**
—This is applicable where the prolapse is only partial. It is especially useful in children, and for slight cases in adults where there is no hæmorrhoidal condition of the mucosa. The object of the cautery is to cause limited sloughing of the mucosa, and thus narrowing of its circumference, and also to promote adhesions of the mucosa to the muscular coat. With the bowel protruding, the point of the Paquelin cautery at a dull-red heat is drawn from its base to its apex, in a series of radiating lines. In healing, cicatrices will contract in both the longitudinal and the transverse direction. A second application may be necessary.

2. **Excision of the mucous membrane.**—In prolapse of slight degree, and particularly in children in whom the cautery has failed to effect a cure, **V**-shaped portions of the mucous membrane may be excised. It will generally suffice to remove two such pieces, one anteriorly and the other posteriorly. The cut edges of the mucosa are united by sutures. The extent of removal depends upon the proportions of the prolapse.

The whole circumference of the mucous membrane may be excised and the cut edges of the mucosa united to those of the skin—Whitehead's operation. This procedure is suitable for prolapse caused by a hæmorrhoidal condition of the mucosa of the rectum, for any partial prolapse, and for some cases of complete prolapse of very moderate degree. In the latter class, when the mucosa has been united to the skin the muscular wall of the bowel will be folded, and adhesions of the mucosa to the pleated muscular wall will prevent a further tendency to prolapse.

3. **Excision of the prolapsed portion.**—This method is suitable for all cases of complete prolapse. It is attended with a greater risk and, according to some, a less promising after-result than the method described next. The protrusion is covered with sterile gauze and drawn well down, and an incision is made about ¾ in. from the anal margin, and parallel to it, into the prolapse. This will in all probability be below the level of the internal sphincter muscle. The incision is deepened through all the layers of the gut and the peritoneal cavity opened. When this is done, care must be taken to avoid injury to any herniated intestine, which, if present, should be returned into the pelvic cavity. The incision should then be carried through the whole circumference of the protruded gut. The latter may now be unfolded, as it were, by pulling the cut edge of mucosa downwards and turning it inwards. The gut can then be drawn taut and clamped close to the anal margin, the part distal to the clamp being cut away. All

hæmorrhage must be arrested. The edges of the proximal portion of the gut are now sutured to those of the distal portion surrounding the anal margin. The patient should be kept under observation for some time, for fear of contraction necessitating dilatation.

4. Fixation of the gut within the abdomen.—This procedure is an alternative to the foregoing, and opinion is by no means unanimous as to which operation gives the better results. The method is, of course, only applicable to cases of complete prolapse. Its object is to anchor the pelvic colon within the abdomen, and so long as the anchorage remains prolapse cannot recur.

There are two places at which the colon may be fixed—(a) the peritoneum of the anterior abdominal wall and underlying transversalis fascia, and (b) the iliac fascia and peritoneum of the iliac fossa. In either case, after the abdomen is opened the colon is drawn upwards as far as possible and fixed in this taut position by sutures. In the former case the peritoneum is raised from the anterior abdominal wall on either side of the incision and its two edges sutured to the walls of the colon, and the longitudinal band upon the latter is sewn directly to the transversalis fascia. Thus a broad surface for adhesion is secured. In the latter case the principle is similar; the peritoneum having been lifted from the iliac fossa, the bowel is sewn to the iliac fascia, and the peritoneum to the walls of the bowel. In all probability this gives a firmer anchorage than the former method, and it is certainly less likely to cause, at a later date, intestinal obstruction or pain from the dragging of the adhesions, both of which have been known to follow the anterior fixation.

BENIGN TUMOURS

ADENOMA OF THE RECTUM

Adenoma of the rectum is common in childhood, but less frequent in later life. It originates in the mucosa, at first is sessile, but usually becomes pedunculated; it forms a firm, bright-red swelling with a smooth or lobulated surface. It is composed of glandular tissue similar to the glands of Lieberkühn; occasionally it may undergo cystic degeneration. In children it is invariably pedunculated, and rarely exceeds the size of a cherry, whereas in adults it is relatively more frequently sessile, and may attain much larger dimensions (Fig. 507). It is usually single in the child, but in the adult it is relatively more commonly multiple (Fig. 508). In children the adenoma invariably remains a simple tumour, but in later life it by no means infrequently becomes malignant. Many instances are recorded in which the removal of an adenoma by cutting through the base of attachment has been followed by a malignant growth. Simple

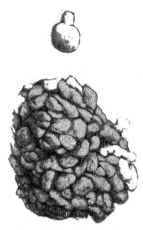

Fig. 507. — Adenomatous polypi from a child and an adult.

adenoma and carcinoma may be present simultaneously.

The **symptom** is painless hæmorrhage; sometimes this is accompanied by mucoid discharge. If the adenoma originate low in the rectum, or if the pedicle be sufficiently long, the polyp may protrude through the anus. Rarely will the pedicle become gripped by the sphincters, and the tumour slough off. An adenoma is seldom (probably never in the child) of sufficient size to cause impediment to the passage of fæces. A simple neoplasm may be the starting-point of an intussusception of the rectum.

Diagnosis.—When the tumour is pedunculated the diagnosis is easy, as by digital examination the pedicle can usually be felt; if the tumour be high-lying a sigmoidoscopic examination will always reveal the true condition. The diagnosis of a sessile adenoma can often only be made by microscopy.

Treatment.—An adenoma should always be removed. In the child it is sufficient to cut it off after ligaturing, cauterizing, clamping, or twisting the pedicle. In the adult similar treatment will suffice for an obviously pedunculated and undoubtedly innocent tumour. If there exist any suspicion of malignant disease, the base of attachment and the adjacent mucosa should be removed, and submitted to microscopy; and if malignant transformation be found, the case must be treated accordingly.

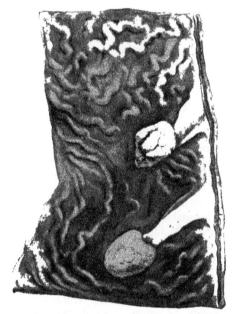

Fig. 508.—Two pedunculated adenomas.

PAPILLOMA OF THE
RECTUM

The so-called villous tumour of the rectum is rare; it resembles the villous tumour of the bladder and the pelvis of the kidney, and consists of a lobulated spongy mass, sessile or pedunculated, with long villous tufts studding its surface; these tufts are composed of mucous membrane and are very vasonlar (Fig. 510). The villous tumour is

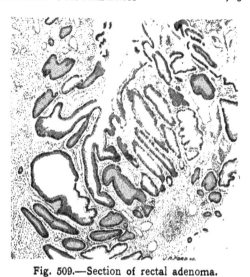

Fig. 509.—Section of rectal adenoma.

confined to adult life, and is very liable to become malignant; it may be single or multiple; if pedunculated it always has a short and broad pedicle. The

symptoms are hæmorrhage and a glairy white discharge which seems characteristic. Occasionally the tumour may protrude through the anus, or portions may become detached and be passed in the motions. The **treatment** is always removal. The tumour, the pedicle if present, and the adjacent mucosa should be removed, the edges of the mucosa being sutured. Microscopical

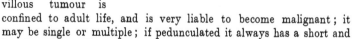

Fig. 510.—Section of rectal papilloma.

examination is essential, and if malignant transformation has taken place the case must be treated accordingly.

PAPILLOMA OF THE ANUS

Papillomatous masses occasionally arise in the anal canal, or in the skin immediately surrounding the anus. .They are typical papillomas, covered with squamous epithelium. They resemble the venereal warts of the genitals, and are probably always caused by the irritation of discharges, either from the genitals or from the rectum. These warts must be treated by attention to their causes, strict cleanliness and the application of a dry powder. If no improvement follows, they may be removed by the knife or by the application of carbonic dioxide snow.

FIBROMA

Swellings consisting of fibrous tissue are frequently seen in the rectum and anal canal, but the majority of these are not tumours in the true sense of the word ; they are inflammatory in origin. Occasionally a true fibroma occurs ; it may be single or multiple, sessile or pedunculated, and is usually of small size, although a few instances are recorded in which the tumour reached large proportions. Mixed fibromas, such as fibro-myoma and fibro-myxoma, have been recorded but are very rare. The symptoms are similar to those of adenoma.

LIPOMA OF THE RECTUM

Rectal lipoma is rare ; in many of the cases recorded as such the tumours really originated in the pelvic colon either as submucous or subserous growths ; when the latter, the pedicle has contained a protrusion of peritoneum—a point to bear in mind when operating upon these tumours through the rectum. The symptoms are very indefinite. If large, lipomas may cause obstruction ; they have been known to become extruded and cast off.

Vascular nævi, lymphomas, and tumours consisting in part of *bone* and *cartilage* have been described as occurring in the rectum, but they are all exceedingly rare.

MALIGNANT TUMOURS

SARCOMA OF THE RECTUM

Rare anywhere in the intestinal tract, sarcoma attacks the rectum slightly more frequently than the bowel above. It affects the two sexes equally ; it has usually been recorded in middle-aged or elderly subjects.

All types of sarcoma have been recorded—round-celled, spindle-celled, alveolar, lympho-, and melanotic. The spindle-celled is the most frequent variety. The growth usually originates in the sub-mucosa, but is said to commence sometimes in the muscular wall. It forms a sessile mass projecting into the lumen of the bowel; occasionally it may become more or less pedunculated, and has been known to prolapse during defæcation. It may involve only a limited portion of the rectum, but occasionally tends to grow extensively both circumferentially and vertically, clinically resembling chronic inflammatory conditions, for which it has not infrequently been mistaken. The mucosa covering a sarcoma may sooner or later ulcerate. The growth tends to invade parts surrounding the bowel; glandular involvement is not uncommon, but visceral deposits are rare.

The melanotic variety has usually occurred at the anus, but has been seen also in the rectum. It is very malignant, visceral deposits occurring early.

The **symptoms** are similar to those of carcinoma (p. 718). The lumen of the bowel is, however, less encroached upon, and the obstruction less marked.

Diagnosis.—A sarcoma has to be differentiated from carcinoma, from chronic inflammatory affections, and from the diffuse ano-rectal syphiloma. In the early stages its submucous position will distinguish it from carcinoma; but later, when ulceration is present, clinical diagnosis may be impossible. Similarly, differentiation between an ulcerating sarcoma and chronic inflammatory ulceration may be clinically impossible, and even extremely difficult microscopically.

The **treatment** is similar to that of carcinoma (p. 720). The ultimate prognosis is bad, recurrence nearly always taking place shortly after removal.

CARCINOMA OF THE RECTUM[1]

A carcinoma may originate in the rectum, the anal canal, or the skin at the verge of the anus. About 3 per cent. of primary cancers occur in the rectum. Carcinoma is four or five times as frequent in the rectum as elsewhere in the intestine. Cancer of the anal canal is much less common.

Carcinoma of the rectum occurs most frequently between 40 and 60 years of age. Youth is not exempt; the youngest patient in my series was 13. The younger the patient, the more rapid and malignant the growth.

The growth is nearly always single. A few cases are recorded in which two primary growths were present in the rectum, and rarely two primary growths have been reported, of which one was in the rectum and one elsewhere. The tumour may originate in any part, but a common starting-point is low down, within reach of the finger;

---

[1] *See also* Vol. I., p. 553.

another favourite site is at the junction with the pelvic colon. Figs. 511, 512, 513, and 514 illustrate different appearances of cancer in different parts of the rectum.

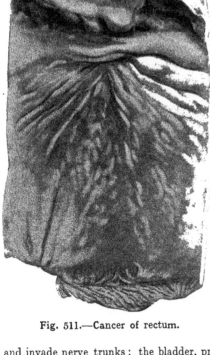

Fig. 511.—Cancer of rectum.

Pathology.—The growth is columnar-celled (Fig. 515), and originates in the glands of the mucosa. It spreads by (1) direct extension, (2) the lymphatic channels, and (3) the blood stream.

1. Direct extension.—The vertical and circumferential extent of rectal cancer varies greatly. When first seen, it may be a small nodule involving a very limited surface of the bowel wall; in other cases it may have surrounded the entire bowel—the annular type. Between these two all possible varieties exist.

The growth, originating in the mucosa, early invades the muscular coats (Fig. 516), and sooner or later the perirectal tissues. Thus the tissues of the ischiorectal fossæ may be invaded, the presacral and precoccygeal tissues may be infiltrated, and the growth may become fixed to the pelvic walls and invade nerve trunks; the bladder, prostate, and seminal vesicles, or uterus and vagina, according to sex, may be infected, and in high-lying growths the peritoneum may be involved. Rarely the growth extends down the anal canal, and may protrude at the anus. There is evidence to show that in some cases cancer cells extend in the submucous tissues far beyond the naked-eye limits of the growth.

2. **Lymphatic spread.** —The lymphatic vessels of the rectum accompany the hæmorrhoidal veins, and pass backwards and upwards to the pararectal glands, which lie in close connexion with the lateral and posterior surfaces of the bowel from just above the attachment of the levator ani muscle to the upper limits of the rectum. Their efferent vessels accompany the veins in the pelvic mesocolon,

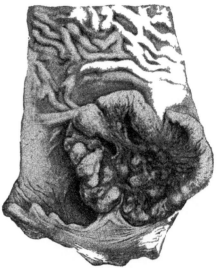

Fig. 512.—Cancer of rectum.

and enter glands adjacent to the superior hæmorrhoidal vessels. The lowermost of these glands are situated immediately in front of the sacral hollow, but higher up as the mesentery increases in length they become farther removed from the sacrum, whilst at the upper limit they are not far distant from the pelvic brim, and in some cases may communicate with the glands along the iliac vessels. Efferent vessels from these enter glands situated around the inferior mesenteric vessels, which are practically continuous with the lumbar glands. Experimental injection of the lymphatics of the rectum shows that in some cases

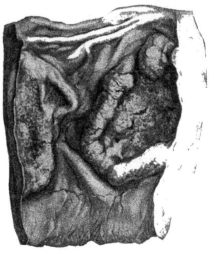

Fig. 513.—Cancer of rectum.

those from the lower portion of the bowel may pass to the oblique inguinal glands. This, however, is not confirmed by clinical experience, since these glands are not invaded by a rectal cancer.

A rectal cancer may involve any or all of these glands. The duration and extent of the cancer is no criterion of the extent of the glandular involvement. In a comparatively small primary growth extensive glandular involvement may be present, and vice versa.

Enlarged glands in association with cancer of the bowel are not necessarily cancerous. There is always the possibility of mere septic absorption from the ulcerating growth.

3. Spread by the blood stream.—We are entirely ignorant of the processes which govern the spread of cancer by this route. Visceral metastases are not necessarily a late occurrence. We have insufficient data to judge of their frequency; in fifty consecutive autopsies upon persons dying from the disease, at very varying intervals after the appearance of symptoms, I found metastases were recorded in seven only. In all the liver was involved, and in one the spleen. In three,

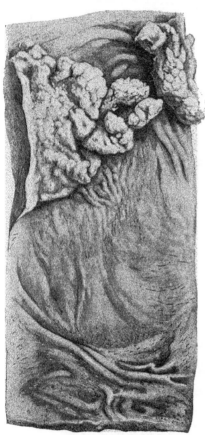

Fig. 514.—Cancer of rectum.

secondary growths were scattered over the peritoneum, but possibly in these the spread was by the lymphatics.

Symptoms.—The typical symptoms are those of ulceration combined with stricture (*see* pp. 699 and 704). In intensity each symptom varies within wide limits. Hæmorrhage and the teasing diarrhœa may be absent for some time; clinical evidence of material narrowing of the lumen of the bowel may be long delayed, and indeed in a few cases the disease may run its course without symptoms of obstruction appearing; in others again, symptoms of obstruction may be the initial manifestation, and in such the disease has advanced insidiously and assumed large proportions without symptoms of rectal ulceration.

If untreated, rectal carcinoma leads to a fatal issue in about one and a half to two years on the average. Not infrequently life is terminated by acute intestinal obstruction, arising in various ways. Most commonly the bowel above the constriction becomes exhansted, and the colon progressively dilates. Occasionally the distended pelvic colon may undergo torsion around its mesenteric axis. In any obstruction of the large bowel. the cæcum may be the most distended part, and occasionally an acute dilatation of the cæcum may be the initial evidence of failing compensation. Should such a cæcum have retained its original peritoneal relationships, and be suspended by a mesentery, a volvulus around its mesenteric axis may occur. Rarely the diseased part becomes intussuscepted into the lower bowel. Very infrequently the small·lumen left by the invading growth may be occluded by a fæcal mass or foreign body, such as cherry- or plum-stones.

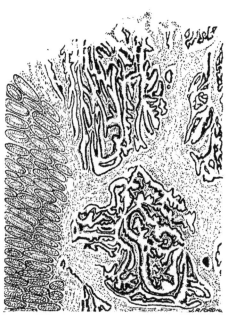

Fig. 515.—Edge of a malignant ulcer of rectum, showing typical appearance of columnar-celled cancer.

In a few cases peritonitis may cause death. Bowel distended by mechanical obstruction is predisposed, partly by virtue of its impeded circulation, to infection. In cancer of the rectum the pelvic colon or cæcum may thus become acutely infected, and necrosis of the walls may result, with local or diffused peritonitis, which is practically always fatal.

·In the absence of these complications, factors which aid in the fatal termination are exhaustion from repeated hæmorrhages, pain, especially when the large nerve trunks are involved, sleeplessness from the incessant diarrhœa and pain, and absorption of toxins.

Diagnosis.—It should be a cardinal rule thoroughly to examine every case presenting the slightest symptom of rectal trouble. If this rule were followed, and patients encouraged to present themselves on the first evidence of rectal disease, cancer would generally be recognized without difficulty at an early stage. The irregularly hard growth projecting into the lumen of the bowel is quite characteristic. Investigation under anæsthesia and with the sigmoidoscope may be necessary.

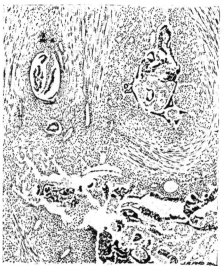

Fig. 516.—Section of rectal cancer, showing infiltration of the muscular wall.

Although in most cases the cancer is typical to sight and touch, it may sometimes be confused with other diseases. Chronic septic and tuberculous ulcerations, especially when associated with polypoidal masses of swollen and œdematous mucosa, are apt to be mistaken for carcinoma. The history, the flat and comparatively superficial ulcer, and the absence of induration will generally serve to differentiate these conditions. If any doubt remains, a portion of the swelling must be submitted to microscopy without delay. At times diagnosis between a benign and a malignant neoplasm of the rectum may be difficult (p. 712). The rare sarcoma may usually be distinguished by noting that it is a submucous rather than a surface growth.

Treatment of removable cancer.—A growth may be considered removable when confined to the rectum (to determine this, examination under anæsthesia may be necessary), when invaded glands are operable and visceral deposits are absent. Exceptions naturally occur. For instance, slight invasion of the prostate has been successfully dealt with by ablating a portion of the gland ; similarly, the posterior vaginal wall, and indeed the uterus in a few chosen cases, have been successfully removed ; so has an adherent loop of small intestine. Fixation to the bony pelvis contra-indicates operation, but invasion of the perirectal cellular tissue does not necessarily do so. Each case must be judged upon its own merits, and the age and general condition of the patient must be fully considered. No attempt at removal must be made during the phase of acute obstruction.

The principle to be observed in operation is that the primary growth and the lymphatic drain (whether there be obvious invasion or not) must be removed in continuity, for if this be interrupted the wound may become infected with cancer cells. It is obvious that the perirectal cellular tissue, including the pararectal glands, and the mesentery of the pelvic colon, including the glands along the hæmorrhoidal vessels, must be removed.

The operations may be classified under two headings, according to whether the growth is removed (1) entirely from the perineal aspect, or (2) partly through the abdomen and partly through the perineum—the *combined abdomino-perineal operation.*

1. **Perineal approach.**—There are two methods of perineal approach—(*a*) through the true perineum, and (*b*) from behind, after removing the coccyx, and as much of the sacrum as is necessary.

(*a*) *Removal through the true perineum.*—By dissection from the perineum, the rectum is severed from its connexions, and the upper rectum or pelvic colon drawn through the perineal wound and sutured to the skin. In order to mobilize the rectum sufficiently to permit approximation to the perineum without undue tension, it is necessary to sever the muscular (levatores ani), the fascial (visceral prolongations of the pelvic fascia), the peritoneal (the peritoneum of the recto-vesical or recto-vaginal pouch) and the vascular (branches of the superior hæmorrhoidal vessels) connexions. The lower pelvic mesocolon must also often be divided.

An endeavour may be made to preserve the external sphincter by commencing the incision, after thoroughly stretching the muscle, at the muco-cutaneous junction, raising the mucous membrane as in Whitehead's operation, and deepening the dissection into the perirectal tissues at the upper level of the sphincter. Owing to the limited space this attempt often fails, and the great stretching and possibly tearing necessitated may render the muscle impotent. Only very limited dissection is possible by this route.

When no effort is made to preserve the sphincter the incision encircles the anus and is prolonged anteriorly and posteriorly in the mid-line. Through this wound a much more thorough dissection may be performed.

(*b*) *Exposure of the rectum from behind.*—Kraske introduced this

2 u

route for high-lying growths, and, although the operation has been modified by many surgeons, it still bears his name. The bone is exposed by a median or slightly left lateral incision terminating a little behind the anus. Some surgeons remove the coccyx only, others a piece of the left border of the sacrum, others (following Rydygicr) turn back a flap of the sacrum and coccyx, which is replaced at the close of the operation. The levatores ani are divided on either side, the rectum separated by blunt dissection with as much of the perirectal tissues as possible, the peritoneal cavity opened, and the pelvic mesocolon divided piecemeal until sufficient bowel has been freed to permit approximation of the proposed site of section to the anal margin without undue tension. The further steps are modified to meet the requirements of the case. When the colon can be brought well down to the anus the best procedure is to divide the rectum just above the internal sphincter muscle, and the bowel above at a point which will allow it easily to reach the anus ; the mucous membrane of the anal canal is removed, the bowel drawn through the sphincteric orifice and sutured to the skin of the anal margin. If some extent of the lower bowel is healthy, this may be left and the upper cut end anastomosed to it. This is not so good a method, as it may tempt the surgeon to encroach too near to the growth ; moreover, the stitches nearly always give way, and fæcal extravasation results, followed by prolonged suppuration and probably some constriction. Neither procedure may be applicable, from inability to free the upper bowel sufficiently. In such case, a perineal anus is established. The many attempts that have been made, by means of various treatments of the bowel, to gain some control over such an anus have been uniformly unsuccessful.

The main arguments against all operations from the perineal aspect are these : (i) The branches of the superior hæmorrhoidal vessels are cut close to the bowel wall, that is on the distal side of the junction of the anastomotic loop between the lowest sigmoid and superior hæmorrhoidal arteries ; hence, gangrene of the transplanted bowel is liable to occur, followed by prolonged suppuration, and constriction. Similarly, if the bowel is united to the anal skin with any tension, the sutures give, the bowel retracts, and a stricture results in the healing process. (ii) Not infrequently, owing to the fact that the bowel cannot be brought to the anal margin, the operation has to be terminated by a perineal anus. This can never be foretold previously to operation. An inguinal is better than a perineal anus. (iii) Little, if any, of the mesentery of the pelvic colon is removed ; hence the glandular lymphatic drain is very imperfectly eradicated.

Although some surgeons claim encouraging ultimate results from these perineal operations, the majority agree that recurrence is very frequent. Indeed, one surgeon reports recurrence within periods from six months to three years in no fewer than 54 out of a total of 57 cases. The recurrences are found to be in the lymphatic glands of the pelvic mesocolon, in the pelvic peritoneum, and in the bowel ends. That is, recurrence takes place above the level of previous operative inter-ference, and in tissues which might have been removed by a more extended operation.

2. The combined abdomino-perineal operation. — This procedure attempts to remove more thoroughly the tissues invaded by the upward spread of the cancer. There are two methods of executing it:

(a) The greater part of the pelvic colon and its mesentery are removed and a permanent iliac colostomy established.

(b) Only the lower part of the pelvic colon is removed and a corre-sponding length of mesentery, the cut end of the pelvic colon being brought to the anus and stitched to the skin there, or if circumstances permit the lower rectum is left and anastomosed to the pelvic colon.

In both cases the removal is commenced through the abdomen.

In (a) merely a sufficient loop of the pelvic colon is left to permit establishment of a permanent iliac colostomy. The pelvic colon and its mesentery are divided, the vessels ligatured and the peritoneum incised on either side of the bowel to the level of the recto-vesical or recto-vaginal reflexion. All the tissue is removed from the front of the sacrum. The peritoneum is divided at the base of the bladder or vagina, and the rectum separated from the parts in relation to it anteriorly and laterally. The ureters will probably be seen and must be carefully avoided. When the bowel has been freed as far as is possible, i.e. to the base of the bladder anteriorly and to the levatores ani laterally, it is pushed to the bottom of the pelvis and the peritoneal covering of the pelvic floor is repaired as far as possible. In the exaggerated lithotomy or the prone position the coccyx is excised, and the rectum, and as much as possible of the surrounding tissues, including a considerable portion of the levatores ani, the sphincter muscles, and the tissues of the ischio-rectal fossæ, together with the colon, are removed.

In (b) the object of the operation is to remove the disease exten-sively and to bring the pelvic colon to the anal margin. The superior hæmorrhoidal vessels, even when the bowel is otherwise freed, will from their comparative shortness prevent the colon being brought to the anus. Hence these vessels must be isolated from all connexions and ligatured cleanly, no surrounding tissue being included in the ligature. If the artery be ligatured immediately above the origin of the lowest sigmoid branch, there is probably little danger of gangrene of the bowel to be brought to the anus, for collateral circulation is established through the arch formed by it and the lowest sigmoid artery. The hæmorrhoidal vessels having been ligatured and divided, the peritoneum is severed as in (*a*), and the separation of the rectum from its connexions is also conducted in a similar manner. The operation is completed from the perineum after removing the coccyx, but the sphincters are preserved, or by some surgeons the lower rectum. In the former method the bowel is drawn down and removed so that the portion within the grasp of the sphincters is without tension, and it is there sutured ; in the latter, the pelvic colon is anastomosed to the rectum. In this operation, less bowel will generally be removed, and hence less of the mesentery of the pelvic colon, than in (*a*).

Choice of methods.—When weighing the respective values of the operation performed entirely from the perineal aspect, and that by the combined abdomino-perineal method, two points have to be considered, viz. the relative mortalities and the end-results.

Mortality.—All operations for rectal cancer are prolonged and severe, and accompanied by considerable shock. The immediate mortality, therefore, is by no means slight. In addition, the prolonged suppuration in the perineal wound which sometimes occurs may lead to a fatal issue in persons already enfeebled by a rectal cancer and its complications. The mortality of the Kraske operation is probably greater than that of the one performed entirely through the true perineum. Statistics of mortality given by different surgeons vary widely. The mortality must obviously be influenced by the general condition of the patient, and the extent of operative removal necessary. There is no doubt, however, that at the present day the immediate mortality of the combined method of operating is greater than that of any operation performed from the perineal aspect only, and this is one great argument against the routine performance of the abdomino-perineal operation.

End-results.—These, again, are very various as given by different authorities, but the majority of surgeons agree that recurrence after perineal excision and the Kraske operation is very frequent. We have not yet sufficient statistics to show that the combined operation is followed by a more lasting freedom from recurrence.

The combined method is theoretically superior to any perineal operation, but its relatively higher mortality necessitates careful selection of the subjects. They should be moderately spare, not too old, free from arterial degeneration or pulmonary disease, and otherwise sound in constitution.

In favour of the abdominal approach it may be urged : (1) That the liver and other viscera may be palpated for metastases, in the presence of which the patient may be spared any mutilating operation. (2) That glandular enlargement may be observed and feasibility of removal decided. (3) That the pelvic peritoneum may be seen and felt (and, of course, the whole peritoneum, for it sometimes happens that secondary nodules may be scattered over the peritoneum without clinical evidence of their presence). (4) That an inspection of the mesentery of the pelvic colon will generally enable the operator to determine whether it is sufficiently extensive to permit of the colon being brought to the anal margin if it is intended to adopt this method ; if this seems to be impossible, an iliac colostomy may be established, thus abolishing any possibility of having to terminate a perineal operation by the formation of a perineal anus. (5) That it is the only way in which the pelvic colon can be sufficiently freed and its blood supply safely preserved in order that it may be brought to the anus if this method be thought desirable, for by ligating the superior hæmorrhoidal artery immediately above the origin of the lowest sigmoid artery, the arterial arch between the two vessels is preserved and the blood supply to the bowel is ensured. (6) That as gangrene of the transplanted bowel does not occur, as it not infrequently does in the perineal method of operating, convalescence is much shortened and stricture is less liable to follow. (7) That a far wider severance and removal of perirectal tissues can be performed than by either of the perineal methods of operating.

If it be proposed to perform the combined operation, it has still to be determined which is the better of the two methods to pursue. Time alone will decide whether the end-results of the more extensive removal of the tissues are a sufficient compensation for the loss of the normal anus. Theoretically, the former operation would seem to offer the best results, but naturally there will be great aversion on the part of a patient to have to submit to any artificial anus when the other alternative seems possible.

An iliac colostomy is preferable to any perineal anus. In the latter an infection of the mucosa frequently occurs from the surrounding wound. The escape of the discharges from the inflamed mucosa are very annoying. An artificial anus in the iliac region can be attended to by the patient himself, and a daily irrigation will render him comparatively comfortable.

Treatment of irremovable cancer. — Discovery of an irremovable rectal cancer does not always demand immediate performance of colostomy. A few cases of rectal cancer will run their course without any necessity for the operation. There is little evidence to show that the rate of growth is delayed by diverting the passage of fæces over it, but symptoms may be very much relieved. The indications for a palliative colostomy are—

Intestinal obstruction, acute or chronic.

Hæmorrhage apparently caused by fæces passing over the growth.

Pain caused by the presence of fæces in the bowel.

The teasing diarrhœa.

Hæmorrhage and diarrhœa may be relieved by curettage and cauterization, but the symptoms will almost surely recur, when the process may be repeated.

Carcinoma of the Anal Canal

Anal cancer (Fig. 517) originates from the lining of the anal canal or the skin of the anal margin. There is evidence to show that in a few cases it has grown from the edge of a chronic fissure or ulcer.

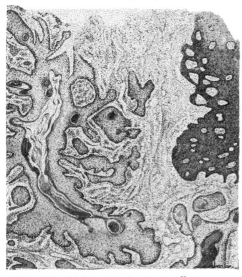

Fig. 517.—Section of squamous-celled cancer of anal canal.

Generally speaking, the squamous-celled tumour is of slower growth than the glandular cancer, and usually cancer of the anal canal conforms to this rule. Anal cancer is, however, of more rapid growth than many forms of skin cancer. The disease spreads (1) by *continuity of tissue* to the skin of the perineum (though it does not tend to infiltrate the rectal wall to any extent), (2) by *the lymphatic system*. The glands invaded are those in the groin—the oblique set of the inguinal glands.

Symptoms.—Since the growth is at the anal margin, pain is present from the outset. At first only experienced when the bowels move, it later becomes more or less constant. Some blood-stained discharge occurs early, and this is constant, and independent of the bowel action. Pruritus ani may be severe. Symptoms of intestinal obstruction may or may not be present, depending upon the degree of occlusion of the anal canal. As the growth infiltrates the sphincters, incontinence of fæces results. On examination there will be seen the typical appearance of a squamous-celled carcinoma.

Diagnosis.—The disease has to be differentiated from a chronic indolent fissure, condylomata and gummatous ulceration at the anal margin, and also from tuberculous infiltration of the anal canal.

Treatment.—This consists in early and free removal. In all cases, whether obviously enlarged or not, the inguinal glands of both groins must be freely removed. It is impossible, for anatomical reasons, to remove the primary growth and lymphatic drain in one piece. The glandular operation is naturally performed first. The removal of the primary growth is conducted in a manner similar to that described already (p. 721) for the removal of a rectal cancer through the true perineum. The cut ends of the bowel are sutured to the perineal skin. No attempt can be made, of course, to preserve the external sphincter muscles.

PRURITUS ANI

An affection of the perianal skin, in which the one symptom is itching. There are two distinct clinical conditions—(1) that due to some obvious source of irritation, (2) that occurring independently of any lesion in the rectum or the anal canal.

1. The irritation may be set up by oxyurides or by the discharges from internal hæmorrhoids, fistulæ, ulcers within the anal canal, or from tumours, simple or malignant. It may arise from the unconscious escape of mucus, owing to weakness of the sphincters, whether natural to the patient or due to prolapse or to previous operation. It may also result from lack of local cleanliness, or the presence of redundant circumanal folds which allow of the collection of secretion or fæcal matter. In advanced cases the itching is intolerable, rendering the patients very depressed and at times suicidal. It varies from day to day, and from week to week; it is worse at night-time and when the body is thoroughly warmed. When the condition has been present for some time the skin of the perineum shows evidences of prolonged and forcible scratching; the dermatitis extends backwards over the coccyx, forwards over the scrotum or vulva, and outwards over the buttocks.

The primary cause must be removed. After this, when the condition is of long standing, itching will not be relieved at once, and local treatment may be necessary. No one application will suit all cases. The changes must be rung between powders, ointments, and lotions. If the itching is acute a soothing application is preferable, but if chronic a stimulating remedy is more efficacious. Before any application the parts should be washed with some non-irritating soap, e.g. Castile soap, or oatmeal and water, and carefully dried. The powders may contain boric acid, starch, zinc oxide, calomel, calamine, bismuth, etc. Ointments may contain any of these, or chloroform, morphia, cocaine, salicylic acid, aconite, subacetate of lead, balsam of Peru, belladonna, ichthyol, etc. Many of these substances may be used in lotions.

2. This variety is regarded as a nervous manifestation, possibly associated with the gouty, the neurotic, or some other constitutional diathesis. The patients are often of the nervous irritable type, and the pruritus is rendered worse after any excitement or nervous strain.

The skin involved is an elliptical area, supplied by the 3rd and 4th sacral nerves, immediately surrounding the anus, and extending up the anal canal, back nearly to the coccyx and anteriorly along the perineum; it becomes dry, thin, and atrophic.

The condition may be relieved by one or other of the drugs already mentioned, but often only temporarily. Good results from the employment of radium are reported by Sir Malcolm Morris and others. In cases in which all other methods fail, operative treatment must be advised, if the symptoms are severe. The object of the operation is to cut all the nerves going to the affected skin.

A curved incision is made on each side of the anus, just externally to the affected part, and prolonged forwards and backwards, leaving the diseased skin attached by two pedicles in the mid-line, anteriorly and posteriorly. The flaps of skin are dissected from subjacent tissues, and anteriorly and posteriorly where it remains attached it is undercut so that it is entirely severed from its deep connexions. Hæmorrhage is arrested most carefully, as the occurrence of a hæmatoma may endanger the vitality of the flaps, which are replaced and retained by sutures. Sensation returns, but not the pruritus. Occasionally a spot or two of skin does again suffer from pruritus, but this may be treated in a similar way.

BIBLIOGRAPHY

Anderson, " The After-Result of the Operative Treatment of Hæmorrhoids," *Brit. Med. Journ.,* 1909.

Bastianelli, " Principles of a Radical Treatment for Procto-Sigmoiditis," *Ann. of Surg.,* 1909.

Blake, " Excision of Carcinoma of the Rectum by the Combined Method," *Ann. of Surg.,* 1908.

Bruce, " The Treatment of Ulcerative Proctitis by Zinc Kataphoresis," *Proc. Roy. Soc. Med.,* 1908.

Buchanan, " Excision of the Rectum for Cicatricial Stricture by the Combined Method, with Preservation of the Sphincter," *Surg., Gyn., and Obstet.,* 1907.

Cunningham, " Procidentia Recti : Treatment by Excision," *Ann. of Surg.,* 1909.

Discussion on the Operative Treatment of Cancer of the Rectum, *Proc. Roy. Soc. Med.,* 1911.

Gaudiani, " Beiträge zur Aetiologie und Behandlung der entzündlichen Mastdarmstenosen," *Deuts. Zeits. f. Chir.,* Bd. xcvi.

Handley, " Surgery of the Lymphatic System," Hunterian Lectures, *Brit. Med. Journ.,* 1910.

Hartmann, " Some Considerations upon High Amputation of the Rectum," *Ann. of Surg.,* 1909.

Keith, " Malformations of the Hind-End of the Body," *Brit. Med. Journ.,* 1908.

Lusk, " Excision of the Rectum for Cancer," *Surg., Gyn., and Obstet.,* 1908.

Lusk, " A Technique of Resection of the Male Rectum," *Surg.,Gyn.,and Obstet.,* 1909.

Lusk, " Resection of the Male Rectum for Cancer, by the Combined Method in Two Stages," *Ann. of Surg.,* 1910.

Mayo, " Removal of the Rectum for Cancer : a Statistical Report of 120 Cases," *Ann. of Surg.,* 1910.

Miles, " A Method of performing Abdomino-Perineal Excision for Carcinoma of the Rectum and of the Terminal Part of the Pelvic Colon," *Lancet,* 1908.

Miles, " The Radical Abdomino-Perineal Operation for Cancer of the Rectum and of the Pelvic Colon," *Brit. Med. Journ.,* 1910.

de Muls, " Hæmorrhoids in Children," *Arch. of Pediatrics,* 1905.

Ronchet, " De l'Amputation Abdomino-Périnéale du Rectum Cancéreux," *Arch. Gén. de Chir.,* 1908.

Schumann, " Ueber des Sarcoma recti," *Deuts. Zeits. f. Chir.,* Bd. cii.

Sheldon, " The Technique of Resection for Prolapse of the Rectum," *Surg., Gyn., and Obstet.,* 1910.

Wood-Jones, " The Nature of the Malformations of the Rectum and Uro-Genital Passages," *Brit. Med. Journ.,* 1904.

Zésas, " Les Hémorroïdes chez l'Enfant," *Arch. Gén. de Chir.,* 1908.

THE LIVER, GALL-BLADDER, BILE PASSAGES, AND PANCREAS

By G. GREY TURNER, M.S.Durh., F.R.C.S.Eng.

Anatomy of the liver and of the biliary apparatus.
—The liver measures a little more than 6 in. in the greatest vertical direction, and a little less than 6 in. antero-posteriorly. Its
summit reaches to the upper border of the right 5th rib at a point
1 in. internal to the mammary line, and, therefore, is not directly
accessible without traversing the pleura, lung, and diaphragm. Some
part of each of the 6th, 7th, 8th, 9th, 10th, and 11th ribs lies over

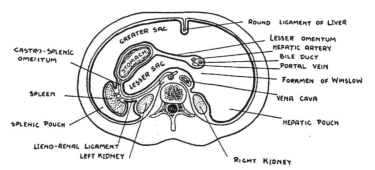

Fig. 518.—Transverse section of the peritoneal cavity at level of
foramen of Winslow.

the liver, as well as the cartilages from the 6th to the 9th, while the
pleura extends to within 2 in. of the costal margin.

The peritoneal space just below the liver—the hepatic pouch (Fig.
518)—is important, for here collections may form when the gall-bladder
leaks.

The gall-bladder (Fig. 519) is usually pear-shaped, and has a capacity
of 1½ oz. At its junction with the cystic duct there is often a lateral pouching
called the pelvis, or Hartmann's pouch, which, when distended, may be
mistaken for the commencement of the cystic duct.

The cystic duct is about 1½ in. in length and runs downwards and to
the left to join the common hepatic duct. Its lumen, normally only ⅛ in. in

diameter, is further narrowed by spiral folds—Heister's valves—so that,
unless dilated, it does not permit the passage of a probe.

The cystic artery lies to the inner side of the duct, and is not in
direct contact with it. In the angle between the cystic and the hepatic ducts
one or more lymphatic glands are constantly present, and, when
enlarged, may closely simulate calculi.

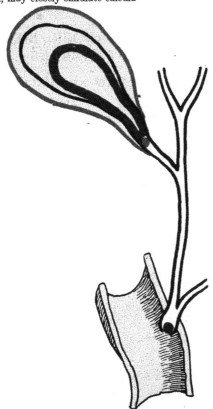

Fig. 519.—Diagram of the gall-bladder and bile-ducts.

The *black* outlines represent the normal conditions ; *red* indicates a calculus impacted in the
cystic duct, with consequent distension of the gall-bladder and no jaundice ; and *green*, a
stone in the lower end of the common duct, with a contracted and thickened gall-bladder,
and deep jaundice.

The common hepatic duct is about 1¼ in. in length, while the
common bile-duct is about 3 in. long and ₁⁷₆ in. in diameter, and may
conveniently be divided into three portions.. The *first or supraduodenal
portion* extends to the upper border of the duodenum, in the free edge of the
gastro-hepatic omentum. Behind it runs the portal vein, and to its inner side

the hepatic artery. This portion of the duct is often in relation with one or two lymphatic glands, and small veins or an arterial twig may cross it and be the source of serious hæmorrhage if wounded. The *second or retroduodenal portion* is 1 in. to 1¼ in. long, and in two cases out of three is more or less surrounded by pancreas. The *third or transduodenal portion* passes obliquely through the duodenal wall and ends in the ampulla of Vater, which opens into the bowel on a papilla. The common duct gradually diminishes in diameter from 8 mm. at the beginning to 2·5 mm. at its orifice.

THE LIVER

MALFORMATIONS AND MISPLACEMENTS

As a result of constriction by corsets and belts, the liver may be pushed up, or may be flattened antero-posteriorly with downward elongation of the whole of the right lobe, or of its lower border.

Sometimes a definite, very mobile, tongue-like lobe arises by a broad attachment or a thin pedicle from the lower border, without elongation of the whole lobe. Such a process (" floating lobe " or " *Riedel's lobe* ") is often associated with gall-stones. It is distinguishable from an enlarged kidney by the facts that it can be pushed beyond the middle line, and that the kidney can be felt separately.

HEPATOPTOSIS, OR MOVABLE LIVER

Dislocation of the normal liver is only commonly met with in association with general visceroptosis (Glénard's disease). The liver is displaced downwards and rotated so that the upper surface looks forwards, and the heavier right lobe is advanced inwards as well as downwards. It may be loose and replaceable, or may be fixed in its abnormal position. Total hepatoptosis, a rare condition, is commonest in women between 40 and 60.

Etiology.—Ptosis may be due to congenital weakness of the hepatic supports, and has been met with in children. The exciting cause may be trauma, but is usually the general weakening associated with rapid child-bearing or with neurasthenia.

Treatment.—When the visceroptosis is general, most benefit is likely to accrue from abdominal massage and exercises (Swedish), combined with a well-fitting abdominal belt or corset. For hepatic displacement alone, attempts have been made to support the organ by forming adhesions between the liver and the parietes, by shortening the suspensory ligament, or by stitching the edge of the liver to the abdominal wall.

INJURIES

The liver is more often injured than any other solid abdominal organ. Usually the violence is direct and considerable. The injury may be entirely subcutaneous, or associated with an open wound.

Morbid anatomy.—The right lobe is involved six times as often as the left, and the convexity twice as often as the concavity. The actual injury to the liver may take the form of a contusion, a subcapsular rupture, or a laceration. In the subcapsular variety the liver may be very extensively torn, leaving a gap an inch or more wide beneath its capsule (Fig. 520). Whatever the type, the most serious feature is hæmorrhage, either into the peritoneal cavity or into the liver or ducts.

Injuries to the diaphragm, lung, stomach or bowel, kidney or spleen are often serious complications.

Clinical features.—With the slighter injuries there may be only mild shock with rigidity and tenderness over the liver and limitation of respiratory movement. Later, there may be some jaundice and glycosuria ; and later still, perhaps, evidence of infection. As a rule, there is severe pain with great tenderness over the liver, and extreme general rigidity, the chest being held almost still. Marked pallor suggests grave internal hæmorrhage, and it may be possible to detect free fluid in the abdominal cavity. In cases that survive,

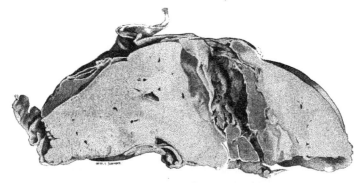

Fig. 520.—Old subcapsular laceration of the liver.

distension soon ensues, and jaundice commonly occurs some days after the injury.

Diagnosis.—The cases may be arranged in three groups : (a) Those with signs of overwhelming internal hæmorrhage, but with nothing to indicate its source ; (b) those with evidence of severe hæmorrhage, with injury to the parietes, fracture of ribs, or localized pain and tenderness over the liver region ; (c) those in which the site of the injury suggests a possible rupture of the liver, but in which there are no signs of hæmorrhage; but only localized tenderness and rigidity, with subsequent enlargement of the liver and some slight jaundice.

Prognosis.—Injuries sufficiently serious to demand surgical interference are attended with a mortality of 60 or 70 per cent. The lesser degrees of contusion or laceration may recover spontaneously, but the possibility of late death from secondary hæmorrhage, infection, or pulmonary embolism must be remembered.

Treatment.—In open wounds it is always wise to operate.

In subcutaneous injuries, evidence of severe hæmorrhage, or in the milder cases an increasing pulse-rate or persistence of tenderness and rigidity, indicates interference.

In operating it must be borne in mind that the hæmorrhage is partly controlled by the rigidity of the abdominal muscles, and that as soon as this is relaxed the bleeding may become furious.

The best incision is a median one from the xiphisternum to the umbilicus. Exposure of a laceration far back on the convexity may require a cross-cut to the right or division of the suspensory and right lateral ligament. Hæmorrhage may be temporarily checked by grasping the portal vein and hepatic artery between the fingers in the foramen of Winslow and the thumb in front. Lacerations should be sutured, if possible, but if the site of injury cannot be easily exposed, reliance should be placed on immediate packing with gauze. Sometimes a combination of the two methods is useful.

Often in stab wounds the diagnosis can only be confirmed by laparotomy, which may have to be combined with a transpleural incision along the track of the knife.

In the after-treatment of liver injuries, secondary hæmorrhage, abscess—intrahepatic or perihepatic—and biliary fistula must be watched for.

SURGICAL INFECTIONS

LIVER ABSCESS

Multiple liver abscesses may result from infection conveyed by (a) the hepatic artery, (b) the portal vein, (c) the bile-ducts, or (d) direct continuity.

Single liver abscesses.—The most typical is the tropical dysenteric abscess. This generally results from infection by the *Amœba dysenteriæ*, only occasionally complicating the bacterial form of the disease. The white races, especially males over 40, furnish 90 per cent. of the cases. The abscess may occur at any stage of the disease, or long after all dysenteric symptoms have disappeared. Alcohol, free living, and exposure are all exciting causes.

Morbid anatomy.—In about 70 per cent. of cases the abscess is confined to the right lobe, the posterior and upper part being the favourite site. Though usually spoken of as "solitary," in about 40 per cent. of cases there is more than one abscess. (Fig. 521.) The contents of the abscess cavity are usually chocolate-coloured, very viscid, and not offensive. The abscess may extend into the surrounding healthy liver, may burst into the peritoneum, the lung, or more rarely externally, or may shrivel up and its contents become inspissated.

Clinical features.—The symptoms are characteristically vari-

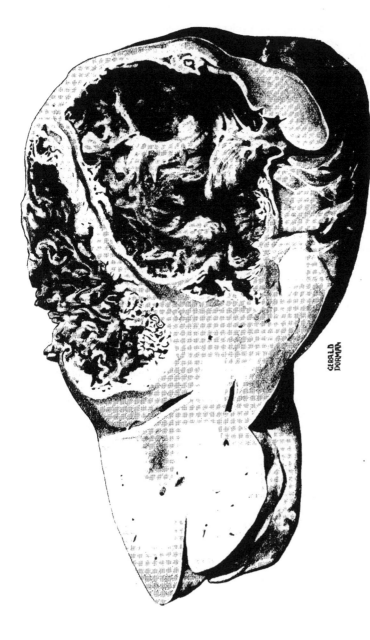

Fig. 521.—Tropical abscess of the liver, showing two distinct cavities separated by a strong septum. The uppermost abscess extended to the surface, giving rise to fatal peritonitis.

able. There may be dull pain over the liver region, or sometimes over the acromion, a tendency to stoop to the right, and perhaps coughing on deep inspiration. The temperature may be continuously elevated or regularly variable, simulating malaria ; or it may be very little elevated, and in some chronic cases may be normal or subnormal. Sweating is usually profuse, the skin yellowish and "earthy," and wasting marked.

Physical signs.—The liver is enlarged, usually upwards, producing dullness almost as high as the scapular angle. The whole hepatic region is commonly bulged and, later, tender on deep pressure.

Diagnosis.—From malaria diagnosis is made by blood examination and by the effect of quinine. The upward enlargement of the liver is unlike that seen in suppurating gall-bladder and in cancer, but it may be very difficult to distinguish the condition from suppurating hydatid, gumma, or subdiaphragmatic abscess. The fluorescent screen may give valuable help, as also may an examination of the fæces for amœbæ. The diagnosis is rendered certain by the use of the exploring needle. It is necessary to emphasize the ease with which even a large abscess may be missed unless a thorough exploration of the liver be made. A constant vacuum should be kept in the syringe attached to the needle, which may with safety be $3\frac{3}{4}$ in. long. The finding of the abscess should be immediately followed by operation, the needle being left *in situ* as a guide. Amœbæ may be found in the fluid, but prolonged search is often necessary, though they are usually numerous in the discharge from the abscess on the days following the operation.

Prognosis.—Without operation the prognosis is very bad, and even surgical treatment has a mortality of about 20 per cent.

Treatment.—In the few cases in which the abscess is actually invading the skin a simple incision, followed by drainage through a very large tube, will effect cure. Many successful results have been reported from cannula drainage carried out immediately after the presence and site of the abscess have been determined by exploratory puncture, but for surgeons who have no special experience of this class of cases the open operation is undoubtedly the best.

An abscess in the hepatic dome is best approached by excision of part of the 9th or 10th rib, just behind the mid-axillary line. It may be necessary to approximate the costal to the diaphragmatic pleura, either by stitching or by packing, and to incise the diaphragm. In very many cases the pleura and peritoneum along the operative track are found to be already adherent.

When the principal enlargement is downwards the abdomen should be opened by a vertical incision over the prominent part through the right rectus muscle. If the adhesions are not sufficient, the peritoneum should be protected by gauze packing. The abscess is then opened by forceps, and the finger introduced and any secondary abscesses opened. Drainage is secured by a large rubber tube, 1 in. in diameter, wrapped round with gauze to prevent pus oozing up by its sides before the liver adheres to the parietes. During the first two days the pus should be sterile, and after that should only contain amœbæ. Every care must be taken to avoid secondary infection if the abscess is to close rapidly. As a rule the cavity rapidly contracts, but the hepatic enlargement may only slowly decrease. It is often necessary to aid drainage of large cavities by initiating a siphon action through the tube. Sometimes there may be a considerable discharge of bile, which only ceases gradually.

INFECTIVE GRANULOMATA

Tuberculosis of the liver is rare. It may take the form of solitary masses, and localized abscesses have been operated upon successfully. The liver may be enlarged, but usually there are no distinctive diagnostic features.

SYPHILIS

Only the tertiary manifestations are of surgical interest.

Gummata, either single or multiple, may occur, often as late as five to twenty years after infection. They form yellowish masses, accompanied by perihepatitis, and sometimes by diffuse sclerosis and lardaceous disease. The dome of the right lobe is most commonly affected, and the diaphragm often invaded. Another common site is near the portal fissure. They may become absorbed, leaving scars which by their contraction tend to cause syphilitic cicatrization or even lobulation of the liver, or they may break down, become infected, and simulate abscesses. Jaundice is rare, but ascites may be present if the gumma obstructs the portal vein.

Treatment.—Exploration may be advised in cases that have resisted medical treatment. If the diagnosis is confirmed the abdomen may be closed and remedies persevered with, but when there is doubt the mass may be excised or opened and some tissue scooped out for examination. This interference may hasten the effect of the appropriate therapeutic measures, described in Vol. I.

CIRRHOSIS

For the treatment of the ascites an operation, now generally known as omentopexy, was devised independently by Talma of Utrecht, and Drummond and Morison of Newcastle-upon-Tyne, and first successfully practised by Morison in 1895. This operation aims at establishing an efficient collateral venous circulation between the abdominal wall and the omentum and viscera, thus helping to carry off the portal blood.

That this does actually occur is proved by the great development of the subcutaneous veins some time after the operation. (Fig. 522.)

The operation can only be recommended for ascites depending on alcoholic cirrhosis and due to portal obstruction, and not merely the result of toxæmia. The patients selected should have withstood several tappings, should be free from pulmonary, cardiac, or renal disease, and should become absolute teetotalers after recovery.

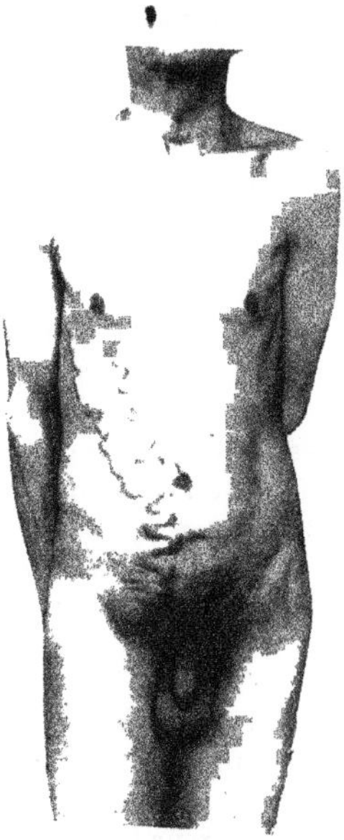

A supra-umbilical incision is made to expose the liver and spleen and confirm the diagnosis. Then through a small suprapubic opening a Keith's tube is introduced into Douglas's pouch, and the abdomen emptied of fluid. The surfaces of the liver and spleen are scrubbed with gauze to set up some peritoneal reaction, and the omentum is fixed at two or three points to the parietes, especially to the peritoneal edges of the wound. Afterwards the parietes are kept in contact with the liver and spleen by carefully strapping the abdomen from above downwards. Continuous drainage is secured by Keith's tube. Reaccumulation of fluid may demand one or more tappings. Some operators dispense with drainage and depend on subsequent tapping.

Results.—In properly selected cases the mortality is very low and the after-results are uniformly good, patients remaining alive well for 2, 3, 5, 6, and over 11 years. (*See* Fig. 522.) The operation has been used for ascites due to a great variety of causes, but usually with unsatisfactory results.

Drainage into the subcutaneous tissue has been suggested by Essex Wynter, and carried out by Sampson Handley.

Fig. 522.—Photograph of a patient alive and well 11 years after omentopexy for alcoholic cirrhosis.

The great development of the epigastric veins is well shown on the right side. That a similar condition did not arise on the left side was probably due to the fact that the patient always wore an inguinal truss.

(*Photograph kindly lent by Professor Rutherford Morison.*)

SIMPLE TUMOURS

Angiomas of the liver have several times been successfully removed. Though usually quite small, this species of tumour may attain the size of a child's head. As operative interference may be

2 *v*

very dangerous, and as there is no special tendency to become malignant, these tumours are best left alone unless there is some distinct indication for removal.

MALIGNANT TUMOURS

Of the malignant tumours, the only important variety from an operative point of view is that which arises as an extension from malignant disease of the gall-bladder (*see* p. 760).

Primary carcinoma and **sarcoma** of the liver, though rare, are important, because they may occur in the form of massive growth which may degenerate and simulate a cyst, an abscess, or a gumma. The right lobe is usually the one affected, the growth forming a single large tumour. Sarcoma is even rarer than carcinoma.

Secondary carcinoma and **sarcoma** are more common, and the growths are generally multiple and of various sizes.

Treatment.—When the diagnosis of secondary malignant disease is established, operative interference is out of the question, but exploration is certainly justified with a doubtful localized tumour, for many inflammatory conditions are indistinguishable from new growth. If, as is usual, radical operation is not feasible, the patient should be given the chance that a course of iodide and mercury may offer.

CYSTS

Simple single cysts are rarely found. Though usually small, they may attain the size of a child's head. They are, as a rule, situated near the free margin of the liver, and have been found in connexion with the round ligament.

Cystadenomas and *multiple cystic disease* also rarely occur.

HYDATIDS

These cysts occur in the liver more frequently than in all other situations put together (63·4 per cent.). The disease manifests itself between the ages of 20 and 40, but, though uncommon, cases do occur in children, usually from 8 to 10 years of age.

Pathology; morbid anatomy.—The tumour is usually situated in the right lobe, either deeply embedded or pointing towards the upper surface. The cyst may be single; there may be two of about the same size; or numbers of small cysts may be present (the multilocular variety).

The true cyst is composed of two layers, an outer, whitish, firm cuticle, and an inner cellular layer from which the scolices develop. These are surrounded by a fibrous capsule formed by an alteration of the adjoining parts. The scolices possess suckers and hooklets, and, though at first attached to the capsule, later float free in the cyst fluid. The fluid is clear, often opalescent, of specific gravity 1002 to 1010, and, when the cyst shows active growth, contains no albumin. Hooklets may be found in the fluid, but are not numerous.

Secondary changes.—Hydatids may die, the cysts usually shrivelling up and the contents becoming less fluid and more gelatinous, and, later, may become converted into a cheesy mass, sometimes with calcareous deposits. Rupture may follow slight trauma or gradual erosion. Suppuration is common and may be determined by injury. The infection may come from the bile or some adjacent hollow viscus, or may be hæmic as in typhoid fever.

Clinical features.—Hydatid cysts usually obtrude themselves on account of their size, but they may be very large without giving rise to injurious pressure on neighbouring organs. The patient may complain of dragging or a feeling of weight, or of attacks of pain depending on peritonitis or suppuration.

Physical signs.—As a rule the liver is enlarged upwards and may compress the lung, and also cause bulging of the costal arch. When the cyst can be felt below the costal margin it is dull and usually very tense and elastic, so much so that it may resemble a solid tumour ; it rarely presents the so-called hydatid thrill. Marked tenderness, jaundice, and ascites when present are usually due to inflammatory changes, or to pressure on bile-ducts, portal vein, or inferior vena cava. Jaundice is rare.

Diagnosis.—Malignant disease and cirrhosis, syphilis, suppuration and hepatoptosis may all be mistaken for hydatids, and even on operation multilocular hydatids may be difficult to diagnose from cancer. When the hydatid enlarges the liver upwards, pleural effusion or hydatid disease in the lung may be simulated. In these circumstances skiagraphy may help, the fluorescent screen clearly showing the diaphragm and its movements. Exploratory puncture should *not* be done when the presence of hydatids is suspected.

Prognosis.—Although natural death of the parasite may occur at any time, the cyst may burst and disseminate, or become infected. Perforation into the peritoneum or pleura may occur with fatal results ; but rupture into the stomach, duodenum, or bile passages is less rapidly disastrous and may even result in cure.

Treatment.—The essential treatment is to remove the mother cyst and to deal with the adventitious capsule as best possible. Cysts that project downwards are most safely reached through an abdominal incision, while for those that occupy the dome of the liver, and that cannot be satisfactorily reached from the abdomen, the thoracic route must be chosen, an incision being made in the 8th or 9th interspace. It is necessary to protect the surrounding parts from contamination by the fluid, for fear of secondary implantation. This may be done by gauze packing, or by stitching the sac to the abdominal wound before opening it. Some surgeons prefer to divide the operation of evacuation into two stages, leaving the opening of the sac to a second operation ten days later.

Whenever possible, complete excision is the ideal operation. As, however, the adventitious capsule is intimately associated with the surrounding parts, this can seldom be carried out; but enucleation of the true cyst may be combined with partial excision of the capsule. The large area left after excision or enucleation may be completely or partially closed by tier sutures, any part not so closed being treated by gauze packing. In any case, drainage must be provided.

If excision is not expedient, the cyst should be opened and emptied, and every part of the lining membrane removed by forceps or by gauze scrubbing. The remaining cavity must be packed if there is much hæmorrhage, and in all cases freely drained.

Very large tumours, of which the whole interior cannot be reached, should be marsupialized by stitching the edges to the peritoneum or fascia of the parietal wound. The interior may then be packed and drained.

GALL-BLADDER AND BILE-DUCTS

MALFORMATIONS

Congenital Obliteration of the Bile-Ducts

This condition is probably due to antenatal descending cholangitis. Clinically, there is jaundice, either at birth or very soon afterwards; this rapidly increases and becomes associated with cholæmia and tendency to hæmorrhage, life seldom being prolonged beyond six months.

Treatment.—In cases that have survived infancy an operation may be undertaken. If the gall-bladder is not distended with bile, cholecystenterostomy will be useless, and an attempt will have to be made to unite a dilated duct or a free surface of the liver to the small intestine.

Cystic Dilatation of the Common Bile-Duct

There are two classes of cases: (a) those with a free opening into the duodenum; (b) those with definite obstruction in the common duct. The condition is most frequent in children, but may first show itself about middle life. Clinically, there is a large cyst below the liver, associated with jaundice. The onset is gradual and the whole condition painless.

Treatment must be operative, usually by anastomosing the cyst and some part of the intestine, preferably the duodenum.

INJURIES

The gall-bladder may be ruptured subcutaneously or wounded by a stab or a bullet. A large bile-duct may be damaged, and there may be associated injuries to the liver or other viscera, or to some large vessel such as the portal vein.

Morbid anatomy.—The rent in the gall-bladder is usually at the fundus, and may be a mere puncture or a tear an inch or more in length. The ducts may be completely torn across, but more usually only part of the circumference is involved, so that healing occurs, though stricture may follow.

Clinical features.—Either accident may be early fatal from associated injury, and, in any case, will be attended with shock. When the shock passes off, the patient may appear to recover completely, or the abdomen may become distended, painful, tender, rigid, and dull in the right side, especially about the iliac region. Jaundice is almost invariable, and is of diagnostic importance, for it is present in 65 per cent. of injuries to the bile passages, and only in 4·75 per cent. of injuries to the liver. After a time the general abdominal distension diminishes, but is followed either at once or in two or three weeks by the development of a localized collection of fluid in the right side.

Treatment.—If an injury to the bile passages is diagnosed early, an operation should be carried out. A rent in the fundus of the gall-bladder may be closed by suture or used for purposes of drainage, or the viscus removed altogether. If one of the larger ducts be injured the treatment will depend on the size of the tear. A small hole may be treated by stitching a tube to the margin of the rent, thus providing for external drainage, but almost complete division demands an attempt at suture, combined with external drainage.

In complete rupture of the common duct it may be possible to reunite the ends or to implant the proximal one into the duodenum, but it will usually be safer and easier to ligature both and to perform cholecystenterostomy (Terrier).

In cases not seen until a localized collection has formed, it is best merely to establish external drainage without attempting to find the hole in the duct.

INFECTIVE GRANULOMATA

Tuberculosis, whether of the gall-bladder or of the ducts, though found after death in a fair proportion of cases of intestinal tuberculosis, is undoubtedly very rare as a clinical entity. The gall-bladder has been opened for suspected calculi, but found to contain only tuberculous granulation tissue.

Diagnosis is practically impossible, though, singularly, jaundice has always been absent. The **treatment** consists either in excision of the gall-bladder, or in thorough curettage with use of pure carbolic acid, etc.

Calcareous tuberculous glands along the cystic or common ducts may simulate gall-stones.

Syphilis.—Sometimes gummata or syphilitic cicatrices have caused obstruction of the common duct, and given rise to symptoms of gall-stones, while a gumma in the margin of the liver may suggest a similar diagnosis. Cases with a strong syphilitic history should be given a course of mercury and iodide before operation is contemplated.

INFECTIONS

CHOLECYSTITIS

Cholecystitis is much commoner than cholangitis, owing to the readier drainage of the ducts into the intestine.

Cholecystitis, though usually associated with gall-stones, may occur independently, and there is evidence to show that such infections may exist for quite a time before the gall-stones appear.

This is borne out by a series of the Mayos' cases of cholecystectomy. In 365 cases, all inflammatory, gall-stones were found in only 69 per cent. of the specimens in an acute catarrhal condition, in 76 per cent. of the chronic catarrhs, and in 93 per cent. of the advanced chronic cases.

Pathology of non-calculous cholecystitis.—The causative organism may reach the gall-bladder either directly from the bowel and ducts, or through the blood stream. The commonest infections are probably by B. typhosus, Bacillus coli, B. influenzæ, and the pneumococcus, in that order.

The **different varieties of cholecystitis,** apart from the special type of causative organism, are really only different stages of the ordinary processes of inflammation.

Clinical features.—The milder cases merely present indistinctive dyspeptic symptoms. In the more severe varieties there may be continuous or paroxysmal local pain and tenderness, with nausea and vomiting, catching of the breath, a very slight tinge of jaundice, and rise of temperature to 101° or higher. As the local rigidity disappears, the enlarged and tender gall-bladder may be felt.

In the most acute cases the onset is very sudden, with rigors, high temperature, and often peritonitic symptoms. Chronic cases so closely simulate chronic cholelithiasis that the same description will serve (*see* p. 752).

Diagnosis.—Gall-stones and acute appendicitis are the conditions most likely to be confused with cholecystitis. In the former the attacks of colic are more sudden and pass off more abruptly, and the temperature is seldom maintained so high as in cholecystitis. In appendicitis the pain is lower, vomiting is more likely to be prominent, and breathing is not interfered with. It may be impossible to differentiate the very acute cases from acute pancreatitis, intestinal obstruction, or pneumonia.

Treatment.—The milder cases may completely recover on rest, limitation of diet, and the exhibition of alkalis. Persistent tenderness with fever, or obvious enlargement of the gall-bladder, necessitates surgical interference, which in the very severe cases must be prompt. The operation will usually consist in drainage of the gall-bladder. Cholecystectomy adds to the operative risk, and fails to provide drainage of the deeper ducts, and is therefore not generally advisable.

CHOLANGITIS

Cholangitis is nearly always associated with the presence of gall-stones, and it may persist even after the calculi have been passed. The ducts are full of bile-stained pus.

Clinical features.—The condition may be preceded by the symptoms of gall-stones, and may follow directly on an attack, or be ushered in by a rigor, with perhaps uneasiness about the hepatic region ; the patient feels ill and generally looks poisoned, and is more or less drowsy. Chills may be repeated irregularly, while the temperature between them is either a little raised or subnormal. Jaundice is usual, but not invariable, and, if well developed, probably depends on some causative obstruction. The liver is enlarged and tender, and the spleen may be palpable. The disease is subject to remissions.

Treatment.—Operation for calculi is unwise during an attack of cholangitis. Free purgation, abundance of fluid by the mouth, infusion of saline, and the exhibition of urotropin in 10-grain doses are the most useful therapeutic measures ; opium should be studiously avoided. If improvement does not follow, the ducts must be drained, usually through the gall-bladder.

GALL-STONE DISEASE

Pathology ; etiology.—Experimental research has proved that, though mild inflammation due to attenuated infections is a potent etiological factor, a virulent infection is not followed by calculus formation.

When gall-stones cause symptoms, organisms, especially bacilli of the colon group, are generally found, not only in the bile, but in the calculi themselves. Their presence leads to a mild catarrh of the mucous membrane, and, therefore, to an increased production of cholesterin.

According to Aschoff, mere stagnation of bile in the gall-bladder, without an infective catarrhal process, may lead to the formation of cholesterin stones by simple deposition from the bile. When infection is added, there is an increased production of cholesterin, and also of calcium salts, which are deposited on the cholesterin nucleus. These, in conjunction with bile pigment, constitute the pigmented calculi.

Though usually formed in the gall-bladder, calculi may originate in any of the extrahepatic or even intrahepatic ducts. Some authorities state that very small calculi deposited in the ducts may be washed into the gall-bladder by the normal bile current.

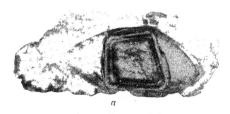

a

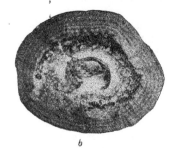

b

Fig. 523.—Gall-stones, showing nuclei.
(Actual size.)

a, Calculus from the common duct. The quadrilateral stone forms the nucleus around which an oval stone has formed, this in turn being covered by amorphous material.
b, Calculus from the gall-bladder, a catgut suture forming the nucleus. (*From a specimen kindly lent by Hamilton Drummond.*)

The gross forms gall-stones usually take are illustrated in Plate 99.

As a rule, no nucleus can be found, but without doubt small gall-stones often form the centres on which larger ones are built (Fig. 523, *a*). It is important to recognize that unabsorbable ligatures and sutures may later form the starting-point of calculi (Fig. 523, *b*). Inspissated mucus, degenerated epithelium, and more rarely masses of bacteria, may constitute a nucleus round which bile pigments, etc., may be deposited.

Pathological consequences of gall-stones.—Gall-stones are often found post mortem which have exhibited no previous evidence of existence, but they may cause inflammation and sometimes obstruction.

Inflammation depends on organisms which may be similar to those associated with the gall-stone origin, or may be the result of a secondary invasion. The Bacillus coli is most frequently found.

In slight cases or very early stages the gall-bladder may show very little beyond microscopic changes in its walls, though the bile may be turbid or flocculent, and later the contents may become purulent, forming an "acute empyema of the gall-bladder." After a time the

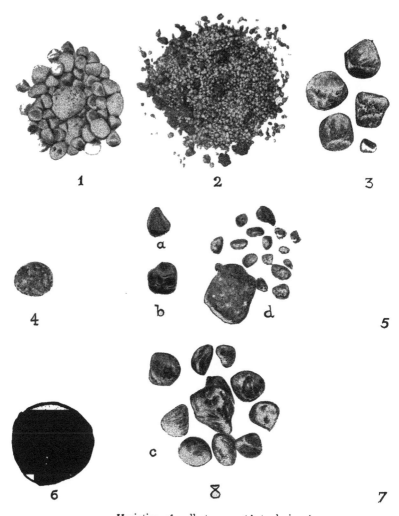

Varieties of gall-stones. (Actual sizes.)

1 and 3. Clusters of calculi as ordinarily met with in the gall-bladder.
2, The very small type of gall-stone, of which there were 3,654 removed from a case of acute disten:
    the gall-bladder, one of the larger stones being impacted in its neck.
4 and 5, Examples of single calculi from the gall-bladder, such as produce ball-valve obstructions.
6, A calculus which was impacted in the ileum, producing acute obstruction.
7, A typical stone from the common duct.
8, A group of calculi from one case: (a) from the gall-bladder, (b) from the right hepatic duct, (c
    the common duct, (d) from the common hepatic duct.

PLATE 99.

mucous membrane is reddened and the whole wall thickened (Fig. 524), while still later there may be ulceration or localized gangrene, though this usually only occurs when obstruction coexists. Hæmorrhage may take place into such an inflamed gall-bladder. When the inflammation becomes chronic the gall-bladder is thickened and exhibits fibroid changes, while the contents are in most cases purulent, forming "chronic empyema of the gall-bladder."

Peritoneal adhesions commonly form and persist, and rarely they may cause trouble.

Obstruction is most commouly produced by the impaction of a calculus in the neck of the gall-bladder, in its pelvis, or in the first compartment of the cystic duct. In the acute eases the consequences depend on the condition of the gall-bladder at the time of the impaction. If its contents be infected, the viscus rapidly becomes inflamed and acutely distended, and its peritoneal coat soon becomes reddened and lymph-covered. The mucous membrane ulcerates, and gangrene may supervene (Plate 100) and lead to perforation or to extensive sloughings. An inflamed gall-bladder usually acquires adhesions to the stomach, duodenum (Fig. 525), or hepatic flexure of the colon. It may suppurate and burst into one of the adherent viscera, or more rarely through the belly wall, leading to the formation of an external biliary

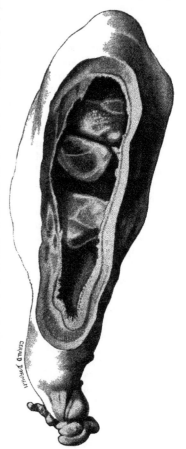

Fig. 524.—Acute inflammation of the gall-bladder, following impaction of a calculus in its neck.

fistula. When perforation occurs into one of the hollow viscera, calculi as well as pus may thus escape, but not uncommonly the calculus is of the large, single variety, and in these circumstances the gall-bladder contracts upon and firmly grasps the calculus, no further distension occurring, as the secreting glands in its wall have been destroyed by the inflammation. Such a calculus, tightly grasped by the contracted and functionless gall-bladder, is apparently safely imprisoned, but it may be potent for evil, for, as a result of the slow contraction of the gall-bladder, the stone may be constantly pressed against the neighbouring viscus until it finally erodes through into the stomach or intestine. Thus, large calculi, capable of causing intestinal obstruction, may find their way into the bowel. (Plate 99, 6, and Figs. 525 and 526.) Moreover, the resulting cicatrization and adhesions may produce pyloric obstruction or hour-glass stomach.

When the obstruction is gradual, or the contents of the gall-bladder are not infected at the time of impaction, "hydrops" of the gall-bladder ensues, the viscus undergoing gradual distension with watery or sometimes inspissated jelly-like mucus, and its wall becoming thinned without inflammatory changes. (Fig. 527.)

These greatly distended gall-bladders may give rise to little inconvenience, but they may be ruptured by violence, or may develop cholecystitis due to secondary infection (p. 741). A hydrops may also result from an acute obstruction with infection, the latter gradually dying down, or lighting up from time to time, but always with lessened virulence. Sometimes relief of obstruction alternates with recurrences, and gives rise to an "intermittent hydrops."

Gall-stones in the ducts.—Calculi either reach the ducts from the gall-bladder, after which they probably increase in size (Fig. 523, a), or they are formed in the ducts themselves. Commonly, they give rise to symptoms from obstruction, and to this infection may be superadded.

Obstruction is due to the size of the stone, the resultant contraction of the duct, and the associated inflammatory changes. It may be temporary, and simply lead to slight dilatation of the ducts above, which disappears with the passage of the stone into the duodenum. Or the stone may act like a ball valve, falling back into the dilated portion of the duct above, only to be forced down again at some future time. In each successive attack the ducts become more and more distended.

The obstruction is seldom complete for long, and such a calculus may permit free passage of the bile, gaining increment by gradual deposition until it may reach the great size sometimes seen. (Fig. 523, a.) But the impaction, though rarely absolute, may be practically permanent; then the ducts above become uniformly dilated, to form large channels all through the liver (Fig. 528), the common duct itself being sometimes as large as the small intestine if the dilatation is cylindrical, or like a huge cyst if it is saccular.

When a stone is impacted near the lower end of the common duct it may dilate the orifice and escape into the intestine *per vias naturales*,

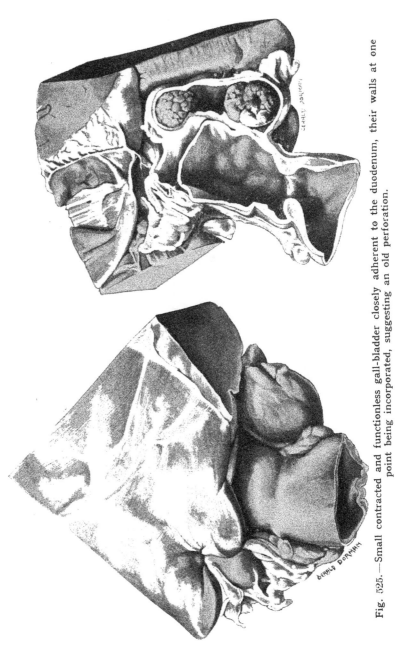

Fig. 525.—Small contracted and functionless gall-bladder closely adherent to the duodenum, their walls at one point being incorporated, suggesting an old perforation.

but more usually it ulcerates through the duct and bowel wall just above the duodenal papilla (Fig. 529).

A calculus in the ampulla of Vater may obstruct the opening and throw the bile and pancreatic duct into a continuous channel; it is then a potent cause of pancreatitis. (Fig. 519.)

Remote consequences of gall-stones. — Fistulæ may be external or internal; spontaneous or the result of surgical

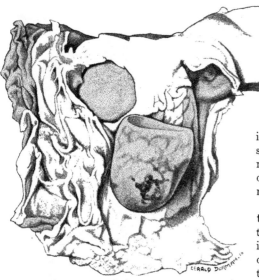

interference; constant or recurring; and biliary or mucoid or muco-purulent.

External fistulæ, when spontaneous, almost invariably depend on suppuration of the gall-bladder associated with an obstruction in the cystic duct. They usually open just above the umbilicus, but sometimes appear over the normal

Fig. 526.—The first part of the duodenum is laid open, showing a large opening into the gallbladder, which is occupied by a faceted calculus. Lying free in the bowel is the sister calculus, which became impacted in the ileum and caused the death of the patient from acute obstruction. The facets on the two calculi exactly correspond.

(From a specimen in the Museum of the University of Durham College of Medicine.)

situation of the gall-bladder, in the iliac fossa, the loin, or even between the lower ribs.

External fistulæ, secondary to surgical interference, may be mucoid or biliary. In the former, either an obstruction in the cystic duct has been overlooked, or the gall-bladder has been fixed to the skin of the abdominal wall instead of to the peritoneum. The latter depend upon some obstruction remaining in the common duct, due to calculus, stricture, or involvement by pancreatitis.

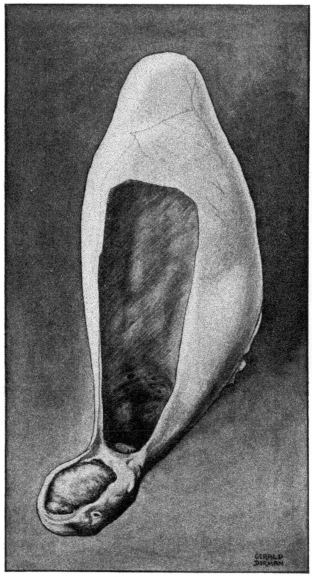

Fig. 527.—Chronic distension of the gall-bladder (hydrops)
from impaction of a calculus in its neck.

The *treatment* is expectant if the obstruction is certainly only temporary, as in pancreatitis. An obstruction may be removed or

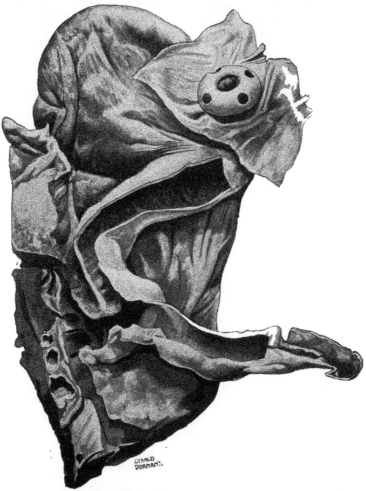

Fig. 528.—Dilatation of the bile-ducts throughout the liver, the result of long-continued calculous obstruction. Cholecystenterostomy had been performed with the Murphy button.

cholecystenterostomy performed; or an attachment of the gall-bladder to the skin may be separated and the viscus closed by suture.

Internal fistulæ are probably commoner than external, but remain unrecognized owing to their frequent lack of symptoms. They usually pass between the gall-bladder and the stomach, duodenum, or colon, but they may be between the gall-bladder and the kidney, the lung, or even the bladder or uterus.

Stricture of the ducts.—This condition is only common in the *cystic duct*, where it frequently follows the impaction of a calculus. It is best treated by cholecystectomy.

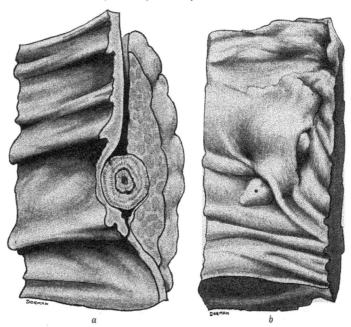

a   *b*

Fig. 529.—Diagrams made from actual specimens of calculi in the common duct.

a, Calculus impacted in the pancreatic portion of the duct, in a position suitable for removal by transduodenal choledochotomy.

b, Showing how a calculus impacted in the same situation has ulcerated into the duodenum, the papilla remaining intact.

In the *common duct* stricture is much more important, but, fortunately, rarer. It usually follows long impaction of a calculus, and presents the symptoms of obstructive jaundice with or without attacks of pain.

Treatment.—Plastic restoration of the duct may be possible, but in most cases, if the gall-bladder is available for the purpose, cholecystenterostomy is the wiser procedure.

Intestinal obstruction in connexion with gall-stones may be due to (a) impaction of a calculus in the lumen of the bowel ; (b) adhesions or deformity associated with an internal biliary fistula ; (c) involvement of the hepatic flexure of the colon by an inflamed gall-bladder.

Clinical features of gall-stone disease.—Gall-stones are probably three or even four times as common in the female as in the male sex, and, on the average, begin to cause trouble at about the age of 35. In many cases they are quiescent for long periods ; in others they only cause indefinite symptoms, such as "indigestion," or "windy spasms," often erroneously attributed to other causes. Jaundice is infrequent in cholelithiasis.

The **symptoms** that gall-stones may cause are pain, tenderness, nausea and vomiting, and jaundice, to which may be superadded the symptoms of infection. The physical signs are those of local peritonitis, with or without enlargement of the gall-bladder.

Pain may or may not take the form of " an attack of colic." Colic starts abruptly in the epigastrium or right hypochondrium, frequently after a meal and usually during the daytime. The onset may be accompanied by collapse, vomiting, and profuse perspiration. The pain may be agonizing, doubling the patient up, but after a time, varying from a few minutes to several hours, it passes off, leaving the patient exhausted and sore. Other patients suffer from dull aching or sharp pains in the liver region, usually aggravated by food and relieved by vomiting. The pain may be referred to the back, shoulder, neck, front of chest, or down the arm. During an attack there may be rigidity of the whole abdomen, especially marked in the upper right quadrant, which is excessively tender. The tenderness, at first superficial, later is only elicited by deep pressure, or better by Naunyn's test, which depends on the inability of the patient to take a full inspiration while the examining fingers press deeply down beneath the right costal arch. Sometimes tenderness is found posteriorly, two or three finger-breadths from the 10th to the 12th dorsal spines, either alone or with the anterior tenderness.

Nausea and vomiting may occur independently of pain. Nausea is often extreme. When vomiting occurs it is at first of greenish, watery fluid, but afterwards no bile is seen, merely watery fluid and mucus.

Jaundice is found only in about 20 per cent. of all cases, and even with stones in the common duct only in $33\frac{1}{2}$ per cent. When definite and long-continued, it depends on impaction of a stone in the common duct ; when slight and transient, it may result from catarrh associated with obstruction in the cystic duct. In any case, this symptom does not appear until the day after the attack, but if the block is in the common duct it may afterwards vary from day to day, until it either disappears or gradually assumes an olive-green tint. Even with recent and slight jaundice, severe bleeding may follow any wound, and in long-standing cases spontaneous hæmorrhages may occur. Itching is another very distressing symptom.

Slight fever occurs apart from any marked infection, and instability of temperature is almost characteristic of gall-stones. A high temperature or repeated rigors suggest severe infection. Stones in the common duct and bile infection, ague-like paroxysms with rigors, and temperature running up to 104° or 105° and as suddenly coming down, make up the clinical picture of Charcot's "intermittent hepatic fever."

General symptoms such as depression and anorexia, with sour breath and coated tongue, are invariably accompaniments. There may be considerable abdominal distension and marked constipation. Sometimes gall-stones are found in the fæces.

Local physical signs.—Rigidity of the upper segment of the right rectus and deep tenderness have already been mentioned. The presence of a local tumour, when discoverable, is important. Generally, this tumour is the distended gall-bladder (Fig. 519), perhaps augmented by surrounding inflammatory complications; but sometimes an inflammatory mass around the common duct, or, rarely, even a mass of stones, may be felt.

A palpable gall-bladder appears as a smooth, rounded, pear-shaped tumour which moves up and down with respiration, cannot be held down, is continuous with the liver above, and can be slightly rocked from side to side. When such a gall-bladder enlarges, it usually does so in a direction downwards and inwards towards the umbilicus, but quite commonly it enlarges directly downwards and may even reach the right iliac fossa. Just after an attack the gall-bladder is usually tender, and this may persist, but chronic enlargements are neither painful nor tender.

The cases as seen by the surgeon may be arranged in the following groups :—

1. Acute cases without jaundice.—There is sudden onset with severe pain, general disturbance, and elevation of temperature. At first the right hypochondrium is rigid and tender, but at a later stage the enlarged gall-bladder may be easily felt. The neck of the gall-bladder or the cystic duct will be found blocked by a calculus.

2. Acute cases with jaundice.—The jaundice follows an attack of colic, and there is much general disturbance, often with rigors. The right hypochondrium is tender and rigid, but at no stage can the gall-bladder be felt. A calculus is impacted in the common duct.

3. Quiescent (interval) cases without jaundice.—The patient

2 w

may suffer from vague abdominal discomfort, or may be entirely free from symptoms, with merely the history of an attack. The gall-bladder may be felt distended or there may be simply deep tenderness. There are stones in the gall-bladder or common duct or both.

4. Quiescent (interval) cases with jaundice.—The patient has the general symptoms of jaundice. The gall-bladder is not enlarged though the liver may be palpable. There are stones impacted in the common duct.

Diagnosis.—If, after an attack of pain in the upper abdomen, the enlarged and tender gall-bladder can be felt, or there is definite tenderness over the region of the gall-bladder or common duct, the diagnosis of gall-stones is straightforward. In the absence of these signs the diagnosis may have to be made from the history alone. When there is colic, the abrupt seizures, the nausea and vomiting, and the shivering are most suggestive. In cases without colic, the constant local discomfort with shivering, and the alternation of soreness with periods of complete relief, distinguish the trouble from gastric or duodenal ulcer. Marked shivering, constant slight jaundice, and wasting suggest lodgment of calculi in the common duct, without impaction, so that most of the bile escapes into the bowel. Chronic jaundice, varying in intensity, and free from an olive-green tint, associated with attacks of colic, is in favour of gall-stones. The combination of distension of the gall-bladder with obstructive jaundice renders the diagnosis of gall-stones improbable (Courvoisier's law). (Fig. 519 and Plate 102.)

The **prognosis** is very uncertain. Gall-stones are always dangerous. Acute obstruction may develop in the first attack, and proceed to gangrene, perforation, and peritonitis; or countless attacks of colic may culminate in the passage of all the stones, perhaps after years of suffering; or, not infrequently, malignant disease or pancreatitis may supervene.

Treatment.—Unless some condition, such as diabetes, extreme obesity, or cardiac or renal disease, renders operation unduly dangerous, gall-stones should be removed as soon as diagnosed.

Palliative treatment during an attack consists in enjoining absolute starvation. Excessive nausea or vomiting demands gastric evacuation and lavage with an alkali. Pain may be alleviated by hot poultices over the hepatic region, while thirst may be relieved and elimination stimulated by the rectal administration of a pint of half-strength saline every four hours. This plan will often obviate the necessity for morphia, with advantage to the rapidity of recovery and the subsequent condition of the patient. Between the attacks, if operation is not to be undertaken, ample exercise, abundant drinks of water, and gentle but efficient laxatives should be advised.

Operative treatment. The time to operate.—An interval between attacks should be chosen, unless spreading inflammation, acute pancreatitis, or sudden perforation and acute peritonitis demands immediate operation. Even in the presence of localized suppuration some preparation is usually advisable, and long-continued jaundice requires a period of probation owing to the danger of hæmorrhage and of toxæmia.

Preliminary treatment.—Obesity should be reduced by the prohibition of starches, sugars, and fats, combined with free purgation and abdominal massage.

In the presence of jaundice or symptoms of cholangitis, thorough clearance of the alimentary canal and the liberal use of saline solution with small doses of urotropine are the most valuable preparatory measures. To obviate the hæmorrhagic tendency, calcium chloride has been much vaunted, but its value is doubtful; a far better method is the free flushing of the system with normal saline. Bleeding has also been prevented and checked by alien serums; fresh horse or rabbit serum is best, ox serum being unsuitable. Antidiphtheritic serum is often the readiest to hand, and may be given subcutaneously or intravenously in doses of 10 to 30 c.c.

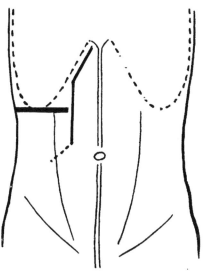

Fig. 530.—Incisions used in gall-bladder surgery. The vertical incision is that usually employed. The transverse is recommended by Rutherford Morison.

The operation.—In acute gall-stone conditions, ether by the open method affords the safer anæsthesia owing to the risk of acetonuria after chloroform.

A convenient incision is a vertical one extending 4 in. downwards from the costal margin, through the outer half of the right rectus muscle. Freer access may be gained by carrying the cut upwards and inwards to the costo-xiphisternal notch (Robson); and still further room can be obtained by adding a similar extension obliquely outwards below (Bevan) (*see* Fig. 530). The deeper ducts can be brought nearer the surface by placing a long, narrow sand-bag transversely beneath the lower thoracic region. Then by drawing on the gall-bladder, lifting forward the liver and rotating it on its transverse axis, the surgeon can straighten out the ducts and approximate the deeper parts still further to the surface. The operator must remember to remove the sand-bag before attempting to suture the wound. A transverse incision may be used instead; this affords excellent exposure of the gall-bladder, ducts, and hepatic pouch (Fig. 531). Before opening the gall-bladder, careful examination must be made of the whole biliary apparatus, and of the liver, pylorus, duodenum, pancreatic head, and hepatic flexure. The ducts are palpated by passing the fingers along the right side of the gall-bladder, over its neck, down the cystic duct, and through the foramen of Winslow. Here the common duct can be felt between the fingers behind and the thumb in front of the gastro-hepatic omentum. The lower parts of the duct must be felt

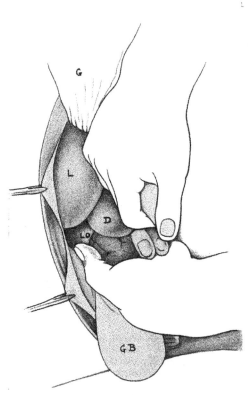

Fig. 531.—Exposure obtained by the transverse incision for gall-stones advocated by Rutherford Morison.

L., Liver ; D., duodenum ; G.B., gall-bladder : L.O., free edge of lesser omentum ; G , a gauze pack. The fingers of the operator are in the foramen of Winslow, steadying and thrusting forward the lesser omentum, while the thumb is free to palpate the common duct.

(*Brit. Med. Journ., Nov. 8, 1902 ; by permission of the Editor and of Professor Rutherford Morison.*)

for through the duodenal wall. Finally, the hepatic ducts are to be explored right up to the liver. It must be remembered that sometimes, in a very tense gall-bladder, small calculi cannot be felt; also that enlarged glands near the neck of the gall-bladder and at the junction of the cystic and common ducts may be mistaken for calculi. After removal of the stones, another examination of the ducts is necessary to ensure that no calculi have been overlooked. In every case the interior of the gall-bladder should be carefully explored by the surgeon's finger.

Before opening the viscus the rest of the abdomen must be shut off by gauze-packing. The subsequent steps depend on the conditions found. *If calculi are found only in the gall-bladder, are free, and not associated with inflammatory signs,* they should be removed, and the gall-bladder should then be drained (cholecystostomy). Cholecyst-endesis, by which the opening in the viscus is sutured and the abdomen closed, perhaps with a small drain down to the sutured gall-bladder, is generally inadvisable, for it makes no provision for the escape of a possibly overlooked tiny stone, or for drainage of the infected biliary canal.

In *cholecystostomy* a drainage-tube is fastened into the open gall-bladder by an invaginating sero-muscular purse-string suture of No. 1 chromicized catgut, placed ⅔ in. from the cut edge, and the fundus is then fixed to the parietal peritoneum. In simple cases, with free flow of bile, the tube may be removed in from four to seven days.

If calculi are impacted in the neck of the gall-bladder or in the cystic duct, with or without suppuration or gangrene, an attempt must be made to dislodge them back into the viscus with the fingers working from outside. The gall-bladder must then be opened, its contents removed, and the interior carefully dried with a strand of gauze. If bile at once flows, the duct is free, but in inflammatory conditions the thickening may delay the appearance of bile for some days. In acute conditions, the surgeon need not fear for the ultimate patency of the duct, and may perform cholecystostomy; but in chronic cases, if bile does not flow, he must assure himself that the duct is patent, or he must remove the gall-bladder (cholecystectomy).

If the obstructing calculus cannot be removed by manipulation, an incision may be made directly over it (cysticotomy), or removal of the gall-bladder may be necessary. In cases of great urgency the gall-bladder may simply be drained, and if the calculus does not come away it may be removed at a second operation.

When inflamed and suppurating the gall-bladder and its surroundings are very vascular, and its removal may be attended by troublesome hæmorrhage. In these circumstances excision is much more dangerous than simple drainage.

The same remarks apply to gangrene of the gall-bladder. This is rarely total, and nearly always first reaches the peritoneal surface at the fundus (Plate 100). In most cases drainage is safest and best ; in a few the fundus only may be excised ; and, even for total gangrene, ample drainage and isolation by gauze packing is probably the wisest course, for in these cases the shortest possible operation, with little loss of blood, is essential.

If the gall-bladder is firmly adherent to surrounding structures as the result of chronic inflammation, it may be impossible even to see the viscus until the adhesions are separated. To avoid peritonitis or fistula, great care is necessary in separating the stomach, duodenum, or colon, for where the gall-bladder has leaked into these viscera communications frequently exist. After exposure, these densely adherent gall-bladders are often found to be quite small and closely contracted. on a mass of stones. They are frequently very thick-walled, and often white and shiny (Fig. 532). Such gall-bladders should be removed, for a certain proportion of them turn out to be the seat of malignant disease.

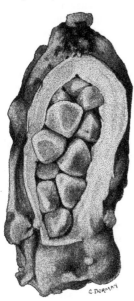

Fig. 532.—Chronically inflamed and thickened gall-bladder with calculi. Such a gall-bladder is often the seat of malignant disease.

Sometimes the greater part of the gall-bladder has been destroyed, only the neck and cystic duct remaining. After removal of the calculus, a tube must be led out from the duct and the cavity walled off by gutta-percha tissue or gauze. The omentum is. useful as a covering for the involved area.

Cholecystectomy.—The removal of a moderate-sized gall-bladder, if the region of the cystic duct is free, may be commenced by catching and dividing the cystic artery and duct, and then separating the gall-bladder from the liver from below upwards. A very large viscus must sometimes be emptied to secure a view of the region of the neck. When the gall-bladder is shrivelled, or when the parts about its neck are obscured (Fig. 525), then it is best to separate the organ from the liver as a first step, and to use it as a tractor while the cystic duct and artery are carefully exposed.

As a rule, the gall-bladder is not removed when drainage of the ducts is necessary, but if thought desirable a tube may be brought

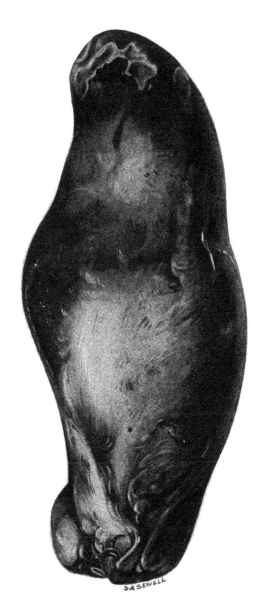

Acute cholecystitis, the result of calculous obstruction of the cystic
duct. There was extensive gangrene of the mucous membrane,
which had extended to the peritoneum at the fundus. (Actual size.)

PLATE 100.

out from the end of the duct. In any case, it is wise to insert a small tube down to the region of the divided and ligatured duct. The raw area on the liver may sometimes be covered with peritoneum reflected from the sides of the gall-bladder, but any oozing from it must be treated by gauze packing.

If calculi are present in both gall-bladder and common duct, they can but rarely be pushed from the duct into the gall-bladder, and, therefore, this condition necessitates the opening of both. The duct should be opened first, the intact gall-bladder being a useful tractor. The calculi may be free in the duct or impacted in the lower end. Whenever possible, the calculi should be pushed into the supraduodenal portion of the duct, which can be safely opened and the stones removed. Direct drainage of the common duct is usually advisable. The stones are now removed from the gall-bladder, which may be afterwards closed if healthy, or may require to be separately drained.

Calculi impacted in the lower end of the duct may rarely be pushed on into the duodenum, or pushed back into the duct above, but, as a rule, the duct must either be opened behind the duodenum or by the transduodenal route (Fig. 529, *a*). When calculi are also present in the hepatic ducts they may be forced down into the common duct, or removed by direct incision, or broken up and extracted in fragments.

If any doubt exist as to the complete removal of the fragments, not only must ample external drainage be provided, but a good-sized metal probe must be passed from the duct into the duodenum, so dilating the papilla that the fragments may pass.

After-treatment.—If vomiting be troublesome, a pint of hot water should be drunk; and if this fail, the stomach should be washed out. Even in the absence of vomiting, eructation of mouthfuls, or hiccup with fullness and epigastric distress, demands gastric lavage, repeated if necessary; for these symptoms may be premonitory of acute dilatation of the stomach, a very grave complication.

The rectal injection of half-strength normal saline should be used in all but the simplest cases, for it combats any tendency to shock, relieves thirst, and, most important of all, greatly aids elimination.

Results of operations.—The removal of gall-stones that have not left the gall-bladder or set up dangerous complications should not cause a mortality of more than 2 per cent.; and even taking all gall-stone operations together the death-rate is probably but 5 per cent.

The percentage of recurrences in simple cases is small (not more than 2 or 3 per cent.), but it rises *pari passu* with increasing complications. There is not yet sufficient evidence to show which type of operation is most successful. Cholecystostomy appears to have been attended by a large proportion of recurrences, but this operation has often to be used when there is infection of the deeper ducts. It is important to recognize that recurrence takes place after complete removal of the gall-bladder. Overlooked malignant disease or progressive pancreatitis may lead to disappointing results after otherwise successful operations.

NEW GROWTHS

Simple growths of the gall-bladder and ducts are very rare; fibromas, lipomas, and cystic adenomas have been met with; papillomas are the most frequent, but here apparently they are not so closely associated with cancer as elsewhere.

CARCINOMA OF THE GALL-BLADDER

Etiology.—In over 80 per cent. of cases gall-stones and cancer are associated. Cancer is commoner in women than in men in the same sex proportion as calculi. The average age is just over 50, the disease being uncommon before 40 years.

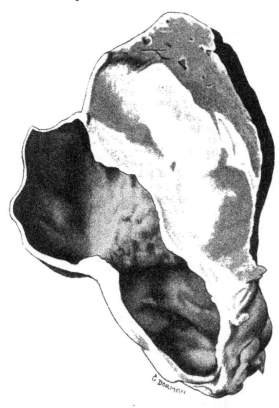

Fig. 533.—Primary carcinoma of the gall-bladder producing hour-glass deformity, and involving the liver by direct extension. (Actual size.) Case of successful excision by Rutherford Morison.

Morbid anatomy.—The disease is met with in three forms: (1) As a definite localized tumour, usually at the fundus, though sometimes in the body, producing an hour-glass constriction, or at the neck, causing obstruction (Fig. 533); (2) as a diffuse thickening of the whole wall of the gall-bladder, which is white, glistening, and tightly contracted on a mass of calculi (Fig. 532); (3) rarely as a fungating growth, filling the gall-bladder and perhaps causing hæmorrhage (Fig. 534).

Microscopically, the growth is usually columnar or spheroidal-celled. It tends to spread down the ducts and to involve the liver by direct extension; later it may extend to the colon, duodenum, or peritoneum.

Clinical features.—The early history is usually that of cholelithiasis, gradually followed by long-continued illness, with constant hepatic pain and progressive emaciation, disproportionate to gall-stone disease. Jaundice appears late in about half the cases.

Physical signs may be entirely absent, or there may be a hard, nodular tumour in the gall-bladder region.

Diagnosis. — Gall-stones, especially with inflammatory complications, malignant disease of the liver, carcinoma of the stomach adherent to the liver, or a growth in the hepatic flexure, most commonly lead to confusion. The history and symptoms rather than the physical signs are likely to aid in differentiation.

Prognosis. — Death usually occurs within six months.

Operative treatment. — Unless the pre-

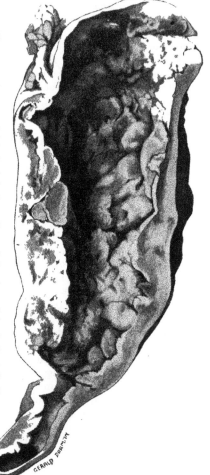

Fig. 534.—Carcinoma of the gall-bladder of the fungating type. The viscus was greatly distended with hæmorrhage.' (Actual size.)

sence of unequivocal secondary deposits renders operation useless, exploration should always be made, for inflammatory masses may closely simulate cancer. The diagnosis confirmed, and the possibility of complete clearance ascertained, the surgeon should freely remove the gall-bladder, with a wedge of healthy liver tissue.

Direct extension to the liver does not necessarily preclude successful operation, but careful examination is required to determine the absence of associated secondary deposits in that organ. If complete excision be impossible, operation should be abandoned, for the mere removal of calculi never does good. Even in apparently favourable cases, early recurrence in the liver or peritoneum is very frequent. Cases in which a chronically inflamed gall-bladder is found microscopically to harbour cancer present better results.

CARCINOMA OF THE BILE-DUCTS

Primary malignant disease of the bile-ducts occurs more frequently than is supposed. The disease differs from cancer of the gall-bladder in that it is usually without gall-stones, and that males are more commonly affected than females, though it occurs at the same period of life.

Pathology.—The growth may affect any duct, but usually attacks one or other end of the common duct. It forms a columnar-celled carcinomatous ring and appears as a stony, hard, white nodule, not larger than a cherry, easily mistaken for a calculus. Obstruction is absolute, the ducts above become greatly dilated and the liver bile-logged, death occurring from cholæmia or cholangitis.

Clinical features.—Jaundice commences insidiously and gradually deepens without intermissions until the skin may assume a dark bronzed or olive-green tinge. Pain is inconstant ; there may be an attack of colic, but this is seldom repeated. There are no physical signs beyond enlargement of the liver, and of the gall-bladder when the common duct is involved.

The **diagnosis** is suggested by painless, persistent, and otherwise unexplained jaundice in a patient between 50 and 60. Gall-stone obstruction is nearly always attended by a history of repeated attacks of pain and sudden onset ; cancer of the pancreatic head may be palpable, or may be indistinguishable ; while catarrhal jaundice so surely clears up as to render diagnosis certain.

Prognosis.—Death inevitably occurs from cholæmia, hæmorrhage, or infection, in from six months to a year from the onset.

Treatment.—It may be possible to excise the growth, either with end-to-end union, implantation into the peritoneal surface of the duodenum, or ligature of both ends and cholecystenterostomy. Generally, however, cholecystenterostomy without excision will be the only available measure. This may enhance the patient's comfort by relieving pruritus ; and it ensures against a possible mistake in diagnosis.

THE PANCREAS

Anatomy.—The pancreas lies in the epigastric and left hypo-chondriac regions, crossing the posterior abdominal wall at the level of the first lumbar vertebra, its head nestling in the duodenal hollow opposite the 2nd and 3rd lumbar vertebræ, and its tail abutting on the spleen (Fig. 535). The greater part lies behind the stomach, the lesser sac forming its most important anterior relation. The main

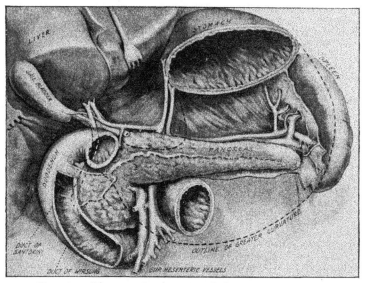

Fig. 535.—Diagram showing the relations of the pancreas.

(From " Surgery, Gynæcology, and Obstetrics," Dec., 1908, by permission of Dr. W. J. Mayo.)

duct (Wirsung's) opens into the second part of the duodenum, 3 or 4 in. from the pylorus, either directly or through the ampulla of Yater.

The pancreas is a compound tubular gland, resembling the parotid, but more loosely arranged and possessing interacinous islands of small polygonal cells known as the islands of Langerhans.

Abnormalities.—The head of the pancreas may completely surround the duodenum. An accessory pancreas, varying in size from a hempseed to a bean, may lie in the wall of the stomach, duodenum, jejunum, or ileum, and has been found at the apex of a gastric or intestinal diverticulum. Rarely the pancreas is abnormally movable, and has been found in both diaphragmatic and umbilical hernias.

INJURIES

Though more rarely injured than the other viscera, the pancreas suffers slight traumatisms not infrequently. The injury may be penetrating, or, much oftener, subcutaneous, and, though commonly confined to the viscus, may be associated with lesions elsewhere. There may result extensive and perhaps fatal hæmorrhage, or escape of juice with retroperitoneal inflammation, or acute pancreatitis due to bruising. In slighter injuries the peritoneum covering the pancreas is often torn, and blood and pancreatic juice escape into the lesser sac, leading to the development of an inflammatory effusion or pseudo-cyst (see p. 771) and the production of fat necrosis.

Clinical features.—The symptoms vary with the severity of the trauma. In some cases there is profound shock or hæmorrhage without localizing signs other than the site of the injury. In others, shock is less severe, and is accompanied by pain, vomiting, tenderness and rigidity of the upper abdomen, and the rapid accumulation of free fluid; in such a case, subsidence of symptoms and resolution may occur, or the development of local peritonitis or of pancreatitis may be indicated by increasing symptoms and a rising temperature and pulse-rate. Permanent recovery may ensue or temporary amelioration be followed by signs of an inflammatory effusion into the lesser sac. Glycosuria rarely occurs, but when present is of valuable diagnostic significance.

Treatment must at first be expectant, unless there are evidences of severe internal hæmorrhage. If the symptoms steadily become accentuated, while the tenderness and rigidity persist or a mass develops, operative interference is necessary. The pancreas can best be exposed by tearing through either the gastro-hepatic omentum or the gastro-colic omentum. The object of the operation is (1) to stop hæmorrhage, (2) to prevent leakage, and (3) to provide drainage.

If the pancreas is found torn it may be possible to tie bleeding vessels, and then to suture the laceration—in this way a pancreas completely torn in two has been repaired. Bleeding having been stanched and any associated injury treated, all clots must be removed and the lesser sac either irrigated or thoroughly mopped out. A large rubber tube must be inserted and packed round with gauze to control hæmorrhage and to soak up escaping juice.

In dealing with penetrating wounds, associated injuries, especially of the stomach, must be carefully sought. In some few cases, fluid with the characteristics of pancreatic juice has been removed from the chest in convalescence.

PANCREATITIS

Etiology.—Experimental injection of a variety of substances into the duct of Wirsung produces acute inflammation with hæmorrhages, and glycosuria, and, later, abscesses or chronic inflammation. In man, gall-stones frequently coexist with pancreatitis, while sometimes possibly stones have been passed after causing the inflammation. When endeavouring to correlate these facts, Opie found that in 62 per cent. of subjects the termination of the bile-duct was so arranged that a small stone lodged there would dilate the ampulla and permit retrojection of bile into the pancreatic duct; this retrojected bile may have the same effect in producing pancreatitis as the various substances used experimentally.

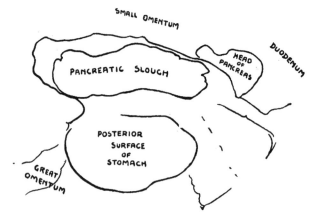

ILLBLADDER

UNDUS OF
STOMACH
LAID
OPEN

SMALL OMENTUM

DUODENUM

HEAD
OF
PANCREAS

PANCREATIC SLOUGH

POSTERIOR
SURFACE
OF
STOMACH

GREAT
OMENTUM

Key to Plate 101.

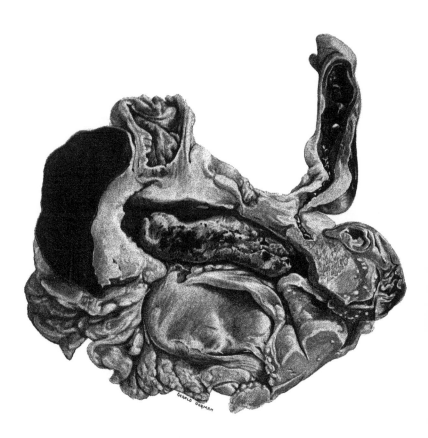

Sloughing of the pancreas, the result of acute inflammation of seven weeks' duration. The blackened slough is lying completely separated from the head, the only part of the gland to be spared. Gall-stones are seen in the pancreatic portion of the common duct, and fat necrosis is well shown. The parts are exposed from behind.

PLATE 101.

As the same agents may cause acute or chronic pancreatitis, some explanation for the incidence of the two classes must be sought. Flexner concludes that the sudden retrojection of fresh, unaltered bile causes acute changes, while the bile that is found in cases of chronic obstruction, containing a diminished amount of salts and an excess of colloid material, sets up chronic changes. Causal agents carried by the blood-stream, such as alcohol or tuberculous toxins, are more likely to give rise to chronic than to acute mischief.

Varieties of pancreatitis.—Pancreatitis may consist (1) in inflammation of the *ducts ;* or (2) in inflammation of the *parenchyma.*

" Fat necrosis " and hæmorrhage are two features so strikingly characteristic of pancreatitis that they must be separately discussed.

Fat necrosis was first properly described by Balser in 1882. The appearance is quite characteristic (Plate 101), and consists in small localized whitish or yellowish necrotic blotches scattered over the fat, varying in size from a pin's head to areas $\frac{1}{4}$ in. or more in diameter. The process is most marked near the pancreas, but is often widely distributed over the omentum and mesentery and may sometimes even be seen in the preperitoneal fat. This phenomenon results from splitting up of the fatty molecule into its fatty acid and glycerine by the escaped pancreatic juice. It is common in acute, but uncommon in chronic pancreatic lesions.

The **hæmorrhage** may either show itself in the substance of the gland, as a bloody peritoneal effusion, or as a general tendency to bleeding. Hæmorrhage into the gland may take the form of a massive bleeding—the so-called " pancreatic apoplexy," which has been recorded in vascular and blood diseases, sepsis, and poisoning, usually in fat people. Hæmorrhagic peritoneal effusion is seen in acute pancreatitis, and when associated with fat necrosis forms a striking picture.

The general tendency to bleeding is seen in the chronic varieties, with or without jaundice. In these cases, remote spontaneous hæmorrhages may occur under the skin, but, of course, the tendency to bleeding is principally observed after operations.

Morbid anatomy.—The slighter changes in the pancreas are not visible to the naked eye. This is especially true of the changes following catarrhal inflammation of the ducts and of those in chronic pancreatitis.

In **acute pancreatitis** the pancreas may be embedded in blood, or may be but a little larger and, in the early stages, firmer than normal. There may also be areas of softening of the pancreatic substance with definite evidence of gross infection. · Later, necrosis of considerable areas of the gland is obvious, and may involve either scattered patches or, more commonly, an extensive portion of the body, but the head and extreme end of the tail are often spared. In very acute cases the pancreas may become a disintegrating mass associated with retroperitoneal cellulitis, but, when time permits, the parts around form the walls of an abscess cavity in which a large slough may lie completely separated from the rest of the gland (Plate 101). Such an abscess may burst into one of the hollow viscera, or even externally, and in this way part of the pancreas may be discharged, and the patient recover.

In all cases peritonitis is considerable, most marked about the pancreas, and sometimes localized in the lesser sac (inflammatory effusion into the lesser sac). The effusion may be serous, hæmorrhagic, or deeply bile-stained.

In chronic inflammation few changes may be apparent to the naked eye; but sometimes the whole gland is a little enlarged and uniformly hard, looking like a " waxen cast "; or, again, the head only may be enlarged, irregular, and knobby, like a malignant tumour.

Microscopically, there are two forms of chronic pancreatitis—(1) the interstitial interlobular variety, in which the normal connective tissue is converted into a dense fibrous stroma compressing and gradually replacing the gland, and (2) the interacinous variety, in which the fibrous tissue separates the glandular acini and even sometimes the separate cells. In this form the cell islands are soon involved and diabetes often supervenes.

Clinical features. Catarrhal pancreatitis. — Catarrhal inflammation probably often precedes the more acute processes and may arise after influenza, or as a complication or sequel of mumps, and probably is the active feature in many cases of so-called catarrhal jaundice.

Suppurative catarrh of the ducts resembles suppurative cholangitis, with which it is usually associated. It may also occur with pancreatic calculi. The treatment is external drainage via the common bile-duct.

Acute pancreatitis usually occurs about middle life, the period of election being between 35 and 50, though it has occurred in a child of only 5, and in a man of 75. Males are affected twice as often as females. Although the disease may attack healthy patients, there is frequently a history of antecedent dyspepsia and of seizures of pain in the upper abdomen, and in about 25 per cent. of the cases the victims are stout people of alcoholic habits.

The onset is always sudden, and usually very acute, with epigastric pain so severe and collapse so profound that perforation of the stomach is closely simulated. Epigastric tenderness and muscular rigidity in the supra-umbilical zone are associated with violent belching and vomiting. The pulse is small and thready, and cyanosis may be marked. Such cases may end fatally within twenty-four hours.

In those that survive the early collapse, inflammatory symptoms supervene ; usually the pulse now becomes accelerated, but it may remain slow.

Constipation is generally obstinate, but there may be diarrhœa and even melæna. Albuminuria is common ; glycosuria is rare, but, if found, helps to confirm the diagnosis. Slight jaundice occurs in about one-fifth of the cases.

Locally, there are at first great tenderness and rigidity in the upper abdomen, and in from twelve to twenty-four hours an indefinite mass may be felt in the epigastrium or sometimes in the left lumbar region. Later still the signs of epigastric or diffuse peritonitis with fluid or of retroperitoneal cellulitis may be superadded ; or evidence of inflammatory effusion into the lesser sac may indicate a tendency to localization and subsequent recovery.

In some cases, after an acute onset the symptoms may apparently disappear for a time, but the pulse-rate remains fast, and a mass gradually develops in the pancreatic region ; this is followed by localized suppuration or sloughing of the gland (Plate 101). In others, ultimate recovery after a prolonged illness may follow rupture of an abscess into the bowel, or temporary improvement may end in late death from pancreatic insufficiency. In cases of another class, changes are seen similar to those of acute pancreatitis, but of a milder character. This form may only be revealed during operations for cholelithiasis, and, though recovery often results from removal of the calculi and drainage, is of grave prognosis.

Hæmorrhage from neighbouring vessels is especially liable to occur in acute pancreatitis.

Diagnosis of acute pancreatitis.—Most of the cases have been mistaken for acute intestinal obstruction. visceral perforation, or gall-stones. The most important features are the agonizing pain, often unrelieved by morphia, the tendency to cyanosis, and the very marked epigastric tenderness, soon followed by the development of a mass. These symptoms, with evidence of epigastric peritonitis and a subsequent inflammatory swelling posteriorly, particularly if in the left lumbar region (Körte), are suggestive of acute pancreatitis. The discovery of fat necrosis on opening the abdomen is strongly confirmatory. The Cammidge test is unreliable in the early stages of acute pancreatitis. A diagnosis of gall-stone disease is often correct, but a more serious pancreatitis may accompany it.

The **prognosis in acute pancreatitis** is always very grave, the mortality being probably 75 per cent.

Treatment of acute pancreatitis.—Whenever acute pancreatitis is suspected an operation is demanded : (1) to remove the cause, which will usually mean removal of gall-stones and drainage of the bile passages ; (2) to relieve tension about the pancreas by dividing its peritoneal covering; (3) to remove fluid from the peritoneum; and (4) to provide drainage. Körte, however, holds that under no consideration should the gall-bladder be incised and drained at the primary operation while the patient is collapsed.

The gland is best exposed by a free median incision. Probably, most benefit follows free external bile drainage, and many cases are cured by this alone. The pancreas should be exposed by tearing through the small omentum, and then through the overlying peritoneum. Any accumulation of fluid in the lesser sac will thus be evacuated and an escape provided for retroperitoneal extravasation. Incision of the substance of the pancreas itself is of doubtful value; if it be done, a dissector should be employed for the purpose, owing to the risk of severe hæmorrhage. If the general peritoneal cavity contain much fluid, it should be emptied and drained. When there is a definite localized mass the surgeon may find a considerable retroperitoneal collection, which may be drained from the front. When the case is of longer duration and the symptoms indicate sloughing of a considerable part of the gland, the sloughs must be sought and removed. Holes into the bowel for natural evacuation must not be overlooked.

Relapses after operations for acute pancreatitis.—The majority of cases that survive operations for acute pancreatitis appear to be completely cured, though a proportion develop chronic pancreatitis or diabetes, so that the prognosis after operation must be uncertain. Recurring attacks of pain are probably due to overlooked gall-stones or to concomitant duodenal ulcer. Sometimes a cyst develops as a late result, or slight recurrence may follow insufficiently prolonged drainage.

Chronic Pancreatitis

This group includes all cases that come on gradually and that are attended by an increase of fibrous tissue. The etiology, pathology, and morbid anatomy have been already described. The disease is rarely primary, but once initiated it tends to increase progressively, and to end in death.

Changes in the fæces.—(1) The stools are unusually bulky, soft, light-coloured, and offensive, while there may be a spurious diarrhœa; (2) there may be an abnormal amount of fat (steatorrhœa); (3) sometimes there may be faulty digestion of meaty food, as shown by the discovery of undigested muscle fibres (azotorrhœa).

Changes in the urine.—(1) Glycosuria is rare and unreliable as a diagnostic symptom; (2) alterations may be detected by the Cammidge reaction, which depends on the fact that in inflammatory lesions of the pancreas the kidneys excrete a substance with a glyco-nucleo-proteid content which on hydrolysis yields a body giving the reactions of a pentose.[1] This

---

[1] For the successful performance of this test an absolutely reliable chemist is necessary, as all the manipulations must be conducted with extreme care.

reaction is only a link in the chain of evidence. Some reject it as valueless and misleading in diagnosing pancreatitis. But a typical positive reaction with a negative control is strongly suggestive of inflammatory disease of the pancreas.

Moynihan sums up thus : " If azotorrhœa and steatorrhœa are simultaneously present, the evidence in favour of pancreatic disease is strong ; if also the pancreatic action is present, the evidence is conclusive."

Clinical features.—The cases vary very much in their onset, and may usually be divided into the following groups :—

1. Those in which attacks of pain are the main feature.
2. Those in which the first definite symptom is jaundice.
3. Those with general failure of health and possibly glycosuria.
4. Cases accidentally discovered at operation, in which the symptoms of gall-stones have masked those of the pancreatitis.

In the first group the condition probably begins as a subacute infection, which quietens down as it becomes chronic. The attacks of pain may be due to little outbursts of inflammation or to the gall-stones, the original cause. In these cases there are often attacks of shivering, and in the later stage there are apt to be the general symptoms mentioned in the third group.

The second group includes the cases in which the condition is most commonly mistaken for cancer. Jaundice may gradually deepen without intermission, and the patient rapidly waste. If, in these circumstances, the gall-bladder be distended, cancer is closely simulated.

In the third group there is extreme weakness and emaciation, with loss of appetite and loathing of food. The skin assumes an earthy hue, there are alterations in the urine and fæces, and there may be diabetes.

Many cases, undoubtedly, fall into the fourth group, and are discovered during operations. But the surgeon must not be led into diagnosing chronic pancreatitis from undue hardness of the gland without the confirmatory evidence afforded by an examination of the fæces and urine.

Physical signs.—In any of these groups an enlargement of the pancreas may be felt, the gland being swollen and tender. The enlargement varies from time to time, and may even vanish and reappear. There may be no tumour, but tenderness in the epigastrium or just above and to the right of the umbilicus. In cases with jaundice the gall-bladder is usually felt to be distended.

Prognosis. — Chronic pancreatitis is rarely a direct cause of death, but often leads to fatal diabetes.

Treatment.—The presence of a definite mass with or without jaundice indicates the necessity for operation. Such a mass may be malignant or inflammaory ; if the latter, it may disappear after mere exploration, after drainage of a retroperitoneal collection, or after

2 x

cholecystenterostomy. This latter operation is desirable, if possible, and may even sometimes prove of benefit in malignant disease. If a satisfactory anastomosis be found very difficult, external drainage should be substituted. When painless jaundice is the only symptom, operation should be deferred for at least six weeks to give time for spontaneous clearance, lest the jaundice be only catarrhal. If there be merely attacks of pain confidently attributable to pancreatic involvement, operation is necessary, for the attacks may proceed from gall-stones or pancreatic calculi. If there be no removable gross lesion, it is a moot point whether anything further than simple laparotomy can be of service, though some recommend routine cholecystenterostomy.

When a general failure of health or glycosuria can be traced to pancreatic involvement, without an acute onset or without any enlargement of the organ, surgical intervention is to be avoided.

SYPHILIS AND TUBERCULOSIS

Syphilis rarely affects the pancreas. It may take the form of an indurative pancreatitis or of a gumma. Isolated gummata have been recorded sufficiently often to justify administration of iodide and mercury in any case of irremovable pancreatic tumour, without unequivocal signs of cancer.

Tuberculosis is equally rare, but may occur in the miliary form, or as an isolated tuberculoma.

PANCREATIC CYSTS

Classification.—Cysts of the pancreas may be classified as follows :—

1. *True cysts.*
    Acinous.—(i) Retention cysts ; (ii) Cystadenomas, (a) multilocular, (b) papillomatous, (c) congenital cystic.
    Interacinous.—(i) Lymphatic, (ii) Parasitic.
2. *Pseudo-cysts.*
    Intraperitoneal.—Inflammatory effusions into lesser sac, (a) the result of injury, (b) secondary to pancreatitis.
    Retroperitoneal.—The result of (i) old hæmorrhage or necrosis of pancreas, (ii) breaking down of a new growth.

Donoghue has drawn attention to certain parapancreatic cysts which spring from the neighbourhood of the tail and probably originate in the remains of the Wolffian body.

Pathology.—Of the true cysts, those due to *retention* are the commonest. For the most part, they have been observed post mortem, and have presented no symptoms during life. Though usually the size of an orange, they may be as large as a man's head, or even attain enormous proportions necessitating surgical interference. The obstruction is in most cases a consequence of chronic interstitial pancreatitis.

The *cystadenomas* are still more rare. They may give rise to no symptoms during life, and only be discovered at necropsy, as in the case shown in Fig. 536, or one or more of the loculi may attain large size, giving rise to all the signs of pancreatic cysts.

Sometimes these tumours contain papillomas, while in other cases their structure suggests cystic epithelioma or carcinoma.

Congenital cystic disease also very rarely occurs, and is associated with the same condition in other organs.

Interacinous cysts.—Hydatids bear this relation to the gland, but are rare in the pancreas.

All the varieties of true cyst occur most commonly in the tail, though they may be found in any part of the gland.

Pseudo-cysts.—If we dismiss the cystic conditions due to the softening and breaking down of malignant new growths, there are two principal conditions to be discussed under this head—(1) the retroperitoneal collection of fluid in association with the breaking up of the pancreas from old hæmorrhage or inflammation; (2) inflammatory effusions into the lesser peritoneal sac.

Jordan Lloyd first drew attention to the cases which follow on injury. Laceration of the pancreas is combined with tearing of the overlying peritoneum, so that there is an escape of blood and pancreatic juice into the lesser sac. This leads to an inflammation, which results in the closing of the foramen of Winslow, and further adds to the effusion distending the lesser sac. Sometimes even gall-stones, bile, and pancreatic fluid have been found in this situation.

The **content of pancreatic cysts** is an alkaline albuminous fluid, having a specific gravity of 1010 to 1020. It is either clear or a reddish-brown, or definitely blood-stained, and usually, though not invariably, contains one or more of the pancreatic ferments.

Secondary changes.—In some cases hæmorrhage occurs into a cyst, either from injury or from erosion of vessels, and may later lead to the suggestion that such a cyst has arisen in an old hæmorrhage. Secondary infection may take place, and may lead to acute symptoms. Malignant disease may also arise.

Anatomical relations.—A pancreatic cyst sufficiently developed to be recognized may present in a variety of situations: (a) above the stomach, between it and the liver; (b) behind the stomach; (c) below the stomach, between it and the transverse colon; (d) below the transverse colon; (e) behind the stomach and colon; (f) between the layers of the mesocolon. The relations of a pancreatic cyst also depend on whether it springs from the head, the body, or the tail of the gland.

An effusion into the lesser sac of the peritoneum (pseudo-cyst) causes a general bulging of the epigastric and left hypochondriac regions with prominence of the lower part of the chest on that side; as it increases, the umbilical and left renal regions may be similarly invaded. The stomach is

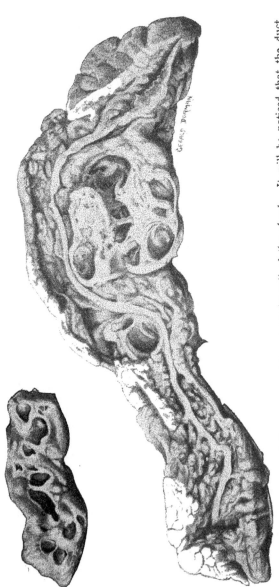

Fig. 536.—Cystadenoma of the pancreas, lying near the tail of the gland. It will be noticed that the duct of Wirsung courses round the tumour. The smaller drawing is part of the tail of a pancreas the subject of chronic inflammation, and shows dilatation of the duct.

lifted forwards and pushed upwards, while the colon is thrust downwards and forwards against the belly wall. On the left the swelling impinges on the parietes just below the costal margin, the spleen being pushed up and the splenic flexure down, so that in this situation such an effusion can easily be reached by the surgeon.

Clinical features.—Cysts are generally found in adults, though they may occur even in infants. Whereas true cysts commence gradually, and are often discovered accidentally, pseudo-cysts invariably follow injury or some acute inflammatory disturbance.

In the true cysts the symptoms usually depend on the size of the tumour, and may merely be those of epigastric fullness or distress, or there may be nausea and vomiting, symptoms of intestinal obstruction, or jaundice from pressure on the bile-ducts. Pain, when present, often heralds secondary changes. As a rule, there are no characteristic urinary changes. The cysts feel soft and cystic when large, but firm and solid when small.

The history of the pseudo-cysts that arise as the result of injury is usually that of a blow or crush of the upper abdomen, followed by severe pain, with signs of collapse, and with tenderness and rigidity in the epigastrium. These symptoms usually subside in the course of a day or two, but later there is a return of the pain, accompanied by a sense of fullness in the upper abdomen ; here a swelling soon becomes obvious, and often so rapidly increases in size as to cause dyspnœa within a very few days. The history is not always so rapid, and there may be an interval of a week or even some months before a recurrence of pain and the appearance of a swelling reveal the nature of the case.

Diagnosis.—The diagnosis is usually a question of the differentiation of a cystic tumour in the upper abdomen, because, as a rule, evidence of interference with the pancreatic function is absent ; if present, however, urinary or fæcal changes may be of great confirmatory value.

Prognosis.—In true cysts of the pancreas a spontaneous cure never occurs. The inflammatory effusions into the lesser sac may disappear without treatment, but generally tend to get rapidly worse.

Treatment.—Puncture or aspiration should never be employed, as it involves a grave risk of sepsis or hæmorrhage, without any compensating advantage. Complete extirpation, though an ideal method, can seldom be satisfactorily carried out.

Drainage is the treatment most generally applicable and satisfactory. The parietal abdominal incision should be made over the most accessible part of the cyst, usually in the middle line above the umbilicus. After protecting the general peritoneal cavity by gauze packing or by slightly withdrawing the cyst, if possible, from the abdomen, the surgeon evacuates the cyst and carefully examines its interior for secondary cysts or calculi. If the cyst can be brought to the surface, he then marsupializes it by stitching the edges of the opening to the abdominal wall; if not, he must fix a dressed tube into the cyst by means of a purse-string suture, or, failing this, must rely on careful packing to prevent leakage. The discharge will probably be scanty at first, but it soon becomes abundant and proteolytic. In an ordinary case the track will close in about four to eight weeks.

Sometimes lumbar drainage has been found necessary, but as a primary operation this can only be necessary in deep-seated cysts.

NEW GROWTHS

With the exception of cysts, all tumours of the pancreas are comparatively rare. Of the simple tumours, *adenomas* and *cystadenomas* have been most often observed. Such tumours have been successfully removed.

CARCINOMA

May be primary- or secondary. Primary cancer may be masked by the resultant enlargement of the liver. The growth may commence in any part, but is commonest in the head, where it may form a hard, nodular, rounded mass the size of an orange, or it may be diffuse. A striking feature is the enormous dilatation of the gall-bladder which occurs when the bile-duct is compressed (Plate 102). Very often a cancer involving the head of the pancreas has had its origin in the glands, and not in the pancreas itself.

Clinical features.—The disease is more common in males, and usually occurs between the ages of 40 and 60. The cases can be separated into three groups, according to whether the bile-duct, the portal vein, or the duodenum is most involved. In the first group, jaundice is the most prominent symptom—it comes on gradually, and stealthily deepens until the patient is of an olive-green colour, with a marked tendency to hæmorrhage and an intolerable itching; in the second group, ascites is the prominent feature; and in the third, gastric symptoms, depending on obstruction of the duodenum; but, in any case, jaundice is almost certain to appear at some stage of the illness. Pain may be present, usually above the umbilicus and through to the back. Unaltered fat or undigested muscle fibres may be found in the fæces. Glycosuria is only present when the whole gland is involved, or when there is chronic pancreatitis. The absence of urobilin points to cancer.

Diagnosis.—In gall-stones there is nearly always a history of previous attacks, an onset attended with pain, intermissions in the jaundice, and an absence of palpable tumour or enlarged gall-bladder. (Fig. 519.) Chronic pancreatitis may exactly simulate cancer, but there is usually a history of coincident gall-stone attacks. The jaundice is

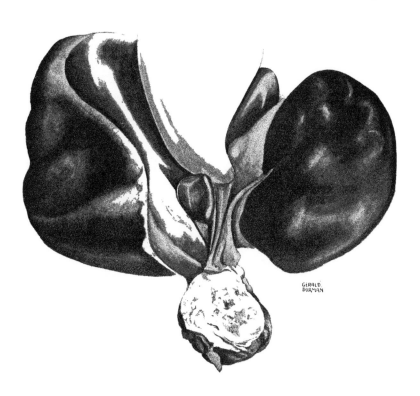

Enormous distension of the gall-bladder, secondary to malignant disease of the head of the pancreas.

PLATE 102.

not so deep, nor is wasting so marked, while characteristic changes are more likely to be found in the urine, and the duration is longer.

Prognosis.—The disease seldom lasts longer than six to twelve months, and may end fatally in a much shorter period.

Treatment.—New growths limited to the tail, and even some in the body of the gland, have been successfully removed. Tumours arising in the head of the gland have occasionally been shelled out, but Desjardins, in 1907, worked out experimentally an operation for complete excision of this part of the gland which gives promise of success. As a palliative measure, cholecystenterostomy is sometimes available, and may be worth while merely to relieve the intense itching.

If the signs of cancer are not unequivocal this operation should certainly be performed, for it may cure a doubtful case.

PANCREATIC LITHIASIS

Pancreatic calculi are very rare. Though usually only discovered after death, they have been found during life, either in the fæces or in the course of operation, and have occasionally been diagnosed and deliberately removed.

The calculi are long and oval, or resemble coral, and vary in size from material like sand to masses as big as a hazel-nut. Chemically, they are composed of carbonate and phosphate of lime or magnesia, and are, therefore, opaque to the Röntgen rays.

Symptoms may be entirely absent; and, in any case, none can be claimed as pathognomonic. In some cases, after attacks of pain like gallstone colic, but most intense under the left costal arch and in the left shoulder, pancreatic calculi have been found in the stools. There may be symptoms of a concomitant pancreatitis, and a positive pancreatic reaction has often been obtained.

Treatment.—If diagnosed by the X-rays, the location of the calculi will be indicated. Those in the main duct may be removed through the duodenum by enlarging the papilla, otherwise the pancreas may be directly incised.

PANCREATIC FISTULA

This is usually a sequel to some operation on the pancreas, either for injury, inflammation, or the treatment of a cyst.

The constant escape of secretion leads to digestion of the surrounding skin, which soon becomes extensively excoriated. Such a fistula may be very chronic, and may even resist treatment for years. Beyond the local inconvenience and the loss of secretion, the condition may be a source of septic absorption and of subsequent lardaceous disease. The amount of discharge varies with the character of the food taken, in response to the physiological excitation of the organ.

Treatment.—It is first necessary to see that there is no cause likely to keep the fistula active, such as a mass of sloughing pancreas. Drainage must not be hampered by too small an opening in the parietes; it must be allowed to be free, and the surrounding skin protected by bland dusting powders and ointments. To lessen the discharge, Wohl-gemuth recommends a carbohydrate-free diet, with frequent small doses of bicarbonate of soda. Fats should be given plenteously.

To encourage closure of the fistula, Beck's bismuth paste may be used. or, as a last resource. thorough cauterization may be employed. Excision of the track is not advisable. Sometimes when the fistula closes the cyst re-forms.

BIBLIOGRAPHY

Bland-Sutton, Sir John, *Gall-Stones and Diseases of the Bile-Ducts.* 1910
Desjardins, *Rev. de Chir.,* 1907, xxxv. 945.
Drummond and Morison, " A Case of Ascites due to Cirrhosis of the Liver, cured by Operation," *Brit. Med. Journ.,* Sept. 19th, 1896.
Halsted, William S., " Retrojection of Bile into the Pancreas a Cause of Acute Hæmorrhagic Pancreatitis " ; and **Eugene L. Opie,** " The Etiology of Acute Hæmorrhagic Pancreatitis," *Johns Hopkins Hosp. Bull.,* Nos. 121-3.
Handley, W. Sampson, " Hunterian Lectures on Surgery of Lymphatic System," *Brit. Med. Journ.,* April 16th, 1910.
Kehr, Prof. H., " Injuries and Diseases of the Liver and Biliary Passages," Berg-mann's *System of Practical Surgery,* vol. iv.
Körte, W., " Surgical Treatment of Acute Pancreatitis," *Ann. of Surg.,* Jan., 1912.
Lejars, Félix, trans. by W. S. Dickie, *Urgent Surgery.*
Maccarty, William Carpenter, " Pathology of the Gall-Bladder and some Associated Lesions," *Ann. of Surg.,* May, 1910.
Mayo, William J., " A Review of Fifteen Hundred Operations upon the Gall-Bladder and Bile Passages, with especial reference to the Mortality," *Ann. of Surg.,* Aug., 1906.
Mayo, William J., " Surgical Treatment of Pancreatitis," *Surg., Gyn., and Obstet.,* Dec., 1908.
Morison, R., *Brit. Med. Journ.,* Nov. 3rd, 1894.
Moynihan, Sir Berkeley, *Gall-Stones and their Surgical Treatment.* 1905.
Robson (Mayo) and Cammidge, *The Pancreas, its Surgery and Pathology.* 1907.
Rolleston, H. D., *Diseases of the Liver, Gall-Bladder, and Bile-Ducts.* 1905.

THE UPPER AND LOWER URINARY TRACT

By J. W. THOMSON WALKER, M.B.Ed., F.R.C.S.Eng.

THE KIDNEY

Anatomy of the kidney.—The kidney extends obliquely from the level of the middle of the 11th dorsal vertebra to that of the transverse process of the 3rd lumbar vertebra. Behind it lie the diaphragm, and the anterior layer of transversalis aponeurosis, which separates it from the quadratus lumborum muscle, the costo-vertebral ligament, and, at the lower pole, the psoas. The pleura is in relation with the kidney between the diaphragmatic origin from the external arcuate ligament and the 12th rib. The anterior relations are shown in the accompanying diagram. (Fig. 537.)

The kidney lies embedded in a fatty capsule contained within the fascia propria or perirenal fascia. The perirenal fascia appears between the transversalis fascia and peritoneum, and divides at the outer renal border into an anterior layer which crosses in front of the kidney and great vessels, and a stronger posterior layer, the fascia of Zuckerkandl, which, after supplying a fine covering to the renal vessels, becomes attached to the vertebral bodies. Above, the layers, after enclosing the suprarenal, become attached to the diaphragm : below, the anterior layer lines the peritoneum, while the posterior layer is gradually lost in the extraperitoneal fat. The perirenal fascia thus forms an envelope open on its internal and inferior aspects. The true renal capsule closely invests the organ and enters the hilum, but is easily stripped from the surface.

The renal pelvis is the trumpet-shaped upper expansion of the ureter which enters the sinus of the kidney. It usually presents two primary divisions, each divided into calyces, and on the average can hold $3\frac{1}{2}$ drachms, though distension with more than 2 drachms causes pain.

The renal artery divides at the hilum; two or three branches pass in front of and one behind the pelvis. One of the anterior branches passes to the upper pole, sometimes without entering the hilum. The arterial supply is divided into an anterior and a posterior system, independent of each other. The least vascular line, or exsanguine line of Hyrtl, runs parallel to and a little *behind* the convex border, and separates the anterior and posterior arterial systems.

An additional renal artery is present in about 20 per cent. of bodies, more commonly on the left side.

Lymphatics of the kidney.—The glands earliest affected in renal malignant disease are those at the hilum, those along the vena cava, and those between the aorta and the spermatic vein. The lymphatics from the hilum to the glands, along the great vessels, do not anastomose with neighbouring plexuses.

Attachments of the kidney.—The following structures, which prevent displacement, but allow free movement (3 to 5 cm.) with respiration, combine to support the kidney: (1) The renal vessels; (2) the peritoneum; (3) the attachment of the retroperitoneal surfaces of the duodenum, colon, and pancreas; (4) the adhesions to the suprarenal capsule; (5) the perirenal

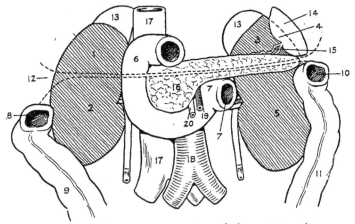

Fig. 537.—To illustrate the anterior relation of the kidneys (diagrammatic).

1 and 2, Peritoneum-covered surface of right kidney in apposition, respectively, with liver and small intestine; 3 to 5, peritoneum-covered surface of left kidney in apposition, respectively, with stomach, spleen, and small intestine; 6, duodenum; 7. duodeno-jejunal junction; 8, hepatic flexure of colon; 9, ascending colon; 10, splenic flexure; 11, descending colon; 12, attachment of transverse mesocolon; 13, suprarenals; 14, gastric surface of spleen; 15, splenic vessels; 16, pancreas; 17, inferior vena cava; 18, aorta; 19, superior mesenteric artery; 20, superior mesenteric vein; 21, ureters.

fascia and the network of fine fibres which pass to it from the renal capsule; (6) the perirenal fat; (7) the fascia of Toldt, which connects the perirenal fascia on the right side with the hepatic flexure and the duodenum, and on the left with the splenic flexure; and (8) the intra-abdominal pressure.

THE RENAL FUNCTION

The function of the kidneys in disease may be estimated by observing symptoms of renal failure, by the examination of the urine, and by certain tests.

1. **Signs and symptoms of renal failure.**—Thirst is the most frequent symptom, and is more severe at night. The tongue is dry, at first along the centre, and later over the whole surface. It becomes red, glazed, and cracked. In the later stages of urinary septicæmia it is covered with a dry brown fur ("parrot tongue"). There are loss of appetite and inability to

take solid food. Nausea and vomiting are late symptoms. There is frontal headache. The skin is dry and harsh, and the face has a peculiar yellow earthy look in the late stages. Emaciation is often present. Hiccup and drowsiness are grave symptoms. The temperature is subnormal in all aseptic cases and in chronic septic pyelonephritis.

2. **Examination of the urine.**—A persistently low specific gravity (1010 or less) is a grave symptom, and continuous reduction in the urea output shows a seriously impaired renal function. In some cases polyuria, in others oliguria or anuria, may be evidence of renal inadequacy.

3. **Special tests of the renal function.** (a) Cryoscopy. —Cryoscopy consists in determining the freezing-point (Δ) of the urine or of the blood and urine. By this means the amount of solids held in solution by each fluid is ascertained, and an estimate of the work performed by the kidney can be made. The Δ of the urine lies between −1·30° and −2·20° C., and of the blood at −0·56° C. There are many fallacies in this method, and it is unsuitable for general clinical use.

(b) **Methylene-blue test.**—If 15 minims of a 5 per cent. aqueous solution of methylene blue are slowly injected into the gluteal muscles, chromogen (transformed into blue by boiling with acetic acid) appears in the urine in from fifteen to twenty minutes, and blue itself is detected half an hour after the injection. The urine rapidly becomes olive green, emerald green, bluish-green, prussian blue, and finally a deep blue colour. The colour may not, however, pass beyond emerald green. The excretion of blue is at its height in four or five hours, remains stationary for several hours, and then gradually declines. It has usually disappeared in from forty to sixty hours, the chromogen disappearing some hours earlier. In pathological conditions of the kidneys the appearance of the blue is delayed, the excretion prolonged, and the total quantity reduced.

(c) **Indigo-carmine solution** is also used. An intramuscular injection of 4 c.c. of a 4 per cent. solution of indigo-carmine is given, and the urine is stained in twenty minutes. The elimination reaches its maximum half an hour later, and should be complete in two hours. This method is specially useful for chromocystoscopy, the depth of staining of the efflux of each ureter being observed with the cystoscope.

(d) **Phloridzin test.**—If a subcutaneous injection of 10 mg. of phloridzin be given, sugar can be detected in the urine in fifteen or sometimes thirty minutes. The glycosuria is at its height from three-quarters of an hour to an hour after the injection, and has usually ceased in two to two and a half hours. It amounts to 1 to 2 grm. of glucose. Delay in the appearance and reduction in the total quantity of sugar indicate a reduced renal function. The lowest limit of normal glycosuria lies between 50 cg. and 1 grm., and the highest between 2 and 2·50 grm.

(e) **Phenol-sulphone-phthalein test.**[1]—This test is at present under trial. Half an hour previous to the injection the patient drinks 300 c.c. of water. A subcutaneous injection of 1 c.c. of a solution containing 6 mg. of phenol-sulphone-phthalein is given, and the urine collected in a test-tube containing a drop of 25 per cent. NaOH solution. The commencement of elimination is noted, and the quantity excreted during the first and second hours is estimated by comparing the urine with a standard solution in a Dubosq's colorimeter. Elimination should commence in from five to eleven minutes; 40–60 per cent. of the drug should be excreted in the first hour, 20–25 per cent. in the second hour.

[1] Geraghty, *Trans. Amer. Assoc. of Genito-Urinary Surgeons*, vol. v., 1910.

EXAMINATION OF THE KIDNEYS BY INSPECTION, PALPATION, AND PERCUSSION

A greatly enlarged kidney forms a rounded, unilateral, abdominal swelling a little above the level of the umbilicus and more prominent in the recumbent posture. There is fullness in the flank, but no projection backwards. Where the renal pelvis is greatly distended with fluid a vertical groove may be seen on the surface of the swelling.

On palpation a renal tumour presents rounded borders, without any sharp edges, and frequently retains a reniform shape. It projects forwards into the abdomen, and backwards into the posterior kidney area at the angle between the ribs and the spinal muscles. With the fingers in the loin, the kidney tumour, if small, can be projected against the anterior hand by a sudden push (" ballottement "). Unless fixed by adhesions, renal tumours descend with inspiration, though rather less freely than tumours of the spleen, liver, or suprarenal body. The tumour can usually be separated from the liver, and seldom reaches the middle line.

Percussion gives a dull note, merging into that of the spinal muscles behind. Anteriorly there is a zone of comparative resonance, when the colon lies on the front of the tumour. If the colon is collapsed and dull on percussion, it can be rolled beneath the fingers. On the right side there is usually an area of resonance between the renal dullness and that of the liver.

EXAMINATION OF THE URINE OF EACH KIDNEY— EXPLORATION

Examination of the urine of each kidney.—The urine of each kidney may be obtained by the following methods :—

(a) **Separators.**—The principle of the separators is the formation of a septum in the middle line of the bladder, so that one ureter opens on each side of it, and the draining of each of these compartments separately. The separators of Luys and Cathelin are those most commonly used, but they have largely been superseded by ureteral catheterization. In the former, the patient lies on the back on an operating chair, and the urethra is cocainized. The bladder is washed, and 6 or 8 oz. of fluid injected. The instrument is passed ; in the male, deep depression between the patient's thighs is necessary in order to make the curved portion of the separator ride over the posterior lip of the internal meatus. The patient is now fully raised into a sitting posture and the screw turned to render the chain taut and form a membrane. The urine is collected in tubes, and the examination continued for twenty or twenty-five minutes.

(b) **Catheterization of the ureters.**—A fine catheter, 30 in. in length, is introduced into the ureter either through a specially constructed cystoscope or through an open tube under the guidance of a reflected light. The bladder is washed and distended with 10 oz. of clear fluid, and the cystoscope, loaded with a catheter, is introduced. The window is manœuvred into a position close to the ureter, the catheter is gently inserted into the opening, and pushed gently on for 12 in. Then the other ureter is catheterized if a double-barrelled instrument is being used ; or if a single-barrelled cystoscope is being employed it is withdrawn—leaving the first catheter in position—reloaded and reintroduced, and the second ureter catheterized. In direct catheterization of the ureters (Kelly's method), which is only applicable to the female bladder, the urethra is dilated sufficiently to permit the introduction of a short wide speculum. The patient is then placed in the knee-chest position, so that the bladder becomes distended by atmospheric pressure. Any fluid which remains in the bladder is mopped up with pledgets of wool. Light is projected into the bladder either from an electric head-lamp or reflected from a forehead mirror. The manipulation is made directly through the open tube.

Exploration of the kidney.—Exploration of the kidney by operation may be necessary in the following cases: (1) To diagnose abdominal tumours of doubtful nature. Laparatomy will be the best method. (2) To ascertain the nature of disease already localized to the kidney. An oblique lumbar incision and extraperitoneal examination of the kidney is advisable for this purpose.   (3) To ascertain the extent and connexions of the tumour and the condition of the lymphatics in a large malignant growth of the kidney.   Either a lumbar extraperitoneal examination of the kidney combined with an exploration through an opening in the peritoneum in front of the colon, or a laparotomy alone, may be used.   (4) To ascertain the presence and condition of the second kidney when one is diseased and nephrectomy is proposed.   For this purpose cystoscopy and ureteral catheterization have replaced nephrotomy, which is only required in the rarest cases, when these methods are rendered impossible by cystitis. Access is obtained through a lumbar incision, and the kidney is examined extraperitoneally by inspection, palpation, and incision, and, if necessary, a slip of the kidney substance is removed and examined microscopically. The abdominal route only permits of palpation, and has proved worthless.

POLYURIA

Continuous polyuria (80 to 100 ounces in twenty-four hours) is observed in those forms of chronic interstitial nephritis which result from urinary obstruction or from other conditions, such as calculus and tuberculosis, that cause gradual destruction of renal tissue. The total quantity of urea and other urinary solids is much diminished. Nervous polyuria may be transient or may continue for some weeks or months; it is accompanied by indefinite abdominal pain and frequent micturition. The renal function is not impaired in nervous polyuria.

OLIGURIA AND ANURIA

Oliguria is a diminished secretion of urine, anuria a total cessation of the secretion. The types of oliguria and anuria may be classified thus:—

1. Hysterical anuria.
2. Anuria due to changes in the general blood pressure.
3. Reflex anuria:
    (i) Urethra.
    (ii) Bladder.
    (iii) Ureter.
    (iv) Kidney.
4. Infective anuria:
    (i) Hæmatogenous $\begin{cases} (a)\ \text{toxic.} \\ (b)\ \text{bacterial.} \end{cases}$
    (ii) Ascending urinary.
5. Urinary-tension anuria:
    (i) Obstruction $\begin{cases} (a)\ \text{gradually increasing.} \\ (b)\ \text{sudden.} \end{cases}$
    (ii) Sudden relief of hypertension.

6. Anuria from destruction or removal of renal tissue :
   (i) Gradual destruction.
   (ii) Sudden complete destruction or removal.

1. **Hysterical anuria.**—Anuria may last for several hours or even days, but no symptoms of uræmia supervene. A copious polyuria immediately follows the anuria.

2. **Circulatory anuria.**—After severe, prolonged operations temporary oliguria or anuria may result from the low blood-pressure of shock, and also from the effect of the anæsthetic and the absorption of antiseptics. If the kidneys are diseased, this may initiate continuous and fatal anuria. In shock caused by grave injuries to the body, and in the collapse of cholera, anuria is present.

3. **Reflex anuria.**—The passage of urethral instruments, especially if roughly used, or if necessitated by disease in the deeper part of the canal, may be followed by suppression of urine. The urethra may be healthy and its mucous membrane intact. The kidneys may show chronic nephritis or deep congestion, but sometimes they appear normal. There is usually a rigor with rise of temperature to 103° or 104° Fahr. In the majority of cases the symptoms are due to septic absorption, and in some to a combination of septic absorption and a reflex effect on the circulation of the kidneys, while in a few they are purely reflex in nature.

Surgical interference with the bladder may be followed by suppression of urine.

Reflex impulses from a ureter, started by a catheter or stone, may inhibit the secretion of the corresponding kidney. The function of both kidneys may be suppressed and complete anuria result owing to the lodging of a stone in one ureter or the kinking of the ureter of a movable kidney. The second kidney is always diseased. (*See* Calculous Anuria, p. 837.) Disease of one kidney, such as pyelonephritis, may reflexly cause oliguria or temporary attacks of complete anuria.

4. **Infective anuria.** (i) *Hæmatogenous.*—In acute nephritis caused by a hæmatogenous infection, in septicæmia, influenza, pneumonia, typhoid fever, and in auto-intoxication from gastro-intestinal infection, suppression of urine is frequently present, and may be fatal. Anuria following urethral operations is toxic in nature in many cases. In hæmatogenous infection of the kidney with the Bacillus coli communis complete suppression may occur. (*See* Hæmatogenous Pyeionephritis, p. 802.)

(ii) *Ascending.*—An acute ascending infection of the kidneys may cause fatal anuria. Chronic septic pyelonephritis secondary to disease of the lower urinary organs is accompanied by oliguria, and complete anuria may supervene. (*See* Ascending Pyelonephritis, p. 802.)

5. **Urinary-pressure anuria.**—Complete anuria may follow the sudden relief of urinary tension such as is caused by the quick emptying of an over-distended bladder. Rapid occlusion of both ureters by stone or malignant disease also leads to complete suppression of the renal function. (*See* Calculous Anuria, p. 837.)

6. **Anuria from destruction or removal of renal tissue.**—The removal of a solitary kidney, or of the only working kidney, is followed by anuria, and death in a few days. If the second kidney is active, but incompetent from disease, the patient may survive the operation and die some months afterwards. Where the kidney is slowly destroyed by disease there are attacks of partial or complete anuria, and finally complete suppression.

Treatment of anuria.—Hysterical anuria is treated by bromides, valerian, etc. Diuretics should bo administered, and care exercised to prevent fraudulent disposal of any urine that is passed.

Circulatory anuria is treated by raising the blood pressure by means of strychnine, ergot, adrenalin, and pituitary extract, and by saline infusion. In *reflex* anuria the cause of the reflex inhibition should be removed (*see* Calculous Anuria, p. 837, *and* Pyelonephritis, p. 801). In *infective* anuria it may be necessary to incise one or even both kidneys (*see* Pyelonephritis). Sudden relief of long-established severe obstruction, as, for example, the complete emptying of a chronically over-distended bladder in a case of enlarged prostate, should be avoided.

The following measures should be adopted in cases of anuria : Diuretics are administered such as caffeine (5 gr.), diuretin (10 gr.), theocin sodium acetate (5 gr.), hot Contrexéville water, and citrate of potash (15 gr.). Hot fomentations and poultices are applied over the loins, or the kidneys may be dry-cupped. The patient is placed in a hot pack or a vapour bath. In severe cases the introduction of one to two pints or more of glucose solution (2½ per cent.) into a vein has a powerful diuretic effect.

In urgent cases a pint of glucose solution (25 per cent.) is infused into a vein. This solution is hypertonic and increases the molecular content of the blood. In less urgent cases the injection may be given subcutaneously or intramuscularly, or introduced into the rectum. Jeanbrau recommends an isotonic solution of glucose (47 grm. per 1,000), or of saccharose or lactose (90 grm. per 1,000).

BACTERIURIA (BACILLURIA)

Bacteriuria (bacilluria) is a condition of the urine in which bacteria are present in so great abundance that they render the fluid cloudy to the naked eye, yet inflammatory products are almost or entirely absent. Bacterial growth is excessive, and reaction minimal. Bacteriuria is found in infants and children, as well as in adults. Women are more frequently affected than men.

Pathology.—The Bacillus coli is present in pure culture in over 80 per cent. of cases. The bacillus of typhoid is next most frequent ; less frequent are the Staphylococcus albus, the Proteus vulgaris, the Streptococcus, and the Bacillus subtilis. These bacteria are usually present in pure culture. Bacteriuria may arise spontaneously, or it may complicate some urinary disease.

In spontaneous cases a history of constipation or indigestion can usually be obtained, and pronounced phosphaturia may precede the bacteriuria. Other predisposing causes are chronic septic conditions of the mouth and throat, operations upon the rectum or anus, boils or carbuncles, appendicitis, and dysentery. Typhoid fever precedes the typhoid form, and other fevers, such as smallpox, diphtheria, scarlet fever, and measles, may be accompanied by bacteriuria.

Bacteriuria may supervene during the course of chronic prostatitis or seminal vesiculitis, or it may immediately follow the passage of a sound or catheter. The bacteria gain admission to the urinary tract through the kidneys (hæmatogenous infection), or may be introduced into the urethra or bladder by instrumentation, or may ascend from the urethral opening in women and female children (urinary or ascending infection). The statement that they may pass directly through the rectal and bladder walls is unsupported by direct evidence. In uncomplicated cases, post-mortem examination has shown a complete absence of any lesion of the urinary mucous membrane.

Symptoms.—When passed the urine is hazy and frequently opalescent from the suspension of myriads of bacteria. On rotating a glass beaker, so as to circulate the fluid, a peculiar and characteristic appearance like drifting mist or smoke is seen. The reaction is usually acid, occasionally neutral, and rarely alkaline. On centrifugalization, no deposit is obtained and the fluid remains cloudy. The urine has usually a strong fishy odour and contains a trace of albumin. Under the microscope the field is crowded with bacteria, usually the motile Bacillus coli. A few leucocytes may be found, and epithelial cells from the renal pelvis, ureter, and bladder, or the prostatic urethra. The only constant sign is the bacterial emulsion in the urine. The urine may remain constantly cloudy for months or years, or it may suddenly clear, perhaps to become clouded again with equal suddenness.

There may be no symptoms at all, but signs of localized inflammation are seldom entirely absent. These consist in increased frequency of micturition, and urgency or scalding on passing water. In children, nocturnal enuresis may result. Frequently, if the prostatic urethra or the prostate is the seat of the bacterial growth, the last few drops of urine are milky with bacterial emulsion, while the rest is merely hazy. In other cases the focus of bacterial growth is confined to the renal pelvis.

Prognosis.—In some cases bacteriuria is transient and appears for a few days only, rapidly disappearing under treatment. Usually, however, it continues with exacerbations and remissions for months or years. During this time the health of the patient may be uninfluenced, but there is the constant danger of a virulent bacterial inflammation arising in some part of the urinary tract.

Treatment.—This consists in the administration of urinary antiseptics and diluents, and in local treatment of the focus of inflammation and removal of the source of bacterial infection. Of urinary antiseptics the best are urotropine (15–30 gr. daily), oil of turpentine (15–30 minims daily) in capsule, hetraline or helmitol (30 gr. daily), and salol (30 gr. daily). The administration of diuretics and alkaline waters with these antiseptics renders the urine less suitable for bacterial growth. Contrexéville, Vichy, or Evian water may be given, or the patient directed to drink large quantities of distilled water or barley-water.

Rovsing advises that a catheter should be retained in the urethra for a week or more while salol is administered by the mouth and large quantities of distilled water are drunk.

Where the focus of bacterial growth is confined to the prostatic urethra, washing the bladder and urethra by Janet's irrigation method may quickly relieve the symptoms and suppress the bacterial growth. The solutions suitable for this irrigation are permanganate of potash (1 in 10,000 to 1 in 5,000), oxycyanide of mercury (1 in 10,000), and nitrate of silver (1 in 10,000).

It is of the utmost importance to empty and regulate the bowel and prevent further absorption. A course of artificially soured milk may be continued for several months.

Anti-coli horse serum has been administered with some success in acute cases of Bacillus coli infection of the urinary tract, and may be tried. A dose of 25 c.c. of the serum should be injected subcutaneously on three successive days. If improvement has not taken place at the end of that time, the treatment should be abandoned. Calcium lactate (20 gr. thrice daily) should be administered by the mouth to prevent the unpleasant effects of the serum.

Treatment by vaccines gives varying results. In some cases the bacteria in the urine rapidly diminish in quantity and in a few cases disappear. Vaccines should be autogenous. In Bacillus coli infections small doses of vaccine up to 10 or 15 million bacteria are less efficacious than higher doses of from 30 to 50 or even 100 million, which should be given at intervals of a week.

Where the bacteriuria is superimposed on some pre-existing disease of the urinary tract, the latter should be suitably treated.

HÆMATURIA

An appearance resembling blood is given to the urine in hæmoglobinuria, and after the ingestion of some drugs, such as senna, rhubarb, sulphonal, etc. The final test for hæmaturia is the microscope. The urine in hæmoglobinuria has a peculiar purple colour, it contains no clots, and shows no blood corpuscles, even after centrifugalizing.

Localization of the source of hæmaturia.—Blood from an area anterior to the compressor urethræ escapes from the meatus independently of micturition; that from any part behind this muscle is mixed with the urine and is only discharged with it.

Hæmaturia may be the solitary symptom, or it may be accompanied by localizing symptoms.

Severe pain in one kidney and ureteric colic will localize the hæmorrhage to this kidney, renal pelvis, or ureter; but dull aching in one kidney may be present in vesical disease such as papilloma and malignant growth.

Pain at the end of the penis on micturition points to an affection of the base of the bladder, or of the prostatic urethra; while pain at the base of the sacrum, in the rectum, or in the perineum suggests the prostate.

Frequent micturition localizes the point of hæmorrhage to the prostatic urethra or bladder. Copious bleeding from the kidney may, however, cause vesical irritation and frequent micturition.

The combination of obstruction and hæmaturia is most frequently due to prostatic or urethral disease, but may result from a papilloma of the bladder near the internal meatus, or with a long pedicle, or even from temporary impaction of a clot in the urethra.

The longer the blood remains in contact with the urine, the more likely is it to be discoloured. The higher the source of blood in the urinary tract, the better the admixture with the urine. Blood in a highly acid urine is brownish, and in an alkaline urine bright red.

A brownish or smoky appearance of the urine indicates that the blood is small in quantity, well mixed with the urine, and the reaction acid. Such bleeding is usually renal in origin, and only forms a sediment after several hours. In coffee-coloured urine the source of bleeding is frequently the kidney or kidney pelvis, but may be the bladder or the prostate, especially if there is urethral obstruction. A purple tinge denotes venous bleeding, which may be derived from any part of the urinary tract. If the urine has a delicate pink colour, the blood usually comes from the bladder or the prostatic urethra. Bright-red blood indicates copious bleeding from an arterial source, and may arise in any part of the urinary tract, most frequently in the bladder or prostate.

Blood appearing at the beginning of micturition (initial hæmaturia) usually comes from the prostatic urethra. Terminal hæmaturia (appearing at the end of micturition) is derived from the prostatic urethra or the bladder. No inference can be drawn as to the source of blood mixed with the whole of the urine (total hæmaturia).

2 y

Slender worm-like clots, 10 or 12 in. in length, are sometimes passed, and indicate the kidney or renal pelvis as the source of bleeding. More frequently, however, the clots passed from the ureter are small plugs, ½ in. in length. The blood may be rapidly passed into the bladder and there form irregular masses or flat clots, which indicate the position of coagulation, but not the source of the hæmorrhage. Urethral bleeding may form a cast of the urethra, which is discharged with the urine.

Albumin is present even where the amount of blood is very small. In cases of renal hæmaturia, however, the quantity of albumin exceeds the amount corresponding to the admixture of blood. If, on estimation, excess of the albumin over the proportion of 1·6 to 1 of hæmoglobin be found, this points to a renal cause of the hæmaturia (Newman).

In renal hæmaturia the corpuscles often appear as pale discs almost devoid of colouring matter, while those added to the urine in the lower urinary tract are less changed.

Casts of the renal tubules, if present, indicate a renal lesion. Epithelial cells from the kidney, pelvis, and ureter, bladder, or urethra may be discovered and help to localize the source of the hæmorrhage.

The kidneys, ureters, and bladder should be examined by abdominal palpation, and the prostatic and membranous urethra, the prostate, seminal vesicles, bladder base, and lower ureters examined from the rectum.

Cystoscopic examination supplies a means of certain localization. The bladder is thus examined for growths or ulcers, and the ureteric orifices for evidences of disease or staining of the efflux. Finally, the ureters should be catheterized, and a sample of urine obtained from each kidney for microscopical examination (p. 780).

The **diagnosis of the cause of hæmaturia** will be described under the various diseases, but one form which cannot be referred to any single disease must be discussed here.

Essential renal hæmaturia.—This name has been given to a group of cases where hæmaturia has been localized to one kidney. Careful microscopical examination of these kidneys frequently gives evidence of some degree of chronic nephritis; this occurs in scattered patches, however, and may therefore easily be overlooked. A few cases have been recorded in which hæmaturia without other symptoms and without albuminuria has been caused by a more extensive unilateral chronic nephritis (Poirier, Loumeau).

A varicose condition of one or more of the renal papillæ as a cause of hæmaturia has been described by Fenwick, Whitney, Pilcher, and others. Its origin is doubtful; possibly it may result from a patch of interstitial nephritis similar to the condition just described. Profuse unilateral renal hæmaturia unaccompanied by other symptoms may be met with as a premonitory or early symptom of chronic Bright's disease.

Essential hæmaturia is spontaneous, strictly unilateral, and is not affected by rest or movement. The blood is abundant and well mixed, and gives the urine a dark, port-wine colour. Clots are very rarely formed. The bleeding may suddenly cease after some weeks or months, and may as suddenly reappear and become persistent. In the intervals no albumin can be detected nor tube casts found. No bacteria are present in the urine. On the affected side there is occasionally a dull aching pain, uninfluenced by movement. The kidney is not tender or enlarged.

In 13 cases of unilateral symptomless hæmaturia in which I explored the kidney and removed a portion for examination, the microscope showed cortical patches of fibrosis in all, of varying size. Newman has recorded a case of severe renal hæmaturia which preceded other symptoms of tuberculous disease by two years. Symptomless hæmaturia may occur in some growths of the kidney at a very early stage of their development.

Treatment of hæmaturia.—Only exceptionally is treatment for hæmaturia, apart from operative measures, required. Morphia, ergot, ergotine, tincture of hamamelis, and calcium chloride or lactate may be used.

Local treatment.—In *renal hæmaturia* dry cupping and ice-bags may be applied over the kidney. Adrenalin has been injected into the renal pelvis through a ureteric catheter, 1 drachm of 1-in-5,000 solution being used.

In *vesical hæmaturia* a catheter should be passed and the bladder washed out with large quantities of hot boric solution or of a hot, very weak solution (1 in 15,000) of silver nitrate. Afterwards 10 or 12 oz. of a solution of anti-pyrin (10 per cent.), or 1 or 2 drachms of adrenalin solution (1 in 2,000), are injected into the bladder, left for a few minutes, and then run out. Any clots in the bladder may be washed out through a large catheter, or, better, through a large evacuating catheter such as is used in lithotrity. The rubber lithotrity bulb may be attached and the clots sucked out. These methods should not be persisted in for long; if the clots are large, and distending the bladder, suprapubic cystotomy should be performed, the clots cleared out, and a stream of hot boric solution (115° to 120° F.) passed through a catheter in the urethra, and allowed to well out of the suprapubic opening.

In a case of *unilateral renal hæmaturia* nephrotomy is necessary, and if a papilla of the kidney shows congestion it may be cut away with a sharp spoon. Where nephrotomy fails to discover any lesion in the renal substance the wounds in the kidney and renal pelvis should be closed with catgut sutures. The hæmaturia in the majority of cases ceases after the exploration, apparently as a result of pressure upon the bleeding vessel by the sutures. Nephrectomy should not be performed for this reason, and also because bilateral nephritis may give rise to unilateral hæmaturia. Very rarely recurrence of hæmorrhage necessitates a second operation.

Decapsulation may be combined with nephrotomy, but the results are similar to those of nephrotomy alone, the hæmaturia recurring in rare cases.

PYURIA

Pyuria indicates inflammation in one or more parts of the urinary tract. Bacterial infection may occur in an otherwise healthy urinary tract, or may be superadded to stone, stricture, growth, or other gross lesions. Further, one bacterial inflammation may be superimposed upon another of a different character.

Apart from acute inflammation of the urethra, the position of which will be evident from the discharge of pus at the meatus, the largest quantities of pus are derived from purulent collections in the kidney. In cases of long-standing bladder inflammation the total quantity of deposit may be large, but the proportion of pus is not so great. The fluffy muco-purulent deposit of urethritis settles quickly to the bottom of the glass, while that of cystitis forms billows in the urine, which is usually highly coloured and concentrated. In severe old-standing cystitis the urine may be like coffee with milk. The sediment, after standing for an hour or two, is viscous and clings like slime to the bottom of the vessel. Pus from the renal pelvis, or from a dilated kidney, produces a milky urine when passed, but later lies at the bottom as a heavy, flat, yellowish layer, which rolls heavily to the lowest part when the vessel is canted. The supernatant fluid is cloudy with suspended pus or bacteria.

The urine is usually pale and of low specific gravity. Suppurative renal disease combined with cystitis produces a solid layer of pus at the bottom of the glass, and above this a layer of billowy, fluffy muco-pus.

In chronic cystitis the urine has a pungent ammoniacal odour. As a rule, purulent urine from the kidney has no characteristic odour, but a purulent collection in a dilated kidney may be offensive, and a pyelitis with excessive bacterial growth may possess a very strong disagreeable and penetrating smell. Bacillus coli, the gonococcus, and Bacillus typhosus produce acute cystitis, in which the purulent urine remains acid. The tubercle bacillus produces a subacute or chronic cystitis with an acid urine. The staphylococcus, streptococcus, and Bacillus proteus cause ammoniacal decomposition of the urine. The urine from a case of suppurative pyelitis is usually acid, but ammoniacal decomposition may take place.

Pus appearing at the beginning of micturition has a urethral origin. When the urine is clear at the beginning of micturition and purulent at the finish, the pus comes from the prostate or bladder.

Intermittent pyuria is found in pyonephrosis, and also when an abscess or an infected vesical diverticulum repeatedly discharges into the urethra or bladder.

Albumin proportional to the quantity of pus present is found in the urine of all uncomplicated cases of pyuria. If it be present in excessive quantities, renal complications may be suspected.

Epithelial elements may be present in the urine, but have less significance in regard to localization here than in hæmaturia. Tube casts are only found in the slighter forms of pyelonephritis.

Localizing symptoms may be present which point to the source of the pyuria. The cystoscope will frequently localize the otherwise obscure origin of pyuria. The examination of the ureteric orifices should never be neglected. Disease of the bladder exclusively surrounding one ureteric orifice, changes at the orifice itself, and the observation of murky or purulent urine coming from one ureter will show that there is disease of the kidney, whether renal symptoms be present or not. When the quantity of pus in the urine is small and the bladder inflamed it may be very difficult to distinguish the pyuria by examining the ureteric efflux, and ureteral catheterization will then become necessary. When the pus is present in quantity with little urine, pipes of semi-solid pus are observed issuing from the ureteric orifice.

In some cases of long-standing pyuria, radiography shows the presence of stones in one or both kidneys, when no symptoms of their presence have been observed.

PNEUMATURIA

In this condition gas is discharged with the urine at the end of micturition. Pneumaturia may result from the introduction of air into the bladder during instrumentation, from the escape of intestinal gas through a vesico-intestinal fistula, or rarely from spontaneous development of gas in the urinary tract. This may be due to liberation of CO_2 by fermentation of sugary urine through the action of Bacillus coli, or occasionally Proteus vulgaris; in non-glycosuric cases the gas has been said to be derived from the blood or from gaseous decomposition of the urine by gas-producing bacteria such as the colon bacillus.

Treatment.—When no fistula exists, treatment consists in removing the cause of the fermentation by washing the bladder and administering urinary antiseptics. Glycosuria should be treated. The treatment of fistula of the bladder will be discussed later (p. 878).

CONGENITAL ABNORMALITIES OF THE KIDNEY AND URETER

Fœtal lobulation of the kidneys occasionally persists throughout life. Complete absence of both kidneys has been found in acephalic fœtuses. Supernumerary kidneys are rare. A third kidney has occasionally been found.

ABSENCE OR ATROPHY OF ONE KIDNEY

In 93 cases which I collected of death from uræmia or anuria after an operation on one kidney, the second kidney was absent in 10 and completely "atrophied" in 8. Unsymmetrical kidney and extreme congenital atrophy of the kidney occurs in 1 in 2,400 bodies (Morris). The left kidney is more frequently absent than the right, and male subjects are more often affected than female in the proportion of 2 to 1. The renal vessels on the affected side are absent or rudimentary, and the ureter is absent (93 per cent.) or is represented by a solid fibrous cord attached to the bladder. The corresponding half of the vesical trigone is atrophied. The ureteric orifice may be undiscoverable, but occasionally shows as a small dimple or even as an opening into a lumen extending from 1 to 2 cm. In 70·8 per cent. of cases there is some associated congenital malformation in the genital system, almost always on the same side. Other congenital malformations have also been noted, such as hare-lip, web-fingers, etc.

The solitary kidney is usually larger than normal, lobulated, and often globular or irregular in shape. The single ureter enters the bladder in the usual position, or is displaced towards the middle line or to some abnormal position such as the urethra.

Extreme congenital atrophy is very rare, but a less complete form is more frequently observed. The condition is usually due to loss of function of the kidney from blocking of the ureter or disease of the kidney itself. In congenital atrophy some rudiment of the kidney is always found, and the ureter is present, although sometimes merely as a fibrous cord.

Dangers and diagnosis of solitary kidney.—A single kidney is prone to be attacked by disease such as calculus, malignant growths, tuberculosis, and chronic nephritis. Apart from this, however, the condition does not shorten life.

It is imperative that proof of the presence of an active second kidney be obtained whenever nephrectomy is proposed. Congenital malformation of the generative organs is present in 70·8 per cent. of these cases, and should lead to a thorough investigation of the second kidney.

On cystoscopy the ureteric orifice is absent in 33 per cent. of cases. When a ureteric orifice is present the ureter should be catheterized. Finally, lumbar exploration of the kidney should be carried out when the previous methods have failed. Abdominal exploration has proved fallacious.

FUSED KIDNEYS

Fusion of the kidneys into one mass gives rise to an organ presenting a great variety of sizes and shapes. The lowest degree of fusion is when two kidneys are united by a fibrous band, and the highest when two kidneys are indistinguishably fused in a single mass. The following names have been applied to the various shapes, viz. horse-shoe kidney, S-shaped kidney, long kidney, shield-like kidney, discoid kidney.

The *horse-shoe kidney* is the most common degree of fusion—1 in 1,000 bodies (Morris). The kidneys are united by a band passing between the lower poles across the aorta and vena cava. The fused kidneys lie nearer the middle line than normal, and are displaced downwards, the uniting band frequently lying as low as the bifurcation of the aorta. The bond of union varies from a flat band of fibrous tissue to a definite bridge of renal tissue. The blood-vessels of each kidney are frequently increased in number and abnormal in distribution; the ureters pass down in front of the uniting band. Diagnosis depends upon the discovery of a horse-shoe-like swelling in front of the lumbar vertebræ, and the discovery of a hydronephrosis or of shadows of calculi which lie nearer the middle line than usual. This malformation has been mistaken for a malignant growth.

In unilateral fused kidney the ureters may open in the normal position and lead to the view that two normal kidneys are present.

The course of the ureters can be demonstrated by passing into each a bougie opaque to the X-rays.

Fixed Misplacement of the Kidney

The fixed misplaced kidney is occasionally normal in size and contour, but usually shows considerable malformation. The remaining kidney, if not fused, is sometimes absent or atrophied.

The misplaced kidney is found at the bifurcation of the aorta, on the promontory of the sacrum, over the sacro-iliac synchondrosis, in the iliac fossa, or the hollow of the sacrum. The suprarenal capsule accompanies it.

If one kidney only is misplaced, it is usually the left. The renal vessels are, as a rule, abnormal in origin, number and distribution; malposition of the colon and rectum and genital malformations are frequently present.

Symptoms and diagnosis.—Disease of a misplaced kidney frequently gives rise to pain in the corresponding lumbar region, and this may distract attention from the real cause of the symptom. Renal misplacement seldom causes symptoms *per se*. In women a pelvic kidney may disturb menstruation, pregnancy, and parturition. The diagnosis will rest upon the discovery of a tumour on the promontory or in the pelvis, the absence of the kidney from the same side, and sometimes upon signs of renal disease in the urine. Tumours of the pelvic organs, especially ovarian cysts, and also hydatid cysts must be excluded. The rectum may be shown by air inflation to pursue an abnormal course. A very short ureter has been observed on catheterization. Psychic disturbances have been noted. A doubtful tumour in this situation usually necessitates a laparotomy for diagnosis.

Treatment.—When the existence of a second efficient kidney has been certainly ascertained, the presence of pronounced symptoms justifies removal of the misplaced organ.

CONGENITAL ABNORMALITIES OF THE RENAL PELVIS AND URETER

The renal pelvis may bifurcate into its upper and lower branches before entering the renal hilum, or may even sometimes show a third primary division. Unilateral duplication of the ureter occurs in 4 per cent. of bodies; it may affect a part or the whole length of the tube, which may open into the bladder by one or two apertures.

The ureter which drains the upper part of the kidney usually crosses that from the lower part, and opens lower on the trigone.

Bilateral double ureters are of less frequent occurrence. Five and even six ureters have been found in one individual.

The ureter may be congenitally misplaced and open into the male prostatic urethra or seminal vesicle, into the female urethra or vagina, or into the rectum. The misplaced ureter is usually a supernumerary one, and the ureteric orifice is narrowed and sometimes ends blindly in the form of a cyst in some part of the bladder wall. In the female subject, incontinence of urine while the patient could pass a quantity of water voluntarily has been noted when a ureter opened into the urethra. The ureter should be transplanted into the bladder in such cases.

Congenital narrowing of the ureter leads to hydronephrosis or to atrophy of the kidney.

MOVABLE AND FLOATING KIDNEY

The normal respiratory excursion of the kidney varies from $\frac{1}{2}$ to $1\frac{1}{2}$ in.

Pathological anatomy.—A *floating* kidney is entirely surrounded by peritoneum, which also clothes its pedicle and forms a mesonephros. It is a very rare congenital malformation, and cannot be diagnosed from a movable kidney without operation; an intraperitoneal operation is required for its relief. A *movable* kidney moves within the thickened perirenal fascia behind the peritoneum. The delicate perirenal fat is diminished or entirely absent, and the fibrous threads connecting the fibrous capsule of the kidney with the perirenal fascia are thickened. Milky patches of thickening are frequently observed on the fibrous capsule. The renal vessels are elongated, the artery more so than the vein. The suprarenal body does not move with the kidney. The attachments of the kidney to the duodenum and the ascending colon on the right side and to the pancreas and the descending colon on the left are usually separated. Thick bands of adhesions between the kidney and colon may, however, be found. The kidney occasionally becomes adherent in an abnormal position such as the iliac fossa.

Torsion of the vascular pedicle may occur even when the excursion of the kidney is moderate. The renal vein is obstructed, and the organ becomes engorged with blood, enlarged, and dark purple with subcapsular hæmorrhages.

Kinking or twisting of the ureter may be caused by swinging of the kidney, or by its rotation on its transverse axis and twisting of the ureter over the renal vessels. The pelvis becomes distended with urine. Repetition of such attacks induces hollowing of the kidney and intermittent hydronephrosis.

Undue mobility of the kidney may exist alone or may be merely part of a general visceroptosis. The stomach is frequently dilated. Movable kidney may be the seat of interstitial nephritis, stone, tuberculosis, or new growth.

Etiology.—The average age is $33\frac{1}{2}$ years (McWilliams). Movable kidney occurs in from 5 to 10 per cent. of women and from $\frac{1}{2}$ to 1 per cent. of men. The right kidney is affected in 8 out of every 10 cases. Both kidneys are affected in 5 per cent. of cases. No single cause satisfactorily explains the occurrence of abnormal mobility of the kidney in all cases. The following factors are of importance :—

1. *Congenital mobility* is rarely observed.

2. *Anatomical factors.*—The kidneys lie in shallow recesses, one on each side of the vertebral bodies, the paravertebral fossæ. Wolkow and Delitzen state that persons with movable kidneys have shallow paravertebral fossæ which are open at the lower end. In women they are shallower and more open than in men, and on the right side more than on the left.

Mansell-Moullin holds that there is a slight rotation of the vertebræ to the right in a large number of right-sided people, and this makes the right lumbar recess shallower.

The liver does not cause downward displacement of the right kidney.

3. *Atrophy of the perirenal fat* is found in many cases.

4. *Weakness of the abdominal walls.*—Glénard states that general visceroptosis always accompanies movable kidney and results from weakness of the abdominal wall. This is disproved by statistics and experience.

5. *Injury and pressure.*—In 11·4 per cent. of cases there is a distinct history of a blow, severe muscular strain, or other injury in the region of the kidney. The wearing of corsets does not produce movable kidney.

6. *Drag of adhesions between kidney and bowel.*—Bands of adhesions, probably the result of chronic constipation, pass between the kidney and the colon, and the drag of these is a cause of movable kidney (Arbuthnot Lane).

7. *Pathological conditions of the kidney.*—Tumours, hydronephrosis, calculus, and other diseases may coexist with movable kidney, and in some cases appear to be a factor in the causation of the· mobility.

Clinical features.—Mobility of the kidney, even with wide range of movement, may be unaccompanied by symptoms.

1. **Symptoms referred to the kidney.** (a) *Pain and discomfort.*—There is renal pain of a heavy, aching character, and attacks of acute pain may occur, followed by enlargement and tenderness of the kidney. The pain is initiated and aggravated by movement and relieved by rest ; it is increased during the menstrual period.

(b) *Undue mobility.*—In slight degrees of mobility the kidney usually moves parallel with the vertebral column, but it may swing round so that the lower pole approaches the bodies of the vertebræ— " cinder-sifting movement " (Morris). In another form the upper end of the kidney falls forward, while the lower end remains in contact with the posterior abdominal wall. In the wider ranges of movement the kidney descends below the costal margin, at first vertically, and then the lower pole swings towards the vertebral column so that the hilum faces upwards. Exceptionally, the pedicle is so long that the kidney may be found in almost any part of the abdomen, and may descend into the true pelvis.

The movable kidney is uninfluenced by respiratory movements, and escapes from the grasp with a sudden slip that is characteristic, the patient experiencing a sickening sensation. The tumour can be reduced into the loin, and is then no longer palpable.

(c) Some *lack of resistance* is detected in the loin of the affected side when the patient is examined on her hands and knees.

(d) *Enlargement of the kidney.*—Intermittent hydronephrosis not infrequently results from abnormal mobility.

(e) *Changes in the urine.*—Hæmaturia is rare, but it may follow muscular exertion. Albuminuria is frequently observed, and disappears on resting. Tube casts due to venous congestion are present in the urine in 8 out of 180 cases (Newman). Transient polyuria coincides with the relief of an attack of hydronephrosis. Anuria may result from torsion of the renal pedicle, and has been known to last for nine days without ill after-effects.

Frequent micturition may be reflex during an attack of pain, or the result of polyuria after an attack of hydronephrosis.

2. **Symptoms referred to other organs.** (a) *Gastro-intestinal symptoms.*—There may be epigastric pain and burning unconnected with the taking of food. The patient complains of a sinking sensation, loss of appetite, nausea, eructations, a feeling of distension, and vomiting, and becomes thin and anæmic. In such cases the stomach is usually distended, and may be displaced ; the right kidney is movable and the condition is due to the drag of adhesions on the second part of the duodenum or of a thickened band of peritoneum on the pylorus. Recurrent attacks of flatulent distension of the colon and constipation, perhaps resembling intestinal obstruction, may be caused by adhesions between the kidney and large intestine. Jaundice, epigastric pain, and distension of the gall-bladder may repeatedly occur ; they have been ascribed to pressure of the kidney on the common bile-duct, or to dragging of the kidney upon the second part of the duodenum.

(b) *Nervous symptoms.*—Mobility of the kidney is often accompanied by neurasthenia of various degrees, and is considered by Suckling to be a cause of some forms of insanity.

Dietl's crises.—The patient is liable to crises which may be due to dragging on adhesions connected with the pylorus or bowel or to torsion of the vascular pedicle or kinking of the ureter. The attack may follow a muscular effort. (a) When the stomach or bowel is affected there is severe epigastric or general abdominal pain. Vomiting and collapse are usual. The abdominal muscles are rigid, especially on the side of the movable kidney. Later, the abdomen becomes distended and tympanitic. The bowels are constipated, and the temperature may be raised. (*b*) When the ureter is obstructed the kidney becomes large and tender, the urine is diminished, and there may be complete anuria. The attack lasts some hours or even days. (*c*) With torsion of the renal pedicle there are again acute abdominal symptoms. In addition the urine becomes scanty, albuminous, and sometimes bloody, and complete suppression may supervene. The kidney is painful, large, and tender. Polyuria may follow the attack, and the urine contains blood, and hyaline, granular, and blood casts.

Diagnosis.—The following conditions may give rise to difficulty in diagnosis :—

1. *A distended gall-bladder.*—The presence of jaundice, the constantly palpable tumour, the restricted range of movement, the area of dullness blending with that of the liver, the absence of a bowel note in front of the tumour, are characteristic of the distended gall-bladder.

2. *Riedel's lobe of the liver.*—The respiratory movement is the same as that of the liver, and greater than that of the kidney, the dullness is continuous with that of the liver, and the edge of the swelling is sharp.

3. *Small ovarian tumour with a long pedicle.*—This can be reduced into the pelvis, but not into the loin ; the pedicle is attached below and can be demonstrated from the vagina.

4. *Malignant growth of the intestine.*

5. *Scybalous masses in the intestine.*

In doubtful cases an opaque catheter should be passed up the ureter, the pelvis of the kidney filled with collargol (10 per cent.), and a radiogram obtained.

Treatment.—Operation is imperative—(1) where the mobility is causing disease of the kidney ; (2) where the kidney is exerting harmful traction on other organs ; (3) where the kidney lies below the waist line and is uncontrolled by a mechanical apparatus ; (4) when the patient is going to reside in tropical and uncivilised countries ; (5) where the patient has to perform manual labour and cannot afford an expensive apparatus. But in most cases palliative treatment may be tried before resorting to operation.

Operative treatment is likely to fail—(1) where general visceroptosis is present ; (2) where there is severe neurasthenia and no symptoms can be referred to the kidney.

In a few cases of movable kidney with neurasthenia, control of the renal movements by a mechanical apparatus will alleviate or cure the neurasthenia, and in these cases also operation will be followed by a similar result.

Palliative treatment. 1. *By rest and by increasing the body* *fat.*—It is hoped to obtain an increased deposit of fat around the kidney, but this does not obtain in practice. This treatment is, however, a useful adjunct to other methods. In severe cases the full Weir-Mitchell treatment should be insisted upon.

2. *By mechanical apparatus.*—The kidney truss exerts pressure upwards and outwards by a thin padded metal plate (Ernst). It must be applied lying down.

The kidney belt is an abdominal belt coming down over the iliac crest and accurately moulded to the hips. The lower border follows the curve of the groin and overlaps the pubic bones. There is an elastic inset on each side, and perineal straps are attached. An oval or horse-shoe-shaped kidney pad is added. The belt must be applied when the patient is lying down. It may be fitted to the lower part of a corset.

The corset for movable kidney (Gallant) is accurately fitted. Below the waist it is inflexible and elastic; above the waist it permits free play of the trunk.

Operative treatment.—The kidney is exposed by an oblique lumbar incision or by a vertical incision along the outer border of the erector spinæ muscle. The kidney is then fixed—(*a*) By sutures passing through the kidney capsule or through the kidney substance, carried through the muscles of the abdominal wall at the upper edge of the wound, and tied. (*b*) By stripping the capsule of the kidney (decortication). (*c*) By stitching the stripped capsule to the parietes; the capsule may be rolled up on the anterior or posterior surface, or split into wedges or strips. (*d*) By partial stripping and by sutures through the substance of the kidney. (*e*) By placing strips of gauze below the lower pole to promote granulation and cicatrization. (*f*) By the formation of a shelf of peritoneum or fibrous capsule; this may be done by stitching through the parietal peritoneum and abdominal muscles below the kidney after opening the peritoneal cavity (Bishop), or by reflecting a strip of fibrous capsule and stitching it below the kidney without opening the abdomen (Watson Cheyne).

Results.—The operative mortality is stated at 1 per cent., but it is lower than this in skilled hands. In 116 cases examined not less than three months after operation, Keen found that 57·8 per cent. were cured and 12·9 per cent. improved, while in 19·8 per cent. the operation had failed. Failure consisted either in recurrence of the mobility or in persistence of the pain.

INJURIES TO THE KIDNEY

1. Injuries without External Wound

The right side is more often affected than the left, and the injury is rarely bilateral.

Etiology.—Rupture of the kidney may be due to a direct blow, kick, or squeeze, or to indirect violence, as in a fall from a height on to the buttocks, or in forcible acute flexion of the body, when the kidney may be injured by impact against the 12th rib or the transverse process of a vertebra.

Pathology.—There may be tearing of the fatty capsule alone, with perirenal hæmorrhage and subsequent formation of fibrous tissue, or a slight subcapsular rupture of the kidney, with accumulation of blood beneath the fibrous capsule, or a laceration of both fibrous capsule and kidney substance which may reach the renal pelvis. The tears radiate transversely from the hilum, and affect especially the anterior surface and lower pole, but may be complete. Sometimes the ureter or a large branch of the renal artery is ruptured. Laceration of the renal pelvis or of a calyx is common. The peritoneum may be torn, and blood and urine poured into the peritoneal cavity. This occurs more frequently in children, since the protective layer of perinephric fat is not developed before the tenth year. Ribs may be fractured, or the spinal column, pelvic girdle, bowel, liver, spleen, bladder, or lungs injured. Repair takes place rapidly in slight injuries. Infection and suppuration causing perinephritic abscess, suppurative nephritis, pyonephrosis, and peritonitis occur in 11·8 per cent. of cases.

Symptoms.—Shock is present in all severe grades of rupture. It may be delayed for some hours, so that the patient may walk a considerable distance after the accident, and only collapse when he sees blood in the urine. Pain radiates along the ureter and is accompanied by retraction of the testicle. It is especially severe when clots are passing along the ureter. There is also dull, heavy, deep-seated pain, increased by pressure and movement. The abdominal muscles are rigidly contracted. Soon after the injury, or some days later, a tumour due to perirenal effusion of blood appears in the loin. It is dull on percussion and tender on palpation, and may be movable (pseudohydronephrosis). It is usually diffuse and obscured by rigidity of the muscles. If the swelling is clearly outlined and "ballottement" can be obtained, the renal pelvis has been distended with blood and a hæmatonephrosis formed.

Hæmaturia is present in 91·5 per cent. of cases. It is absent when the rupture does not penetrate the renal pelvis or calyces, when the ureter is plugged with clot or ruptured by the violence. Blood may be delayed for some days. In half the cases it has disappeared in a week, but it may persist and appear intermittently for several weeks and may be fatal after two to three weeks. In copious bleeding there is clotting in the bladder with retention of urine.

Secondary hæmorrhage due to suppuration and necrosis of the kidney occurs. Temporary or persistent anuria is sometimes observed, and is due to previous disease or atrophy of the uninjured kidney.

Discoloration of the skin at the external abdominal ring, scrotum, or labium may appear, after a fortnight or three weeks, as the result of blood tracking along the spermatic vein. Intraperitoneal effusion of blood and urine may be detected in the pouch of Douglas on rectal examination.

The possible **complications and sequelæ** are—(1) anuria, (2) intraperitoneal hæmorrhage, (3) pseudo-hydronephrosis, (4) retention of urine, (5) septic complications, (6) traumatic hydronephrosis, (7) movable kidney, (8) traumatic nephritis.

Course and prognosis.—In favourable cases the urine clears in a few days, and the symptoms disappear in ten days. In severe cases the immediate dangers are shock and hæmorrhage, and the remote, septic complications and anuria. The later the onset and the less acute the progress of the septic process the better the prognosis. Prognosis is chiefly affected by hæmorrhage and by injury to other organs. Recovery takes place in 70 per cent. of uncomplicated cases.

Treatment.—Slight and moderately severe uncomplicated ruptures are treated by efficient strapping of the side and a covering broad bandage. by ice-bags over and under the loin, and by absolute rest in the recumbent position. The food should be fluid. Calcium lactate is given in doses of 10–15 gr. every four hours. for forty-eight hours, and morphia administered hypodermically. Shock. if not profound, should not be too energetically treated. lest bleeding be encouraged. If there is retention the bladder should be emptied under the most rigid aseptic precautions. An evacuating cannula and bulb may be used to empty the bladder of clot; but if this measure is not quickly successful the bladder should be opened suprapubically. the clots cleared out, and a large drain inserted.

Operation on the kidney may be required for—(1) immediate severe hæmorrhage, (2) delayed severe hæmorrhage, (3) suppuration of the injured kidney, (4) septic peritonitis, (5) hydronephrosis or pyonephrosis. The kidney is exposed by an oblique lumbar incision, the clots are cleared away, and a search made for the bleeding-point. Tears of the kidney are closed with catgut sutures. and extensive laceration and bruising by packing with strips of gauze. A distended renal pelvis should be incised. the clots turned out, and the pelvis packed with gauze. Detached portions and shreds of kidney tissue are removed, and primary nephrectomy may be necessary. Rectal and intravenous infusion of glucose solution (1 per cent.) should be given after the operation.

Suppuration should be treated by free incision and drainage, and laparotomy may be necessary for septic peritonitis. Persistent anuria is treated by nephrotomy and packing (*see also* p. 783).

Results.—The results have greatly improved in recent years with early aseptic operations. Operative interference in septic complications should not be too long delayed. In uncomplicated cases the death-rate is 18·9 per cent. In cases treated expectantly the mortality is 21·1 per cent. ; in conservative operations, 11·7 per cent. ; and in nephrectomy, 17·9 per cent. (Riese).

2. Injuries with External Wound

Wounds of the kidney are much less frequent than subcutaneous injuries. The intestine, spleen, liver, or pleura may also be wounded. The blood escapes by the external wound, and, unless there is a long sinuous track, no accumulation takes place around the kidney. The kidney may prolapse from a large wound. Primary union is rare, prolonged suppuration common. Urinary fistulæ occur, but seldom persist.

Symptoms.—There is external hæmorrhage, and urine escapes through the wound after a few days when the hæmorrhage is subsiding. Hæmorrhage from stab wounds may be severe and rapidly fatal. In bullet wounds the external hæmorrhage is seldom severe, but it may be intermittent. Pain is persistent, but does not radiate along the ureter. Occasionally, flatus from laceration of the intestine may be passed from the external wound. Septic complications occur on the fourth or fifth day, and portions of clothing and sloughs may be discharged.

Prognosis.—This is comparatively good, and operation is frequently successful. Wounds of other organs increase the gravity of the prognosis. The mortality of incised wounds is as low as 15 per cent. (Albarran), but bullet wounds have a high mortality—53 per cent. (Küster).

Treatment.—If the external hæmorrhage is moderate and diminishing, it will be sufficient to clean and drain the wound. A careful watch must be kept for recurrent hæmorrhage and septic complications. If a foreign body has lodged, or hæmorrhage is severe, the track should be freely enlarged, and the kidney exposed and examined. In complicated cases exploratory laparotomy is necessary.

ANEURYSM OF THE RENAL ARTERY

[Only 25 cases of this rare condition were found in the literature by Skillern in 1906. It is most often caused by trauma in active men, but may occur spontaneously in either sex in association with endocarditis or arterial degeneration. The size varies from that of a hazel-nut to a large swelling occupying the whole loin and extending inwards as far as the middle line. When the aneurysm is large, and especially when a false aneurysm has formed, the kidney tissue is extensively destroyed by pressure, the colon displaced forwards and inwards, and the liver or spleen pushed upwards.

Clinical features.—A small aneurysm produces no symptoms; a large one forms a swelling in the kidney region. The tumour usually appears some days or weeks after an injury, but two or even fourteen years may elapse. The swelling is smooth, slightly movable or fixed, and does not move with respiration; it is rarely painful or tender. Hæmaturia is early, and usually precedes the discovery of the swelling. Profuse and rapidly fatal hæmorrhage follows rupture into the renal pelvis or peritoneal cavity. Pulsation has rarely been observed. Morris found a loud systolic bruit over the tumour in one case.

Treatment.—The condition will usually be diagnosed during an exploratory laparotomy. A small opening in the sac should be sufficient to permit recognition of the laminated character of the contents. If severe hæmorrhage takes place the wound should be plugged with gauze, the abdomen opened in the semilunar line, and the pedicle of the kidney exposed and ligatured. The aneurysmal sac and kidney are then removed. In three cases operation has been successful.

PERINEPHRITIS

Chronic perinephritis leads to the formation around the kidney of a layer of inflammatory tissue, either fibro-sclerotic or fibro-lipomatous, and tough adhesions are formed with surrounding structures.

Some form of chronic inflammatory disease of the kidney is invariably present, such as pyelonephritis, pyonephrosis, calculus, or tuberculosis.

In the sclerotic form the fatty capsule of the kidney is replaced by a dense layer of fibrous tissue, sometimes of cartilaginous hardness. In the more common fibro-lipomatous form the delicate perirenal fat is replaced by coarse nodular fat with a tough fibrous stroma. The fibro-lipomatous mass may develop principally around the pelvis or at one pole.

The symptoms and treatment are merged in those of the underlying renal disease. The movements of the kidney are not appreciably limited.

PERINEPHRITIC ABSCESS

A perinephritic abscess may occur at any age, and may be primary or secondary. Men are more frequently affected than women, and the right side more often than the left.

Etiology.—The primary form may follow injury. More frequently it develops during the course of typhoid, scarlatina, measles, or pneumonia, tonsillitis, carbuncle, or even eczema. The secondary form complicates suppuration in some neighbouring organ, such as the kidney (25 per cent.), liver, gall-bladder, appendix, pelvic organs, or vertebræ. Tuberculous perinephritic abscess is especially found in tuberculous disease of the vertebræ, and is very rarely secondary to tuberculosis of the kidney. Pus from an empyema or an abscess of the lung may track through the costo-lumbar hiatus of the diaphragm and form a perinephritic abscess.

Bacteriology.—The bacteria found, in their order of frequency, are Bacillus coli, streptococcus, staphylococcus. The gonococcus and pneumococcus are rare.

Pathology.—The collection is usually unilocular, but occasionally multilocular. It is situated outside the fibrous capsule, and may be inside or outside the perinephric fascia. In the former case the pus will spread along the ureter into the bony pelvis, while in the latter it will appear on the surface of the body over the iliac crest or pass into the iliac fossa. Four varieties are distinguished according to situation:

1. Above the kidney, or subphrenic, which is frequently connected with intrathoracic suppuration. The kidney is pushed down and may be felt below the mass.

2. Below the kidney, which tends to pass downwards to the iliac fossa and may rupture into and pass along inside the psoas sheath and appear in Scarpa's triangle, or pass into the pelvis and escape at the sciatic notch.

3. In front of the kidney, limited by peritoneum; this is rare. It may rupture into the peritoneal cavity, bowel, bladder, or vagina.

4. Behind the kidney, a much more common variety which may pass through the lumbar muscles at the triangle of Petit.

Symptoms.—When perinephritic abscess complicates some other disease the symptoms are superadded to those of the primary disease. When the perinephritic suppuration is primary the onset is usually insidious and the pain slight and insignificant. The general condition of the patient is bad, and there is high remittent fever, though in rare cases the temperature is not raised. Occasionally the onset is sudden and heralded by a rigor. Pain and tenderness over the kidney become marked. The pain may radiate to the shoulder or arm, but more frequently passes downwards to the scrotum or labium. It is increased by movement, respiration, coughing and sneezing. The abdominal muscles are rigid on the diseased side.

The corresponding thigh is stiff and becomes flexed and rotated slightly outwards. Extension is restricted, but flexion unlimited. There may be transient paralysis of the lower limb.

The whole loin bulges outwards and backwards. The anterior swelling is less than in kidney tumours. The tumour does not move on respiration, and there is little movement on palpation. In suprarenal perinephritic abscess there may be jaundice, ascites, and œdema of the legs, and persistent vomiting when the right side is affected. In infrarenal abscess there are symptoms of involvement of the psoas muscle, neuralgic pain in the groin and genitals, retraction of the testicle, and constipation. Œdema in the loin may be present, especially if the abscess be behind the kidney. When the kidney is diseased there is pyuria. In acute cases, pus forms in from ten to twelve days ; in subacute, in three or four weeks.

In tuberculous cases acute symptoms are absent, and pain and tenderness are slight.

If no operation is performed, either the patient dies of septicæmia or the abscess ruptures on the surface or into the pleura, bronchi, colon, peritoneum, bladder, or vagina.

Diagnosis.—The condition may be mistaken for typhoid fever in the early stage, and for hip-joint disease or pyonephrosis at a later period. When only fever and general symptoms are present, leucocytosis will show that suppuration is going on in the body, a negative Widal reaction will exclude typhoid fever, and examination of the blood will eliminate malaria. Against hip-joint disease there are freedom of flexion and rotation of the thigh and absence of local tenderness.

A pyonephrosis is regular and well defined ; it moves with respiration, projects forwards rather than laterally or backwards, and does not cause œdema of the skin. A pyonephrosis may be present and be concealed by a perinephritic abscess.

Prognosis.—Good results are obtained by prompt operation in primary cases. The longer the operation is delayed the worse is the prognosis. In secondary perinephritic abscess the prognosis depends upon the original cause.

Treatment.—Early operation is the only successful method. The kidney is exposed by an oblique incision, and all pockets of the abscess drained, care being taken not to overlook iliac and subphrenic collections of pus.

If the kidney is the seat of abscess, pyelonephritis, or pyonephrosis, it should be freely incised and drained. If nephrectomy be necessary it should be postponed to a later date. When the abscess has originated in an empyema, this should be drained.

In old-standing cases with persistent sinuses a diseased kidney or an imperfectly drained empyema may necessitate nephrectomy, resection of portions of ribs, or other secondary operations.

The mortality of cases treated without operation is 80 per cent., and of operated cases 7·1 per cent. (Watson).

SURGICAL INFLAMMATIONS OF THE KIDNEY AND PELVIS

These may be bacterial or nonbacterial, and caused by mechanical ꭐeans or by the excretion of irritants.

ASEPTIC PYELONEPHRITIS

This form of pyelonephritis occurs under the following conditions :—

1. *In acute retention of urine.*—Guyon and Albarran have shown that in retention of urine there may be acute congestion of both kidneys, progressing to interstitial and intratubular hæmorrhages with desquamation of tubular epithelium. The quantities of urine and of renal salts are reduced, and blood, renal cells, and epithelial and blood casts are present. Polyuria follows relief of the retention, and the urine contains casts for several days. If the obstruction is completely relieved and sepsis is absent, the symptoms entirely disappear.

2. *Due to excretion of irritants.*—A mild catarrhal pyelonephritis may be induced by the elimination of certain balsamics, such as sandalwood, copaiba, and turpentine.

3. *In chronic urinary obstruction.*—In this condition the ureters and renal pelvis become dilated and thickened, and chronic interstitial nephritis develops. Both kidneys are affected, but usually unequally.

The **symptoms** are slight and easily overlooked. Dull aching pain in one or both kidneys, constant thirst, especially at night, and anorexia are associated with frontal headache and appreciable loss of weight. The temperature is slightly subnormal, and the tongue dry. There are no cardiac or vascular changes ; the kidneys cannot be felt and are not tender.

The urine is pale and clear, free from tube casts and cells, and contains a low percentage of urea and other urinary constituents. The polyuria amounts to 80–100 ounces per diem, and is more marked at night.

INFECTIONS OF THE KIDNEY AND PELVIS

Bacteriology.—The Bacillus coli is the commonest cause of renal infection ; next in frequency come the staphylococci (especially aureus), streptococci, Proteus vulgaris (Hauser), and B. pyocyaneus ; the pneumococcus and the gonococcus are rare. The B. coli is usually found in pure culture, but sometimes is mixed with proteus, staphylococcus, or streptococcus. Anaerobic bacteria are occasionally found,

2 z

especially in pyonephrosis. The staphylococcus and Proteus vulgaris cause ammoniacal decomposition ; in the rare pure streptococcal and in the common B. coli infections the urine remains acid.

Pyelonephritis occurs in two forms—(a) primary or " hæmatogenous " pyelonephritis, appearing without previous urinary disease, and believed to be caused by blood-borne bacteria ; and (b) secondary or " ascending " pyelonephritis, which follows infection of the lower urinary tract.

(a) **Primary or hæmatogenous pyelonephritis.** — This disease occurs in infants, children, and adults. In infants and young children it is comparatively common, and affects the pelvis more severely than the kidney. In adults it exhibits a predilection for the right kidney, for the most active period of life, and for the female sex, especially during pregnancy (see p. 808).

Etiology.—Usually there is a history of chronic constipation, and sometimes of recent diarrhœa ; in such cases the colon is probably the chief source of the bacteria.   Tonsillitis, boils, or carbuncles may be the primary focus, while the renal infection occasionally complicates influenza or typhoid fever.

(b) **Secondary or ascending pyelonephritis.**—This disease results from extension of infection from the lower urinary organs. It is the last phase of many chronic vesical and urethral diseases, and sometimes follows surgical interference with the bladder or urethra (" surgical kidney "). Although at first often unilateral, later it is invariably bilateral, affecting one side more than the other.   As seen by the surgeon, the disease is bilateral in 83 per cent. of cases.

Etiology.—Bacteria are introduced into the bladder by faulty instrumentation, or rarely are carried from a previously infected urethra by a sterile instrument. The predisposing causes are urethral obstruction, prolonged cystitis, vesical new growths, operations on the bladder involving the ureteric orifice, and stone in the bladder or ureter.

Pathology of infective pyelonephritis.—In the *acute* forms there may be extensive hæmorrhages in the renal substance, with irregular pale or yellowish purulent areas in the cortex and medulla.   Sometimes small bosses on the surface correspond to the position of these areas. Microscopically, definite abscesses are seen, with destruction of kidney tissue, and cloudy swelling of the secretory epithelium is a prominent feature.   There are patches of dense infiltration with leucocytes.

In the most *fulminating* types the kidney is plum-coloured, with dark cortex and paler pyramids, and is engorged with blood.

In the *chronic* varieties the abscesses may be still present, but there is always marked interstitial change, and at points collections of small round lymphocyte-like cells are seen. At places the tubules and glomeruli may be destroyed by the newly formed fibrous tissue. In very advanced cases the kidney may be much reduced in size, very tough, and firmly adherent to the surrounding tissues. It may contain small cysts.

Clinical features. (1) Acute hæmatogenous pyelonephritis.—The attack is often preceded by headache, lassitude, and anorexia, and by diarrhœa or by an exaggeration of habitual constipation. In 6 per cent. of cases there is a sudden desire to micturate, followed by great frequency and strangury lasting a few hours or a day or two.

In a *mild* case there is a rigor followed by rise of temperature to 101° or 102°, aching in one loin, and tenderness, without enlargement, of one kidney. The urine is abundant, pale, with low specific gravity and a stale-fish odour, and bacteruria is present. The attack lasts ten or fourteen days.

In a *more severe* attack the temperature reaches 102° or 103°, the patient is prostrate, drowsy, perhaps delirious, and suffers general abdominal pain, and also backache, especially in one loin. The diseased kidney, which, as a rule, is palpably enlarged, is intensely tender, and the abdominal muscles on that side are rigid. The urine is scanty, acid (very rarely alkaline), and contains bacteria, pus cells, blood corpuscles, tube casts, and epithelia from the rènal pelvis and bladder. The leucocyte count is 18,000 to 20,000. The Bacillus coli has been found in the blood, especially in children.

After two or three weeks the acute symptoms may subside, but may repeatedly recur owing to exacerbations in the first kidney or to fresh infection of the second kidney.

The illness may last for months. Instead of pursuing a benign course, there may be repeated rigors, a high swinging temperature (106° to 107°), and death occurs in four or six weeks from the onset.

In the rare *fulminating* cases a severe rigor and rise of temperature to 104° or 106° is followed by drowsiness and coma. There are abdominal pain and rigidity, vomiting, and scantiness or complete suppression of urine.

(2) Acute ascending pyelonephritis.—During the course of some disease of the lower urinary organs, and usually as a sequel to instrumentation, there is a rigor with a rise of temperature to 102° or 104°. Drowsiness, apathy, and backache, more marked on one side, are frequently associated with nausea, vomiting, absolute constipation, and increasingly distressing hiccup. The tongue is dry, red, and glazed, and later becomes covered with brown or black fur ("parrot tongue"). The abdomen shows flatulent distension and rigidity, especially on one side. At first both kidneys are tender,

but after twenty-four hours this is confined to one organ, which is enlarged. Polyuria has frequently been present beforehand, but now is replaced by partial or complete suppression. The temperature may remain at 102° or over, or may be high and swinging with recurring rigors. Labial herpes is common.

The symptoms increase in severity, muttering delirium supervenes, and the patient becomes comatose and dies. Uræmic dyspnœa and Cheyne-Stokes breathing may be present, but convulsions are extremely rare. In less severe cases the secretion of urine becomes re-established, the temperature falls, flatus is passed, and the symptoms subside.

Some cases are characterized by recurrent hæmorrhages.

(3) Chronic suppurative pyelonephritis. — Chronic pyelonephritis may follow acute pyelonephritis, whether hæmatogenous or ascending, or may be engrafted on a chronic aseptic pyelonephritis; when fully developed it gives rise to " urinary septicæmia." The complexion is sallow, the skin dry and harsh, the mouth and throat dry, the tongue dry, and later glazed, red, and cracked. There are dyspepsia, nausea, frontal headache, and constant drowsiness, with persistent loss of weight and appetite.

The urine is abundant (80–100 oz. per diem), pale, neutral or faintly acid, of sp. gr. about 1006, and hazy with pus or with flakes. Bacteria are plentiful, but bacteriuria only occasionally occurs. Nocturnal polyuria and vesical irritation are the chief subjects of complaint. In the ascending variety the symptoms of the primary lower disease are also present. Acute exacerbations are probable from time to time, especially after surgical intervention.

Prognosis.—(1) In mild cases of **hæmatogenous** pyelonephritis the prognosis is good, but relapses may occur, and in a large percentage of cases bacteriuria or slight chronic pyelonephritis persists. In acute cases the outlook is grave, and operation is frequently necessary. Fulminating cases frequently terminate fatally.

(2) Many patients die during the acute attack of **ascending** pyelonephritis, and most of those that recover suffer from chronic pyelonephritis. Removal of the urinary obstruction will probably arrest the disease, but the kidneys are permanently damaged.

(3) Chronic pyelonephritis persists for years, and eventually destroys the kidney. The dangers of secondary stone formation in the kidney and of ascending pyelonephritis in the other kidney are ever present.

Treatment. (1) Acute hæmatogenous pyelonephritis. (a) *Medicinal.*—Mild and early cases may be suitably treated by confinement to bed, and the application of cupping or of hot fomentations and turpentine stupes over the loins, combined with the administration of urinary antiseptics such as urotropine, hetraline, or helmitol, and the free use of alkalis and diuretics such as theocin sodium acetate, potassium citrate, and Contrexéville water. A smart purge, followed by small doses ($\frac{1}{20}$ to $\frac{1}{6}$ gr.) of calomel, should be given.

(b) *Serum treatment.*—The suitable anti-serum, usually the anti-ba'cillus coli serum, may be hypodermically injected in daily doses of 25 c.c. for three days, accompanied by calcium lactate in 20-gr. doses thrice daily by the mouth to prevent joint pains and serum rashes. This treatment is only suitable for acute cases, and should be abandoned if not effectual in three days.

(c) *Vaccine treatment.*—Graduated doses of dead bacteria are injected from autogenous cultures, or from stock vaccine if time prevents the preparation of an autovaccine. Beginning with small doses of 2 or 3 millions, repeated in four or five days, the dose rises rapidly to 10, 15, 20, 25, 30 millions, and so on to 100, 150, and 200. These injections should be made once a week ; if any reaction occurs, the doses should be reduced and a longer interval allowed. This treatment is only suitable for chronic cases where no complication such as growth or stone is present.

(d) *Operative treatment.*—Only nephrotomy and nephrectomy need be considered. I have collected 20 cases of nephrotomy with 7 deaths ; these include 5 personal cases, all of whom survived nephrotomy. The after-results of nephrotomy are unsatisfactory ; chronic pyelonephritis persists, and nephrectomy may be required later. Nephrectomy gives the best results in acute cases ; of 17 collected cases, all recovered. ·

(2) **Acute ascending pyelonephritis.**—(a) *Prophylactic measures* consist in rigid asepsis and the utmost gentleness in all urethral manipulations.

(b) *Non-operative treatment* is conducted on the lines laid down for acute hæmatogenous pyelonephritis (above). Sweating may be induced by a hot pack or hot vapour bath, and by hypodermic injection of pilocarpine. Suppression of urine demands rectal or intravenous infusion of glucose solution (*see* Anuria, p. 783).

(c) *Operative treatment.*—This is necessary if non-operative measures fail ; it aims at two objects—removal of urinary obstruction if present, and relief of congestion and drainage of the kidney. Any unrelieved urinary obstruction first receives attention. Suprapubic cystotomy rapidly performed, and the insertion of a large tube, gives the best drainage with the least shock. The obstruction can be more permanently treated later if the patient survive. For relief of the renal congestion and sepsis, the kidney should be freely incised along the convex border and a large rubber drain introduced into its pelvis ; another large drain is placed outside the kidney.

Nephrectomy may become necessary in the hæmorrhagic type of pyelonephritis.

(3) **Chronic pyelonephritis.**—Prophylaxis consists in all measures directed against chronic obstruction and sepsis in the lower urinary organs.

When chronic pyelonephritis has become established, operative interference with bladder or urethra must be undertaken with the utmost caution. Suprapubic drainage should precede prostatectomy by a week or more, and external urethrotomy should be preferred to dilatation or internal urethrotomy for stricture. Urinary antiseptics and diuretics should be freely administered.

If the second kidney is proved to be healthy by examination of its urine, nephrectomy may be performed. Circumstances, however, rarely render this possible.

In chronic hæmatogenous pyelonephritis operation may be necessary for recurrent exacerbations, persistent cystitis, secondary calculus, or, rarely, anuria.

Vaccine treatment, at any rate in cases complicated by stone, growth, or obstruction, has not given satisfactory results.

PYELITIS

The intimate relation between the kidney and the renal pelvis precludes absolute limitation of severe inflammation to one or other, but there are cases of mild subacute or chronic inflammation where the pelvis is affected and the kidney but slightly involved.

Etiology.—Mid adult life is most frequently affected. The infection may be hæmatogenous, or may ascend from the lower urinary organs. A calculus may be present in the renal pelvis.

Pathology.—The mucous membrane is hyperæmic, and in severe forms is thickened, velvety, and may show petechiæ and superficial ulceration. In old-standing pyelitis the wall is thick and leathery, the mucous membrane is opaque and may show small colloid-filled cysts (pyelitis cystica) or tiny sago-grain lymph-follicles (pyelitis granulosa). The condition may be unilateral or bilateral.

Symptoms.—These are usually insignificant in non-calculous pyelitis. The temperature may rise to 100° F. at night, and there is slight constant renal aching with occasionally some tenderness on pressure. The kidney is not enlarged.

Polyuria is present, most markedly at night. The urine is pale, opalescent, acid, of low specific gravity (1008), and usually odourless, but occasionally it has a fishy smell. On standing, it deposits a flat creamy layer of pus which moves heavily on tilting the glass. Microscopically, bacteria and tailed and overlapping epithelial cells are seen, but no tube casts.

Cystoscopically the ureteric efflux is copious, frequently repeated, and cloudy. The lips of the ureteric orifice are reddened and thick and surrounded by a halo of congestion. Urethral catheterization demonstrates the characteristic urine, which may be alkaline on the diseased side.

The symptoms of pyelitis may be obscured by those of cystitis.

Diagnosis.—In cystitis the diagnosis depends upon the presence of renal aching, the observation of a cloudy efflux and changes at the ureteric orifice, and the examination of a specimen drawn by the ureteric catheter. It is incomplete until calculus has been found or excluded.

Treatment.—Any cause of local irritation such as stone should be removed, and diseases of the lower urinary tract such as stricture and enlarged prostate treated.

Urinary antiseptics (urotropine, hetralin, helmitol) and diuretic waters (Contrexéville, Evian, Vittel) should be given.

Vaccine treatment should be tried in chronic cases (*see* Pyelo-nephritis, p. 805).

Instillations of argyrol and other silver preparations may be made through the ureteric catheter, but are only justifiable in expert hands.

In severe cases, where all methods of treatment have failed, the kidney should be exposed, the pelvis opened, drained by a rubber tube and washed with nitrate of silver solution.

PYELITIS OF INFANCY AND CHILDHOOD

Many cases are met with in infants and older children, especially girls. There is frequently a history of constipation, and sometimes of diarrhœa.

The **symptoms** begin suddenly with a rigor, followed by rise of temperature (104° to 106° F.), which becomes remittent in type. The child is pale, restless, and distressed. Anorexia is marked, and delirium, squinting, and vomiting follow. Emaciation is slow. There may be repeated chills.

The local symptoms are insignificant. Attacks of screaming due to colic occur, and there may be tenderness on palpation of the kidney. There is occasionally pain during and increased frequency of micturition. Yellowish staining of the diapers may be the first sign.

The urine is strongly acid and contains pus, some albumin, red blood-corpuscles, epithelial cells from the renal pelvis and sometimes from the bladder, and occasionally hyaline and finely granular casts. Bacteria are present, usually the Bacillus coli, occasionally the staphy-lococcus or the streptococcus.

Diagnosis.—This depends upon the examination of the urine.

Pyrexia with extreme distress and rigors without other symptoms in a child under two years where malaria can be excluded are usually due to pyelitis (J. Thomson).

The condition has been mistaken for malaria, typhoid, and general tuberculosis.

Prognosis.—Rapid improvement under treatment and recovery is the rule, but a fatal termination occasionally occurs.

Treatment.—Citrate of potash is given in doses of 24 gr., or in severe cases 36–48 gr., per day, in infusion of digitalis, and continued till the danger of relapse is past ; urotropine and salol may be added.

Operative measures are rarely necessary. Nephrotomy may be performed if the child is steadily losing ground.

Pyelitis (Pyelonephritis) of Pregnancy

Pyelonephritis not infrequently develops during pregnancy, when it has special characteristics.

Pathology.—The bacteriology is similar to that of other renal infections. The right kidney is nearly always attacked (93 per cent.), and the disease most frequently appears about the fourth month of pregnancy. It has been ascribed to compression of the ureter by the gravid uterus, but at this early stage the uterus is hardly likely to cause pressure. The infection may have followed the passage of a catheter (ascending), or may be hæmatogenous.

Symptoms.—There is a rigor and the temperature rises, with severe paroxysmal unilateral renal pain and frequent painful micturition. The urine contains pus and bacteria, but may be almost clear even in severe cases. The general condition usually remains good, although the temperature is high and swinging. In a few cases the disease is bilateral, and there are rapid emaciation, drowsiness, burning thirst, dry tongue, and other signs of uræmia. The abdomen is rigid on one side, and the kidney tender and enlarged.

Diagnosis.—This depends on the position of the pain and tenderness, and on the examination of the urine. A mistaken diagnosis of appendicitis may easily be made.

Prognosis.—Premature labour occurs in 25 per cent. of cases, and the child dies in one-third of these (Legueu). When the attack occurs early in pregnancy the puerperium is usually apyretic, but if the onset is late there is usually fever during the puerperium. If the pyelitis is late and the pregnancy goes on to full term the child is healthy and well nourished.

Bacilluria and slight pyelonephritis frequently persist, and there are exacerbations during succeeding pregnancies.

Treatment.—Prophylaxis consists in careful asepsis in catheterization, and in the treatment of constipation during pregnancy.

If bacilluria or chronic pyelonephritis is present, this should be energetically treated. The production of abortion or the induction of premature labour is seldom necessary, but may be called for in a severe case. Urinary antiseptics and vaccine treatment should be given. Nephrotomy has yielded good results in severe cases. In acute bilateral pyelonephritis, premature labour should be induced.

Nephrectomy may be necessary in grave unilateral pyelonephritis. It is well borne in the early months of pregnancy, but less so after the fifth month. The mortality is 9·5 per cent. (Cova).

PYONEPHROSIS

Pyonephrosis is distension of the kidney and its pelvis with pus or purulent urine. There are two forms—(1) pyonephrosis secondary to hydronephrosis, or uro-pyonephrosis ; (2) pyonephrosis from acute pyelonephritis.

Etiology.—The etiology of uro-pyonephrosis is similar to that of hydronephrosis. The condition is unilateral, most frequent on the right side and in women. The obstruction is usually situated high in the ureter and is due to stone, stricture, or ureteral duplication. The superadded infection is either ascending, from recent cystitis, or hæmatogenous.

Pyonephrosis developing in acute pyelonephritis may complicate chronic disease of the lower urinary organs, and is more frequent in men.

The bacteria are those of other renal infections. A pyonephrosis is "open" when the obstruction is incomplete, and "closed" when it is complete.

Pathology.—When the infection ascends, the pelvis is greatly dilated. In other cases the kidney is transformed into a large multilocular sac, and the pelvis is small and hidden. The kidney is frequently firmly adherent to its surroundings, and may be surrounded by a thick .fibro-fatty layer. The interior is lined with smooth, tough, thick membrane, and the wall contains sclerosed and infiltrated renal parenchyma.

Partial pyonephrosis may occur from blocking of one section of a dichotomous pelvis or of one or several calyces by stone. In uropyonephrosis the contents are urine with a varying admixture of pus. In pyonephrosis there is pus with little urine. Primary or secondary calculi may be present. (Fig. 538.) The ureter is dilated, thickened, and tortuous when the obstruction is low down.

Clinical features.—The symptoms of cystitis may obscure those of pyonephrosis. In the ascending variety there are usually symptoms of pyelonephritis. Suppuration in a hydronephrosis is shown by a rigor and a rise in temperature.

The symptoms of pyonephrosis are pain, tenderness, swelling, and pyuria. The pain is constant, heavy and boring in character, and tenderness is pronounced at first. There may be severe colic and also flexion of the thigh. The tumour has the characteristics of a renal tumour, and is large, firm, smooth, and non-fluctuating.

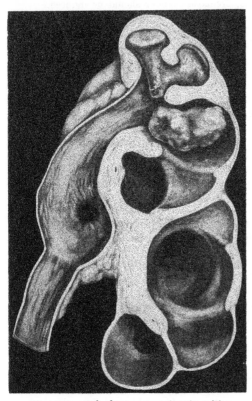

Fig. 538.—Calculous pyonephrosis with dilatation of ureter.

Pyuria is the cardinal symptom. It forms an abundant thick, heavy deposit, subject to pronounced variations in quantity. There are recurrent attacks of complete retention of pus, during which the urine becomes clear, the tumour larger, more tender, painful and tense, and the temperature rises.

On cystoscopy, cystitis is usually found, and the orifice of the ureter is seen to be open, round, and immobile, and to have thick and in some instances œdematous or ulcerated margins.

In a closed pyonephrosis an efflux is absent; in an open pyonephrosis it consists of semi-solid pus, watery pus, or purulent urine.

Diagnosis.—The diagnosis of a closed pyonephrosis depends upon the history of pyuria, and the presence of a renal tumour with symptoms of septic absorption.

If pyuria is present, this and cystoscopy will lead to a diagnosis. Large intermittent discharges of pus in the urine are found in three conditions, viz. pyonephrosis, a suppurating vesical diverticulum and a purulent collection communicating with the ureter. The cystoscope will distinguish a diverticulum of the bladder, and pyonephrosis has a characteristic tumour.

In pyelonephritis without retention there is a small quantity of pus in the urine, and catheterization of the ureter reveals no obstruction.

In tuberculous pyonephrosis there are tubercle bacilli in the urine and often tuberculous lesions elsewhere ; the tuberculous ureter is thick and hard, and the general tests for tuberculosis are positive.

Treatment.—1. Continuous drainage by ureteral catheters of increasing calibre and daily lavage of the pelvis are seldom practicable.

2. Plastic operations are referred to under Hydronephrosis (p. 818), but they are usually rendered worthless by the extensive functional destruction of the kidney.

3. Nephrotomy may be confined to incision and drainage of the kidney, or an attempt may be made to re-establish the lumen of the ureter. The pyonephrotic sac is opened through an oblique lumbar incision, the contents evacuated, septa broken down, search made for interstitial abscesses and for stone, and a large tube placed in the nephrotomy wound and another outside the kidney. This operation is rapid and devoid of shock, and is suitable for the worst cases. The mortality is 17–23 per cent. After the operation the general health and the function of the second kidney show great improvement. In 27 per cent. of cases (Küster) the wound closes, the sac shrinks, and the patient is cured.

A fistula remains in from 45·6 to 56 per cent. of the cases (Küster). Attempts to obviate it have been made by passing sounds from above downwards (Bazy) or from the bladder upwards (Albarran), and by tying a catheter in the ureter. A fistula may be cured by removal of its fibrous wall, the opening up of the sac, removal of calculi, and free drainage.

Should these fail, a urine-collecting apparatus may be fitted, or nephrectomy may be performed.

4. Secondary nephrectomy is indicated where septicæmia persists or exhaustion is following the prolonged suppuration. The mortality is 5·9 per cent., but to this must be added the mortality of nephrotomy (23·3 per cent.), making the total mortality 29·2 per cent.

Primary nephrectomy may be partial in rare cases. Total nephrectomy is performed by the lumbar route, and the best method is subcapsular nephrectomy, the mortality of which is 17 per cent. (Küster). The chief danger is the inadequacy of the second kidney from disease—in 40 per cent. of cases (Legueu). Nephrectomy should not be performed until the condition of the second kidney has been thoroughly investigated.

RENAL AND PERIRENAL FISTULÆ

Of these fistulæ the great majority follow an operation; a few appear spontaneously or result from injury.

1. **Perirenal fistulæ unconnected with the urinary organs.** —Perirenal fistulæ unconnected with the urinary organs may take origin in an empyema, appendicitis, or other purulent collection. The original seat of the suppuration is shown by the history of the case or the presence of scars. Much information can be obtained by radiography after injection of a bismuth emulsion.

Examination of the urine, cystoscopy, and catheterization of the ureter on the fistulous side demonstrate that there is no urinary infection, and that the ureter on this side is patent and the kidney active.

2. **Spontaneous renal fistulæ.**—These are rare. A fistula may follow wounds of the kidney, but is rarely permanent. Pyonephrosis may rupture into the perinephric tissue and burrow to the surface of the body or open into the pleural cavity, a bronchus, the stomach, duodenum, or elsewhere. Calculi may be discharged on the surface from a spontaneous fistula.

The discharge is purulent or uropurulent. Diagnosis is usually difficult. To symptoms of pyonephrosis there are superadded those of rupture of a large abscess into a bronchus or elsewhere. The escape of pus is usually intermittent.

3. **Postoperative renal fistulæ.**—There is usually a single fistula opening at the posterior part of the operation scar, but in tuberculous disease several intercommunicating fistulæ may be present. The discharge may be pus, pus and urine, or pure urine. The fistulous track is narrow and usually straight. The walls are thick, fibrous, and rigid. The factors which cause a permanent fistula may be obstruction of the ureter or pelvis, tuberculous infection of the track, a thick, hard, unyielding track wall or kidney, or calculi or concretions in the lumen of the fistula.

A fistula after nephrectomy may be due to necrotic portions of the kidney being left in the pedicle, to an infected pedicle ligature, or to septic or tuberculous infection of the wound.

Diagnosis.—Usually the cause of the fistula and the condition of the kidney are well known, but it may be uncertain if the fistula is urinary or not. The discharge should be examined for urea. After an intramuscular injection of methylene blue a urinary discharge will be tinged with blue. The presence of stricture of the ureter and the quantity of urine that escapes down the ureter are ascertained by ureteral catheterization.

Treatment.—In some cases nephrostomy has been performed with the view of producing a permanent fistula. A modification of Hamilton Irving's suprapubic drainage apparatus should be fitted to receive the urine from the fistula. In postoperative purulent non-urinary fistulæ the track should be dissected out, and all side tracks and pockets opened up and drained.

In urinary fistulæ, when the ureter is patent, drainage by a catheter *en demeure* has been recommended.

Injection of the fistula with a bismuth paste may be tried for three weeks. If the ureter is impassable and the kidney retains a considerable part of its function, a plastic operation on the renal pelvis is necessary. If the functional value of the kidney is low and the second kidney healthy, nephrectomy should be performed.

SURGICAL TREATMENT OF NON-SUPPURATIVE NEPHRITIS

Acute nephritis.—In 1896, Reginald Harrison recommended incision of the renal capsule and puncture of the kidney for *acute* nephritis when associated with delayed convalescence, with suppression, or with cardiac and circulatory complications. Others have recommended nephrotomy with the same object.

Chronic Bright's disease.—1. Edebohls, Pousson, Casper, and others have treated *acute exacerbations* of chronic Bright's disease by operation when medical treatment has failed. Cases with advanced cardiovascular and pulmonary complications are unsuitable. Decapsulation and nephrotomy have been recommended. Except in the rare cases of proved unilateral disease, decapsulation is rapidly performed on both sides. The immediate mortality is 25 per cent., partly due to the patients being moribund when the operation was performed. Some cures have been claimed, but improvement is usually temporary.

2. In 1901, Edebohls suggested decapsulation for *chronic* Bright's disease, in the belief that thus a collateral anastomosis would be established, and provide a free flow of blood through the kidney; he hoped to cause absorption of the interstitial fibrous tissue, and, by removal of the pressure upon the tubules, obtain regeneration of the renal epithelium. According to Edebohls, experiments show that, although the fibrous capsule invariably re-forms in a few weeks, the new capsule is composed of loose connective tissue which does not compress the kidney. A parietal anastomosis has actually been observed, which was not strangled by contraction of the new capsule. The kidney has also been transplanted into the peritoneal cavity, and formed adhesions with the serous membrane or the omentum.

Although the course of the disease is generally uninfluenced, improvement is undoubted in some, and a cure has been claimed in a few cases. The operative mortality is 5 per cent.

HYDRONEPHROSIS

Hydronephrosis is chronic aseptic retention of urine in the kidney and renal pelvis due to ureteral or urethral obstruction.

Etiology.—Hydronephrosis is slightly more frequent in the female sex and on the right side. It may be bilateral, especially when the obstruction is urethral.

Ureteral obstruction may be caused by—(a) changes in the wall of the ureter (valves, folds, strictures); (b) obstruction of the lumen

by calculi, tumours, foreign bodies, blood-clot; (c) pressure from
without by tumours, fibrous bands (Fig. 539), purulent collections,
an aberrant renal vessel (Fig. 540); (d) kinking of the ureter from
undue mobility of the kidney; (e) torsion of the ureter.

Urethral obstruction may be caused by a congenital fold or diaphragm or obliteration, or more
frequently by stricture and enlarged
prostate.

Congenital hydronephrosis occurs
before or soon after birth, and when
unilateral may be due to valves or
folds in or stenosis of the duct,
or to bending or kinking of a
ureter misplaced in the bladder,
urethra, ejaculatory duct, seminal
vesicle, vas deferens, or vagina.
More frequently congenital hydronephrosis is bilateral, and is due
to urethral obstruction caused by
a septum or imperforate portion, a
cyst, torsion of the penis, or phimosis.
In some cases no obstruction can
be found, but the bladder, ureters,
and kidneys are greatly dilated. In
these cases there may be dilatation
of the colon, and the condition is
probably due to changes in the
sympathetic nervous system.

Pathology. — Hydronephrosis
is said to be due to the persistence of folds of the mucosa and
muscle found in the fœtal ureter,
and to twisting that occurs during
development from the Wolffian duct.

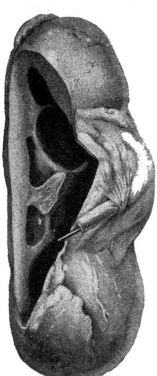

Fig. 539.—Hydronephrosis due
to bands of adhesion between
ureter and renal pelvis.

Hydronephrosis due to abnormal vessels passing to the lower
pole in front of or behind the ureter
may cause obstruction by pressure upon that duct.

Hydronephrosis due to movable kidney is intermittent, and is
the result of kinking of the ureter. It is also held that the mobility
may be consequent upon the increased size of the kidney already
hydronephrotic.

Adhesions between the colon and the pelvis resulting from chronic
constipation may be the cause of hydronephrosis.

When a tense hydronephrosis is found soon after an injury it has usually preceded the injury. Late traumatic hydronephrosis results from stricture caused by injury to the ureter.

In hydronephrosis due to calculus the stone may lie at the outlet of the pelvis or at the lower end of the ureter. Stenosis of the ureter on the vesical side of the stone is frequently present.

A hydronephrosis is " closed " when the obstruction has become complete, and " open " when urine escapes. In an open hydronephrosis

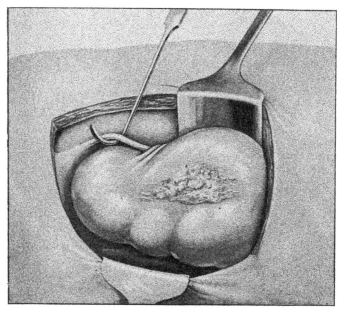

Fig. 540.—Hydronephrosis due to aberrant renal vessels (operation view) : aneurysm needle under normal ureter.

there are attacks of retention due to temporary complete closure of the outlet.

Pathological anatomy.—In the early stage the normal capacity of the renal pelvis (30–60 minims) is increased to 1 oz. or more. The pelvis is sac-like and the kidney hollowed, but the organ is not enlarged. The calyces become dilated, and the pyramids flattened and then hollowed. In the fully developed hydronephrosis the sac is formed from either the pelvis or the kidney. When the pelvis is chiefly affected it forms a large globular sac on which the hollow kidney is set as a cap. When the kidney alone is distended the surface shows rounded bosses corresponding to the hydronephrotic pockets; the pelvis is small and hidden.

The interior of the hydronephrosis shows a single large cyst with pockets (pelvic type) (Fig. 541), or a small central cavity with numerous rounded chambers leading from it (kidney type). The lining membrane is smooth, opaque, and white. If the obstruction is situated at the lower end of the ureter this tube is thickened, dilated, and tortuous.

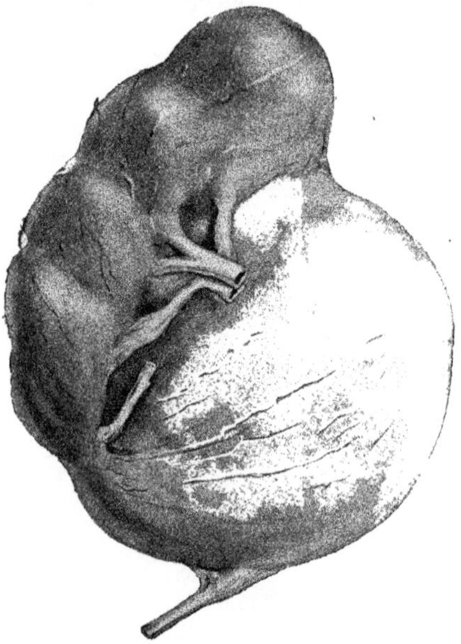

A partial hydronephrosis may be formed by the blocking of one segment of a double pelvis or the malformation of a-calyx.

Even in advanced cases there is a considerable amount of sclerosed kidney tissue present in the wall of the sac. The contents consist of urine with a specific gravity of 1005 or less. The fluid may become mixed with blood and form a hæmatonephrosis.

Symptoms.—In the early stage the kidney is not palpably enlarged, and either there are no symptoms or there is aching pain at the costo-muscular angle with persistent polyuria. Later, a rounded tumour moving with respiration and pre-

Fig. 541.—Hydronephrosis (pelvic type) due to stenosis of uretero-pelvic function.

senting the characters of a renal tumour (see p. 780) is found in the loin and may fill a large part of one side of the abdomen; it is not tender. The tumour may be constant in size and the urine normal in quantity, or there may be "intermittent" hydronephrosis in which the tumour for considerable periods completely disappears. At varying intervals—often after exertion or the drinking of a diuretic fluid—there are attacks of retention of urine in the sac, accompanied by severe pain, diminution in quantity of urine passed, and sometimes complete suppression. At the same time the tumour is large, tense, and tender. After some hours or days a large quantity of urine is passed, the pain subsides, and the tumour disappears.

On cystoscopy there may be in the early stage increased frequency of ureteric contractions from polyuria, and in the later stage diminished frequency from the reduction in quantity of urine. When the block is complete there may be an occasional gaping at the ureteric orifice, and when the muscular power of the pelvis and ureter are completely destroyed the orifice is still.

A ureteric catheter is arrested at some part of the ureter or uretero-pelvic junction, where the obstruction is situated. It usually passes after gentle manipulation, and a rapid flow of urine follows.

Diagnosis.—The symptoms may lead to a diagnosis and the X-rays show the presence of a stone. Frequently the diagnosis is uncertain in the early stages, and commencing dilatation can only be ascertained by one of the following methods :

1. *Estimation of the capacity of the renal pelvis* (Kelly) by passage of a ureteric catheter and injection of a known quantity of fluid after removal of the pelvic contents. A capacity of 30-40 c.c. shows a moderate degree of hydronephrosis.

2. *Pyelography* (Voelcker and Lichtenberg).—The pelvis of the kidney is emptied by ureteral catheter and a warm solution of collargol (10 or 20 per cent.) is slowly injected. A radiogram is taken, and a shadow showing the contour of the renal pelvis and calyces is obtained.

3. *Proportional renal mensuration* (Thomson Walker).—The shadow of the kidney is obtained by the X-rays, and the normal size is shown by the following measurements : The normal outer border of the kidney may be outlined as passing through three points—(*a*), on the horizontal mid-plane of the 12th dorsal vertebra at a distance from its margin equal to double the narrowest transverse measurement of the centrum ; (*b*) and (*c*), corresponding points on the mid-planes of the 1st and 2nd lumbar vertebræ. The size of the kidney can be measured by passing a ureteric catheter opaque in alternate half inches and obtaining a radiogram. On the plate the shadow value of half an inch is obtained, and the kidney shadow is measured with this.

Prognosis.—If sepsis is superadded a pyonephrosis results, and the prognosis is grave. Bilateral hydronephrosis is not incompatible with an active life, but eventually leads to suppression of urine.

Treatment. — Congenital hydronephrosis is rarely operable ; bilateral nephrostomy may be performed if both kidneys are affected, but the infants invariably die.

In cases of urethral obstruction with hydronephrosis, operation for the relief of the obstruction should be undertaken. No direct operative treatment of the hydronephrosis will be necessary.

In cases of movable kidney, early nephropexy should be performed. In advanced cases the uretero-pelvic junction should be examined both outside and within the pelvis. When calculus is present it

3 *a*

should be removed and the lumen of the ureter examined for stenosis. When an aberrant vessel is present, but not closely related to the point of obstruction, it need only be divided if it interferes with the plastic operation for the relief of the obstruction. If the vessel is the cause of the obstruction, it should be divided between two ligatures and the lumen of the ureter examined for stenosis.

Numerous operations are performed for congenital and acquired malformations of the ureter and dilatation of the renal pelvis, such as pyeloplication (Israel), orthopædic resection by removing the part of the pelvis and kidney below the level of the outlet (Albarran), resection of a large triangular flap of the pelvis (Thomson Walker), anastomosis of the ureter, or pyelo-ureteral anastomosis, which may be lateral implantation of the cut ureter (uretero-pyeloneostomy) or direct anastomosis of a hydronephrotic sac with the bladder (nephrocysto-anastomosis). Finally, there are plastic operations on strictures and valves, such as splitting of a valve and uretero-pyeloplasty. Nephrostcmy, i.e. the incision and permanent drainage of the sac, is sometimes performed.

Primary nephrectomy is indicated when the sac is very large and its wall thin and fibroid, but only in cases where it has been proved that a second kidney is present and efficient. Secondary nephrectomy is required when conservative operations have failed.

TUMOURS OF THE KIDNEY

BENIGN GROWTHS

Benign growths form less than 7 per cent. of renal growths. Adenoma is met with as a single, rarely multiple, cherry-sized subcapsular tumour of greyish-white or pink colour and with a well-defined fibrous capsule. It usually occurs in kidneys the seat of chronic interstitial nephritis. The microscopical structure may be acini lined with cylindrical epithelium, and containing papillary formations (papillary adenoma) or solid or hollow masses of cylindrical epithelium (tubular adenoma). Lipoma is a small (very rarely large) single or multiple subcapsular tumour. Fibroma forms fibrous nodules in the cortex or medulla. Leiomyoma is rare, and originates in the smooth muscle of the capsule. Small benign tumours are found post mortem ; large growths are indistinguishable clinically from malignant growths.

MALIGNANT GROWTHS

The varieties met with are—(1) carcinoma, (2) sarcoma, (3) hypernephroma, (4) mixed tumours of embryonic type.

The great majority of renal growths are found under the age of 5 or over 40 years.

The right kidney is more frequently affected ; bilateral growths are rare. Men are more often affected than women (227 to 73, Albarran).

Etiology.—The growths in infancy and childhood are congenital,

There is no direct evidence that injury causes renal growths. Stone may coexist, but is not an important factor in etiology.

Pathology and histology. 1. Carcinoma.—Of recent years it has been shown that carcinoma is a rare growth of the kidney (7 per cent., Garceau). It originates in the renal tubules, and shows the following varieties of structure, viz. (*a*) diffuse infiltration, the cells

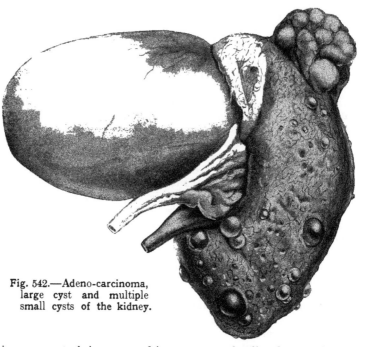

Fig. 542.—Adeno-carcinoma, large cyst and multiple small cysts of the kidney.

in some parts being arranged in masses or alveoli—adeno-carcinoma (Fig. 542); (*b*) tubules lined with epithelium closely resembling the structure of normal kidney—adenoma-carcinoma; (*c*) acini containing papillary growths—papillary adeno-carcinoma.

The tumours are usually small, and on section are grey, yellow, or brown in colour, with tracts of fibrous tissue.

2. **Sarcoma** is most common in children, and is more often bilateral than carcinoma. It may reach enormous proportions (33 lb., Van der Byl). The growth may arise from the capsule, from the perivascular connective tissue, or in the substance of the kidney.

On section the surface has a greyish, brain-like appearance, and an alveolar arrangement in parts, and there is an ill-defined capsule. These tumours are of the spindle- and small round-celled varieties.

3. **Hypernephroma.**—These tumours in some respects resemble the cortex of the suprarenal gland in structure, and Grawitz showed that they take origin in small aberrant nodules of suprarenal tissue found in the cortex of the kidney beneath the capsule. Stoerk has recently disputed their suprarenal origin, and looks upon them as papillomatous in structure. More recently, Wilson and Willis have shown that they arise from the Wolffian body.

The growths are most frequently found under the capsule and in the upper pole of the kidney, the right being more frequently affected than the left, and male subjects more often than female. They are very rarely bilateral, and are the most common form of renal growth. The growth may become active at any age. It is surrounded by a firm fibrous capsule, and its substance is broken up by fibrous bands. The presence of a large quantity of fat in the cells gives the growth a characteristic yellow-red colour. Patches of necrosis and hæmorrhages are common. Microscopically there is a network of capillary vessels, and set directly upon these, in one or several rows, are large polyhedral cells with clear protoplasm containing fat droplets. (Fig. 543.)

4. **Mixed tumours.**—These tumours usually arise during the first four years of life. There is a basis of immature connective tissue, the cells being round, oval, or spindle-shaped. In this are found embryonic striped muscle fibres, also non-striped muscle fibres, cartilaginous nodules, fatty and elastic tissue, and epithelial tubules. When striped muscle fibres are abundant the growth is termed a " rhabdo-myo-sarcoma "; when the epithelial elements are numerous the name " embryonic adeno-sarcoma " is used. These growths arise from the tissues of the sinus of the kidney and distend the organ (Bland-Sutton).

Extension and metastasis.—New growths of the kidney spread along the renal veins to the vena cava, and extend to the perirenal tissues, suprarenal gland, lymph-glands, along the aorta and vena cava, renal pelvis, and ureter. The most frequent seats of metastatic deposit in renal growths are the lungs, liver, lymph-glands, bones, and rarely the second kidney, the pleura, omentum, suprarenal gland, and brain.

Concomitant disease of the kidney, such as movable kidney, tuberculosis of the kidney, or calculus, occurs, but has no etiological value.

Symptoms.—The cardinal symptoms are hæmaturia and tumour. Hæmaturia is present in over 90 per cent. of adult cases, and is the first symptom in 70 per cent. In children it is much less frequent (15 per cent.), and occurs late. The hæmaturia is spontaneous, intermittent, and capricious, and is but little influenced by rest. The blood is well mixed and varies in quantity. Ureteral clots like long, slender worms are sometimes found, or there may be small maggot-like clots in blood-stained urine.

Clots may cause ureteric colic in passing, and copious bleeding may fill the bladder with clotted blood and cause strangury and retention of urine.

Palpable tumour is present in the advanced stage of nearly all

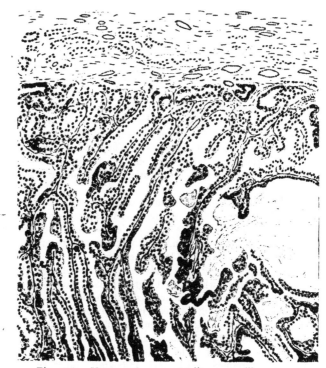

Fig. 543.—Hypernephroma of kidney, papillary type.

growths. In children it is the initial symptom in one-third of the cases. The tumour moves with respiration until it is fixed by adhesions.

Pain may be due to the passage of clots along the ureter, or there may be renal aching from tension, which is unaffected by movement and only temporarily relieved by drugs. Costal neuralgia and radiating pain or sciatica from invasion of nerves by the growth may be present.

Portions of the growth may occasionally be passed in the urine. Albuminuria is due to toxic nephritis. Polyuria is sometimes observed. Varicocele may develop suddenly or slowly, and is usually a late symptom. It is due to pressure of enlarged glands or of the growth, or to engorgement of the capsular vein which anastomoses with the spermatic vein. It disappears after nephrectomy, and should not be considered a contra-indication to operation. The development of a varicocele in a man past 35 should always lead to careful examination for renal tumour. Cachexia appears late. A specific fever of a remittent or recurrent type is observed in 8 per cent. of cases (Israel). Increased arterial tension has been noted, and in hypernephroma an abnormally rapid pulse is not uncommon.

The X-rays give a dense shadow with indefinite outline, and metastatic nodules in the lungs can be clearly demonstrated by this means.

Course and prognosis.—The average duration of the disease from the appearance of the first symptom to the fatal issue is three and a half years (Garceau).

Diagnosis.—Where hæmaturia is the only symptom the disease can be localized to one kidney by the cystoscope. Portions of the growth may be found in the urine, but exploration of the kidney is the sole certain method of diagnosis. Where tumour is the only symptom an exploratory laparotomy may be necessary to establish the diagnosis. Tumour with hæmaturia, without other symptoms, is characteristic of growth.

Treatment.—Palliative treatment consists in the administration of ergot, adrenalin, or calcium lactate to control hæmorrhage, and of opium and morphia to soothe pain. Nephrectomy is sometimes justifiable for the relief of pain, even when secondary growths are known to be present, but is seldom necessary.

Early total nephrectomy alone holds out a prospect of cure. Operation is contra-indicated where (a) the growth has spread beyond the kidney, (b) the second kidney is functionally inadequate, (c) the patient is weak and cachectic, or (d) the heart is dilated and feeble.

In all large growths the peritoneum should be opened and the peritoneal aspect of the tumour examined. The liver and lymph-glands should be examined. The efficiency of the second kidney must be previously determined, and thoracic radiograms taken to exclude pulmonary metastases.

The ideal operation should remove the kidney and growth, adipose capsule, the lymphatic vessels, and the suprarenal capsule. Nephrectomy is performed by the lumbar route. The mortality of this operation for renal growth has fallen during recent years from 76 per cent. (1885) to 22 per cent. (1902).

Recurrence takes place in 60 per cent. of cases, and in over 70 per cent. of these it occurs during the first year. Recurrence is rare after the third or fourth year, but has been described after four and a half years (Abbe) and five years (Witzel).

From 7 to 10 per cent. of cases survive at the end of the fourth year without recurrence. In children the operative mortality is higher (25 to 30 per cent.), and recurrence is more rapid and certain (67 to 81 per cent. of survivals). Cases are recorded in which the patients were alive and well eighteen years (Malcolm), five years (Israel), and four years (Döderlein, Abbe) after operation.

TUMOURS OF THE RENAL PELVIS AND URETER

Primary growths of the renal pelvis are very rare. Calculi have been present in the pelvis in some cases.

Pathology.— Epithelial tumours (papilloma and epithelioma) are most frequent, while mesoblastic tumours (sarcoma, myxoma, rhabdo - myoma, and lipoma) are rare.

Papilloma is the commonest form, and is situated at the uretero - pelvic junction or in the ureter, and may protrude into the bladder. The tumour closely resembles vesical papilloma and tends to become malignant. (Fig. 544.) The growths spread into the kidney and

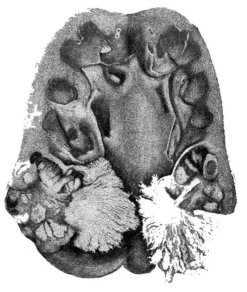

Fig. 544.—Malignant growth of kidney and papillomatous growth of renal pelvis.

along the ureter. Columnar-celled carcinoma is less frequent, and forms a nodular growth which rapidly spreads to neighbouring structures and forms metastases.

Obstruction at the outlet of the pelvis may cause hydronephrosis, which may become hæmatonephrosis or pyonephrosis.

Symptoms.—The symptoms are hæmaturia, pain, and tumour. Attacks of renal retention occur, accompanied by intense renal and ureteral pain and rapid enlargement of the kidney. On cystoscopy a tumour may be seen projecting from the ureter, and the ureteral catheter may draw blood and urine from the renal pelvis.

Treatment.—Nephrectomy, combined if necessary with ureterectomy, is the only radical method. It may be necessary to remove the lower part of the ureter through the bladder after suprapubic cystotomy, and to take with it an area of bladder wall around the ureteric orifice. Recurrence almost invariably takes place.

CYSTS OF THE KIDNEY

Apart from retention cysts of the kidney due to obstruction in the renal pelvis (hydronephrosis, pyonephrosis), there are several varieties of cysts, some of doubtful origin. These are as follows:—

Multiple cysts in chronic nephritis.
Dermoid cysts.
Polycystic kidney and congenital cystic kidney.
Solitary cysts or serous cysts.
Hydatid cysts.

Dermoid cysts are very rare, only five or six examples having been recorded.

Polycystic Kidney (Congenital Cystic Kidney)

In this condition the kidney is transformed into a collection of cysts, and has an appearance almost like a bunch of grapes. The disease may occur in several members of the same family. Although probably always congenital, if not obvious at birth it may not conspicuously develop till adult life. It is most commonly observed during infancy, or between the ages of 40 and 50. Women are more frequently affected than men. The disease is practically always bilateral, though it may be more advanced in one kidney than in the other. The organ may reach enormous proportions, and is converted into a mass of cysts varying from a pin's head to a cherry in size.

The contents are a clear yellow, sometimes brownish, fluid which holds in suspension cortical and columnar epithelial cells, tube casts, red blood-corpuscles, leucocytes, and occasionally uric-acid and calcium-oxalate crystals. Urea is present in small quantities, and albumin, phosphates, chlorides, and cholesterin.

The intercystic kidney tissue may be invisible to the naked eye. The wall of the cysts consists of connective tissue lined by columnar, cubical, or flattened epithelium.

Cystic changes are present in the liver in 18 per cent. of cases. The liver cysts are due to dilatation of biliary canals, and are not usually numerous.

In a few cases cystic changes have also been found in the pancreas, spleen, thyroid, ovaries, uterus, and seminal vesicles. Hypertrophy of the heart and arterio-sclerosis are frequently present.

Symptoms.—If the cystic condition is very advanced in the infant, the large size of the kidney may cause difficulty in labour, and the child usually soon dies with uræmic symptoms.

In the adult, many cases present no symptoms at all. Frequently, however, after a long latent period, a renal tumour appears with somewhat indeterminate symptoms, which ultimately progress to those of renal failure.

In the second or tumour stage a large swelling presenting the renal characteristics appears on one side, the second kidney not yet being enlarged on palpation. Tenderness is rare; pain is late, and consists of a dull aching in the loin, with an occasional colic due to the passage of clots. There may be albuminuria and pronounced polyuria, interrupted by periods of oliguria. Hæmaturia, when present, is slight and intermittent. In the last stage there is bilateral tumour, the urine becomes scanty and anuria supervenes.

Treatment.—From the fact that the disease is practically always bilateral, surgical intervention is ill advised. Nephrotomy with the evacuation of large cysts has been performed for pain and pyuria. Nephrectomy is useless owing to the bilateral distribution.

SOLITARY CYSTS

Large cysts of the kidney, sometimes wrongly termed " serous " cysts. are very rare. (Fig. 542.) They are usually unilateral. Generally single, and of the size of an orange or larger, the cyst has a thin, transparent fibrous wall incompletely lined with flattened or cubical epithelium, and is filled with a clear amber fluid containing albumin, chlorides, phosphates, and traces of urea, and occasionally blood. The interior frequently shows the remains of septa. Very rarely the cysts communicate with the pelvis. They are generally held to be retention cysts from blocking of tubules.

Symptoms.—Only the largest cysts cause symptoms. Dull aching pain, or more rarely sudden severe lumbar pain and vesical tenesmus, has been noted. A large cyst may produce pressure on the great veins and on the bowel. The urine is normal. The tumour has the characteristics of a renal tumour, and is most likely to be confused with hydronephrosis or new growth. The fixed volume, even after ureteral catheterization, and the normal outline of the renal pelvis on injection of collargol (pyelography), show that there is no dilatation of the pelvis. A cyst of large size may be mistaken for an ovarian cyst. A correct diagnosis is made in only 8 per cent. of cases.

Treatment.—The cyst may be brought up to the surface and opened, and the cyst wall stitched to the skin. This is followed by fistula in half the cases.

Resection of the pouch should be carried out whenever possible. The salient part of the cyst wall is cut away, and the portion of cyst wall within the kidney cauterized.

Partial nephrectomy may be performed if the cyst is at one pole. Total nephrectomy is the usual treatment for very large cysts.

HYDATID CYSTS

The kidney is only affected in .065 per cent. of cases of hydatid disease (Thomas).

Pathology.—The embryo is arrested in the capillary plexus of the convoluted tubules, usually at one pole. The growth is slow, but the cyst may finally increase rapidly in size. The neighbouring kidney tissue is destroyed by pressure. Active growth sometimes ceases and the cyst dies, shrinks, and the walls become calcified, the fluid being absorbed and the contents converted into a putty-like mass. A large cyst may rupture into the pelvis of the kidney, and the daughter cysts be passed in the urine. The cyst may now collapse and die, or it may refill and rupture again after some years. Rupture into the stomach, intestine, lung, or peritoneal cavity may take place. Suppuration frequently follows rupture, and is a grave complication.

Symptoms.—A painless, globular tumour not moving with respiration is found in the position of the kidney, which may be detected attached to the tumour. Percussion is dull or tympanitic on the anterior surface. The cyst is hard and fluctuation is seldom detected. The urine is normal.

Rupture occurs very frequently, and is accompanied by renal pain and ureteric colic, vomiting, and collapse. The urine becomes turbid, is alkaline, and contains small hydatid cysts (complete or ruptured), scolices, hooklets, fat droplets, and sometimes blood. Frequent micturition, strangury, and even retention of urine may be caused. Rupture may be followed by toxæmia, high temperature, urticaria, and occasionally convulsions.

Diagnosis.—Hydatids grow very slowly, are painless, and show no variations in size. Ureteral catheterization and pyelography exclude dilatation of the kidney. Polycystic kidney is bilateral, while hydatid and solitary cysts are unilateral. Exposure of the individual to contagion, a hydatid thrill, hooklets or cysts in the urine, when rupture has taken place, assist in diagnosis. Eosinophilia is present, and recently the diagnostic reaction known as " fixation of the complement " has been successfully employed.

Treatment.—Nephrectomy should only be performed when conservative measures are impossible, or when suppuration or rupture has taken place. The mortality is 19 per cent. Resection or partial nephrectomy is only applicable in small cysts.

The pouch may be " marsupialized," and washed daily with iodine solution. After removal of as much of the cyst as possible, the opposing surfaces may be stitched together with catgut.

PERIRENAL TUMOURS

These are rare, but of wide variety. Lipoma, fibroma, fibro-myoma, and mixtures of these, may grow from the capsule or at the renal hilum, but are usually small; sarcomas are also found. Mixed tumours are rare; they arise from Wolffian remains and resemble renal mixed tumours in structure. Perirenal cysts are believed to arise in Wolffian remains or in detached portions of embryonic peritoneum (Rambaud).

Perirenal tumours may be large and cause pressure-atrophy of the kidney or obstruction of the ureter.

Tumour formation, slow except in sarcomas, is the only constant symptom, but pressure symptoms may be present. The urine is normal. Early removal is required, by the lumbar route for small tumours, transperitoneally for large ones. The kidney should be saved, if possible, except when the growth is sarcomatous.

TUMOURS OF THE SUPRARENAL GLAND

These growths are rare; they resemble the structure of the gland, and are grouped under the name hypernephroma. Isolated examples have been described of glioma, neuroma, glio-fibroma, angioma, lymphangioma, lipoma, and cysts. About one-third of the new growths of the adrenals are found in infancy and childhood. Females are more frequently affected than males, and the left side more often than the right. Hypernephroma may be benign or malignant, and has the histological characters of the cortex of the suprarenal gland. There is a framework of capillary blood-vessels upon which large, polygonal, frequently vacuolated cells are regularly arranged. In the meshes of the vascular network the cells become arranged in alveolar form or in long columns. The vacuoles in the cells frequently contain fat, and pigment granules may be found in the protoplasm. The tumours are single or multiple. They are rounded, possess a fibrous capsule and a characteristic yellow colour, and frequently show hæmorrhages. In the benign hypernephroma the cells are smaller, more uniform in size, and regular in arrangement. Transition between simple and malignant forms is seen in the same tumour. In malignant growths metastases take place by the blood-stream, and deposits are found in the lungs, bones, and liver.

Symptoms.—Hæmaturia is very rare, and is due to passive congestion of the kidney from invasion of the renal vein. Progressive emaciation with profound anæmia is the most characteristic feature; anorexia, vomiting, constipation, and sometimes œdema are observed. Pigmentary changes very rarely develop. In children there may be arrest of mental development. There may be unilateral hypertrophy, precocious puberty, and excessive genital development. At first hidden under the ribs, the tumour is later detected in the hypochondriac region behind the bowel. The kidney may sometimes be recognized below it. Pain is frequent and is sometimes referred to distant parts. The growth is often only discovered post mortem.

Diagnosis.—The majority of cases are diagnosed as renal growths. The characteristic features are the absence of changes in the urine, early and extreme emaciation, pigmentary and developmental changes, the level of the tumour at the 7th or 8th costal cartilages, the lower border of the suprarenal growth being broad and almost horizontal. Pyelography may aid in distinguishing the origin of the growth.

Prognosis and treatment.—The average duration of life after symptoms appear is from six to ten months (Ramsay). Early removal of the growth with the kidney is the only radical method. There is danger of severe hæmorrhage and of opening the pleural cavity during separation of adhesions. Rapid recurrence after removal is the rule.

TUBERCULOSIS OF THE KIDNEY AND URETER

Tuberculosis of the urinary organs may exist alone, or may be secondary to tuberculosis of the genital system or to tuberculosis of some other organ such as the lung. The combination of genital and urinary tuberculosis is very frequent in the male, rare in the female.

Tuberculosis of the kidney is said to be primary or secondary. The term "primary" is used in the narrow sense that the kidney is the primary focus in the urinary system.

Renal tuberculosis occurs—(1) as a part of acute miliary tuberculosis, both kidneys being strewn with miliary tubercles; (2) as a tuberculous infiltration of the kidney. Miliary tuberculosis is met with, especially in early childhood, as an insignificant part of a general tuberculous infection. It has no surgical interest.

Method of infection.—The bacilli reach the kidney by one of three paths—(1) ascending. (secondary renal tuberculosis) ; (2) hæmatogenous (primary renal tuberculosis) ; (3) lymphatic.

Although ascending tuberculosis has been proved experimentally to be possible, it is doubtful if it ever occurs clinically.

Hæmatogenous infection is the method by which the kidney is attacked in the great majority of cases. Lymphatic infection from the mediastinal lymph-glands infected from a bygone pleurisy is said to occur frequently (Brongersma), but proof of this is lacking.

Etiology.—Renal tuberculosis is most frequent between the ages of 20 and 40 ; it is uncommon in childhood and rare in old age. Women are the more frequently affected, and the right kidney more often than the left. Tuberculous disease is unilateral in from 85 per cent. (Legueu) to 92 per cent. (Krönlein) of cases in the early stage. In the late stage it is bilateral in 53·3 per cent. In children it is bilateral in 53 per cent. of cases. Secondary infections with Bacillus coli, the streptococcus, and the staphylococcus may occur.

Pathological anatomy.—The following varieties may be enumerated :—

1. **Miliary tuberculosis.**

2. **Ulcero-cavernous form.**—This, the common form, commences with congestion and ulceration at the apex of a pyramid at one pole, and progresses from the pelvis outwards until the pyramid is entirely hollowed out. Other pyramids are attacked, and the pockets may unite to form larger cavities. (Plate 103.)

Tubercles may dot the cortex, singly or in groups, or may entirely permeate it. At the mouth of a calyx or of a large branch of the pelvis into which the ulcerated calyces open there is thickening of the wall and narrowing of the outlet, which may temporarily shut off this part from the urinary tract.

3. **Tuberculous hydronephrosis.**—Where thickening and contraction of the wall of one part of the pelvis or of a single calyx continues to the point of obliteration, or where the same process develops at the outlet of the ureter, a partial or total tuberculous hydronephrosis results. The fluid content is pale and turbid with white flakes, and the lining irregular and greyish-white.

Parenchymatous and interstitial nephritis and waxy disease are observed in the kidneys of tuberculous patients, and are due to the poisons produced by the tubercle bacillus.

Tuberculous lesions are found in the renal pelvis and ureter. Stenosis of the pelvic outlet causes hydronephrosis. The fatty capsule and fat around the renal vessels are greatly thickened, coarse, fibrous, and densely adherent. Enlarged lymph-glands are present. Giant-cell systems may be found in the perirenal fat.

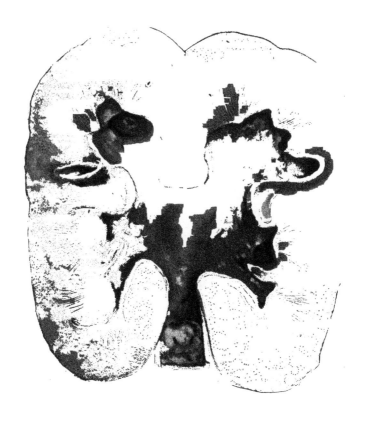

Tuberculous disease of the kidney.

PLATE 103.

Symptoms. 1. Vesical symptoms.—The symptoms may be entirely confined to the bladder. The onset is insidious, with gradually increasing frequency of micturition, at first during the day, and later at night also.

2. Changes in the urine.—Polyuria is an early symptom. It exists only on the diseased side, and is more marked at night. The urine is abundant, very pale and opalescent, faintly acid or neutral, and hazy, with a small amount of pus well mixed with the urine. The urea and chlorides are reduced. Hæmaturia may be entirely absent, or only present in microscopic amount. There may be slight persistent terminal hæmaturia or a considerable outburst of hæmorrhage, which may precede other symptoms by many months and recur during the course of the disease. Albuminuria may be present independently of pyuria or hæmaturia.

3. Pain.—The kidney may be completely destroyed without pain, but renal aching is sometimes present, and the patient may be unable to lie on the affected side. Ureteral colic may be caused by the passage of clots or débris. Pain at the neck of the bladder and at the end of the penis is due to cystitis.

4. Other symptoms.—On examination the tuberculous kidney is not usually enlarged. If palpable it may be hard and irregular. It is frequently tender. In the late stage it may be small, shrunken, and not palpable, or it may be hydronephrotic and enlarged.

There is frequently tenderness along the line of the ureter, which can be felt as a thick cord on deep palpation of the abdomen, or on rectal or vaginal examination.

The second kidney may be enlarged, painful and tender from hypertrophy, with or without commencing tuberculosis.

There is progressive loss of weight and lassitude.

Course and prognosis.—The course is slow, and remission of the symptoms for weeks and even months may be observed. The disease gradually advances until death takes place some years (seven or even ten) after the onset of the symptoms. The disease progresses until the kidney is completely destroyed; during this time the bladder and the second kidney become affected. Septic infection may be superadded either by hæmatogenous infection or, more frequently, by ascending infection from septic cystitis caused by catheterization or bladder washing. General tuberculosis rarely follows. Death takes place from anuria when both kidneys are invaded, or from exhaustion due to septic infection.

Diagnosis.—The diagnosis can usually be made by the discovery of tubercle bacilli with pus or blood in the urine, but when the ureter is completely blocked no changes may be observed in the urine. In doubtful cases von Pirquet's and Calmette's tests may be useful.

It is necessary to localize the disease to the kidney and to ascertain which kidney is affected. The presence of symptoms such as pain and enlargement of the kidney is not always reliable, for a hypertrophied healthy kidney may be enlarged and ache, while a kidney destroyed by tubercle may not be palpable, painful, or tender.

On cystoscopy general cystitis without typical tuberculous appearances may be found, or there may be tubercles or ulceration of the vesical mucous membrane or a collection of tiny cysts grouped around one ureteric orifice. The orifice may be open, trumpet-shaped, and extensively ulcerated. In old-standing tuberculosis of the kidney the ureteric orifice may be dragged upwards and outwards, and appear like a tunnel (Fenwick).

The urine of each kidney should be obtained by means of the ureterio catheter and examined for tubercle bacilli, pus, blood casts, etc.

Treatment. 1. **Tuberculin.**—Amelioration of symptoms, and in some cases disappearance of pus and tubercle bacilli from the urine, may be observed, but recurrence of the symptoms may take place after some months or years. Tuberculin treatment is recommended in —(a) cases of unilateral renal tuberculosis where nephrectomy has been refused, (b) vesical tuberculosis after nephrectomy, (c) bilateral renal tuberculosis, (d) renal with active extra-urinary tuberculosis, and (e) renal tuberculosis in children, on account of the great frequency of bilateral disease.

2. **Climatic and medicinal.**—A warm equable climate is most suitable (Egypt, Morocco, South Africa). Nourishing diet, with plenty of milk and fats, should be recommended. Urotropin is unnecessary if no septic infection be present, and it may irritate the hypersensitive bladder. Sandalwood oil soothes the vesical irritation. Washing the bladder is useless therapeutically, and involves great danger of introducing sepsis.

3. **Operative.** *Nephrectomy.*—Nephrectomy in the early stage of renal tuberculosis is the only method by which a cure can be assured, and the operation is indicated whenever the diagnosis of unilateral renal tuberculosis is made.

Nephrectomy is contra-indicated in—(i) Bilateral renal tuberculosis ; but nephrectomy of the more advanced organ is sometimes advocated to diminish the toxæmia.

(ii) Non-tuberculous nephritis of the second kidney ; but if the tests for the function of this kidney be satisfactory, nephrectomy should be performed.

(iii) Tuberculous lesions of the bladder ; although these do not contra-indicate nephrectomy if the second kidney can be proved healthy. After nephrectomy the cystitis either subsides spontaneously or disappears under tuberculin.

(iv) Tuberculous lesions of other organs ; but obsolete tuberculous foci such as spinal curvature, ankylosed joints, healed tuberculous disease of bones, etc., do not contra-indicate nephrectomy. Moreover, in active but limited tuberculous disease of the genital organs, nephrectomy may be performed. In active disease of the lungs or other organs, nephrectomy is contra-indicated.

(v) A generally enfeebled state of the patient.

The following procedures may be carried out in regard to the ureter : (i) The upper end may be fixed in the lumbar wound. This usually leads to tuberculous infection of the wound, and is not recommended. (ii) The ureter may be ligatured, cauterized, and dropped into the retroperitoneal space. The ureteral disease usually subsides and gives no further trouble, but occasionally cystitis is kept up. (iii) The ureter is excised. This is done at the time of the nephrectomy by prolonging the incision. The ureter is stripped from the peritoneum and followed into the pelvis, where it is ligatured and cut across. Some inches of the tube usually remain and give rise to no trouble. Kelly suggests removing the lower end through the vagina with a portion of the bladder wall.

Results of nephrectomy for primary tuberculosis.—Brongersma has shown an immediate mortality of 7·18 per cent. in 513 cases of nephrectomy by ten surgeons. Where the modern methods of diagnosis were used to exclude unsuitable cases the mortality fell to 2·85 per cent. There is a risk, amounting to 10·6 per cent., of the patient dying of tuberculosis during the first two years, and a risk of 3·12 per cent. of a fatal result from tuberculosis after that.

Nephrotomy.—This is a preliminary or a palliative operation when the patient is much enfeebled from toxæmia, and very rarely for great pain or severe hæmorrhage.

SYPHILIS OF THE KIDNEY

Nephritis due to *secondary* syphilis is rare, and always bilateral. In slight cases there is a trace of albumin in the urine and slightly marked œdema. In severe cases there is oliguria, pronounced albuminuria, with epithelial casts and a few leucocytes in the urine, nausea, vomiting, anasarca, and eventually uræmia, and in such cases interstitial nephritis with changes in the glomeruli and blood-vessels are usually found.

Tertiary syphilis may give rise to subacute or chronic interstitial nephritis, or less frequently a parenchymatous nephritis. The disease may be unilateral. and may affect only one part of the kidney. Scarring of the kidney is sometimes found. Gummata are single or multiple. When a large gumma is present the kidney is enlarged; hard, and irregular. Such kidneys have been removed for malignant growth or tuberculous disease. Amyloid degeneration may occur in tertiary syphilis. Congenital syphilis may affect the kidney during fœtal life, and, as Stoerk has shown, cause arrest or delay of development, so that at birth the outer layer of the cortex contains imperfectly developed tubules and glomeruli. During infancy and childhood acute or chronic interstitial nephritis is the usual form of the disease. This condition is usually bilateral, but one kidney or a part of a kidney may be affected.

Treatment.—The diet and general management of these cases differ in no way from those of other forms of nephritis. Mercury should be given in small doses and with caution, and in tertiary lesions it should be combined with iodides.

BILHARZIOSIS OF THE KIDNEY AND URETER

Bilharzial lesions of the *kidney* are very rare. Ova have been found in the renal pelvis and parenchyma in cases of advanced pyelonephritis and interstitial nephritis, and in subcapsular cysts; they may form calculous nuclei. In the pelvis there are hæmorrhages and ulceration. The mucous membrane of the pelvis is covered with prominent grey-yellow plaques formed by blood pigment, uric-acid crystals, and ova.

The lower end of the *ureter* is most frequently affected, but the whole duct may be involved. The lumen may be contracted and obliterated, and dilatation of the ureter and hydronephrosis results.

ACTINOMYCOSIS OF THE KIDNEY

Renal actinomycosis presents the general characteristics of the disease (*see* Vol. I., pp. 873-9).

RENAL CALCULUS

Stones formed in the kidney may remain lodged in a calyx or in the pelvis, or they may pass down the ureter and either become arrested in the duct or pass into the bladder.

Etiology.—A urinary calculus is an agglomeration of crystals held together by a cement substance. The crystalline element is produced by the precipitation of certain salts as a result of their excess, or of changes in reaction, or as a consequence of bacterial action. In this way crystalline forms of phosphates, oxalate of lime, and uric acid are deposited in the urine.

In infants, masses composed of urates and uric acid are frequently found in the convoluted tubules soon after birth. These disappear when the flow of urine is fully established, but may remain to form the nucleus of a true calculus.

The presence of a colloid cement substance is the second essential factor. The colloid bodies of the normal urine (mucin, urochrome) are "reversible"—that is, they may be dissolved again—and therefore they do not form a calculus even when crystals are deposited from the urine. An "irreversible" colloid—that is, one which is insoluble when once precipitated (e.g. fibrin)—is necessary.

The average age at which renal calculi occur is 38 years (Watson). Operations for renal calculus are rarely necessary in children under 10. Men are more frequently affected than women; the kidneys are equally affected. In the early stage the disease is unilateral, but later it is bilateral in over 50 per cent. of cases.

Heredity, sedentary habits, certain foods, and hard drinking-water

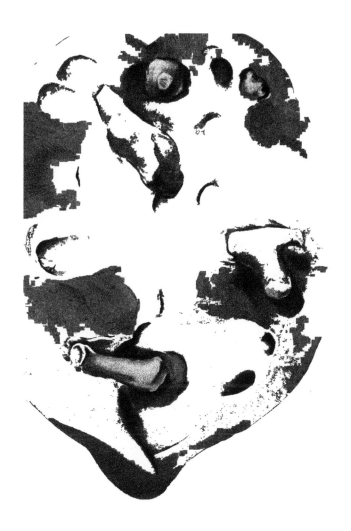

Multiple calculi of the kidney.

PLATE 104.

are important etiological factors. Calculous disease is common in India both in Europeans and in natives. In Europe calculus is specially prevalent in Central Russia, Hungary, Holland, Italy, Northern Germany, Western France, and the eastern counties of England.

Structure and chemical composition.—The calculus consists of a central nucleus surrounded by laminæ of varying composition. The nucleus generally consists of urate of ammonia in infants, of uric acid in adults, and of oxalate of lime after the age of 40. In rare cases a fragment of blood clot forms the nucleus, and the ova of bilharzia have been found in countries where bilharziosis is rife. Frequently there are alternate layers of uric acid and oxalate of lime or triple phosphates or calcium carbonate. The following substances enter into the composition of renal calculi, viz. uric acid, ammonium and sodium urate, calcium oxalate, calcium phosphate, calcium carbonate, ammonium and magnesium phosphate, cystin, xanthin, indigo, blood.

Calculi are rarely composed of a single salt. Phosphatic deposits take place where the urine becomes alkaline. Oxalate of lime is much the most frequent component, 44 per cent., and uric acid next, 22 per cent. (Morris). Oxalate-of-lime calculi are usually single, very hard, dark-brown or black, with a nodulated surface, or covered with fine or coarse clear crystalline spicules, and are laminated on section. Sometimes they form small multiple seed-like bodies. Uric-acid calculi are single or multiple, hard, smooth, sometimes highly polished, and yellow or red-brown in colour. Ammonium and sodium-urate calculi occur in children, and are small, soft, friable, and pale fawn in colour. Calcium-phosphate calculi are greyish-white, hard, with irregular and sometimes crystalline surface, and are found in neutral or slightly alkaline urine. Calculi of mixed phosphates (fusible calculus) are whitish-grey, non-laminated, mortar-like friable masses, which grow rapidly in alkaline urine. Cystin calculi are yellow, smooth, and soft, assume a greenish waxy appearance after removal, and have a radiating structure. Xanthin calculi form smooth, hard, reddish or cinnamon-coloured stones. Indigo calculi are blue-black with a grey, polished surface, and leave a blue mark on white paper. Blood or fibrin calculi form faceted masses of putty-like consistence, and have a brown colour and laminated structure.

The majority of calculi removed by operation are single, but multiple calculi are not uncommon. (Fig. 545.) Small calculi may form in a pouch in the pelvis or a calyx, and pass down the ureter at intervals for many years. Larger calculi are rounded or oval, and may be freely movable in the pelvis or firmly fixed. Large calculi are branched, and the branches fill the calyces. (Plate 104.) Calculi of $1\frac{1}{2}$ lb. (Shield) and 3 lb. (Le Dentu) have been found. A calculus has very rarely been found embedded in the substance of the kidney.

3 *b*

Changes in the kidney.—When a large stone is present the kidney is destroyed by pressure and there is extensive perinephritis. Complete or partial hydronephrosis or pyonephrosis may develop.

Symptoms.—Occasionally a calculus lies quiescent for many years. Persistent cystitis may be present, but no symptoms of renal disease. In some cases there are signs of profound toxæmia due to pyelonephritis, without symptoms of stone. The cardinal symptoms are pain (70 per cent.) and hæmaturia. Pain may be fixed renal

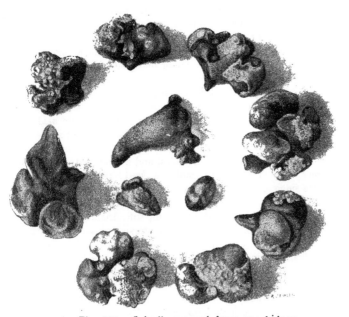

Fig. 545.—Calculi removed from one kidney.

pain or renal colic. The former is a constant ache of varying intensity, increased by movement and relieved by rest. In walking, the body may be inclined to the diseased side, and when lying the thigh is flexed. The greatest pain is produced by a small round or oval, rough, crystalline stone free in the renal pelvis.

Renal colic commences over the kidney, and radiates along the line of the ureter to the external abdominal ring or into the testicle, which is retracted, or it may shoot along the urethra to the tip of the penis. In a severe attack the patient rolls in agony, the face is pale, the skin clammy and sweating, and vomiting occurs. The abdo-

minal muscles are rigid and the thigh flexed. There may be intense
desire to micturate, but anuria may be present. If unrelieved by
treatment, the attack lasts for one or several hours, and then ceases
suddenly or gradually. After an interval a quantity of blood-stained
urine may be passed. Referred pain may be observed in the testicle,
labium, thigh, leg, sole of the foot, or heel. There may be bladder
pain and irritation when the bladder is healthy. Pain may be referred
to the second kidney, but if that organ is healthy the referred pain is
always accompanied by pain in the diseased kidney.

Hæmaturia is present in less than half the cases. It is microscopic, moderate, or copious, and is intimately connected with
movement and exertion.

Pyuria may be moderate, but if there is pyonephrosis it is
abundant and intermittent.

The urine is usually acid, rarely alkaline and decomposing. It
may contain hyaline casts, crystals of calcium oxalate, or uric acid.
Phosphaturia may be present.

Polyuria is a late symptom, and calculous anuria may supervene.
The kidney is occasionally tender, and the abdominal muscles rigid.
An abdominal tumour may be formed, and rarely a large collection
of stones is felt as a hard, irregular, craggy, grating mass.

On cystoscopic examination there is unilateral hæmaturia
or pyuria. Elongation of the ureteric orifice and inflammation
surrounding the opening may be observed. Radiography shows a
calculus shadow.

Course and complications.—As the stone increases in
size the pain diminishes. Renal calculus may exist for years without
causing grave inconvenience. The complications that may occur are
—(1) migration with renal colic, (2) obstruction with calculous hydronephrosis or calculous anuria, (3) infection causing pyelitis, pyelonephritis, pyonephrosis, perinephritis, and perinephritic abscess.

Diagnosis.—The most important symptoms are the severity of
the pain and the effect on it and on hæmaturia of movement and
jarring. The previous passage of a calculus and the presence of
numerous crystals in the urine are important.

Apart from stone, renal colic may result from undue mobility of
the kidney, from ureteritis, or from the passage of blood clot, débris,
or large quantities of uric-acid or oxalate crystals. Renal pain may
be caused by nephritis, and simulated by the crises of locomotor
ataxy, by hysteria, by osteo-arthritis of the lumbar vertebræ, and by
hepatic colic.

The final test is the X-ray examination.

In cases where cystitis is the prominent feature the cystoscope will
show a purulent efflux on one side, which will lead to a diagnosis.

Before operation is undertaken it is necessary to ascertain the presence and health of the second kidney by cystoscopy, chromocystoscopy, and examination of the urine drawn from the ureter of the second kidney by the ureteral catheter.

Prophylactic treatment.—This consists in the treatment of oxaluria, phosphaturia, and lithiasis, and the removal of local conditions which may assist the formation of stone, viz. urinary infection and obstruction.

Treatment of symptoms. *Renal colic.*—The patient is placed in a hot bath and a hypodermic injection of morphine sulphate ($\frac{1}{4}$ to $\frac{1}{2}$ gr.) with atropine sulphate ($\frac{1}{200}$ gr.) administered. Hot fomentations or poultices are applied over the loin and abdomen. Very rarely it is found necessary to keep the patient lightly under the influence of chloroform for an hour or more.

Renal hæmaturia.—This is occasionally severe after a fall or blow. The patient should rest in bed with an ice-bag over the kidney. A hypodermic injection of morphia should be given, and 10 to 15 gr. of calcium lactate administered by mouth every four hours. For persistent and severe hæmaturia, operation is necessary.

Calculous anuria. (See later.)

Operative treatment.—When the diagnosis is made the stone should, unless in some exceptional cases, be removed without delay.

Cases of extensive bilateral calculous disease with progressive renal failure or with widespread sepsis, and cases in which small calculi are frequently passed and the X-rays do not show a large single shadow or a collection of small shadows in the kidney, are unsuitable for operation.

1. Nephrolithotomy.—The kidney is exposed by a lumbar incision, and the stone removed by incision through the convex border. The pelvis and ureter are also examined.

The nephrotomy wound is closed with catgut in rounded needles. When there is sepsis and dilatation of the kidney a medium-sized drain should be placed in the kidney wound. The dangers of nephrolithotomy are hæmorrhage and septic infection. Postoperative hæmorrhage is usually due to sepsis or to tearing out of ligatures. When slight it may be controlled by morphia and calcium lactate; but if copious and persistent, exposure and packing of the kidney may be necessary, and sometimes nephrectomy is required.

Results.—In aseptic kidneys, when dilatation is not present, the mortality is 2·2 per cent (Watson). In infected cases the death-rate is as high as 20·3 per cent. (Schmieden). In infected cases a fistula may persist, and this may also result from calculi having been left in the kidney, or from ureteral or pelvic obstruction. Fistulæ occur in 8·1 per cent. of all cases (Watson) and in 22·2 per cent. of infected cases (Schmieden).

2. **Pyelolithotomy.**—The calculus is removed through an incision in the pelvis of the kidney. The kidney is drawn out of the lumbar wound and turned forwards and upwards, a longitudinal incision made in the wall of the pelvis, and the stone removed. The edges of the opening are then stitched with fine catgut. I turn down a flap of kidney capsule and cover the closed incision to prevent leakage. Mayo recommends a flap of fatty tissue for the same purpose.

Results.—The mortality in 54 uncomplicated cases was 11·1 per cent., and a fistula remained in 22·2 per cent. (Schmieden).

3. **Nephrectomy.**—Primary nephrectomy is rarely performed for calculus. It may be necessary—(1) in severe uncontrollable hæmorrhage during nephrolithotomy, (2) when the kidney is atrophied or destroyed by suppuration, (3) when calculi are so numerous and large that they cannot be removed without destroying the kidney, (4) when a malignant growth is present.

Secondary nephrectomy may be called for in—(1) urinary fistula causing great discomfort and irremediable by other means, (2) recurrence of stone with atrophy of the kidney, (3) prolonged renal suppuration.

Results.—Primary nephrectomy for calculus has a mortality of 30·1 per cent., and secondary nephrectomy 18·1 per cent. (Watson).

Bilateral calculi and calculi in a solitary kidney. —It is unwise to remove the stones from both kidneys at the same operation. The less affected kidney should first be operated upon, in case it may become necessary to perform nephrectomy on the second kidney later.

Statistics show a mortality of 35 per cent. in operations on double calculi (Küster). In operating on a solitary kidney, pyelolithotomy should be preferred to nephrolithotomy.

CALCULOUS ANURIA

Calculous anuria occurs usually in men between the ages of 40 and 60. The calculus is small and single, and the exciting cause is violent exercise, shaking, or jarring.

Pathology.—There is usually only one calculus, which is arrested at the upper end of the ureter (61 per cent.), the lower part (28 per cent.), or the middle (11 per cent.). The obstructed kidney is large and deeply congested with ecchymoses on the surface, and the pelvis contains 2 or 3 drachms of blood-stained urine under considerable tension. The second kidney is always the seat of organic disease, usually interstitial nephritis. In a few cases this ureter is also blocked by calculus, and rarely there is congenital absence of the second kidney.

The suppression on the affected side is due to sudden, complete obstruction by the impacted calculus ; that on the opposite side is usually reflex.

The following conditions may be found :—

1. The ureter of a single functional kidney blocked by stone ; the second kidney absent, atrophied, or completely destroyed by disease.

2. The ureters of two functional kidneys simultaneously blocked by stones.

3. The ureter of one functional kidney blocked by stone, and the function of the second kidney, which is diseased, suppressed by reflex influences.

Symptoms.—The kidney on the recently affected side is frequently enlarged and tender, and there is rigidity of the abdominal muscles, especially marked on this side. There may be tenderness per rectum along the line of the ureter and of the lower end of the ureters. The calculus can sometimes be detected by the finger in the rectum or vagina. On cystoscopic examination the ureteric orifice on the recently diseased side is congested or even ecchymosed.

A severe attack of ureteric colic usually precedes the onset of the anuria, but suppression may supervene without pain or other symptom.

The course of calculous anuria is divided into two stages :

1. **A period of tolerance.**—The average duration of this stage is five or six days, and the longest sixteen days. The anuria may be absolute, but frequently a little urine is secreted or there are one or more intervals of copious polyuria.

After some days, digestive disturbances appear and the appetite fails. There are nausea, constipation and flatulence sleeplessness, irritability, headache, and lassitude.

2. **A period of intoxication.**—This stage commences about the fifth or seventh day. Drowsiness and, eventually, hallucinations and muttering delirium supervene. The pupils are contracted and twitchings of the muscles occur, but convulsions are absent. There may be inability to move one or both legs, and the knee jerks are slow or abolished. The pulse and respiration are slow and irregular, and eventually Cheyne-Stokes respiration develops. The temperature is subnormal. Œdema is usually absent. Hiccup and vomiting are frequent symptoms. The bowels are constipated. The patient dies either during an attack of dyspnœa or from increasing coma and gradual heart failure.

Diagnosis. 1. **What is the cause of the anuria ?**—Previous attacks of colic, and the history of calculi, or the detection of a calculus in the ureter by the finger in the rectum or by radiography and cystoscopy, may aid diagnosis. The absence of fever excludes pyelonephritis as a cause.

Other forms of obstruction, such as bladder or pelvic growths, must be excluded. The history and examination readily exclude anuria resulting from advanced tuberculous disease, polycystic disease, or chronic nephritis, and the symptoms are unlike those of acute nephritis.

2. **Which side is affected?**—When there is a history of bilateral ureteral colic the side of the recent pain is that of the active kidney and recently blocked ureter. The abdominal muscles are rigid on the affected side. The kidney is tender and may be enlarged, and the ureter also is tender.

Extensive radiographic shadows in one kidney show that this organ was previously destroyed, and a shadow in the line of the opposite ureter would indicate and localize the cause of the anuria.

Catheterization of the ureter may demonstrate the affected side and the position of the stone.

Prognosis.—Death occurs in 71 per cent. of unoperated cases (Leguen), usually on the tenth or twelfth day. In cases which recover spontaneously, relief is usually obtained on the fifth to the tenth day.

Treatment.—Operation should be performed at the earliest possible moment in all cases. The mortality rises each day the operation is delayed, from 25 per cent. before the fourth day to 42 per cent. before the sixth day. In addition, other means should be adopted to re-establish the secretion. Diuretics such as Contrexéville water, tea, theocin sodium acetate (4 gr. every four hours) combined with digitalis, should be given. Two pints of normal saline or a $2\frac{1}{4}$ per cent. solution of glucose should be infused into a vein during or after the operation. A purge should be administered, and every means taken by hot packs and vapour baths to obtain a free action of the skin. The nature of the operation depends on the position of the obstructing stone, the possibility of localizing it, and the ease or difficulty with which it can be removed. It is more important to relieve the obstruction quickly than to remove the calculus. Nephrotomy should be performed when the stone is localized to the pelvis, when no accurate localization has been possible, or when it has been localized to the ureter but its position would necessitate a prolonged operation for its removal. If the stone is found it should be removed; if it is not found a large drainage-tube is placed in the renal pelvis and the kidney wound lightly packed with gauze. The obstructing calculus can be removed later.

Pyelotomy or ureterotomy may be substituted for nephrotomy when the stone is readily accessible.

The mortality of cases treated by operation is 46·3 per cent.

THE URETER

Anatomy.—The ureter narrows at its junction with the renal pelvis near the lower pole of the kidney, again at the pelvic brim, and again at its entrance into the bladder.   As seen in radiography, the upper end of the ureter lies at the tip of the transverse process of the 2nd lumbar vertebra; thence the duct descends across the tip of the transverse process of the 3rd and the transverse processes of the 4th and 5th lumbar vertebræ, and passes vertically across the pelvic brim, internally to the sacro-iliac synchondrosis.   It then curves outwards across the outer border of the sacrum and ischial spine, and turns inwards above the shadow thrown by the horizontal ramus of the pubic bone.

The ureter is adherent to the peritoneum, and, when the membrane is raised, remains attached to it.   In the male its terminal extravesical portion is crossed by the vas deferens.   In the female it crosses beneath the broad ligament, and alongside and then in front of the lateral fornix of the vagina and the cervix uteri.   Here it passes below and behind the uterine artery, and is surrounded by a dense venous plexus.

The intramural portion is ¾ in. long, and passes very obliquely through the bladder.   The ureteric orifices open on the bladder base, ¾ in. to 1 in. apart.

Examination.—On deep palpation, in a favourable subject, a thickened ureter can be felt lying alongside the vertebral column.

On rectal palpation, in the male the ureter is felt above and outside the base of the prostate, and in the female it may be felt in the anterior wall at the junction of the middle and upper thirds of the vagina.

The appearance, movements, and efflux of the vesical orifice of the ureter are examined by cystoscopy or by Kelly's tube.

The urine of each kidney is obtained by ureteral catheterization (p. 780).

The X-rays sometimes show the shadow of a much dilated or greatly thickened ureter.   Calculi impacted in the ureter throw a radiographic shadow in the line of the duct. (Plates 38–41, Vol. I.)

It is sometimes necessary to pass an opaque bougie up the ureter in order to define the line of the duct and the position of a doubtful shadow.   The ureter may be sounded by passing a ureteric catheter or a wax-tipped bougie.

PROLAPSE

There may be unilateral or bilateral prolapse of the whole thickness of the ureteral wall or of the mucous membrane alone.   A globular or sausage-shaped cyst is formed, varying in size from a pea to a walnut or larger.   The wall consists of a double layer of mucous membrane, and at the summit of the swelling the stenosed ureteric orifice opens.   Calculi are sometimes found in the sac.   The condition may result from a congenital narrowing of the ureteric orifice or an acquired stenosis from ureteritis.   The symptoms are irregular.   There may be pain in the kidney or ureter, or symptoms of vesical irritation or of urethral obstruction.   Occasionally there is complete retention. Attacks of hæmaturia may be the only symptom.   The cyst may appear at the external meatus in the female subject.   The cystoscope shows a pink, semitranslucent, globular or sausage-shaped swelling over which fine blood-vessels course.   The cyst may slowly fill and slowly collapse under observation.   Treatment consists in cutting off the pouch at its base with scissors and removing any calculi that are present.

INJURIES

1. SUBCUTANEOUS INJURIES AND PENETRATING WOUNDS

Injuries of this nature are rare. The peritoneum is simultaneously ruptured in 8 per cent. of cases. The duct is injured by impact against the transverse process of a lumbar vertebra or by overstretching. Urine accumulates in the retroperitoneal space or leaks into the peritoneum.

Symptoms.—There are pain and tenderness, which pass off in a few days if the injury is uncomplicated. A swelling appears in the loin in a few days or after some weeks. It is rounded or elongated and well defined, and may assume a large size. Suppuration takes place and the temperature rises. It is impossible to diagnose between a rupture of the ureter and rupture of the renal pelvis. A urinary fistula follows penetrating wounds of the ureter. The prognosis is good when early operation is performed.

Treatment.—Operation should immediately follow diagnosis. It is difficult to find the end of the ureter when it is completely torn across, and a catheter should be passed up the duct from the bladder before commencing the operation. The ends, when identified, should be anastomosed. Nephrectomy may be required in rare cases for septic complications, or for the cure of intractable fistula.

2. SURGICAL WOUNDS

Injury to the ureter is occasionally caused by forceps during delivery, but more frequently occurs during pelvic operations, especially on the ovaries and uterus. It may be partly or completely cut, or its wall or blood supply damaged, so that it sloughs and a fistula forms after some days. The fistula may open in the vagina or in the cervix, if a subtotal excision of the uterus has been performed, or it may open at the abdominal wound.

Treatment.—When the ureter has been partly cut or lacerated the edges of the wound should be sutured with fine catgut.

A ureteral catheter should be retained in the ureter for a week. A covering of areolar tissue or even of peritoneum greatly assists healing of the ureteral wound. An irregular tear or a complete laceration is better treated by resection of a portion of the tube, followed by anastomosis by one of the following methods:—

1. End-to-end anastomosis.
2. End-to-end anastomosis with invagination.
3. Anastomosis by means of a button or a tube of magnesium.
4. End-to-side anastomosis with or without invagination.
5. Lateral anastomosis.

When a portion of the ureter has been torn away, one of the following procedures may be carried out:—

1. Implantation of the upper part of the ureter into the bladder (ureterocysto-neostomy).
2. Uretero-ureteral anastomosis, the torn ureter being grafted with the sound ureter.
3. Formation of a cutaneous fistula.
4. Implantation into the intestine.
5. Immediate nephrectomy.

Nephrectomy should, if possible, be avoided; cystitis is frequently present, and thus there is danger of ascending pyelonephritis of the remaining kidney.

Results.—In 60 cases of ureteral anastomosis there were 43 complete recoveries, 9 recoveries after temporary fistula, and 8 deaths (Alksne).

FISTULA

Fistula of the ureter may be cutaneous or vaginal, and may be congenital, or result from surgical operation, or follow parturition. On the vesical side of the fistula there is usually stenosis of the ureter, and above the fistula the ureter and kidney are frequently dilated. Infection of the fistula, ureter, and kidney invariably occurs.

When the ureter is completely severed, cystoscopy shows no movement at the ureteric orifice, but in partial division rhythmic contraction is observed. Methylene-blue solution injected into the bladder will escape by the fistula if it communicates directly with the bladder, but does not escape when the ureter only is affected. It is sometimes difficult to ascertain which ureter is fistulous. This information is obtained by cystoscopy, when the orifice of the affected ureter is motionless and without efflux, and the subcutaneous injection of indigo-carmine is followed by a coloured efflux from the healthy ureter and none from the fistulous ureter.

The position of the fistula is ascertained by sounding the ureter with an opaque bougie and obtaining a radiogram.

Treatment.—The introduction of a catheter *en demeure* is impossible in many cases on account of the stricture. When it has been practicable the result has not been permanently satisfactory, the stricture recontracting and the fistula again appearing.

Several methods of transplantation of the ureter have been tried. Exposure of the upper end of the ureter and implantation into the bladder is occasionally successful.

Implantation into the cæcum or sigmoid has been practised with an operative mortality of 58 per cent. in bilateral implantation, and of 29 per cent. in unilateral implantation. Death usually occurs within a short time from ascending pyelo-nephritis.

Plastic operations on the vagina and obliteration of the vagina have been successful in a few cases.

Nephrectomy should only be performed after other methods have failed.

STONE

The great majority of stones found in the ureter have been formed in the renal pelvis. Rarely a calculus forms around a foreign body such as a silk stitch (Fig. 546, 3). Impaction usually takes place at the outlet of the renal pelvis, at the entrance of the ureter into the bladder, or at the level of the brim of the bony pelvis. In rare cases the position of the calculus varies with the attitude of the patient.

There is usually only one calculus (90 per cent.), but there may be two, three, or as many as twenty-seven. Ureteral calculi are bilateral in only 3·6 per cent. of cases.

In shape they resemble a date or a coffee-bean. When large they may be round or sausage-shaped. Ureteral calculi weighing 816 gr. (Bloch), 803 gr. (Carless), and 780 gr. (Fedcroff) have been recorded. The surface may be smooth, bossy, or spiculated. (Fig. 546.) There is frequently a stricture below the point of impaction. In old-standing cases the ureter above the calculus is dilated, and the kidney hydronephrotic. There are calculi in the corresponding kidney

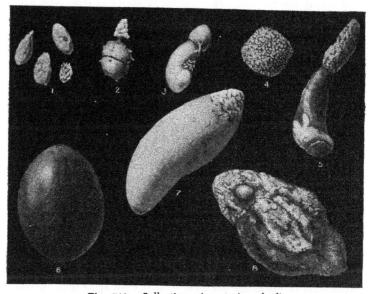

Fig. 546.—Collection of ureteric calculi.

1, Calculi passed after temporary impaction ; 2, calculus impacted at ureteric orifice, mush-room-shaped portion in bladder ; 3, calculi formed on silk sutures ; 4–8, impacted calculi removed by operation.

in 13 per cent. of cases. Pyonephrosis may be found ; sclerosis and atrophy of the kidney are rare.

Symptoms.—When the calculus passes along the ureter there is an attack of renal colic, repeated at frequent or at long intervals. The pain may commence at a spot in the line of the ureter lower than the kidney, and it may remain fixed at this spot. There may also be fixed, dull aching pain over some part of the ureter. This pain is aggravated by movement or straining, or on taking diuretics. The attacks of colic may be frequent and severe till the calculus is expelled into the bladder. The patient frequently feels something drop into the bladder, and the pain ceases. After some hours or days the calculus is discharged from the urethra.

At the upper part of the ureter the symptoms are rarely distinguishable from those of calculus in the renal pelvis. When the stone lies just outside or in the wall of the bladder, symptoms of bladder irritation become prominent, and there is pain along the urethra to the end of the penis. Genital symptoms also appear, such as painful emissions, hæmospermia, and testicular pain, and there may be constant pain in the rectum, aggravated by defæcation. Hæmaturia may be severe, and usually follows renal colic. During an attack of colic there may be oliguria or temporary anuria, and under certain conditions calculous anuria becomes established.

Pus, bacteria, crystals, and tube casts may be present, and phosphaturia is sometimes observed.

The complications that may occur are calculous anuria, infection (usually hæmatogenous), and chronic obstruction. As a result of infection, pyelonephritis or pyonephrosis may develop, and as a result of obstruction, hydronephrosis.

Examination—There may be tenderness over the impacted calculus; if the stone is at the lower end of the ureter it may be felt per rectum or per vaginam. On cystoscopy the ureteric orifice is unaltered, or shows surrounding congestion and thick and gaping lips; sometimes it is puckered and surrounded by heaped-up velvety mucous membrane or by œdematous bullæ. Occasionally the trigone is hidden with œdematous mucous membrane. A stone impacted in the intra mural portion of the ureter is seen as a red swelling outside and above the ureteric orifice; its brown or white tip may project from the opening.

The efflux may be rapid and forceful, and may be tinged with blood or cloudy with pus. If a stone be impacted low down, the movements of the orifice are often slow, and the efflux is discharged feebly.

The ureter may be sounded by means of a ureteral catheter or a solid bougie. In female subjects Kelly has used wax-tipped bougies which show scratches on the wax when a calculus is present.

Radiography is the most reliable method of diagnosis. Stones as small as a split pea, or even smaller, can be demonstrated. Very minute calculi may be overlooked, and pure uric-acid calculi, which are rare, do not throw a shadow. The diagnosis of small stone shadows may be confused by the shadows of the vertebral transverse processes, the sacrum, ischial spine, and the horizontal ramus of the pubes, or by calcified lymph-glands, calcified appendices epiploicæ, opaque bodies in the appendix, atheromatous arteries, phleboliths, calcareous deposits in old scars or chronic inflammatory tissue or on ligatures, calcareous deposits in the seminal vesicles, intestinal contents (Blaud's pills, bismuth-covered fæces, etc.), or enteroliths. A differential diagnosis is made by the position of the shadow, the shape, number, and clinical history. In doubtful cases stereoscopic radiograms should be taken after passing an opaque bougie up the ureter.

1. **Diuretic treatment.**—If small stones have recently passed into the ureter with recurring attacks of renal colic, and especially if a calculus has previously been passed, diuretics such as potassium citrate and acetate, theocin sodium acetate, Contrexéville, Evian, or Vittel water should be administered, together with antispasmodics such as atropine or belladonna.

The treatment should be limited to four or six months. When dilatation of the kidney is commencing (as shown by the collargol pyelographic method), operation should be undertaken without delay.

2. **Instrumental treatment.**—The passage of a bougie up the ureter, or of a special ureteric catheter with a distensible balloon, and the injection of oil and eucaine into the ureter, have been used in special cases.

3. **Operative treatment.**—This is indicated—(1) in calculous anuria, (2) where medicinal treatment has failed, (3) where infection has occurred, (4) where dilatation of the kidney is commencing.

A calculus situated in the lumbar segment of the ureter is exposed by an oblique lumbar incision; one impacted at the pelvic brim is reached by a curved incision commencing at the level of the anterior superior iliac spine, and passing downwards and inwards parallel to Poupart's ligament and about 2 in. above it. The peritoneum is raised and the ureter is found adhering to it. A calculus arrested in the pelvic portion of the ureter may be removed by the same route, or by the sacral extraperitoneal route of Morris. The latter operation is carried out by an incision parallel to the sacral spines, 2 in. from the middle line, and carried down beyond the coccyx. The gluteus maximus muscle and the sacro-sciatic ligament are divided. In a third method the abdomen is opened in the middle line and the peritoneum incised over the ureter. The vaginal route is used when the stone can be felt from the vagina. A calculus in the intramural portion of the ureter is removed from within the bladder after suprapubic cystotomy. In all cases stricture of the ureter should be sought and treated.

Results.—Excluding cases of calculous anuria, extraperitoneal ureterolithotomy has an operative mortality of 5·5 per cent. Recurrence is rare.

THE BLADDER

Anatomy.—The bladder normally holds 8 to 10 oz. In moderate distension about 1½ in. of the anterior wall of the viscus above the symphysis pubis is uncovered by peritoneum. In front of the bladder, behind the pubic symphysis, is the space of Retzius, filled with areolar tissue. The internal meatus of the urethra is on a level with the middle of the symphysis pubis and about 2 cm. behind it. This is the most fixed part of the bladder. The base in the male is in relation to the prostate, which underlies the anterior half of the trigone, and behind this lie the seminal vesicles, above which is the peritoneum of the recto-vesical pouch.

In the female bladder the base is in relation to the anterior vaginal wall, to which it is adherent. The anterior fornix of the vagina is in relation to the bladder for about 1 in. behind the base of the trigone, and behind this the anterior surface of the uterus lies upon the posterior wall of the bladder almost to the apex. At the apex of the bladder the peritoneum covers it for a short distance before being reflected on to the uterus. In the child, about one-half of the bladder lies above the pubic symphysis (Symington). The anterior surface is entirely uncovered, and the posterior completely covered by peritoneum.

The trigone of the bladder is a structure distinct from the rest of the organ, and the muscular fibres are derived from the internal longitudinal layer of the ureters, which unite to form the interureteric bar of Mercier, and also pass forwards to the internal meatus, interlacing to form a thick muscular layer, and passing into the internal longitudinal muscular layer of the urethra.

The bladder sphincter consists of non-striped muscle fibres continuous with the muscle of the trigone lying on the upper surface of the prostate.

The mucous membrane is composed of transitional epithelium, and there are no papillæ. The mucous membrane of the trigone is thick and adherent, that over the rest of the bladder thinner and freely movable.

The lymphatics from the anterior surface pass to glands along the external iliac vessels, those of the upper part of the bladder pass to the external iliac and hypogastric glands, and those of the lower part and posterior wall pass to the sacral ganglia at the bifurcation of the aorta.

The nerve supply is derived from the 2nd, 3rd, and 4th sacral nerves. The sympathetic nerves are derived from the hypogastric and hæmorrhoidal plexuses. The lowest reflex centre for the bladder is contained in these sympathetic plexuses.

Examination.—A greatly distended bladder forms a prominent rounded suprapubic swelling, which can be felt as a smooth, round, elastic mass, and is dull on percussion.

On rectal examination about 1½ in. of the bladder base just behind the trigone can be felt above the prostate, and a bimanual examination can be made with the other hand above the pubes. A distended bladder forms a soft cushion which tends to bury the prostate. The infiltration of a malignant growth at the base of the bladder may be detected in this situation.

On vaginal examination the short urethra can be felt in the anterior vaginal wall, and the trigone of the bladder can sometimes be defined. Behind this the bladder base can be palpated from the anterior fornix.

Examination by catheters and sounds.—The passage of a catheter is required to withdraw the urine in vesical atony or urethral obstruction, to ascertain the presence and quantity of residual urine, or to obtain an uncontaminated specimen of urine from the bladder. A calculus is sometimes felt on passing a catheter, and a portion of growth may be caught in the eye of a catheter.

The most stringent antiseptic precautions must be used in passing instruments into the bladder. The method of passing instruments is described at p. 893.

For sounding the bladder the organ should contain 6-8 oz. of fluid. The stone sound is introduced in the same way as a metal catheter, and when the beak engages in the prostatic urethra the handle is fully depressed between the thighs and then pushed onwards so that the beak rides over the posterior lip of the internal meatus. The bladder should be systematically searched by turning the handle from side to side while slowly withdrawing.

Exploration by operation.—When necessary the bladder may be opened suprapubically and the patient placed in the Trendelenburg position. With bladder retractors and the help of a head-lamp the interior of the bladder can be thoroughly searched.

The perineal route in the male and the urethral and vaginal routes in the female are unsatisfactory and inadequate methods of exploration.

Radiography is discussed elsewhere (Vol. I., p. 629).

Cystoscopy.—There are two methods of cystoscopy—(1) indirect, (2) direct.

1. *Indirect cystoscopy.*—This is carried out by means of a cystoscope after distension of the bladder with fluid. The various forms of cystoscope are described in special works on the subject. For routine use an " irrigation " cystoscope is most useful. This consists of a hollow tube with an angled beak which carries a small electric lamp. At the proximal end of the tube there is a valve which prevents the escape of the fluid until required. A telescope with a prism and lenses fits the interior of the tube and is slipped in after the bladder is washed and distended. The patient lies on a couch with a sand-pillow beneath the pelvis, or sits in a special chair with the knees and hips flexed and the thighs widely apart. The urethra is anæsthetized by instilling 15 minims of a 2 per cent. solution of cocaine into the prostatic urethra by means of a Guyon's syringe. The catheter portion of the cystoscope is lubricated with glycerine and introduced, and the bladder filled with warm boric solution. The telescope is now introduced, the light switched on, and the window turned to the base of the bladder. Careful and prolonged washing may be necessary to obtain a clear medium when hæmaturia or pyuria is present, and a weak solution of silver nitrate (1 in 10,000) or a small quantity of adrenalin may be used in order to stop oozing.

2. *Direct cystoscopy.*—This method was perfected by Kelly, and has been modified by Luys and others. Kelly's specula are used for women only, and are plated metal cylinders 3½ in. long with a funnel-shaped expansion and a handle at the outer end. The instrument is introduced with an obturator after dilatation of the urethra. General anæsthesia may be necessary. The patient is placed in the knee-chest position, the speculum is introduced and the obturator withdrawn. Air rushes in and distends the bladder, and light is projected through the tube from a head-lamp. Luys has modified this method, and uses it in the male also. His instrument consists of a metal tube 10 cm. long for female, and 18 cm. for male subjects. The patient is placed in the Trendelenburg position with local or general anæsthesia.

The direct methods are inferior to the indirect where examination only is desired. There is frequently difficulty in obtaining the proper distension of the bladder with the atmospheric pressure, and the position of the patient is irksome and embarrassing. Urine tends to collect in the bladder during the examination, and must be removed with a suction apparatus. Where applications to the interior of the bladder are necessary, or foreign bodies have to be removed, the direct methods are invaluable.

The methods of collecting urine from each kidney have already been considered (p. 780). The tests of the function of each kidney should be used. The most suitable are the phloridzin and the phenol-sulphone-phthalein tests (p. 779).

INCONTINENCE OF URINE

Incontinence of urine may be false or true.

In *false incontinence* the bladder is full, as in chronic retention from prostatic or urethral obstruction, and the escape is the over-flow from the distended organ.

In *true incontinence* the bladder is not distended. Of this there are two types, passive and active. In the *passive* type the sphincter is paralysed and the urine dribbles away without distending the bladder and without the assistance of contraction of the bladder. In the *active* type the urine is expelled by contraction of the bladder. Here there is sphincter action, but it is either too weak to resist normal contractions of the bladder, or the contractions are so strong as to overcome a normal sphincter.

INCONTINENCE DUE TO MECHANICAL CAUSES

This occurs more frequently in women than in men. It may be observed in a very slight degree on exertion in otherwise normal individuals. Parturition is a frequent cause. In older women in-continence occurs in combination with cystocele. Forcible dilata-tion of the urethra for digital examination of the bladder was at one time a frequent cause of incontinence in women. In men, perineal prostatectomy or the perineal drainage of the prostatic cavity after suprapubic prostatectomy may cause incontinence.

Treatment.—In slight cases strychnine and ergot should be given. The use of a vaginal pessary is of service. A cystocele should be excised.

For urethral dilatation Duret has transplanted the urethra for-wards to the neighbourhood of the clitoris, and Gersuny operates by dissecting up the female urethra and twisting it on its long axis. Paraffin has been injected around the urethra and vesical orifice in incontinence of urine in the female. If treatment fails a urinal must be worn.

INCONTINENCE DUE TO NERVOUS DISEASE

Incontinence occurs in organic diseases of the spinal cord. In some cases there is false incontinence (i.e. chronic distension and overflow), especially in the early stages of the bladder affections of tabes and transverse lesions of the cord. After a time the bladder regains some of its contractile power, the residual urine is reduced to 8 or 10 oz., and the patient can expel the rest voluntarily. Incon-tinence in these cases is first noticed at night; bed-wetting which develops in adult life without other symptoms should lead to a careful examination of the central nervous system.

In multiple sclerosis a different type of incontinence is met with, the bladder being contracted and urine spasmodically ejected without control.

Treatment.—The over-distended bladder should be slowly emptied by the catheter at regular intervals under the strictest aseptic precautions. If there is complete retention this should be done three times in twenty-four hours. The bladder should be washed with silver-nitrate solution (1 in 10,000) if any sign of infection is observed. Urinary antiseptics (urotropine, etc.) are combined with strychnine and ergot, and the bowels carefully regulated. For continual incontinence a urinal must be worn.

Incontinence due to Bladder Spasm

In multiple sclerosis, incontinence is due to spasm. In acute inflammation of the bladder and prostatic urethra, uncontrollable spasm may cause active incontinence. This is usually nocturnal. Tuberculosis of the bladder is a frequent cause.

Treatment.—In acute cases hot fomentations should be applied suprapubically and on the perineum, morphia and belladonna suppositories used, and a hot-water enema, to which 30 gr. of antipyrin have been added, given.

Contrexéville or Vittel water and sandalwood oil may be administered, and hot sitz-baths are useful. In chronic cases diuretics and sandalwood, belladonna and hyoscyamus, and small doses of opium should be given, and the cystitis simultaneously treated. In tuberculous cystitis the bladder should not be washed.

Incontinence of Childhood—Nocturnal Enuresis—Essential Enuresis

Up to the end of the first year the bladder acts automatically. About that time mental control by inhibition of the act of micturition begins, and by the end of eighteen months, or at most two years, it is fairly established, although there may still be occasional lapses up to the age of 3 years. After that age constant or frequent bedwetting must be regarded as abnormal. The onset of enuresis is usually observed between the ages of 5 and 8, but the nocturnal control may never have been established. Enuresis is usually nocturnal, sometimes it is also diurnal, rarely it is diurnal only. Boys and girls are equally affected.

Etiology.—In certain cases some source of irritation is present, such as thread-worms, anal fissure, vulvitis, phimosis, and balanitis, and the incontinence is looked upon as reflex. Enlarged tonsils and

3 c

adenoids are present in some cases, and enuresis is said to be due to partial asphyxia during sleep.

In other cases there is some abnormality in the urine or bladder, such as highly acid urine, uric-acid crystals, phosphaturia, bacilluria, cystitis, vesical calculus, or tuberculous cystitis. In some cases no source of irritation, no alteration in the urine or disease of the bladder can be found. These cases are called " essential enuresis." In these children there is frequently an heredity of nervous disease, such as epilepsy, neurasthenia, alcoholism, insanity, etc. The child may be nervous, quiet, sensitive, and furtive, and often suffers from stuttering and habit spasms. The enuresis is always worse after excitement. In a small number of cases the enuresis occurs during a minor epileptic attack.

Prognosis.—Where some abnormality amenable to treatment is found, the prognosis is good. In the majority of cases of essential enuresis continence becomes complete with or before the advent of puberty. Most cases get well under treatment, but in a small percentage the enuresis persists, sometimes into adult life.

Treatment.—All sources of irritation, such as thread-worms, phimosis, or anal fissure, hyperacid urine, phosphaturia, bacilluria, cystitis, stone, etc., should receive appropriate treatment.

When no source of irritation is found, treatment along the following lines is indicated : Mental excitement and late hours should be avoided, and sometimes even school and lessons temporarily stopped. The principal meal should be at mid-day, and fluids prohibited after five o'clock. Tea, coffee, ginger-beer and ginger-ale, highly seasoned foods, sugar, and pastry should be avoided, and meat taken only in moderation. The child is trained to hold water as long as possible during the day, and to empty the bladder before bedtime. He should be wakened to micturate after about one and a half hour's sleep. Belladonna is given in doses suitable to the patient's age and idiosyncrasy. In a child of five years or over the dose should commence with 3 minims of the tincture, and slowly increase up to 30 or 40 minims three times a day unless symptoms of poisoning appear. If the enuresis is controlled the dose is kept a little beyond the point of control for a fortnight, and then gradually reduced. Tincture of lycopodium may be combined with belladonna. Nux vomica and ergot in small doses are sometimes useful, and potassium bromide, antipyrin, and fluid extract of *Rhus aromatica* have been recommended.

Local treatment should, if possible, be avoided ; but it is successful in some cases where other methods have failed. This consists in the instillation into the prostatic urethra of nitrate of silver (1 per cent.), and treatment with the continuous current applied by means of a urethral electrode.

Cathelin has suggested the injection of fluid into the sacral canal with the object of causing pressure on the sacral nerves. He claims 80 per cent. of cures, but the treatment has not been so successful in other hands.

RETENTION OF URINE

Etiology.—The causes of retention of urine may be classified as follows :—

1. **Retention with obstruction.** (*a*) *Prostate.*—(1) Simple enlargement, (2) malignant disease, (3) stone, (4) acute prostatitis and prostatic abscess. (*b*) *Urethra.*—(1) Rupture of urethra, (2) acute urethritis, (3) stricture, (4) stone and foreign bodies, (5) pressure from without, pelvic tumours, etc.

2. **Retention due to atony.**—(*a*) With symptoms of nervous disease ; tabes and other spinal lesions. (*b*) Without symptoms of nervous disease ; idiopathic atony.

3. **Retention in acute and chronic intoxications.**—Typhoid, appendicitis, salpingitis, arsenical, mercurial, belladonna, or lead poisoning, and syphilis.

4. **Retention from inhibition or spasm.** — Hysterical retention ; retention after anal and rectal operations.

Diagnosis.—It is necessary to distinguish between anuria and retention and between atonic and obstructive retention. In obstructive retention the form of obstruction must be ascertained.

In anuria there have been previous signs of renal disease, but no symptoms of disease of the bladder or urethra. There is no pain, no distension of the bladder, and an instrument passes easily into the bladder but draws no urine. In retention of urine there is usually a history of increasing difficulty of micturition and other signs of obstruction. Symptoms of renal disease are absent or insignificant. The bladder is distended.

In retention due to atony there is no pain and no desire to micturate. In obstructive retention there are recurrent spasmodic attempts to empty the bladder ; these are sometimes absent in old men.

A large-sized instrument enters the bladder easily if retention is due to atony, but is arrested if retention is due to obstruction ; the presence of signs of spinal disease clinches the diagnosis.

In young men the most frequent cause of acute retention is gonorrhœa, and there is a history of an acute discharge. In adult life retention is usually due to stricture, and there is a history of gradually increasing difficulty of micturition, culminating in complete retention after alcoholic excess or exposure to cold. The passage of an instrument confirms the diagnosis.

In old men enlargement of the prostate is the most frequent cause of retention. There is a history of nocturnal frequency and increasing difficulty, and rectal examination shows that the prostate is enlarged.

Treatment.—The following is the treatment suitable to the chief types :—

1. *Acute inflammation of the urethra (gonorrhœa, etc.).*—Every means should be tried to relieve the retention without the passage of a catheter. A hot bath or sitz-bath, followed by a rectal injection of hot water and a suppository containing belladonna and opium, should be given. If relief is not obtained in half to three-quarters of an hour an anæsthetic should be given, the urethra thoroughly washed out with potassium permanganate (1 in 5,000), and then a rubber catheter passed. The bladder should be washed with permanganate or protargol (1 in 10,000) solution and a little of the solution left in the bladder. If acute prostatitis and prostatic abscess is present early operation is indicated.

2. *Obstruction of the urethra by stone, foreign bodies, pedunculated bladder growths, blood clot, etc.*—Relief by catheter should be given without delay. Spasm of the compressor muscle may hinder the passage of the catheter and may necessitate the use of several metal sounds before the catheter can be introduced.

If the bladder is distended with blood clot an attempt may be made with a large metal catheter to break up the clot and wash it out, or a lithotrite may be used and an evacuating cannula. Should these methods fail, the bladder must be opened suprapubically, the masses of clot removed, and a large rubber drain inserted.

3. The *distended atonic bladder of spinal disease* should be regularly catheterized with the same precautions as in enlarged prostate.

4. *Retention from reflex spasm after operations, and retention due to hysteria.*—In operation cases the catheter is passed without delay. In other cases hot baths and other means of relieving spasm (*see* Acute Inflammation) should first be tried. A metal catheter is the best instrument for these cases.

5. *Retention with enlarged prostate.*—The preliminary measures detailed above may be tried, but recourse to the catheter will nearly always be necessary. The following points are of the utmost importance :—

    i. The most rigid asepsis must be practised.

    ii. The delicate handling of instruments is essential.

    iii. All the urine of an over-distended bladder must not be withdrawn at once, or must be drawn off very slowly.

Coudé and bicoudé catheters are most suitable. When obstruction is felt the greatest gentleness is exercised ; sometimes twisting to one side or another, or withdrawing a little and pushing on, will be successful. In cases of enlarged prostate the urethra is greatly elongated, and may require deep insertion of a metal prostatic catheter with a large curve and a long beak; a gum-elastic catheter bent into a full curve or into some other shape may be successful when other catheters have failed.

These methods failing, suprapubic puncture will be necessary (*see* below).

The vesical or renal hæmorrhage, or the suppression that may follow sudden emptying of an over-distended bladder, are avoided by keeping the patient warm in bed, and by drawing off only 10 or 15 oz. at intervals of half an hour until the bladder is empty. Another method is to tie in a catheter of very fine calibre and allow the urine to dribble slowly away. When the bladder is empty a few syringefuls of silver nitrate solution (1 in 10,000) should be injected and allowed to escape, and the catheter tied in. Stimulants and a mixture containing urotropine, strychnine, citrate of potash, and infusion of buchu should be given.

After several days of continuous bladder drainage the decision will have to be made as to whether " catheter life " is to be commenced or an operation performed.

6. *Retention with stricture.*—A hot sitz-bath and rectal injections, followed by a suppository of morphia ($\frac{1}{4}$ gr.), should be tried. This failing, a catheter should be passed, preceded by a No. 7 or 8 French bougie if necessary. When a filiform bougie only will pass, it should be tied in place. After half an hour the urine begins to trickle alongside the bougie; a few hours later a larger instrument, and eventually a catheter, can be introduced.

A more rapid method is to use a metal catheter with a conical end which screws on to a filiform bougie. The bougie acts as a guide, and the catheter is forced through the stricture. Harrison's whip bougies are useful, especially if laterally grooved to facilitate escape of urine. There is less danger of completely emptying a distended bladder in a case of stricture than in enlarged prostate.

If instruments fail, the bladder must be emptied by suprapubic puncture an inch above the upper margin of the pubic symphysis in the middle line. The skin is incised, and then the aspirating needle introduced. There is little risk of injuring the peritoneum when the bladder is distended and the percussion note dull. The aspirating needle should not be large, lest leakage at the point of puncture of the bladder take place. There is a danger of prevesical abscess if the urine is septic. Usually after a single aspiration an instrument can be introduced through the stricture and tied in, but in rare instances the puncture must be repeated.

Operation for the relief of the stricture should be performed as soon as possible.

EXTROVERSION

In this rare condition the anterior vesical wall is congenitally absent, so that the mucous membrane is exposed and the urine discharged on the surface. Male infants are more frequently affected than female.

At birth there is a dark-red, plum-sized suprapubic swelling. The mucous membrane becomes folded, irregular, and excoriated; at its margin there is a zone of scar tissue with irregular epithelial ingrowths into the mucosa. The umbilicus may be normal and separated from the open bladder by healthy skin, or the bladder may fill the entire space from the umbilicus to the root of the penis. The ureters, which are frequently dilated, open on two nipples close together, and the trigone is undeveloped. The penis is undeveloped and epispadiac; at its base in a small pocket are the sinus pocularis and ejaculatory ducts. The foreskin is well developed in the form of an apron. The scrotum is split or rudimentary, and rarely contains the testicles. The prostate is absent or rudimentary. The pubic bones do not unite in the middle line, and may be separated by 3 in. or more. Associated deformities, such as hare-lip, cleft palate, and spina bifida, are sometimes observed. The perineal muscles may be defective, and the anal sphincter ill developed. Less extensive degrees of this maldevelopment may be observed. The condition is ascribed either to an arrest of development or to an intra-uterine rupture of the bladder following obstruction.

Symptoms and prognosis.—The conditions of existence are extremely miserable. There is constant escape of urine, saturating the clothes and leading to inflammation and excoriation of the skin. The mortality from ascending pyelonephritis is very high, but occasionally the patients attain adult life and even old age.

Treatment.—Of the many operations suggested, the following are the chief types:—

I. Formation of a reservoir in the body.

A. *From the bladder.*
    i. Closure of the defect by osteoplastic operation (Trendelenburg).
    ii. Closure of the defect by flaps.
        (*a*) Autoplastic methods, of skin (Woods) or of intestine.
        (*b*) Heteroplastic methods.

B. *From the rectum.*
    i. By transplantation of the ureters.
    ii. By vesico-rectal fistula.

C. *From the sigmoid flexure.*

D. *From the vagina.*

II. No reservoir formed in the body.

    i. Implantation of ureters (*a*) in the urethra (Sonnenberg), (*b*) in the skin.
    ii. Nephrostomy.

The operation that has given the most successful results is transplantation of ureters and trigone into the sigmoid flexure by Maydl's method. The danger of ascending pyelonephritis is much reduced by retaining the sphincter action of the bladder base. Peritonitis and fistula are also dangers. The immediate mortality of this operation varies from 5·5 to 26·7 per cent. Soubottine's operation consists in making a fistula between the bladder and the rectum. By a horse-shoe incision surrounding the rectal aspect of the fistula an area of rectum is marked out, and this is folded so as to form a small bladder, the lower open end of which is controlled by the anal sphincter. The suprapubic gap in the anterior bladder wall is then closed.

DIVERTICULA

A diverticulum is a pouch lined with vesical mucous membrane, surrounded by fibrous tissue, coarse fat, and often some non-striped muscle, and communicating with the bladder by a narrow opening. Diverticula should be distinguished from the pouches or saccules of a sacculated bladder commonly seen in prostatic obstruction. They are single or multiple, small as a pea, or as large as or larger than the bladder cavity. Small diverticula are frequently multiple. The orifice has sharply defined edges, may admit a crow-quill or the point of the forefinger, and frequently is surrounded by trabeculation. The ureteric orifice sometimes opens in the wall of the diverticulum or close to its orifice. (Fig. 547.)

Diverticula are most frequently found in the lateral walls or on the posterior wall. Rarely they open on the trigone. They may occur in infants, but are most frequently found in male adult life.

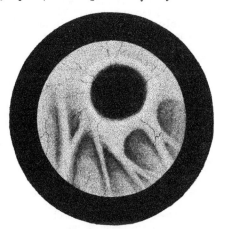

Fig. 547.—Diverticulum of bladder (cystoscopic view).

Symptoms.—The symptoms are usually puzzling and irregular. There may be apparently causeless attacks of frequent micturition at varying intervals or almost continuously, or recurrent attacks of difficulty and retention of urine.

Symptoms are sometimes entirely absent, and the diverticulum is discovered accidentally. Micturition in two parts may be present in large diverticula. Sometimes the second supply is purulent when the first is clear. On passing a catheter the bladder is apparently emptied, when the point of the catheter slips onwards and a large quantity of urine is passed. The edge of the diverticulum may sometimes be felt with a sound. A large diverticulum can be felt as a tumour in the lower part of the abdomen when the bladder is distended. Diagnosis is made with the cystoscope. The dimensions and position of a diverticulum are demonstrated by skiagraphy after distending the bladder with a bismuth emulsion.

Complications.—These are—(1) dilatation of one or both kidneys, (2) infection, (3) calculus in the diverticulum, (4) malignant growth at or near the opening.

Prognosis and treatment.—The prognosis is grave when infection has taken place or when malignant growth exists. After infection, washing the bladder has little effect on the diverticulum. In the female subject a Kelly's tube may be passed, and a catheter introduced through this into the orifice, and the diverticulum washed out. The following operations have been performed :—

1. Drainage outside the bladder.—This is only applicable to large diverticula, and leads to a permanent urinary fistula.

2. Closure of the orifice of the diverticulum from within the bladder, and drainage of the diverticulum outside the bladder.

3. Drainage into the bladder.—The walls of the bladder and diverticulum are split upwards or downwards, and the edges stitched together, so that the cavity of the diverticulum is thrown into the bladder.

4. Excision of the sac and repair of the bladder wall.—This operation is the most radical, and gives good results. Where the diverticulum lies low in the pelvis and is extensive the excision is very difficult and may be impossible.

HERNIA

This is rare, occurring in only 1 per cent. of hernia operations. It is more frequent in men, and in advanced life. The great majority of bladder hernias are inguinal; femoral are less common; and the obturator, sciatic, and perineal varieties are very infrequent.

Etiology.—The bladder · is thin-walled and distended, and the abdominal wall weak. Urethral obstruction, old age, coughing, straining, traction of an extraperitoneal lipoma, traction on the peritoneum-covered area of the bladder by a large hernia, adhesions between the bladder and the omentum and intestine, are recognized causes.

Pathological anatomy.—There are three varieties : (1) *Extra-peritoneal :* The bladder is prolapsed without a hernial sac of peritoneum. (2) *Intraperitoneal :* The peritoneum-covered portion of the bladder is drawn into a hernial sac with bowel or omentum. (3) *Paraperitoneal :* A sac of peritoneum is present, and adherent to this is the bladder. The large majority are of this nature.

The communication between the prolapsed portion and the bladder is temporarily narrowed, but there is no permanent constriction. Cystitis may be present, and a phosphatic stone has been known to form in the prolapsed portion.

Symptoms.—A swelling is present at one of the sites of hernia, and has the following characteristics : (1) It is irreducible. (2) It is large when the bladder is distended, and small when it is emptied. (3) Pressure on the swelling causes a desire to micturate. (4) Fluctuation may be detected. (5) The swelling is dull on percussion.

Micturition in two parts is a common symptom. There is difficulty in micturition, and sometimes complete retention, and the patient may only be able to pass water by pressing on the swelling, or in a certain posture. If a catheter is introduced it may pass into the hernia and be felt under the skin. Strangulation of a bladder hernia has occurred in several cases.

Diagnosis.—In 67 per cent. of cases diagnosis is made at hernia operations. Injury of the bladder seldom occurs if the neck of the sac is carefully inspected during the radical cure of hernia.

Treatment.—The bladder should be stripped from the hernial sac (paraperitoneal variety), or reduced with the other hernial contents (intra-peritoneal variety). If the bladder is opened during an operation it should be carefully dissected off the sac, closed, and returned to the pelvis, and a catheter tied in the urethra. The hernia operation is concluded in the usual manner.

INVERSION AND PROLAPSE (URETHRAL CYSTOCELE)

This condition occurs in women and female children. The whole thick-ness of the bladder wall, including the peritoneal investment, is inverted through the urethra, or the mucous membrane alone is prolapsed. The exciting cause is straining due to coughing, sneezing, constipation, or diarrhœa. There is a round swelling at the meatus, the size of a walnut or an orange, covered with reddened, easily bleeding, mucous membrane, on which the ureters are sometimes visible. The tumour is tender, increases in size on straining, and is irreducible or only reduced with difficulty. A probe passes along the urethra alongside the tumour, and can be swept round it, but is not free in the bladder. There is incontinence of urine. The tumour may not recur after reduction. Melted paraffin has been injected around the lax urethra. Cysto-ureteropexy and plastic operations on the urethra have been successful.

PERIVESICAL HYDATID CYSTS

Hydatid cysts in the pelvic subperitoneal tissue may be primary or, more frequently, secondary. The cyst becomes adherent to the bladder, prostate, and rectum, and mounts above the brim of the pelvis. There is bladder irritation, pain on micturition, and later retention of urine. Sciatica may be present. A firm, rounded, dull swelling appears above the pubes and closely resembles the distended bladder. On passing a catheter the swelling remains, and on bimanual examination fluctuation can be detected. Hydatid fremitus is rarely elicited. The diagnosis is greatly assisted by the "complement-fixation" reaction. The cyst is opened suprapubically, and the contents completely removed. The cavity is drained if septic, and closed if aseptic.

INJURIES

RUPTURE

This may involve the inner coat alone, but generally it is complete. Fully 90 per cent. of cases occur in male subjects, and usually between the ages of 20 and 40. The bladder is invariably distended at the time of the rupture. A considerable proportion of ruptures occur during alcoholic intoxication, and follow kicks, blows, or crushes. In fracture of the pelvis a splinter of bone may penetrate the bladder. Rupture may also result from indirect violence, such as falls from a height, muscular effort or straining, and it has followed the forcible injection of fluid into a diseased bladder. Spontaneous rupture has occurred in an ulcerated or cancerous bladder.

Pathology.—The rent is most frequently situated on the postero-superior wall, and opens the peritoneal cavity. Extraperitoneal rupture is less common, and affects the anterior or lateral walls. Rupture of the base or lateral walls usually results from fracture of the pelvis, but has been observed without fracture. The rupture is single and usually small in size, with clear-cut or bruised margins. When the rupture is intraperitoneal the urine escapes into the peritoneal cavity and general peritonitis supervenes. Aseptic urine does not necessarily cause peritonitis, although it is toxic when absorbed. The urine very readily becomes infected, usually from the passage of instruments. In extraperitoneal rupture the urine infiltrates the cellular planes and suppuration follows.

Clinical features.—Shock is present and may be severe, but occasionally it is absent and symptoms are delayed.

There are pain, urgent desire to micturate, and straining, but inability to pass water. The abdomen is rigid and tender, there is no dullness corresponding to a distended bladder, and the patient has not passed water for several hours. On passing a catheter a little bloody urine is withdrawn. Rarely, the catheter passes through the rent, and a large quantity of urine is obtained. If a catheter is passed several times the quantity of urine is always the same; and if the patient is set upright after withdrawal of the urine a large quantity can be obtained, although immediately before this the bladder had been emptied. When the rupture is *extraperitoneal*, dullness appears above the pubes, and there is tenderness and rigidity.

Infiltration spreads in the pelvis, and escapes by the sciatic notch into the buttock, by the obturator foramen into the upper part of the thigh, or along the inguinal canal into the scrotum. Abscess formation and the development of fistulæ follow, and then thrombosis and septicæmia. In *intraperitoneal* rupture peritonitis appears within the first twelve hours. Death, due to the toxic effect of the urine, may take place without peritonitis,

Diagnosis.—The diagnosis is made from the clinical features detailed above. In rupture of the urethra, blood appears at the meatus and the passage of a catheter is obstructed. In rupture of the kidney the blow is in the lumbar region, the loin is tender, and bladder irritation is absent. In fracture of the pelvis, retention of urine may be present without rupture, the diagnosis being made by passing a catheter.

The injection of fluids into the bladder in order to ascertain if a smaller quantity is returned, and the inflation of the bladder with air which will escape into the peritoneal cavity and obliterate the liver dullness, are to be deprecated as they disseminate infection. Except in the rare case of partial rupture, cystoscopy is not of diagnostic value since it is impossible to distend the bladder. Suprapubic exploration of the bladder is the most satisfactory diagnostic method.

Treatment.—Operation should be performed immediately, unless the shock is too profound, when a few hours' delay is permissible. When the diagnosis of *intraperitoneal* rupture is established, laparotomy is performed, the urine and blood are removed, the patient placed in the Trendelenburg position, and a search made for the rupture. If it is accessible it is closed by catgut sutures, a catheter tied in the urethra, and the peritoneum drained. If the wound is inaccessible it will only be possible to drain the peritoneum and tie a catheter in the urethra. When the rupture is *extraperitoneal* a suprapubic incision is made, the rent sutured, and the bladder drained.

Results.—Cases operated on in the first twelve hours have a mortality of 38 per cent., while those operated on after this time have a mortality as high as 71 per cent.

Collected cases of extraperitoneal rupture with urinary infiltration have a mortality of 83 per cent. (Mitchell).

WOUNDS

Bullet wounds of the bladder are not common, and stab wounds with a bayonet or dagger are rare. Accidental wounds during surgical operations are met with when the bladder is drawn into a hernial sac, in operations on the uterus, and in symphysiotomy. Falls from a height and impaling of the bladder from the perineum are not uncommon. The wound is complete and frequently double; it may be intra- or extraperitoneal. Bladder wounds are usually complicated by injury to the bony pelvis, rectum, uterus, vagina, urethra, and intestine.

Foreign bodies—e.g. fragments of clothing, pieces of wood, bullets —are frequently carried into the wound, and infection is constant.

Symptoms.—Shock is usually present, and may be profound. There are pain, tenesmus, frequent desire but inability to pass water ; a few drops of blood may be passed after much straining. Urine mixed with blood may escape from the wound, but this may be prevented by a coil of small intestine plugging the wound or by the flow of the urine into the peritoneal cavity. There may be profuse hæmorrhage from the wound. When the rectum is injured, fæces and flatus escape from the wound. Spontaneous closure is very rare, and peritonitis almost invariably supervenes, although it may be delayed until the separation of sloughs on the seventh or eighth day.

In extraperitoneal wounds where the wound is small and oblique there is perivesical and periurethral extravasation of urine, which becomes infected, and this is followed by thrombosis in the vesical and prostatic veins.

Recto-vesical or vesico-vaginal fistula, or fistula on the surface of the abdomen, scrotum, perineum, thighs, or buttocks, is very common.

Diagnosis.—The escape of urine from the wound and the presence of blood in the urine with tenesmus are sufficient to establish the diagnosis. The intra- or extraperitoneal nature of the wound will usually be decided by operation.

Treatment.—Laparotomy should be performed as soon as possible when there is a wound of the lower part of the abdomen. Wounds of the bladder and intestine are searched for and sutured. An extraperitoneal wound on the anterior surface of the bladder may be used for draining the bladder, or it may be closed and a catheter tied in the urethra. When the bladder has been wounded from the perineum the wound should be carefully examined and free drainage provided. If symptoms of peritonitis supervene the abdomen should be opened.

CYSTITIS

Inflammation of the bladder is due to the combination of a bacterial infection with some factor producing lowered resistance. Rarely, a virulent type of bacteria may alone cause cystitis, but usually some predisposing factor collaborates by producing congestion or injury of the bladder wall, or stagnation of the urine ; the most common are masturbation, affections of the female genital organs, pregnancy, stricture, enlarged prostate, calculus, foreign bodies, malignant growths, operations upon the bladder, atony from nervous disease.

Bacteriology.—Mixed infection is frequent. The Bacillus coli occurs more frequently than any other bacterium, and is often found in pure culture. The following bacteria may also occur, alone or in mixed infections, viz. streptococcus, staphylococcus, proteus, gonococcus, pneumococcus of Fränkel and of Friedländer, Bacillus pyocyaneus, and the typhoid bacillus. In chronic cystitis, anaerobic bacteria are frequently present. The bacteriology varies during the course of either an acute or a chronic attack. The urine is acid in cystitis due to Bacillus coli and the gonococcus.

Infection may occur from the kidney by bacteria borne in the urine or from the urethra by direct spread (gonorrhœa) or by the passage of instruments ; bacteria may also reach the bladder through a cystotomy wound or a fistula, or by the rupture of an abscess or the formation of a fistula with the bowel.

Pathological anatomy and cystoscopic appearances.—The whole surface of the bladder is seldom involved in acute cystitis. The base is frequently affected alone, or, less often, an area of cystitis is situated at the apex or some other part of the organ. Numerous patches may be distributed over the bladder. In severe cystitis and in chronic cystitis the whole surface is inflamed.

The capillary vessels are engorged, the mucous membrane becomes reddened, spongy or woolly, and the outline of the vessels is obscured. The surface is bright red, and the mucous membrane is thrown into stiff folds and ridges, with shreds of muco-pus or desquamated epithelium adhering to it. Hæmorrhages into the subepithelial tissues may occur. If the hæmorrhages are numerous the condition is known as hæmorrhagic cystitis.

In bullous cystitis the surface is covered with yellow semitransparent bullæ. Small closely grouped granules in the inflamed mucous membrane are characteristic of follicular cystitis. In cystic cystitis there are yellow sago-grain-like follicles which are either scattered or grouped together, and may be surrounded by a halo of inflammation. Extensive phosphatic deposit may take place. Necrosis of the superficial layers of mucous membrane mixed with fibrin forms a membrane which is cast off in the condition known as croupous or diphtheritic cystitis. The infection in these cases is usually streptococcal.

In very virulent infections exfoliation of the mucous membrane may take place and the necrosed membrane come away as a cast of the bladder. Ulceration is usually confined to the superficial layers, especially along the summits of ridges and folds. Less frequently there is a circumscribed deep round or oval ulcer with a heaped-up, sharply cut edge. A spreading ring-like ulcer is rarely observed. Leucoplakia is found in chronic cystitis. In chronic cystitis the submucosa and muscular layers are infiltrated and sclerosed, and the perivesicular fat becomes fibrous, adherent, and greatly increased. The bladder contracts and the cavity is permanently diminished. Calculi frequently form in the bladder in chronic cystitis, especially where there are sacculi or residual urine.

Symptoms.—The symptoms are frequent micturition, pain, and changes in the urine. In slight cases the urine is passed every two hours and there is some urgency. In severe cases a few drops of urine are passed every few minutes, active incontinence may be present, and the frequency is as great during the night as during the day. Polyuria is often present. There is pain on attempting to hold water, and scalding pain in the urethra during micturition ; in severe cases, cramping pain may radiate from the neck of the bladder down the thighs at the end of micturition. Pyuria is always present. The pus is mixed with mucus and forms a slimy, tenacious deposit which clings to the bottom of the receptacle. Blood is present in severe cases and appears at the end of micturition.

Complications.—Retention of urine may occur, especially where obstruction (stricture, enlarged prostate) is already present. Ascending infection of the kidneys is a serious and fatal complication. Abscess of the walls of the bladder or in the perivesical tissue may complicate chronic cystitis.

Diagnosis.—1. Vesical symptoms may be caused by extra-urinary conditions such as tabes, hæmorrhoids and anal fissure, pregnancy, ovarian or uterine tumours, and prolapse of the uterus. Pyuria is absent in these cases.

2. Urinary conditions other than cystitis may cause frequent micturition, such as the passage of large quantities of urine in diabetes insipidus, diabetes mellitus, and hysterical polyuria. In highly acid urines, oxaluria, and phosphaturia, frequent and urgent micturition with pain is often present, but pyuria is absent. In enlarged prostate, stricture, and urethral polypi, frequency of micturition may be present

without cystitis. In certain diseases of the kidney, notably tuberculous disease, calculus, and pyelitis, frequent micturition and pyuria may occur without cystitis.

Is the cystitis primary or secondary ? Renal calculus, pyonephrosis, renal tuberculosis, pyelonephritis, and urethral or prostatic disease may all cause secondary cystitis. The diagnosis is made by the history of the primary infection and the use of the cystoscope and urethroscope.

Prognosis.—In uncomplicated cystitis the attack lasts from two to five weeks, and recovery is usually complete. When a diverticulum or sacculi of the bladder are present, recurrent attacks and eventually chronic cystitis may be expected. When there is urethral obstruction the cystitis rarely disappears until the obstruction is completely removed. Cystitis in a paralysed bladder is permanent. When the cystitis is secondary to renal disease it will persist until this is cured.

Treatment. Acute cystitis.—The patient is confined to bed and placed on low diet. Diuretics are administered, such as Contrexéville water, barley-water, parsley-tea, and buchu. When the urine is acid, citrate of potash, potassium bicarbonate, magnesium sulphate, and liquor potassæ should be given, and sandalwood oil added.

To relieve spasm, belladonna, hyoscyamus, opium, and bromide of camphor are given, and hot fomentations applied to the lower abdomen and perineum. Hot sitz-baths are recommended twice or thrice a day, and relief may be obtained by means of a hot rectal enema or a vaginal douche containing antipyrin. The bowels should be opened with a saline purge.

No attempt should be made to wash the bladder at this stage.

Subacute cystitis.—The patient is allowed up and a less restricted diet permitted, but all highly spiced foods, curries, much meat, coffee, and all alcoholic drinks are forbidden.

Urinary antiseptics such as urotropine, hetralin, helmitol, urodonal, and salol should be administered, and sometimes benzoate of soda and ammonia and boric acid will be found valuable. If the cystitis is due to Bacillus coli or other bacteria which flourish in acid urine, alkalis should be given, but if the urine is alkaline from ammoniacal decomposition, dilute mineral acids, boric acid, benzoate of soda and ammonia, and especially sodium acid phosphate, are indicated. Bladder-washing should be commenced, and vaccine treatment with an autogenous vaccine will be found useful (*see* below).

Chronic cystitis.—If renal, prostatic, or urethral disease is present, this must be treated. The treatment is similar to that of subacute cystitis. Bladder-washing plays a prominent part in the treatment ; a visit to one of the Continental spas, such as Wildungen,

Contrexéville, or Vittel, is frequently of great service. Vaccine treatment is occasionally beneficial (*see* below), while drainage of the bladder with daily flushing or continuous irrigation may become necessary.

In acid cystitis a preliminary washing with a weak alkali such as bicarbonate of soda (1 or 2 per cent.) is useful, while in very alkaline cystitis a weak solution of acetic acid ($\frac{1}{2}$ per cent.) may be employed. The following solutions are useful, viz.: potassium permanganate, 1 in 5,000 or 10,000 ; oxycyanide of mercury, 1 in 1.000 or 5,000 ; biniodide of mercury, 1 in 10,000 or 20,000 ; tincture of iodine, $\frac{1}{2}$ to 1 drachm to the pint ; nitrate of silver, 1 in 2,000 or 10,000.

The instillation of small quantities ($\frac{1}{2}$–2 drachms) of more powerful solutions is sometimes useful. These are introduced by means of a small syringe and catheter. Iodoform in sterilized liquid paraffin (5 per cent.), gomenol (5 to 20 per cent.), silver nitrate (2 per cent.), and protargol (2 per cent.) may be used.

In intractable subacute and chronic cystitis the bladder may be drained by catheter in the urethra, or by the perineal or suprapubic routes.

Serum and vaccine treatment.[1]—In acute cystitis, especially if due to the Bacillus coli or the streptococcus, serum-therapy may be useful. The serum is injected subcutaneously, and a large initial dose is given (20 c.c.), followed by smaller doses (10 c.c.). Calcium lactate should be given at the same time to prevent serum rashes and joint troubles.

Vaccine treatment is most suitable for cases of subacute and chronic cystitis. The patient is inoculated with an autogenous vaccine, commencing with small doses at intervals of three or four days, rising slowly to higher doses, and extending the interval to a week or longer. A reaction should be avoided. The vaccine of Bacillus coli is that most frequently used, the dosage commencing with 3 millions or less of dead bacteria, and rising to 4, 5, 10, 15, 20, and so on to 100 and eventually to 200 millions. The staphylococcus is given in doses commencing at 100 millions, and rising to 500 or 1,000 millions ; and the streptococcus commences at 2, 3, 5, and 10 millions, and rises gradually to 50 and 100 millions. The treatment may extend over several months.

TUBERCULOUS CYSTITIS

Tuberculous cystitis may be "primary" in the bladder, or secondary to a tuberculous focus in the kidney or the male genital system.

Etiology.—Vesical tuberculosis occurs in youth and early adult life, very rarely in old age, and is more common in men than in

---

[1] *See also* Vol. I., pp. 90-108.

women. It is doubtful whether primary tuberculous cystitis ever exists. It was held that when the bladder and kidney were affected the infection was primary in the bladder and secondary in the kidney (ascending); but it is now recognized that the early symptoms of cystitis are usually reflex, the bladder being non-tuberculous. In cystitis secondary to tuberculosis of the kidney there is either direct spread by continuity along the ureter or deposit of bacilli from the urine. In cystitis secondary to genital tuberculosis in the male the tuberculous process either passes directly through the bladder wall from the seminal vesicles or prostate, or spreads from a tuberculous prostatic urethra into the bladder.

Pathology.—Greyish tubercles form in the mucosa, caseate, and break down into a tiny superficial ulcer with sharply cut edges. Several of these ulcers may run together, and a large area of bladder wall may thus be ulcerated. Deep ulcers may also form. They are round, oval, or serpiginous, with a greyish-red granular base and a deeply undermined edge. Irregular masses of granulation tissue are occasionally seen. In old-standing tuberculosis the bladder is contracted and adherent to the rectum and female genital organs, and there is tuberculous deposit in the pelvic lymph-glands. Tuberculous lesions of the kidney on one or both sides, or of the seminal vesicles or prostate, are also present. Tuberculosis of the female genital organs is rare.

Symptoms.—Cystitis arises spontaneously and insidiously in a young patient, and progresses gradually but persistently. Frequent micturition is the earliest symptom; at first diurnal and moderate, later it becomes nocturnal also and the intervals much less. Micturition becomes urgent, and urine is passed every quarter- or half-hour, day and night, sometimes involuntarily during heavy sleep. There are vesical pain, urethral scalding, and cramp-like pain at the end of the penis. A little bright blood often appears at the end of micturition. Severe attacks of hæmaturia may occur at intervals.

Polyuria is present and is due to tuberculous changes in the kidneys. The urine is pale and opalescent, faintly acid, of low specific gravity, and contains a small quantity of pus well mixed. The symptoms are unaffected by movement, but are influenced by dietetic indiscretion and cold damp weather.

Course and prognosis.—If septic complications are avoided the disease is slowly progressive, and death takes place after some years from renal failure due to bilateral renal tuberculosis. Frequently, however, septic complications arise, almost invariably as the result of catheterization, and occasionally secondary stone formation follows. Subacute or chronic septic pyelonephritis eventually supervenes.

Vesical tuberculosis secondary to unilateral renal tuberculosis may disappear after nephrectomy. When the disease is secondary to tuberculosis of the seminal vesicle or prostate the prognosis is unfavourable.

Diagnosis.—The spontaneous development of subacute cystitis in youth or early adult life should raise the suspicion of tuberculosis. The appearance of the urine, the discovery of the tubercle bacillus, and the result of inoculation of animals are important in diagnosis. Tuberculous disease may be found in the genital system or elsewhere in the body. The cystoscope shows discrete greyish-yellow opaque tubercles or deep tuberculous ulceration. Changes at the ureteric orifice and grouping of tuberculous inflammation round it show disease of the corresponding kidney.

Treatment.—Tuberculous cystitis secondary to unilateral renal tuberculosis generally diminishes or disappears after nephrectomy. In other cases further or different treatment is necessary.

General treatment.—Residence in a warm, dry climate, such as Egypt, Algiers, the French or Italian Riviera, has a very beneficial influence. The food should be plain and nourishing; highly spiced foods and alcoholic drinks should be avoided. If the infection is mixed, urinary antiseptics should be used, but in pure tuberculosis they have no effect. Guaiacol (5 minims in a capsule thrice daily), cacodylate of soda ($\frac{1}{2}$–1 gr. hypodermically), and disodium methyl arsenate ($\frac{1}{2}$ gr. hypodermically) have been recommended. Sandalwood oil is useful for its soothing effect, and belladonna and hyoscyamus for reducing the spasm of the bladder.

Tuberculin should be given in all cases, and very striking results are frequently obtained. Pain, frequency, and irritability diminish, the blood disappears from the urine, and the patient increases in body weight. When the bladder alone is affected the tuberculous process may disappear completely. When the cystitis is secondary to renal tuberculosis, marked improvement is observed in early cases, but relapses occur. In genito-urinary tuberculosis the results are less favourable, but amelioration of the symptoms may be anticipated. The treatment should begin with small doses ($\frac{1}{4000}$ mg. T.R.) and be very slowly increased by weekly injections to $\frac{1}{1000}$ mg. The treatment extends over one or several years.

Local treatment.—I am opposed to local treatment by means of bladder-washing and instillations. Temporary improvement is observed in many cases, but septic complications almost invariably supervene.

The following local treatment has been used: The bladder is washed with boric acid, and other solutions containing antipyrin or opium to soothe pain. Instillations of $\frac{1}{2}$–1 drachm have been given with Guyon's syringe: corrosive sublimate (1 in 10,000 up to 1 in

3 d

5,000), iodoform or guaiacol in liquid paraffin (5 per cent.), gomenol (5 to 20 per cent.), picric acid ($\frac{1}{2}$ to 1 per cent.) have been used.

Treatment by direct application of nitrate of silver, etc., may be made in either sex through Luys' direct cystoscope.

In the very rare cases of a solitary ulcer it is excised by suprapubic cystotomy. In other cases ulcers have been curetted, or cauterized with silver nitrate, chloride of zinc, and other caustics, and the bladder drained. .

SYPHILIS

Syphilitic disease of the bladder is very rare. In secondary syphilis symptoms of acute or chronic cystitis may develop. On cystoscopic examination there is congestion and swelling of the mucous membrane, and multiple small superficial ulcers with indurated edge may be present. In tertiary syphilis there may be gummata or ulceration of the bladder wall. The gummata may form papillomas which are indistinguishable from other forms of papilloma except that they disappear under antisyphilitic treatment. In other cases the gumma is a round nodular swelling covered with ulcerated mucous membrane. The symptoms resemble those of new growth. The lesions disappear rapidly under antisyphilitic treatment.

ACTINOMYCOSIS

Actinomycosis very rarely affects the bladder, and is always secondary to intestinal actinomycosis, spreading directly to the bladder from the appendix or rectum. Extensive perivesical inflammation is present, and there is usually a perivesical abscess. The symptoms are those of cystitis, and an indurated mass is found in the perivesical tissue and round the appendix or rectum. The diagnosis can only be made by the discovery of the yellow actinomycotic granules in the urine. The treatment consists in administering large doses of iodide of potash and opening collections of pus if they exist. The bladder is washed with urinary antiseptics.

TUMOURS

Men are more frequently affected by tumours of the bladder than women, usually between the ages of 40 and 60. Vesical growths are rare in children and are of the connective-tissue varieties.

Secondary growths result from the spread of malignant growths from the pelvic organs. In the rare papillomatous tumours of the renal pelvis or ureter new growths may become implanted on the bladder mucous membrane or spread from the ureteric orifice.

EPITHELIAL GROWTHS : PAPILLOMA—VILLOUS PAPILLOMA

Pathology.—These tumours are covered with villi, and are either sessile or pedunculated. They vary in size from a split pea to a Tangerine orange, and are single (60 per cent.) or multiple (40 per cent.). They may affect any part of the bladder, but are usually situated at the base, behind and to the outer side of one ureteric orifice and frequently concealing it. Although rarely situated on the trigone,

·they frequently surround it and sometimes the urethral orifice. The papilloma has a central trunk of fibrous tissue, elastic and plain muscle fibres, and blood-vessels, from which branches spread out and subdivide. (Fig. 548.) The epithelial covering is transitional in type, the deeper cylindrical cells radiating in characteristic manner. The nuclei show karyokinetic figures, and there is abundant vacuolation of the cells. Small villous tumours spring up on the mucous membrane around the first papilloma, and others become scattered over the bladder.

These growths are histologically benign, but many of them, in spite of their histological characters, must be regarded as malignant for these reasons: (1) They spread by implantation. (2) They frequently recur after removal; the recurrent growth is multiple, although the primary growth may have been single. (3) Multiple growths become sessile and irregular, and in a large number of cases eventually infiltrate the bladder wall.

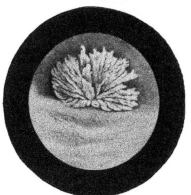

Fig. 548.—Papilloma of bladder (cystoscopic view).

Symptoms. — Hæmaturia is the characteristic and usually the only symptom. It appears suddenly without an apparent cause, is little affected by rest, continues for one or two micturitions, or for a day or a week, and suddenly ceases. The blood is copious and well mixed with the urine, and flat or irregular clots may be present. After a few weeks, months, or several years there is a similar attack of hæmorrhage. The attacks recur with increasing duration and diminishing intervals. Slight aching pain in one kidney is frequently present.

A pedunculated papilloma may obstruct the internal meatus and cause retention of urine, or become engaged in the prostatic urethra and cause strangury. Clot retention from excessive hæmorrhage is rare.

Course and prognosis.—The duration may extend over many years (ten to twenty-five years), during which there is increase in size and multiplication of the growth. The papilloma may remain single and attain a large size; usually, however, multiple tumours are found. Recurrence after operation is common, and malignant transformation frequently takes place.

Diagnosis.—Symptomless hæmaturia in a young or middle-aged adult is usually due to papilloma of the bladder, to " essential " renal hæmaturia, or to early renal growth.

The presence of tube casts and renal colic from the passage of clots indicates a renal source. Portions of vesical papilloma may be passed in the urine, or may be removed in the eye of a catheter. The diagnosis is made with the cystoscope.

Cystoscopy.—A papilloma is seen as a sessile or pedunculated, round or irregular tumour, with tendrils of varying length, which float in the fluid medium. A leash of vessels passes up to the growth from the trigone. A large growth may obscure the cystoscope light.

Treatment. 1. Non-operative.—Daily instillations for six months of 2 oz. of nitrate of silver solution (1 in 3,500 at 100° F.) or resorcin (2 per cent.), by means of a Guyon's syringe, have been advocated by Casper and others. Necrosis of the tumours has apparently occasionally followed.

2. Operative. (a) *Removal through the urethra* (" *intravesical opera-tion* ").—This is carried out by means of a Nitze operating cystoscope or by Luys' direct cystoscope, or in the female through the Luys or Kelly cystoscope. The papilloma is snared by a fine platinum wire, and left in the bladder to be expelled with the urine. Many sittings may be required, small portions being snared at a time. The growths must be favourably situated for easy access. Subsequent hæmorrhage is sometimes severe. Good results have been obtained with small easily accessible growths by some surgeons. The mortality in Weinrich's collected cases was 1 in 150, and 71 per cent. had no recurrence after three or four years.

(b) *Removal by open operation.*—This should be adopted in all cases. If multiple papillomas are present a chart showing their number and position should be drawn at a preliminary cystoscopy. Suprapubic cystotomy is performed, and the patient placed in the Trendelenburg position. The growths are fully exposed by proper retractors and a powerful head-lamp. With special scissors and forceps the growth is removed with the mucous membrane on which it is set, the cut edges stitched together, and the interior of the bladder treated with silver nitrate solution (4 to 6 per cent.), and drained with a large suprapubic tube.

For some years after the operation the bladder must be inspected at intervals for recurrence. At the earliest appearance of a recurrent bud of papilloma it should be destroyed with the electric cautery through Luys' direct cystoscope.

When the bladder is filled with large masses of papillomatous growth the contents should be cleared out, and the hot douche, cautery, adrenalin, or other means used for stopping the bleeding.

In some cases total cystectomy after ureterostomy is the only operation which holds a prospect of cure. Owing to the high immediate and remote mortality, cystectomy can [only be adopted in very rare cases.

Results.—The mortality of open radical operations for papilloma of the bladder is very small under modern conditions. In Rafin's statistics there was a mortality of 3·8 per cent. in 156 cases. Recurrence of papilloma took place in 28 per cent. With more thorough operations better results can be obtained.

Adenoma of the bladder is a rare tumour arising in the glands at the base. It may be diffuse or circumscribed.

Cholesteatoma consists in a great thickening of the epithelium, which becomes squamous and pearly in appearance. It is very rare.

CARCINOMA

A number of malignant growths differing widely in their gross and microscopic characters are grouped under this head, viz. malignant papilloma, nodular and infiltrating growths.

1. *Malignant papilloma.*—A papillomatous tumour may be malignant from an early stage of development, or it may have the characters of a simple villous tumour for many years and then become malignant.

In a malignant growth the villi are stunted and irregular in size and shape, and the tumour is irregular in contour and sessile. The bladder wall becomes infiltrated and the mucous membrane at the base of the tumour adherent to the submucous tissue. Microscopically there is rapid and irregular proliferation of the epithelium, and the base shows the invasion of lymphatic spaces and veins by irregular masses of cells.

2. *Nodular growths.*—These are sessile, rarely pedunculated, irregular, nodular or smooth, and varying in size from a hazel-nut to a Tangerine orange. Occasionally there is a round tumour with a flat or depressed surface showing stunted villi. These tumours belong to the papillomatous group, and consist of a mass of irregular villi closely matted together, and sometimes necrotic on·the surface. In the deeper part, masses of cells infiltrate the muscular planes, passing along the lymphatic vessels.

3. *Infiltrating growths.*—The growth forms flat nodules on the surface, but its greatest extent is intramural. It may take the form of a hard, depressed ulcer surrounded by nodules or by a raised hard ring of growth. The histological structure varies as follows, viz. :—(*a*) Epithelioma : Squamous epithelioma (chancroid) with cell nests develops in a patch of leucoplakia. (*b*) Cylindrical epithelioma or adeno-carcinoma develops in the tubular glands at the base of the bladder and is rare. (*c*) Spheroidal-celled carcinoma : This forms a soft or hard tumour·

according to the proportion of fibrous stroma. It consists of alveoli of varying sizes, filled with spheroidal cells.

Malignant growths of the bladder remain for a long time localized to the viscus. Perivesical spread may be extensive, and early penetration is a feature of some growths. Adhesions to the vagina, uterus, rectum, and intestines form, and perforation may occur. Spread along the lymphatics follows the lymphatic trunks. In the latest stages metastatic deposits are found in the lungs, pleura, liver, spleen, and kidneys.

Symptoms.—Hæmaturia is the most frequent (90·2 per cent.) and the earliest symptom. A little blood appears at the end of micturition; at first intermittent, it later becomes constant, and there may be intercurrent severe attacks of hæmorrhage.

Frequent micturition occurs in 68 per cent. of cases, and may be the initial symptom. It is nocturnal as well as diurnal, and is usually due to cystitis, although it may occur without cystitis and with a clear urine.

Pain is due to cystitis, to obstruction by blood clot, or to pressure on nerves. It is felt along the urethra, at the end of the penis, in the suprapubic region and groin, in the perineum, anus, and down the thighs or along the sciatic nerve. The urine sometimes contains a persistent excess of epithelial bladder cells, and portions of the growth may be passed. Flat or limpet-shell-shaped phosphatic concretions may form on ulcerated patches and be discharged with the urine. Emaciation is present in advanced cases.

Diagnosis.—There are two clinical types—(1) cystitic (40 per cent.), (2) hæmaturic (60 per cent.). Cases belonging to the cystitic type may be mistaken for stone, simple enlargement of the prostate, or malignant disease of the prostate. The diagnosis is made by rectal examination and cystoscopy. The hæmaturic type must be distinguished from simple papilloma or tuberculous disease by examination of the urine for the tubercle bacillus and by cystoscopy.

Course and prognosis.—The average duration of life after the first appearance of symptoms is under three years. Septic cystitis and ascending pyelonephritis is the usual cause of death. Radical operations in the early stages give an increasingly favourable prospect of cure (see below).

Treatment.—Radical operation should be undertaken if the growth is confined to the bladder and the patient sufficiently robust. It is contra-indicated by renal, pulmonary, or circulatory inadequacy. The radical operations are—(1) resection of the bladder wall, (2) cystectomy.

1. **Resection** is preferred wherever possible, as the mortality is 10 per cent. compared with 46 per cent. in cystectomy. The follow-

ing conditions are unsuitable for resection, though they do not contra-indicate cystectomy, viz. (1) very extensive growths confined to the bladder, (2) rapidly growing malignant papilloma, (3) growths involving both ureters, the trigone or urethra, (4) intractable cystitis.

Free exposure, the Trendelenburg position, and good illumination are necessary. The area of the bladder wall with the perivesical fat giving a margin of an inch all round the growth is removed. If this includes the ureteric orifice the ureter is implanted into the upper part of the bladder wound.

2. **Cystectomy.**—The ureters must first be transplanted and the bladder removed at a subsequent operation. Implantation into the rectum, large intestine, urethra, vagina, skin of the loin, or suprapubic wound, or bilateral nephrostomy, has been performed. Implantation into the vagina in the female and into the skin in the male has given the best results. In the male, cystectomy is performed by a combined perineo-abdominal method. The posterior surface of the prostate and seminal vesicles is first exposed by a curved prerectal incision. The patient is then placed in the Tredelenburg position, and the bladder exposed suprapubically. The peritoneum is stripped off, the ureter and large vessels exposed and clamped, and the bladder raised and detached from the prostate. The prostate may be removed with the bladder (cysto-prostatectomy).

In the female (Pawlik's operation) the ureters are exposed from the vagina, cut across and implanted in the vaginal wall, and after some weeks the bladder is exposed and removed by a suprapubic operation. The urethra is implanted into the vagina, the outlet of which is closed. The vagina forms a reservoir for the urine.

Results of operation.—In 30 cases in which I resected the bladder wall for malignant growth, there were 3 deaths (10 per cent.). In 10 of these, one ureter was transplanted. Watson collected 96 cases, with a mortality of 21·8 per cent. Kümmel found that of 47 cases 10 were well sixteen, fifteen, eight, and six and a half years after operation. In 39 cases of cystectomy collected from the literature the operative mortality was 46·1 per cent. Only 10 cases could be traced, and in but 2 of these was the period longer than fifteen months; one was above five years (Hogge) and one sixteen years (Pawlik).

Palliative treatment.—This is adopted when radical operation is contra-indicated.

Hæmaturia.—The patient is confined to bed, and the foot of the bed is raised. Opium, ergot, and calcium lactate are given. The bladder is washed with large quantities of hot silver-nitrate solution (1 in 10,000), continuous irrigation being made through a double-way catheter. This is followed by the instillation of a little adrenalin solution (1 in 1,000). If the bladder is distended with clot an attempt should be made to remove the clot by means of an evacuating cannula and bulb, and, this failing, the bladder should be opened suprapubically, the clots cleared out, and a large rubber drainage-tube inserted. Partial operations sometimes relieve severe bleeding.

Pain.—Suppositories of extract of belladonna ($\frac{1}{4}$ gr.) and morphia ($\frac{1}{8}$ gr.), to which cocaine ($\frac{1}{4}$-1 gr.) may be added, or the injection of tincture of opium (20 minims) with antipyrin (30 gr.) in hot water as an enema, may give relief. Washing the bladder with silver-nitrate solution may be beneficial, and if the urine is alkaline and phosphatic material is being deposited, sodium acid phosphate (20 gr. thrice daily) and urinary antiseptics should be given. Washing with a very weak solution of acetic acid often gives relief. Supra-pubic cystotomy may become necessary, and is followed by continuous irrigation, a permanent suprapubic drain being established.

Partial operations may relieve pain, but should be avoided when severe cystitis is present.

Nephrostomy after ligature of the ureter (Watson), ureterostomy, or implantation of the ureter in the loin on one side with nephrectomy (Harrison), or on both sides (Fenwick), may be used in inoperable carcinoma of the bladder with great pain.

CONNECTIVE-TISSUE NEW GROWTHS

Sarcoma of the bladder is found in infancy and late adult life, but is rare. The growth arises in the submucous or in the perivesical areolar tissue, or rarely from the intramuscular connective tissue; it is situated on the posterior or lateral walls. The tumour is pedun-culated or sessile and infiltrating. The bladder cavity may be filled with polypoid masses, and the wall infiltrated with growth. The urethra is sometimes blocked, and the polypoid masses may appear at the external meatus in the female.

The varieties are spindle-celled, round-celled, melanotic, myxo-sarcoma, rhabdo-myoma, and chondro-sarcoma.

Other connective-tissue tumours, such as myoma, myo-fibroma, and myxoma, are only rarely found. Dermoid cysts have been described.

VESICAL CALCULUS

Etiology.—The etiology of stone formation in the urinary tract is discussed under Renal Calculus (p. 832).

Stone in the bladder is less frequent in children than in adults, and much more frequent in men (especially old men) than in women. Calculi are " primary " when they form in an aseptic urine, and " secondary " when they result from bacterial changes in the urine. The nucleus may be formed by a small oxalate-of-lime or uric-acid calculus descended from the kidney, or a portion of blood clot, a fragment of a catheter, a pin, a silk ligature, a fragment of necrosed bone, or other foreign body in the bladder. The two important predisposing factors in the production of secondary calculi are bacterial action and stagnation of urine. This combination is frequently found in old men with enlarged prostate and cystitis.

Pathology.—Vesical calculi are formed of uric acid, phosphates, or oxalate of lime, in that order of frequency, and rarely of cystin, indigo, or calcium carbonate.

Uric-acid calculi (Fig. 549, 1-3) may consist of pure uric acid or of ammonium or sodium urates. They are single or multiple, rounded, oval, or flat. The surface is smooth or finely nodular and easily polished. They are sandy-yellow to dark-brown, show regular concentric lamination, and are of hard consistence. *Oxalate-of-lime* calculi (Fig. 549, 6) are usually single, vary from a pea to a chestnut in size, and have a dark-brown colour. The surface is covered with closely set conical bosses (mulberry calculus) or a few sharp projecting spines (star form). They are very hard, and on section show irregularly disposed laminæ. *Phosphatic* calculi (Fig. 549, 4, 7) consist of basic calcium phosphate, alone or mixed with ammonio-magnesium phosphate, and perhaps with ammonium urate. They are soft and crumbling, but when crystalline are very hard. On section, they are granular and rarely show lamination. *Cystin* calculi are oval, granular, yellowish-brown, have a soapy appearance, and turn greenish-yellow when exposed to air. *Xanthin* stones are smooth and yellow, and *indigo* are blue, while *calcium carbonate* are greyish-white, earthy-looking, hard stones. Calculi are rarely composed of a single ingredient.

Phosphatic stones develop rapidly, a large stone forming in a few weeks. Uric-acid calculi form less rapidly, and oxalate stones require some years to reach moderate size.

Vesical calculi may be movable or may be fixed in diverticula (Fig. 549, 8) or saccules, or in the ureteral or urethral orifices. A stone may be spasmodically grasped in the upper part of the bladder, or may be wedged behind an enlarged prostate.

Multiple stones may be present to the number of 400 or 500.

Cystitis may precede the development of a calculus, or result from its presence. Papilloma or malignant growth rarely complicates stone. Chronic pyelonephritis is the usual cause of death.

Symptoms.—There may be preceding attacks of renal colic when the stone or its nucleus has descended from the kidney. Fixed and very large calculi are " latent."

Frequent micturition and discomfort after micturition are the earliest and most common symptoms. The frequency of micturition is absent at night unless severe cystitis is present. Pain is felt in the neck of the bladder and is referred to the end of the penis ; it is sharp and cutting, and is experienced at the end of micturition. Hæmaturia is frequently present. It is slight, and appears at the end of micturition, and the blood is bright. An intermittent stream is sometimes observed, and complete retention may occur. All the symptoms of stone are aggravated by jolting movements and improved by rest.

The urine contains crystals of oxalate of lime, uric acid, or

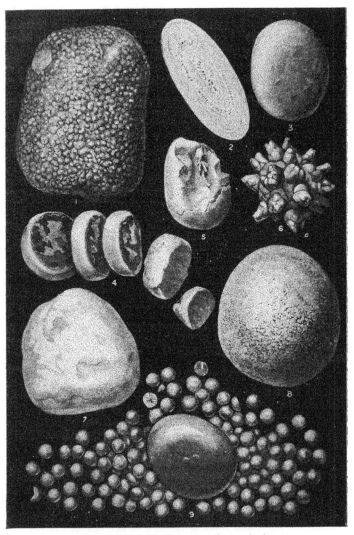

Fig. 549.—Collection of vesical calculi.

1-3, Large uric-acid calculi; 4, collection of disc-shaped phosphatic calculi; 5, calculus
formed on silk suture; 6, mulberry calculus (oxalate of lime); 7, large phosphatic
calculus; 8, phosphatic calculus from diverticulum; 9, collection of vesical calculi in
enlarged prostate

phosphates. microscopic quantities of blood, an excess of leucocytes, and usually some epithelial cells. In children, screaming on mieturition and retention of urine are not infrequent, or there may be active incontinence of urine. In small boys "milking" of the penis to ease the pain leads to an enlarged, turgid, semi-erect condition of the organ which is very characteristic. When cystitis complicates stone the frequency of micturition becomes nocturnal as well as diurnal, the pain is increased, and pus and mucus appear in the urine, which frequently becomes alkaline and stinking.

In old-standing cases symptoms of ascending pyelonephritis appear, and the patient shows signs of "urinary septicæmia."

Diagnosis.—The severity of the pain and its sharp character, the diurnal frequency, and the pronounced effect of movement and jarring on all the symptoms, are characteristic of calculus. The previous passage of a stone or past operations for stones are important points. Fixed stones do not produce the characteristic symptoms. Rectal and vaginal examination usually fails to detect the stone. When the calculus is large it may be detected bimanually, especially in children.

The bladder is examined with a sound after introducing a few ounces of fluid, and the impact of the metal instrument on the stone gives a characteristic sensation and sound. In children the stone lies at the neck of the bladder, in adults behind the trigone, and in old men frequently behind an enlarged prostate. The ridges of a trabeculated bladder, phosphatic deposit, and new growths may give rise to difficulties in diagnosis with the sound, and care should be taken that the handle does not come in contact with a ring or button.

A small stone may be detected by using a lithotrity evacuator and bulb.

Cystoscopy is the most certain method of detecting a calculus, and is especially useful in fixed calculi. Radiography shows a shadow in the vesical area.

Treatment.—A small calculus may sometimes be removed by means of the cannula and aspirator used in litholapaxy.

The operations performed for stone in the bladder are of two classes, viz. : (1) Crushing (litholapaxy or lithotrity), (2) cutting (lithotomy).

Litholapaxy or lithotrity.—The modern operation of litholapaxy (Bigelow, 1878) consists in crushing a stone and removing the fragments at one sitting. Four or five ounces of boric solution are introduced into the bladder ; the lithotrite is passed, the handles are raised, the blades separated. The stone rolls in between the blades and is caught. The blades are now locked and the male blade screwed home, and this manœuvre is repeated until all the fragments are crushed, when the lithotrite is removed. A large cannula is now passed,

and the aspirator bulb applied. By alternate compression and relaxa
tion the fragments are swept into the bulb and fall by their weight
into the glass bulb. When all the fragments have been removed the
bladder is washed with weak nitrate-of-silver solution and a catheter
tied in the urethra for a few days.

Litholapaxy has been performed upon young children. The
youngest child on whom it has been done, a boy of fifteen months,
was under the author's care.

Difficulties and contra-indications.—Litholapaxy is contra-indicated
by (1) severe and persistent cystitis, (2) considerable enlargement
of the prostate, (3) advanced sacculation, (4) fixed calculi, (5) spasmodic contraction of the bladder, (6) new growths of the bladder
complicating stone, (7) very large and hard stones.

Urethral stricture or a narrow meatus should be treated before
litholapaxy is performed.

Perineal litholapaxy, through a median external urethrotomy
wound, has been performed, but it is inferior to litholapaxy and to
suprapubic lithotomy.

Dangers.—Ascending pyelonephritis and perforation of the bladder
wall are rare. A rise of temperature may occur when cystitis is present, and is avoided by careful .preparation of the bladder and by
tying in a catheter and washing the bladder after the operation.

Suprapubic lithotomy.—The bladder is distended with fluid
and opened suprapubically, and the stone removed by lithotomy
forceps or a scoop. If the prostate is enlarged, prostatectomy is
now performed.

Median perineal lithotomy.—The patient is placed in the
lithotomy position, and the membranous urethra opened on a staff
by a median perineal incision.

The forefinger is introduced along a gorget into the bladder, and
a pair of lithotomy forceps or a scoop passed alongside this and
the stone removed. A rubber perineal drainage-tube is tied in the
bladder for some days.

Lateral lithotomy is now abandoned in favour of one of the
methods here described.

Vaginal lithotomy consists in opening the bladder base behind
the trigone on an instrument introduced through the urethra, and
removing the stone with lithotomy forceps. Vesico-vaginal fistula is a
frequent sequel.

Results of operation.—The results in 1,670 cases of stone in the
bladder operated on at St. Peter's Hospital in the years 1864–1910 showed
a mortality in the first decade of 15·25 per cent., and of 3·36 per cent. in the
last decade.

The death-rate of litholapaxy varies from 2 per cent. (Legueu) to 3·6 per
cent. (Zuckerkandl).

In the practice of surgeons who perform lithotrity, suprapubic or perineal lithotomy shows a high death-rate, as all the gravest cases are treated in this way. Thus, Freyer's statistics show a perineal lithotomy mortality of 18·2 and a suprapubic lithotomy mortality of 12·75 per cent. When, however, the *same* cases are treated in the two operations, the results are less disproportionate. Assenfeldt, in 460 cases of suprapubic lithotomy, found a death-rate of 3·6 per cent.

FOREIGN BODIES

Foreign bodies reach the bladder by the urethra or through the bladder wall. They may result from surgical operations. Silk ligatures used in operations upon the bladder or pelvic viscera, or the flexible guide of a urethrotome, are examples. Foreign bodies are frequently introduced by the patient. The mucous membrane becomes inflamed at the points of contact with the foreign body, and ulceration and even penetration of the bladder wall may follow. The foreign body becomes encrusted with phosphatic deposit, and a large phosphatic stone is formed. The symptoms are similar to those of stone in the bladder, and the diagnosis is made from the history, by radiographic examination, and by cystoscopy.

Treatment.—Urethral operations are most suitable in the female subject, but are also feasible in some cases in the male. In the female a large Kelly's tube is used after dilatation of the urethral orifice, and the patient placed in the Trendelenburg position. The foreign body is seized with fine forceps and removed, a finger in the vagina assisting the manœuvre. In the male, Luys' direct cystoscope should be used. When these methods fail (50 per cent.) the bladder is opened suprapubically, the foreign body removed, and, unless severe cystitis with ulceration is present, the wound is closed.

PERICYSTITIS AND PERIVESICAL ABSCESS .

Etiology.—Pericystitis may be secondary to disease or injury of the bladder, or it may arise in the neighbouring organs or structures, such as the urethra, rectum, prostate, appendix, or pelvic bones. Men are more frequently affected than women. Two forms are recognized : (1) Chronic fibro-lipomatous pericystitis with or without points of suppuration ; the bladder is surrounded, especially at its base and around the seminal vesicles and lower ends of the ureters, by a thick fibro-lipomatous mass. (2) Perivesical suppuration and abscess ; in the diffuse form the areolar tissue is widely infiltrated, in the circumscribed form the pus is thick and foul. The abscess may rupture into the bladder, rectum, peritoneum, or bowel, and a recto- or entero-vesical fistula follow.

Symptoms. 1. *Pericystitis from bladder disease.*—There is a greatly thickened bladder wall, and perhaps an abdominal tumour. When a diverticulum is present it may be demonstrated by radiography after distension of the bladder with bismuth emulsion.

Localized perivesical suppuration may develop slowly and escape recognition. An acute abscess may rupture into the bladder, causing an acute cystitis. The temperature is high, the patient is seriously ill and may have repeated rigors. A tumour is found on suprapubic or bimanual palpation. which may be mistaken for malignant growth, or a boggy mass can be felt from the rectum. The abscess may rupture into the rectum or bowel, and a recto- or entero-vesical fistula forms with discharge of fæces and gas by the urethra.

Prevesical abscess, or abscess of the space of Retzius, may be acute or chronic. In acute prevesical abscess, in addition to the symptoms of abscess, there are suprapubic pain and tenderness, dullness on percussion, and above the pubes appears a prominent rounded swelling, which closely resembles a distended bladder. but remains unchanged on emptying the bladder. In chronic prevesical abscess there are obscure pain and a moderate degree of cystitis.

2. *Pericystitis from disease of other organs.*—When an appendicular abscess invades the pelvis it may open into the bladder. There are signs of cystitis, and later the discharge of a quantity of fetid pus in the urine, followed by acute cystitis, and a fistula may form between the cæcum or appendix and the bladder. The urine remains clear till the abscess has ruptured into the bladder, when it becomes purulent and fetid, and if a fistula forms it contains fæcal material and gas is passed with the urine. There is a hard mass in the region of the bladder, extending suprapubically or confined to the pelvis.

Similar symptoms are produced by pericystitis originating in the rectum, sigmoid flexure, or small intestine.

There may be intermittent discharge of pus with pain and fever in the intervals of retention of pus, or continuous discharge of pus without general symptoms.

The diagnosis is made from the intermittent discharge of large quantities of pus in the urine, and the absence of pyonephrosis. Cystoscopy shows a patch of thickened inflamed mucous membrane, and a round or irregular opening may be seen in this area.

Treatment.—No radical treatment for chronic fibro-lipomatous cystitis is possible. In acute cases the perivesical areolar planes should be freely drained. A prevesical abscess or an interstitial abscess may be accidentally opened in exploring the bladder by suprapubic operation. Chronic abscesses are opened by a vertical or transverse suprapubic incision and blunt dissection. Great care should be taken not to open the peritoneum.

FISTULA

1. Suprapubic Vesical Fistula

The orifice of the fistula is usually situated at the lower end of a suprapubic operation scar. It is small, and may be surrounded by a collar of granulation tissue, or it may lie at the bottom of a depressed scar. When the urine is decomposing and constant cleanliness is not observed the scar is thick and red and the surrounding skin inflamed and excoriated.

All the urine may escape, or it may be discharged partly by the urethra. The leak may be intermittent.

Etiology.—A permanent fistula may be intentionally formed by the surgeon for incurable urethral obstruction or other disease. Fistula resulting from accidental wounds or from extension of malignant growths or tuberculous disease is rare. The most frequent form of fistula results from the non-healing of a suprapubic cystotomy wound. This is caused by septic cystitis, too long retention of drainage-tubes, adhesion of the cystotomy wound to the back of the pubic symphysis, prolapse of a peritonea sac, spread of malignant growth or tuberculous infection along the track, unrelieved urethral obstruction, or delay in healing due to old age or extreme debility or nervous disease.

Treatment.—Sepsis is energetically treated by daily washing the bladder, a catheter being tied in the urethra. Should these measures fail, the track of the fistula should be dissected down to the bladder wall and removed, care being taken not to open the peritoneal cavity. The bladder is dissected free from the pubic symphysis, and the cavity explored for phosphatic débris and calculi. If the bladder is very septic it will be wise to drain it, and follow the operation with constant or repeated irrigation. Any urethral obstruction present must be removed. If cystitis is not severe the wound in the bladder should be closed by a double row of catgut sutures and the prevesical space drained for a few days. A catheter is tied in the urethra.

2. VESICO-INTESTINAL FISTULA

Etiology.—The fistula may be spontaneous or traumatic. Spontaneous fistula may take origin in the bladder in chronic cystitis, malignant growth, or some other condition which will cause perivesical abscess. The abscess forms adhesions and ruptures into the bladder and bowel. Simple, typhoid, tuberculous, or malignant ulceration of the rectum or intestine may lead to the formation of a fistula.

Pathology.—The vesical opening is most frequently high up on the posterior wall; it is rarest on the anterior wall. A fistula on the right side of the bladder usually communicates with the cæcum or appendix, and one on the left side with the sigmoid flexure.

The opening in the bladder is small and is surrounded by an area of inflammation. The communication with the bowel may be direct, but there is usually either a tortuous track or an intermediate cavity. The rectum is most frequently affected, then the sigmoid flexure, ileum, and cæcum, in that order. The coils of intestine are matted together in a dense mass.

Symptoms.—When the bladder is previously healthy, spontaneous cystitis develops, and may persist for some weeks before a fistula is formed. There are symptoms of deep-seated suppuration. A history of rectal or intestinal disease or of chronic cystitis can usually be obtained. There is occasionally evidence of rupture of an abscess into the bladder. .

Pneumaturia (*see* p. 788) is a constant and characteristic sign, and may be the first intimation that perforation has occurred. The passage of fæcal material in the urine may be constant or intermittent, and varies from a few brown shreds to considerable masses of fæcal matter. The urine is hazy with mucus and bacteria, and contains irregular white flakes. The odour may be distinctly fæcal. Fragments of undigested food may be recognized. When the fistula is enteric the urine is yellow with bile. Cystitis is present to a varying degree, and may be remarkably slight. Urine is frequently passed by the bowel, and the whole of it may be discharged in this way, giving rise to frequent watery stools.

On cystoscopy, cystitis is found, but this may be slight, and confined to the immediate neighbourhood of the fistulous opening. The opening may be hidden by a fold, but is usually seen as a small round opening in which lies a plug of fæcal matter. It may be surrounded by œdematous bullæ.

Prognosis.—The condition may exist for many years (three, four, twenty) without affecting the general health. The dangers are retention of pus and fæcal matter in an intermediate cavity, peritonitis, ascending pyelonephritis, intestinal obstruction.

Treatment.—The fistula may close spontaneously if the bladder and rectum are washed.

Surgical treatment consists in deflecting the fæces from the intestinal orifice, or in attempting to close the fistula. The portion of bowel may be excluded by short circuit or by colostomy when the rectum is involved.

A rectal fistula may be attacked through the rectum or across the bladder after suprapubic cystotomy. These methods are inferior to the perineal operation. In fistula originating above the rectum the abdomen is opened, the coils of intestine separated, the fistulous portion excised, and the ends anastomosed. The fistula is then closed.

3. Vesico-Vaginal Fistula

Etiology.—Traumatic vesico-vaginal fistula is rare, apart from surgical operation or parturition. It may follow operation on the genital organs, vaginal drainage of the bladder for cystitis, or ulceration due to a pessary or to malignant or tuberculous disease.

Pathology.—The common form opens directly from the bladder into the anterior fornix, less frequently into the cervix uteri. The ureter may be implicated and a vesico-utero-vaginal fistula result. There is usually extensive scarring and prolapse of the vesical mucous membrane.

The vagina, vulva, and skin of the thighs are irritated and excoriated by the escaping urine. There is cystitis, and sometimes vesical calculus.

Symptoms and diagnosis.—The vaginal escape of alkaline and decomposing urine is the chief symptom. In vesico-uterine fistula the urine is seen to issue from the os uteri, and coloured fluid injected into the bladder appears at the os.

In vesico-utero-vaginal fistula the discovery of the ureteric orifice is assisted by the intramuscular injection of methylene blue or indigo carmine.

Treatment.—Before undertaking a plastic operation the urine must be rendered aseptic, calculi removed, and vulvo-vaginitis treated. Suprapubic cystotomy should be established for at least a week before the operation. There are three methods of approach—(1) vaginal, (2) vesical, (3) peritoneal. The vesical and vaginal should be combined. Various plastic operations have been practised. For a week after the operation the bladder is kept dry by means of a White's suction apparatus.

NERVOUS DISEASES

The nervous diseases which affect the bladder are principally spinal lesions. Cerebral disease seldom affects the organ so long as consciousness is retained, and it is doubtful if it is influenced by changes in the peripheral nerves. Nervous disease of the bladder gives rise to the following symptoms :—

1. *Pain.*—There may be either constant aching in the bladder, unaffected by micturition, or attacks of acute pain (vesical crises).

2. *Increased desire and bladder spasm.*—This may be the only symptom or may be one symptom in a group. It is not infrequently combined with partial retention. Spasm of the bladder may lead to active incontinence.

3. *Absence of desire* may result in the patient passing water only once or twice in the twenty-four hours. With this there is residual urine in varying amount. There is diminished sensibility of the bladder.

4. *Difficult micturition.*—This is present in almost all cases of nervous disease of the bladder in spinal lesions, and is combined with residual urine. There are delay in commencing micturition, a feeble stream, straining, and dribbling.

5. *Complete retention of urine* is due to paralysis of the bladder muscle. This may be present at the onset of the bladder affection, and the tone of the muscle improves later, so that micturition can be performed, but the bladder is incompletely emptied.

6. *Incontinence of urine* (see p. 848).

The following varieties of nervous affections of the bladder are observed :—

1. *Active incontinence.*—(*a*) Reflex micturition. (*b*) Incomplete reflex micturition.

2. *Passive incontinence.*—(*a*) Distension with overflow. (*b*) Collapse with outflow.

When the bladder is cut off from the control of the cerebrum it acts automatically. A quantity of urine collects, the reflex of micturition is initiated, and the bladder empties itself. This is repeated at intervals ("flushing-tank action "). The condition occurs in lesions above the lumbar centre, and, as Müller has shown, in lesions involving the lumbar centre also. There is sometimes uncontrollable spasm of the bladder.

The bladder may be fully or partly distended, and the urine is passed involuntarily by bladder contraction from time to time. In passive incontinence the contraction of the bladder is abolished and the outflow is purely mechanical. The bladder may be fully distended or it may be collapsed, but it is seldom, if ever, completely empty, a certain amount of urine collecting before the elastic resistance of the urethra is overcome.

Changes in the bladder in nervous diseases.—Cystitis is frequently present, the infection being usually introduced by the catheter. The cystitis becomes chronic, and the urine is frequently alkaline and ammoniacal. Phosphatic calculi form rapidly. Trabeculation of the bladder is observed in tabes dorsalis, and I have found it also in atony from postero-lateral sclerosis and from spina bifida, but it was absent in cases of multiple sclerosis and supralumbar myelitis. It also occurs in idiopathic atony of the bladder. In my opinion, the trabeculation in these cases is due to atrophy and not to hypertrophy of the bladder muscle.

Rarely, in spinal disease, ulceration of the bladder may develop and rapidly perforate.

Bladder symptoms in special nervous diseases.—The bladder is more frequently affected in tabes than in other forms of nervous disease, and the vesical symptoms may appear when the symptoms of spinal disease are only partly developed. There is gradually increasing difficulty in micturition—delay in commencing, loss of power of projection, intermittent flow, and after-dribbling ; there may be a diminished desire. A varying quantity of residual urine is found, and there is widespread trabeculation. The atony increases until there is complete retention, or this may rapidly develop at the commencement of the bladder symptoms. Nocturnal enuresis is usually present. After a varying period of weeks or months the tone of the bladder frequently improves, so that there are 8 or 10 oz. of residual urine, and the rest is passed voluntarily. Vesical and urethral crises are rare. In acute and chronic spinal meningitis and acute and chronic myelitis, and in multiple sclerosis, the characteristic change is gradually increasing atony of the bladder, and eventually complete retention develops, and dribbling of urine from overflow follows. This may continue, but usually the bladder acts automatically after a time. Spasmodic contraction of the bladder is occasionally observed, but this later passes into the atonic condition described. In spina bifida affecting the sacral canal, atony of the bladder may be observed.

Atony of the bladder without obstruction or signs of nervous disease.—I have described a series of cases under this title. The condition occurs in young and middle-aged patients, and is unconnected with venereal disease. There is gradual onset of difficulty in

3 *e*

micturition, delay, feeble and intermittent stream. Chronic distension of the bladder with voluntary micturition may be present, or residual urine amounting to 4 to 10 oz. There is loss of sensibility of the bladder in some cases and increased sensibility in others. Well-marked trabeculation (atrophy) of the bladder is present in all.

Urethral obstruction and spinal disease are eliminated.

The disease was present in cases for eight to eighteen years without the development of nervous lesions. The lesion is probably localized in the hypogastric and hæmorrhoidal plexuses of the sympathetic.

Injury to the nervous system.—Corner gives the following table of the state of the bladder in various injuries:—

Concussion of the brain.
1. Reflex or unconscious micturition.
2. Active retention: (a) active overflow; (b) passive overflow; (c) absolute retention.

Compression.
1. Passive retention.
2. Active paralytic overflow.
3. Passive paralytic overflow.

Spinal injuries.
1. Supralumbar lesions: (a) active retention; (b) reflex micturition; (c) exaggerated reflex micturition.
2. Lumbar lesions: (a) passive retention; (b) active paralytic overflow; (c) passive overflow.

Treatment. 1. Relief of retention and removal of residual urine.—Rigid asepsis must be observed. For complete retention the catheter must be passed thrice in twenty-four hours. The tone of the bladder frequently improves with regular catheterization, and the frequency of catheterization may be reduced. When the residual urine does not exceed 6 or 10 oz., the catheter should be passed once a day, and if less than that, once a week. If urethral obstruction is present it must be removed.

2. Prevention and treatment of cystitis.—Urinary antiseptics should be given from the commencement of the bladder symptoms, and constipation prevented. If infection has occurred the bladder is washed out (see under Cystitis, p. 862). The bladder should be examined from time to time to ascertain if a phosphatic calculus has formed.

3. Treatment of atony.—The patient should be encouraged to try to expel all the urine, he should be regularly catheterized, and should be given ergot (liquid extract, 20–30 minims thrice daily) and strychnine (liquor, 5 minims). Mercury and iodides have no effect. The electrical current may be used with advantage, one terminal being placed over the suprapubic region or the sacrum and the other over the perineum, or an electrode may be introduced into the bladder or into the rectum. A weak interrupted current should be used, and at first the sittings are short. The galvanic current may also be employed.

THE URETHRA

Anatomy (Figs. 202, 203, Vol. I., pp. 806, 807).—The male urethra is divided anatomically into three parts—the prostatic (1¼ in.), the membranous (¾ in.), and the spongy urethra (about 6 in.); a *pars intramurales* is also described.

Clinically, the canal is more conveniently divided by the compressor urethræ muscle into the posterior urethra (corresponding to the prostatic urethra) and the anterior urethra, which, again, is divided into the bulbous or perineal and the penile urethra.

The urethra has an S-shaped curve. The internal meatus is situated on a level with the middle of the pubic symphysis and about 2 cm. behind it. Thence the canal passes vertically downwards for about ½ to ¾ in. to the level of the verumontanum; there it turns slightly forwards and maintains a forward and downward direction to the junction of the membranous and bulbous urethra. The canal now turns sharply upwards and forwards along the under surface of the triangular ligament. At the peno-scrotal junction it turns downwards in the flaccid penis to the meatus. The fixed curve of the urethra extends from the peno-scrotal junction to the internal meatus, the deepest part of the curve lying at the termination of the bulbous urethra, the *cul-de-sac du bulbe*. This is 4 cm. from the internal meatus and 3 cm. from the peno-scrotal junction. The angle formed by these two segments is one of 93 degrees. The walls of the urethra lie in contact. Its calibre and musculature are described elsewhere (Vol. I., p. 805). The lining epithelium is columnar, except at the fossa navicularis, where it is squamous.

On the posterior wall of the prostatic urethra is the verumontanum, on which the sinus pocularis and ejaculatory ducts open. On each side of this ridge is a gutter-like prostatic sinus, into which the prostatic ducts open.

The membranous urethra, which is surrounded by the compressor urethræ muscle, has numerous mucous glands. On each side of this lie Cowper's glands. In the mucous membrane of the anterior urethra there are mucous glands (glands of Littré), the ducts of which open obliquely forward. There are also 10 or 12 larger lacunæ on the roof, and the largest of these (lacuna magna) opens on the roof of the fossa navicularis. The ducts of Cowper's glands open on the floor of the bulbous urethra, 1 in. in front of the membranous urethra. The lymphatics of the prostatic urethra pass to the glands along the internal iliac vessels, those of the membranous and bulbous urethra to the glands along the external iliac vessels and internal pudic vessels, those of the spongy urethra to the inguinal and femoral glands.

Female urethra.—The female urethra is 1½ in. long, has a slight anterior concavity, and is intimately united with the anterior vaginal wall. The external meatus is the narrowest part. The epithelium is squamous at the external and columnar near the bladder.

Examination.—On rectal examination the membranous urethra can be felt in the middle line below the prostate, and the prostatic urethra lies in the vertical sulcus between the lobes of the prostate.

For examination of the urethra with sounds, an acorn-tipped bougie or *bougie à boule* is used. If it is arrested, the distance from the external meatus is noted and a smaller instrument is tried. There may be creaking on passing through a cartilaginous stricture, grating in passing over a stone or a phosphatic deposit, or a tearing sensation when a false passage is made. Resistance is felt 5½ or 6 in. from the meatus at the contracted membranous urethra; this is overcome by gentle pressure on the perineum. There is slight resistance at the entrance of the bladder.

Urethroscopy.—There are two varieties of urethroscope. In one the light is reflected from a lamp at the proximal end of the tube, and in the other the lamp is placed in the lumen of the tube at its distal end. For the anterior urethra the tube is 5½ in. long, and straight, being provided with a metal obturator. For the posterior urethra the tube is 8½ in. long and has a curved beak, the distal opening being on the convexity of the beak.

For anterior urethroscopy the patient lies on a high table, and the tube with the obturator in position is oiled and introduced. The instrument sinks as far as the membranous opening, the obturator is removed, and a pledget of cotton-wool on a carrier introduced to remove the moisture. The lantern is applied to the tube and the light switched on. The urethra is examined as the tube is slowly withdrawn. The tap of the air-bulb, which has previously been distended, is now opened, and the urethra distends like a tunnel. Air-distension is especially useful in examining a stricture.

For examination of the prostatic urethra the pelvis of the patient is raised on a cushion, or the patient is placed in a special chair with the hips and knees well flexed.

The posterior urethra is anæsthetized by introducing 20 minims of a 1 per cent. cocaine solution by means of a Guyon's syringe. The posterior urethroscope tube is well depressed when the beak reaches the membranous urethra, so that it passes on into the prostatic portion. The obturator is withdrawn, a tampon of wool introduced to remove the moisture, and the lantern is applied.

The female urethra can be palpated on the anterior wall of the vagina. The urethroscope is used in the same manner as in the male, but without air-distension.

Urethral shock.—On the first instrumentation a nervous patient may feel faint, but quickly recovers on the application of the usual remedies. True urethral shock is rare, and is a much more serious condition. During or immediately after the passage of an instrument the patient gives a few short gasps, becomes unconscious, and after one or two inspiratory stridors stops breathing. The pupils dilate, the pulse becomes imperceptible, and the heart sounds cease. A loud expiratory effort may occur after breathing has stopped. The condition is fatal in a large proportion of cases. Energetic stimulation and artificial respiration may be tried, and are occasionally successful.

URETHRAL, URINARY, OR CATHETER FEVER

The rise of temperature that sometimes follows instrumentation has been ascribed on one theory to nervous influences, and on another to sepsis. It is now generally accepted that urethral fever is septic in origin, the infection originating either in a septic instrument, in an already infected urethra, or in septic urine. Infection is more likely to take place when an obstructive lesion is present than in an unobstructed urethra, in lesions of the bulbous than of the penile urethra, and in those of the prostatic than of the anterior urethra. A rough inexperienced hand is more likely to produce urinary fever than a gentle educated touch.

Types of urethral fever. 1. Urethral fever without suppression of urine.—(a) The temperature may rise to 100° F. or 101° F., with slight malaise, but falls again in a few hours to normal.

(b) A single severe rise to 102° F., or higher, accompanied by a rigor, may occur a few hours after the passage of an instrument. The patient is restless and ill, the tongue dry, the mouth parched, the urine scanty and high-coloured. In twenty-four to thirty-six hours, after profuse perspiration, the temperature falls to normal.

(c) The fever is prolonged (acute remittent type). After an initial rigor the temperature rises to 102° F. or higher, remaining high for several days, then falling gradually to normal. sometimes with a short recurrent rise.

(d) A rigor follows internal urethrotomy, and the temperature rises to

103° F. or 104° F., and falls in a few hours. A second rigor occurs with another rise of temperature, and the rigors are repeated at irregular intervals. Venous thrombosis, pneumonia, or other complications eventually supervene, and the patient dies after several weeks.

2. **Urethral fever with suppression of urine.**—(a) There is a rigor a few hours after internal urethrotomy, and the temperature rises to 104° F., or even higher. A few ounces of bloody urine are passed, and the secretion becomes completely suppressed. The patient is restless and wanders. He becomes rapidly comatose, and dies within eighteen to thirty-six hours of the operation.

(b) After the passage of a catheter in a case of enlarged prostate there is a rise of temperature, and the tongue is dry and glazed. The patient is drowsy and heavy, and wanders at night. The temperature remains high; buccal dysphagia, hiccup, and vomiting follow; the quantity of urine diminishes and complete suppression supervenes, and death results in a considerable proportion of cases.

Treatment.—Prophylactic treatment consists in the sterilization of all urethral instruments, washing the bladder and urethra with nitrate of silver when the urine is already septic, and the administration of urinary antiseptics and diuretics before and after instrumentation. When infection has occurred a smart purge is administered, diuretics such as Contrexéville water or barley-water are freely given, and urinary antiseptics administered. If the infection is due to the Bacillus coli, large doses of alkalis should be given. A catheter is tied in the urethra, and in some cases suprapubic drainage is installed. Vaccine and serum treatment may be tried.

The treatment of suppression of urine is discussed elsewhere (p. 783).

CONGENITAL MALFORMATIONS

CONGENITAL ABSENCE OR OBLITERATION OF THE URETHRA

This is rare. The penis is absent or rudimentary, and other malformations are present. The bladder may communicate with the rectum, uterus, or umbilicus. The children are usually still-born or die soon after birth.

PARTIAL OBLITERATION OF THE URETHRA

This may be found in the glans, in the bulbous, membranous, or prostatic urethra. The anterior urethra is most commonly and the prostatic urethra least often affected.

If no outlet is present, there is distension of the bladder with dilatation of the ureters and kidneys. The kidneys may be the seat of congenital malformation and be inactive, so that distension of the urinary passages does not take place. The urine may find an outlet through a patent urachus, a vesico-rectal fistula, a vesico-utero-rectal fistula, a penile or vaginal fistula. In the majority of cases the child is still-born or dies soon after birth. If life is prolonged, fatal ascending infection occurs after a few years.

Treatment.—Suprapubic puncture and cystotomy are emergency operations to relieve distension. In atresia of the glans urethræ the dilated urethra should be opened and a penile fistula established, a plastic operation being carried out later on the urethra.

DOUBLE URETHRA

This is rare, and may be combined with double penis, double scrotum, double bladder, atresia ani, and other congenital malformations.

The second urethra may open on the perineum or in the inguinal region. A more frequent condition is where a canal opens on the glans or below the penis and runs backwards on the upper or under surface of the penis. The track varies in length from ¼ to 5½ in., and usually ends blindly. In a few cases the canal joins the urethra, and rarely it passes back into the bladder.

A double urethra has been described in the female subject.

When the second canal communicates with the urethra or bladder, urine escapes from both orifices. The penis may swing from side to side during micturition. In gonorrhœal infection there is discharge from both orifices, but the infection may attack the abnormal canal while the urethra escapes. When the abnormal canal is the seat of chronic inflammation it may be laid open in its entire length and the lining membrane destroyed with the cautery. A thick scar may result which interferes with erection. Extirpation of the unopened tract by dissection is more difficult, but the after-result is better.

Congenital Narrowing of the Urethra

The points most frequently affected are the external meatus, the junction of the fossa navicularis and the penile urethra, the membranous urethra, and the prostatic urethra. The external meatus is most frequently the seat of stenosis. The symptoms are those of stricture.

Treatment.—In stenosis of the meatus the urethra is slit downwards, and the mucous membrane and skin are brought together by catgut sutures. In deeply situated stenosis, dilatation with graduated bougies should be tried, and, that failing, external urethrotomy, followed by the regular instrumentation.

Congenital Dilatation of the Urethra

This is independent of stenosis. The dilatation affects the under surface of the penile urethra, rarely the bulbous urethra. A similar condition may occur in the female urethra. Symptoms may appear soon after birth, or may be delayed. Micturition is frequent and painful, the stream is poor and is followed by dribbling. A swelling appears on the under surface of the penis during micturition, and the penis may be twisted to one or other side, or becomes erect. Incontinence is a late result.

Treatment.—The sac should be excised, the urethra repaired, and the skin stitched separately. A catheter is tied in after the operation.

Hypospadias and Epispadias

These conditions are considered at pp. 966, 967.

PROLAPSE

About 170 cases of this rare condition are on record, more than half of them in girls under 15, and most of the rest in elderly women. (*See* p. 985.)

URETHROCELE

This condition—a pouching of the urethral mucous membrane, filled with decomposing purulent urine—is considered at p. 985. A similar condition may occur in men.

INJURIES AND RUPTURE

Injuries

The urethra may be injured from within the lumen by the passage of instruments (*see* p. 883), or from without by cutting weapons, bullets, etc. The penile urethra is most frequently affected. Hæmorrhage is usually severe. When free exit for the urine is afforded no extravasation takes place, but when the urethral wound does not correspond to the skin wound, or when the wound is in the perineum, widespread extravasation is likely to occur. Immediate exploration and suture of the urethra should be carried out, and a catheter tied in the urethra for four days. When suppuration and extravasation have already taken place, a catheter should be tied in and the wound thoroughly cleansed.

RUPTURE

There may be bruising of the mucous membrane (interstitial rupture), rupture of the fibrous sheath (partial external rupture), of the mucous membrane (partial internal rupture), or of the mucous membrane, corpus spongiosum, and fibrous sheath (total rupture). A part of the circumference of the urethra (partial rupture) or the whole circumference (complete rupture) may be affected. In complete rupture the severed ends retract and may be widely separated.

Rupture of the *penile* urethra is rare, and results from injuries during erection. The seat of election is the peno-scrotal junction.

Rupture of the *bulbous* urethra is more frequent, and results from a kick, or blow, or fall on the perineum. The rupture is usually complete and total, and the severed ends retract some distance. The position of the rupture depends upon the attitude of the body at the time of the injury. A force striking the perineum from before backwards injures the bulbous urethra, but one striking the perineum from behind forwards damages the membranous urethra. The urethra is crushed between the injuring body and the pubic arch and triangular ligament. Rupture of the *membranous* urethra occurs in severe injuries with fracture of the pelvis or dislocation of the pubic bones. The *prostatic* urethra is rarely ruptured.

Symptoms.—In *penile* rupture there is hæmorrhage from the meatus for a few days, pain on micturition, but rarely retention of urine. Extravasation of urine does not occur, but stricture invariably follows. Rupture of the *bulbous* urethra is the most common form. After a blow on the perineum there is sharp pain, increasing in severity, and blood appears at the meatus. A tumour rapidly forms in the perineum, which becomes tense and tender. In slight cases where the fibrous sheath is not ruptured this swelling is absent. Retention of urine frequently follows the injury. *Membranous* or *prostatic* rupture is associated with fracture of the pelvis, and may escape observation at first. Hæmorrhage is slight, and bruising appears in the perineum after some days. There is retention of urine. A tender swelling is felt on rectal examination, and the abdominal muscles are frequently rigid. The bladder is distended.

Diagnosis.—The history and symptoms are usually sufficient to make the diagnosis easy. Differentiation between rupture of the posterior urethra and extraperitoneal rupture of the bladder is difficult. In the former, tenderness and swelling are present around the membranous and prostatic urethra on rectal examination, and on passing a catheter there is obstruction at the posterior urethra. The bladder is distended in rupture of the urethra.

Prognosis.—In *penile* rupture the symptoms rapidly subside, but a stricture forms within a few months. In *bulbous* rupture extravasation and infection follow the attempted passage of urine, and the patient may succumb if operation is delayed. In less severe cases the hæmatoma breaks down and fistulæ form in the perineum. Stricture usually follows in a few weeks, but may be delayed for some years.

Treatment. — In rupture of the *penile* urethra the canal is washed with silver-nitrate solution (1 in 10,000) and a soft catheter is tied in for four days. Metal instruments are passed after a fortnight, and this is continued regularly. In *bulbous* rupture a metal catheter is passed gently along the urethra, keeping to the roof. If it enters the bladder the urine is drawn off and the instrument kept in position. If it does not pass the rupture it is left in the urethra. The patient is placed in the lithotomy position and the hæmatoma incised. A curved transverse incision is preferable for membranous rupture, and a median incision for bulbous. The clots are turned out and the oozing stopped by irrigation with hot lotion. If the urethra is only partly severed the torn edges are readily found and are trimmed and sutured with catgut over a catheter which is tied in position. If the urethra is completely severed the vesical end is difficult to find. The two ends are united with catgut and the perineum repaired. If the ends cannot be approximated the cavity is lightly packed and drained and a catheter fixed in place. Suprapubic drainage should be established and continued for a fortnight. Should the vesical end not be found, suprapubic cystotomy must be performed and the end identified after retrograde catheterization.

Results.—The mortality of uncomplicated rupture of the urethra was 14·15 per cent. in 205 cases (Kaufmann). Treatment by retained catheter has a mortality of 18·17 per cent., and rupture of the urethra with fracture of the pelvis a mortality of 40 per cent.

In a large number of cases, immediate operation has prevented the formation of stricture or reduced the contraction to a linear scar readily amenable to treatment.

CALCULUS

There are two varieties of this condition—(1) primary, when the stone originates in the urethra ; (2) secondary, when a migrating calculus is arrested in the canal.

Etiology.—Primary calculi originate in phosphatic crusts that are deposited on raw surfaces in the urethra, especially when stricture is present, or in a para-urethral pocket.

Pathology.—Primary urethral calculi are composed of calcium and magnesium phosphate, ammonio-magnesium phosphate, or calcium carbonate. Secondary calculi have a nucleus of uric acid, calcium oxalate, or other ingredients found in renal or vesical calculi. As the calculus grows it is moulded by the shape of the urethra, and the urethra itself becomes dilated. Several faceted calculi may be found. When a urethral calculus projects into the bladder it takes a mushroom or umbrella shape. In the majority of cases one or several strictures coexist, and the calculus lies behind a stricture or between two strictures. Perineal fistulæ may be present. A calculus may lie in a pouch communicating with the urethra, and project into the canal.

Symptoms. 1. Impaction of a migrating stone.—There is frequently a preliminary attack of renal colic, when the stone descends from the kidney. The stone is felt to enter the urethra during micturition, and there is sudden arrest of the stream, intense pain, and continuous ineffectual straining, with the passage of a few drops of blood, followed by complete retention of urine. On passing a metal catheter the membranous urethra is found spasmodically contracted, and the click of a stone is felt in the prostatic urethra. The calculus may be felt from the rectum. Recurrent attacks of difficult micturition or complete retention occur when the stone becomes impacted behind a stricture of the bulbous or penile urethra, and the calculus can be felt on palpating the urethra.

2. Stone lodged in the urethra.—There are pyuria and a urethral discharge, difficult and frequent micturition, discomfort, and a feeble, twisted stream. Urinary fistulæ may be present, and there is usually a stricture. The stone is felt on palpation and seen on urethroscopic examination.

Treatment.—A migrating calculus of the prostatic urethra is usually pushed back into the bladder on passing a catheter. It should be evacuated with a lithotrity bulb or crushed and removed. If the calculus is not pushed back into the bladder the catheter may be tied in position for a few days ; on its being removed the stone will probably be expelled.

Small calculi in the penile and bulbous urethra can sometimes be removed with urethral forceps or a snare if no stricture is present. If they lie behind a stricture, external urethrotomy is necessary. A fixed calculus in the prostatic urethra should be removed by median perineal section, and the bladder explored for other stones. When calculi are embedded in para-urethral pockets the wall of the pocket should be carefully destroyed.

FOREIGN BODIES

A large variety of foreign bodies may be found in the urethræ of erotic individuals, and portions of surgical instruments may be accidentally left in the canal. The foreign body does not remain for long in the urethra. It is either forced out by the urine or removed by the surgeon, or it may pass backwards into the bladder. When it remains in the urethra there are purulent discharge, pain, burning, and hæmorrhage, increased by erections. Frequent micturition, difficulty, dribbling, and sometimes complete retention of urine occur. The foreign body quickly becomes encrusted with phosphates. Periurethritis and periurethral abscess may result. The situation is usually the fossa navicularis or bulbous urethra, rarely the prostatic urethra.·

Treatment.—The body may be swept out by the stream of urine if the meatus is compressed during the flow and then suddenly relaxed. A long firm body may be pressed out from the perineum or penis. Meatotomy is frequently necessary.

A pin with a round head lies in the urethra with the head bladderwards and the point buried in the mucous membrane. The point should be manipulated through the urethra and skin, and the pin drawn out, the head reversed, and then pushed out of the meatus. Small bodies or portions of catheter may be withdrawn by means of long fine urethral forceps, and a magnet has been employed to remove an iron foreign body.

The urethroscope is used to diagnose and remove foreign bodies, urethral forceps being passed along a large urethral tube.

If these measures fail, external urethrotomy should be performed and the foreign body removed. When the foreign body lies in the prostatic urethra it will be easier to push it back into the bladder and deal with it as a foreign body of the bladder.

STRICTURE

Stricture of the urethra is congenital, inflammatory, or traumatic. The congenital variety has already been described (p. 886).

Etiology.—The female urethra is very rarely affected. Acquired stricture has been observed in male infants, but the age is usually between 20 and 40 years.

Inflammatory stricture results from chronic urethritis, which has a gonorrhœal origin in 90 per cent. of cases. Any condition which tends to prolong the inflammation in chronic urethritis, such as a narrow meatus, phimosis, injudicious treatment, alcohol, or exposure, acts as a predisposing cause. Rarely, chronic urethritis due to tuberculosis of the urethra or diabetes produces stricture. Stricture has followed a urethral chancre or a gumma.

Pathological anatomy.—In traumatic stricture, fibrous tissue develops between the severed ends of the ruptured urethra, the extent of which depends upon the distance they lie apart, necrosis from the injury, or subsequent sloughing from septic complications. The lesion develops rapidly, is single, and the seat of election is· the bulbous urethra. A thick tough mass of fibrous tissue involves the mucous and submucous coats and the cavernous tissue, and sometimes also the perineal tissues and skin.

Gonorrhœal strictures are usually multiple, and most frequently affect the bulbous urethra. The prostatic urethra is very rarely affected in gonorrhœal stricture. The strictured portion of the wall is confined

to a narrow circular band, but it may measure an inch or more in
old-standing cases, or rarely almost the whole length of the anterior
urethra is sclerosed. Complete obliteration of the lumen has been
recorded, but is very rare.

The following terms have
been applied, viz.: "annular" stricture, a fine band
involving the whole circumference (Fig. 550); "bridle"
stricture, an isolated band
stretching across the lumen;
"resilient" stricture, an
elastic stricture which recon-
tracts quickly after dilatation; "cartilaginous" strie-
ture, a hard fibrous mass,
usually of considerable extent.
In an "irritable" stricture
there is a rise of temperature
or even a rigor after each
instrumentation. An "im-
passable" stricture is one
through which no instrument
can be passed. A stricture
may affect the whole circumference of the urethra or
only the floor, roof, or lateral
walls. The lumen is central
or excentric, and it may be
tortuous.

The histological changes
consist in proliferation of the
epithelium, which becomes
squamous, and sclerosis of
the subepithelial tissue, the
fibrous tissue invading the
submucous tissue, and the
erectile tissue of the corpus
spongiosum.

The urethra behind the
stricture shows chronic inflammation and dilatation.
Vegetations and ulcerations
are frequently present. The

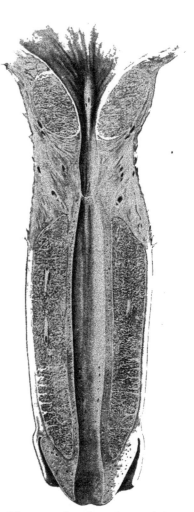

Fig. 550.—Annular stricture of the
bulbous urethra.

bladder muscle is hypertrophied, and cystitis is common. There may be acute retention of urine or chronic vesical distension. The ureters and eventually the kidneys become dilated, and ascending septic pyelonephritis is usually present in old-standing cases.

Symptoms.—In stricture of large calibre the only symptom may be a persistent purulent discharge (gleet). In stricture with small lumen the stream is small, thin, twisted, forked, or sprayed, or it may appear in small jets or only in drops. The projection is feeble, there may be a pause before micturition commences, and the stream finishes in a dribble. Frequent micturition is usually due to chronic urethritis of the prostatic urethra or to cystitis. Pain may be felt at the seat of the stricture during micturition, at the external abdominal rings, or in the back over the kidney on one or both sides. Pain on ejaculation and backward flow of semen into the bladder occur and are a cause of sterility.

Retention of urine may be transient, lasting a few minutes or half an hour. Acute total retention of urine is caused by a chill, dietetic or alcoholic indiscretion, or sexual excess. There is severe suprapubic cramping paroxysmal pain, the patient is pale and sweating, and the bladder is felt as an oval suprapubic swelling. No urine escapes, or only a few drops from time to time. In some cases there is a remarkable absence of pain. Retention of urine is due to spasm of the compressor urethræ muscle or congestion of the mucous membrane at the stricture. Incontinence of urine is observed in narrow strictures. A small quantity of urine may be retained in the urethra behind the stricture and dribble away after micturition. Involuntary dribbling of urine is observed when the bladder is chronically overdistended.

In the later stages chronic cystitis is present, and there is frequent and painful micturition day and night. In long-standing stricture dilatation and septic infection of the ureters and kidneys lead to symptoms of urinary septicæmia and of renal failure.

Examination.—A cartilaginous stricture can be felt on palpation, and becomes more distinct when a bougie is passed.

To detect a stricture a large gum-elastic bougie (No. 20 F: or 21 F.) should be introduced along the urethra ; it is arrested by the stricture. Spasm of the compressor rarely causes obstruction sufficient to resist gentle pressure with a bougie of this size. Smaller instruments are now passed until one is found which will enter the lumen of the stricture. In strictures of comparatively large calibre an acorn-tipped bougie is used. The acorn tip passes through the stricture, and on being withdrawn the shoulder of the acorn hitches at the stricture and the length of the stricture can be ascertained. The aero-urethroscope is useful in diagnosing strictures of wide calibre.

Diagnosis.—1. Spasm of the compressor urethræ (spasmodic stricture) is caused by acute or chronic inflammation of the prostatic urethra. The difficult micturition is here intermittent in character ; the obstruction lies in the position of the membranous urethra, gentle continuous pressure succeeds in overcoming this resistance, and the aero-urethroscope shows the contracted membranous urethra.

2. Malignant disease of the prostate gives rise to increasing difficulty of micturition. The onset of symptoms in stricture dates from a much earlier age, and the position of the obstruction and rectal examination are sufficient to make a diagnosis.

Complications.—The following are complications that may be observed :—

1. Retention of urine.
2. Septic complications (acute or chronic urethritis, periurethral abscess, acute or chronic prostatitis, epididymitis, cystitis, pyelonephritis, pyonephrosis).
3. Extravasation of urine.
4. Fistula.
5. Stone in the urethra.
6. Malignant growth of the urethra.

Treatment by dilatation.—Metal instruments or flexible bougies of silk or cotton web are used. The surgeon stands on the left of the patient and handles the instrument with his right hand while he manipulates the penis with the left.

In introducing a metal instrument the tip is inserted into the meatus while the shaft lies transversely across the left Scarpa's triangle. The handle is carried towards the patient's abdomen and onwards to the middle line, and gradually raised. The left hand leaves the penis and is used to support the perineum. The handle is now raised to the vertical and swings down between the thighs, being transferred to the left hand. In passing elastic bougies the penis is grasped behind the glans and the organ kept on the stretch. The bougie is introduced and lightly held by the forefinger and thumb of the right hand. If the bougie is arrested it is withdrawn a little and again pushed gently on. If this fails, progressively smaller instruments should be used until the size that will pass is reached. A filiform bougie should only be used after larger instruments have failed ; if it does not pass, the end may be bent to an angle and the face of the stricture searched around its periphery. Assistance may be obtained by introducing a syringeful of oil into the urethra and gripping the meatus to retain the oil. If this is unsuccessful a number of filiform bougies may be passed together down to the stricture and each tried in succession. An instrument sometimes passes readily when the patient is placed under an anæsthetic, or under spinal analgesia, when all other methods have failed. · If these attempts fail and no retention is present, the patient is replaced in bed and a brisk purge administered. A further trial will usually be successful.

Most strictures are amenable to instrumental dilatation. Dilata-

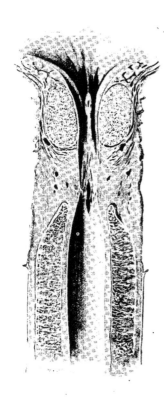

tion is carried out in three ways—(a) as intermittent dilatation, (b) as rapid dilatation, (c) as continuous dilatation. Intermittent dilatation is the method of treatment of the majority of strictures. A bougie which fits the stricture is found, and progressively larger instruments, rising one size at each interview, are passed at intervals of at first four or five days, and then a week, and when the size reaches 18 or 20 F. a fortnight's, and then three weeks', interval is allowed. As the larger sizes are reached, the intervals are extended to two, three, four months, and finally six months and a year. Above the size of 22 F. steel instruments should be employed.

The urethra should be washed before and after the passage of an instrument, and urinary antiseptics administered. Strictures which have not become tough and leathery from long duration, irregular treatment, or chronic inflammation will be completely relieved by this method.

Fig. 551.—Stricture of the bulbous urethra, with recent false passage.

Continuous dilatation is useful in cases where retention of urine has complicated a very narrow stricture. The patient is confined to bed, a filiform bougie passed and fastened in, and the urine trickles alongside. At intervals of twelve hours a progressively larger instrument is substituted until the stricture permits the entrance of a medium-sized bougie. Intermittent dilatation is then substituted.

Rapid dilatation consists in passing bougies of increasing size in quick succession through the stricture until a large size is reached. This method ruptures the stricture, although the epithelial covering may remain intact, and leads to the development of a denser stricture at a later date.

Complications of dilatation. 1. *False passage* (Fig. 551).— Blood appears at the meatus, and a peculiar sensation of grating is felt. The urethra should be washed with warm boric lotion to which tincture of hamamelis is added. Further instrumentation should be postponed for a week.

2. *Infection.*—This is prevented by the sterilization of instruments, the lubricant, the hands, the washing of the penis and urethra, and the administration of urinary antiseptics before the passage of instruments. Urethral lavage with permanganate-of-zinc solution (1 in 5,000) quickly cures the urethritis.

Cystitis and Ascending Pyelonephritis are considered under those headings (pp. 860, 802).

3. *Syncope.*—Faintness or actual syncope may occur. The patient should be recumbent when instruments are passed.

The usual remedies for syncope are adopted. On succeeding instrumentations a solution of eucaine (8 per cent.) should be injected into the urethra before the instrument is passed.

Operative treatment.—In a certain number of cases a cutting operation becomes necessary. The following are the indications for operation :—

A. *Gradual dilatation may have failed.*
   1. Cartilaginous stricture.
   2. Resilient stricture.
   3. Irritable stricture.
   4. Hæmorrhage.
   5. Recurrent epididymitis.
   6. Recurrent retention of urine after instrumentation.
   7. Periurethral abscess and extravasation during the course of dilatation.

B. *Cases unsuitable for dilatation.*
   1. Impassable stricture.
   2. Urethral complications such as stone, periurethral abscess, extravasation of urine, fistula.
   3. The stricture complicates enlargement of the prostate, stone, tuberculosis, chronic cystitis, and new growths of the bladder.
   4. Renal complications.

C. *The patient is unable or unwilling to carry out dilatation.*
   1. Residence beyond reach of regular medical aid.
   2. Want of time.

Internal urethrotomy.—This consists in cutting the stricture by means of a specially guarded knife (urethrotome) introduced along the urethra. A filiform guide is passed through the stricture, the fine grooved staff is screwed on to it and follows it. A triangular knife is run along the groove and cuts the stricture. A catheter is tied in the urethra for forty-eight hours. Large metal instruments are passed at increasing intervals after the operation.

Results.—Of 1,018 patients treated for stricture by internal urethrotomy at St. Peter's Hospital, 8 died (0·78 per cent.). The causes of death were: (1) exacerbation of old-standing pyelonephritis (50 per cent.); (2) anuria and uræmia; (3) septicæmia; (4) hæmorrhage.

Internal urethrotomy usually affords complete relief if followed by the passage of instruments at long intervals. If after-dilatation is neglected, recontraction of the stricture is common.

External urethrotomy with a guide (Syme's operation).—The stricture is dilated to a No. 4 English gauge and a Syme's staff introduced. The patient is placed in the lithotomy position, and an incision made on the staff just above its shoulder and carried back through the stricture to the membranous urethra. A gorget is introduced and guides a perineal drainage-tube into the bladder.

External urethrotomy without a guide. — The following operations are undertaken when the surgeon has failed to pass an instrument through the stricture :—

(*a*) *Wheelhouse's operation.*—A Wheelhouse staff is passed down to the stricture and an incision made upon it about 1 in. from the end. The staff is hooked in the upper end of the wound, the mucous membrane picked up on each side, and careful search made for the opening. When this is found a probe is passed through the stricture, which is then slit up and the operation finished as in Syme's method.

(*b*) If Wheelhouse's operation fails, the incision is carried back and exposes the dilated urethra behind the stricture; a probe is passed through the stricture from behind forwards, and the scar tissue slit on this.

(*c*) *Cock's operation* was originally introduced for cases of acute retention in impassable stricture. The tip of the left forefinger is placed in the rectum on the apex of the prostate, and a knife entered in the middle line of the perineum ½ in. in front of the anus and pushed straight for this point. The dilated urethra behind the stricture is opened.

(*d*) *Suprapubic cystotomy* and retrograde catheterization followed by perineal section has little to recommend it over the perineal dissection (*b*).

Results of external urethrotomy.—The mortality was 8 per cent. in 100 cases at St. Peter's Hospital. Gregory found a mortality of 8·8 per cent. in 992 cases. Bougies should be passed at regular intervals after the operation.

Excision of strictures.—A single stricture of moderate dimensions may be resected. The whole thickness of the spongy body is removed with the stricture, and the severed ends carefully united. The urine is drained for a fortnight through a suprapubic opening. Satisfactory results have been obtained, but the operation is limited in applicability.

PERIURETHRITIS AND PERIURETHRAL SUPPURATION

The source of infection is the urethra, and the inflammation takes various forms, such as abscess, masses of fibrous tissue, gangrenous or phlegmonous inflammation (" extravasation of urine ").

Etiology.—The urethra is usually the seat of stricture, but injury during instrumentation or internal urethrotomy, new growths of the urethra, foreign bodies, calculi, or a retained metal catheter may be the predisposing cause. There is usually a mixed infection of Bacillus coli, streptococcus, and staphylococcus ; rarely one of these is present in pure culture. Anaerobic bacteria are usually found mixed with aerobic bacteria, but occasionally alone. They are especially frequent in phlegmonous periurethritis (" extravasation of urine "), Inflammation spreads either by thrombosis in the corpus spongiosun or by the spread of inflammation along the urethral gland ducts.

PERIURETHRAL ABSCESS (URINARY ABSCESS).

The abscess may develop in relation to the penile or bulbous urethra during the course of acute gonorrhœa or chronic urethritis. A tender swelling appears on the under-surface of the penis, and by rupture both externally and into the urethra may establish a urinary fistula.

Abscess around the bulbous urethra may develop insidiously and form a hard, tender nodule, or may commence with a rigor and run an acute course with fever, local tenderness and pain, and rapid formation of a swelling. The swelling is limited posteriorly at the middle of the perineum by the fascia of Colles, but passes forwards under cover of the scrotum. Partial or complete retention of urine is frequently present.

Treatment.—A penile periurethral abscess in the anterior part of the canal should be opened through the urethra with the help of a wire speculum or a short urethral tube. A perineal periurethral abscess is opened by a free median perineal incision, and the cavity flushed with biniodide solution. All pockets are opened, counter-openings made if necessary, and the cavity freely drained and lightly packed with iodoform gauze. When a narrow stricture and cystitis coexist a median perineal cystotomy with drainage of the bladder should be performed.

3 *f*

DIFFUSE PHLEGMONOUS PERIURETHRITIS (EXTRAVASATION
OF URINE)

This is a virulent, rapidly spreading infection, with sloughing of the urethra. Stricture is usually present, but is not necessarily narrow, and may even be absent. The condition rarely commences as a periurethral abscess. Usually the onset is sudden, and the symptoms at once become severe. After a rigor the temperature rises to 102° F., or higher, and profound toxæmia rapidly develops. The patient is pale, and the skin clammy; the tongue and mouth are dry, and delirium quickly appears. The urine is passed with difficulty and in small quantity. A dull-red, brawny induration appears in the perineum and rapidly increases. The spread is limited by the attachment of Colles's fascia behind the transverse perineal muscle posteriorly and to the rami of the pubes laterally. The scrotum becomes red and œdematous, the penis swollen and distorted, and the infiltration rapidly mounts on to the pubes and abdominal wall. Crepitation from the formation of gas is sometimes detected. A fatal result from toxæmia is not uncommon, and may occur after operation.

Treatment. — Immediate multiple incisions should be made wherever the infection has spread, and washed through several times in the twenty-four hours with hydrogen peroxide or biniodide solution (1 in 2,000). Hot fomentations should be applied, stimulants freely administered, and subcutaneous and rectal saline infusions given. Sloughing of the urethra occurs, and fistulæ form and later require treatment.

CHRONIC INDURATIVE PERIURETHRITIS

There is a stricture of the bulbous urethra, usually of the irregular cartilaginous type, and large masses of fibrous induration form in the perineum and scrotum. There are usually several urinary fistulæ, and the indurated mass frequently contains one or several small abscesses. Calculi may form in the fistulæ and behind the stricture, and a malignant growth has been known to develop.

Treatment.—Internal urethrotomy should be performed and a catheter tied in as a preliminary to operation on the periurethral induration a week or more later. If the stricture is impassable, external urethrotomy is performed at the time of the perineal operation.

A staff is placed in the urethra, and, with the patient in the lithotomy position, the indurated mass is split down the centre to the corpus spongiosum and each half dissected away, removing fistulæ and small abscesses in the substance of the mass. The opening in the urethra is repaired with catgut sutures and a catheter tied in the urethra.

FISTULA AND ACQUIRED DEFECTS

Urethral fistulæ may open on to the skin of the penis, scrotum, perineum, groin, gluteal region, or into the rectum.

Etiology.—Congenital defects may take the form of hypospadias or epispadias (pp. 966, 967). The most common congenital form is a fistula of the membranous or prostatic urethra, and is combined with atresia ani, and the perineal muscles may be atrophied. Acquired fistula arises from trauma, inflammation, or new growth. Traumatic fistula arises from within the urethra from false passages and sloughing due to tying in a metal catheter, and from without by stabs, impaling, bullet wounds, etc., or after surgical operations such as external urethrotomy (Fig. 552), perineal prostatectomy, and after opening or rupture of a periurethral abscess or the incision of gangrenous periurethritis. Tuberculous disease and bilharziosis are rare causes.

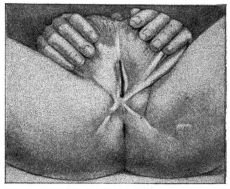

Fig. 552.—Acquired defect of urethra after removal of large urethral calculus.

Symptoms.—Urine escapes from the fistula during micturition. The symptoms of stricture are also present. Fistula of the penile urethra usually opens directly into the urethra, and is surrounded by a firm ring of fibrous tissue. In perineal fistula there may be one or several openings. The fistulæ are surrounded by hard, fibrous induration. In urethro-rectal fistula the urine is dis-

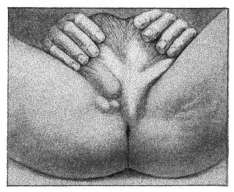

Fig. 553.—Result of plastic operation for repair of defect: same case.

charged into the rectum at each micturition, and produces a watery motion. Gas may be passed along the urethra and fæcal matter escape with the urine. Urethritis and cystitis are usually present.

Treatment.—The treatment of fistula with massive induration has already been discussed. In cases without induration the stricture is dilated, or internal urethrotomy performed and a catheter tied in the urethra for a week. The fistula is scraped and cauterized, or dissected down to the urethra, the opening in that canal closed, and the bladder drained suprapubically for a fortnight. In larger defects, plastic operations are necessary (Fig. 553). For fistula at the base of the glans penis the edges of the fistula are excised, and the raw surfaces united with catgut and covered with a flap of skin from the penis (Dieffenbach's operation). For fistula on the undersurface of the penis various flap operations have been used. For the repair of extensive urethral defects the operations are autoplastic or heteroplastic. In the former a defect in the floor of the bulbous urethra is repaired by uniting longitudinal flaps over a catheter and covering these by undercutting and approximating the skin. The latter methods are suitable for cases where portions of the urethra have been completely destroyed or removed.

Portions of tissue from other parts of the patient's body have been used, such as the foreskin, mucous membrane from the lower lip, or the long saphenous vein. Mucous membrane has also been transplanted from other human beings, such as the mucous membrane of a prolapsed uterus, and from bullocks, goats, and birds. The results of these operations have varied, but the autoplastic have been more satisfactory than the heteroplastic.

In urethro-rectal fistula, stricture, calculi, and other complications should first be treated, and the bladder drained suprapubically. A curved prerectal incision is made, and the urethra and rectum dissected apart. The fistula is cut across and the openings sutured. The rectum may be twisted so as to remove the sutured fistulæ from immediate proximity.

NEW GROWTHS

Growths are comparatively rare, the male urethra being more frequently affected than the female. The benign growths met with are papilloma, fibroma, caruncle, myoma, adenoma, and cysts; the malignant, carcinoma and sarcoma. Gonorrhœa is said to play an important part in their etiology. In the male papilloma and adenoma, and in the female caruncle, are the most frequent forms of growth.

Benign Growths: Papilloma

Papillomas are found in the anterior urethra, rarely in the prostatic urethra, and resemble those met with on the glans penis and foreskin. There is a purulent discharge, and sometimes a peculiar sensation during micturition. The diagnosis is made with the urethroscope. The growths bleed very readily, and are easily torn by the passage of instruments. There may be a few isolated growths, or the urethra may be choked with papillomatous masses. The warts should be removed through the urethroscope. Urethral forceps or a specially constructed urethroscope tube is used for the purpose, and the bases are touched with nitrate of silver.

Polypi

Urethral polypi usually occur in the prostatic urethra, springing from the verumontanum or close to it, rarely in the anterior urethra. Two forms are found—(1) fibroma, which consists of loose fibrous tissue covered by a thin layer of mucous membrane; (2) adenoma, in which there are numerous gland follicles having appearances identical with those of the "hypertrophied" prostate. Myoma and fibro-myoma have also been described. A chronic urethral discharge is usually present, but may consist of only a few shreds or may be absent. Tickling and crawling sensations are sometimes experienced, and hæmorrhage follows instrumentation. The polypus is discovered by the urethroscope, and is removed by fine alligator forceps or the electro-cautery.

CYSTS

Small cysts are produced by blocking the urethral lacunæ. Cysts of the sinus pocularis are rare. A cyst of Cowper's gland or ducts may form a considerable swelling which ruptures into the urethra. The treatment consists in incision with the electric cautery through the urethroscope tube.

CARUNCLE

Urethral caruncle is discussed at p. 989.

MALIGNANT GROWTHS OF THE MALE URETHRA

Malignant growths of the male urethra are rare. Hall collected 48 examples. In addition to these, Barney records 2 cases, and I have had 4 under my care. The condition usually occurs between the ages of 50 and 60, rarely before 40. Trauma and leucoplakia from chronic urethritis are important factors in the etiology, and stricture is present in half the cases. The bulbous urethra is usually affected, less often the penile urethra, and rarely the prostatic portion. The growth takes the form of a squamous epithelioma, very seldom a sarcoma. It infiltrates and destroys the mucous membrane and invades the corpus spongiosum. Eventually fistulæ form in the perineum.

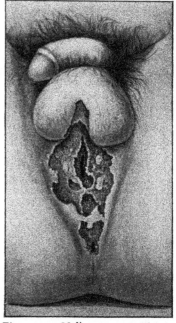

Fig. 554.—Malignant growth of urethra ulcerating on perineum and scrotum, and round anus.

Symptoms.—The symptoms vary considerably. There is increasing difficulty, partly due to the fibrous stricture already present. Hæmorrhage follows the passage of an instrument, and there may be a bloody discharge without instrumentation. A purulent discharge is frequently present.

A swelling appears in the perineum in some cases, the skin becomes red, and either a fistula forms spontaneously, or the swelling is incised for a simple periurethral abscess. The growth then fungates, and progressive destruction of the perineal tissues takes place (Fig. 554). In the penile urethra hard induration of the wall of the canal is felt, which slowly increases and spreads. The penis is ventrally curved during erection, and becomes swollen into a club-like form. Urethral examination shows a fibrous stricture through which .the instrument may enter an irregular cavity with friable, readily bleeding walls. Urethroscopy may give a view of the growth. Lymph-glands are affected later, those along the iliac vessels and in the groins being first involved. Metastases occur in the bones, liver, and lungs.

The **diagnosis** from stricture is usually difficult. Spontaneous hæmorrhage from the urethra, repeated severe hæmorrhage after instrumentation, and persistent hæmaturia are important symptoms. From subacute and chronic periurethritis and from periurethral abscess the diagnosis is sometimes only made by exploratory operation.

Treatment.—Resection of the urethra has been performed in the early stage, and amputation of the penis has given good results, but when the growth is extensive, complete removal of the penis (Thiersch-Gould operation) is necessary.

MALIGNANT GROWTHS OF THE FEMALE URETHRA

These are periurethral or urethral. The former occur after the age of 50, and the latter earlier. The urethral variety may be pedunculated or sessile, appearing as a dark-red grape-like polypus or a nodular ulcerated area. The growths are squamous or rarely columnar epithelium, or sarcoma. There is pain on micturition, on coitus, and on sitting and walking, frequent micturition, difficulty, and occasionally complete retention. Incontinence is rare, hæmaturia is usually present. The urethra may be excised by a longitudinal incision on the anterior wall of the vagina. The vesical end is, if possible, preserved and implanted in the vaginal wall.

TUBERCULOSIS OF THE URETHRA AND PENIS

Tuberculosis of the urethra is rare. Primary tuberculosis has been observed, but the infection is almost invariably secondary to tuberculosis of the urinary or genital system. The female urethra is seldom affected. In the male, the posterior urethra is usually attacked by spread from the prostate or the bladder. A deep tuberculous cavity may open from the substance of the prostate into the posterior urethra, or there may be superficial ulceration or tuberculous granulation tissue. The anterior urethra may show small superficial ulcers. If the penis is affected the urethral mucous membrane is involved in the tuberculous infiltration. A periurethral cold abscess may form, and eventually fistulæ appear in the perineum.

Stenosis of the urethra is occasionally observed in the bulbous or female urethra in cases of urinary or genital tuberculosis. There is seldom a localized stricture, but the wall is infiltrated, and an irregular fibrous thickening results.

A urethral discharge is always present, usually thin and pale, but occasionally so abundant and purulent and associated with symptoms so acute as to suggest gonorrhœal urethritis. Hæmaturia, frequent and difficult micturition, and occasionally complete retention may be present. There is irregular periurethral induration.

Tuberculosis of the penis may be confined to ulceration of the glans, usually on the under surface, or the corpora cavernosa may be invaded.

Treatment.—Urethral tuberculosis is so seldom an isolated lesion that separate treatment is rarely necessary. Stricture should be treated by internal urethrotomy and dilatation. A cold abscess is opened and tincture of iodine applied. Fistulæ are treated by scraping and injection of iodoform emulsion, bismuth paste, or iodine.

Conservative treatment should be adopted when the penis is involved but amputation may become necessary for extensive lesions. Tuberculin may be administered.

BIBLIOGRAPHY

HÆMATURIA

Klotzenberg, *Zeits. f. Urol.*, 1908, p. 125.
Pilcher, *Ann. of Surg.*, 1909, p. 652.
White, Hale, *Quart. Journ. of Med.*, 1911, p. 509.

CONGENITAL ABNORMALITIES OF THE KIDNEY

Albarran, *Ann. des Mal. des Org. Gén.-Urin.*, 1908, p. 1601.
Ballowitz, *Virchow's Arch.*, 1895, cxli. 309.
Heiner, *Folia Urol.*, Oct., 1908.

MOVABLE KIDNEY

Billington, *Movable Kidney.* London, 1910.
Cheyne, Sir W. Watson, *Lancet*, April 24, 1909.
Lane, Arbuthnot, *Lancet*, Jan. 17, 1903.
Walker, Thomson, *Lancet*, Aug. 11, 1906.
Wolkow und Delitzen, *Die Wanderniere.* Berlin, 1899.

INJURIES OF THE KIDNEY

Curschmann, *Münch. med. Woch.*, 1902, xlix. 38.
Riese, *Arch. f. klin. Chir.*, 1903, vol. lxxi.
Watson, *Boston Med. and Surg. Journ.*, July 9 and 16, 1903.

PERINEPHRITIS

Guiteras, *N.Y. Med. Journ.*, 1906, lxxxiii. 169.
Townsend, *Journ. Amer. Med. Assoc.*, 1904, xliii. 1626.
Zuckerkandl, *Wien. klin. Woch.*, Oct. 13, 1910.

PYELONEPHRITIS AND PYELITIS

Brewer, *Surg., Gyn., and Obstet.*, June, 1908, p. 699.
Cova, *Ann. di Obstet. e di Ginecol.*, 1903, p. 692.
Dudgeon, *Lancet*, 1908, i. 616.
Legueu, *Ann. des Mal. des Org. Gén.-Urin.*, 1904, p. 1441.
Morse, *Amer. Journ. of Med. Sci.*, 1909, p. 313.
Pousson, *Folia Urol.*, Jan., 1909, p. 445.
Sampson, *Johns Hopkins Hosp. Bull.*, 1903, No. 153, p. 336.
Thomson, *Scot. Med. and Surg. Journ.*, 1902, p. 7.
Walker, Thomson, *Pract.*, May, 1911.

PYONEPHROSIS

Cahn, *Münch. med. Woch.*, 1902, xlix. 19.
Greaves, *Brit. Med. Journ.*, July 13, 1907.
Morris, Sir Henry, *Lancet*, 1910, i. 1597.
Watson, *Ann. of Surg.*, 1908, No. 3.

RENAL AND PERIRENAL FISTULÆ

Heitz-Boyer et Moreno, *Ann. des. Mal. des Org. Gén.-Urin.*, 1910, No. 11.

NON-SUPPURATIVE NEPHRITIS

Edebohls, *Med. News*, April 22, 1899, and *Med. Rec.*, May 4, 1901.
Pousson, *Chir. des Néphrites*, Paris, 1909.
Walker, Thomson, *Pract.*, June, 1903.

HYDRONEPHROSIS

Israel, *Deuts. med. Woch.*, 1906, p. 22.
Mayo, *Journ. Amer. Med. Assoc.*, 1909, p. 1383.
Schloffer, *Wien. klin. Woch.*, 1906, p. 50.
Volcker und Lichtenberg, *Beitr. z. klin. Chir.*, 1907, p. 1.
Wagner, *Folia Urol.*, June, 1907.
Walker, Thomson, *Lancet*, Aug. 11, 1906.

TUMOURS OF THE KIDNEY, RENAL PELVIS, AND URETER

Garceau, *Tumours of the Kidney.* 1909.
Grégoire, *Presse Méd.,* 1905, p. 49.
Heresco, *Ann. des Mal. des Org. Gén.-Urin.,* 1901, p. 655.
Israel, *Deuts. med. Woch.,* 1911, p. 57.
Schmieden, *Deuts. Zeits. f. Chir.,* 1902.
Stoerk, *Beitr. f. path. Anat. u. allgem. Path. von Ziegler,* 1908, p. 393.
Taddei, *Folia Urol.,* 1908, pp. 303, 638.
Walker, *Ann. of Surg.,* 1897, p. 549.
Willis and **Wilson,** *Collected Papers of the Mayo Clinic,* 1910, p. 419.

CYSTS OF THE KIDNEY

Gardner, *Intercol. Quart. Journ. of Med. and Surg.,* 1894, i. 147.
Roche, *Ann. des Mal. des Org. Urin.,* 1895, p. 1139.
Seiber, *Deuts. Zeits. f. Chir.,* 1905, p. 495.
Stromberg, *Folia Urol.,* 1909, p. 541.

TUBERCULOSIS OF THE KIDNEY AND URETER

Albarran, *Ann. des Mal. des Org. Gén.-Urin.,* 1908, p. 81.
Brongersma, *I. Congrès de l'Assoc. Internat. d'Urol.,* Paris, 1908, p. 533.
Casper, *Deuts. med. Woch.,* 1905, p. 98.
Hallé et Motz, *Ann. des Mal. des Org. Gén.-Urin.,* 1906, i. 162.
Krönlein, *Folia Urol.,* 1908, p. 245.
Kümmel, *Arch. f. klin. Chir.,* 1906, p. 270.
Lichtenstein, *Zeits. f. Urol.,* 1908, p. 219.
Walker, Thomson, *Pract.,* May, 1908.
Zuckerkandl, *Zeits. f. Urol.,* 1908, p. 97.

TUMOURS OF THE SUPRARENAL GLAND

Ferrier et Lecéne, *Rev. de Chir.,* 1906, p. 325.
Garceau, *Tumours of the Kidney.* 1909.
Israel, *Deuts. med. Woch.,* 1905, p. 746.

SYPHILIS AND BILHARZIOSIS OF THE KIDNEY

Delamore, *Gaz. des Hóp.,* 1900, p. 553.
Madden, *Bilharziosis. London,* 1907.
Stoerk, *Wien. med. Woch.,* 1901.
Sutherland and **Thomson Walker,** *Brit. Med. Journ.,* April 25, 1903.

RENAL CALCULUS

Bevan and **Smith,** *Surg., Gyn., and Obstet.,* 1908, p. 675.
Brödel, *Johns Hopkins Hosp. Bull.,* 1901, p. 10.
Faltin, *Folia Urol.,* 1908, Hefte 3, 4.
Gage and **Beal,** *Ann. of Surg.,* 1908, p. 378.
Israel, *Arch. f. klin. Chir.,* 1900.
Kümmel, *Zeits. f. Urol.,* 1908, p. 193.
Newman, *Lancet,* 1909, p. 8.

PROLAPSE OF THE URETER

Kapsammer, *Zeits. f. Urol.,* 1908, p. 800.
Portner, *Monats. f. Urol.,* 1904, Heft 5.

INJURIES OF THE URETER

Alksne, *Folia Urol.,* 1908, p. 280.
Barnasconi et Colombine, *Ann. des Mal. des Org. Gén.-Urin.,* 1905, ii. 1361.
Boari, *Il Policlinico,* July 15, 1899.
Bovee, *Ann. of Surg.,* 1900, p. 165.
Markoe and **Wood,** *Ann. of Surg.,* 1899.
Morris, Sir Henry, *Hunterian Lectures,* 1898.
Poggi, *XIX. Congrès de Chir.,* Paris, 1906, p. 188.
Scharpe, *Ann. of Surg.,* 1906, p. 687.

BIBLIOGRAPHY

905

Fistula of the Ureter
Boari, *Ann. des Mal. des Org. Gén.-Urin.*, 1909, ii. 1332.
Payne, *Journ. Amer. Med. Assoc.*, 1908, p. 1321.

Stone in the Ureter
Bloch, *Folia Urol.*, April, 1909.
Jeanbrau, *Des Calculs de l' Uretère.* 1909.
Kolischer and **Schmidt,** *Journ. Amer. Med. Assoc.*, Nov. 9, 1901.
Rigby, *Ann. of Surg.*, Nov., 1907.
Walker, Thomson, *Lancet*, June 17, 1911.

Examination of the Bladder
Kapsammer, *Nierendiagnostik u. Nierenchirurgie.* 1907.
Walker, Thomson, *Renal Function in Urinary Surgery.* London, 1908.

Extroversion of the Bladder
Maydl, *Wien. med. Woch.*, 1894, 1896, 1899.
Peters, *Brit. Med. Journ.*, 1902, ii. 1538.
Petersen, *Med. News*, Aug. 11, 1911.
Trendelenburg, *Ann. of Surg.*, 1906, p. 281.

Diverticula of the Bladder
Berry, *Proc. Roy. Soc. Med.*, Surg. Sect., 1911, p. 158.
Young, *Johns Hopkins Hosp. Repts.*, 1906, p. 401.

Inversion and Prolapse of the Bladder
Hirokawa, *Deuts. Zeits. f. Chir.*, 1911, p. 575.
Leedham-Green, *Brit. Med. Journ.*, 1908, i. 976.

Injuries of the Bladder
Dambrin et **Papin,** *Ann. des Mal. des Org. Gén.-Urin.*, 1904, p. 641.
Goldenberg, *Beitr. z. klin. Chir.*, 1909, p. 356.
Morel, *Ann. des Mal. des Org. Gén.-Urin.*, 1906, p. 801.
Quick, *Ann. of Surg.*, 1907, p. 94.

Syphilis of the Bladder
Asch, *Zeits. f. Urol.*, 1911, p. 504.
von Engelmann, *Folia Urol.*, 1911, p. 472.
Frank, *II. Deuts. urol. Kongress*, Berlin, 1909, p. 356.

Actinomycosis of the Bladder
Ruhrah, *Ann. of Surg.*, 1899, p. 417.
Stanton, *Amer. Med.*, 1906, p. 401.

Cystitis
Hallé et **Motz,** *Ann. des Mal. des Org. Gén.-Urin.*, 1902, p. 17.
Lichtenstein, *Wien. klin. Woch.*, 1907, No. 40.
Newman, *Lancet*, 1912, i. 490.
Stoerk und **Zuckerkandl,** *Zeits. f. Urol.*, 1907, p. 3.

Tuberculous Cystitis
Hallé et **Motz,** *Ann. des Mal. des Org. Gén.-Urin.*, 1904. p. 16.
Karo, *Med. Rec.*, Oct. 2, 1909.
Rovsing, *Arch. f. klin. Chir.*, 1907, p. 1.
Walker, Thomson, *Pract.*, May, 1908.

Tumours of the Bladder
Casper, *Berl. klin. Woch.*, 1908, No. 6.
Paschikis, *Folia Urol.*, 1908, ii. 450.
Rovsing, *Arch. f. klin. Chir.*, 1907, p. 1047.
Stoerk und **Zuckerkandl,** *Zeits. f. Urol.*, 1907, p. 1.

Walker, Thomson, *Lancet*, Nov. 12, 1910 : and *II. Congrès de l'Assoc. Internat. d' Urol.*, London, 1911.
Watson, *Ann. of Surg.*, Dec., 1905.
Wilder, *Amer. Journ. of Med. Sci.*, 1905, p. 63.

VESICAL CALCULUS
Histon, *Brit. Med. Journ.*, 1904, ii. 833.
Kasarnowsky, *Folia Urol.*, 1909, p. 469.
Know, *Zeits. f. Geb. u. Gyn.*, 1911, Heft 7.

PERICYSTITIS
Schmidt, *Surg., Gyn., and Obstet.*, 1911, p. 281.

NERVOUS DISEASES OF THE BLADDER
Böhme, *Münch. med. Woch.*, Dec. 15, 1908.
Corner, *Ann. of Surg.*, 1901, p. 456.
Müller, *Deuts. Zeits. f. Nervenheilk.*, 1901, p. 86.
Walker, Thomson, *Ann. of Surg.*, 1910, p. 577 ; and *Zeits. f. Urol.*, 1911, p. 1.

CONGENITAL MALFORMATIONS OF THE URETHRA
Beck, *N.Y. Med. Journ.*, Jan. 29, 1908.
Bucknall, *Lancet*, Sept. 28, 1907.
Dubot, *Ann. des Mal. des Org. Gén.-Urin.*, 1902, No. 1.
Gutmann, *Zeits. f. Urol.*, 1910, p. 575.
Keith, *Brit. Med. Journ.*, 1908, ii. 1805.

INJURIES AND RUPTURE OF THE URETHRA
Legueu, *Ann. des Mal. des Org. Gén.-Urin.*, 1907, ii. 1090.
Rutherfurd, *Lancet*, Sept. 10, 1904.
Sczcypiorski, *Ann. des Mal. des Org. Gén.-Urin.*, 1907, ii. 1033.

STONE IN THE URETHRA
Fenwick, *Trans. Path. Soc.*, 1890, vol. xli.
Pasteau, *Ann. des Mal. des Org. Gén.-Urin.*, 1901, p. 416.

STRICTURE OF THE URETHRA
Groves, Hey, *Bristol Med.-Chir. Journ.*, 1910, p. 325.
Rutherfurd, *Lancet*, Sept. 10, 1904.
Sawamura, *Folia Urol.*, 1910, iv. 683.

NEW GROWTHS OF THE URETHRA
Barney, *Boston Med. and Surg. Journ.*, 1907, p. 790.
Bonzani, *Folia Urol.*, 1909, p. 491.
Hall, *Ann. of Surg.*, 1904, p. 375.
Preiswerk, *Zeits. f. Urol.*, 1907, p. 273.

TUBERCULOSIS OF THE URETHRA AND PENIS
Asch, *Zeits. f. Urol.*, 1909, iii. 174.
Chute, *Boston Med. and Surg. Journ.*, 1903, p. 361.
Hallé et Motz, *Ann. des Mal. des Org. Gén.-Urin.*, 1902, p. 1464.
Sawamura, *Folia Urol.*, 1910, iv. 683.

THE MALE GENITAL TRACT

BY RUSSELL HOWARD, M.S., F.R.C.S.

THE PROSTATE

Anatomy.—The prostate is a glandular organ shaped like a chest-nut and weighing from 15 to 20 grm. It surrounds the first part of the urethra, the base of the bladder rests on it, and it is situated between the symphysis pubis and the rectum.

The anterior aspect of the gland is attached to the posterior surface of the symphysis pubis by specialized bands of the anterior fibres of the recto-vesical fascia forming the pubo-prostatic or anterior true ligaments of the blad-der, while the lateral as-pects are covered with a reflection from the recto-vesical fascia under which a large plexus of veins (the plexus of Santorini) is found. The posterior aspect is attached to the rectum by dense fibrous connective tissue in which no large vessels are found.

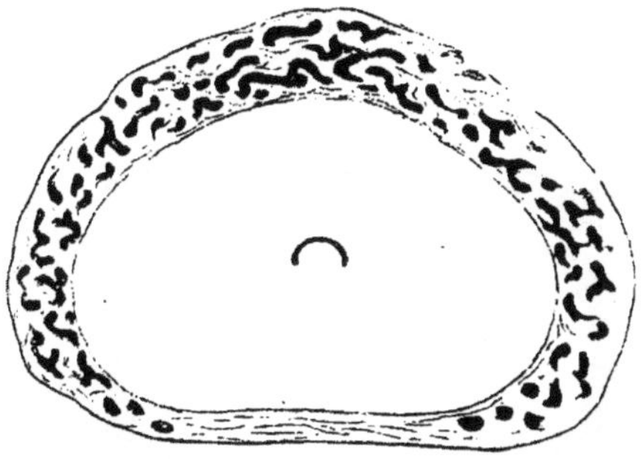

Many of the fibres of the levator ani muscle end

Fig. 555.—Section of normal prostate, show-ing the prostatic plexus of veins and the capsule.

on the prostate, which thus lies outside the pelvis but in the tissue that forms the pelvic diaphragm.

The prostatic urethra is $1\frac{1}{4}$ in. long, crescentic on section, and pene-trates the prostate in such a way that a large segment of the gland lies below and a small one above it. The common ejaculatory ducts pierce the prostate, and, like the sinus pocularis and prostatic glands, open into the prostatic urethra.

The arteries of the prostate are derived from the interior vesical artery ; and the veins, which form a large plexus round the gland, enter the dorsal vein of the penis and the veins of the urethra. (Fig. 555.)

ACUTE PROSTATITIS

Acute prostatitis in the vast majority of cases follows gonorrhœal urethritis or urethritis due to instrumentation of the urethra, but it may occur occasionally in the course of one of the infectious fevers. The gonococcus enters the prostate through the prostatic ducts and initiates an acute inflammation, ending either in resolution, chronic prostatitis, or suppuration. (*See* Vol. I., pp. 808, 841.)

CHRONIC PROSTATITIS

Chronic inflammation of the prostate is most frequently secondary to a chronic urethritis, usually gonococcal, but may follow an acute prostatitis. The condition is a very common sequel to gonorrhœa, and has far-reaching consequences. The morbid anatomy shows a chronic suppuration occurring in the ducts of the prostate with interstitial fibrosis, the pus escaping into the urethra and appearing in the urine as comma-shaped white threads. It is one of the causes of gleet.

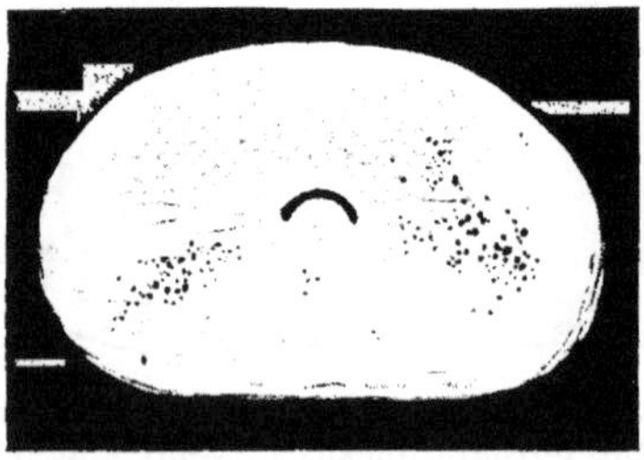

Fig. 556.—Section of prostate, showing the corpora amylacea.

The condition is discussed in Vol. I., p. 842.

PROSTATIC CALCULI

It is important to distinguish two separate conditions which have been described under this term. They are (*a*) calculi in the prostatic urethra, (*b*) calculi in the prostate. The first are formed either in the kidney, the bladder, or locally in the prostatic urethra, and becoming impacted, cause difficulty of micturition. They will not be further discussed here. Calculi of the second variety, the true prostatic calculi, are formed in the prostate itself. In every adult prostate small bodies known as corpora amylacea are found (Fig. 556), which consist of inspissated secretion, epithelial cells, and lecithin. They are multiple, and of a colour varying from light grey to black. These bodies are scarcely pathological, but become so when by infiltration with lime salts they form prostatic calculi (Fig. 557). Stones in the prostate are therefore usually multiple, over a hundred having been met with in some cases, and are usually small, but they may weigh as much as 120 grm. They consist of phosphate, oxalate, and carbonate of lime round an organic nucleus, and so give a good shadow with the X-rays.

Symptoms.—Calculi may exist for years in the prostate, and only be discovered on autopsy. In some cases they are passed per urethram without other symptoms. When symptoms are present they are those of cystitis of the base of the bladder, viz. pain, difficulty and frequency of micturition. The symptoms arise when the calculus protrudes into the prostatic urethra either through one of the ducts or by ulceration of the mucous membrane. Hæmaturia may occur, but is usually slight, and urethral discharge may be present. Suppuration may take place round the calculi and lead to formation of an abscess, which may burst into the urethra, the perineum, or the rectum.

The **diagnosis** is made by—(1) Feeling the stones per rectum, if they are large enough. In some cases the stones may be felt to grate on one another. (2) Feeling the stones in the urethra by the passage of a sound. The grating characteristic of a calculus is always felt in the same place just as the sound enters the bladder. In some cases combined rectal and urethral examination may lead to a correct diagnosis. (3) Radiography, only a positive result being of value.

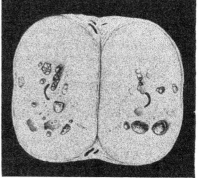

Fig. 557.—Prostate with prostatic calculi *in situ*.

Treatment.—In cases of accidental discovery of prostatic calculi no treatment is necessary, but if symptoms are present the prostate should be incised from the perineum and all the stones removed. Calculi in the prostate may also be reached through the bladder. This viscus is opened by the suprapubic route, the prostate incised, and the stones removed.

Abscesses should be treated by perineal incision, removal of the calculi, and drainage.

TUBERCULOSIS

As in tuberculosis of the other parts of the genito-urinary tract, tuberculosis of the prostate is most commonly seen in young adults and in those who are disposed to the disease by heredity. Chronic inflammation of the prostate due to infection by the gonococcus is another very important predisposing condition, and one on which too little stress has been laid. The disease in the prostate is frequently associated with tuberculosis of the kidney, bladder, vesiculæ, and testis, and it is often difficult in a given case to distinguish the primary focus. The pathological anatomy of the disease does not differ from that of tuberculosis elsewhere. The tuberculous process usually commences at the periphery of the gland, and then invades the centre ; the tubercles coalesce to form soft caseous areas in the gland, which may burst into the urethra, the perineum, the bladder, or the rectum.

Symptoms.—Tuberculosis of the prostate may be latent for months or years, and is frequently discovered during a routine examination of the prostate and vesiculæ in the investigation of a case of testicular, renal, or vesical tuberculosis. Even when symptoms are present they are not pathognomonic, for they closely resemble those of any form of inflammation of the base of the bladder.

The symptoms are pain, frequency, and difficulty of micturition, unrelieved by treatment ; a burning, aching pain in the perineum and round the anus, and the presence of blood in the urine and semen. The hæmaturia is usually seen at the end of micturition, and is slight, but is increased by instrumentation of the urethra. The hæmospermia is also slight, and may be absent. A urethral discharge may be present, but its diagnostic importance is minimized by the difficulty of establishing its prostatic origin and of demonstrating tubercle bacilli in it.

Diagnosis.—This depends on rectal examination combined with evidence of tuberculosis elsewhere in the body, but especially in the genito-urinary tract. On examination the prostate is found to be somewhat enlarged and feels nodular, the nodules being small and isolated and more uneven than in any other disease. The gland is tender ; in advanced cases fluctuation is present, and the seminal vesicles can frequently be felt to be affected.

Tuberculosis of the prostate may not be suspected until a fluctuating swelling is found in the perineum or bulging the anterior rectal wall.

Examination of the urethra by the sound and endoscope, or examination of the bladder by the cystoscope, is of little value in the diagnosis. These examinations are unnecessary, and may result in severe hæmaturia or cystitis.

The **prognosis,** as in all other forms of genito-urinary tuberculosis, is not very favourable, but cure may result if other parts of the tract are not seriously involved.

Treatment.—The treatment consists, for the most part, of general hygienic measures and vaccine inoculation. All local applications to the deep urethra are to be avoided, as they can do no good to the tuberculous process in the substance of the gland.

Catheterization for the relief of pain and difficulty of micturition is useless as a lasting resource, and continuous catheterization cannot be borne. When the pain and urgency of micturition become intolerable, the bladder should be opened and permanently drained by a suprapubic incision.

Radical treatment, consisting of removal of the entire prostate with the vesiculæ seminales, has been attempted with some measure of success, but is only appropriate in a minority of cases—those in which tuberculosis is not advanced in other organs, but is primarily localized to the prostate.

If an abscess forms, it should be opened from the perineum, the walls thoroughly scraped to eradicate the disease, and the cavity injected with iodoform emulsion. Fistulæ should be treated by thorough curetting. The prognosis of this operation is not good, fistulæ usually remaining.

CHRONIC ENLARGEMENT

Pathology.—The pathology of the increase in volume and alteration in shape of the prostate that occurs so frequently after middle life is not finally settled, so that the term chronic enlargement is to be preferred to another term which would imply a more exact pathological condition. From histological examination alone authors have differentiated (a) a diffuse fibro-myomatous overgrowth (myomatosis), (b) a form with multiple localized fibro-myomas, (c) a diffuse adenomatous overgrowth, (d) a form with localized adenomas; but there is much evidence that these variations are merely stages of the same pathological change.

Etiology.—The cause of chronic enlargement of the prostate is quite unknown, but the following theories have been held :—

1. The disease is a new formation either of fibro-myomas, similar to those in the uterus, or of fibro-adenomas.

2. It is a part of a general arterio-sclerosis, or of a localized arterio-sclerosis affecting the urinary organs.

3. It is an inflammatory hyperplasia of the elements of the gland due to alcoholism, sexual excess, constipation, sedentary life, etc.

4. It is a terminal result of chronic gonorrhœal inflammation of the gland.

But none of these theories is satisfactory, and it is best at present to consider the condition as a chronic enlargement of the prostate occurring for unknown reasons in men after the age of 50. Cases, however, have been known before this age.

Enlargement of the prostate is of no more intrinsic importance than a lipoma of the shoulder ; its seriousness depends upon the interference with the act of micturition, due to the position of the gland at the outlet of the bladder.

Condition of the prostate.—The prostate, if normal, weighs about 20 grm., but when chronically enlarged has been found to weigh as much as 250 grm., or more ; it may be enlarged as a whole or in parts, and the enlargement may be symmetrical or asymmetrical.

If enlarged as a whole it becomes more spherical, and the groove between the lateral lobes is obliterated. The enlargement may be slight and hard, or very great and soft. In partial enlargements the middle lobe (i.e. that part between the mucous membrane of the bladder and the common ejaculatory ducts) is the part usually affected, and projects into the bladder as a spherical mass or as a collar surrounding the orifice of the urethra. Such an enlargement of the middle lobe cannot be felt per rectum, although it may attain the size of a large walnut and block the entrance of the urethra. The anterior commissure is rarely affected. (Fig. 558.)

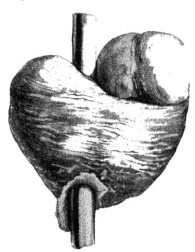

Fig. 558.—An enlarged prostate after removal by the suprapubic route. The median lobe is particularly affected.

Results. (a) **Effects on the urethra.**—The enlargement of the prostate takes place in an upward direction, owing to the resistance of the triangular ligament, and carries the base of the bladder with it. This produces a lengthening of the prostatic urethra, so that an ordinary catheter may not be able to reach the bladder. The total urethra may increase in length from the normal 8 in. to 12 in. The calibre of the urethra may be altered in two ways: either it may be narrowed by the pressure inwards of the enlarged lateral lobes, or it may be widened by being stretched over the mass; the latter is the more common. Deviation of the urethra may also occur from excessive enlargement of one or other lateral lobes. The shape of the prostatic urethra is frequently altered by enlargement of the middle lobe, so that it is more curved than usual and requires the use of a catheter with a special bend.

(b) **Effects on the bladder.**—With the increasing difficulty in expelling the urine, the muscular wall of the bladder becomes hypertrophied; but this change soon reaches its limit in elderly men, and is followed by dilatation of the bladder, fasciculation and vesiculation, with fibrosis of the muscle bundles. The projection into the bladder of the enlarged prostate causes the orifice of the urethra to be no longer the lowest part of the bladder, and there is the formation of a steadily enlarging postprostatic pouch behind the enlarged middle lobe. (Fig. 559.)

(c) **Effects on ureters and kidneys.**—The effects on these structures are similar to those following other causes of urethral obstruction, e.g. stricture. The lumen of the ureter becomes dilated, and its muscular coat atrophied, till the tube may reach the size of a piece of small intestine. The pelvis of the kidney becomes dilated, and there is an interstitial fibrosis of the kidney which destroys the secretory tubules and leads to renal insufficiency.

(d) **Inflammatory effects.** —Sooner or later a cystitis develops, either from direct infection by instrumentation or by infection from the bowel, and there will follow ureteritis, pyelitis, and pyelonephritis.

(e) **Effects on the circulation.**—The veins of the periprostatic plexus, with

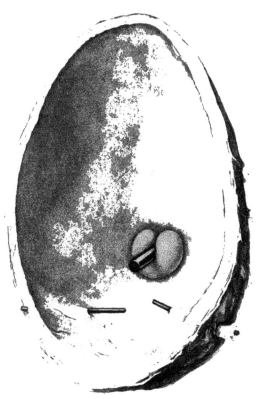

Fig. 559.—Bladder laid open, showing the obstruction caused by enlargement of the prostate. A bristle is seen in each ureter and a stylet in the urethra.

which the dorsal veins of the penis communicate, become dilated and varicose. Rupture of one of these may even lead to profuse hæmaturia.

(f) **Effects on the sexual organs.**—The common ejaculatory ducts which pass through the prostate may be distorted and compressed so that semen can no longer pass along them. This will lead to dilatation of the vesiculæ seminales and to aspermia.

3 g

(*g*) **Effects on the act of micturition.**—The increasing obstruction at the orifice of the urethra leads to increasing difficulty of micturition, the chief difficulty being experienced in starting the act. With enlargement of the middle lobe, straining to pass urine drives the lobe still farther into the orifice of the urethra, and the patient learns that straining is futile. The absence of effort and the weakening of the bladder wall lead to diminished force of the stream, which is hardly projected beyond the feet. The bladder is not completely emptied by the act, and urine will accumulate (residual urine).

Symptoms.—The patient in the early stage of enlargement complains of increasing *difficulty* and also of *frequency* of micturition. The difficulty is most marked at the commencement of the act, and the patient finds that micturition is most easily performed by waiting without straining. Frequency is often first noticed at night, the patient rising two or three times to empty the bladder ; the amount of urine voided at night is increased (nocturnal polyuria). There is loss of projection of the stream, and the patient frequently cannot micturate in the recumbent position. The difficulty of micturition is increased by cold, alcoholic or venereal excesses, constipation, or by holding the urine longer than is desirable. Increased sexual excitement and persistent erections, which may induce acts of impropriety, are common. The difficulty and frequency of micturition may steadily increase until the bladder becomes constantly distended, and incontinence with overflow results, but any of the following complications may supervene and alter the clinical picture :—

1. Complete retention of urine. This is due to congestion of the prostatic plexus of veins and the urethral mucous membrane, induced by cold, by venereal excess, or more frequently by prolonged holding of the urine, such as may occur on long railway journeys or at public meetings. This complication may be the first serious intimation to the patient that he has prostatic enlargement.

2. Severe hæmorrhage from rupture of a prostatic vein.

3. Cystitis, causing pain on micturition, frequency, and pyuria.

4. Calculus in the bladder, causing pain on micturition and hæmaturia.

5. Prostatic abscess—a rare complication.

Effects on the general health.—The general health may remain good for years, but with increasing frequency and difficulty there is impairment due to pain and loss of sleep. As the bladder becomes distended and the effects of back pressure on the kidneys are felt, the patient suffers from headaches, thirst, polyuria, and anorexia, and there is loss of flesh and strength. These effects are more marked if sepsis is added to the mechanical effects of the enlarged prostate.

Examination.—Examination per rectum may reveal a large soft prostate pressing backwards into the rectum, or a firm, slightly enlarged prostate. In both cases the enlargement is smooth and the mucous membrane of the rectum moves easily over it. One or other lateral lobe may be chiefly enlarged, but the condition of the middle lobe cannot be examined through the rectum.

Examination of the urethra with a catheter reveals an obstruction to the passage of the instrument at the entrance to the bladder. The urethra is found to be lengthened, and the curve of the instrument has to be altered to allow it to slip past the obstruction. The catheter is not gripped on removal, as it is by a stricture.

The endoscope is not of much value in examination of the enlarged prostate, but the cystoscope will permit examination of an enlarged middle lobe, besides showing the condition of the bladder walls, the mouths of the ureters, and the presence or absence of pouches and calculi.

Residual urine is examined for by making the patient micturate until he thinks the bladder is emptied, and then passing a catheter; but several examinations are necessary, as the condition fluctuates.

The condition of the kidneys can be ascertained by a careful analysis of a twenty-four hours' specimen of urine, by examining the blood pressure, the hæmo-renal index and the electrical conductivity of the urine. The urine should also be examined for pus and bacteria.

General treatment.—The patient should carefully avoid all causes of prostatic congestion, such as alcoholic and venereal excess, constipation, bicycling, horseback riding, the use of highly spiced food, and the prolonged holding of the urine. He should avoid late meals, drink freely of non-alcoholic fluid, and take as much exercise as his general condition will allow. By following the rules of a regular, simple life, a prostatic patient may live for years in comfort, and avoid both catheterization and operation.

Catheterization.—This should only be resorted to when absolutely necessary, and then under strict aseptic precautions. For acute retention the catheter must be passed (*see* later); for chronic retention also this instrument must be employed, but the frequency of its use varies considerably. It may only be necessary to empty the bladder at long intervals (months intervening), when some slight prostatic congestion is present, but the frequency with which catheterization is required generally increases. A patient with a large bladder rarely has to pass the catheter more than twice a day, but if the bladder be small and spasm of the muscle be present, more frequent catheterization is necessary. "Catheter life," with the infrequent or regular passage of a catheter, may be lived for years with comfort, and is consistent with great bodily and mental activity.

The catheters (which, of course, must be carefully sterilized) should be soft and large-bored, the coudé or bi-coudé being the most convenient shape. Metal catheters should only be used if soft ones cannot be passed, and then only by the surgeon. A gum-elastic catheter, of which the curve can be altered whilst in the urethra by partially withdrawing the stilette, is often serviceable.

Permanent catheterization is indicated if with cystitis catheterization is difficult, painful, or associated with hæmorrhage. A soft, self-retaining catheter, such as Casper's, should be passed, and, if the bladder is washed out twice daily, may be retained for a month and then changed. At first the patient should be kept in bed, but later he may be allowed up with a suitable apparatus; he should empty the bladder every two or three hours. A urethritis is always caused at first, but this soon ceases, and the catheter may be worn with comfort.

Cystitis should be treated by the administration of urinary antiseptics, and by washing out the bladder; and strict asepsis is essential in all instrumentation.

Operative measures.—The modern operative treatment of the chronically enlarged prostate consists of removal of the organ, either by the suprapubic or the perineal route. Whether the prostate is removed in its entirety from its sheath, or whether fibro-myomatous or adenomatous growths are shelled out from the prostate, is a matter of dispute, and is of little interest from the clinical point of view, but the question of the selection of cases suitable for this operation is of vital importance.

There can be no doubt that some patients with prostatic enlargement live for years in comfort by careful attention to their mode of life and the occasional passing of a catheter, but, on the other hand, many cases do badly. Difficulty in passing a catheter, hæmorrhage, cystitis, attacks of acute retention, and the formation of calculi are common, and lead to much misery; while the back-pressure effects on the kidneys with ascending pyelitis tend to shorten life, and render some radical treatment necessary.

Complete prostatectomy in the majority of cases relieves the patient of all his symptoms and is a most successful operation, but it is not without serious risk of death from shock or hæmorrhage, and important sequelæ and complications may deduct from the value of the result. It must also be remembered that in some cases—10 per cent., according to some observers—the diagnosis should be carcinoma of the prostate, and the early removal may possibly result in cure, which is most unlikely if the patient is left till the diagnosis is certain. The condition of the prostate must also be considered, the large soft prostate being much more readily removed, with less fear of complications, than the hard small prostate.

Above all, the general condition of the patient must be taken into account, and more especially the state of the kidneys, as shown by the patient's symptoms and a careful analysis of his urine. A weak heart, atheroma of the vessels, urine of persistent low specific gravity containing albumin and of low molecular concentration, contra-indicate the operation, as do wasting, thirst, headache, polyuria, and a low hæmo-renal index. Pyuria from cystitis, or unilateral pyelitis, is not a barrier to operation if the urine is of high specific gravity, many cases of cystitis clearing up after the operation.

To sum up, complete prostatectomy is indicated if a patient with a chronically enlarged prostate has to pass a catheter frequently or passes it with difficulty, if the use of the instrument causes pain and hæmaturia, if cystitis supervene or a calculus form in the bladder, or if attacks of acute retention are common, provided that the general condition is good and the kidneys are shown to be doing their work well. The operation is more especially indicated if the prostate is large and soft. The question of the route, suprapubic or perineal, to be adopted is not yet settled, but the balance of evidence at present is in favour of *suprapubic prostatectomy*, and most surgeons adopt this route for all their cases. It is the easier operation, and permits a more thorough exposure of the bladder ; its great disadvantage, difficulty of drainage, seldom arises.

The operation consists in opening the bladder by an incision above the pubis after the viscus has been distended with fluid, incising the mucous membrane over the prostate, and then enucleating the organ with the fingers, aided by the fingers of the other hand in the rectum pushing the prostate upwards and forwards. The prostatic urethra and the common ejaculatory ducts are usually torn across. After the prostate has been removed, hæmorrhage is stopped by sponge pressure, and the bladder drained by a large tube. The after-treatment consists in washing the bladder out daily, the tube being removed on the third day. The suprapubic wound should be closed at the end of the third week.

Perineal prostatectomy.—This operation may be performed in many ways, and the primary incision in the perineum may be either a median longitudinal or a transverse one. In the median perineal incision the membranous urethra is opened, the prostatic urethra dilated, and a retractor passed into the bladder, so that when it is pulled upon the prostate is drawn into the wound ; the fibrous sheath of the prostate is then incised, and the gland enucleated with the finger in one or more pieces. The bladder is drained by a tube, and the cavity, left by removal of the prostate, packed with gauze. During healing a bougie must be passed at regular intervals to maintain the patency of the urethra.

Complications of complete prostatectomy.—*Hæmorrhage* may be severe, but will usually yield to sponge-pressure and adrenalin. It may, however, be necessary to pack the cavity left by removal of the prostate.

Sepsis.—Acute epididymo-orchitis may occur, especially if cystitis have existed before the operation. The condition frequently ends in suppuration. Ascending pyelitis may also occur. *Cellulitis* of the pelvic tissue is an occasional sequela. Stricture, incontinence of urine, and suprapubic fistula may all follow the operation.

The *sexual power* may be lost, but this is more common after the perineal operation than after the suprapubic. Power of erection may remain, but without ejaculation of semen. In some cases, lost sexual power may be regained.

Uræmia with *suppression of urine* may speedily follow operation.

Calculi may form in the pouch left after removal of the prostate.

Treatment of acute retention of urine due to enlarged prostate.—A full dose of urotropine should be given, and an attempt made to empty the bladder by catheterization. If this succeeds, the bladder must be emptied regularly until the power of spontaneous micturition is regained. A second attack of retention should not be allowed to occur. If regular catheterization is impossible, a catheter should be tied into the bladder for a day or two.

If catheterization fails, the bladder should be aspirated above the pubes, and then another attempt made to pass and tie in a catheter. If, after two or three suprapubic aspirations, attempts to catheterize fail, the bladder should be drained through a suprapubic incision, and a day or two later the prostate removed by this route.

NEW GROWTHS

Benign growths of the prostate only exist as the adenomas and fibro-myomas of chronic enlargement, and have been considered under that heading (p. 913).

Malignant growths of the prostate consist of sarcoma and carcinoma, of which the latter is by far the more common.

SARCOMA[1]

Sarcoma of the prostate is rare, but it occurs at all ages, even sometimes in infants; it is invariably primary.

Symptoms.—There is an increasing difficulty in passing urine, with more or less sudden complete retention. Occasionally hæmaturia and pyuria are present, and fragments of growth may be passed per urethram. On rectal examination the growth is felt projecting backwards into the rectum as a large, firm mass, over which the mucous

---

[1] *See also* Vol. I., p. 509.

membrane does not move freely. Involvement of the pelvic glands is late, but metastasis in the lungs and other organs is common, the disease being invariably fatal.

Treatment.—This is similar to the palliative treatment of carcinoma of the prostate (p. 923). Attempts at removal can be made, but are usually followed by rapid local recurrence.

CARCINOMA [1] (Fig. 560)

Etiology.—In the prostate, as in other parts of the body, the cause of carcinoma is unknown. It has been stated that malignant disease not infrequently commences as chronic enlargement, but proof of this is wanting, and it is more likely that the cases were carcinomatous from the first. Chronic gonorrhœal inflammation has also been assigned as a cause, but on insufficient evidence.

Pathologically, the disease can be divided into soft (medullary) and hard (scirrhus) types, according to the amount of fibrous tissue in the growth ; but of more importance is the clinical division into—

(a) Growths which for a long time resemble innocent enlargements, and are frequently removed under that idea, the diagnosis being established by the microscope and the after-history.

(b) Growths which, having rapidly infiltrated the surrounding tissue, fungate into the bladder and rectum and involve the pelvic glands early, so that the pelvis soon becomes filled with a carcinomatous mass. These cases are the diffuse prostato-pelvic carcinomas of Guyon.

(c) A rare form of growth which is followed by general carcinomatous invasion of bone, the primary growth in the prostate being small and often difficult to discover. The secondary growths occur in the bone marrow, especially of the vertebræ, of the lower end of the femur and of the humerus, and gradually destroy the bone, leading, in some cases, to multiple spontaneous fractures. Secondary growths in internal organs are rare, but carcinoma of the prostate in man is sometimes associated with general carcinomatosis.

Secondary carcinoma of the prostate is rare, and it is unusual for bladder growths to invade the prostate, although invasion of the bladder by prostatic carcinoma is the rule.

Symptoms.—In an early stage of carcinoma of the prostate the symptoms are similar to those of chronic enlargement, viz. difficulty and frequency of micturition, loss of projection of the stream, retention of urine, and finally the incontinence of overflow ; but there are

[1] *See also* Vol. I., p. 536.

important differences, and afterwards other symptoms are added. In the first place, it may be stated briefly that the symptoms of carcinoma are much more rapidly and steadily progressive than those of chronic enlargement, and that the interference with micturition is more pronounced than the physical signs would lead one to expect.

Pain is a more marked and earlier feature in malignant disease than in chronic enlargement. It is referred to the end of the penis,

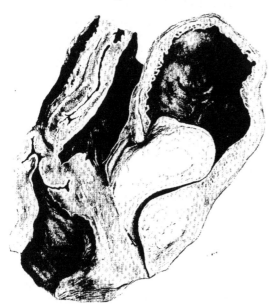

to the hypogastrium and the perineum, and, although increased by micturition, is not relieved by it. It is also very resistant to treatment, being due to infiltration of the nerve plexus by the carcinomatous growth. With involvement of the sciatic nerves, pain extending down the leg occurs.

True incontinence of urine may be set up in carcinoma, due to destruction of the

Fig. 560.—Section of the bladder, prostate, and rectum, showing carcinoma of the prostate ; the bristle is in the common ejaculatory duct.

bladder sphincters, but only towards the end of the disease.

Hæmaturia is rare unless there is ulceration of the growth, but it has nothing to distinguish it from the other causes of bladder hæmorrhage. As a rule it is slight. Pieces of growth may be passed per urethram.

Pyuria is always present when the growth has ulcerated into the bladder, but the cystitis rarely reaches a severe degree.

Interference with defæcation is similar to that occurring in cases of simple enlargement, but may go on to complete obstruction. Ulceration into the bowel leads to hæmorrhage and discharge per rectum.

Cachexia is marked and occurs early. It is not relieved by feeding and by treatment of the symptoms of urinary infection, as in cases of simple enlargement.

Physical signs.—The prostate should be examined per rectum after taking the precaution to empty the bladder. It is always considerably enlarged, and the surface presents marked irregularities, which are usually hard and nodular. Hard, conical projections can often be felt extending along the vesiculæ seminales or along the wall of the pelvis; the glands in the pelvis can frequently be felt to be enlarged and hard. The rectal mucous membrane is not freely movable over the tumour.

Examination of the urethra and the bladder by the catheter, sound, or cystoscope is contra-indicated, if the diagnosis can be made by rectal examination, as likely to cause severe hæmorrhage and cystitis. If examination of the urethra is carried out, only soft instruments should be used. The cystoscope is difficult to pass, and gives little information, especially as bleeding rapidly obscures the view. In a few cases the growth resembles a vesical tumour, but a differential diagnosis is at once made on rectal examination. Late in the disease complete retention of urine, rectal obstruction, involvement of the ureters, with subsequent hydronephrosis and pyonephrosis, anæmia, and secondary deposits, occur, whilst hypostatic pneumonia is frequently the direct cause of death.

Treatment.—In the great majority of cases palliation of the symptoms is the only treatment possible. The pain should be relieved by morphia, antipyrin, hot bottles and hot applications. For the retention of urine, catheterization with *soft* catheters is permissible if their passage does not cause severe pain and hæmaturia, but if it does so a permanent suprapubic opening should be made. All local treatment should be put off as long as possible, as it will only hasten retention of urine, cystitis, and hæmaturia.

The radical treatment of removal is sometimes carried out, under a mistaken diagnosis of chronic enlargement, by the suprapubic route, but rapid recurrence is inevitable, and the danger of death from hæmorrhage considerable.

Lately, attempts at radical cure have been made by removing the entire prostate, the seminal vesicles, the vasa deferentia, and the trigone of the bladder as far as the entrance of the ureters, but it is too early to speak of the results of this treatment, although patients have been reported as being alive three years after operation.

NEUROSES

Nervous disturbances of the prostate are of three kinds—hyperæsthesia of the gland, hyperæsthesia of the mucous membrane of the prostatic urethra, and spasm of the muscular fibres of the prostate causing difficulty in micturition. All three are usually found combined in the same patient.

Prostatic neuroses usually occur in young adults who have either had an inflammatory condition of the urethra and prostate, and often much treatment for it, or who are neurasthenic and have indulged in masturbation or sexual excesses.

In the first variety of neurosis the patient complains of a feeling of fullness or weight in the perineum, often occurring in attacks. On examination of the urine no prostatic threads or abnormal contents are found, but rectal examination shows the prostate to be very tender.

If the neurosis affects the prostatic urethra, similar symptoms are present, and the passage of a catheter causes severe pain as the instrument enters the bladder. The urethra, however, shows no sign of inflammation, and there is no discharge.

The spasmodic variety of neurosis of the prostate is the most frequent of the three, and is characterized by difficulty in micturition, especially in the initiation of the act, which varies from time to time. As a rule, this difficulty is exaggerated by the presence of others, but it may be present and necessitate straining even when the patient is alone. The passage of a catheter after the bladder is supposed to have been emptied will often demonstrate residual urine, but presents no difficulties except a slight one at the neck of the bladder. The spasmodic obstruction is distinguished from those due to organic stricture of the urethra, or to prostatic enlargement, by the facts that there is no lengthening of the urethra, that the difficulty varies from time to time, and that a large catheter passes more readily than a small one. The condition may be associated with attacks of spasm of the detrusor muscle of the bladder, causing urgent micturition without pain or difficulty.

Treatment.—Any inflammatory condition of the urethra or prostate should be attended to, and the patient assured of the absence of serious disease. Too much local treatment, especially if it be painful, is harmful as tending to increase the neurosis. Passage of a large sound daily, with the general treatment of neurasthenia, will often result in cure.

THE VESICULÆ SEMINALES

ACUTE VESICULITIS (SPERMATO-CYSTITIS)

Acute vesiculitis is most commonly secondary to acute urethritis, the usual cause being infection by the gonococcus, but it may follow septic urethritis induced by instrumentation of the urethra. Other causes are prostatitis, cystitis, and suppuration after removal of the prostate. The symptoms and treatment are dealt with under Gonorrhœal Spermato-Cystitis, Vol. I., p. 843.

CHRONIC VESICULITIS (SPERMATO-CYSTITIS)

Chronic vesiculitis may be gonorrhœal, septic, or tubercular. The first two may be considered together.

CHRONIC SEPTIC OR GONORRHŒAL VESICULITIS

This condition usually follows a urethritis of a similar nature, and is not infrequently preceded by an acute attack.

Symptoms.—There is a feeling of weight and pain in the perineum, and frequently also a chronic urethral discharge which on endoscopic examination is found to come from the ejaculatory ducts. There may be frequeney and pain on micturition, and sexual irritability, leading at first to increased sexual desire and power, and later to diminution of the sexual appetite and to impotence. On rectal examination the vesiculæ are found to be enlarged and painful, and pus can frequently be squeezed from them into the urethra. Chronic urethritis and prostatitis are often concomitants.

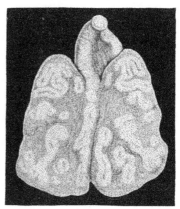

Fig. 561.—Section of a vesicula seminalis, showing advanced tuberculosis.

Treatment.—The only rational treatment for this condition, besides the administration of urinary antiseptics, is the emptying of the vesiculæ of their abnormal contents by digital manipulation. The vesiculæ are stroked from above downwards, their contents being squeezed into the urethra. This is repeated daily until relief of all symptoms is obtained ; but the condition is very rebellious to treatment.

In old-standing cases it may be justifiable to remove the vesiculæ through a perineal incision.

TUBERCULOUS VESICULITIS (Fig. 561)

Tuberculous vesiculitis is usually associated with tuberculous disease in other parts of the genito-urinary tract, especially in the epididymis and the prostate. It has, however, been stated that primary disease is not uncommon, and that the tuberculous disease of the epididymis is secondary to vesiculitis.

Symptoms.—The condition is usually discovered during routine rectal examination in cases of tuberculosis of the testis, prostate, or bladder, but in some cases the first symptom may be the appearance of a chronic abscess in the perineum. There are frequency of micturition, a feeling of weight in the perineum, and occasionally a urethral discharge.

On rectal examination the vesicula in the early stages feels hard and nodular, but later the nodules soften, and in advanced cases a soft fluctuating swelling is felt.

Treatment.—The form of treatment is largely determined by the condition of the other parts of the genito-urinary tract. In cases of tuberculous disease of the testis submitted to epididymectomy or castration the corresponding vesicula, if diseased, should be removed at the same operation by perineal section, and this plan should also be followed if primary disease of the vesicula is diagnosed. In cases of advanced genito-urinary tuberculosis, general treatment is all that is indicated. Tuberculous abscesses should be opened from the perineum and the contents carefully scraped out.

CYSTS, CONCRETIONS, AND NEW GROWTHS

Cysts of these organs have been described, and are usually considered to be retention cysts due to stricture of the duct. Stricture of the common ejaculatory duct is very rare, and it is probable that most cases of alleged cysts of the vesiculæ have little to do with these receptacles.

Concretions have been found in connexion with chronic vesiculitis, but they are very rare.

New growths are usually secondary to disease of the prostate; primary new growths are so rare as to be pathological curiosities.

THE TESTIS

CONGENITAL ABNORMALITIES

POLYORCHISM

The majority of reports of cases of polyorchism are untrustworthy, but several definite cases of this rare condition have been described. Only cases verified by dissection and microscopical examination should be admitted, for encysted hydroceles, omental hernia, etc., have all been described as supernumerary testes.

ANORCHISM—MONORCHISM

These cases are more frequently met with than cases of polyorchism, but the condition still remains very rare. The testis alone may be absent, or any or all parts of the sexual apparatus, on one or both sides. The condition is usually associated with abnormalities of the external sexual apparatus.

ANTERIOR INVERSION

Several forms of inversion of the testis have been described, but anterior inversion is the only one of interest. It is said to occur in one in every twenty males. With anterior inversion the body of the testis and the tunica vaginalis are posterior, whilst the epididymis is anterior. If not recognized, the condition may lead to errors of diagnosis, or, more important still, to injury of the testis in the tapping of a hydrocele, if the position of the testis has not been carefully ascertained beforehand.

IMPERFECT DESCENT

In the early stages of development the testis is situated in the abdomen, below the kidney, and it is only in the seventh and eighth months of foetal life that it descends into the scrotum. The descent of the testis is governed by the gubernaculum testis, a fibro-muscular bundle with attachments above to the lower pole of the testis, the globus minor of the epididymis, and the caecum, and below to the skin at the bottom of the scrotum and over the perineum, the symphysis pubis, and the anterior superior spine of the ilium. In the course of its normal descent the testis passes through the inguinal canal: its arrest at any point constitutes *the imperfectly descended testis ;* its departure from the normal direction, into that of some of the non-scrotal fibres of the gubernaculum, *the ectopic testis.*

The testis may therefore be situated in the abdomen, in the inguinal canal, just outside the external ring, or in the perineum, over the symphysis pubis or near the anterior superior spine. The testis has also been found in Scarpa's triangle, having passed into the thigh over Poupart's ligament after it had issued from the external abdominal ring. The cause of imperfect or abnormal descent is unknown, but it is probably intimately connected with development of the testis, as the incorrectly placed organ is nearly always undeveloped and functionless as far as the secretion of spermatozoa is concerned ; even if spermatozoa are found in the semen of a cryptorchid it will only be at puberty or soon after, the imperfectly descended gland under-going premature atrophy.

In all cases of imperfectly descended testis the processus vaginalis is to be found in the scrotum, but the upper end does not become shut off from the general peritoneal cavity, and the patient always has a potential or an actual inguinal hernia. Fluid may collect in the peritoneal pouch and form a congenital hydrocele.

Diagnosis.—The diagnosis of imperfectly descended testis is made by finding the scrotum empty, and, unless the gland is actually intra-abdominal, by feeling the organ in its abnormal position. Obvious as such a condition would appear to be, mistakes are made in the case of young children with very mobile testes. In these children the slightest stimulus, such as slight coldness due to removal of the clothing, will cause the testis to be retracted into the inguinal canal, and casual examination will lead to error. In imperfect descent the organ cannot be made by manipulation to reach the bottom of the scrotum, but the merely extremely mobile testis can readily be pressed down into its proper place.

Treatment.—In considering treatment, the value of the organ and the dangers of the condition must be taken into consideration. It has already been pointed out that the imperfectly descended testis is an ill-developed gland usually incapable of spermatogenesis, but this does not necessarily mean that it has no function. As is well known, removal of both testes in a young subject prevents the development of the secondary male characteristics, probably owing to lack of the internal secretion of the testes ; but development of these characteristics does occur in cryptorchids, showing that the internal secretion is normal. At the same time, it is also well known that one testis is sufficient for the purposes of development, and therefore the loss of the internal secretion of one imperfectly descended testis may be ignored. From the physiological point of view, consequently, there is no benefit to be gained from saving one imperfectly descended testis, nor will the placing of such a testis in the scrotum lead to its developing active spermatogenesis. Further, the imperfectly placed organ is specially liable to certain accidents and diseases. In the perineum, in the inguinal canal, in front of the pubis, or in Scarpa's triangle, it is particularly liable to injury from blows and subsequent inflammation and atrophy. The abnormal attachments of the epididymis and its mesentery may lead to torsion, whilst malignant disease is relatively more common in the imperfectly descended than in the normally placed testis.

The fact that imperfect descent is complicated by a patent processus vaginalis, and that radical cure of hernia is easier and more certain after removal of the testis, must also be taken into account. At the same time it must be remembered that at puberty a testis that has remained in the inguinal canal will sometimes descend into its normal situation in the scrotum.

In all cases except those in which the organ is in the abdomen, operation is indicated, and the organ can either be (a) fixed into the scrotum, (b) removed, or (c) returned to the abdomen.

(a) **Orchidopexy** is only possible in the exceptional cases in which the spermatic vessels are long enough to reach the bottom of the scrotum without tension, whilst attempts to increase the length of the spermatic cord by division of structures and inversion of the testis usually lead to atrophy of the organ. The operation of orchido-pexy is therefore only indicated in exceptional cases. Complete atrophy and re-ascent of the testis are common, and the results of the operation are usually disappointing. The steps of the operation are as follows : An incision is made over the external abdominal ring, as in Bassini's operation for inguinal hernia, and the external oblique aponeurosis divided and opened. The processus vaginalis testis is then identified and opened, and the testis exposed. The peritoneal process is divided above the testis, and the upper end carefully separated from the structures of the spermatic cord and ligatured as in a hernia operation. The testis and spermatic cord are then lifted from their bed, pulled downwards, and all bands of fascia carefully divided until the cord is so long that the testis will lie on the thigh, three or four inches below Poupart's ligament. If this lengthening cannot be obtained by division of the fascia only, the spermatic vessels must be divided, and the testis left attached merely by the vas and artery of the vas. The forefinger is then passed into the scrotum, and a pocket for the testis made there. Into this pocket the testis is placed, and held in position by a purse-string suture passed through the tissues above it. The conjoined tendon of the internal oblique and trans-versalis is then sutured to Poupart's ligament above the vas, and the other layers of the abdominal wall closed as in a radical cure of hernia.

(b) **Removal of the testis.**—This is the operation usually per-formed for imperfect descent on one side, especially if the case is complicated by hernia or torsion ; but when these complica-tions do not exist, little harm is likely to result from waiting for the onset of puberty, on the off-chance of descent occurring at that time.

(c) **Returning the testis to the abdomen.**—This can be done when both testes are imperfectly descended, so that the internal secre-tion may not be lost; but it must be remembered that torsion and malignant disease are more apt to occur in these organs, and that the extension of any inflammation from the urethra is more dangerous in an abdominal than in a scrotal testis.

The hernia which so frequently complicates imperfect descent of the testis should always be treated by radical cure ; trusses designed to allow the descent of the testis whilst retaining the hernia are useless. When the radical cure is performed the testis should be removed, to permit more complete and more secure closure of the inguinal canal. If the condition is bilateral, one or both testes should be returned to the abdomen.

TORSION OF THE SPERMATIC CORD (AXIAL ROTATION OF THE TESTIS)

Torsion of the spermatic cord (Fig. 562) is associated with developmental errors of attachment of the epididymis and the common mesentery to the testis, and these errors are more frequently found in the imperfectly descended organ than in one normally placed in the scrotum. The rotation usually takes place at the globus minor, and is of such

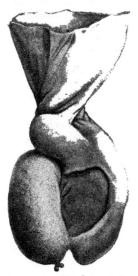

a nature that the testis is inverted and the globus major and hydatid are found below. The twist may be half a turn, but as many as four turns have been described. Although this condition is always associated with errors of development, the exciting cause of the rotation is unknown, some cases occurring during violent exercise, others during sleep. Clinically, the cases may be divided into acute and recurring.

ACUTE TORSION

Symptoms.—The patient, usually the subject of an imperfectly descended testis, is suddenly seized with violent pain in the groin, vomits, and becomes collapsed, the symptoms and physical signs closely resembling those of acute strangulated hernia. In the groin a firm, tender, oval lump is felt, which cannot be separated from the abdomen, and which has no impulse on coughing. The scrotum

Fig. 562.—Torsion of the spermatic cord.

on the side of the lump is empty, and the skin usually red and œdematous. Fluid, which is generally blood-stained, may be found in the vaginal cavity.

Results.—If the testis be removed and examined it will show extreme congestion, extravasation of blood into every part, and a purple or black colour. This extravasation of blood destroys the testicular substance, so that atrophy, which may be complete, always follows. In a few cases the organ becomes infected with the colon bacillus, and suppuration with sloughing results.

Treatment. (a) **With testis in the scrotum.**—If the case is seen soon after the rotation has occurred, an attempt should be made to untwist it. This has been successful in a certain number of instances, but success does not always avert subsequent atrophy. If the attempt to untwist is not successful, the testis should be exposed and removed, although if the twist is slight and the extravasation of blood not excessive an attempt to save the testis may be made.

(*b*) **Wiih imperfectly uescended testis** (Fig. 563).—In these cases the testis should always be removed, the processus vaginalis separated and ligatured, and the internal abdominal ring closed.

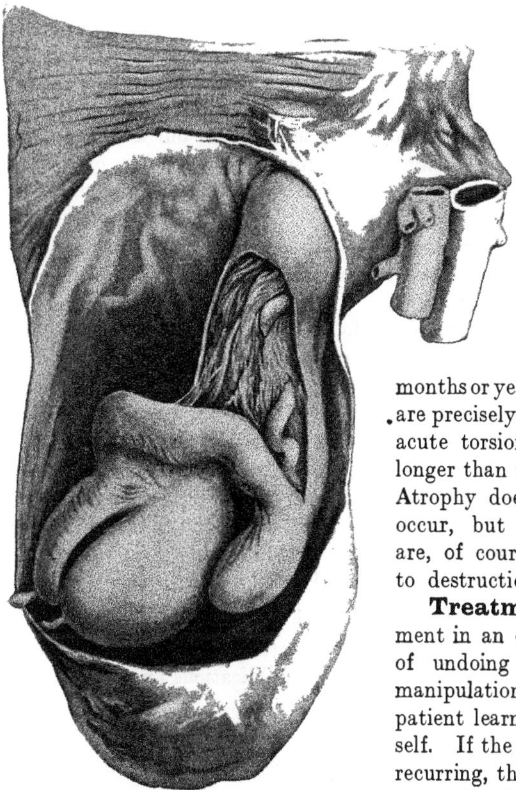

RECURRING TORSION

This term has been given to cases in which the symptoms of torsion occur at varying periods over a course of months or years. The symptoms are precisely similar to those of acute torsion, but rarely last longer than twenty-four hours. Atrophy does not necessarily occur, but frequent attacks are, of course, liable to lead to destruction of the organ.

Treatment.—The treatment in an early case consists of undoing the rotation by manipulation; sometimes the patient learns to do this himself. If the condition is really recurring, the testis should be exposed and fixed in the scrotum by suturing, but if the testis is imperfectly descended it should be removed.

Fig. 563.—Dissection of an imperfectly descended testis, showing the condition which is liable to result in torsion.

INJURIES OF THE TESTIS

CONTUSED WOUNDS

These wounds are due to blows or squeezes of the testis, and result in extravasation of blood. The extravasation may occur into the tunica vaginalis (traumatic hæmatocele), into the testis (hæmatocele

3 *h*

of the testis), or, very rarely, into the epididymis. There is always accompanying ecchymosis of the scrotum. Severe contusions of the testis are rare, owing to the mobility of the organ.

Symptoms.—The general symptoms are often severe, and include collapse and vomiting. Locally there is severe pain, especially if hæmorrhage is taking place inside the tunica albuginea, with swelling and ecchymosis of the scrotum. The swelling in severe cases may extend up the spermatic cord to the internal abdominal ring (hæmatocele of the spermatic cord). The initial symptoms in slight cases do not last long, and the patient may resume work, but in a few hours orchitis results, and the pain and swelling increase. This orchitis, in which the epididymis may share, lasts for some days, and is frequently followed by atrophy of the testis.

In very severe contusions the tunica albuginea may be ruptured ; marked extravasation of blood into the testis without rupture of the tunica albuginea is very rare.

Results.—Mild injuries are followed by complete recovery, but after severe injuries some amount of atrophy is the rule and may be complete. Suppuration rarely follows. In a large number of cases of malignant disease a history of injury is obtained, but it is doubtful whether there is any direct connexion between the two.

Treatment.—After slight injuries, rest with elevation and support of the scrotum is all that is necessary ; but if the pain is severe, an incision to let out the blood is advisable, and a timely incision may possibly in some cases prevent atrophy.

Suppuration, if it occur, should be treated by incision and drainage.

INCISED WOUNDS

Incised wounds require the same treatment as similar wounds in other parts of the body, and have like complications and results.

DISEASES OF THE TESTIS

INFLAMMATION

Inflammation of the testis may be mainly limited to the body (orchitis) or to the epididymis (epididymitis), but in the majority of cases both parts of the organ are affected, and the condition will be described under the term epididymo-orchitis. Those cases in which the body of the testis is mainly involved will be indicated after epididymo-orchitis has been described.

EPIDIDYMO-ORCHITIS

Epididymo-orchitis may be divided into acute, subacute, and chronic forms, but a classification on etiological grounds is of more importance. The condition may be caused by—

(a) Infection of the testis by micro-organisms which have reached the organ by way of the vas deferens from the urethra, prostate, and vesiculæ seminales. By far the most frequent of these organisms are the gonococcus, staphylococci, and streptococci, but in some cases the tubercle bacillus reaches the testis by this route.

(b) Infective micro-organisms which reach the testis by means of the blood-stream. These cases are secondary to the general infective diseases, such as mumps, typhoid fever, scarlet fever, smallpox, etc., or are due to invasion by the tubercle bacillus or the spirochæte of syphilis.

(c) Gout.

(d) Injury and strain.

GONORRHŒAL EPIDIDYMO-ORCHITIS

This important variety of Epididymo-Orchitis is discussed in Vol. I., p. 839.

EPIDIDYMO-ORCHITIS OF URETHRAL ORIGIN OTHER THAN GONOR-RHŒAL URETHRITIS—SEPTIC EPIDIDYMO-ORCHITIS

The most frequent causes of non-gonococcal urethritis are septic organisms which invade the urethra after instrumentation, operations on the urethra, and prostate, the passage and impaction of calculi in the urethra, or the bursting of abscesses from the vesiculæ, prostate, and Cowper's glands into the urethra. Urethritis due to septic organisms is not infrequently followed by an epididymo-orchitis which has the same symptomatology and physical signs as that due to the gonococcus, and at first demands the same treatment.

Prognosis.—Although the majority of cases of septic epididymo-orchitis end either in resolution or in fibrosis, a large number go on to suppuration. This pus formation may occur in one of three places:

(a) *In the tunica vaginalis.*—This is perhaps the most common place, the fluid present in the tunica in all cases of acute epididymo-orchitis becoming more or less purulent. The redness and œdema of the skin are most marked in front of the testis, where a fluctuating swelling forms, from which pus is evacuated. This condition does not lead to fungous testis or to atrophy unless it is coexistent with suppuration in the testis.

(b) *In the body of the testis.*—Owing to the dense tunica albuginea, suppuration in the body of the testis is frequently associated with gangrene and sloughing of the organ. The body is much enlarged, and if incisions are not made into it the pus bursts externally, frequently through several fistulæ. Complete atrophy of the testis is a common sequel.

(c) *In the epididymis.*—If suppuration occur in the epididymis a fluctuating swelling forms at the lower and posterior part of the scrotum. After the discharge of the pus, healing occurs by fibrous tissue, and the secretion of the testis is usually lost to the semen.

Treatment. 1. The urethritis.—The patient should be given urinary antiseptics and sedatives such as urotropine, hetralin, buchu, acid sodium phosphate, etc., and encouraged to drink freely of bland fluids. If injections of astringents and antiseptics into the urethra are being used, it is probably wise to discontinue them.

2. General treatment.—While the condition is acute the patient should be confined to bed on a light diet and the bowels freely opened ; the more complete the rest in bed the sooner will resolution occur. Drugs such as morphia, antimony tartrate, anemone pulsatilla, salicylate of soda, etc., may be given for the relief of pain. Vaccine-therapy has also been employed with some success.

3. Local treatment.—The testis should be well supported either by a good suspensory bandage or, if the patient is in bed, on a small pillow. For the first forty-eight hours cold may be applied either by means of an ice-bag or by evaporating lead lotion, but warmth in the shape of fomentations equally relieves the pain, and probably is of more value in promoting resolution.

If a hydrocele be present and the pain intense, relief can frequently be obtained by puncturing with a tenotomy knife and allowing the escape of fluid. Counter-irritation by painting the scrotum with silver nitrate (3i ad 3i) till smarting is complained of will often relieve the pain and allow the patient to get about if this is necessary. Bier's method of passive congestion can also be tried. As soon as the acute stage is over, the testis should be carefully strapped to promote absorption of the inflammatory products, and the strapping with suspension of the testis should be continued until all thickening has disappeared. This treatment, combined with the giving of potassium iodide and injections of fibrolysin, should also be carried out for simple chronic epididymo-orchitis.

If suppuration occur the abscess should be carefully opened over the most prominent part. Great care should be taken in opening an abscess in front of the scrotum, as the pus is frequently confined to the cavity of the tunica vaginalis, and a careless incision may open the tunica albuginea and infect the testis.

Incision into the testis with a tenotomy knife has been advised in the early stages of epididymo-orchitis, even in gonorrhœal cases. The proceeding is not without danger, and is probably useless. Excision of the fibrous nodules of chronic epididymo-orchitis has been done, but the results as regards sterility are doubtful. In cases of gangrene the organ should be excised and the scrotum drained.

ORCHITIS

Orchitis may occur as a secondary affection to epididymitis, or the inflammation may primarily affect the body of the testis, the epididymis being only slightly involved. Orchitis is much rarer than epididymo-orchitis, and is due to injury, gout, or infection by one of the organisms of the specific diseases, particularly epidemic parotitis (mumps), typhoid fever, smallpox, scarlet fever, and possibly rheumatism and influenza.

Traumatic orchitis has been considered under Injuries of the Testis (p. 932).

GOUTY ORCHITIS

Inflammation of the body of the testis due to gout is very rare, but the possibility of its occurrence may be considered settled. An acute or subacute orchitis develops without any apparent cause, usually in a patient who is middle-aged and gives a history of attacks of articular gout. The course of the disease is tedious, as relapses are apt to occur. The epididymis is only slightly affected; but a condition of epididymo-orchitis secondary to gouty urethritis has also been described.

Treatment.—The treatment consists in supporting the testes and in the local application of warmth, combined with the medicinal treatment of the gouty diathesis.

ORCHITIS OF EPIDEMIC PAROTITIS

This variety of orchitis usually develops between the sixth and the eighth day of the parotitis, and is much more common in some epidemics than in others. It occurs in boys and young adults, being almost unknown in childhood or old age. It may occur in an epidemic without the development of parotitis, or it may precede the parotitis; in some cases it has developed after inflammation of the submaxillary gland, without any involvement of the parotid. The condition is mainly an orchitis, but cases of epididymitis have been described.

Symptoms.—The body of the testis becomes tender, hard, and painful. The skin of the scrotum is red, and there may be a secondary hydrocele. The condition, though usually unilateral, may be bilateral. The orchitis usually rapidly clears up, four days being the average duration of the disease, but in some cases atrophy follows. This is particularly apt to occur in older patients, and is more common in some epidemics than in others. Should it occur in both testes, impotence or even infantilism may result.

Treatment consists in rest in bed, warmth, and support of the testes. The patient should remain in bed till all the swelling has disappeared.

Orchitis of Typhoid Fever

Orchitis occurring in typhoid usually appears during the height of the disease, but it has been known as early as the seventh day, or it may occur during convalescence. It is a rare complication. The inflammation is usually subacute, and may not be noticed owing to the general condition of the patient. The body of the testis becomes hard, tender, and swollen, and then gradual resolution takes place ; suppuration and atrophy, although not unknown, are rare. One testis only is usually attacked.

Orchitis of Smallpox

Orchitis is a rare complication of smallpox, but it occasionally terminates in suppuration. It has also been described following vaccination for smallpox.

Orchitis of Scarlet Fever, Influenza, and Malaria

Orchitis is an extremely rare complication of these diseases, but its possibility should be remembered in seeking for the origin of an otherwise unexplained orchitis.

Orchitis and Rheumatism

The cause of rheumatism is still uncertain, and it is doubtful if rheumatic orchitis really exists. Polyarthritis is very frequently of gonorrhœal origin, and it is possible that cases described as rheumatic are really cases of epididymo-orchitis secondary to gonorrhœal urethritis which is complicated by gonorrhœal arthritis.

Orchitis has also been said to have complicated tonsillitis, but the latter affection may be due to such different causes that discussion of the subject is unnecessary.

Epididymo-Orchitis and Strain

The connexion, if any, between epididymo-orchitis and strain is one of great importance, as it is not infrequent for workmen to claim compensation for an attack of epididymo-orchitis which is alleged to have followed the lifting of a heavy weight. Whether epididymo-orchitis is ever due to strain is doubtful. It has been suggested that violent contraction of the cremaster muscle due to great muscular effort may cause the testis to strike so forcibly against the pillars of the external ring as to produce an acute epididymo-orchitis, but this is difficult of proof. Cases of epididymo-orchitis of obscure origin are not very uncommon, and it is easy to attribute them, in the absence of an obvious cause, to an alleged strain, but great care should be taken to exclude all other possible causes before this is suggested. Many cases are due to gonorrhœal urethritis, the discharge ceasing for a time when the testes are attacked. Others are cases of acute tuberculosis, or are due to subacute torsion of the spermatic cord. This last condition was not recognized by the older writers on diseases of the testis, and accounts for many cases of acute epididymo-orchitis of apparently unknown cause. Acute torsion of the spermatic cord may follow a muscular effort, which may thus be the exciting cause of the torsion, the predisposing cause being a congenital abnormality of the attachments of the testis (*see* p. 930).

Some cases of epididymo-orchitis may be due to thrombosis of the veins of the pampiniform plexus. I have a specimen of this condition. The onset was acute, with symptoms of acute epididymo-orchitis, and after this had subsided a hard lump was left in the scrotum just above the body of the testis. The testis was excised under the impression that the lump was a malignant tumour, but after removal the condition of thrombosed veins of the pampiniform plexus was obvious.

TUBERCULOUS EPIDIDYMO-ORCHITIS

Tuberculous epididymo-orchitis is usually associated with tuberculosis in other parts of the genito-urinary tract, especially the vesiculæ seminales and the prostate. The disease may, however, be most advanced in the testis, and it is probable that in some cases the tuberculosis is localized in this organ, the organisms reaching the affected part by the blood-stream. The epididymis is usually attacked before the body of the testis (Fig. 564), perhaps for months before the body is affected. Infection of the epididymis can occur in one of two ways—either the organism has infected the vesiculæ, prostate, or urethra, and reaches the testis by spreading along the lymphatics of the vas deferens ; or it reaches the testis by the blood-stream. Both these methods may occur, but probably the infection is most commonly conveyed along the vas from the vesiculæ, which can usually be shown to contain tubercle bacilli in cases of tuberculous epididymitis.

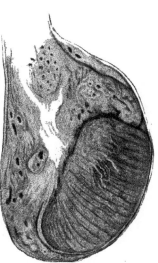

Fig. 564.—Early tuberculosis of the epididymis.

The disease occurs at all ages, but is most common in young adults between the ages of 20 and 30 years, and it has the usual etiology of tuberculosis.

Varieties.—Clinically it is possible to distinguish two forms, an acute and a chronic. The *acute* variety has a sudden onset, with severe pain and swelling of the epididymis, the symptoms and physical signs closely resembling those of acute epididymo-orchitis of gonorrhœal origin. From this it can be diagnosed by the absence of urethral discharge, or, in the rare cases in which this is present, by isolating the tubercle bacillus from the exudate.

The *chronic* variety of tuberculous epididymo-orchitis is the more common (Fig. 565), and is insidious in its onset. Usually the first thing noticed by the patient is a small painless nodule in the back part of the testis, associated with a slight aching pain in the part. On examination this nodule is usually found to be in the globus minor of the epididymis, but not infrequently it is situated in the globus major. This difference of situation may be explained by the two modes of infection. Thus, if the infection spreads along the vas, the globus minor is first affected; but in blood-borne infection the globus major suffers first, the spermatic artery entering the epididymis near the upper end.

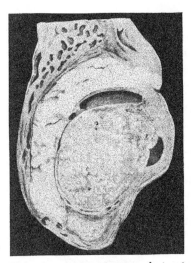

Fig. 565.—Advanced tuberculosis of the epididymis and body of the testis.

Signs.—When the disease is moderately advanced it presents the following physical signs: The skin of the scrotum tends to be adherent to the lower and posterior aspect of the testis; later a fluctuating swelling will form at this point, burst, and discharge pus. The epididymis is enlarged and nodular, the nodules at first being firm, but later becoming softened in the centre. The vas is often normal, but sometimes small nodules can be felt in it, giving it a beaded feel. The rest of the cord is normal, but is sometimes infiltrated with inflammatory products, especially in cases of mixed infection. The body of the testis appears on clinical examination to be normal, but after removal small tubercles can usually be seen in it. These tubercles are most numerous near the mediastinum testis.

A small hydrocele is present in about 30 per cent. of the cases, but is not a prominent feature of tuberculous disease of the testis. On rectal examination, nodules of tubercular deposit can frequently be felt in the vesiculæ and prostate, and there may be evidence of tuberculous disease of other parts of the genito-urinary tract, especially in the other testis. The disease, if not treated, usually becomes bilateral, although it is generally more advanced on one side.

Prognosis. — The prognosis of *acute* tuberculous epididymo-orchitis is bad, the inflammation, as a rule, rapidly terminating in suppuration and sinus formation. In the acute cases also the body of the testis is affected early and severely.

The prognosis of the *chronic* variety is better, the inflammation frequently terminating in fibrosis (Fig. 566), but in the majority of

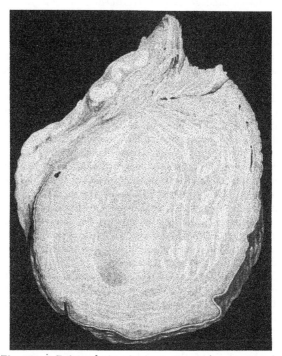

Fig. 566.—Tuberculosis of the testis ending in fibrosis.
It is difficult to distinguish epididymis from body, and both are firmly adherent to the skin.
The condition closely simulates malignant disease.

cases suppuration occurs sooner or later. The prognosis as regards the life of the patient depends on the involvement of other parts of the genito-urinary tract.

Treatment. Acute cases.—The prognosis in the really acute case is so bad as regards saving the testis that castration should be advised as soon as the diagnosis is made, provided the disease is not advanced in other parts of the genito-urinary tract.

If the patient will not agree to this he should be put to bed, the testis well supported, and the general treatment of tuberculosis carried out. If suppuration occur, consent for removal of the testis will often be given, but if not the abscess should be opened and the disease eradicated as far as possible. Epididymectomy is not indicated in acute cases, as the body is invariably affected.

Chronic cases.—The usual constitutional treatment for tuberculosis should be carefully carried out, and beyond supporting the testis in a suspensory bandage no local treatment is necessary. Treatment. by injection of tuberculin has proved of value, and should always be tried in chronic cases. Bier's method of passive congestion has also been used with success in cases of tuberculous testis, and may be given a trial before more radical methods are tried. If general treatment fails, and the condition goes on to suppuration, one of the three following operations may be advised :—

(*a*) The abscess is opened and the diseased parts are thoroughly scraped with a sharp spoon so as to remove, as far as possible, all tuberculous tissue. This may be followed by healing, and the testis is saved, although its function is lost. Frequently, however, a sinus persists, and further treatment becomes necessary.

(*b*) *Epididymectomy.*—In this operation the diseased epididymis is dissected off the body of the testis, care being taken to save the vessels, and an attempt made to obtain healing by first intention. The procedure has the advantage of leaving the patient his testis, but the advantage is a sentimental one, as the organ is functionless. Consent for this operation can often be obtained when castration is refused. Its chief value is in those cases where the second testis has already been removed or is the seat of advanced disease.

(*c*) *Orchidectomy.*—It is a question for consideration, in all cases of tuberculous epididymo-orchitis in which the disease is limited to the testis, whether early castration is not the best treatment. The loss of one testis is no real disadvantage to the patient, while the risk of a general genito-urinary tuberculosis is a matter of supreme importance. It cannot be gainsaid that a large number of patients with chronic tuberculosis of the epididymis recover and remain well if general constitutional treatment for tuberculosis is efficiently carried out ; but in many cases the disease progresses to other parts of the genito-urinary tract, leading ultimately to the death of the patient. This result may be prevented by an early orchidectomy.

When castration is performed for tuberculous disease the cord and vas should be removed as high as possible, and it is. usually advisable to remove the vesicula seminalis at the same operation.

TUBERCULOUS EPIDIDYMO-ORCHITIS IN CHILDREN

Tuberculous disease of the testis is rare in children, only nine cases being diagnosed in the London Hospital in children under the age of 12, out of 11,493 patients under that age. The disease has been seen a few weeks after birth. It is usually insidious in onset, and presents the same physical signs as in the adult, but associated disease of the vesiculæ and prostate is uncommon. The disease starts in the epididymis, which it probably reaches through the blood-stream. It is, however, frequently associated with tuberculous peritonitis, and according to some authors with tuberculosis of the vertebræ (Pott's disease).

Prognosis is bad, the inflammation usually ending in suppuration and sinus formation.

Treatment.—This does not differ from the treatment of the disease in the adult, but early castration is to be advised, to prevent, if possible, infection of the peritoneum. Local scraping and epididymectomy are unsatisfactory in these small testes.

Syphilitic Epididymo-Orchitis

Syphilis affects the testis in the secondary, intermediary, tertiary, and inherited varieties of the disease, but is most commonly met with in the intermediary stage, i.e. two to four years after infection.

During the early secondary stage the epididymis is chiefly affected, the patient suffering from a symmetrical subacute epididymitis which is painless and mainly localized to the globus major. The condition is rare, but probably frequently passes unnoticed among the other manifestations of secondary syphilis.

In the intermediary and tertiary stages the body of the testis is chiefly affected, the lesion being a chronic orchitis ending either in gumma formation or in diffuse fibrosis and later atrophy of the testis. These two conditions frequently occur together, the organ on section showing a general fibrosis with small gummata.

Physical signs.—In a well-marked case of syphilitic orchitis (*see* Plate 79, Vol. I., facing p. 746) the following physical signs are present : The skin of the scrotum, at first normal, becomes adherent to the front of the testis ; and later, if the disease is untreated, a large piece of the skin sloughs away, exposing the characteristic wash-leather slough of a gummatous ulcer. Through the hole in the skin thus made the testis may fungate. The body of the testis is at first uniformly enlarged and painless, but later, if multiple gummata form, it may become nodular. The organ feels light if weighed in the hand, and testicular sensation is lost early. The epididymis, vas deferens, and spermatic cord are usually normal, but thickening of the vas and gummata of the epididymis have been described. If the epididymis is unaffected it is frequently difficult to differentiate it from the enlarged body. Rectal examination reveals no lesion of the vesiculæ and prostate, and there is no enlargement of the abdominal glands. A hydrocele is present in the early stages in the majority of cases (Plate 105, Fig. 1), and it may be necessary to draw off the fluid before the physical signs of syphilitic orchitis can be made out. Later the fluid may be absorbed, and the cavity of the tunica vaginalis completely obliterated by adhesions. If a gumma forms and softens, fluctuation may be obtained in the front of the swelling. When fibrosis follows, the body of the testis becomes hard and is frequently smaller than normal, the epididymis may be distorted, and a large hydrocele is frequently present. With atrophy of both testes sexual desire is diminished and, later, impotence may follow.

Diagnosis.—The diagnosis has to be made from malignant disease of the testis, and is often so difficult that it can only be settled either by the effects of treatment or by an exploratory incision. Wassermann's serum diagnosis (Vol. I., p. 32) is valuable in these cases.

Treatment.—This consists in giving mercury in the secondary stage and mercury and iodide of potassium in the intermediary and tertiary stages. Resistant cases with ulceration and fungous testes may be treated by castration combined with a course of mercurial treatment.

INHERITED SYPHILIS OF THE TESTIS

Inherited syphilis of the testis is rarer than tuberculous disease of that organ in children, but is met with in children a few months old and up to 10 and 12 years. After that time it is extremely rare, but Fournier has described a case in a young man of 24 years.

The body of the testis is usually affected, although cases limited to the epididymis have been described. The disease usually presents itself as a diffuse, painless orchitis ending in fibrosis and atrophy of the testis, and, if bilateral, as it generally is, may result in infantilism. Gumma formation, leading to ulceration and fungous testis, may occur, but is rare. The physical signs are similar to those of the acquired variety, but hydrocele is not so common.

Treatment.—As in the acquired form, this consists in giving mercury and iodide of potassium.

ATROPHY OF THE TESTIS

A diminution in the size and functional power of the testis may be either the result of inflammation affecting the gland (orchitis), or a degeneration of the glandular elements without supervening fibrosis.

Inflammatory atrophy may follow orchitis from any cause, such as injury, syphilis, tuberculosis, mumps, etc., and the fibrosis and atrophy may be partial or complete; usually they are partial. The testis becomes harder and smaller than usual, and is frequently nodular.

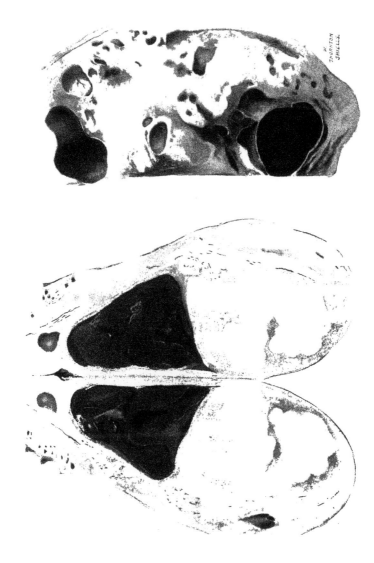

W THORNTON SHIELDS

Fig. 1.—Tertiary syphilis (gumma) of the testis with a localized hydrocele. (*Specimen 20130, London Hospital Museum.*)

Fig 2 Teratoid tumour of the testis (fibro cystic disease). (*Specimen 20530, London Hospital Museum.*)

The tunica albuginea is thickened and wrinkled, and the gland on section shows bands of fibrous tissue running in all directions, the normal testicular substance having disappeared. The epididymis shares in the fibrosis and atrophy, and there is frequently a vaginal hydrocele. The condition may be either unilateral or bilateral.

Degeneration atrophy of the secretory tubules of the testis may occur from various causes. It may be due to interference with the blood supply by injury to the vessels of the cord, either by accident or operation; to lesions of the central nervous system, either cord or brain; to pressure from an old-standing hydrocele or hernia; or it may be associated with some grave constitutional disease, such as diabetes or leukæmia. The testis in this form of atrophy feels soft and flabby, and on microscopical examination shows fatty degeneration of the essential cells without increase in the fibrous connective tissue. The epididymis shares the atrophy.

Both forms of atrophy of the testis, if bilateral, are associated with complete or relative sterility. In advanced cases, spermatozoa are completely absent from the semen (azoöspermia), or are few in number (oligospermia); and if the atrophy is complete, and especially in degeneration atrophy, the patient is impotent.

Atrophy of one testis has no effect on sexual life, provided the other testis is healthy.

Treatment must be directed to the cause; for the condition itself nothing can be done.

ARREST OF DEVELOPMENT

Arrest of development of the testis must be carefully distinguished from atrophy. It is usually found associated with malposition of the testis; in fact, all misplaced testes are maldeveloped testes. This arrest of development of the testis is congenital, and may affect both the internal and external secretions. Usually it interferes with the external secretion only, for cryptorchids generally develop the secondary sexual characters of the male, although as a rule they are sterile. There is no treatment for this condition.

NEW GROWTHS OF THE TESTIS

INNOCENT NEW GROWTHS

Innocent new growths of the testis are so rare as to be pathological curiosities.

The following varieties have been described :—

(a) *Fibroma.*—A few cases have been reported, but the descriptions of nearly all of them suggest that the disease was inflammatory in origin.

(b) *Osteoma.*—It is doubtful whether true bony tumours are ever found in the testis.

(c) *Myoma.*—This tumour, of which two at least have been reported, is believed to arise in the remains of the gubernaculum testis.

(d) *Adenoma.*—Ticene and Chevason have described small nodules, never larger than a pea, occurring in ectopic testes, which they think are true adenomas. They have never seen them in the normally placed organ.

MALIGNANT NEW GROWTHS

Malignant growth of the testis, whether primary or secondary, is rare, only about ·06 per cent. of all male patients admitted to the London Hospital suffering from this disease. These growths will be considered from a clinical point of view.

Malignant disease of the testis may occur at any age, and may even be congenital. It usually occurs in one testis, but French writers have described a special variety which has a tendency to attack both testes at the same time. It appears to be relatively more common in the imperfectly descended testis than in the normally placed organ, but some writers have denied this statement. In a large proportion of cases the disease appears to follow injury to the testis, but this trauma may only be the means of calling the patient's attention to what is a symptomless disease.

Clinical symptoms.—These at first are absent, but later there is a dragging pain in the groin and pain across the loins. Later still, with secondary deposits in the lumbar glands, there may be sharp attacks of abdominal pain, and the usual signs and symptoms of malignant cachexia.

Physical signs.—The disease nearly ·always affects the body of the testis, primary malignant disease of the epididymis being rare. The body becomes uniformly enlarged, the growth for a long period being confined by the tunica albuginea. Later there is appearance of localized nodular bulgings of the tunica albuginea, of a softer consistency than the rest of the tumour. If the tumour contains much cartilage it is exceedingly hard, but the rapidly growing fleshy growths with a large amount of degeneration of the tumour tissue feel soft and semi-fluctuant.

Testicular sensation may be either absent or present, depending upon the stage of the disease and the amount of normal testicular substance remaining. If the testicle is supported in the hand it feels heavy. The epididymis becomes greatly stretched and thinned out over the enlarged body to such an extent that in the majority of cases it is not possible to differentiate between the body and the epididymis.

A general or localized effusion may be present in the tunica vaginalis, but this is not common. In a few cases this effusion is blood-stained. The spermatic cord is usually unaffected, except that it is a little thick-

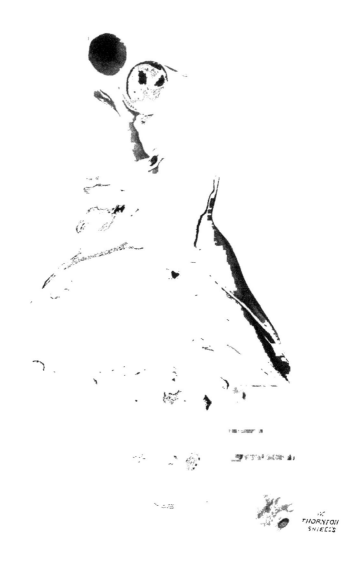

Rapidly growing malignant tumour of the testis, with secondary
nodules in the spermatic cord.

(*Specimen 2039, London Hospital Museum.*)

PLATE 106.

ened by the increase in the size of the vessels necessary to supply the vascular tumour and by the hypertrophy of the cremaster muscle that follows the increase in weight. The cord may, however, be infiltrated by the new growth and become nodular (Plate 106), the nodules varying in size from that of a pea to a growth as large as the normal testis. The vas deferens remains unaffected.

The skin of the scrotum is at first normal, but later large dilated veins can be seen in it. With advance of the disease the skin ceases to move freely over the testis, and finally becomes firmly adherent at one part; through this the tumour, if not removed, will eventually fungate. The glands affected first are the lumbar glands, situated on the front of the lumbar vertebræ and surrounding the aorta and the vena cava just below the level of the renal arteries and veins. A large deep-seated mass is felt on one side of the spinal column near the umbilicus. This mass is fixed and nodular, and does not move on respiration. Pressure on the vena cava may lead to dilatation of the superficial veins of the abdomen, and later to ascites and to œdema of the lower extremities. Occasionally the inguinal and external iliac glands are affected. Metastasis may occur to any part of the body, but is most common in the lungs.

Diagnosis has to be made from hæmatocele, hydrocele, chronic orchitis, and tuberculous disease. From hæmatocele the diagnosis is often extremely difficult, especially if there is no history of accident; in such cases exploratory incision is advisable before orchidectomy is performed.

Prognosis.—The prognosis is extremely grave, largely owing to the late stage of the disease at which the patient usually comes under observation. Early removal sometimes results in complete freedom from recurrence.

Treatment.—The treatment is removal of the organ as soon as the diagnosis is made. This should be done even if there is evidence of secondary enlargement of the lumbar glands, as the patient will certainly be rid of a source of inconvenience and the danger of the growth fungating will be avoided. Local recurrence is not usual.

Operation is contra-indicated in cases of advanced disease with a large lumbar swelling and with infiltration of the cord, as the growth will fungate through the wound and there may be serious difficulty in stopping hæmorrhage at the operation.

The question of the removal of the lumbar glands at the time of removal of the primary growth is an important one, as the modern operative treatment of malignant growth demands the removal of the nearest set of lymphatic glands as well as of the growth itself. Attempts, more or less successful, have been made to remove the lumbar glands, and there can be no doubt that this is the correct line of treatment, but whether it can usually be done with safety to the patient has yet to be decided.[1]

Pathology.—The difficulty of classification of new growths is perhaps more marked in connexion with the testis than with any other organ, in consequence of their great variety and complexity of structure. Recent researches and observation have, however, done much to simplify the confusion, and the following growths can now be differentiated by the microscope :—

1. **Sarcoma.** (a) *Round-celled.*—These tumours show in every part masses of small round cells invading the normal testicular substance. They are the most common form of sarcoma.

(b) *Spindle-celled.*—These tumours are much rarer than the round-celled growths, but show the same structure in every part of the growth.

(c) *Lympho-sarcoma.*—These tumours show the reticular structure of lymph-glands, but are hardly to be differentiated from the small round-celled sarcomas.

2. **Endothelioma.**—Endotheliomas are rare, but show the same histological characteristics in the testis as in other organs.

3. **Carcinoma.**—These tumours may be either columnar-celled or spheroidal-celled, according as they arise in the ducts or in the glandular substance of the testis, or frequently the cells may be of comparatively undifferentiated type. Like the sarcomas, they are uniform in structure, and are exactly comparable with carcinomas in other glandular organs.

4. **Teratoid growths.** (*See* Teratomas, below.)

TERATOMAS [2]

These tumours have been described under various names; of these the most common are fibro-cystic disease (Plate 105, Fig. 2), adenoma, chondroma, chondroma complex, chondro-sarcoma, chondro-carcinoma, embryoma, chorion-epithelioma. These names indicate the complex nature of the growths and the extraordinary diversity of the tissues found in them; examination of single specimens has led to great difference of opinion as to their nature. Clinically they may show every type, from a slowly growing encapsuled and apparently innocent tumour to a highly malignant growth destroying life by metastasis in a few weeks. They are most common between the ages of 30 and 40.

In all cases examination of some part of the tumour shows a simple

[1] Since writing the above I have removed the glands lying along the aorta, the common iliac, and the external iliac artery, in a boy of 11, with complete success.

[2] *See also* Vol. I., p. 586.

fibro-cystic structure, the cysts being lined with a columnar or flattened epithelium. Here and there in the stroma masses of true cartilage are nearly always found, but other parts of the tumour may show a sarcomatous, carcinomatous, endotheliomatous, or chorionepitheliomatous structure. The metastasis may also show the simple fibro-cysto-chondromatous structure, but in other cases it may be sarcomatous, carcinomatous, or chorion-epitheliomatous.

It is probable that these growths arise in sex cells which are attempting to develop under some unknown stimulus.

Clinically the only diagnosis possible is malignant disease of the testis, and early removal of the testis is indicated in all cases, no matter how slowly growing the tumour may be.

DERMOID TUMOURS

Under this term several entirely different conditions have been described :—

(a) Cases of malignant teratoma which are described above.

(b) Pilo-sebaceous dermoids arising in the skin of the scrotum and attached to the testis, but not in or of it.

(c) Tumours encapsuled in the testis and containing hair, teeth, bone, etc.

If the term dermoid of the testis is to be retained, it should indicate this last variety only. These tumours are very rare, not more than three or four having been described in England in the last five-and-twenty years. They are congenital in origin, but may not be recognized until the patient has reached adult life, and are of very slow growth. At any time during their existence, but particularly at puberty, they may become inflamed and suppurate, discharging hair, teeth, pieces of bone, etc., and so making the diagnosis easy. They should be removed as soon as diagnosed.

MALIGNANT DISEASE OF THE EPIDIDYMIS

Malignant disease of the epididymis is rare, only five cases being found in the London pathological museums. The growth is usually a sarcoma, either round- or spindle-celled, but a case of primary squamous-celled carcinoma has been described.

The treatment is removal of the testis as soon as the diagnosis is made.

CYSTS OF THE EPIDIDYMIS

Cysts of the epididymis have been divided into two classes : (a) small superficial cysts, frequently multiple and bilateral, occurring in men over 40, rarely growing larger than a pea, and seldom containing spermatozoa ; (b) large cysts growing in the substance of the epididymis, usually single, occurring in men under 40, growing slowly, perhaps reaching the size of a small orange, and frequently containing sperma-

3 *i*

tozoa (spermatoceles). It is doubtful, however, if these two classes are distinct from one another, and, as the exact pathology of cysts of the epididymis is uncertain, it is unnecessary to make the division.

Pathology.—Probably these cysts do not all arise in the same way ; the following views of their origin are held :—

1. They are retention cysts of the tubules of the epididymis or vasa efferentia. 2. They arise in fœtal remnants such as the paradidymis (organ of Giraldès), the vas aberrans, the remains of Müller's duct, or the pronephros (hydatid of Morgagni). This view would make them analogous to some cysts of the ovary and embryonic in origin. 3. They are due to bursting of an excretory tubule into the connective tissue round the epididymis. 4. They form in the connective tissue and have a secondary connexion with the excretory tubules.

Pathological anatomy.— Cysts of the epididymis most commonly occur in the region of the globus major and extend upwards into the cord, depressing the body of the testis so that it lies more horizontally than usual. (Fig. 567.) They are frequently bilateral, and may be multiple and loculated. They vary in size from a pin's head to a cyst containing five or six ounces of fluid, and are usually of very slow growth. The fluid contained in them is either

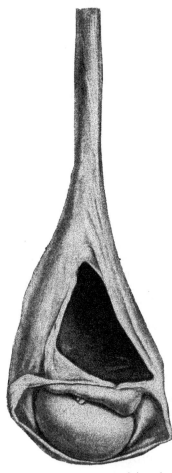

Fig. 567.—Cyst of the epididymis.

(a) a pale limpid fluid with only a trace of albumin, or (b) a milky-white opalescent fluid containing some albumin and many spermatozoa, either living and active or dead and disintegrating ; it is usually the large cysts that contain spermatozoa. The cyst may persist in spite of several tappings, or may disappear after tapping.

There is usually a connexion between these cysts and the tubules of the epididymis or vasa efferentia, but in many cases no such connexion can be demonstrated by injection or dissection.

Symptoms.—As a rule symptoms are absent, although there may be some pain. Usually attention is drawn to the cysts by chance, or by their gradual enlargement. They have frequently been mistaken for extra testes. They mostly occur in middle life or old age, and are of no importance. When of medium size, such a cyst presents on examination a rounded or lobulated, translucent, and painless cystic swelling in the globus major; it is attached to and moves with the body of the testis, which is more horizontal than usual.

In small cysts, difficulty in the recognition of translucency and apparent solidity owing to tenseness may confuse the diagnosis; large cysts may envelop the testis and simulate hydroceles of the tunica vaginalis, but may be distinguished from them by the fact that on careful examination the testis can usually be found below and free from the cystic swelling. The cyst may suddenly increase in size and become painful after a slight blow; this may be the first intimation to the patient that he has a pathological condition in the scrotum.

Treatment.—These cysts are of slow growth and painless, and therefore may be left alone. If, however, they increase in size so as to cause inconvenience, they may be tapped from time to time, or, if the patient should desire it, they may be removed by dissection.

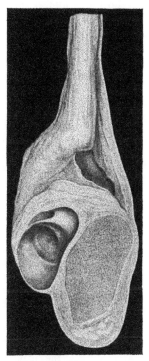

Fig. 568.—Cyst of the tunica albuginea.

CYSTS OF THE TUNICA ALBUGINEA (CYSTS OF THE TESTIS)

These cysts are exceedingly rare, only one or two specimens having been described. They arise between the layers of the tunica albuginea, and are probably due to injury and extravasation of blood. So rare are they that the diagnostic points are unknown. If necessary, the treatment is removal. (Fig. 568.)

OTHER CONDITIONS OF THE TESTIS

NEURALGIA

This term is applied to a painful condition of the testis usually occurring in paroxysms.

The cases have been classified as follows :—

(a) *Cases without an obvious lesion.*—These cases, though rare, exist. The testis is the seat of paroxysms of acute pain, although examination *in situ* or after removal fails to show any apparent abnormality. The pathology is quite unknown, but there may be a history of sexual irregularities or excesses.

(b) *Cases with a lesion in the body or epididymis.*—The most common of these lesions are small nodules of fibrous tissue in the globus minor of the epididymis, the result of a gonorrhœal epididymo-orchitis. The nodule is usually acutely tender, and the pain radiates from it. Other lesions are small cysts of the epididymis, fibrosis of the body, atrophy of the testis, and the results of injury to the testis. In the case of chronic epididymo-orchitis the pain is perhaps due to retention of semen behind the blocked tubules of the epididymis.

(c) *Lesion in the adnexa of the testis and elsewhere.*—The two most common lesions of this variety are varicocele and renal or urethral stone. Pain in the testis in varicocele is not an uncommon symptom, although it may be entirely absent ; whilst pain radiating to the testis is one of the classical symptoms of renal colic. Other conditions with which intense testicular pain is sometimes associated are hydroceles, small fibrous and cartilaginous tumours in the tunica vaginalis, and pressure on the nerves by a new growth of the spine.

Symptoms.—In most cases there is constant tenderness of the testis, exaggerated during the paroxysms of pain, and usually extremely marked in any nodule that may be present either in the testis proper or in the epididymis. The paroxysms are frequently caused by exercise, slight injury, and changes of temperature. Coitus in some cases relieves the pain, but in others it appears to induce the paroxysms. The pain starts in the testis, and may radiate along the spermatic cord to the lumbar region. It is usually so severe that the patient is incapacitated, and it has sometimes induced self-mutilation. During the paroxysms, which may last from a few minutes to several hours, the testis is frequently retracted owing to spasm of the cremaster muscle.

Treatment.—The first step in treatment is to remedy any pre-existing disease in the testis and its adnexa. A varicocele should be ligatured, cysts of the epididymis removed, a hydrocele operated upon, and so forth. The removal of the pathological condition is frequently followed by complete relief of all symptoms, and no further treatment of the neuralgia is necessary. In other cases relief of the pain does not follow the treatment of the underlying condition, or there may be no apparent organic lesion in the testis. The prognosis in these cases is not good, as the condition is very rebellious to treatment, which is mainly empirical. Relapses after apparent cure are common. During the attacks of pain the patient should be put at rest in the horizontal position and the testis be supported by a suspensory bandage. Local application of cold or heat should be tried, or mild counter-irritation of the scrotum employed. In severe attacks it is necessary to give morphia to relieve the pain ; quinine and aconite have been employed for the same purpose.

Firm pressure of the spermatic cord against the symphysis pubis for fifteen minutes has been followed by relief of pain.

The general health should be considered, and especially the question of sexual hygiene, as some cases are dependent either upon sexual excesses and irregularities or upon sexual continence.

Operative treatment.—The operative treatment, other than relieving any obvious pathological condition, consists in removal of the testis. Its advisability is doubtful. Cases are recorded by the older writers, such as Cooper, Curling, and Blizard, but the results were not all satisfactory. In some of the cases in which relief followed, the testis was the seat of obvious disease and the operation was justifiable ; but when no lesion exists, removal of the testis has been followed by recurrence of the pain in the spermatic cord or even in the other testis. Castration may therefore be recommended if an obvious lesion of the testis is present, which cannot be remedied in any other way ; but if no lesion exists the operation is unlikely to effect a cure. In all cases the patient should be warned of the uncertainty of relief following castration.

SPERMATORRHŒA

This term implies a frequent escape of seminal fluid at other times than during a sexual orgasm. As a pathological condition, if it exists, it is exceedingly rare. Escape of seminal fluid not infrequently occurs during defæcation, especially if there is much straining at stool with the passage of hard fæces. It occurs in men who lead a continent life, and is a purely mechanical effect, the fæcal mass squeezing against the contents of the seminal vesicles, which are between the rectum and the bladder. It is a perfectly natural and harmless phenomenon. Spermatozoa may also be found in the urine which is first passed after coitus or an emission.

Patients who have for a long time indulged in sexual excesses or masturbation not infrequently increase the irritability of the sexual organs to such an extent that emission takes place on very slight provocation, and often with incomplete erection of the penis and a minimum of pleasurable feeling; but this is a condition of irritability of the sexual apparatus with frequent emissions, not spermatorrhœa.

Some patients also suffer from frequent nocturnal emissions; but here again the term spermatorrhœa is not applicable, erection and orgasm being present.

The alleged disease is one that is firmly believed in by the laity, and the following conditions frequently give rise to the fear that the patient is suffering from a dreaded disease which only exists in his imagination :—

1. Escape of a little prostatic fluid after sexual excitement accompanied by complete or partial erection of the penis.

2. Frequent nocturnal emissions.

3. Escape of muco-pus in a patient who has a general or localized urethritis, prostatitis or vesiculitis, or Cowperitis.

4. Deposits of urates or phosphates from the urine, more especially the latter, which sometimes appear as a "milky" deposit at the end of micturition.

5. The normal mucous cloud in urine.

Amongst the insane, complaints of spermatorrhœa are frequently made, and they may be attributed by the patient to past masturbation or sexual excesses; but the condition only exists in the diseased imagination.

To sum up, the term spermatorrhœa is a misnomer, and should be discarded from medical literature.

Nocturnal Emissions

The occurrence of emission of semen during sleep may be either physiological or pathological. In healthy adult men, living well as regards food and drink, and leading a continent life, nocturnal emissions accompanied by voluptuous dreams and erection of the penis are natural if they do not occur more frequently than once in ten days or a fortnight, and are not accompanied by any bad reaction on the general health. They are pathological if they occur more frequently —for example, several nights in succession or several times in the same night; if they are not accompanied by full erection of the penis; or if they cause the patient to feel weak, irritable, and easily tired. Pathological nocturnal emissions usually follow sexual excesses, habitual masturbation, irritation from a tight prepuce or inflamed prostate, or unhealthy sexual excitement; or they may be the result of organic disease such as myelitis, tabes dorsalis, or general paralysis of the insane.

Treatment.—If, on careful consideration of the history and the effects of the emissions, the condition is considered physiological, the patient should be frankly assured that the condition is natural and no treatment is necessary. For frequent emissions with bad after-effects, the treatment consists in careful sexual hygiene after treatment of any local condition such as phimosis. The diet should be spare and unstimulating, and alcohol is to be avoided, especially in the evening. Mental occupation, with a sufficiency of healthy outdoor exercises, the avoidance of prurient thoughts and literature, are all-important. Engorgement of the prostate in the early morning, due to the full bladder, is a source of irritability, and can be readily removed by emptying the bladder immediately on waking. Cold sponging of the genitals or cold baths are also useful. Drugs other than aperients are of little use, but general tonics may be useful. Sedatives such as bromide of potassium, hyoscyamus, cannabis indica, or opium may be tried, but they are of little use without careful regulation of the sexual life.

THE SPERMATIC CORD AND TUNICA VAGINALIS

HYDROCELE

Hydroceles may be either primary or secondary, and it is advisable to discuss the latter first.

SECONDARY HYDROCELE

This form of hydrocele may be divided into acute and chronic.

1. *Acute secondary hydroceles* are generally due to inflammations or injuries of the testis, the most common being gonorrhœal epididymo-orchitis, but they also occur with the orchitis of the specific infective fevers. These hydroceles are cases of *vaginalitis*, the inflammation of the tunica vaginalis being secondary to the inflammation of the testis, and the effusion inflammatory in origin and nature. The condition is frequently unnoticed, as it is masked by the symptoms of the acute inflammation of the testis, and the treatment is identical with the treatment of the primary inflammation. Resolution is by far the commonest result, but suppuration occurs in a certain number of cases, and the tunica has to be drained (*see* Acute Epididymo-Orchitis, p. 933). Acute hydroceles also occur with acute inflammation of the scrotum or spermatic cord, or they may be secondary to acute torsion of the testis. In this latter condition the fluid is usually blood-stained.

2. *Chronic secondary hydrocele* is also generally due to a chronic vaginalitis secondary to chronic inflammation of the testis, as in tubercular epididymo-orchitis and syphilitic orchitis.

In some cases chronic hydroceles are passive effusions into the cavity of the tunica vaginalis, as in cases secondary to neoplasm of the testis.

The **treatment** of secondary hydrocele is that of the primary condition, but in the case of hydrocele secondary to syphilitic orchitis tapping or radical cure may be necessary.

PRIMARY HYDROCELE

The primary form of hydrocele may be acute or chronic. Acute primary hydrocele due to an acute vaginalitis is rare, but cases have been described of acute pneumococcic and acute septic infection of the tunica vaginalis, with effusion of inflammatory lymph into the tunical cavity; and it is possible that acute rheumatic vaginalitis occurs.

Chronic primary hydrocele may also be due to a chronic vaginalitis such as tuberculous infection of the tunica, which is most common in children, and is frequently associated with tuberculous peritonitis; but the pathology of the common vaginal hydrocele is unknown, and it will be described under the title of primary idiopathic hydrocele.

1. *Primary Idiopathic Hydrocele of the Tunica Vaginalis*

Two views are held as to the causation of this disease : (1) that it is secondary to a chronic inflammation of the testis or epididymis ; (2) that it is a passive effusion into the cavity of the tunica vaginalis from unknown causes.

Of these two views the latter is the one most generally held by English surgeons, while the former is favoured by French surgeons.

The condition is most frequently met with in elderly patients, and especially in Europeans resident in the tropics, but it may occur at any age.

A preceding or accompanying history of inflammation of the testis or epididymis is unusual, the patient rarely giving any cause for the disease.

Pathological anatomy. Fluid.—The usual amount of fluid in a hydrocele is about half a pint, but occasionally hydroceles are seen containing quarts of fluid. The fluid closely resembles blood serum ; its specific gravity is about 1022, and it contains about 6 per cent. of albumin, the fluid becoming solid on boiling. It is generally straw-coloured, but may be brownish from admixture of blood, or may sparkle from the amount of cholesterin in it. It contains fibrinogen, and therefore coagulates on the addition of blood or other source of fibrin ferment.

Tunica vaginalis.—The tunica vaginalis even in old-standing cases may be simply thinned owing to the pressure of the fluid, and show no other feature. On injection with soft paraffin, long finger-like processes may sometimes be seen projecting into the connective tissue of the scrotum. In other cases thickening of the tunica occurs, causing the hydrocele to be constricted in places, or even loculated. In old cases, especially those that have been tapped many times, fibrosis of the tunica may be present, and in some instances the walls of the sac are as much as half an inch in thickness. Calcification of these thickened sacs, which are often of cartilaginous hardness, is not infrequent. In rare instances, projecting from the walls of the sac or lying free in the cavity are small cartilaginous or fibrous bodies. In a few specimens, inflammatory adhesions may partially obliterate the cavity of the tunica and localize the hydrocele to one part.

Testis.—In long-standing cases, thickening of the tunica albuginea with atrophy of the testis may be present, due to the pressure of the fluid, but this is rarely important. In some cases the distension of the digital fossa of the tunica with fluid lifts the epididymis away from the body of the testis, and thus thins out the vasa efferentia, which may be so pressed upon as to prevent escape of spermatozoa from the gland, and in this way double hydrocele in a young subject may lead to sterility. In some long-standing cases the testis is so squeezed out and incorporated with the wall of the hydrocele that it is not immediately discoverable on opening the hydrocele.

Spermatic cord.—This is sometimes a little thickened from hypertrophy of the cremaster fibres.

Penis.—In large hydroceles the skin of the penis and scrotum may be so dragged forward that the penis is lost in it, and only represented by a dimpled fold of skin resembling the umbilicus.

Symptoms.—The patient rarely complains of pain, but only of the discomfort and weight of the distended scrotum or the difficulty of micturition and inconvenience if the penis is buried.

On examination, a pear-shaped swelling with base downwards is found distending one-half of the scrotum. The skin of the scrotum is unaffected, and the fingers can get above the swelling and grasp the cord, showing that there is no communication with the abdomen. Usually the scrotum can be readily folded up on to the abdomen. The swelling is found to be translucent, but several fallacies in connexion with this sign may occur. In the first place, translucency is absent if the walls are very thick or calcareous, or if hæmorrhage has occurred (hæmatocele); in the second place, translucency may be present in a hernia of a child if it contains gut distended with gas.

The testis, when distinguishable, is usually found below and behind the fluid, but in cases of inversion of the testis it is found in front—a point of great importance when the hydrocele has to be tapped. The swelling is usually plainly cystic to the touch, and has no expansile impulse on coughing. The affections most likely to cause errors in diagnosis are hæmatocele, cysts of the epididymis or testis, scrotal hernias, and neoplasms of the testis; and the condition may be complicated by the presence of cysts of the epididymis, hydrocele of the cord, or hernia.

Complications. (a) Rupture.—This may be traumatic or spontaneous ; in the latter case it may occur while the patient is quietly resting, and is probably due to the giving way of one of the finger-like processes described above, or of the wall at the site of a previous tapping. There is a sharp sudden pain, followed by alteration in the condition of the scrotum, the definite cystic swelling changing to a diffuse œdematous condition, often with evidence of blood extravasation. The penis, prepuce, and the other half of the scrotum usually become swollen. The pain, as a rule, steadily increases, and causes the patient to seek relief. Spontaneous cure, suppuration, or recurrence of the hydrocele may follow.

(b) Inflammation and suppuration.—These terminations are rare, and are usually due to definite injury, although this is not absolutely necessary.

(c) Transformation into hæmatocele may be due to either tapping or injury, or may occur spontaneously and insidiously.

Treatment.—Treatment may be palliative by tapping, or curative by radical operation. Treatment by injection of various irritants into the sac is obsolete.

Tapping.—A hydrocele may be tapped as often as it becomes inconvenient on account of its size. The position of the testis should always be ascertained before tapping, either by marking its position when the translucency test is applied, or in the case of small hydroceles by feeling it. The skin of the scrotum is cleaned in the manner usual for all operations, and drawn tensely over the swelling with one hand whilst with the other the aseptic trocar and cannula is plunged through it into the cyst, the puncture being usually made in front, but always away from the testis. Care should be taken to avoid any superficial scrotal veins. The fluid is then drawn off, the cannula removed, and the small puncture closed with a little collodion. In a few cases no recurrence follows tapping, but as a rule it has to be repeated at intervals.

Radical cure.—This can be advised in all cases except when the patient is elderly or debilitated in health, and it is usually completely successful, though recurrence has been recorded. Two operations are advised, and it is immaterial which is chosen—(a) excision of the tunica vaginalis lining the scrotum, or (b) inversion of the sac.

(a) *Excision of the tunica vaginalis lining the scrotum.*—It is doubtful if the old division into a parietal and a visceral layer of the tunica vaginalis can be maintained. Some authorities consider that the body of the testis is uncovered by a serous membrane, but that the organ projects into the cavity of the tunica vaginalis in the same way that the ovary projects into the peritoneum. (Fig. 569.) If this is so, excision of the tunica vaginalis lining the scrotum means complete excision of the tunica, and recurrence is most unlikely.

The operation is a simple one, and is easily performed through a two-inch incision in the scrotum. Care should be taken to arrest all hæmorrhage, even from the smallest bleeding-points, otherwise a troublesome hæmatoma may result.

(b) *Inversion of the sac.*—The tunica is opened, the fluid allowed

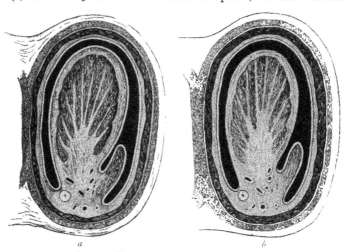

Fig. 569.—Diagram illustrating the two theories regarding the relationship of the tunica vaginalis to the testis.

a, Tunica vaginalis covering the testis and lining the scrotum ; *b*, tunica vaginalis lining the scrotum, but not covering the testis.

to escape, and the sac simply inverted, with or without suture. Recurrence is rare.

Treatment of rupture.—Rupture may either be treated by rest and support until the œdema has disappeared, when a radical cure may, if necessary, be performed, or the operation may be done as soon as the patient comes under observation. The former, as less liable to be followed by complications, is probably the better course to pursue.

Treatment of suppuration.—As in cases of suppuration elsewhere, the abscess cavity should be opened and drained.

2. *Infantile Hydrocele* (Fig. 570, 1)

In this variety of hydrocele the processus vaginalis is closed above at the internal abdominal ring, but the part lying in the cord, that normally should be obliterated, remains patent and becomes filled with fluid. The condition is common, and appears soon after or at birth.

Physical signs.—A fluid swelling extending from the inguinal canal to the bottom of the scrotum, translucent, and not reducible.

Treatment.—If left alone the hydrocele frequently disappears spontaneously, or it may not return after tapping several times. It is very seldom necessary to perform a radical cure by dissection.

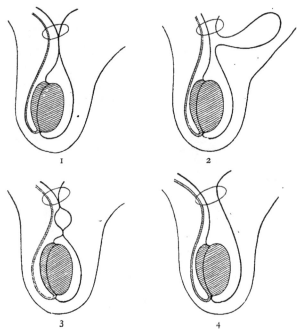

Fig. 570.—Diagrams of varieties of hydrocele.

1, Infantile; 2, bilocular; 3, encysted hydrocele of the cord; 4, congenital.

3. *Bilocular Hydrocele* (Fig. 570, 2)

The bilocular hydrocele shows two pouches—one running down into the scrotum and having the relationships of an infantile hernia, and the other extending up into the abdomen either behind or in front of the peritoneal cavity. The abdominal pouch may be very large and extend above the umbilicus and down into the pelvis. The condition is rare. Hæmorrhage may occur into the sac and form a bilocular hæmatocele.

Symptoms.—The diagnosis will be made by finding an infantile hydrocele which has a communication with a cyst lying above Poupart's ligament.

Treatment.—The hydrocele may be tapped, but it is better to remove it by dissection. The constriction between the two sacs usually occurs at the inguinal canal.

4. *Diffuse Hydrocele of the Cord*

This is a very rare condition, the cause of which is unknown. It is a collection of fluid, resembling blood serum in composition, in the meshes of the connective tissue of the spermatic cord.

Symptoms.—The patient exhibits a pyriform swelling, the base of which rests on the top of the testis, whilst the apex disappears into the external abdominal ring. The swelling is painless and disappears under slight continuous pressure, but reappears directly the pressure is removed. The condition is somewhat difficult to diagnose from an omental hernia.

Treatment.—The hydrocele may be tapped and the fluid withdrawn, but it soon returns. Radical cure consists of incision and drainage.

5. *Encysted Hydrocele of the Cord* (Fig. 570, 3)

Although cysts may arise in the spermatic cord from several causes, the above term is given to a cyst formed by fluid collecting in an unobliterated portion of the processus vaginalis which is closed above and below. These cysts are usually found in children, but may be discovered at any age.

Symptoms.—The condition presents itself as a small, rounded, freely movable, translucent cystic swelling, situated in the cord between the testis and the external abdominal ring. The cyst moves with the testis and cannot be completely reduced into the abdomen. In some cases the cysts are multiple and may communicate with the peritoneal cavity. Hæmorrhage may occur into such an encysted hydrocele, converting it into an encysted hæmatocele of the cord.

Treatment.—In young children the cyst may disappear spontaneously or after tapping, but if a radical cure is considered advisable the cyst should be dissected out.

6. *Congenital Hydrocele* (Fig. 570, 4)

A congenital hydrocele, which is not necessarily manifest at birth, is an effusion of fluid into an entirely unobliterated processus vaginalis. It may be present on one or both sides; if bilateral, causes for increase of fluid in the peritoneal cavity, such as tuberculous peritonitis and cirrhosis of the liver, should be sought, the hydrocele merely representing an overflow from this cavity.

Physical signs.—There is a translucent pyriform swelling in the scrotum, lying in front of the testis and running up into the abdomen. There is frequently an impulse when the patient coughs or cries. By steady pressure the fluid can be returned into the abdomen, but the sac soon refills when the patient stands upright. The diagnosis has to be made from congenital hernia, with which, however, it may be complicated.

Treatment.—As the condition always represents a potential hernia, it should be treated as a hernia. A truss must be worn constantly for two years, and the hydrocele must be tapped occasionally. As this treatment is irksome, a radical cure as for a congenital hernia is better and surer.

HÆMATOCELE OF THE TUNICA VAGINALIS

By this term is meant an extravasation of blood into the cavity of the tunica vaginalis. The condition is not common.

Etiology.—In the majority of cases a hæmatocele is preceded by a hydrocele, but this is by no means necessarily so, although French writers generally believe that previous inflammatory conditions of the tunica vaginalis are nearly always present before the onset of the hæmatocele.

1. **Spontaneous origin.**—In some cases of hæmatocele the condition appears to arise without any cause. The most careful questioning both before and after the diagnosis is established fails to elicit any history of injury, strain, or previous disease of the testis or its covering, and examination of the testis after removal gives no clue to the origin of the hæmatocele. It is possible in these cases that the blood-vessels are primarily at fault, but this has still to be proved.

2. **Injury.**—The great majority of cases of hæmatocele are due to a definite injury, perhaps the most frequent being in the tapping of a hydrocele. It follows in one of two ways: (a) During the tapping a vessel is injured in the tunica vaginalis, which rapidly fills with blood. A warning of this may be given at the time of tapping, by the escape of blood-stained fluid from the cannula. (b) A vessel may rupture after the tapping, owing to the sudden relief of pressure due to the removal of the hydrocele fluid. In these cases the swelling will rapidly return after tapping, but the physical signs will alter from those of hydrocele to those of hæmatocele. Hæmorrhage into a hydrocele may also be due to a blow, or to the strain of muscular effort or even coughing; and for the same reason a hæmatocele may occur in the tunica vaginalis without the previous formation of a hydrocele.

3. A hæmatocele may in rare instances be secondary to a malignant new growth either of the testis or of the tunica vaginalis.

This condition is rare, although small localized hydroceles are not uncommon with malignant tumours of the testis.

4. With acute torsion of the spermatic cord a small hæmatocele always forms in the cavity of the tunica vaginalis.

Symptoms.—Clinically, hæmatoceles may be divided into two classes : (1) acute cases, which usually have a very definite history of injury and in which diagnosis is generally easy ; and (2) chronic cases without a definite history, and in which diagnosis is always difficult and often impossible without exploratory incision.

Acute hæmatocele.—The onset of these cases is sudden, and follows a blow on the scrotum or a muscular strain, the patient usually being the subject of a hydrocele ; or it follows the tapping of a hydrocele.

The scrotum rapidly swells, and there is generally marked cechymosis of the scrotal skin. The swelling is painful and tender, semi-fluctuant and non-translucent. As a rule the position of the testis cannot be made out, but it is usually situated below and behind the swelling. Tapping causes escape of blood and diminution, but not disappearance, of the swelling. If left the ecchymosis of the scrotum disappears, the pain diminishes, and the swelling gets smaller, but in a few cases inflammation terminating in suppuration may occur, the physical signs changing to those of a scrotal abscess. Complete resolution of a hæmatocele is rare, some thickening of the tunica vaginalis and blood-clot remaining.

Chronic hæmatocele.—The onset in these cases is insidious, the patient giving no history of a cause. The swelling grows slowly, but usually there are irregular increases in size, followed by retrogression, suggesting small and repeated hæmorrhages. It may be months before the hæmatocele grows to a size that is inconvenient to the patient.

The swelling is firm, and feels solid, and is not tender or translucent. It is often irregular and nodular, and testicular sensation cannot be obtained. It is frequently impossible to ascertain the position of the testis or to differentiate between body and epididymis. The cord may be thickened, and the skin of the scrotum may not be freely movable over the swelling. If tapping is resorted to, no fluid may escape from the cannula, but usually there issues some dark-brown or black fluid containing degenerated blood-corpuscles and cholesterin. In these chronic cases as in the acute, inflammation and suppuration may occur and cause a scrotal abscess.

Pathological anatomy.—If a recent case be examined there may be no definite changes in the tunica vaginalis or in the testis, the only pathological condition found being blood, partly coagulated and partly fluid, in the cavity of the tunica vaginalis and in the scrotal tissues outside the tunica. In old-standing cases the tunica vaginalis is thickened sometimes to the extent of three-quarters of an inch, and is covered internally with a membrane formed by organization of a layer of the blood-clot. (Fig. 571.) The cavity is filled with dark-brown, or greyish clot and a dingy-brown fluid consisting of serum, blood pigment, degenerated corpuscles, and cholesterin. The tunica albuginea testis is

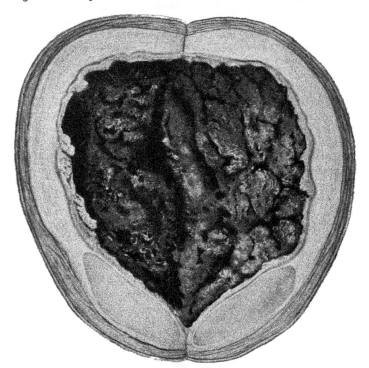

Fig. 571.—A large hæmatocele.

thickened, and there may be marked degeneration and fibrosis of the body of the testis and the epididymis, although a hæmatocele may exist for years without causing any considerable damage to the gland. The spermatic cord may be much thicker than normal.

Diagnosis.—The diagnosis in acute cases is usually very easy, but in old-standing cases, especially those without history, the diagnosis from syphilitic orchitis and new growth, and especially the latter, is very difficult or impossible. In many cases castration has been performed for hæmatocele under a mistaken diagnosis of malignant disease, or hæmatocele has been diagnosed instead of neoplasm and valuable time has been wasted.

The diagnosis can often be settled by watching the case and noting the steady increase in size of a malignant tumour; but time is wasted in this way, and it is much better to employ an exploratory incision.

The diagnosis from syphilitic orchitis is made by the history and by noting the effect of the administration of large doses of iodide of potassium and mercury, or by the employment of Wassermann's serum test (Vol. I., p. 32).

Treatment.—In acute cases with small hæmatoceles, or when the condition or wishes of the patient do not permit of more radical methods, the treatment consists of rest in bed, support of the scrotum, and tapping with a large-sized trocar. If the case is seen soon after the hæmatocele forms, an ice-bag or evaporating lead lotion may be applied to the scrotum.

When the hæmatocele is very large or old-standing, or has been preceded by a hydrocele, an operation is indicated, and this results in rapid and permanent cure of the condition. Three operations may be considered :—

1. **Incision and removal of the blood-clot,** with or without drainage. This may be done to recent large hæmatoceles not preceded by hydrocele or associated with well-marked changes in the testis.

2. **Excision of the tunica vaginalis** lining the scrotum, with removal of the clot. This operation is similar to that performed for the radical cure of a hydrocele, and is the one usually to be advised in hæmatocele; it generally results in permanent cure. In cases with a greatly thickened or calcareous tunica it may be difficult to perform, and great care must be taken to arrest all hæmorrhage.

3. **Castration.**—In many cases the subjects of hæmatocele are elderly men, and, as has been stated, the testis may be very atrophic. Before operating on old-standing hæmatoceles with very thick walls it is well to obtain permission to remove the testis, and to do this without hesitation if the operation prove long and tedious. It has the advantages of speedy recovery after the operation, and a certain freedom from recurrence.

If suppuration occur in a hæmatocele, the swelling should be freely opened and drained, or in old-standing cases orchidectomy should be performed and the scrotum drained.

HÆMATOCELE OF THE SPERMATIC CORD

Hæmatoceles of the spermatic cord are divided into encysted and diffuse varieties; both are rare.

3 *j*

Encysted Hæmatocele of the Spermatic Cord

Is produced by hæmorrhage occurring into an encysted hydrocele of the cord. It is exceedingly uncommon, and the diagnosis is only made on exploring a swelling of the spermatic cord. The treatmenr is removal.

Diffuse Hæmatocele of the Spermatic Cord

Is caused by rupture of one of the veins of the pampiniform plexus, with hæmorrhage into the cellular tissue of the cord. The cause of the rupture may be a blow on the cord, but more usually it is a result of violent muscular exertion, such as severe straining at stool.

Symptoms.—During muscular exertion a severe cutting pain is felt in the inguinal region, and this is followed by the appearance of a diffuse semi-solid swelling in the cord, extending from the inguinal canal to the top of the testis, which can usually be plainly differentiated below. Ecchymosis of the scrotum often follows.

Treatment.—A small hæmatocele may be left to be absorbed, but if it is large the swelling should be incised, the clot removed, and the bleeding-point secured.

VARICOCELE

A varicocele consists of a varicose enlargement of the veins of the pampiniform plexus and the spermatic cord. The disease rarely, if ever, affects the spermatic vein in the abdomen, nor are the veins accompanying the artery to the vas affected. The superficial veins of the penis and scrotum are frequently enlarged and tortuous. The condition is much more frequently seen on the left side than on the right, but both sides may be affected.

Varicocele is most frequently met with in adolescents, and is rarely seen in middle-aged or old men, although a varicocele present in youth may persist throughout life.

Etiology.—The cause is unknown, but the condition is probably a congenital abnormality of the spermatic veins exaggerated by the feeble flow of the blood through them on account of the long, narrow, tortuous course of the spermatic artery and the assumption by man of the upright posture. Dilatation of the veins of the pampiniform plexus may, however, be entirely due to back-pressure. This is seen in the varicocele that sometimes accompanies neoplasms of the left kidney, as the result of invasion of the renal vein and blocking of the left spermatic vein. A varicocele arising in an elderly subject should always lead to examination of the kidney.

The reason of the greater frequency of varicocele on the left side is unknown, in spite of many ingenious theories, the chief of which are —the entrance of the left spermatic vein into the left renal vein at a right angle ; the presence of the iliac colon on the left side pressing on the vein ; the greater contraction of the muscles on the left side of the abdomen owing to the more extensive use of the right arm.

Pathological anatomy.—The veins of the pampiniform plexus are lengthened, dilated, tortuous, and increased in number (Fig. 572). Their muscular coats become atrophied, and there is fibrosis of the adventitia, so that the walls are thickened and the veins stand open like arteries when cut across. Phleboliths may be present in them. The skin of the scrotum is lax, thin, and moist, and is deficient in the power of healthy contraction. The testes are very pendulous, and the patient may complain that the left testis is atrophic. It is extremely doubtful if varicocele ever leads to serious atrophy of the testis, and certainly in the great majority of cases there is no loss of sexual power even with a very large varicocele.

Symptoms.—The disease is most frequently discovered on medical examination prior to entering one of the public services, the patient being unaware that he has any pathological condition. In some cases there is a feeling of weight and discomfort, increased by standing, exercise, or hot weather, and in others there are attacks of pain which may be severe (neuralgia of the testis). The condition is readily recognized from the long, lax condition of the scrotum, the characteristic feel of the distended veins,

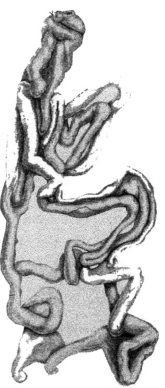

Fig. 572.—Dilated veins from a varicocele.

"like a bag of worms," and the dilated and tortuous veins of the scrotum. On recumbence it is less marked, but it is aggravated by standing, warmth, and exercise. To the patient the testis may feel more flabby than on the normal side, but, as stated above, atrophy is rare.

Treatment.—This may be either *palliative* or *operative*. The former consists in wearing a suspensory bandage, the best variety being

Keetley's. The patient should be assured that atrophy of the testes and loss of virility will not occur, and should be treated on general lines for neurasthenia, if present. Operation should be reserved for very large varicoceles which cause severe discomfort and pain or interfere with the patient's work or exercise, and is contra-indicated when neurasthenic symptoms are well marked. By far the most usual object of operating is to enable the patient to enter one of the public services. The wisdom of rejecting candidates because they have a varicocele is doubtful, as the condition is in itself seldom a source of trouble.

The operation consists in removing an inch or so of the anterior group of veins of the spermatic cord, the small posterior group running with the artery to the vas being carefully preserved. The veins should be exposed just where they are entering the external abdominal ring, and it is useless to attempt to separate the spermatic artery from the veins. This artery is nearly always included in the ligature, but if the artery to the vas and its veins are preserved, as well as the sympathetic plexus of nerves running with it, atrophy of the testis does not ensue. The operation is frequently followed by an epididymo-orchitis, but if suppuration does not occur the condition soon disappears. Pain from the inclusion of the ilio-inguinal nerve in a ligature may follow the operation, and neurasthenics may complain of pain, atrophy of the testis, and loss of virility.

ENDEMIC FUNICULITIS

Endemic funiculitis is an acute inflammation of the spermatic cord which occurs in certain tropical and subtropical countries.

The **cause** is unknown, but it is undoubtedly due to bacterial infection, and a diplococcus has been isolated from the affected tissue.

The **pathological anatomy** is that of an acute inflammation of the cellular tissue of the cord with a thrombosis of the veins of the pampiniform plexus. Suppuration is the common termination.

Symptoms.—The onset of the disease is sudden, with constipation, vomiting, and a raised temperature. These symptoms, with the physical sign of a painful swelling in the scrotum extending up to the abdominal rings, suggest strangulated hernia, but the signs of inflammation are more marked, while the general symptoms are not so severe. The skin over the swelling is red and œdematous, and there is no impulse on coughing. With suppuration, the swelling becomes soft and fluctuating, and there is sloughing of the testis.

Treatment.—The whole of the cord and the testis should be excised and the scrotum drained in severe cases, but in the milder forms free incision, drainage, and fomentation will suffice.

THE PENIS

CONGENITAL ABNORMALITIES

ABSENCE OF THE PENIS

Absence of the penis is very rare, and in reported cases the urethra has opened into the rectum. Apparent absence is more common, a small penis being hidden in the pad of fat over the symphysis pubis. In a case under my care the penis in a healthy child was represented by a small depression above

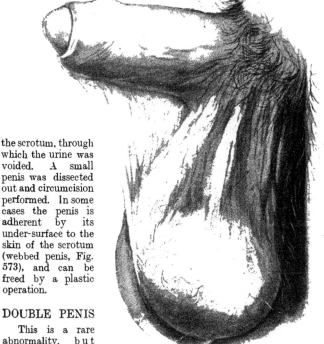

the scrotum, through which the urine was voided. A small penis was dissected out and circumcision performed. In some cases the penis is adherent by its under-surface to the skin of the scrotum (webbed penis, Fig. 573), and can be freed by a plastic operation.

DOUBLE PENIS

This is a rare abnormality, but authentic cases have been reported. Both penes may be functional and void urine and semen.

Fig. 573.—Webbed penis.

Epispadias and hypospadias are usually accompanied by deformity of the penis, which in hypospadias of the complete and peno-scrotal varieties is usually small, curved downwards, and fastened to the scrotum by bands of skin.

HYPOSPADIAS

Hypospadias is a congenital abnormality of the urethra and penis in which the external opening of the urethra is on the under surface of the corpus spongiosum. It is the result of arrested development of the penis occurring in early fœtal life, so that the differentiation from the female condition is not complete, and in cases of complete hypospadias the diagnosis of the sex may be difficult. Such a condition is termed pseudo- or external hermaphrodism.

Depending upon the situation of the urethral orifice and the amount of deformity of the penis, three varieties are distinguished —(1) hypospadias of the glans penis, (2) penile and peno-scrotal hypospadias, (3) perineo-scrotal hypospadias.

1. *Hypospadias glandis.*—This variety is due to the failure of the invagination of the surface epithelium forming the urethra in the glans to join the genito-urinary sinus which forms the urethra in the body of the penis. The opening, which may be double, is situated just at the attachment of the glans penis to the body of the organ. The penis is usually well formed, and the prepuce, which is generally redundant, forms a kind of hood over the glans. If the opening of the urethra is sufficiently large, the condition causes no difficulty in coitus or micturition.

2. *Hypospadias penis.*—The external opening of the urethra is in the body of the penis, and usually at the junction of the penis and scrotum (peno-scrotal variety). It is due to failure in development of the uro-genital sinus and the corpus spongiosum. The penile urethra is represented by a moist red furrow, and the corpus spongiosum by two dense fibrous bands lying on either side of the under surface of the penis, and representing the sides of the original cloaca. These two bands cause the penis to be curved downwards and incapable of normal erection. The glans penis and the corpora cavernosa are usually ill developed. The patient suffers from difficulty in micturition, and is unable to project the stream beyond the scrotum, which is therefore liable to become eczematous. Coitus is in most cases incomplete or impossible.

3. *Hypospadias perinealis.*—This form of hypospadias is rare, and is usually associated with cleft scrotum and undescended testes, making differentiation of the sex difficult or even impossible. The opening of the urethra is in the perineum (Fig. 574). The penis and glans are ill developed, the corpora cavernosa being very small, and the scrotum is bifid. Coitus is impossible, and the patient has to micturate in the squatting position. There is never incontinence of urine in any degree of hypospadias, as the opening is always below the constrictor urethræ. The diagnosis of the condition is obvious on examination.

Treatment.—Hypospadias glandis usually requires no treatment; but if the opening of the urethra is too small it should be enlarged. The condition is often compatible with full sexual vigour and efficiency. Hypospadias penis and hypospadias perinealis are unsatisfactory to treat, and in many cases it is probably best to leave the condition untreated. Many plastic operations have been devised, but the patient is rarely satisfied with the results of any of them. It is probably best to defer operation till puberty, or till the patient can take an intelligent interest in his cure and give all the help in his power to the after-treat-

ment. Several operations are necessary in severe cases, and not too much should be attempted at one time. The penis should first be freed from the two fibrous bands which cause its downward curve, and an attempt then made to form a urethra

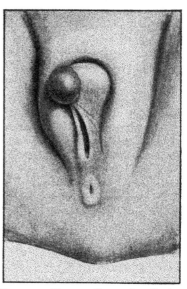

Fig. 574.—Hypospadias perinealis (external pseudo-hermaphrodism).

EPISPADIAS

Epispadias is a congenital abnormality of the urethra and penis in which the penis is cleft above and the urethra opens on the upper surface. Like hypospadias it may be divided into three degrees, according to the position of the opening—(1) The opening is just behind the glans; (2) the opening is on the body of the penis; (3) the cleft extends the whole length of the penis, and is frequently complicated by ectopia vesicæ. The third degree is by far the most common.

In the first two degrees the corpora cavernosa are present, and the penis is short but large, with a tendency to turn upwards; but in the third degree the penis is stunted and practically represented by the glans, while the corpora cavernosa are very defective.

Cleft scrotum, imperfectly descended testis, congenital hernia, non-union of the symphysis pubis, and ectopia vesicæ are frequently present in association with the third degree of epispadias.

It is difficult to explain this deformity, but the explanation which appears to be most in accordance with facts is that the condition is really one of hypospadias in which torsion of the penis has occurred at an early age of fœtal life so that the under surface becomes the upper.

Symptoms.—In the common form with complete cleft of the penis the chief trouble is the dribbling incontinence of urine which occurs owing to the division of the sphincter muscles. This leads to eczema of the surrounding parts and the usual miserable condition of patients suffering from urinary incontinence. Coitus is difficult or impossible.

Treatment.—The treatment of epispadias consists either in uniting the edges of the fissure of the urethra or in performing plastic operations. The same difficulties are present as in hypospadias, but after several attempts it may be possible to get a fairly satisfactory result. Incontinence of urine will continue in cases of complete epispadias, however satisfactory a penis may be formed.

HERMAPHRODISM

This subject may be conveniently discussed here, owing to its close association with malformations of the penis.

The only true criterion of sex is the structure of the genital gland, the male gland producing spermatozoa and the female ova. A true hermaphrodite, therefore, would be an individual who possessed both kinds of genital glands, an ovary and a testis on either side, or two of each kind. Such an individual has never been known to survive birth, even if the condition has occurred amongst prenatal monsters, which is doubtful. Cases of true hermaphrodism are reported from time to time, but the descriptions are always lacking in essential details, and the only true scientific proof would be obtained from microscopic sections of the genital glands. True hermaphrodism therefore probably does not exist in human subjects.

PSEUDO-HERMAPHRODISM

In early fœtal life there is no distinction between the sexes either in the internal or in the external sexual organs, and rudiments of the sexual apparatus of the opposite sex persist in all individuals throughout life. In the external organs the male genitals are merely a further development of the female. The penis is a large clitoris enclosing the urethra, the scrotum the coalescence of the labia majora, while the descent of the testes is frequently simulated by the descent of the ovaries into the sacs of inguinal herniæ. The female breast is represented by the rudimentary, functionless male breast. In the internal organs of generation, the male retains in the uterus masculinus the representation of the uterus, Fallopian tubes, and vagina of the female, both being developed from Müller's duct ; whilst in the female the duct of Gartner represents the vas deferens, both having their origin in the Wolffian duct.

It is not, therefore, surprising that individuals are met with in whom the rudiments of the sexual apparatus of the opposite sex become more developed than normal, and a condition results in which it is not easy to determine the sex of the patient without microscopical examination of the genital gland. Such an individual is termed a pseudo-hermaphrodite, and two varieties, external and internal, are differentiated, according as the internal or the external genital glands are chiefly or wholly affected.

Careful examination in recent years of these pseudo-hermaphrodites has shown that about 95 per cent. of them possess testes, and are therefore males. It might be expected that at puberty the sexual instincts of the pseudo-hermaphrodite would indicate the sex, but this is not always so, and instances are known of individuals with congenital abnormality of the external sexual apparatus living happily as married women although microscopical examination of the genital gland has revealed the presence of spermatozoa.

Internal Pseudo-Hermaphrodism

In these cases the external organs of generation are normal and well developed, the secondary sexual characters—breast, distribution of pubic hair, and voice—are of the normal type, but the individual possesses a large uterus and Fallopian tubes. The condition is only discovered during operation or post-mortem examination. The reason for operation is frequently the presence of an inguinal hernia, in the sac of which the uterus is found, having been dragged there by the descent of the testis, which in these cases is attached to the uterus. In such individuals imperfect descent of the testes is common.

Treatment.—It is only when the uterus is found in the sac of an inguinal hernia that treatment is required ; then the uterus should be removed, and the canal closed as in the usual radical cure.

External Pseudo-Hermaphrodism

In the course of development of the external genitalia the male passes through a stage which closely resembles the female. The testes are not yet descended, the folds of the scrotum have not formed, and the penis is represented by the small genital eminence. Arrest of development at this stage will give rise to an individual with external genitalia resembling those of the female, although the genital glands are testes. The opposite condition, in which in an individual with ovaries the development continues till the male external organs are formed, is unknown, although cases of hypertrophy of the clitoris are recognized. The testes not infrequently descend later, and are sometimes removed during an operation for supposed hernia, and the sex of the patient becomes recognized on microscopical examination of the genital gland.

Patients with external pseudo-hermaphrodism therefore resemble females, and are often named and educated as girls; but, in view of the fact that 95 per cent. of all pseudo-hermaphrodites are males, the patients should always be educated and treated as boys.

External pseudo-hermaphrodism is sometimes complicated with ectopia vesicæ.

The condition of the secondary sexual characters in these patients and their sexual instincts vary. In some cases the secondary characteristics are undoubtedly masculine, and no doubt of the sex exists after puberty; but in others the secondary characters which in the human race are almost confined to the male do not develop, and the sexual instincts may be so perverted that the patient, although a male with testes, may live happily as a married woman. Determination of the sex may be impossible in some cases without microscopical examination of the genital gland.

The psychology of these patients is important from the medico-legal standpoint, and the condition may account for some cases of sexual coldness or perverted sexual instincts met with in apparent females who are really males.

Fortunately, pseudo-hermaphrodites are usually sterile, either from obvious reasons or because the undescended testes are malformed and non-functional.

PHIMOSIS

In phimosis the prepuce cannot be retracted freely over the glans owing to its length, to smallness of its opening, or to adhesions. These conditions are frequently combined, and the phimosis may be either congenital or acquired.

Congenital Phimosis

In the newly-born infant the prepuce is normally slightly adherent to the glans penis, but these adhesions disappear as the child gets older, so that inability completely to retract the prepuce in the newly born should not be called phimosis and does not necessarily call for circumcision. Apart from complications, circumcision is necessary—(a) if the preputial orifice is so small that the end of the glans and the orifice of the urethra cannot be easily uncovered; (b) if the prepuce is long and projects well beyond the glans (this may be associated with a narrow preputial orifice or not); (c) if the prepuce is closely adherent to the whole of the glans penis; (d) if, although the prepuce can be retracted behind the corona, there is difficulty in getting it back—in other words, if there is a tendency to paraphimosis.

Symptoms.—Children with phimosis are brought to the surgeon for two reasons—because the parents think that circumcision is required, or because some complication has arisen.

Complications.—The complications of phimosis are—

(*a*) Difficulty and pain on passing urine.

(*b*) Retention of urine, with its sequelæ on the bladder, ureters, and kidneys.

(*c*) Incontinence of urine.

(*d*) Retention of secretion or formation of calculi under the prepuce.

(*e*) Inflammatory conditions. Balano-posthitis.

(*f*) Hernia or prolapsus ani, due to straining.

(*g*) Sexual excitement. Masturbation and its effects.

(*h*) Difficulties in coitus.

(*i*) Paraphimosis.

(*j*) Malignant disease.

An important associated condition which should always be looked for, and, if found, treated when circumcision is performed, is a small (pin-hole) urinary meatus. If this condition is overlooked, difficulty of micturition may continue after the operation.

Treatment.—Cases in which the prepuce in a child cannot be freely retracted owing to *slight* adhesions between the prepuce and the glans should be treated by separating the adhesions with a probe, retracting the prepuce, and smearing the glans with vaseline. Retraction should then be practised daily till the prepuce retracts easily and without pain. These cases are the exception ; all other cases of congenital phimosis should be treated by circumcision unless surgical interference is contra-indicated by some disease, e.g. hæmophilia.

In doing the operation care must be taken to remove a sufficiency of both layers of the prepuce, otherwise the condition will not be remedied ; but at the same time too much should not be removed. When the wound has healed, the corona glandis should be covered. The operation in adults can be readily performed under local anæsthesia.

ACQUIRED PHIMOSIS

Acquired phimosis may be transitory or permanent, and the former may pass into the latter.

Transitory acquired phimosis is due to inflammatory conditions of the prepuce or glans, such as soft sores, hard chancres, balano-posthitis of gonorrhœa, septic sores, etc. In these conditions the inflammatory œdema of the prepuce prevents retraction. The treatment is cleanliness and relief of the primary affection. The patient should sit in hot baths, syringe with hot weak antiseptic lotion under the prepuce, and endeavour to retract it so that it may be thoroughly cleaned. If it is found impossible to secure freedom from foul secretion, the prepuce should without delay be freely slit up dorsally as far as the corona in order to avoid sloughing and to establish an exact diagnosis.

Permanent acquired phimosis is the result of inflammatory lesions ending in the formation of scar tissue, such as the healing of ulcers and chancres, or fibrosis supervening on a chronic balano-posthitis. The condition is of special importance in elderly men, as it may pre-dispose to carcinoma, and it will be more fully dealt with in considering malignant diseases of the penis.

PARAPHIMOSIS

This term indicates inability to draw the prepuce forward again after it has been retracted behind the glans penis. It is always associated with phimosis, which may be congenital or the result of an inflammatory condition of the prepuce or glans penis.

Acute paraphimosis is frequently seen in boys and young men who have retracted a tight prepuce from curiosity or when mas-turbating, but is also common after coitus or as a complication of chancre or gonorrhœa. The condition is usually recognized at a glance. The glans penis is swollen and congested, and behind the corona is a red œdematous roll of tissue, most marked underneath, which represents the returning layer of the prepuce. Behind this is a deep sulcus which corresponds to the narrow preputial orifice, and behind this again is a second œdematous collar of skin corresponding to the outer layer of the prepuce. The whole penis is swollen and congested, and frequently twisted. If the condition is not treated, ulceration of the constricting band formed by the preputial orifice takes place, and the congestion is relieved, but the paraphimosis may become permanent. Very rarely sloughing of the glans penis may occur.

Treatment.—Treatment consists in immediate reduction. In order to reduce the swelling the penis is bandaged firmly from the glans backwards with a cold-water bandage. The bandage is left in position for a few minutes and then removed. The penis is then grasped between the index and middle fingers of both hands while the thumbs rest on the glans. A combination of steady pulling forwards with the fingers and pushing backwards with the thumbs will usually effect reduction. When the œdema has disappeared circumcision should be advised. If reduction is not accomplished in this way, the con-stricting band should be cut across without delay; reduction is then easy.

Chronic paraphimosis is an occasional sequel to acute para-phimosis with moderate constriction, or the condition may be chronic from the first and due to inflammation. It is rare.

Treatment.—Inflammatory conditions should be treated on general principles, but if the condition is permanent from organization of the exudate, as in a case under my care, a plastic operation may be considered advisable.

CALCULI UNDER THE PREPUCE

Preputial calculi are rare, and are only found in association with marked degrees of phimosis. They may be single or multiple, and have been known to reach the size of a man's fist. They arise in three ways: (*a*) deposits of lime salts in retained smegma; (*b*) deposits of urinary salts, chiefly phosphates from decomposing urine retained under a long prepuce; (*c*) bladder-stones which have passed along the urethra and are there retained by the phimosed prepuce. The condition gives rise to a purulent discharge from the prepuce, and the diagnosis is readily made by examination.

Treatment consists in slitting up the prepuce, removing the calculi, and then circumcising the patient.

SHORTNESS AND RUPTURE OF THE FRÆNUM

This is usually of little importance, but the frænum may be so short that the glans penis curves downwards during erection, and so renders coitus painful. Of more importance is rupture of the frænum, a not infrequent accident during coitus, which may lead to severe hæmorrhage, and the small wound is liable to venereal infection.

Treatment.—If the frænum is so short as to interfere with coitus, it should be divided and the artery secured.

INJURIES TO THE PENIS

Contusion of the penis is an uncommon accident, and usually occurs during erection. It may be due either to violent attempts at coitus, or to acts of resistance or revenge on the part of the woman. In some cases the sheaths of the corpora cavernosa are ruptured, causing so-called *fracture of the penis.* In the graver injuries there is severe pain, followed by great swelling of the organ due to extravasated blood, and the urethra is usually injured at the same time. Retention of urine is a common consequence.

Treatment.—In the slighter injuries the treatment consists in wrapping the penis in evaporating lead lotion and waiting for the absorption of the extravasated blood. If the penis is fractured, with laceration of the urethra, the treatment is operative. The wounded part should be freely laid open, the lacerated urethra sutured, all blood clots removed, and the sheaths of the corpora cavernosa sutured.

In some cases contusion of the penis is followed by alteration in the normal erection of the penis. The part in front of the fracture remains flaccid, whilst the posterior end is rigid. This condition is due to the fibrosis that has occurred in the corpora cavernosa in the healing of the lesion. This serious result is best prevented by careful suturing at the time of the accident.

DISLOCATION OF THE PENIS

In this rare accident the prepuce is torn away from its attachment to the glans penis, and the penis itself with the glans is dislocated into the subcutaneous tissue of the groin, abdomen, or scrotum. The skin of the penis hangs down empty in its usual position.

Treatment.—The wound must be freely opened up so as to arrest all hæmorrhage, and the penis brought back into position and sutured. Laceration of the urethra should always be examined for and appropriately treated.

CONSTRICTING BODIES

Constriction of the penis by thread, string, rings, and other foreign bodies is not infrequent. The constricting band is either placed round the penis to satisfy morbid sexual impulses, or in children and young adults to prevent nocturnal enuresis or emissions. In a few cases it is a form of practical joke of the patient's companions.

The penis in front of the constricting band becomes swollen, congested, and œdematous, so that the band cannot be removed, and in a few cases gangrene results. The swelling may be so severe that the constricting band is completely hidden, and the diagnosis can only be made by the history and the swelling.

Treatment.—In most cases an anæsthetic is necessary, and the band is then removed as ingenuity suggests. The use of a director and a Gigli saw is sometimes necessary for the division of metal rings.

NEW GROWTHS OF THE PENIS

INNOCENT GROWTHS

Angiomas (nævi) of the penis have been described, but are rare, the only common innocent growths of the penis being papillomas.

PAPILLOMA

Warts of the penis may be divided into hard and soft varieties.

Hard papillomas are usually single, and are less common than the soft variety. They resemble warts in other parts of the body, and if left untreated or irritated may become carcinomatous. In some cases a horny growth develops in them, and horns of several inches in length have been described. In elderly men, hard warty growths should be looked upon with suspicion as the commonest starting-point of carcinoma of the penis. The growth should be carefully microscoped after complete removal.

Soft papillomas are frequently associated with venereal disease or retained secretion from phimosis, but may occur independently of either of these two causes. They are usually found in the sulcus behind the corona, or on the glans, are multiple, bleed readily, and have a foul secretion. They may be either pedunculated or sessile, and there is frequently associated enlargement of the inguinal glands.

Treatment.—Papillomas both of the hard and of the soft variety should be removed with scissors and their bases cauterized. Absolute cleanliness and the careful treatment of any accompanying venereal disease are necessary to prevent their recurrence.

HORNS

On the penis may arise in connexion with suppurating sebaceous cysts or papillomas. They are rare, but the diagnosis is obvious. Ulceration progressing to carcinoma may occur at the base of a horn. The treatment is complete removal.

MALIGNANT GROWTHS

CARCINOMA

This, the common form of malignant growth affecting the penis, may occur in one of two varieties. The more common is a squamous-celled carcinoma arising from the superficial epithelium, the other variety being a glandular carcinoma springing from the few glands that are found near the corona, the glands of Tyson. The latter variety is said to be more malignant than the former.

Etiology.—The disease is rare before the age of 40, most cases being seen in men of 50 to 70, and usually nearer the latter age. It is predisposed to by phimosis, congenital or acquired, want of cleanliness, venereal sores, papillomas and gummata of the penis. There is also a precancerous condition similar to that met with in the tongue, and called eczema of the glans, Paget's disease of the penis, and leucoplakia, but which is really a chronic superficial inflammation of the glans penis and under-surface of the prepuce. This disease occurs in elderly men, and leads to acquired phimosis, with a tendency to hæmorrhage if the prepuce is forcibly retracted. The condition is recognized by white patches (leucoplakia), which are found on the under-surface of the prepuce and on the glans penis, resembling the white patches of the tongue in chronic superficial glossitis. Raw red patches with a tendency to bleed may also be present. Carcinoma usually develops if the condition is neglected.

Pathological anatomy and clinical features.—Carcinoma of the penis usually starts as a warty growth on or just behind the glans penis. (Figs. 575, 576.) The growth has the usual indurated base and spreads rapidly over the glans, but ulceration does not occur early. The growth is at first limited to the surface of the penis by the fibrous capsules of the corpora cavernosa and the corpus spongiosum, but when it invades these it grows with great rapidity, destroying their structure and often enlarging the penis to three or four times its usual size. The urethra is not involved as a rule, and there is no obstruction to the passage of urine, but ulceration may occur behind the growth and a urinary fistula develop. (Fig. 577.) When ulceration occurs the growth presents the usual characters of a carcinomatous ulcer, with a hard indurated base and a foul secretion. (Fig. 578.) The glands first to be infected are the inguinal glands, usually on both sides, but with involvement of the body of the penis the lumbar glands may show secondary growths. Metastases in other organs are rare. Pain, and even inconvenience, are absent in the early stages, accounting for the advanced condition in which the surgeon usually first sees the disease.

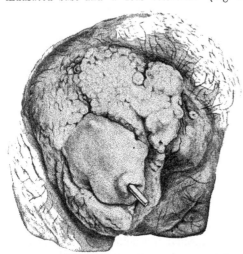

Fig. 575.—Glans penis with carcinoma of the warty type.

In the early **diagnosis** it is important to remember that a carcinoma may be growing unseen behind a tight prepuce; and in every case in an elderly man, where a discharge is present or an induration can be felt under a phimosed prepuce, circumcision should be strongly urged with a view to ascertaining the exact condition of the glans.

The condition which most closely resembles carcinoma of the penis is syphilitic ulceration, which not infrequently occurs in the old scar of a primary chancre, and in some cases the

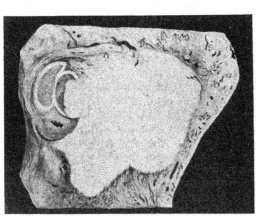

Fig. 576.—Section through the same penis as in Fig. 575.

diagnosis is only established by the effects of treatment or by micro-scopical examination of a small portion of the diseased tissue.

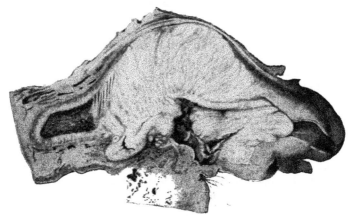

Fig. 577.—Longitudinal section of a penis with advanced carcinoma, showing the formation of a fistula.

Treatment.—The only treatment for carcinoma of the penis is early removal of the growth with a wide margin of healthy tissue, and

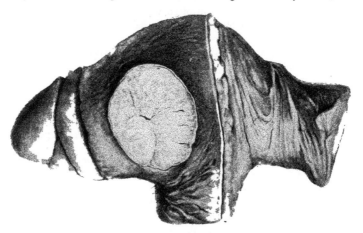

Fig. 578.—Lateral view of a penis with a carcinoma fungating through the skin.

removal of both sets of inguinal glands on the two sides of the body. If the disease is limited to the glans, and the penis is sufficiently long

3 k

partial amputation with removal of the inguinal glands is all that is necessary; but with more extensive disease, and in any case of doubt as to getting clear of the disease, the whole penis should be removed, the crura being detached from the arch of the pubes. The urethra is then brought out into the perineum and fixed just in front of the anus. It is advisable, if this operation is done, to remove the testes at the same time, as this makes micturition more comfortable and prevents excoriation and eczema of the scrotum. Removal of the testes, however, adds to the gravity of the operation, which has frequently to be done in very elderly people debilitated by septic absorption and a fetid discharge. The most difficult part of the operative treatment is the thorough removal of all the inguinal glands, and not infrequently part of the femoral vein must be excised to make the operation complete.

Prognosis.—If the case is seen early and a thorough operation is done, the prognosis is fair, as metastases in distant organs are unusual; but the cases are rarely seen very early, as the condition causes so little pain and discomfort.

SARCOMA

This condition, which may be either primary or secondary, is rare. In the primary cases the growth, which is most often a spindle-celled sarcoma, usually springs from the fibrous sheaths of the corpora cavernosa, and is confined to them for a long time. The penis becomes hard and swollen, and often very painful, whilst interference with micturition or a blood-stained discharge from the urethra may occur.

The only treatment is early amputation, with removal of the glands in both groins.

OTHER CONDITIONS OF THE PENIS
HERPES

Both catarrhal herpes and herpes zoster may attack the penis, the former being by far the more common disease.

Herpes zoster may follow the course of the ilio-inguinal nerve, and does not differ in its course and symptomatology from herpes zoster in other parts of the body. It is extremely rare in the penis. Catarrhal herpes is chiefly seen in the prepuce and glans penis (herpes progenitalis), and the exact cause is unknown. It has been attributed to syphilis, other venereal infections, sexual excess, gout, and other causes, but without much evidence. The disease usually appears shortly after coitus or nocturnal emissions.

Symptoms.—The patient first complains of an itching or burning sensation on the prepuce or glans penis, and a patch of erythema appears at the spot. On this patch of erythema appear a group of small vesicles which soon burst, leaving small ulcers that rapidly heal. The affection usually runs its entire course in a week. In most cases the pain is trifling, but it may be severe (neuralgic herpes).

Prognosis.—The condition rapidly gets well, but recurrence is common, and the excoriated surface may be infected by the *Spirochæte pallida* or other organism if the patient is exposed to infection.

Treatment.—Local cleanliness is all that is needed, but no measures can be absolutely relied upon to prevent recurrence. Arsenic has been strongly recommended. Even if the disease is limited to the prepuce, circumcision may fail to cure, as the disease may reappear on the glans penis.

PRIAPISM

When this condition is pathological there is continued erection of the penis, often accompanied by severe pain, without sexual desire. The condition is rare, and usually only affects the corpora cavernosa, the corpus spongiosum being, as a rule, unaffected. The causes are said to be excessive coitus, injury, alcoholism, leukæmia, gout, and irritation from worms or a tight prepuce. In fracture of the lower cervical or upper dorsal portion of the spine, with injury to the cord, the penis is often turgid but without rigidity.

Symptoms.—The penis is turgid and erect, tender and very painful. Micturition may be interfered with, but this is not usual. The duration of the priapism varies, but it may last for weeks.

Treatment is unsatisfactory, but the drug that has been used with most success is bromide of potassium, whilst morphia may be necessary on account of the pain. Incision of the penis has been tried in some cases with success, and under proper precautions should be given an early trial if bromides fail.

THE SCROTUM

ACUTE SEPTIC INFECTION (CELLULITIS)

Acute septic infection of the scrotal tissues does not differ in cause or course from a similar infection of the skin or subcutaneous tissue in other parts of the body. Locally it is characterized by excessive swelling of the scrotum, and its tendency is to end in gangrene, especially of the anterior part of the scrotum, so that the testes are exposed. The general symptoms are those of acute sepsis.

Treatment.—At first the scrotum should be supported and warmth applied by means of fomentations. If the swelling does not quickly subside, free long incisions on each side of the median raphe should be made, going through the dartos. These incisions should be allowed to gape widely and bleed freely. Afterwards the patient should sit in a hot bath for several hours a day, and in the intervals fomentations should be applied. If sloughing occur, the treatment should be continued, and it will always be found that the testicles are covered without the need of skin grafts.

MALIGNANT GROWTHS

Two forms of malignant growth are met with in the scrotum, squamous-celled carcinoma (epithelioma) and melanotic sarcoma, the former being by far the more common.

SQUAMOUS-CELLED CARCINOMA—

"Chimney-sweep's cancer"—has the same structure and clinical course as similar growths on other parts of the skin. It occurs most frequently in men engaged in occupations in which it is difficult to keep the skin clean, such as chimney-sweeps, tar, gas, and paraffin workers. Not infrequently the disease shows two distinct stages. At first there is a soft warty growth of innocent nature, which may grow for a time and then easily be knocked off, leaving a pigmented eczematous patch (tar-worker's molluscum and tar-worker's eczema). The disease may remain for a long time at this stage, but sooner or later ulceration takes place, and the well-known characters of a squamous-celled carcinomatous ulcer appear. The disease may also start as a papillomatous growth, or as a small subcuticular nodule, as in other parts of the skin.

The inguinal glands become enlarged at first by inflammation, but later they are invaded by the malignant growth, and become hard, matted, and fixed. The disease is limited for a long time to the scrotum and inguinal glands, and metastases in other organs are uncommon. The neoplasm is, as a rule, of very slow growth, and the patient may have given up the dangerous occupation for some years before it appears, but microscopic examination of the skin of the scrotum of a sweep will usually reveal soot in the cells which no amount of washing will remove.

Treatment.—Prophylactic treatment consists of the exercise of great cleanliness by people engaged in the dangerous trades, and the thorough removal of all papillomatous growths as soon as they appear. If squamous-celled carcinoma is diagnosed, the growth should be excised with a large area of the surrounding skin, and at the same time the superficial inguinal glands should be removed from both groins. If the growth has become adherent to one of the testes, the gland should be removed without hesitation.

MELANOTIC SARCOMA

Although the scrotum is, as a rule, deeply pigmented, melanotic sarcoma is not common. If it occur it has the same characters and clinical course as these neoplasms elsewhere, and demands the same treatment. The inguinal glands should always be removed.

INNOCENT GROWTHS

All varieties of innocent new growths are uncommon in the scrotum, and they differ in no respect from similar growths in other parts of the body. The least uncommon are angioma, fibroma, lipoma, and fibro-cellular tumours. Lipoma may attain a huge size, the growth in one reported case weighing 11 lb.

SEBACEOUS CYSTS

∴ Sebaceous cysts of any size are not common in the scrotum. They have the usual features of sebaceous cysts elsewhere, and if necessary should be removed.

LYMPH SCROTUM—ELEPHANTIASIS OF THE SCROTUM

Although thickening of the skin and subcutaneous tissues of the scrotum from lymphatic obstruction may occur from several causes, such as syphilitic ulceration in the groin, sloughing of the inguinal glands, or their complete removal for malignant disease, lymph scrotum and elephantiasis are essentially a manifestation of filariasis, a tropical disease due to invasion of the body by the nematode *Filaria Bancrofti*. Lymph scrotum is the forerunner of elephantiasis, and it is hardly necessary to separate the two conditions. The subject has been sufficiently considered elsewhere (Vol. I., p. 911).

IMPOTENCE

Impotence is a condition in which the ability to have normal sexual intercourse is lost, or very much lessened. This condition must be carefully distinguished from sterility, in which there is a defect in the semen rendering it incapable of fertilizing the ovum. A patient who is impotent is usually sterile, but not necessarily so, for the semen may be ejaculated and be artificially conveyed to the vagina. For example, in cases in which the semen is ejaculated with only partial erection of the penis the patient may be impotent, but should the semen gain entrance to the vagina conception may follow. Impotence may be considered under the following heads :—

1. Impotence due to physical defects in the genital organs.
2. Impotence due to abnormal psychical conditions.
3. Nervous impotence.
4. Paralytic impotence.

1. **Physical defects.**—Under this heading are grouped cases of impotence due to congenital abnormalities such as hypospadias, epispadias, rudimentary penis, to mutilation, elephantiasis of the penis, large hernias and hydroceles, and to induration of the penis and loss of power of erection following fracture of the penis, gonorrhœal and gouty inflammation of the cavernous tissue, periurethral abscesses, etc. Hypospadias and epispadias only cause impotence if present in an advanced degree, many patients with these defects having the power

to copulate, although the semen does not reach the vagina. Impotence due to large hernias, hydroceles, and elephantiasis can usually be cured by suitable operations. In cases of obliteration of part of the cavernous tissue of the penis due to previous inflammation or to trauma, the prognosis is not good, but treatment by iodides, fibrolysin, or local application of mercurials may be beneficial. Excision of the induration is sometimes successful.

2. **Psychical impotence.**—Impotence of this variety may be relative or absolute, and is most commonly found in men who have overtaxed their sexual power either by excessive masturbation or by sexual intercourse. The condition is full of interesting and curious anomalies. The patient, for instance, may be fully capable and active in his intercourse with prostitutes, but cannot have intercourse with his wife. In other cases, something—often of a bizarre nature—is necessary as an extra stimulus before erection or ejaculation can occur. The condition may be congenital, the natural impulse to sexual intercourse being altogether wanting, but it is usually acquired, and, with the exception of excessive venery, mental overwork seems to be the most common cause.

The fear of failure in intercourse may be the cause of psychical impotence, the patient, who may have been a masturbator or may have indulged freely in venery, being persuaded that he has lost, or fearing he may have lost, the power of copulation. This condition not seldom arises when marriage is contemplated, and the fear may be sufficient to inhibit the sexual act. Allied to psychical impotence, and sometimes associated with it, is perverse sexual feeling. The usual stimulus to sexual excitement fails in these patients, but their sexual nature is excited by circumstances that have no such effect on the normal man. In these cases sexual intercourse may fail because of the absence of the abnormal exciting circumstance, although the sexual feelings may be strong. These cases gradually merge with those in which sexual impulses towards persons of the same sex or towards animals are present.

Sexual passion for one's own sex, or pæderasty, may be congenital or acquired. The acquired form is usually seen in elderly people who have indulged in sexual excesses and whose senses have been dulled to normal stimuli. Or again, in large communities of men, such as in monasteries, and in training-ships and boarding-schools, the absence of individuals of the opposite sex, combined with the natural sexual cravings, may lead to acts of perverted sexual intercourse, and these, frequently indulged in, may deprive the patient of the power of intercourse with members of the opposite sex, owing to the absence of the customary stimuli.

The **treatment** of psychical impotence consists in moral control, abstinence for a time from attempts at sexual intercourse, physical exercise, mental occupation, and common sense.

3. **Nervous impotence.**—This condition is one of irritable weakness of the sexual centres in the cord or brain, resulting in imperfect erection of the penis, with premature ejaculation. The patients are usually neurasthenics who may not have indulged in sexual intercourse, but in other cases they have been habitual masturbators. The penis becomes erect or partially erect under the normal stimuli, but the erection passes off before intercourse can be indulged in, or the semen is ejaculated at the moment of intromission into the vagina, or even before. These patients often fear marriage because they feel they are not capable of sexual intercourse, and psychical impotence may be added to the nervous impotence.

The treatment of nervous impotence is similar to that of psychical impotence.

4. **Paralytic impotence.**—This form of impotence differs from the three previous forms in that in them erection of the penis occurs with the ejaculation of semen, but the erection is not properly used, while in this variety of impotence erection does not occur. It may be due to excessive indulgence, especially in the form of masturbation, but is more commonly due to organic disease. It may occur in certain chronic diseases such as diabetes, anæmia, phthisis, morphinism, in certain diseases of the brain and cord such as tabes dorsalis, general paralysis of the insane, or injury or disease of various cerebral centres. The condition may also follow atrophy of the testis from disease or loss by injury or operation, but not necessarily.

Certain drugs such as alcohol, iodine, salicylic acid, and potassium nitrate can also cause diminution of the sexual powers, but the loss is usually recovered directly the use of the drug is stopped.

Treatment in many cases of paralytic impotence is useless, and in others, such as those due to the use of drugs, is obvious. In all cases of impotence, self-control, with a clean, healthy mode of life and thought, is of the utmost importance.

BIBLIOGRAPHY

Casper, *Urinary Surgery.* 1911.
Cooper, Astley, *Diseases of the Testis.* 1830.
Curling, *Diseases of the Testis,* 4th ed. 1878.
Eccles, W. McAdam, *Imperfectly Descended Testis.* 1903
Fenwick, E. H., *Clinical Cystoscopy.* 1904.
Fuller, *Diseases of the Genito-Urinary System.* 1900.
Hutchinson, Sir Jonathan, *Syphilis.* 1909.
Jacobson, W. H. A., *Diseases of the Male Organs of Generation.* 1893.
Mansell-Moullin, C. W., *Enlargement of the Prostate.* 1894.
Manson, Sir Patrick, *Tropical Diseases.* 1907.
Monod et Terillon, *Traité des Maladies du Testicule.* 1889.

THE FEMALE GENITAL TRACT.

BY VICTOR BONNEY, M.S., M.D., B.Sc.LOND., F.R.C.S.ENG.

History.—Note should be taken of the patient's age, her symptoms and their duration, the dates of any pregnancies, the frequency and duration of the menses and *the date of the last one.*

If pain be present, its position and its relation to posture and to the menstrual period should be ascertained.

Examination in the consulting-room is best conducted with the patient lying half on her side and half on her back, but with the shoulders more horizontal than the hips, so that the trunk is somewhat twisted at the waist. This position allows the examiner to apply his weight through his left hand on the patient's abdomen, and materially facilitates bimanual examination. Vaginal examination should be made with one finger, as two may cause pain, and is assisted by turning the patient during its performance, first into the semi-prone and then into the semi-supine position. By this manœuvre the quadrants of the pelvis are successively rendered more accessible.

In bimanual examination, palpation must be chiefly conducted by the hand on the abdomen, the finger in the vagina being held stationary on the cervix or vaginal vault. " Gravity " displacements like prolapse or retroversion should be investigated with the patient standing erect.

Rectal examination is often useful, especially in virgins. The two must be careful not to mistake the projection of the vaginal cervix for a tumour in front of the rectum.

The speculum.—An expert can distinguish almost all diseases of the vagina and vaginal cervix by touch alone, and therefore can frequently spare his patient the discomfort of examination by speculum. Fergusson's speculum is easy to introduce, but shuts up the lips of a lacerated cervix, and fails to demonstrate the condition of the cervical canal. Sims's speculum in a narrow vagina may fail to show the cervix well. The hinged bivalve speculum is better for consulting-room use.

The uterine sound.—This instrument is much less employed than formerly. The direction of the uterus can be estimated by

bimanual examination, while the measurement of the length of the
cavity is of doubtful utility, for great enlargement is obvious by other
means, and small alterations in length (an inch or less), as revealed
by the sound passed without anæsthesia, are often due to the point of
the instrument deviating into a cornu.

The habitual use of the sound in the consulting-room will result
sooner or later in its passage into a pregnant uterus by mistake. Cases
undiagnosable by bimanual examination should be examined under
an anæsthetic and the sound passed then.

Examination under anæsthesia is advisable when serious
symptoms are present and diagnosis by ordinary examination is
obscure. The lithotomy position is the right one for this purpose.

THE VULVA

DEFORMITIES AND DISPLACEMENTS

PSEUDO-HERMAPHRODISM

Malformations of the vulva are rare. The commonest is that seen in a
pseudo-hermaphrodite hypospadiac male. This subject is discussed in the
preceding article (p. 970.)

PROLAPSE OF THE URETHRA

Prolapse of the urethral mucosa occurs in elderly women. The
protrusion is purple-red in colour, with a central aperture, and may
be much inflamed or ulcerated. The patient complains of a very
tender swelling and of difficulty and pain in micturition. The
central orifice in the swelling differentiates it from new growths in
this situation. The redundant mucosa should be amputated ciren-
larly and the cut edge of the urethra united to the surface by fine
silk sutures. Care must be taken not to remove the mucous membrane
of the vestibule, but to limit the excision to that belonging to the
canal, otherwise stenosis may occur.

URETHROCELE

A urethrocele is a protrusion consisting of the lower inch of the
anterior vaginal wall, and containing a pouched portion of the urethra.
The condition is met with in multipara in whom the perineum is
deficient. The patient is conscious of a lump which protrudes on
standing or straining. After the expulsive act of micturition, dribbling
occurs as the distended pouch empties itself.

Treatment consists in excision of the redundant portion of th
vaginal wall, together with the prolonged portion of the urethra,
followed by closure of the openings in the walls of the canals by separate
rows of sutures. Perineoplasty is then performed to prevent recurrence.

INFLAMMATION

STREPTOCOCCAL AND PNEUMOCOCCAL VULVITIS

Infection with the streptococcus or pneumococcus may be primary after wounds, surgical operations, and labour; occasionally it is a secondary infection added to previous lesions, notably soft chancres and syphilis.

When primary, the type is usually erysipelatous with much brawny swelling, but it may be gangrenous, especially in debilitated children (*noma vulvæ*). In secondarily infected venereal sores the inflammation may be most destructive, and terminate in wholesale sloughing of the external genitals (*phagedænic vulvitis*).

Treatment.—Antiseptic fomentations should be applied, stitches removed from operation wounds, and constitutional symptoms met by the injection of an appropriate antitoxic serum, or vaccine. In the rare form of phagedænic inflammation the necrotic tissue should be scraped away with a sharp spoon and the parts well swabbed over with pure carbolic acid.

STAPHYLOCOCCAL VULVITIS (SIMPLE VULVITIS)

Simple vulvitis may occur after any wound of the vulva, or may be due to the irritation of scratching (*pruritus vulvæ*), diabetic urine, ichorous vaginal discharge, rough diapers, or masturbation. The surface is red, sore, and excoriated. In many cases it is associated with vaginitis, as in the vulvo-vaginitis of little children. Antiseptic fomentations and lotions are usually sufficient, combined with the removal of any discoverable cause. In young children vulvitis cannot be cured until the vaginitis is well. These cases are of medicolegal importance, and the pus should be carefully examined for evidence of venereal infection. (*See* Vaginitis, p. 996.)

GONOCOCCAL VULVITIS

Acute gonorrhœa in the female consists of a coincident inflammation of the vaginal cervix, vagina and vulva (*cervico-vagino-vulvitis*). The subject is discussed in Vol. I., pp. 832-34. Owing to the resistant nature of the vulval tissues the inflammation may have entirely subsided in them while still active in the vagina and cervix.

OTHER VENEREAL AFFECTIONS OF THE VULVA

The typical *hard chancre* is rarely met with on the vulva. Instead, the sores are multiple, ulcerative, or sometimes warty. With these is associated much swelling of the labia minora due to lymphangitis, which often hinders a satisfactory view of the parts. Inspection alone will generally fail to determine whether the lesion is syphilitic or merely chancroidal, especially as the two conditions may coincide. In either case the venereal element may be much accentuated by secondary infection with pyogenetic or necrogenetic organisms, leading to great destruction of the parts.

In the *secondary* period of syphilis various manifestations may appear on the vulva, usually taking the form of superficial ulcerations with elevated warty edges. The initial swelling of the labia minora due to lymphangitis may persist, and result in an elephantoid hypertrophy.

Tertiary lesions are rare on the vulva, but when occurring take the form of gummatous masses which by their subsequent changes may occasion much deformity.

Venereal warts, though commonly known as " gonorrhœal," are not due to the gonococcus. They may occur without gonorrhœa, and occasionally in situations other than the vulva (e.g. the umbilicus). Microscopically they are pure papillomas. They are multiple, grow rapidly, and may attain an enormous size, the surface resembling that of a cauliflower. They emit a foul odour and a serous discharge.

Treatment.—Mercury should not, as a rule, be administered until the diagnosis of syphilis is certain. Meanwhile the local condition should be treated by frequent irrigation with biniodide of mercury solution (1–1,000), and by the application of boric ointment on a piece of lint inserted between the labia. After the lymphangitis has subsided the ulcers are best treated with a dusting powder such as aristol. If the inguinal glands suppurate they must be opened.

Secondary lesions may be similarly treated, the patient having been put on a mercurial course or treated by salvarsan. Tertiary lesions require iodide of potassium internally, combined with mercury. Reference has already been made to the local treatment of phagedæna.

Venereal warts should be snipped away with scissors. Oozing may be considerable, but can be checked by sutures or by the light application of a dull-red cautery. Elephantoid hypertrophy of the labia minora is treated by excision.

TUBERCULOUS VULVITIS

This is very rare, and is almost invariably associated with tuberculosis elsewhere. The ulcers are very painful, often foul, and may even be mistaken for malignant disease on account of the granulomatous thickening of the tissues. The diagnosis can only be made by examination of an excised portion of the tissue. The ulcers should be scraped with a sharp spoon until healthy tissue is reached, and carbolic acid then applied. In some cases excision of the diseased area is feasible. Vaccine treatment is of value.

HERPES OF THE VULVA (APHTHOUS VULVITIS)

Occasionally shallow, whitish excoriations are found on the vulva, producing considerable irritation. They are distinguished from venereal disease by the absence of swelling, of labial lymphangitis, and of

glandular enlargement.   Their cause is unknown : clinically they resemble aphthous ulcers of the mouth.   Bathing with a simple antiseptic
lotion suffices.

LEUCOPLAKIC VULVITIS

This very interesting affection has only lately been distinguished
from kraurosis of the vulva.1   Its cause is unknown.   It begins as
a diffuse redness with intense itching, later on the surface becomes
white from epithelial hypertrophy, and the thickened tissues retract,
so that the labia minora and hood of the clitoris almost disappear.
The subepithelial changes consist of diffuse lymphocytosis, the appearance of plasma cells and
complete disappearance
of elastic fibres.   (Fig.
579.)   Painful fissures
may develop, and in
many cases squamous-
celled carcinoma super-
venes.   In others,
extensive subepithelial
fibrosis results, and the
parts present a white
and " ironed-out " ap-
pearance.   This is a
quiescent stage, in
which the characteristic
intense pruritus disap-
pears, while the lia-
bility to carcinoma
diminishes.

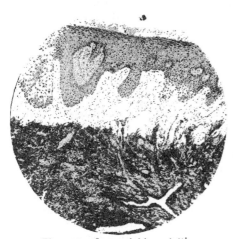

Fig. 579.—Leucoplakic vulvitis.

The epithelium is thickened and the tissue immediately
underlying it is devoid of elastic fibres.

The disease is most
intractable, the pru-
ritus often defying all treatment.   Pathologically it is of great
interest, as, next to X-ray burns, it affords the best example of a
precarcinomatous state.

The parts affected are the labia minora, the hood of the clitoris,
the inner surface of the labia majora, and sometimes the skin as far
back as the anus.   The vestibule and vaginal introit escape.

Treatment.—Of the many applications used for relief of the
pruritus, those most likely to succeed are zymocide lotion and resinol
ointment, but weak alkaline carbolic lotion (phennate of soda) is also
useful.   Iodide of mercury ointment may also be tried.   These failing,
recourse should be had to the X-rays and to zinc-mercury ionization.
In the last resort the affected parts must be excised.

1 See a paper by the author and Comyns Berkeley, Proc. Roy. Soc. Med.

KRAUROSIS VULVÆ

This condition was first described by Briesky. In the early stage multiple red patches are seen around the vaginal introit and on the vestibule. The urethra is usually carunculous. Microscopically, the red patches consist of massive aggregations of plasma cells with many dilated capillaries. The epithelium over them is thinned. Later, shrinkage occurs around the introit, while the whole vulva becomes atrophic and its inner surface smooth and shiny. Great soreness and dyspareunia are early symptoms; later the dyspareunia may also be experienced by the male. The disease is very intractable. In the earlier phases sedative ointments may be tried. Dyspareunia or other distress is best treated by dissecting out the diseased area and at the same time performing a plastic operation to enlarge the vaginal orifice (p. 993). Recurrence is common.

URETHRAL CARUNCLE

A urethral caruncle appears as a bright scarlet " cockscomb-like " protuberance from the posterior edge of the urethral orifice. Occasionally, however the whole orifice may be carunculous without localized protrusion. The formation is entirely inflammatory, and microscopically presents the features of a massive plasma-cell aggregation (*plasmoma*) intermixed with lymphocytes. Its colour is due to numbers of dilated thin-walled capillaries. Embedded in its deeper parts may be found elements of the urethral glands. The condition usually occurs in elderly women, and frequently in association with kraurosis, to which disease it bears a definite histological relation; but it is occasionally seen in the young. The symptoms are those of great soreness, dysuria, dyspareunia and occasional bleeding, but sometimes a caruncle may inexplicably cause no symptoms. The caruncle should be snipped off with scissors and its base well burned with the cautery. Recurrence is extremely likely; if this happens, the lower end of the urethra should be dissected free and removed, and the cut edge of the upper portion sutured to the vestibular mucosa.

ABSCESS OF THE VULVA

The labia majora are occasionally the seat of boils or carbuncles. Suppuration may also occur in one of the numerous glands of the lesser lips. The commonest form of vulval abscess is that of Bartholin's gland at the vaginal introit. Primary infection of this gland is common in gonorrhœa, but may also be due to non-venereal pyogenetic cocci. Frequently a retention cyst of the gland has preceded the infection. Redness, swelling and pain appear in the neighbourhood of the gland, and pus eventually points on the inner surface of the swelling. Where the condition is complicated by previous cyst formation, a persistent sinus leading to the cyst wall is commonly formed. In any case there is a great tendency to repeated recurrence. Boric-acid fomentations should be applied, and the abscess opened and drained. If a cyst is present an attempt should be made to remove the wall, otherwise a sinus will remain.

VULVAL CYSTS

BARTHOLINIAN CYST

A cyst is frequently formed in the duct of Bartholin's gland. The cause is unknown. It presents as an oval swelling bulging inwardly into the introit and outwardly under the lower end of the labia. It is always unilocular, and contains a clear mucus, unless inflamed, when the contents may be brownish and thick or frank muco-pus. Complaint is made of discomfort and the presence of a swelling; if inflammation occurs, pain is severe. The cyst should be excised whole, through an incision over its inner surface. Where suppuration has occurred, this dissection may be impossible. As much as possible of the cyst wall should then be removed and the cavity packed lightly with gauze and allowed to granulate.

LABIAL CYSTS

In the labia majora sebaceous cysts are not uncommon. A cyst of the vestigial "canal of Nuck" (*hydrocele of the canal of Nuck*) is sometimes seen as an elongated swelling extending downwards from the external inguinal ring, and may be mistaken for an inguinal hernia and especially for a hydrocele of a hernial sac. In the labia minora sebaceous cysts are also common. Occasionally thin-walled pedunculated cysts are met with containing a clear fluid. They probably represent distended odoriferous (Tyson's) glands. The cysts, of whatever nature, should be excised. A hydrocele of the canal of Nuck may communicate with the peritoneal cavity, and may be difficult to distinguish from a hernial sac; therefore its interior and contents should always be examined before excision.

URETHRAL CYSTS

Skene's tubules, or the numerous crypts opening through the posterior urethral wall, may occasionally be the origin of cysts. They present as a rounded fluctuating swelling that bulges into the vagina. They resemble a urethrocele, but a sound inverted into the urethra does not pass into the swelling. They may contain pus. If they give rise to trouble they should be dissected out.

OTHER INNOCENT GROWTHS

Venereal warts have already been considered (p. 987). Solitary non-venereal papillomas and soft fibromas, often pedunculated, are occasionally

seen. Lipomas may occur in the labia majora or mons veneris. Very rarely
solid adenomas springing from the sebaceous or odoriferous glands have been
recorded. The treatment in all cases consists in excision.

VULVAL NEW GROWTHS

MALIGNANT GROWTHS

Squamous-celled *carcinoma* of the vulva is not uncommon, and
its almost constant association with a pre-existing leucoplakic vulvitis
(p. 988) has been noted.

There are three common clinical forms—(1) the warty, (2) the
ulcerative, and (3) a superficial erosive, which at first sight does not
perhaps suggest malignancy.

The disease occurs in old women, and may at first run a slow course.
Eventually the inguinal glands become affected, rapidly enlarge, and
soften and break down.

There is a fourth, and rarer, type, viz. that analogous to " sweeps'
cancer " of the scrotum, which usually begins on the labia majora.
Lastly, examples of adeno-carcinoma of glandular origin are on record.

Sarcoma of the vulva is known, and is sometimes of the melanotic
variety.

Treatment.—The whole vulva should be excised, together with
the inguinal glands on both sides.

In excising the vulva, two incisions are required, an outer, which
comprises the whole area, and an inner, to exclude the orifices of the
vagina and urethra. At the conclusion of the operation these latter
are stitched to the skin edges of the wound.

THE VAGINA

DEFORMITIES AND DISPLACEMENTS

In early fœtal life the Müllerian ducts end blindly in the Müllerian
tubercle, an eminence lying in relation with the bladder and Wolffian
ducts in front, the lower bowel behind, and the urogenital sinus
below.

The Müllerian ducts fuse below to form the uterus and vagina, and
the tissue between the Müllerian tubercle and the wall of the urogenital
sinus is gradually hollowed out until the vagina opens on the surface.

IMPERFORATE VAGINA ("IMPERFORATE HYMEN")

Etiology.—This condition is caused by failure of the fused
Müllerian tube to perforate the wall of the urogenital sinus. The
septum represents part of the wall of the urogenital sinus. The hymen
itself is never imperforate, and in these cases it may be seen stretched
out on the septum, but not forming part of it.

Clinical features.—The girl does not menstruate, and after a time complains of periodic attacks of pain lasting for some days. These increase in severity and duration, until in advanced cases the patient is never free from pain. The abdomen becomes swollen and tender, and micturition is difficult. These symptoms are due to the progressive distension with retained blood, first of the vagina (*hæmato-colpos*), and later of the cervix (*hæmatotrachelos*) and Fallopian tubes (*hæmatosalpinx*). The uterus itself is very rarely distended.

The distension of the tubes is soon followed by more or less pelvic peritonitis due to the escape of the blood through the abdominal ostia (*hæmatocele*).

On abdominal examination a definite swelling is felt. If there is much tenderness, distension of the tubes may be inferred. Vaginal examination reveals the stretched septum, bulging, very tender, and of bluish colour owing to the blood behind it.

Treatment.—The retained inspissated blood must be evacuated by free crucial incision of the septum with most rigid aseptic precautions ; if the cervix and tubes are distended there is a peculiar liability to ascending infection which, leading to acute salpingitis, may cause death from general peritonitis.

Where hæmatocolpos alone exists, i.e. where the unenlarged uterus can be felt on the top of the distended vagina, evacuation may be accelerated by flushing out the collapsed vaginal cavity with hot sterile water. If, however, there is any suspicion that the uterus itself is distended, it is better not to douche, lest the fluid be driven up the distended tubes. In these cases the vagina should be simply allowed to drain, the patient being kept in the sitting posture.

ABSENCE OF THE VAGINA, COMPLETE OR PARTIAL

The whole vagina, or its upper, middle, or lower third, may be absent. The defect is due to failure in the complete formation of the Müllerian ducts.

Clinical features.—Patients suffering from this deformity seek advice on one of three grounds—(1) amenorrhœa, (2) symptoms of retained menstrual blood, or (3) marital difficulty.

Treatment.—Since these graver vaginal defects are commonly associated with uterine maldevelopment, symptoms due to retained menstrual blood are not usual. In such circumstances plastic operation attempts are of doubtful value, for, apart from the difficulty of fashioning a serviceable canal, these patients are in nature sexually deficient and unsuited for married life. Where, however, a functional uterus is indicated by the presence of a cystic tumour and recurring monthly pain, completion of continuity of the genital canal is worth attempting, if the defect is not more than 2 in. long.

By careful dissection between the bladder and the rectum the distended cervix or upper part of the vagina, as the case may be, is reached. The retained blood having been evacuated, the wall of the cavity is freed, pulled down, and sutured to the lower part of the canal or to the surface skin. Systematic dilatation must be employed for many months afterwards.

Where the length of vagina to be restored exceeds 2 in. hysterectomy should be performed. Baldwin has successfully constructed a vagina on four occasions by transplanting a portion of the ileum between the bladder and the rectum.

DOUBLE VAGINA

This deformity is due to want of fusion of the vaginal segments and of the Müllerian ducts. It is usually, but not always, associated with a double uterus ; when it is not, the longitudinal septum ends just below the cervix. The deformity may be discovered accidentally, or the patient may complain of marital difficulty. If causing no disability, it should be left untreated ; otherwise the longitudinal septum should be removed and the two halves of the vagina joined by sutures.

VAGINAL SEPTA

Occasionally an annular septum occurs in the vagina, giving rise to dyspareunia. It must be cut away if causing inconvenience ; otherwise it should be let alone.

VAGINAL FISTULÆ

Vesico-vaginal fistulæ occur as a result of prolonged labour or of operative procedures. Uretero-vaginal fistulæ are occasionally met with after total hysterectomy. Recto-vaginal fistulæ result either from laceration during childbirth or from an abscess in the recto-vaginal septum.

Treatment.—A vesico-vaginal fistula may be dealt with either by simply paring the edges and drawing them together by suture, or, when large or intractable, by separating the bladder and vaginal walls and suturing the aperture in each separately. In some cases it may be necessary to deflect a flap from the adjacent part of the vaginal wall to cover the deficiency, or the upper part of the vagina can be detached from the lower portion, closed, and left as an annexe of the bladder (*colpocleisis*). If these methods fail, the abdomen should be opened, the bladder separated from the vagina, and the apertures in each closed. It is absolutely necessary to cure cystitis, if it exists, before performing any operation.

A ureteric fistula, if the communication of the ureter with the bladder is still maintained, may be treated by paring and suturing.

3 *l*

but otherwise must be dealt with by implantation of the injured duct into the bladder or removal of the corresponding kidney. Recto-vaginal fistulæ should be sutured.

CYSTOCELE

A cystocele is a protrusion of the anterior vaginal wall and bladder base between the edges of the two levator ani muscles, which have become divaricated as a result of childbirth.

Etiology.—Inadequacy of the perineum nearly always coexists. The protrusion, though a result of parturition, does not commonly follow that event for some years. It is usually seen, like uterine prolapse and rectocele, with which it is often associated, in women approaching the forties—the stretching of the tissues, which at first is very slow, being accelerated by the loss of muscular tone that accompanies advancing years.

Clinical features.—The patient complains of "something falling," or "the womb falling," though the uterus may not be displaced. The protrusion is a source of soreness or pain, and sometimes of micturitional troubles, usually partial incontinence.

Diagnosis.—The pink rounded protrusion could, after digital examination, only be confused with a lax cyst of the anterior vaginal wall, which is a rarity. A sound in the bladder can be felt under the vaginal wall if the swelling be a cystocele, but not if it be a cyst.

Treatment.—Cystocele may be treated (1) by pessaries, (2) by perineoplasty, or (3) by anterior colporrhaphy.

1. **Pessaries.**—If an operation is not possible or advisable by reason of the patient's refusal, her age or general condition, or the likelihood of further labours, a rubber ring or a Hodge's pessary should be inserted.

2. **Perineoplasty.**—If the patient should not, cannot, or will not wear a pessary, a well-performed perineoplasty (p. 1003) usually suffices to prevent the protrusion. The new perineum must extend forwards so as completely to screen the vaginal orifice. In other cases, though it does not prevent the protrusion altogether, it allows of the retention of a pessary, previously impossible.

3. **Anterior colporrhaphy.**—An oval area of the protruded vaginal wall, with its long axis in that of the vagina, is excised, and the fasciæ (triangular ligaments) underlying it are divided so as to separate the bladder base from the vaginal wall very freely around the margins of the incisions, and allow it to ride upwards before the wound is sutured. The gap in the fasciæ is then sutured transversely, and the gap in the vaginal mucosa longitudinally. A more elaborate procedure consists in dissecting outwards from the margins of the incision until the edges of the levatores ani are reached, and suturing

these together in the middle line under the bladder before the vaginal wound is closed. In either case, perineoplasty must be performed as well, or the condition will recur.

RECTOCELE

A rectocele is a protrusion of the recto-vaginal septum and posterior vaginal wall through the vaginal orifice. It is constantly associated with a deficient perineum, and frequently with cystocele and prolapse of the uterus.

Etiology.—The deformity is due to two factors—(1) deficiency of the perineum, (2) relaxation of the posterior part of the pelvic floor. The rectum falls forwards on the posterior vaginal wall, which, unsupported by a perineum, stretches and protrudes.

Clinical features.—The patient complains of "something falling." In most cases cystocele is present as well. The protruded mass, when large, may become very sore or even ulcerated from the friction of the clothes.

Diagnosis.—On inspection it may be impossible to tell whether the pink swelling is a cystocele or a rectocele, but digital examination will immediately decide the question.

Treatment.—A pessary may be employed to retain the redundant vaginal wall, but if the perineum is deficient it may be impossible to keep the instrument in place. The best treatment is perineoplasty, perhaps combined in severe cases with excision of a portion of the posterior vaginal wall (*posterior colporrhaphy*).

INFLAMMATION OF THE VAGINA

˙VAGINITIS

Inflammation of the vagina is best classified according to its cause, as follows :—

STREPTOCOCCAL AND PNEUMOCOCCAL VAGINITIS (ERYSIPELATOUS OR GANGRENOUS VAGINITIS)

This is chiefly seen in some of the more virulent forms of puerperal sepsis. The appearance varies, the surface being erysipelatous, diphtheroid, or frankly sloughing.

Treatment is that of streptococcal infections generally. Hydrogen peroxide (10 vols.) is the best application if necrosis has occurred, otherwise biniodide of mercury solution (1–2,000) should be used.

STAPHYLOCOCCAL VAGINITIS (SIMPLE VAGINITIS)

Simple vaginitis may be due to injuries, operations, excessive chemical applications, the prolonged wearing of foul pessaries, or the

presence of other foreign bodies. Occasionally it is seen in virgins
without obvious cause.

The surface is red, smarting and painful, and a purulent discharge
flows from the vagina. The cervical canal is often infected as well,
and is apt to remain inflamed long after the vagina has recovered ;
by persistent re-infection it may render treatment directed to the
vagina alone of no avail, particularly in the vulvo-vaginitis of children.

Diagnosis.—This is made absolute by bacteriological examination of the pus. The possibility of gonorrhœal origin must never be
mentioned until bacteriological proof has been obtained. The vulvo-
vaginitis of children, while sometimes gonococcal, is usually staphylococcal, but parents are almost uniformly apt to assume the graver
infection.

Treatment.—Simple antiseptic douching usually suffices. In
virgins, and particularly in children, the hymen may hinder douching,
and, by obstructing drainage, maintain the inflammation. Where an
ordinary douche tube cannot be inserted a glass catheter may be used.

GONOCOCCAL VAGINITIS

The clinical features and treatment of this condition are discussed
in Vol. I., pp. 832–34. The disease runs a more severe course where
the hymen is practically intact, because drainage and medication are
alike interfered with. The hymen becomes swollen, scarlet, and so
sensitive that any attempt to pass a douche nozzle causes severe pain.

Complications.—Bartholin's gland often suppurates. Extension of the infection to the body of the uterus and to the Fallopian
tubes is common, but does not usually occur for several weeks after
the initiation of the attack. Gonorrhœal cystitis is also frequently
met with.

Diagnosis.—No definite statement should be made unless supported by bacteriological proof ; even then caution is to be observed.

The treatment of the complications of gonorrhœa generally has
already been considered (Vol. I., p. 836). During the acute stage,
urinary antiseptics should be given to prevent cystitis.

NEW GROWTHS OF THE VAGINA

CYSTS

Although the vaginal wall normally contains no glands, small
aberrant glandular retention cysts are occasionally found there. They
rarely exceed the size of a pea. A rare condition, *adenomatosis vaginæ*,
in which the whole vaginal wall is beset with glands, has been described
by the author and Glendinning.[1]

[1] *Proc. Roy. Soc. Med.*, vol. iv.

Thin-walled cysts sometimes occur on the lateral or lower part of the anterior vaginal wall. These are Wolffian in origin, and have been found extending up into the broad ligament in the course of Gartner's duct.

The cyst should be excised if it is causing trouble.

SOLID TUMOURS, INNOCENT AND MALIGNANT

Solid tumours of the vagina are very rare. *Myomas* are most often encountered. They appear as rounded hard tumours bulging into the lumen of the canal, and covered by the mucous membrane lining it. *Papillomas* and soft *fibromas* occur occasionally.

Malignant disease is uncommon in the vagina. Squamous-celled *carcinoma* may be primary there or secondary to a growth in the cervix. It assumes the form of a nodular ulceration. Adeno-carcinoma secondary to carcinoma of the corpus is sometimes seen. Metastatic nodules of chorion-epithelioma are relatively common in the course of this interesting disease, and in addition a good number of cases are recorded in which this variety of malignant disease has appeared there primarily.

Sarcoma of the vagina occurs both in children and in adults. In the former it assumes the same " grape-like " appearance that characterizes infantile sarcoma of the cervix. In adults it presents as a soft, red, " velvety "-surfaced mass. Both types are exceedingly rare.

Symptoms.—The innocent growths may give rise to no symptoms, or, by their size, may cause marital difficulty or pain. The malignant tumours present the clinical features common to them elsewhere.

Treatment.—The innocent tumours should be removed. Vaginal myomas are well encapsulated, and shell out easily.

Malignant disease of the vagina is a very serious matter, owing to the readiness with which it spreads to the rectum or bladder, and the frequency with which it is already inoperable when the patient presents herself. Where limited to the vagina, the growth demands total removal of this canal together with the uterus—*total hystero-vaginectomy* (*see* under Carcinoma of the Cervix, p. 1022). Where a small primary growth exists close to the outlet, the lower part of the vagina alone may be excised, and the upper portion pulled down and united to the skin.

THE UTERUS
DEFORMITIES AND DISPLACEMENTS
ABSENCE OF THE UTERUS

The uterus may be absent altogether. Such deformity is usually associated with more or less deficiency of the vagina and maldevelopment of the ovaries.

ATRESIA OF THE CERVIX

The cervix may become imperforate as a result of the application of strong caustics. Rarely it is congenitally so. In either case, if the uterus be functional, retention of menstrual blood occurs. The site of retention varies; if the obstruction be limited to the external os, the cervix is distended first (*hæmatotrachelos*), and later the tubes; if the obstruction be at the internal os, hæmatosalpinx is usually the first event, the uterus distending subsequently. The clinical features are those of retained menses with symptoms of hæmatosalpinx and salpingitis. Communication with the vagina should be established if possible. If, however, this cannot be done, or if the tubes are already disorganized, removal of the uterus and tubes is indicated.

DOUBLE UTERUS (Fig. 580)

The following degrees of double uterus depend on the extent to which the Müllerian ducts have failed to fuse:—

1. *Uterus duplex.*—Two distinct organs. A peritoneal fold from rectum to bladder passes between them.

2. *Uterus bicornis unicollis.*—Two bodies joined to a single neck.

3. *Uterus unicornis.*—A bicornuate uterus in which only one body has developed, the other remaining as a narrow tube.

4. *Uterus septus.*—The uterus is outwardly single and of normal shape, but a longitudinal septum divides its cavity down to the external os.

5. *Uterus subseptus.*—A similar condition to No. 4, but the septum only reaches the internal os.

Clinical features.—The deformity usually causes no symptoms, and is only accidentally discovered. Though any uterine deformity militates against conception, repeated pregnancy has occurred in one half of a double uterus; a decidua is formed in the unimpregnated half, and is expelled after the labour.

Pregnancy sometimes occurs in the undeveloped horn of a unicorn uterus and runs the same course as pregnancy in the Fallopian tube, except that rupture is less common and a greater proportion of the cases go on to term.

Hæmatometra in one half of a double uterus is occasionally met with, the symptoms being those of recurring monthly pain and a cystic tumour to one side of the apparently unenlarged uterus. There is, of course, no amenorrhœa. Septate uteri have been discovered during mechanical dilatation of the organ, the edge of the partition obstructing the passage of the dilator. The half of a bicornuate uterus has been found in the sac of an inguinal hernia, in the male as well as the female (internal pseudo-hermaphrodism).

Diagnosis.—Where two cervices exist, the diagnosis is obvious. With a single cervix, double bodies may be detected by bimanual examination. They sweep outwards in a characteristic manner parallel with Poupart's ligament. The passage of the sound will render the condition clear.

A uterus unicornis may be suspected from the presence of the peculiar outward sweep already mentioned, and only one uterus can be felt.

Pregnancy in an undeveloped horn can only be distinguished from

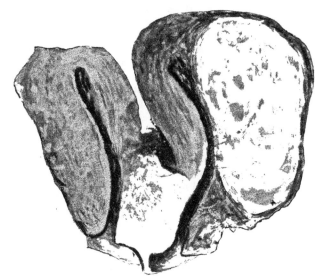

Fig. 580.—Double uterus.

The left horn contains a myoma.   The septum dividing the vagina into two halves is shown.

a tubal pregnancy by noting the relation borne by the tumour to the round ligament, i.e. the ligament terminates in its outer side.

Hæmatometra of an undeveloped horn may be suspected from a consideration of the history, the youth of the patient, and the extreme lateroversion of the recognizable body of the uterus.

Treatment.—If symptoms are absent nothing need be done; otherwise the uterus or the cornu at fault should be removed.

ELONGATION OF THE VAGINAL CERVIX

There are two main types of elongation of the vaginal cervix : (1) a so-called " congenital " elongation, occasionally seen in young women, in which the vaginal cervix, though so elongated as to protrude perhaps from the vulva like a polyp, is extremely thin, and (2) the acquired elongations most commonly due to chronic hyperplastic cervicitis, but more rarely to the development of a myoma, a carcinoma or sarcoma, or large cyst in the cervical wall. In these cases the vaginal cervix is enlarged in every dimension.

Clinical features.—The congenital form may produce no symptoms and may be discovered accidentally. In the acquired variety the patient becomes aware of an abnormal mass filling the vagina or protruding from the orifice, and complains of a sense of dragging or bearing down. If cervicitis be present, there will be leucorrhœa, pain in coitus, and occasional slight blood-stained discharges.

Diagnosis.—The congenital form may be mistaken for a polyp, but inspection of the most dependent part of the protrusion will show the external os, and careful vaginal examination will clinch the diagnosis.

General hypertrophy due to inflammation or new growth could only be mistaken for a tumour extruding through the external os, or for the body of a totally inverted uterus ; careful examination will not fail to distinguish it from these conditions.

Treatment.—The congenital elongation should not be interfered with unless it causes annoyance or produces sterility ; in such case it may be amputated circularly just below the vaginal vault. An acquired hypertrophy must be treated according to its cause. When it is due to cervicitis, circular amputation or tracheloplasty (p. 1011) may be performed ; when it is the result of new growth, the appropriate treatment must be carried out.

PROLAPSE OF THE UTERUS

Etiology.—Rarely prolapse is present at birth, whilst occasionally it is met with in young virgins. In either case the deformity is due to congenital deficiency of the sustentacular apparatus.

In the vast proportion of cases, however, prolapse of the uterus is the result of childbearing. The structures fixing the uterus and vagina in their normal position may be divided into three groups :—

1. *Upper supporting structures.*—These constitute the upper part of the broad ligaments, and comprise the peritoneal folds, the ovarico-pelvic and ovarico-uterine ligaments, the perivascular sheaths of the ovarian vessels and the round ligaments. Though the single elements have no great resisting power, yet taken *en masse* they form a support of considerable strength.

2. *Middle supporting structures.*—These consist of two pairs of fibro-cellular bands uniting the upper part of the vagina and supravaginal cervix to the sacrum and lateral pelvic walls respectively.

The posterior pair, together with their covering peritoneum, form the utero-sacral ligaments ; the very strong lateral pair lie in the base of the broad ligament and are known as Mackenrodt's or the lateral cervico-pelvic ligaments. At their upper edges run the uterine arteries and the ureters.

3. *Lower supporting structures.*—These make up the pelvic floor proper, and consist of the recto-vesical fascia, the levatores ani, and the superficial perineal muscles and fasciæ. The horseshoe-shaped gap between the levatores is filled in by the triangular ligaments, which are perforated by the vagina and urethra, while the fascia of Colles is cleft by the vulva.

The edges of the levatores ani muscles are in relation with the lateral vaginal walls at a point less than an inch up that canal, so that most of the vagina and all the uterus is well above the pelvic floor, which, therefore, only indirectly supports the latter organ.

With the uterus anteverted and the perineal body intact, the genital canal forms a sharp curve, concave forwards. This curve plays a very important part in the support of the uterus, which in the standing posture rests upon the pubis, the bladder intervening, whilst in recumbency it stands nearly vertical on the structures lying in the hollow of the sacrum.

Uterine prolapse is due to weakening more or less of the whole retentive apparatus, for such is the reserve power of its various con-stituents that failure of one group alone is insufficient to cause descent of the organ if the others remain healthy. Thus absolute flaccidity of the upper supports is constantly seen with retroversion, but without prolapse ; and extensive cystocele and rectocele due to bulging of the pelvic floor may coexist with a uterus in normal position.

Prolapse of the female genital canal may be classified under two main types, according to whether the eversion begins (1) *from below upwards*, or (2) *from above downwards*.

In the first, the pelvic floor proper is primarily at fault, and the descent of the uterus is preceded by cystocele and rectocele. The levatores ani are separated and the perineal body and normal vaginal curve are absent.

In the second type, a primary yielding of the upper and middle supports allows the uterus to drop through the vagina, the cervix first protruding at the vulva and being followed by the vaginal walls as they evert from above downwards.

Where the fault primarily lies with the pelvic floor the upper part of the broad ligaments and the utero-sacral and lateral cervico-pelvic ligaments resist the tendency to downward descent, with the result that the vagina is longitudinally stretched ; but if the primary weakness lies with the utero-sacral and lateral cervico-pelvic liga-ments, the upper part of the broad ligament resists the downward pull and the supravaginal cervix becomes elongated, so that the external os may possibly appear at the vulva while the fundus of the uterus remains at its normal level.

Uterine prolapse is aided by high intra-abdominal pressure, and therefore its occurrence often coincides with the adipose and flatulent distension of advancing years.

Theoretically, increased weight of the organ should favour prolapse, but considerable enlargement prevents descent through the pelvis, and, as a matter of fact, many a prolapsed uterus is smaller than normal. Very rarely, large polypoid tumours of the uterus have dragged the organ after them in their descent from the vagina.

Clinical features.—Three degrees of prolapse of the uterus are recognized—(1) where the cervix is still within the vagina, (2) where the cervix protrudes from the vagina, (3) where the whole uterus is outside the vagina, the latter canal being turned inside out.

The symptoms may begin shortly after childbirth, but most commonly not till some years later. A sense of weight, bearing down and backache is complained of, with vesical irritability or partial incontinence of urine. The procident part, when it emerges from the vagina, becomes chafed, scaly and dry, and later ulcerated. The ulcers are typically " callous," with a firm smooth white edge. They cause soreness as a rule, but are liable to acute attacks of inflammation, during which they may suppurate freely, or even slough, with much pain and some constitutional disturbance. Though often mistaken for carcinoma, they very rarely undergo malignant degeneration.

Diagnosis.—The patient should be examined in the standing posture for all " gravity " displacements.

Elongation of the vaginal cervix and complete inversion of the uterus are the only conditions with which prolapse of the uterus could reasonably be confounded. In neither of those cases is the vaginal vault lowered, whereas in prolapse of the uterus this change is constantly observed. The absence of the external os would at once disclose an inversion.

Treatment. Pessaries.—Treatment by pessary is proper for patients in whom age, debility, or the probability of further labours contra-indicates operation, and in those who refuse operation or to whom the time entailed means loss of employment.

The rubber ring is the most generally useful pessary. In a few cases of slight prolapse, the continued retention of the uterus in proper position for some months, or a year or two, may, by allowing the uterine supports to recover themselves, actually effect a cure. In most cases, however, the treatment is merely palliative. Women wearing a pessary must be instructed to douche at least once a day, and to have the instrument changed every three months.

Where no perineal body exists, and also in the coniform vagina
of old age, no ordinary pessary can be retained.   In these cases, if
perineoplasty be contra-indicated or refused, some form of vaginal
stem pessary must be worn, such as Napier's or Maw's.   These are
of great service in feeble, elderly women.

Operative treatment.—Combined *perineoplasty* and *ventro-suspension of the uterus* are the most efficient method of cure, and the
operations may be performed under one anæsthesia.   Perineoplasty
by itself may greatly relieve that variety of prolapse in which the
descent of the uterus is preceded by cystocele and rectocele, and
both in these cases and those in which the uterus primarily descends
it enables a pessary to be worn if this was previously impossible.
Ventro-suspension alone will cure the rare cases of primary uterine
descent without any prolapse of the vaginal walls.   The uterus must
be fixed as high up the anterior abdominal wall as possible, so as to
get a straight pull on the vagina and pelvic floor.   Low fixation of
the uterus increases cystocele, if present.

Many other operations have been designed for the cure of prolapse.
Colporrhaphy, either anterior or posterior, may be combined with
perineoplasty, where great redundancy of the vaginal wall is present.
Intervesico-vaginal fixation of the uterus is much practised on the
Continent and by some American surgeons, when the patient is past
the childbearing age, and various methods of suturing together the
edges of the levatores ani (*myorrhaphy*), of narrowing the vaginal canal,
or of plicating or suturing together the lateral cervico-pelvic ligaments,
have been devised.   All of them, in my opinion, are inferior to ventri-
fixation and perineoplasty in combination.

Success has been reported by Inglis Parsons from injecting into the
bases of the broad ligaments per vaginam a 1-in-5 solution of quinine.
A degree of broad-ligament cellulitis is thereby set up, which fixes the
uterus.   The method may well be tried where a regular operation is
contra-indicated or objected to.

Hysterectomy should never be done for prolapse ; by severing the
connexion between the vagina and the broad ligaments, it facilitates
eversion of that canal so much that the whole vagina turns inside out.
Digital examination of the prolapsed parts in total procidentia will
show how small a proportion of the mass is formed by the uterus itself.
Instead of removing the organ, it should be utilized as an artificial
support of the vagina and pelvic floor by fixing it high up on the anterior
abdominal wall.

Perineoplasty is performed by dissecting up a flap from the posterior
vaginal wall and excising it in the shape of a V.   The edges of the V
are then united by suture to restore the normal forward curve of the
canal.   The skin wound is closed either by a single layer of deep silk-

worm-gut sutures or in layers of catgut uniting (1) the edges of the levator ani, (2) the superficial fascial planes, and (3) the skin. If the rupture extends through the anus the recto-vaginal septum must be split before the vaginal flap is turned up. The gap in the wall of the bowel is closed separately by buried catgut sutures.

RETROVERSION OF THE UTERUS

The uterine axis varies greatly in direction within normal limits, being affected by the state of the intestines and the bladder, and the position of the patient. Various arbitrary degrees of retroversion have been described, which serve no useful purpose, and should be discarded in place of this simple rule : *if, with the patient in the standing posture, the axis of the uterus is directed behind the vertical, the uterus is retroverted.*

Doubtful cases of displacement must *always* be examined with the patient erect, for many a uterus that is retroverted in dorsal decubitus takes up the normal anteverted position when the patient stands. Such patients need no treatment for the retroversion.

Retroflexion is always secondary to retroversion ; the flaccid uterus bends just above the attachment of the utero-sacral and lateral cervico-pelvic ligaments.

Etiology.—Retroversion is caused by yielding of the upper part of the broad ligaments, and this may arise in several ways :—

1. *Gravity.*—An abnormally heavy uterus may retrovert of its own weight, as in some cases of myoma ; on the other hand, a normal organ may stretch ligaments already weak from parturition, maldevelopment, or general debility. The coexistence of a heavy uterus and relaxed ligaments such as occurs in puerperal subinvolution is the commonest cause of retroversion.

2. *Pressure.*—Large tumours lying in front of the uterus may push the organ into retroversion. This often occurs with ovarian cysts and myomas.

3. *Traction.*—The contraction of adhesions may pull the uterus into retroversion. This is often seen in chronic salpingitis, and particularly after bilateral salpingo-oöphorectomy for inflammatory conditions, where the operation has interfered with the normal supporting structures.

4. *Trauma.*—Probably sudden falls or strains may cause retroversion, though this is impossible of proof. It is the most reasonable explanation of the commonly-found cases in virgins, and in many instances the history strongly supports such a view.

Effect of retroversion on the uterus.—It is doubtful if retroversion *per se* has any effect on a healthy uterus, for in virgins this displacement commonly occurs without any signs of uterine disease. Most cases of retroversion are, however, puerperal in origin, and in them the uterus is usually enlarged and often chronically inflamed as the result of the faulty puerperium in which the displacement originated.

Prolonged retroversion of a large uterus frequently causes a white patch of thickened peritoneum on its posterior surface, due to friction. Probably this friction sometimes leads to filamentous adhesions, for these are often found without any evidence of salpingitis. Chronic salpingitis is, however, often associated with retroversion as an extension from the puerperal endometritis present before the displacement.

Clinical features.—Many cases of retroversion exist without symptoms, especially where the uterus is small and only the upper uterine supports are lax. Where the uterus is heavy and the rest of the suspensory apparatus weak, as in most cases of puerperal origin, backache and abdominal pain radiating outwards parallel to Poupart's ligament are felt, due to traction on the utero-sacral and broad ligaments respectively. These pains are worse at the periods, and after standing, but are not entirely relieved by lying down, as is the case in uterine prolapse. Dyspareunia is common, the result either of the accompanying prolapse of the appendages, or of chronic peritonitis and filamentous adhesions at the back of the uterus. Rectal symptoms may occur. Inasmuch as a retroverted uterus is often chronically enlarged by inflammation and subinvolution, leucorrhœa, menorrhagia, and a tendency to sterility are frequent. Should pregnancy occur, it is unlikely to proceed beyond the third month ; indeed, this displacement is the commonest cause of repeated miscarriage. If miscarriage does not take place, the uterus nearly always rises from the pelvis and straightens itself, and may remain in proper position after the labour. In a few cases incarceration results, with retention of urine and severe pressure symptoms. These cases of incarcerated retroverted gravid uterus with a distended bladder have again and again been mistaken for ovarian cysts through neglect to use the catheter.

Treatment.—Retroversion, *per se,* needs no meddlesome interference, especially in virgins. If, however, the displacement is causing definite discomfort it should be treated.

Pessaries.—It is not sufficient that the organ be movable or even replaceable, it must be *retainable,* to justify the use of a pessary. It is often impossible to retain a perfectly movable uterus in anteversion, owing to permanent alteration in the length of the peritoneal folds from prolonged malposition. Before insertion of the appliance, the organ must be brought into complete anteversion, i.e. lying almost parallel with the anterior vaginal wall, for unless all coils of intestine are expelled from the utero-vesical pouch, retroversion soon recurs. Moreover, in this position gravity assists in maintaining the anteversion, whether the patient stand or lie. Such reposition is effected by manipulation, either alone or aided by the uterine sound. If the organ tends to roll back wards immediately the control of the fingers or sound is withdrawn, the introduction of a pessary is contra-indicated, for its slight retaining power is inefficient unless assisted by gravity.

Reposition is most satisfactorily carried out under an anæsthetic ; and where cervicitis or endometritis coexists, the unhealthy mucosa should be curetted at the same time.

Operations.—Of the many operations devised for retroversion, ventro-suspension and shortening of the round ligaments are the two best.

Ventro-suspension consists in fastening the upper part of the anterior uterine wall to the anterior abdominal wall by three or four sutures that, picking up the superficial muscular layers of the former, pass through the peritoneum and aponeurosis on either side of the wound. A strong peritoneal adhesion is thus formed, which gradually stretches into a short artificial ligament about ½ in. long.

Ventro-suspension thus performed is a very satisfactory operation, and does not interfere with subsequent pregnancy. Where, however, real fixation of the uterus has been performed, or where the fundus or posterior wall or one of the cornua has been attached instead of the anterior wall, great difficulties both in pregnancy and in labour have been experienced. Cases are on record of intestinal obstruction by the artificial ligament, but this sequel is very rare.

Shortening the round ligaments.—The original operation devised by Alexander was extraperitoneal, the ligaments being exposed at the external abdominal ring. Since only cases of movable retroversion could be so treated, the operation has been largely given up in favour of *intraperitoneal ligamentopexy.* There are many ways of performing this operation. The most ingenious and best is as follows : The abdomen having been opened, and the uterus anteverted, a ligature is passed under each round ligament about ¾ in. from its uterine attachment, and tied, the ends being left long. A special curved forceps is then inserted through a little slit in the aponeurosis ½ in. outside the edge of the wound, and is pushed outwards, first between the rectus muscle and aponeurosis, and subsequently between the aponeurosis and peritoneum, till the internal abdominal ring is reached. The point of the forceps (still extraperitoneal) is now made to return towards the middle line under the peritoneum of the broad ligament and parallel to and just in front of the round ligament. When it has reached the position of the previously applied ligature it is thrust through the peritoneum and the ligature ends are grasped and withdrawn along the track taken by the instrument.

The forceps being removed, traction is made upon the ligature ends until a knuckle of round ligament appears at the aponeurotic slit.

A similar proceeding having been carried out in the opposite side, each knuckle is fixed by the suture closing the little slit in the aponeurosis on its own side, and the abdominal wound is then sutured.

This proceeding shortens the whole of the front part of the broad ligament on either side and leaves the uterus in a truly normal position. It is, therefore, a better operation than ventro-suspension for retroversion, but is inadvisable where prolapse also exists, as it does not effect a sufficiently direct upward pull on the uterus.

INVERSION OF THE UTERUS

This rare displacement most often occurs immediately after childbirth. Occasionally, however, cases of chronic inversion are seen, with an obscure relation to parturition.

Three degrees of inversion are described —(1) where the inverted fundus is still within the uterine cavity; (2) where it is extruded from the external os; and (3) where the entire body and cervix is turned inside out.

Clinical features.—The accident, when occurring after labour, is marked by severe shock and hæmorrhage. In chronic cases there is bearing-down pain, with bloody discharge, which may be offensive. The everted uterine mucosa becomes ulcerated or may superficially slough. (Fig. 581.)

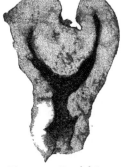

Fig. 581.—Partial inversion of the uterus.

Diagnosis.—The mass might be mistaken for a protruding myoma, but careful examination and the passage of a sound make the condition clear.

Treatment.—A puerperal inversion must be at once reduced by manipulation, but chronic cases can rarely be so treated. The recognized method for these is the use of the Aveling repositor, i.e. a boxwood cup on a rigid stem which is kept pressed against the inverted fundus by indiarubber straps attached to a waistband. It is important to place tampons around the repositor to keep it from slipping off the mass to which it is applied. After twenty-four hours it will usually be found that the displacement has been corrected.

If the repositor fail, the utero-vesical pouch may be opened from below, and the everted anterior wall of the uterus incised from the cervix downwards. The cupped interior of the inversion is thus laid open, the adherent appendages which prevent its reposition are freed, the inversion is reduced, and the wound in the anterior uterine wall and vaginal cervix subsequently closed by sutures. An alternative proceeding is to open the abdomen and incise from above the posterior wall of the cup. Finally, the inverted uterus may be removed by vaginal hysterectomy.

INFLAMMATION OF THE UTERUS

ENDOCERVICITIS AND CERVICAL "EROSION"

Cervicitis may be caused by direct extension upwards of a vaginitis, or may be part of a general uterine infection following labour or abortion. It may also follow obstetric lacerations or operative wounds.

The normal virgin cervical canal is probably bacteriologically sterile. The vagina, on the other hand, always contains organisms. The vaginal epithelium is remarkably thick and resistant, whilst that of the cervix is reduced to a single layer with numerous glandular crypts, from which organisms, once lodged, are with difficulty eradicated.

Cervicitis may undoubtedly occur in chaste virgins from an ascending bacterial infection from the germ-containing vagina, probably due to some lowered condition of resistance.

ACUTE ENDOCERVICITIS

Acute endocervicitis is usually merely a part of a generalized infection of the genital canal, such as that caused by gonorrhœa or puerperal sepsis. The cervical discharge is mucopurulent, or in the most severe cases frankly purulent because the secretion from the cervical glands is inhibited. The internal os tends to bar further ascending infection ; therefore, whilst acute cervicitis is common, acute endometritis is, fortunately, relatively uncommon.

Treatment.—This is considered in the sections on Acute Endometritis (p. 1012) and Vaginitis (p. 995), of which it forms a part.

CHRONIC ENDOCERVICITIS AND CERVICAL "EROSION"

Acute cervicitis is very apt to become chronic, because (1) the tortuous cervical glands harbour organisms, and (2) local treatment is difficult of application.

A cervical erosion is the outward sign of the changes in progress throughout the cervical canal.

Three stages of chronic cervicitis may be distinguished :

Stage 1.—The subepithelial tissue is crowded with cells, chiefly of the lymphocyte type, with some polymorphonuclear leucocytes, which latter are also seen in the gland lumina. The cervical epithelium is irregular and partly desquamated. Around the external os is the area of "erosion." Here the same subepithelial lymphocytosis is seen, while the superficial layers of the squamous epithelium have desquamated. The surface, therefore, is slightly depressed and looks raw and granular (*granular erosion*) (Fig. 582). The discharge is mucous or mucopurulent.

Stage 2.—Subepithelial lymphocytosis is still marked, but other inflammatory cells are appearing (large hyaline cells and plasma cells). The cervical glands are hypertrophied and tortuous, and abnormally muciniferous. In the eroded area the basal layers of the epithelium have ingrown to form new glandular crypts (*glandular erosion*).

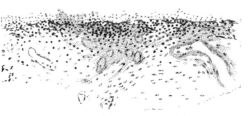

Fig. 582.—Cervical erosion, granular stage.

In some cases definite papillæ of the hypercellular subepithelial tissue project on the surface, giving it a raised velvety aspect (*papillary* or *villous erosion*) (Fig. 583). The discharge is clear mucus, and very profuse.

Stage 3.—Subepithelial fibrosis occurs with disappearance of elastic fibres and a diminution of cellularity. The epithelium of the cervical canal thickens, and becomes almost squamous in places. In the eroded area this hypertrophy is very marked, the epithelium exhibiting interpapillary down-growths like those of the skin. (Fig. 584.) The glandular crypts be-

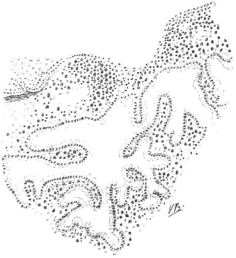

Fig. 583.—Cervical erosion, adenomatous stage.

come occluded by the thickened epithelium and the contraction of fibrous tissue, and numerous slightly raised faintly blue retention cysts present on the surface (ovules of Naboth). The rest of the "erosion area" is whitish (cervical leucoplakia). The discharge progressively diminishes as the glands become occluded,

3 *m*

and the erosion is often said to have "healed." A permanent change is, however, now established in the cervical tissues. (*See* under Carcinoma of the Cervix, p. 1019.)

Clinical features.—The leading symptom of chronic cervicitis is leucorrhœa, popularly known as "the whites." The mucus escaping from the cervix is transparent, but after mixture with the creamy-coloured vaginal secretion it becomes whitish and streaked. It is most copious in the earlier stages of cervicitis, and gradually lessens as the glands become occluded. The cervix is often the seat of old ununited laceration. It is doubtful if chronic cervicitis *per se* can cause pain, but inasmuch as it is often associated with endometritis, retroversion or prolapse, or other abnormal conditions of the genital organs, it is often associated with pain.

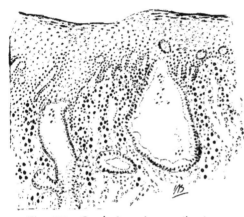

Fig. 584.—Cervical erosion, cystic stage.

Differential diagnosis. — Cervical "erosion" in its earlier phases is readily distinguishable from carcinoma of the cervix, but when severe and old-standing may simulate it so closely that diagnosis can only be made by microscopy. Nor is this surprising, since erosion is the constant precursor of carcinoma.

In general, though slight oozing may follow examination, an erosion never bleeds freely, and though its surface may be irregular and rough, the consistence of the tissues is firm. Carcinoma, on the other hand, always bleeds more or less readily, and its surface, in addition to being irregularly excrescent, is friable. In all cases of doubt a microscopical examination should be made.

Treatment.—Chronic cervicitis may be treated either by applications or by operation.

Applications.—Douches are customarily prescribed for leucorrhœa. Although vaginal irrigation applies chemicals but inefficiently to the cervical canal, it is of use, inasmuch as it washes away the discharge, benefits the surface of the erosion, and allays vaginitis. In the more acute stages antiseptic solutions should be used, such as iodine (1 drachm of the tincture to a pint of water), biniodide of mercury (1–4,000), or lysol (1 drachm to the quart). Later, astringents are employed, such as tannic acid, alum, or sulphate of zinc (2 drachms to the quart).

Soluble vaginal pessaries containing ichthyol or other drugs in a glycerine basis are a more potent method of making applications to the cervical surface.

The direct application of antiseptics such as carbolic acid or "iodized phenol" (iodine 1, phenol 3) on a swab is the most efficient method of direct medication, and if persisted in cures a certain proportion of cases. It is, however, a lengthy, troublesome, and uncertain means of treatment.

Operations.—*Scraping* the diseased cervical mucosa with a sharp scoop is the most rational treatment. Not infrequently it is also necessary to curette the corporeal endometrium, but owing to the depth to which the cervical glands penetrate the tough cervical tissue, nothing short of the vigorous application of a strong, sharp scoop will suffice to eradicate them. The surface of the erosion is similarly treated. In bad cases one of the following operations may be performed.

Trachelorrhaphy is indicated where, in addition to the cervicitis, the cervix is badly split. The lips of the laceration are denuded on their inner and opposed surfaces, except for a narrow strip in the centre of each, and they are then approximated by sutures, so that most of the eroded area is removed and the laceration repaired at the same time. The cervical endometrium above should always be scraped as well.

The operation is faulty, in that a strip of the eroded area is utilized to form the lining of the restored part of the cervical canal.

Tracheloplasty.—The disadvantage attaching to trachelorrhaphy is avoided in tracheloplasty, in which a wedge of the cervix is excised, including the whole of the eroded area. The edges of the two lips thus formed are then sutured to the edges of the cervical canal and to one another on either side of this.

Amputation of the vaginal cervix.—A cuff of mucous membrane covering the cervix is reflected, the cervix amputated circularly, and the edge of the cuff sutured to the edge of the cervical canal. It is the best operation for persistent and severe chronic cervicitis, and is specially indicated where the vaginal cervix is much hypertrophied.

TUBERCULOUS CERVICITIS

This very rare condition usually coexists with corporeal disease. It presents as an ulcerating surface, commonly mistaken for carcinoma, but distinguishable from it by microscopy. It requires hysterectomy.

ACUTE ENDOMETRITIS

Pathology.—Acute infection of the interior of the uterus is most typically seen after labour and abortion. The streptococcus is usually found in the more virulent puerperal infections, but the pneumococcus, staphylococcus, and B. coli also occur. In the absence of recent pregnancy, acute endometritis is most commonly caused by the gonococcus, but it may also arise after operations, in the course of the extrusion of a polypus, or as a consequence of a breaking-down carcinoma.

In acute streptococcal endometritis the mucosa is necrotic, either diphtheroid or foully sloughing, and the whole uterine wall is œdematous, and often presents multiple abscesses. In the less virulent infections, such as the gonococcal, the endometrium is frankly suppurating, the interglandular stroma is packed with polynuclear leucocytes, and much of the epithelium has desquamated.

Clinical features.—The symptoms of puerperal endometritis are those collectively known as " puerperal fever," a full description of which will be found in obstetrical textbooks. Gonorrhœal endometritis usually supervenes some weeks after the initiation of the infection. There is much pain in the lower abdomen and the vagina, and the uterus on examination is very tender. The pulse and temperature are raised. The menstrual period may be suppressed or excessive.

Diagnosis.—The symptoms of acute gonorrhœal endometritis closely resemble those of acute gonococcal salpingitis, with which, indeed, the acute uterine inflammation is often associated.

The presence of a definite swelling on one or both sides of the uterus, coupled with lower abdominal rigidity and distension, is an indication of salpingitis. In the absence of these signs it may be inferred that the affection is limited to the uterus.

Treatment.—Acute puerperal or postabortional endometritis is dealt with by immediately exploring the uterine cavity, removing all gestational fragments, and thoroughly irrigating with a strong antiseptic. Antitoxic serums or vaccines may be tried. The removal of the uterus is a very fatal proceeding in these cases.

In non-puerperal eases, especially if gonorrhœal, no operation is usually indicated. The patient must be kept in bed, and pain alleviated by fomentations to the abdomen and the administration of sedatives. The vagina should be frequently douched with some mild antiseptic in hot solution, and the bowels kept open by saline aperients. Operative interference is to be avoided, for it might precipitate extension to the tubes.

Where a sloughing tumour is the cause, it must be removed if possible.

CHRONIC ENDOMETRITIS

This is very apt to follow acute infection, because the drainage from the uterine cavity is poor, while the numerous glands readily harbour organisms. In many cases of so-called " endometritis," however, endocervicitis is alone present, the internal os forming a natural barrier to infection.

Pathology.—Two stages may be distinguished—(1) the hypertrophic, (2) the atrophic.

1. In the earlier stage the endometrium is swollen and the interglandular stroma crowded with inflammatory cells. At first these are largely polymorphonuclear leucocytes, but later many lymphocytes, with plasma cells and other forms, appear. The glands are elongated and distended, and their lining epithelium is irregular at first and later hypertrophic. (Fig. 585.) The mucosa is hyperæmic, as is the whole uterus. The endometrial surface may be irregular or even polypoid (*polypoid endometritis*).

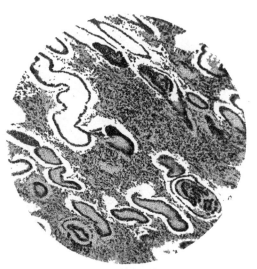

Fig. 585.—Chronic endometritis, hypertrophic stage.

The glands are very large and irregular. The double or treble epithelial contours are due to cross-sections of infoldings of the gland walls. The stroma is full of inflammatory cells.

2. Later the stroma becomes shrunken, fibrous, and much less cellular. The glands atrophy and disappear, or here and there are maintained as retention cysts. (Fig. 586.) The fibrosis extends more or less deeply throughout the whole thickness of the uterine wall, producing the condition known as *fibrotic metritis* (*see* p. 1016).

Clinical features.—The physical signs of the associated chronic endocervicitis are present as well; in addition, the body of the uterus is enlarged, and in the earlier stages is tender and soft, whilst later on it becomes hard and painless.

The menstrual loss is excessive, especially in cases of fibrotic metritis.

Leucorrhœa from the cervix is constant, and the enlarged corporeal glands in the hypertrophic stage also occasion a watery discharge, specially marked just after the " period." The latter is accompanied by an aching, bearing-down pain, referred to the lower abdomen, sacral region and vagina. Dyspareunia may be complained of when the uterus is tender, and conception is unlikely.

There is a variety of the disease known as *senile endometritis*. In old age the uterine mucosa atrophies, nearly all the glands disappear, and the epithelium becomes flattened and often practically squamous. Owing to the absence of glands, the discharge from such a uterus, if infected, is purulent or seropurulent instead of being mucous as usual, and is very apt to become foul. Eventually the endometrium is replaced by a thin layer of red granulation tissue from which occasional small hæmorrhages may occur.

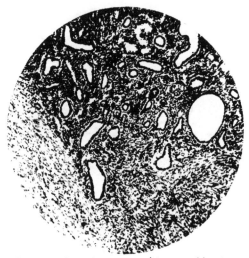

Fig. 586.—Chronic endometritis, atrophic stage.
The stroma is fibrous, and the glands much reduced in size ; some have undergone cystic dilatation.

Treatment. 1. **Drugs and applications.**— Ergot should be given to diminish the hyperæmia of the uterus and to check the excessive menstruation. Applications of iodine, iodized phenol, or carbolic acid may be made to the interior of the uterus, and the general health should be improved by suitable treatment. Soluble vaginal pessaries or tampons soaked in glycerine are sometimes used. Their rationale is doubtful as far as the corporeal inflammation is concerned.

Curettage.—Where definite infection of the uterine cavity is present, the most rational treatment is curettage of the diseased mucosa, the coexistent endocervicitis being treated at the same time, as previously described.

Auvard's self-retaining vaginal retractor having been inserted, the cervix is drawn down with two pairs of volsella forceps, and the direction of the uterine cavity ascertained with the sound. Hegar's graduated uterine dilators up to No. 12 are now passed, the cavity is again sounded, in case the wall has been perforated, the curette inserted, and the mucous membrane erased in strips from above downwards. The cervical canal is then scraped with a sharp spoon and the erosion suitably treated (*see* under Endocervicitis, p. 1011).

Where very marked evidence of infection is present, especially if gonorrhœal, the operation may be concluded by swabbing out the uterus with iodine or iodized phenol.

The dangers of curettage are perforation of the uterus either by a dilator or by the curette, and postoperative sepsis.

Other methods of treatment.—Curettage may fail, or only succeed temporarily. In fibrotic endometritis, and still more in diffuse fibrotic metritis (p. 1016), the curette removes nothing, and does little good. In gonorrhœal cases the infection may be very persistent.

In such circumstances, the operation may be repeated, and the uterus swabbed out with chloride of zinc (30 gr. to an ounce), or with pure nitric acid applied through a glass tube, but these measures are not without risk. To the same end superheated steam has been applied with a special apparatus (atmocausis).

When severe menorrhagia persists in spite of a thorough trial of styptic drugs and properly performed curettage, and particularly when the curette scrapes hard and rough without removing any appreciable amount of tissue, diffuse fibrotic metritis is probably present. In such cases the best treatment is hysterectomy (p. 1022).

PYOMETRA

Distension of the uterus with pus occurs sometimes in senile endometritis, the cervix being stenosed by atrophy. It is also seen in the later stages of cervical carcinoma. The uterus is soft and enlarged, and, viewed from the abdominal aspect, presents a number of dilated capillaries on its surface. Fever and pain may be present, but some cases show very few symptoms. The condition is only discovered on the escape of thick greenish pus when the sound is passed.

Treatment.—Carcinoma, if present, must be eradicated, if possible. In senile endometritis vaginal hysterectomy is the best proceeding, but curettage and strong iodine solution may first be tried.

TUBERCULOUS ENDOMETRITIS

In this rare affection the mucosa is greatly thickened by diffuse cell proliferation, amidst which giant cells are found. The condition is sometimes found post mortem in persons dead of tubercle elsewhere. Often there have been no symptoms. In other cases, irregular bleeding and offensive discharge have led to a diagnosis of carcinoma. Treatment consists in removal of the uterus.

ENDOMETRIAL HYPERTROPHY

Hypertrophy of the endometrium may follow non-infective chronic uterine enlargement and hypervascularity, particularly that caused by myomas. In such cases the mucous membrane exhibits a diffuse hypertrophy, differing from that of endometritis in the absence of inflammatory cells. Cervicitis and cervical erosion are not present. A watery discharge more marked after the menstrual period is the characteristic symptom. It comes from the enlarged uterine glands. Menorrhagia is also present. Removal of the thickened mucosa by the curette is indicated if no tumour of the uterus exists. Where a myoma is present, either myomectomy or hysterectomy is called for. Curettage of a myomatous uterus may produce degeneration or infective necrosis of the tumour, and in any circumstances is likely to fail.

FIBROTIC METRITIS (UTERINE FIBROSIS)

Within the last few years a pathological condition of the uterine wall has been distinguished, characterized by diffuse fibrous overgrowth and corresponding muscular degeneration. Its causation is not known in all cases, but the most marked examples are secondary to long-continued endometritis. In others it is possibly the ultimate outcome of subinvolution after labour or abortion, whilst in a third group a primary cirrhosis of vascular origin appears probable.

Macroscopically, the uterus is usually somewhat enlarged and very hard, and from its cut· surface a number of thick-walled and inelastic vessels project. Microscopically, diffuse fibrosis is seen, especially under and in the endometrium, which is shrunken and hard, and in the worst cases ecchymosed. The vessels have largely lost their muscular tunic, and in places are converted into sinus-like channels without definite coats.

Symptoms.—Profuse and intractable menstrual hæmorrhage from a uterus but slightly enlarged and not deformed is the characteristic symptom. The loss may become almost continuous, and the patient intensely anæmic.

Diagnosis.—Absolute diagnosis is impossible until the uterine cavity has been explored, for similar profuse losses may be caused by intra-uterine polyps, or small sessile myomas or adeno-myomas. In fibrosis the cavity is empty, and the curette scrapes hard and rough on the sclerotic surface. A characteristic feature is the inability of ergot or other styptic drugs to control the hæmorrhage, owing to the degeneracy of the uterine musculature. Many cases are repeatedly and uselessly curetted before the true diagnosis is made.

Treatment.—Hysterectomy is usually necessary, total if the cervix is unhealthy. In doubtful cases a thorough curetting should first be tried.

In young women an alternative to hysterectomy is " utriculoplasty," as practised by Kelly and myself. The operation consists in excising a wedge-shaped portion of the whole thickness of the uterine wall, the base at the fundus and the apex at the internal os, followed by suture of the two moieties to one another, so as to form a miniature uterus or " utriculus." There is a risk, however, of the hæmorrhage returning, which should be explained to the patient before the operation. My first case has had two pregnancies subsequently to the operation.

NEW GROWTHS OF THE UTERUS

CYSTS OF THE CERVIX

Cervical cysts are always inflammatory in origin, and only occasionally attain the size of a walnut. The treatment is that appropriate to chronic cervicitis. When large, the cyst should be excised, or the vaginal cervix amputated.

POLYPUS OF THE CERVIX

Pathology.—Four varieties of cervical polypus are found :

1. The *adenomatous polypus* is a pedunculated, very vascular, inflammatory excrescence of the cervical mucous membrane. It is covered with a short columnar epithelium, and presents a number of racemose glands. surrounded by a cellular stroma. It is bright red in colour and is never larger than an almond.

2. The *cystic polypus* is similarly derived and constructed, but the glands have undergone cystic dilatation. (Fig. 587.) These polypi, therefore, are much larger, often lobulated, and are pale and semi-translucent in appearance. They are uncommon. Both this and the last variety are collectively known as " mucous polyps."

3. The *myomatous polypus* is a sessile submucous cervical myoma which gradually becomes pedunculated. It is hard, smooth, and pink, and may attain a large size.

4. *Sarcomatous polypi* are, fortunately, rare, and such as have been studied have been of the small round-celled or mixed-celled variety. They are soft, irregular in outline, reddish-white in colour, and bleed profusely.

Symptoms.—A glandular cervical polypus gives rise to irregular losses of blood, especially after manipulation or coitus, from the numerous capillaries contained in the tumour. The symptoms of cervicitis are invariably coexistent.

A myomatous polypus of the cervix may occasion no symptoms, and is sometimes discovered accidentally, for since the corpus is uninvolved, menorrhagia is not associated with it, as with myomas higher up. The tumours, when large, may occasion discomfort by their size. They are prone to necrosis, owing to the precariousness of a blood supply conveyed through a narrow pedicle, and may then cause a very foul discharge with constitutional symptoms. They may separate spontaneously.

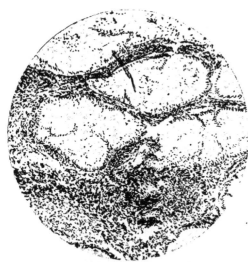

Fig. 587.—Cystic mucous polyp.

The glands are dilated and full of retained secretion. The columnar epithelium lining them is degenerate.

Sarcomatous polypi give rise to continued bleeding, and later to signs of generalized metastasis.

Treatment.–Glandular and cystic polyps should be evulsed and the cervical canal well scraped with a sharp spoon. Myomatous polyps may also be evulsed if small; otherwise they should be treated by the methods described at p. 1042. If the polyp is sarcomatous, radical extirpation of the uterus is indicated.

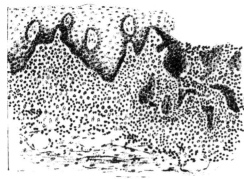

Fig. 588.—Early carcinomatous ulcer of the cervix.

CARCINOMA OF THE CERVIX

Etiology.—Carcinoma of the cervix is commonest between the ages of 40 and 50. It is very rarely seen before 30, and occurs with lessening frequency from 50 up to old age.

The disease bears a remarkable relationship to

childbearing, and is most uncommon in undoubted virgins. This is due to the fact that carcinoma of the cervix is superimposed on cervical "erosion."

Pathology. — Two forms of carcinoma are met with in the cervix, the squamous-celled and the columnar-celled. The first is by far the more common, the malignant epithelial cells being derived from the interpapillary down-growths of the hypertrophied epithelium that covers the erosion. (Figs. 588 and 589.) It is in the third stage of an erosion that carcinoma is most likely to occur (*see* p. 1009).

The columnar-celled growth is derived from the glandular elements of the cervix, and represents about 2 per cent. of the total number of cases.

Histologically, the squamous-celled type presents a number of masses of oval cells closely packed in alveolar spaces between the cervical tissues. These cells usually show no tendency to keratinize, and cell nests are uncommon. (Fig. 589.)

From the primary growth extension occurs both by

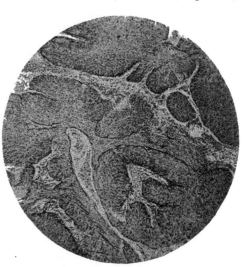

Fig. 589.—Squamous-celled carcinoma of the cervix.

The cells lie in masses closely packed. There is no keratinization or cell-nest formation.

lymphatic permeation and by infiltration. The lymphatic tract first affected, as a rule, is that extending outwards below the uterine artery towards the pelvic wall, from which it ascends to communicate with the lymphatics and glands between the external iliac artery and vein.

These glands, together with others irregularly scattered in the broad ligament, are, therefore, the earliest affected by metastatic growth. It is, however, remarkable that in more than half of the patients dying of the disease no glandular involvement is found on autopsy (Leitch). In this respect, therefore, carcinoma of the cervix is much less malignant than carcinoma in many other parts of the body. Glandular enlargement, when found, is not necessarily carcinomatous, for the invasion of a lymphatic gland by carcinoma is preceded by inflammatory enlargement.[1]

Metastatic growths other than those in lymphatic glands are rare.

Infiltrative growth, as opposed to permeation of trunk lymphatics, occurs in several directions. Anteriorly, the vaginal vault and the bladder become in time involved. Posteriorly, extension occurs along the utero-sacral folds, the posterior vaginal vault, and the recto-vaginal septum. Laterally, the carcinoma spreads into the broad ligament,

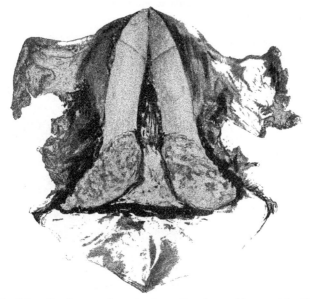

Fig. 590.—Carcinoma of cervix, fungating type. Removed by the radical abdominal operation.

at first displacing the ureter outwards and subsequently involving it. Downwards, the growth involves the vagina.

The disease, even in the latest stages, practically never extends above the internal os. In advanced cases chronic salpingitis is usually found, due to ascending infection. Pyometra is not uncommon.

Symptoms.—The earliest symptom in most cases is hæmorrhage, at first slight or intermittent, and provoked by coitus, examination, or douching, but later continuous, and sometimes very free. Discharge other than blood is then noticed ; it is watery in character, and usually peculiarly offensive. Occasionally it may be the first

[1] *See* the author's Hunterian Lectures, R.C.S., 1900.

symptom. Pain usually supervenes later, is of a continuous gnawing type, and is referred to the lower part of the back and thighs.

Where the hæmorrhage is severe, great anæmia follows, but, apart from this, most patients present more or less cachexia. Occasionally, however, the face is fat and ruddy, almost to the close. In the later stages of the disease, fistulæ form between the vagina and the bladder and rectum. Death is due most commonly to suppression of urine, following blockage of both ureters and bilateral hydronephrosis; in other cases, to exhaustion from loss of blood, or to toxic absorption.

The duration of the disease, from the earliest symptoms to death,

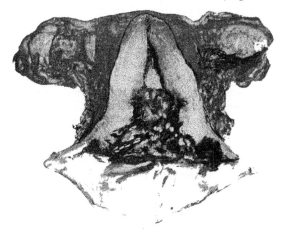

Fig. 591.—Carcinoma of cervix, ulcerative type. Removed by the radical abdominal operation.

in patients unoperated upon, is on an average one year and nine months (Leitch). Its progress is much slower in old women than in the young.

There are four common **clinical types** of the disease:

(1) In the *fungating* variety the growth forms a large irregular excrescence which, sprouting from the cervix, fills the vaginal vault ("*cauliflower excrescence*"). The bleeding is usually profuse, but the tendency to infiltration and lymphatic permeation is less than in the other varieties. (Fig. 590.)

(2) The *ulcerative* form presents as a deep excavation with rugged and friable sides, occupying the position of the cervical canal. In these cases the discharge is particularly foul. (Fig. 591.)

(3) In the *massive infiltrative* type the vaginal cervix is much enlarged and indurated. Little can be seen on inspection, but blood persistently oozes from the external os.

(4) In the *senile atrophic* variety the vaginal cervix has disappeared, and is replaced by a depression at the top of the vagina, from which blood oozes. No mass or ulcer may be felt, and the real condition is easily overlooked.

Diagnosis.—When the disease is well established, the freely bleeding friable mass, fungating or excavated, can scarcely be mistaken. The massive infiltrative form is more difficult to diagnose. The size and induration of the cervix, not less than its tendency to bleed, should awaken suspicion. Allusion has already been made to the slight physical signs of the senile atrophic form.

A quite early case of carcinoma of the cervix is rarely seen. Such cases present either a small reddish nodule or an irregular ulcer, difficult to distinguish from the " erosion " on which the growth is beginning.

The surface of an erosion, though perhaps irregular and hard, is never friable, and though it may sometimes be made to bleed by rough handling, yet any pronounced tendency to hæmorrhage immediately suggests carcinoma. The diagnosis of early cervical carcinoma is often impossible without the aid of the microscope. Therefore, all suspicious cases should be immediately examined under an anæsthetic and a portion of the suspected tissue removed for investigation. The comparative rarity with which patients seek advice in the early stages of the disease is due to their ignorance of the significance of irregular uterine hæmorrhage. The popular delusion that the premenopausal period is normally associated with excessive or continued bleeding cannot be too strongly combated, nor the idea that the absence of pain negatives a malady of any importance. It is, further, of the highest necessity that practitioners should insist on a vaginal examination before treating any case of genital hæmorrhage.

Treatment.—All cases in the operable stage should be promptly dealt with by surgical measures. The disease may be attacked from the vaginal or the abdominal route.

Vaginal hysterectomy. *Standard of operability.*—Simple vaginal hysterectomy is only applicable when the growth is limited to the cervix, when sufficient of the cervix remains to get a hold upon, and when the uterus is sufficiently movable to permit of its being pulled well down towards the vaginal outlet. Induration of the broad ligaments or utero-sacral folds, or extension of the growth on to the vagina, bars the operation.

Not more than 15 per cent. of the cases are seen in this early stage.

The operation.—The growth having been scraped and cauterized, and the limit of the bladder on the vaginal vault ascertained, the mucous membrane covering the cervix is circumcised at its junction with that of the vault. The bladder is then separated from the supra-vaginal cervix by scissors and swab pressure until the peritoneum at the bottom of the utero-vesical pouch is reached. This is then opened. The cervix being now pulled forwards, the utero-rectal pouch is opened behind it. The uterus is then pulled down and, the pulsations of the uterine artery having been defined, the base of either broad ligament is transfixed above the vessel, ligatured and divided. The uterus, now much more mobile, is pulled farther down, and the upper part of the broad ligament with the ovary, ovarico-pelvic ligament, tube and round ligament on either side is included in a couple of ligatures and divided. The vaginal vault is partly closed, and the aperture remaining into the peritoneal cavity lightly plugged with gauze.

When access to the upper part of the broad ligaments is difficult, it may be facilitated by anteflexing the uterine body. Sometimes it is better simply to clamp the broad ligaments in sections before dividing them, and to apply the ligatures afterwards.

Advantages and disadvantages.—The advantages of vaginal hysterectomy are its ease in most cases, and its low mortality (about 6 per cent.). But not more than 15 per cent. of the cases are suitable, and of these a very large proportion suffer from recurrence within a year.

Radical hystero-vaginectomy by paravaginal section. *Standard of operability.*—Access to the pelvis from below can be much facilitated by performing paravaginal section. This consists in making an incision along the junction of the left lateral and posterior vaginal walls, which, dividing the skin of the perineum on the left side, sweeps round the rectum towards the coccyx. The anterior fibres of the left levator ani are severed and a large gap is effected, through which a much more extensive operation is possible.

It is better in carcinoma of the cervix to remove the whole vagina with the uterus, and in this case it is first separated from the skin and its end sewn up so as to exclude the disease from the area of the operation. It is then dissected free of the bladder in front, the rectum behind, and the cellular tissue laterally, before the paravaginal section is performed.

The remaining steps are similar to those of vaginal hysterectomy, except that the ureters are clearly defined and pushed aside, so that the bases of the broad ligaments may be ligatured and divided far out towards the pelvic side wall.

Advantages and disadvantages.—By paravaginal section about 40 per cent. of the cases are operable. Infiltration of the vaginal vault or moderate extension into the broad ligaments or utero-sacral folds does not contra-indicate the operation, but extension to the bladder or rectum or massive infiltration around the ureter renders it impossible. It has the disadvantage that it is impossible to examine the regional glands until the operation has been practically concluded, and in any event they cannot be removed by this route.

The immediate mortality is somewhat lower than that of the radical abdominal operation, but the convalescence is protracted, the deep hole which is left taking weeks to granulate up, and frequently sloughing badly.

Radical abdominal hystero-vaginectomy (Wertheim's operation).—This operation aims at removing the uterus, together with the upper third or half of the vagina, in such a way that the cervix is encapsuled by the latter, across which a clamp has been placed before amputation. Together with the uterus are also removed the appendages, broad ligaments, and as much as possible of the pelvic cellular tissue and regional glands.

Standard of operability.—So long as the growth has not extensively involved the bladder or rectum, or absolutely fixed the uterus in the pelvis, its removal is possible by this method. That the cervix cannot be pulled down is of no moment, if it can be pushed up.

It is often impossible to be certain that the fixation of the uterus is due to carcinomatous infiltration, because similar physical signs may be produced by the chronic salpingitis which commonly accompanies advanced growth. In estimating the degree of involvement of the bladder or ureter, the cystoscope may prove useful. In cases of doubt, examination under an anæsthetic is advisable, and if the possibility of eradication is still undecided the abdomen should be opened and the condition explored from above.

By Wertheim's method between 60 and 75 per cent. of all the cases seen are operable, according to the views of the individual surgeon.

The operation.—The growth, if foul or fungating, is first thoroughly scraped and cauterized. The abdomen is then opened, either immediately or a couple of weeks later, and the ovarico-pelvic and round ligaments on either side are ligatured and divided at the pelvic brim. The peritoneum is now incised across the front of the uterus at the limit of its loose attachment, and by swab pressure, aided by cautious snips, the bladder is pushed off the supravaginal cervix and the upper inch of the anterior vaginal wall.

The ureter of one side is now felt for as it runs in close attachment to the posterior peritoneum of the broad ligament, and its direction onwards having been ascertained, the uterine artery is sought outside this line, is lifted by pressure forceps, and is divided and ligatured as far outwards as possible. By tracing the distal portion of this vessel inwards the point at which it crosses the ureter is attained. From this point onwards the ureter is separated up to its entry into the bladder. Care must be taken not to injure the periureteral sheath. The other ureter is then similarly treated.

The uterus being pulled well forwards, the peritoneum at the bottom of Douglas's pouch is incised and the rectum separated from the vagina. The utero-sacral folds are then divided, the ureter being protected by the fingers during the process. The uterus is now principally tethered by the strong lateral cervico-pelvic ligaments that sweep out on either side under the ureters like a pair of buttresses. The ureters being held out of the way, these ligaments are clamped by angular forceps and divided. The uterus riding up, the bladder is still further separated from the vagina until the latter can be clamped well below the limit of the growth. For this purpose the Berkeley-Bonney vaginal clamp (Fig. 592) will be found the most convenient. The vagina is divided below the clamp either with the cautery knife or with a scalpel. All bleeding-points and previously-clamped tissues are ligatured, and the operator then proceeds to ablate such of the parametric and paravaginal tissue as has escaped removal with the uterus. The most important part of this is a sheet of tissue against the side wall of the pelvis at the upper border of which runs

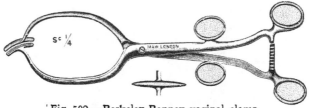

Fig. 592.—Berkeley-Bonney vaginal clamp.

the obliterated hypogastric artery. When this sheet is removed the obturator fossa and the glands there are exposed. The latter should be removed. The glands along the iliac arteries are then stripped off, whether enlarged or not, and all bleeding is finally arrested. The vagina is left open for drainage, and the operation completed by sewing the anterior peritoneal flap to the front of the rectum and back of the pelvis. Inability to empty the bladder always follows the operation for a few weeks, but never persists.

Advantages and disadvantages.—The surgeon can inspect the condition from above, and proceed no further if he finds the operation impracticable; he can excise the whole adjacent lymphatic tract with the primary growth; by removing the growth encapsuled in the upper part of the vagina he minimizes operative cancer infection; the possibility of removal is greater, and the number of patients alive five years afterwards is higher than by any other method.

Against these advantages may be set the high primary mortality of the operation—about 18 per cent. for all cases, and the troublesome complications, such as ureteral, vesical, or rectal fistulæ, that sometimes follow it. In estimating the mortality, however, the enormously

3 n

increased operability rate, as compared with vaginal hysterectomy, must be taken into account. Comyns Berkeley, in an exhaustive paper, has shown that if the cases be classified according to the stage of the disease at the time of operation, the mortality figures are— early, 6·3 per cent. ; advanced, 23·1 per cent. The mortality of the operation, therefore, as applied to early cases, i.e. those which might have been dealt with by vaginal hysterectomy, is about the same as that of the latter operation.

The difficulties of the procedure increase greatly in advanced cases, and are especially formidable in very stout women. Moreover, the hospital patients in whom the disease is most commonly met are from

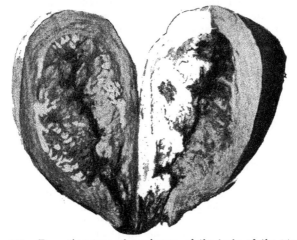

Fig. 593.—Fungating type of carcinoma of the body of the uterus.

the surgical standpoint a most unsatisfactory class, most of them being enfeebled and prematurely aged by a life of hardship and want. In a large proportion the heart is fatty or the kidneys are degenerate.

The ultimate results of the operation must at present be estimated from Continental figures, for it has not been practised sufficiently long in Great Britain. According to Wertheim, nearly 60 per cent. of those operated upon by him were alive five years afterwards. Allowing for a wide margin on results so remarkable as these, British surgeons would be satisfied with 20 per cent. of cures, which would still be an enormous advance on the results of vaginal hysterectomy.

The operation must not, however, be judged solely by the permanent cures effected, for, remembering that these patients, when they first seek advice, have, on an average, less than eighteen unhappy months to live if the disease be left to run its course, the gain of even a year of health and hope is a great boon.

Treatment of inoperable cases.—Where the growth is irremovable, considerable benefit sometimes follows a thorough scraping and cauterization, or the application of pure acetone by a tubular speculum especially in foul, fungating cases. Frequent douching with crude sanitas (1 oz. to a pint) restrains the fetor. To allay pain, aspirin in 10-gr. doses should at first be tried ; later, phenacetin is useful. Morphia should be reserved until the latest possible period.

CARCINOMA OF THE BODY OF THE UTERUS

Etiology.— This disease is rare in women under 45. Its maximum incidence occurs between the years from 50 to 60—i.e. during or soon after the menopause— after which it is met with in lessening frequency. It is much less common than carcinoma of the cervix, and contrasts

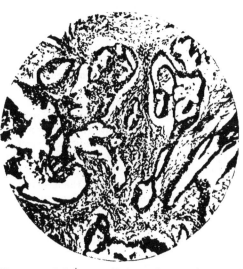

Fig. 594.—Columnar-celled tubular carcinoma of the body of the uterus.

The tubules are irregular, and in many the epithelium is several cells thick.

markedly with it in that it has no relation to marriage and childbearing.

Pathology.—There are two macroscopic forms—the fungating and the ulcerative. In the first, the organ is enlarged and its cavity is filled by a soft pulpy growth sprouting from the wall (Fig. 593); in the second, the uterus may be quite small, though its interior is excavated by a diffuse ulceration, the surface of which is irregular and friable. Microscopically the neoplasm is most often a columnar-celled adeno-carcinoma (Fig. 594), but in senile patients, in whom the corporeal epithelium has undergone degenerative flattening, a keratinizing squamous - celled growth may occur. Lymphatic permeation follows the course of the ovarian vessels, and primarily reaches the lumbar and aortic glands.

Symptoms.—Persistent hæmorrhage and watery discharge are first noticed, but pain is often an early symptom. Fetor occurs relatively later than in cervical carcinoma. On examination the uterus may be found moderately enlarged and soft, whilst in many cases the cervix is so patulous that the finger passed through it detects the soft growth above. In other cases, however, the diagnosis can only be established after dilatation of the canal, digital exploration, and removal of a portion of tissue for microscopical examination.

Later, diffuse peritoneal and omental metastasis occurs, or the patient succumbs to massive growth in the lumbar glands or multiple nodules in the liver or lungs. In either case, irregular nodules and lumps will be felt through the abdominal wall.

Diagnosis.—Corporeal carcinoma is the commonest cause of post-menopausal bleeding. Senile endometritis sometimes gives rise to slight irregular hæmorrhages, but the discharge is principally pus. It is, however, to be remembered that this form of endometritis is the common precursor of carcinoma of the corpus. Before the menopause patients are apt to attribute the symptoms to that event ; the fatal results of this error have already been mentioned (*see* p. 1022). The diagnosis may be obscured by the presence of a uterine myoma, but continuous loss is not characteristic of these tumours. All cases of persistent hæmorrhage at or about the menopause should be immediately investigated, the uterus being explored under an anæsthetic if necessary.

Treatment.—If there is no evidence of metastatic growth the entire uterus with both appendages should be immediately removed. This is best accomplished through an abdominal incision, but in very stout women, with a uterus scarcely or not at all enlarged, the vaginal route may be chosen.

The after-results of hysterectomy for corporeal are far better than those for cervical carcinoma.

For inoperable cases the treatment is similar to that for inoperable carcinoma of the cervix (p. 1027).

CHORION-EPITHELIOMA

This rare and interesting growth is derived from the fœtal trophoblast. It usually follows abortion or labour after an interval of but one or two months, but occasionally does not declare itself for a much longer period. It is peculiarly associated with vesicular moles, and all gradations between that condition and pure chorion-epithelioma have been found. Though usually primary in the uterus, it has originated in the tube after tubal gestation. A number of cases are also on record of primary vaginal growth, elements of the trophoblast having migrated there from the gestation site and initiated the tumour. Its occurrence in teratomas will be referred to later (p. 1074).

Pathology.—The tumour has a characteristic deep blood colour. Microscopically it presents three types of cell—(1) closely set hyaline mononucleated cells identical with the Langhans cells of the normal chorionic villus ; (2) larger cells of the same type laden with granules ; and (3) large multinucleated masses of protoplasm (syncytia) similar to those seen on the periphery of the villus of an early gestation. These cells are embedded in masses of fibrin and extensive blood extravasa-

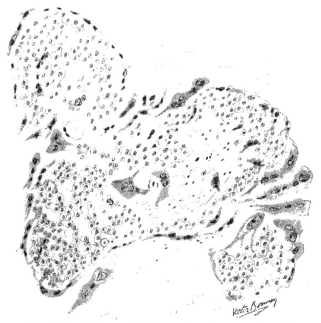

Fig. 595.—Chorion-epithelioma, showing syncytia and Langhans' cells.

tions. The microscopic appearance of a chorion-epithelioma (Fig. 595) is exactly that of the tissues at the growing margin of an early gestation. Modern research shows, indeed, that in the process of the embedding of the human ovum its trophoblast acts practically as a malignant tissue, destroying the maternal tissue with which it comes in contact. Normally, this infiltrative power is arrested after the first few weeks of the life of the gestation ; occasionally, however, it persists and leads to malignant growth.

Metastasis occurs with great rapidity, pulmonary nodules being particularly common.

Symptoms and diagnosis.—The symptoms are hæmorrhage, foul discharge, rapid uterine enlargement, and often fever. Inasmuch as in most cases abortion or labour has occurred quite recently, the symptoms simulate those of retention of conception products, but the true diagnosis should be suggested by the enlargement of the uterus, and confirmed by a microscopical examination of the uterine contents.

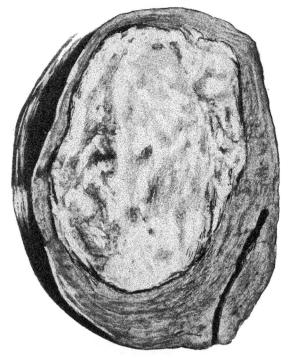

Fig. 596.—Large interstititial myoma undergoing œdematous degeneration.

Treatment.—The fullest possible extirpation of the uterus, adnexa, and broad ligaments, with the upper part of the vagina, is indicated. Cases of spontaneous disappearance are on record, but as a rule the growth is among the most malignant known.

MYOMA (FIBROIDS)

Myomas are by far the commonest tumours affecting the uterus. Rare before 30, after that age they are met with in increasing frequency up to the menopause. It is very doubtful if they ever originate *de novo* after this epoch. Their cause is unknown, but is probably related in some way to sterility, since they are rare in women who have borne children early in life. On the other hand, their presence is in varying degree a bar to conception.

Morbid anatomy.—Myomas occur in three main sites—(1) the uterine body, (2) the cervix, and (3) the broad ligament. They are, however, rarely solitary, so that the various forms are often combined.

1. **Corporeal myomas.**—It is customary to divide these myomas into three groups, according to whether they arise in the midst of the musculature of the uterine wall (*interstitial myomas*), or under its mucosal or peritoneal surfaces respectively (*submucous* and *subperitoneal myomas*).

An interstitial myoma of any size bulges both inwards and outwards. The surrounding uterine musculature is much hypertrophied, so that the organ, quite apart from the tumour, is much larger than normal. The cavity is correspondingly enlarged. (Fig. 596.)

Submucous myomas bulge on the mucosal surface only. The uterus is uniformly enlarged over them and its cavity is much increased. All submucous myomas are at first sessile, but small tumours often become polypoid.

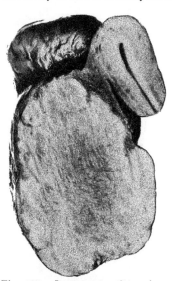

Fig. 597.—Large subperitoneal pedunculated myoma, growing from the posterior wall of the uterus.

Subperitoneal myomas are also at first sessile, but as they grow they tend to become pedunculated, so that a very large tumour is frequently attached to the uterus by quite a narrow stalk. The uterus is not enlarged by a subperitoneal myoma, but, inasmuch as it may form the peduncle of a large tumour, its vascularity may be much increased. (Fig. 597.)

2. **Cervical myomas.**—About 6 per cent. of all uterine myomas grow in the cervix. These tumours, when large and growing interstitially or under the mucous membrane, cause a very characteristic elevation of the uterine body on the top of them. (Fig. 598.) The cervical canal is immensely elongated, and the broad ligaments and bladder are undermined and stretched. A cervical myoma developing on the front of the cervix (Fig. 599) burrows under the bladder and

raises it out of the pelvis; while one growing from its back (Fig. 600) may undermine the peritoneum at the bottom of Douglas's pouch and gradually obliterate the pouch altogether. Cervical myomas growing laterally invade the broad ligament.

3. **Broad-ligament myomas.** — Tumours growing laterally from the side of the corpus or cervix expand the broad ligament. These are not truly *of* the broad ligament. There are several tracts of unstriped muscle in the mesometrium from which true broad-ligament tumours may originate. (Fig. 601.) Thus, myomas of the ovarico·uterine and round ligaments occur. Others are found occasionally springing from the muscle fibres that accompany the ovarian or uterine vessels. These may attain a large size, and, after distending the broad ligament to its fullest capacity, mount up into the abdomen by stripping the peritoneum off its posterior and lateral parietes. The pelvic colon thereby comes to lie sessile on the mass, while the uterus is forced to the opposite side. The ureter is displaced inwards with the peritoneum except in the rare cases of lateral cervical myomas growing very low down, when it may be raised bodily on the top of the tumour.

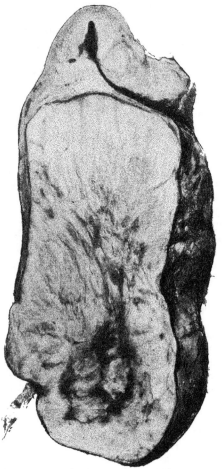

Fig. 598.—Typical central cervical myoma. The body of the uterus is raised on the tumour.

Pathology.—A uterine myoma in its earliest stage presents as a little white nodule embedded in the musculature. Structurally, it consists of densely interlaced unstriped muscle fibres united by some connective tissue. (Fig. 602.) It contains but a few small vessels, derived from the adjacent uterine wall, which surrounds the tumour in concentric layers and forms its capsule.

As the tumour enlarges, the uterine wall around it hypertrophies, and assumes the stratified appearance which characterizes the museulature of the pregnant uterus.

The microscopical structure of a " normal " myoma is identical with that of t h e muscular uterine wall itself, except that it does not contain considerable vessels. Such a tumour takes years to attain large size.

Owing probably to their poor vascular supply, myomas are particularly prone to degenerate ; to this more than to any other factor the serious symptoms are due.

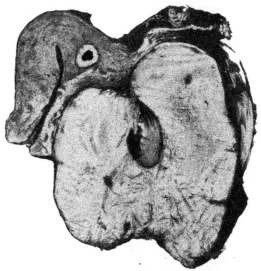

Fig. 599.—Anterior cervical myoma undermining the peritoneum of the utero-vesical pouch. A small interstitial tumour is also present.

These degenerations must be considered in detail, as follows :—

Fibrotic degeneration.—Characterized by increase in the white fibrous elements of the tumour and disappearance of the muscle tissue. The tumour becomes very white and hard, and ceases to grow (*fibro-myoma*).

Calcareous degeneration.—Usually a senile change. The calcific deposit may begin centrally or peripherally. The tumour becomes stony hard and, of course, ceases to grow. The change is most apt to affect pedunculated subperitoneal tumours in old age, and is not entirely beneficent, for the rough surface may set up chronic peritonitis around it.

Œdematous degeneration.—An œdematous swelling affects the interstitial connective tissue, and the muscle fibres degenerate. The tumour becomes pulpy and soft, and rapidly enlarges (*see* Fig. 596).

Myxomatoid degeneration.—This is by some regarded as an advanced stage of the last form. Centrally, the tumour is converted into a yellow-green jelly-like substance. True mucin is not present.

Cystic degeneration.—This, again, is probably a further stage of softening. Usually only one cavity is present, but there may be several. When the change is complete the resemblance to an ovarian cyst is considerable. (Fig. 603.)

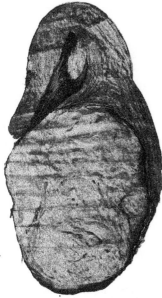

All the last three forms of degeneration are frequently accompanied by chronic peritonitis in the neighbourhood of the tumour.

Red degeneration.—The tumour here exhibits varying tints, from pink up to mahogany-brown. The change is considered due to thrombosis of the vessels supplying the area, and is therefore analogous to " red " infarction. In some cases, however, the coloration is due to free pigment, probably hæmatogenous ; and it is often intensified on exposure to the air. The degeneration has frequently been recorded in connexion with pregnancy, and is characterized by the sudden onset of pain in the tumour.

Fig. 600.—Posterior cervical myoma. The uterus also contains a small submucous polypoid myoma.

Nævoid degeneration.—Occasionally a myoma becomes very vascular, a number of thin-walled blood spaces developing in the tumour. The vessels of the tumour capsule in particular become very large, and the whole uterus is at last covered with large varicosities. These tumours grow very fast, and enlarge at each menstrual period ; on auscultation a murmur is heard over them. The general likeness to pregnancy is often considerable.

"Caseous" degeneration.—A rare change, in which the myoma undergoes a transformation into a substance resembling adipocere. This is not a true caseation.

Sarcomatous degeneration.—About 2 per cent. of all myomas are said to undergo sarcomatous change. Myo-sarcoma, round-, spindle-, and mixed-celled sarcoma, angio-sarcoma, and endothelioma are all on record. The prognosis of these transformed myomas is better than that of primary sarcomas.

Carcinoma of a myomatous uterus.—There is a considerable

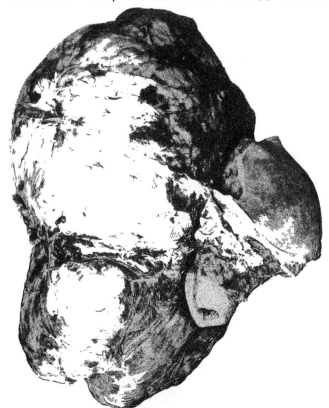

Fig. 601.—Broad-ligament myoma, with the uterus, unenlarged, to the right.

amount of evidence showing that myomas predispose to the development of corporeal carcinoma, but cervical carcinoma complicating a myomatous uterus is very rare. (Fig. 604.)

Symptoms.—The symptoms of uterine myomas may be divided into four groups—(1) menstrual symptoms, (2) pressure symptoms, (3) degeneration symptoms, and (4) symptoms due to certain complications and accidents.

1. **Menstrual symptoms.**—Menorrhàgia is the most constant symptom. It is due partly to the increased size of the menstrual area, partly to the augmented vascularity of the uterus, and partly to unknown causes. For the menstrual period is increased not only in quantity and duration, but often also in frequency, and, further, a small submucous nodule may produce hæmorrhage far in excess of that caused by a much larger mass in exactly the same position in another patient. The menorrhagia usually begins insidiously and steadily increases. Patients have generally so suffered for some years before seeking advice.

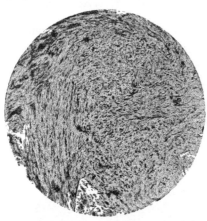

Fig. 602.—Uterine myoma, consisting almost entirely of unstriped muscle fibres running in various directions.

Submucous myomas produce the most severe loss, while the subperitoneal variety may cause no alteration in the periods, the uterus

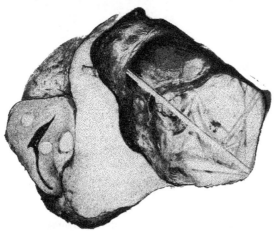

Fig. 603.—Broad-ligament myoma that has undergone cystic degeneration. The uterus is pushed to the left, and contains several smaller tumours.

proper not being enlarged. Menorrhagia with a large subperitoneal myoma suggests the coexistence of a small submucous nodule. Cervical myomas are, however, often associated with very severe loss, although they do not involve the menstrual area proper.

Patients thus afflicted become very anæmic, and eventually develop cachexia associated with breathlessness and cardiac degeneration. Dysmenorrhœa is not a common symptom. When present it is of the

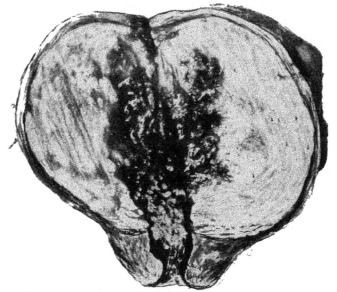

Fig. 604.—Carcinoma of the body of a myomatous uterus.

obstructive variety, and consists in violent spasms of pain associated with the passage of clots from the uterus.

2. **Pressure symptoms.**—These, when severe, are generally due to impaction of the tumour in the pelvis. Cervical myomas are particularly prone to this complication. A myomatous uterus, like a pregnant one, may become retroverted and incarcerated.

The bladder is usually the first organ to exhibit symptoms of pressure, generally in the form of frequency of micturition ; retention is less common and, when present, implies impaction.

Pressure on the ureter is much rarer than might be supposed, but in cases of prolonged impaction these conduits are found dilated.

The bowel is less frequently occluded by pressure than by kinking due to displacement or adhesions. Partial intestinal obstruction is not uncommon, but acute symptoms are comparatively rare.

Very large tumours may press upon the vena cava and produce œdema of the legs, or may distend the abdomen sufficiently to embarrass respiration.

3. **Degeneration symptoms.**—One feature alone is common to most degenerated myomas, viz., tenderness supplants the insensitiveness of the " normal " tumour. If the degeneration be œdematous, myxomatous, or cystic, the tumour rapidly increases in size. The sudden onset of pain characteristic of red degeneration has already been mentioned. In many forms of degeneration slight fever is manifested.

The supervention of carcinoma in the body of a myomatous uterus is characterized by the hæmorrhage becoming continuous instead of periodic.

Sarcomatous degeneration is accompanied by severe hæmorrhage, rapid bossy enlargement of the tumour, ascites, and emaciation.

4. **Symptoms due to complications and accidents.**—*Inflammation* of a myoma is usually caused by infection from the uterine cavity. This very serious complication especially follows labour and abortion, and presents the signs of acute local peritonitis, which later may become generalized. An infected myoma usually undergoes necrosis, and, if submucous, may slough out.

Salpingitis is a common complication, and produces its usual symptoms. It is, as a rule, of the chronic type, the tubes being thickened or distended with clear fluid. Occasionally, owing to regurgitation of menstrual blood, a double hæmatosalpinx is present, and especially with cervical myomas. Pyosalpinx is less frequent (*see* p. 1048).

Ovarian cysts so frequently complicate uterine myomas that no wise diagnostician would often pledge himself that the ovaries were undoubtedly sound. Many masses thought to be purely myomatous are found at operation to be partly ovarian, and vice versa.

Extrusion of a myoma is commonest with a polypoid submucous tumour, but may follow injury or ulceration of the capsule of a sessile one, and is then a septic process from the beginning. Extrusion produces severe, painful, colicky, uterine contractions and free hæmorrhage, accompanied, if the tumour be infected or sloughing, by fever and foul discharge. (Fig. 605.)

Axial rotation of a pedunculated subperitoneal myoma is characterized by sudden violent pain recurring at intervals, tenderness and rapid enlargement of the tumour, and the early development of local peritonitis. Occasionally the uterus itself partakes in the torsion. Such cases present severe shock and profuse external bleeding.

The *supervention of pregnancy* varies in its results. A subperitoneal tumour of moderate size permits a normal termination of gestation.

Interstitial tumours show apparent rapid growth, largely due to hyper-trophy of the pregnant uterus round them ; the net increase in bulk may suffice to produce pelvic impaction or great abdominal distension.

A submucous tumour strongly militates against pregnancy, but if this occurs abortion is probable.

A cervical myoma or a pedunculated subperitoneal mass that has gravitated into the pelvis will obstruct labour, and sessile fundal tumours not infrequently, by their weight, retroflex the soft pregnant uterus and cause incarcer-ation. During the lying - in period a "fibroid" may be extruded or may slough out ; while pu-erperal sepsis affecting a myomatous uterus is a grave disaster.

Physical signs.—The physical signs of a myoma vary with its position. Its connexion with the uterus is usually obvious, but pedunculated subperitoneal tumours may appear to be entirely separate. Submu-cous tumours enlarge the

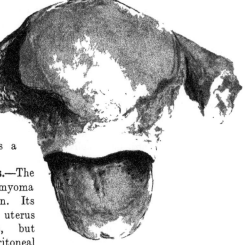

Fig. 605.—Submucous myoma in process of extrusion.

organ uniformly, while those nearer the peritoneal surface stand out as bosses or knobs. A cervical myoma, if interstitial, pro-duces a typical expansion of the cervix like that of the later months of pregnancy ; if submucous, its lower pole may be felt through the external os. Anterior and posterior cervical myomas displace the cervix backwards or forwards, while those in the broad ligament carry the uterus bodily upwards and towards the opposite side. The palpability of a myomatous uterus from the abdomen depends upon the size and position of the tumour. Except in broad-ligament myomas, the swelling is usually central. Cervical myomas, even when large, may not be apparent from above. The abdominal tumour is usually dull on percussion, but that produced by the cervical variety may be partly resonant because the intestines are lifted on the mass. Auscultation may reveal a *souffle*, especially when the uterus is very vascular, as in nævoid degeneration. The sound is produced in the vascular leashes of the broad ligament, and is heard to one side of the mass.

Diagnosis.—If the tumour is obviously connected with the uterus, it only remains to distinguish it from the enlargements due to pregnancy, malignant disease, pyometra, congenital hæmatometra, and uterine fibrosis. Confusion with *pregnancy* can only arise during the early months. Although the fact that amenorrhœa practically never occurs with a myoma unless pregnancy coexists is generally distinctive, immediate diagnosis may be obscured by a false menstrual history, or by the irregular hæmorrhages so often associated with early pregnancy.

In such a case, unless the symptoms are urgent, the surgeon may either watch the rate of tumour growth for a month or two, or place the patient under observation to ascertain beyond doubt the presence or absence of the menses.

Carcinoma of the corpus may produce uterine enlargement comparable with that due to a small submucous myoma, but continuous loss and watery discharge replace the periodic floodings. A sloughing myoma during extrusion may closely simulate malignant disease, but on palpation is firm and hard, quite unlike the friable, almost pulpy, feel of carcinoma. It is to be remembered that carcinoma corporis and myomas frequently coexist, and that the latter very rarely *begin* to give trouble after the menopause.

Pyometra is often due to carcinoma, but in cases secondary to senile endometritis a small sloughing myoma may be simulated. There is, however, little or no bleeding in such cases, and the passage of a sound under anæsthesia decides the diagnosis.

Congenital hæmatometra could only simulate a myoma affecting one horn of a double uterus.

The enlargement and severe periodic hæmorrhages due to *fibrotic metritis* cause close resemblance to a small submucous myoma. In this and the previous case the history and age of the patient may decide, but the diagnosis can often only be clinched by exploratory operation.

If a uterine connexion of the tumour cannot be ascertained, absolute diagnosis is impossible. A myoma may then be mistaken for an ovarian tumour, or for the mass formed by an old hæmatocele, chronic salpingitis, or cellulitis.

Scanty menstrual loss, fluctuation, a smooth contour, and comparatively rapid growth strongly favour a diagnosis of ovarian cyst. The swellings due to encysted blood or inflammatory products are usually distinguishable by their history. The importance of passing a catheter in any case of a doubtful abdomino-pelvic tumour cannot be insisted upon too often.

Prognosis.—Once a myomatous uterus has begun to cause symptoms, no material respite can be expected until the menopause. It must be remembered, however, that myomas postpone this event by several years. At the menopause the patient will be relieved of the blood loss, but symptoms dependent upon the bulk of the tumour, its degenerations and accidents, arc especially liable to supervene about this time. If these dangers arc escaped, the tumour gradually shrinks, though it probably never entirely disappears. The likelihood of carcinoma developing is always present. Although rarely fatal *per se*, a myoma indirectly shortens life by the progressive deterioration of health which the excessive blood-loss produces. In particular, cardiac degeneration is common. A myomatous uterus usually leads to chronic invalidism, but occasionally directly menaces life from excessive bleeding, obstruction to the functions of vital organs, toxic or septic absorption, or the supervention of malignant growth.

General remarks as to treatment.—A small myoma causing no symptoms and discovered accidentally should be let alone.

Where symptoms indicate treatment, two methods present themselves, medical and surgical.

If menstrual hæmorrhage is the *only* symptom, ergot and other styptic drugs may control it. The adoption of non-operative measures must be considered—(a) where, in the absence of urgent symptoms, the patient expresses strong repugnance to operation ; (b) where the menopause is approaching, and moderate hæmorrhage is the only symptom ; and (c) where operation is undesirable on account of cardiac, pulmonary, or other disease.

If, however, the bleeding is severe or the patient's social position interferes with the régime imposed by medical treatment, operation should be advised. Again, if the climacteric is several years distant, medical treatment is contra-indicated, for, apart from the life of invalidism to which the patient is condemned, the habitual exhibition of ergot exercises a deleterious effect on the heart and vessels. Symptoms due to pressure degeneration or any of the accidental occurrences to which these tumours are liable indicate immediate resort to surgery.

Pregnancy is undesirable, except when the myoma is small and subperitoneal ; moreover, conception is unlikely and dangerous in a myomatous uterus ; therefore removal of the tumour is advisable, even if it involve hysterectomy and obligatory sterility.

Medical treatment.—Ergot is the most satisfactory drug for controlling the menorrhagia. The liquid extract (20 to 30 minims three times daily), combined with strychnine and a dilute acid to exalt its effect, should be administered from a few days before the onset of the flow to its end, and then stopped. Sometimes it gives rise to severe uterine-contraction pain, and may be refused on this

3 o

account. Should ergot fail, hydrastis and hamamelis may be tried in doses of 15 and 30 minims of the liquid extract and tincture respectively. The hydrochloride and phthalate of cotarnin (stypticine and styptol) may also give satisfactory results. At the time of the period the patient should rest in bed ; after it is over, iron in some readily absorbable form should be administered. The treatment of myomas by various forms of electricity has deservedly fallen into disrepute.

Surgical treatment.—The ideal treatment of a myoma would at first sight appear to be the removal of the tumour with conservation of the uterus. Collected statistics, however, show that myomectomy is no safer an operation than hysterectomy, and that it sometimes fails to cure the menorrhagia because (1) in many cases a much hypertrophied uterus is left behind ; (2) a small submucous tumour may be overlooked and keep up the excessive loss ; and (3) in a certain number of cases new tumours subsequently develop. At this possible cost is gained the dubious privilege of continued menstruation and the undoubted advantage of possible pregnancy, although not more than 10 per cent. of patients on whom myomectomy has been performed subsequently conceive.

Myomectomy, then, is only to be preferred to hysterectomy (1) where the operation, though equally efficacious, is associated with less risk, as in small solitary submucous tumours causing hæmorrhage, or subperitoneal masses causing pressure or degeneration symptoms ; (2) where, on account of the patient's age and social state, the possibility of future pregnancy justifies an attempt to conserve the uterus, even at a somewhat increased risk ; and (3) where the patient strongly desires the attempted conservation of the uterus after the possible increased risk has been explained to her.

Abdominal myomectomy.—If the tumour is pedunculated, it may be removed by simple ligature of the pedicle in sections. If the tumour is sessile, or its pedicle too massive, it should be enucleated ; the bleeding from the capsule is controlled by under-running with "mattress" sutures, and the peritoneum closed over the uterine wound with Lembert stitches. Interstitial and submucous tumours, unless small and solitary, should not be treated by abdominal myomectomy. Small broad-ligament myomas can be easily shelled out.

Vaginal myomectomy.—Small polypoid submucous myomas can easily be evulsed. If the polyp is contained entirely within the uterine cavity the cervix must first be dilated. Sessile submucous myomas, if not larger than a bantam's egg, can be enucleated and removed through the cervix, their capsule having been first divided. Occasionally these tumours will not enucleate owing to capsular adhesions, and adenomyomas are never enucleable. Enormous submucous tumours can be removed per vaginam piecemeal ("morcellement") with scissors.

Where a solitary myoma is already in process of extrusion, and especially if it is sloughing, vaginal myomectomy should always be undertaken in preference to hysterectomy.

Hysterectomy.—Most gynæcological surgeons hold that where the vaginal cervix is healthy it should be conserved. A few prefer the total operation for all cases, on the ground that the cervical stump may, if infected, cause troublesome discharge, or may develop carcinoma ; but infection is an avoidable fault of technique, and cervical carcinoma in these patients is unlikely because of their sterility. The conservation of the cervix maintains the integrity of the vaginal vault, while the subtotal operation is always easier than the extirpation of the entire uterus. The following are the most important methods of performing hysterectomy :—

Subtotal hysterectomy.—The uterus having been pulled up through a median incision, a pressure forceps is clamped on the tube and ovarico-uterine ligament with its contained ovarian vessels on each side, and a second pair is applied to the round ligaments about an inch from the uterus. The broad ligaments are now divided between the clamps and the uterus as low down as the level of the internal os. A flap of peritoneum on the front of the uterus is then reflected from the upper limit of its loose attachment downwards. The uterine vessels are now in view as they run up either side of the uterus. They are clamped by pressure forceps just above the point where they leave the parametrium to enter the uterus, and the latter is amputated about $\frac{1}{2}$ in. above this line. The uterine vessels on each side are next secured by a ligature which, transfixing the tissue of the cervical stump just within them, is carried round them and tied on their outer side. The clamped broad ligament on each side is transfixed between the forceps holding the ovarico-uterine ligament and tube and the round ligament, and the transfixing ligature divided into two : one half is used to secure the tube and ovarian pedicle with its contained ovarian vessels ; and the other, rethreaded on a needle, is inserted as a puckering suture along the edge of the divided broad ligament as far as its junction with the cervical stump. The two ends of this thread are then made to encircle the round ligament and are tied together.

Any oozing from the cervical stump may be stopped by one or two mattress sutures. The anterior peritoneal flap is then united to the peritoneum on the posterior aspect of the stump, and the operation concluded by closing the abdominal wound in three layers.

Total hysterectomy.—The steps of the total operation are similar to those just described up to the point at which the anterior peritoneal flap is turned down. After this the bladder is gently separated by swab pressure from the supravaginal cervix, sufficiently low to expose freely the anterior vaginal wall. The vagina has now to be opened, either from in front or from behind. In the latter case the step is facilitated by cutting down upon a large uterine dilator previously placed in the vagina. In either case, both walls must be divided transversely in the middle line for about an inch. The fingers can now be thrust across the vagina under the uterus, and the mass pulled up. Each uterine artery having been clamped just before it enters the uterus, the lower part of the broad ligament and the lateral vaginal vault are divided and the organ is removed.

The ovarian vessels and round ligaments are secured as previously described. The uterine arteries are ligatured separately. The lateral vaginal vessels exposed just outside the lateral angles of the divided vagina are treated by mattress suture.

The anterior peritoneal flap is now united to the edge of the cut peritoneum on the posterior vaginal wall, but the latter canal is not further occluded, as it is important in these cases to leave a channel open in case the ligatures on the uterine and vaginal vessels become infected from the vagina. The ureters are liable to damage during total hysterectomy unless their course is clearly defined and the bladder wall separated from the upper part of the vagina.

Hysterectomy for cervical myomas.—The technique just described is not proper for cervical myomas. In such cases the spreading of the broad ligaments, the displacement of the bladder, and the fixity of the mass render the ordinary methods of securing the uterine vessels and amputating the uterus impossible. The difficulty in these cases is the control of bleeding during the removal of tumour and uterus, which, therefore, must be accomplished as quickly as possible. The upper part of the broad ligaments having been clamped and divided, the loose anterior peritoneum and the bladder are pushed off the front of the expanded supravaginal cervix as low as possible. The expanded tissue forming the tumour capsule is now divided transversely in the mid-line for about an inch, and by introducing the finger the plane of cleavage between the tumour and the capsule is defined. The incision is then prolonged to either side, and the lower pole of the tumour enucleated from its bed and pulled up. The incision is now extended around the uterus on each side, the uterine vessels being clamped *en passant.* Subtotal hysterectomy is thus effected, the lower part of the capsule of the tumour (i.e. the expanded supra-vaginal cervix) being left behind. This is trimmed up, or entirely removed, and the vessels are secured.

Hysterectomy for broad-ligament myomas.—After clamping and dividing the broad ligament with its contained ovarian vessels and round ligament, which are stretched over the tumour, the latter is enucleated as far as it will easily separate. The opposite broad ligament is divided in the classical manner, and the uterine artery on that side having been secured, the body of the uterus is amputated towards the tumour, the uterine vessels on that side being clamped as they come into view or spurt. The enucleation of the tumour from its bed in the base of the broad ligament is now easily effected, and the whole mass removed. The difficulty in these cases arises from the danger of hæmorrhage from the uterine vessels on the tumour side.

During the removal of either a cervical or a broad-ligament myoma the greatest care must be taken to avoid injuring the ureters ; this is best done by working inside the capsule of the tumour in the manner just described.

ADENO-MYOMA

These tumours, the " unencapsuled fibroids " of the older writers, have only recently been generally recognized. Macroscopically they form a mass in the uterine wall underneath the mucous membrane, and blending with it ; this may be limited to one part, or may extend right round the cavity. The cut surface has a peculiar honeycombed appearance, shown by the microscope to be due to areas of tissue, exactly resembling the structure of the endometrium, embedded amongst the interlacing muscle bundles which make up the rest of the tumour. The etiology is unknown. The age-incidence and symptoms are indistinguishable from those of myomas. The treatment is that for myomas, from which they can only be diagnosed after removal of the uterus. They cannot be enucleated.

SARCOMA

Sarcoma of the uterus is usually met with as a degenerative complication of uterine myomas, but it may occur apart from those tumours. Histologically it may belong to the round-, spindle-, or mixed-celled types, while myo-sarcoma, endothelioma, and giant-celled sarcoma are occasionally encountered.

Symptoms.—A sarcoma may appear as a rapidly growing intrauterine polyp, which soon recurs after removal ; at other times it forms a large nodular tumour resembling a myoma, but differing from it in its rapidity of growth, its fixity, and the presence of peritoneal fluid. In either case uterine hæmorrhage is likely to be marked.

Diagnosis.—The malignant nature of polypoid sarcoma has often been overlooked from failure to investigate microscopically the tissue removed. When a large mass can be felt from the abdomen a diagnosis of myoma may be made and operative treatment postponed under this error. The rapidity of growth and the signs of ascites should awaken suspicion.

Sarcoma of the cervix is very rare. A peculiar form is occasionally seen in young children, in which the surface of the mass is studded with numerous elevations (grape-like sarcoma). In adults it most commonly assumes a polypoid form. The symptoms are those of hæmorrhage and pain, and the only possible treatment is wide removal, preferably by Wertheim's method (*see* p. 1024).

UTERINE POLYPS

Symptoms.—Five varieties of uterine polyps are found.

1. *Adenomatous and cystic polyps* (*mucous polyps*).—The structure of the growth is similar to that of those occurring in the cervix (*see* p. 1017), except that the glands are tubular, not racemose (Fig. 606). The early symptom is menorrhagia and irregular loss, which later, as the growth extrudes, becomes continuous.

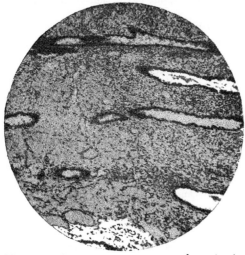

Fig. 606.—Adenomatous mucous polyp, the inflammatory stroma containing elongated hypertrophic glands.

2. *Myomatous polyps*.—The symptoms are those of a submucous myoma, as described at p. 1036. The loss is more strictly periodic than that associated with mucous polyps, the tumour having little vascularity.

3. *Placental polyps*.—Occasionally a portion of the gestation products after abortion or labour remains adherent to the uterine wall and becomes partially organized. Such pedunculated masses occasion more or less continuous loss, dating from the termination of the pregnancy.

4. *Malignant polyps*.—Sarcoma is the only form of malignant growth that commonly becomes actually polypous. The symptoms of these growths have been dealt with already (p. 1045).

Diagnosis.—So long as the polyp is contained entirely within the corpus, its presence can only be discovered after dilating the cervix. It may be suspected, however, when with bleeding and some uterine enlargement the cervical canal is found unnaturally patent.

Treatment.—The cervix having been dilated, the polyp should be removed by torsion and evulsion, except in the case of large myomatous tumours (*see* p. 1041). After the removal of an adenomatous or cystic polyp the mucosa should be curetted. If the polyp be found to be malignant, total extirpation of the uterus and adnexa must be performed.

THE FALLOPIAN TUBE

SALPINGITIS

Pathology.—In the vast proportion of cases the route of tubal infection is through the uterus. Thus salpingitis follows on endometritis of puerperal, postabortional, gonorrhœal, or postoperative origin. Occasionally, however, it is met with in virgins in whom none of these causes are in operation, and in such cases it is either due to the upward extension of a simple cervicitis (*see* p. 1008), or is primary in the tube itself. These primary forms are almost always tuberculous.

Rarely the tube may be infected through the abdominal ostium from an appendicular abscess or a tuberculous peritonitis.

Acute salpingitis may be suppurative or non-suppurative.

1. *Acute suppurative salpingitis.*—The tube is swollen and red ; the peritoneum covering it and the adjacent parts is injected, and soft adhesions unite it to the omentum and to neighbouring coils of gut. The tube wall and plicæ are infiltrated with polymorphonuclear leucocytes, and the lining epithelium is largely destroyed, while the lumen contains pus. The mesosalpinx is thickened by diffuse lymphangitis, the ovary is adherent and may contain thin-walled cysts due to acute serous exudation into the follicles, whilst the peritoneum in the neighbourhood is often raised in irregular blebs by serous exudate. In the most acute cases there is a direct outpouring of pus through the abdominal ostium into the peritoneal cavity. More commonly, however, the tubal fimbriæ, by swelling and adhesion, rapidly occlude the opening, the pus collects in the tube, and thus a *pyosalpinx* is formed. (Fig. 607.)

On account of the fixity of its mesosalpingeal border a distended Fallopian tube assumes a curved shape, curling downwards and inwards. Thus the tube usually almost encircles the ovary, and, as a rule, its lower end is adherent to the floor of the recto-uterine pouch.

Acute salpingitis is commonly bilateral. The subsequent fate of a pyosalpinx varies. It may spontaneously discharge into the rectum to which it has previously become adherent ; more rarely it may empty itself into the vagina, bladder, or uterus ; exceptionally its wall may give way and the pus escape into the peritoneal cavity. More often it becomes surrounded by a mass of adhesions to the uterus, the broad ligament, the bowel, and the omentum, and thus becomes sequestered (*see* Chronic Salpingitis).

Tubo-ovarian abscess.—An acute pyosalpinx is frequently complicated by one or more follicular abscesses of the ovary on the same side. Occasionally the cavity of the pyosalpinx communicates with the cavity of the ovarian abscess, a retort-shaped swelling being formed which tends to burrow in the broad ligament. (Fig. 608.)

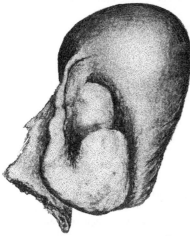

Fig. 607.—Uterus with pyosalpinx attached. The ovary is fairly healthy.

2. *Acute non-suppurative salpingitis.*—In less severe infections, suppuration may not occur. In such cases the tube, if distended, contains a serous fluid, often turbid and discoloured (*acute hydrosalpinx*). Occasionally, considerable hæmorrhage occurs into the tube lumen. The result is a hydro-hæmato-salpinx (*acute hæmorrhagic salpingitis*). In other respects the anatomy of the diseased tube is the same in non-suppurative as in suppurative salpingitis; but so long as suppuration has not occurred, spontaneous resolution is possible.

Chronic salpingitis.—Chronic salpingitis is usually the sequel of the acute variety, but occasionally cases are met with in which no history of the latter is forthcoming. Some of these are due to tuberculous disease.

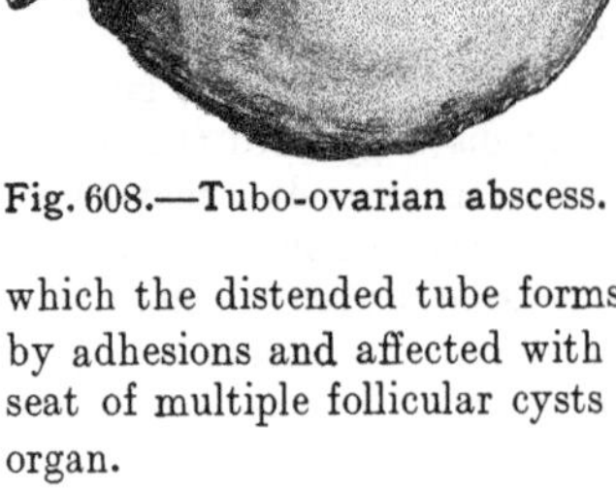

Three conditions may be encountered—(1) chronic pyosalpinx, (2) chronic hydrosalpinx, (3) chronic fibrotic salpingitis.

Fig. 608.—Tubo-ovarian abscess.

1. *Chronic pyosalpinx.*—An old pyosalpinx which has become densely adherent to the adjacent parts, together with the thickened mesosalpinx and infiltrated omentum, forms a conglomerate mass of which the distended tube forms only a part. The ovary, surrounded by adhesions and affected with peripheral sclerosis, often becomes the seat of multiple follicular cysts which in time may totally destroy the organ.

The pus, if secondarily infected by organisms from the bowel, may be very fetid. It is an interesting fact, however, that the pus is often sterile, the bacteria having perished from prolonged sequestration.

2. *Chronic hydrosalpinx.*—The abdominal ostium of an inflamed tube becomes occluded in one of two ways. In the first, adhesion takes place between the fimbriæ and the adjacent ovary or broad ligament. In the second, the œdema of the muscular coat causes the tubal peritoneum gradually to overfold the fimbriæ so that they appear to indraw until they disappear altogether, and the peritoneal surfaces adhere over them. The occlusion soon leads to accumulation in the tube of the secretion from its walls. A pyosalpinx or hydrosalpinx is thus formed. In the latter case the accumulated fluid is clear in colour and odourless.

A hydrosalpinx assumes the same general curve as a pyosalpinx, but even more markedly because, as a rule, it is less tethered by adhesions. (Fig. 609.) It may attain a large size, and is surrounded more or less by adherent omentum and bowel. Both tubes are usually affected.

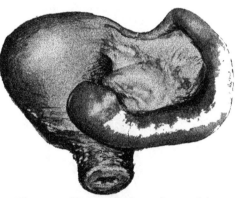

Fig. 609.—Uterus with large **hydrosalpinx** attached.

A hydrosalpinx may intermittently discharge through the uterine ostium, and may on occasions undergo axial rotation, producing symptoms like those of a twisted ovarian cyst.

Tubo-ovarian cyst.—For reasons already stated, the ovary adjacent to a hydrosalpinx frequently contains follicular cysts. Sometimes a cyst in the ovary communicates with the tube, the whole forming a very characteristic retort-shaped swelling. The history and symptoms of a tubo-ovarian cyst are the same as those of a hydrosalpinx.

3. *Chronic fibrotic salpingitis.*—In many cases of chronic salpingitis the inflammatory changes are most marked in the substance of the tube wall, and there is comparatively little exudation into its lumen. The tubal plicæ become much hypertrophied, and the epithelium covering them tends to dip downwards, forming many crypts, and therefore presenting an adenomatous appearance under the microscope (Fig. 610). The wall becomes greatly thickened, at first by cell

proliferation and œdema, and later by fibrosis. The tube curls down-wards and becomes densely adherent to the ovary, the back of the broad ligament, the uterus, the intestine, especially the pelvic colon, and the omentum. The ovary is often cystic as well. The result is a conglomerate mass lying to one side of the back of the uterus, and commonly referred to as a "diseased appendage."

Clinical features. Acute salpingitis. *Symptoms.* — The symptoms of acute salpingitis are those of pelvic peritonitis. The onset is sudden, with severe pain referred to the lower abdomen, the temperature and pulse-rate are high, and there may be some sickness. The bowels are constipated, or when opened occasion much pain. Micturition may also be painful.

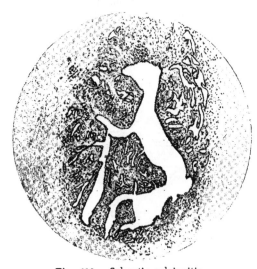

Fig. 610.—Sclerotic salpingitis.

The plicæ are swollen and distorted, and the subepithelial tissues crowded with inflammatory cells. The epithelium lies proliferated, forming many gland-like spaces.

Physical signs.—From the outset there are tenderness and rigidity over the lower abdomen, perhaps more marked on one side. After a day or two an indefinite swelling rises above the pubis. This swelling may be mesial in position, or more marked to one side of the middle line. Resonance is only partially impaired over it, because it is largely made up of adherent coils of gut. At the end of a week it may have attained the level of the umbilicus, and have become much more defined and dull. On vaginal examination nothing but great tenderness to one or both sides of the uterus is first noticed, but later a definite swelling or swellings can be distinguished, extending from the sides of the uterus into the pouch of Douglas. Eventually, in bilateral disease, a large, very tender mass is felt behind and to the sides of the uterus, which it tends to push forwards. The mass is continuous with that felt from the abdomen, and always lies in front of the rectum, which it may compress against the sacrum.

Clinical course.—This varies. In favourable cases the symptoms begin to subside in about three days, and after a period of some week or two complete recovery may ensue. More commonly, however, subsidence is only partial, a permanently tender fixed swelling being left in the region of the appendage, accompanied by the symptoms of chronic hydrosalpinx or fibrotic salpingitis.

· In the more severe cases (*acute pyosalpinx*) the temperature continues to rise after the fourth day, and becomes markedly remittent, indicating the formation of pus in the tube. Rigors may occur. Three courses are now possible. In the first, after some days, a discharge of pus from the rectum may indicate spontaneous evacuation of the retained pus. The symptoms may greatly ameliorate after this event, but since both tubes are usually affected and these spontaneous openings do not drain well, the symptoms after initial improvement frequently recur. In the second course no spontaneous discharge occurs, but the patient gradually passes into a state of chronic fever and pain with recurring exacerbations (*chronic pyosalpinx*).

Finally, in the worst cases, namely, those in which pus escapes through the abdominal ostium into the peritoneal cavity, the symptoms of generalized peritonitis may be present. Except in this event, and the still rarer one of spontaneous rupture of the distended tube into the peritoneal cavity, it is uncommon to find pus actually in the peritoneum in cases of salpingitis.

Chronic salpingitis. *Symptoms.*—The symptoms of chronic salpingitis vary with the condition of the diseased tube.

Where a pyosalpinx is present, the leading feature is continual pain and tenderness over the affected tube or tubes, with recurring exacerbations accompanied by fever and sickness. These exacerbations are often synchronous with the menses and are provoked by exertion or intercourse. Coitus is usually impossible. Intermittent discharges of pus from the tube, via the uterus, may take place. The menses are excessive, prolonged and often anticipated.

In hydrosalpinx and in fibrotic salpingitis these exacerbations are not so marked, but pain is continual in the lower abdomen on one or both sides. Dysmenorrhœa, dyspareunia, and sterility are present.

All forms of salpingitis are almost constantly accompanied by endometritis and cervicitis, the symptoms of which are also present. The uterus is often retroverted, especially in salpingitis of postparturitional origin.

Diagnosis. Acute salpingitis.—The symptoms of ruptured tubal gestation, of axial rotation of an ovarian tumour or a pedunculated myoma, of appendicitis, of a suppurating ovarian cyst, and of acute pelvic cellulitis, all more or less resemble those of acute salpingitis.

The physical signs of *ruptured tubal gestation* are almost identical with those of salpingitis, but there is less tenderness, the pain is markedly unilateral, the patient looks exsanguined, and the temperature at the beginning is either not raised or is actually subnormal. A history of previous amenorrhœa is in favour of tubal gestation, for though the period may be suppressed in acute salpingitis, and particularly in tubo-ovarian abscess, this occurrence *follows* the onset of the symptoms.

Axial rotation of a tumour is distinguished by the presence of a well-defined tumour, often fluctuant and always dull on percussion in the earliest stages of the attack. The mass formed by acute salpingitis is never definite for at least a week, rarely fluctuates, and commonly is partially resonant.

In *appendicitis*, as a rule, the location of the symptoms and physical signs is different. When, however, the appendix lies low down on the brim of the pelvis, inflammation of the right tube may be closely simulated. Sickness, distension, and constipation are greater with appendicitis than with salpingitis. Further, a patient with appendicitis is more ill than one with salpingitis exhibiting the same degree of physical signs. If a definite mass can be felt per vaginam in the position of the right appendage, the case is probably one of salpingitis.

When an *ovarian cyst* in the pelvis suppurates, the signs and symptoms of salpingitis are simulated. Here again the mass is from the beginning well defined, and is, moreover, entirely central in position.

Pelvic cellulitis resembles acute salpingitis in its abrupt onset with fever and pain. The symptoms are less severe, however, and at first there may be little to make out per abdomen ; later, when a swelling appears there it is markedly lateral, and extends outwards towards the iliac fossa. On vaginal examination a typical lateral cellulitis (the only form that could be confounded with salpingitis) stretches outwards from the uterus to the side wall of the pelvis. The induration arches downwards, comes into relation with the lateral vaginal wall, and is not felt through the posterior fornix. It is to be remembered, however, that more or less cellulitis of the upper part of the broad ligament usually accompanies salpingitis.

Chronic salpingitis.—The mass formed by chronic salpingitis, especially an old pyosalpinx, may be so solid and large as to simulate an ovarian tumour, or a myoma attached to the side of the uterus. From these it is distinguished by its tenderness, and by the history and symptoms of inflammation.

A diseased appendage lying behind a retroverted uterus may be mistaken for the retroflexed fundus ; it can be differentiated by careful bimanual examination and the passage of a sound under an anæsthetic.

Tubal carcinoma forms a mass impossible to diagnose from chronic salpingitis except by operation.

In chronic cellulitis and encysted broad-ligament abscess the mass is strictly unilateral, displaces the uterus to the opposite side, and does not extend behind it.

The diagnosis of the *exact condition* of a chronically inflamed tube is important. A *pyosalpinx* may be suspected if recurring attacks of fever are a feature of the case, or if the mass is very large and tender. A *hydrosalpinx* may be felt as a fluctuating elongated swelling, and is much less tender than a pyosalpinx. *Fibrotic salpingitis* is distinguished by the smaller size of the mass, its fixity and hardness, and by the fact that the symptoms are those of chronic pelvic pain without exacerbations. A *tuberculous* origin is to be suspected where, in a virgin, a considerable mass is found, unexplained by the history.

In conclusion, the frequency of diagnostic error in these cases, even by the most expert, must be strongly emphasized; the surgeon's primary duty is to determine the correct treatment, rather than the actual anatomical nature of the swelling felt.

Prognosis.—A patient rarely dies of salpingitis. In acute cases that rapidly subside without the formation of pus the tube may possibly return to the normal, although in most cases the abdominal ostium probably remains permanently sealed up, and so produces sterility.

If pus has formed, the tube is permanently disorganized. In chronic cases all hope of restitution to the normal must be abandoned. The longer the duration, the greater the likelihood of secondary disorganization of the ovary by adhesion, peripheral sclerosis, and follicular cyst formation.

Treatment. Acute salpingitis.—Whenever possible, operative measures should be postponed until the acute stage is passed, (1) because if no pus forms the condition may entirely subside, and (2) because an operation during the height of the attack is much more difficult and dangerous, for the tubal contents are virulent, the tissues are so soft and vascular that ligatures cut through them, the bowel wall is friable and easily tears, and the patient's general condition is unsatisfactory.

Immediate operation is, however, proper—(1) when the severity and extent of the peritonitis suggest a direct outpouring of pus into the peritoneal cavity, and (2) when the cause of the symptoms cannot with reasonable certainty be diagnosed.

If it be decided to temporize, hot antiseptic fomentations should be applied to the lower abdomen, the patient put on a liquid diet, the bowels opened every other day by an enema, and the intestinal distension relieved by the passage every six hours of a long rectal tube. Pain may be met by morphia cautiously given, or better by Bromidia.

Directly the temperature has fallen below 100° F., operation should be undertaken, supposing a considerable mass still remains in the pelvis, for undue delay allows the formation of strong adhesions, and increases the likelihood of ovarian disorganization.

Where the tube alone is affected, *salpingectomy* is generally the operation of choice. It consists in dissecting the tube off the mesosalpinx and dividing it at the uterine cornu; or, if it be desired to remove the entire structure, a wedge-shaped portion of the cornu containing its interstitial segment is excised and the gap closed by sutures.

In some cases the ovary is disorganized, contains collections of pus, or is conjoined to the tube in a tubo-ovarian abscess; then the removal of the whole appendage is required (*salpingo-oöphorectomy*). The tube and ovary having been separated from the surrounding adhesions, the ovarico-pelvic ligament is clamped and divided, and, the inner attachments of the appendage being ligatured in halves, the tube and ovary are removed. The ovarico-pelvic ligament is then ligatured, and all oozing stopped.

Where acute metritis coexists with an acute double pyosalpinx it is sometimes advisable to remove the whole uterus as well, especially if both ovaries have had to be excised, for the uterus is useless after the removal of both appendages, and if conserved may be the source of discharge and pain.

After all operations for acute salpingitis, it is advisable to drain the pelvis for a day or two.

Chronic salpingitis.—The treatment of chronic salpingitis varies with the presumed condition of the tube. A pyosalpinx must, of course, be removed; and the same course must be adopted for any considerable inflammatory enlargement of the appendage, whether the presence of pus be diagnosed or not. A hydrosalpinx should be similarly treated. Fibrotic salpingitis of old standing, and forming but a little mass, need not be interfered with unless it gives rise to sufficient pain and disability to justify the operation.

The ideal operation for chronic salpingitis is *salpingostomy*, which consists in freeing the tube from its adhesions, fashioning a new abdominal ostium by slitting, evacuating the contents, and stitching back the edges of the opening so as to evert the mucous membrane. Unfortunately, this can only be done where the disease is slight and the tube wall relatively healthy, as in many cases of hydrosalpinx.

In all cases of pyosalpinx, and in others where the conservation of the tube is either impossible or, on account of the patient's age, useless, salpingectomy or salpingo-oöphorectomy must be performed. The former should always be preferred if the ovary be reasonably healthy.

In some cases of double pyosalpinx with extensive dense matting of the pelvic organs, removal of the tubes is facilitated by performing subtotal hysterectomy as well. Lastly, where both appendages are so diseased as to require removal, and the uterus is the seat of chronic inflammatory changes, producing menorrhagia and continual discharge, total hysterectomy should, in addition, be carried out.

TUBAL GESTATION

Etiology.—The cause of tubal gestation is unknown. Investigation of early cases shows the tube to be normal except at the site of the pregnancy.

Repeated tubal pregnancy occurs so frequently as to indicate some peculiarity in certain individuals inclining them to this disaster. The event most commonly occurs either in first pregnancies or after some years of sterility.

The suggestions of etiological relationship to salpingitis, to tubal stenosis or diverticula, or to the passage of the ovum from the ovary of the opposite side are not supported by research.

Pathology.—The oösperm burrows through the tubal epithelium and embeds itself in the muscular wall by means of its trophoblast. It develops there in a cavity known as the *gestation sac*, formed in the maternal tissues by the destructive action of the trophoblastic cells. The small track into the tube wall is early occluded by fibrinous deposit, so that the gestation is at first entirely intramural in position. (Fig. 611.)

Primary rupture of the gestation sac.—The continued growth of the ovum leads to rupture of the gestation sac usually within eight weeks of the beginning of gestation. Rupture is brought about (1) by the erosion of the trophoblast and (2) by extravasation of blood into the gestation sac when some large maternal vessel is opened up by the invading trophoblastic cells.

Primary rupture of the gestation sac may occur in one of five directions.

1. *Intraperitoneal rupture.*—The sac perforates through the serous covering of the tube into the peritoneal cavity. This disaster, usually seen in isthmic gestation, because of the small size of the tube there, produces the most severe symptoms. Bleeding is profuse, and may cause death in two or three hours. This is the more striking because the gestation is often less than a month old, the patient bleeding to death from a tubal enlargement not bigger than a marble. (Fig. 612.)

2. *Intraligamentous rupture.*—Occasionally the sac perforates between the layers of the mesosalpinx. A broad-ligament hæmatoma results, and may attain a large size, but the bleeding is much less rapid than in the preceding variety and the symptoms are proportionately less severe.

3. *Intratubal rupture (tubal abortion).*—In ampullary gestation the
sac commonly ruptures into the tube lumen. The blood flows into
the tube and, escaping through the abdominal ostium, drips into the
pelvis, and by its accumulation forms a *hæmatocele*. If the ostium

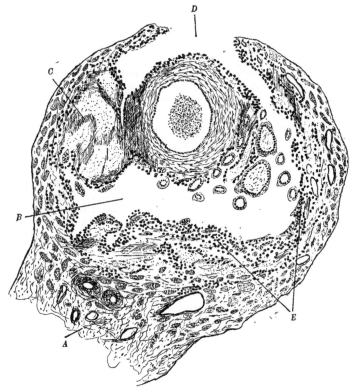

Fig. 611.—Transverse section of a ruptured three-weeks' tubal pregnancy.
The gestation sac is entirely intramural. The lumen of the tube is
somewhat dilated.

A, Mesosalpinx ; B, gestation sac ; C, fibrin mass ; D site of rupture ; E [wall of gestation
sac infiltrated by fœtal cells.

is already closed or becomes blocked by clot the tube is distended
and a *hæmatosalpinx* is formed ; its contents often leak through the
uterine ostium, causing continuous or intermittent vaginal loss.

Occasionally the " blood drip " from the abdominal ostium may
become encysted around this orifice (*peritubal hæmatocele*).

4. *Intramural rupture (tubal mole).*—This form of primary rupture

of the gestation sac is due to its sudden distension by extravasated blood. The sac wall gives way and the blood burrows along the musculature of the tube, forming an intramural hæmatoma, in the midst of which lies the ovum, usually completely separated from its attachment to the maternal tissues. The blood clots, and a "tubal blood mole" is formed (Fig. 613).

This may remain sequestered in the tube wall and possibly eventually become absorbed; more often, however, the sac gives way in a new direction owing to the fact that the trophoblastic cells in the infiltration zone remain active after the fœtal rudiment has perished. This secondary rupture may be intraperitoneal or intratubal. In either case the blood mole becomes extruded, and is found either loose in the peritoneal cavity or in process of extrusion from the tube lumen.

5. *Intra-uterine rupture.*—This can only happen in gestation in the interstitial segment of the tube, and is a rare event. It would produce the signs of miscarriage with severe bleeding, and its occurrence is probably usually overlooked.

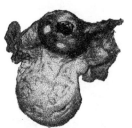

Fig. 612.—Acute intraperitoneal rupture of an early tubal gestation (half actual size).

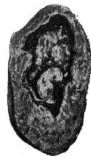

Fig. 613.—Tubal mole in section.

Secondary ruptures.—In most cases of tubal gestation several ruptures of the gestation sac and tube have occurred before operation. Thus, after primary intramural rupture, secondary rupture of the sac into the tube lumen or peritoneum may occur. In other cases the hæmatosalpinx formed by primary intratubal rupture may subsequently give way. This fact accounts for the usual history of several attacks of pain and faintness at intervals of some hours or days. Many of these secondary ruptures produce quite temporary escapes of blood through the apertures being quickly closed by blood clot.

Secondary sacs (*intraperitoneal and intraligamentous gestation*). —Rupture of the primary gestation sac, which always occurs before the third month, usually kills the embryo, but occasionally, if the chorionic villi retain their attachment to the tube wall, the gestation survives and continues to grow in a secondary sac either in the peritoneal cavity or between the layers of the broad ligament. (Fig. 614.) In the first case the sac wall is formed by the tube, the back of the broad

3 *p*

ligament and uterus, adherent intestine and omentum, and the abdominal parietes. In the second, the sac expands the broad ligament, pushes the uterus to the opposite side of the pelvis, and gradually rises into the abdomen by stripping the peritoneum off the side wall of the pelvis and iliac fossa until at term it may lie nearly centrally under the peritoneum in front of the spine and great vessels.

A gestation in a secondary sac may rupture, but it sometimes goes on to term, when " spurious labour " takes place, the uterus expelling a decidual cast. The fœtus then dies, usually within a month, and is

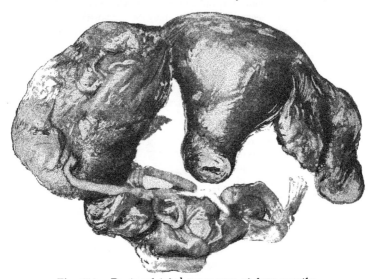

Fig. 614.—Ruptured tubal pregnancy at four months.

The sac is tubo-peritoneal. The opposite tube is in a condition of hæmatosalpinx.

gradually converted into adipocere and subsequently calcified, forming a lithopædion. A sequestered extra-uterine fœtus may remain in the abdomen for forty years without causing trouble. More commonly, however, the sac inflames and suppurates, multiple sinuses are formed communicating in the case of intraperitoneal sacs with the bowel or umbilicus, and in the case of intraligamentous sacs with the skin above the groin, the bladder, or the vagina.

Condition of the uterus.—The uterus in extra-uterine pregnancy enlarges so that at full term it is about the size of a three-months' intra-uterine pregnancy. A decidual hypertrophy of the endometrium also occurs, and may be cast off entire after rupture of the primary gestation sac. This only occurs, however, in a minority of cases ;

in the remainder it is passed as small shreds that escape notice in the general loss.

Symptoms and signs.—Until the gestation sac ruptures, the symptoms of tubal pregnancy are indistinguishable from those of intra-uterine pregnancy. Amenorrhœa and morning sickness are present, and in due course the breasts enlarge.

The symptoms and signs produced by the rupture of the gestation sac are very varied, and can only be interpreted in the light of a full understanding of the pathology of the condition.

1. **Acute intraperitoneal rupture.**—When the primary gestation sac ruptures acutely into the peritoneal cavity the symptoms are most fulminant. The patient is suddenly seized with severe pain and faintness, and soon presents all the symptoms of urgent internal hæmorrhage. The skin is blanched and cold, the pulse very fast and small, the respirations gasping, and the mental condition one of acute anxiety. The pain is referred to the abdomen generally. On examination, localizing signs may be slight or absent altogether, for the tubal enlargement is small and liquid blood in the peritoneum produces no tangible tumour, though after a while abdominal rigidity and slight distension may be noticed. These cases may end fatally in a few hours.

2. **Intramural and intratubal rupture.**—Intramural rupture produces an attack of acute pain due to the rapid swelling of the tubal tissues. If the gestation is destroyed by this event, no further symptoms may occur, and all that can be found is a slight enlargement in the continuity of the tube. More commonly, however, it is followed by a secondary rupture into the lumen of the tube or into the peritoneum, in which case the attack of pain is repeated, with more severity. Faintness and the symptoms of internal hæmorrhage are present, and the signs of a pelvic hæmatocele develop.

Intratubal rupture may, however, be the primary event, in which case the first attack of pain is more violent and faintness more constant. The signs depend upon whether the abdominal ostium is patent or not. In the first case the blood finds its way into the pelvis and, gradually mounting, floats up the intestines and omentum. Blood in the peritoneum acts as an irritant to that membrane, and it has been shown that its presence there is followed in a short time by the appearance of micro-organisms. A plastic peritonitis is thus set up, matting the intestines and omentum around the collection of blood, now known as a *hæmatocele*. In the second event, all the blood collects in the tube lumen, and a large *hæmatosalpinx* is produced. In most cases the double condition obtains, i.e. part of the blood is poured into the pelvis and part is retained in the tube.

Intratubal rupture (tubal abortion), either primary, or secondary to intramural rupture, is the commonest termination of tubal pregnancy, and its symptoms, namely, recurring attacks of abdominal pain and faintness, associated with bleeding from the uterus and the formation of a pelvic mass, are those classically associated with extra-uterine gestation. The recurring pain is produced by the successive ruptures of the tube wall with each fresh outburst of bleeding, while the uterine hæmorrhage is chiefly due to the leakage of the hæmatosalpinx through the uterine ostium, though part of it may be caused by the separation of the intra-uterine decidua.

The mass felt is a conglomerate consisting of the swollen tube, peritoneal lymph and adhesions, the matted intestine and omentum, and the blood free in the pelvis. It appears after the lapse of some days, and becomes increasingly defined and hard as the blood clots.

Where a hæmatocele is formed, the mass lies directly in front of the rectum, and the uterus is pressed forwards on to the bladder, but if a hæmatosalpinx alone is present the swelling is more to one side. Fever is often present after the first day or two, owing to the resultant peritonitis.

3. **Intraligamentous rupture.** — Rupture of the primary gestation sac into the broad ligament is announced by severe pain referred to the lower abdomen on that side, and in a short time an indefinite swelling in the region of the broad ligament is felt. This swelling becomes more defined and enlarged, every increment in size produced by fresh bleeding being accompanied by exacerbation of the pain.

A very large tumour may thus be formed, displacing the uterus to the opposite side, and mounting up into the abdomen behind the peritoneum to one side of the middle line.

4. **Intraperitoneal and intraligamentous pregnancy.**—A living gestation in the peritoneal cavity or between the layers of the broad ligament forms an elastic fluctuating tumour lying either behind the uterus (intraperitoneal) or to one side of it (intraligamentous). Definite uterine enlargement is present, and the signs of fœtal life and active placental circulation may be detected over the tumour.

There is usually a history of an attack of pain in an earlier period of the pregnancy corresponding to the rupture of the primary gestation sac. The severity of the symptoms varies: some patients suffer no more discomfort than is common in the later months of normal pregnancy; others have persistent pain or interference with the intestines amounting to partial obstruction.

Secondary sacs sometimes rupture, the fœtus escaping among the intestines; or the extra-uterine placenta may accidentally separate and cause internal hæmorrhage.

5. **Sequestered extra-uterine pregnancy.**—Where sequestra-

tion has not long occurred the history of an apparent pregnancy terminating in spurious labour will at once indicate the nature of the mass felt. After many years, however, the history may be indefinite, and diagnosis then is difficult or impossible. Most of these cases present themselves because of suppuration round the sac, and in some the extrusion of fœtal bones through the sinuses formed will elucidate the nature of the condition. In others it can only be decided by operation.

Diagnosis.—Acute intraperitoneal rupture of the primary gestation sac may be mistaken for perforation of a gastric or intestinal ulcer, fulminant appendicitis, volvulus and other forms of acutest intestinal obstruction, rupture of a solitary ovarian abscess or ovarian blood cyst, or acute torsion of an ovarian or uterine tumour. In all these catastrophes the striking feature is the suddenness of onset of the symptoms. The two chief points that distinguish acute tubal rupture are the history of preceding amenorrhœa and the signs of internal hæmorrhage, as compared with the signs of shock which characterize most of the other disasters mentioned.

Rupture of an ovarian blood cyst or severe hæmorrhage from dehiscence of a Graafian follicle produces symptoms indistinguishable from acute rupture of a tubal gestation, but the history of amenorrhœa is wanting. Torsion of an ovarian cyst may cause profuse intracystic bleeding, but the presence of a tumour from the outset distinguishes it from the ruptured gestation, in which a mass is only formed after a day or two.

The symptoms of intratubal rupture (tubal abortion), which are often preceded by those of intramural rupture (the formation of a tubal mole), are more likely to be mistaken for salpingitis and pelvic peritonitis, for inflammation or subacute torsion of an ovarian cyst, for subacute appendicitis, or for abortion of an intra-uterine gestation. The recurring attacks of acute pain often associated with a bloody uterine discharge, and sometimes with the passage of a cast, are classically associated with tubal gestation.

The history of preceding amenorrhœa is an important diagnostic feature, for though suppression of a period may occur with acute salpingitis, and particularly with tubo-ovarian abscess, this *follows* the onset of the symptoms.

The mass formed by a hæmatosalpinx and hæmatocele is a conglomerate like that of acute salpingitis—substituting blood for pus—and in neither of them does it appear at once. That of tubal gestation is, however, less tender, and fever, if present, is a late development, whereas in salpingitis it is one of the earliest signs. The patient undergoing a tubal abortion is more or less pallid, and gives a history of fainting attacks with the spasms of pain, while the size of the mass

felt is disproportionate to the slight inflammatory signs. In salpingitis the patient is flushed, the pain is and has been continuous,
and fainting has not occurred.

A twisted ovarian cyst presents as a tumour *from the first*, peculiarly
defined and fluctuating, and there is no preceding amenorrhœa.

A tubal abortion is often mistaken by the patient for abortion of
an intra-uterine gestation, owing to the pain, the blood loss, and (when
it occurs) the passage of the decidual cast. Examination, by revealing
the extra-uterine mass, should point to the nature of the case, but the
diagnosis of postabortional salpingitis is sometimes wrongly made in
these cases. A retroverted gravid uterus when incarcerated and
attempting to abort may be mistaken for tubal gestation with a hæmatocele, and vice versa, but in the former the cervix is characteristically
displaced so that the os points upwards and forwards.

Intraligamentous rupture presents general features resembling
acute pelvic cellulitis, but the absence of inflammatory signs, notwith-
standing the size of the tumour, with the blanching and the history
of pregnancy, should distinguish it.

The diagnosis of later extra-uterine gestation is usually obvious,
but the discrimination from intra-uterine pregnancy may be difficult
if the secondary sac is closely fused to the side or back wall of the
uterus.

Treatment.—All cases up to the sixth month should be immediately operated upon. Some authorities prefer in the case of a hæmatocele to await a possible natural absorption. Apart from its involving
an invalidism extending over two or three months, this practice has
distinct risks : (1) Fresh hæmorrhage may occur, for the trophoblast
continues to grow after the death of the fœtus ; (2) the gestation may
not be dead, but continuing its existence in a secondary sac ; (3) the
hæmatocele may suppurate.

Operation.—In acute ruptures the greatest expedition must be
used, the patient meanwhile receiving saline venous infusion. The
tube should be pulled up, clamped and removed, with or without
the ovary according to the condition of the latter. The blood in the
peritoneum is then rapidly cleared out, and the wound closed. In
hæmatosalpinx cr hæmatocele presenting less violent symptoms the
technique is that of the operations for salpingitis (*see* p. 1054). The
ovary should always, if possible, be conserved. The opposite tube is
found occluded in many cases, but salpingostomy is usually feasible.
Pelvic drainage is not generally necessary after removing the blood
clot, but if definite fever has been present a small tube should be
introduced through the lower end of the wound for a day or two.

If a broad-ligament hæmatoma is found, the blood should be
evacuated, the involved tube removed, and the cavity in the broad

ligament obliterated by sutures, or, if too large for this procedure, brought to the surface and drained.

A ruptured interstitial gestation may be treated either by subtotal hysterectomy—or better, if possible, by exsection of the tube and cornu—and repair of the uterus by sutures.

Intraperitoneal and intraligamentous gestation up to the sixth month should be treated by removal of the sac. In the first case the adhesions to the omentum, back of the uterus and broad ligament, and to the bowel, will have to be dealt with. Where possible, they should be ligatured or clamped before division, but in any circumstances the bleeding will be very free.

In the second case the hæmorrhage will be still more marked, the whole of the sac being commonly placentous. It is frequently best in these circumstances to remove the body of the uterus as well as the tube on the involved side. In either event the operation requires rapid and determined execution.

In the last three months of extra-uterine pregnancy operation may be necessitated by rupture of the secondary sac or separation of the extra-uterine placenta, but the hæmorrhage involved is such that all authorities agree in preferring to await, if possible, the death of the fœtus and cessation of the placental circulation, after which the removal of the gestation is comparatively easy. If compelled to interfere, the surgeon may—(1) remove the fœtus alone and deliberately sequester the placenta by suturing up the sac, (2) remove the fœtus and drain the sac with the placenta *in situ*, or (3) attempt the removal of the entire sac and its contents.

Of these the first plan is the best, but the strictest asepsis must be observed. Drainage of the sac is peculiarly fatal, the patient usually dying of sepsis or of secondary hæmorrhage. The third undertaking is very formidable, unless the placenta is mainly attached to the omentum, when it can be ligatured off successfully.

CARCINOMA

This is a rare disease. The growth assumes a papillary form which, distending the tube, eventually ruptures it into the peritoneal cavity. There is strong evidence that the neoplasm is the outcome of chronic salpingitis in which, as already described, there is a marked tendency for the epithelium to proliferate. A very frequent symptom is a blood-stained watery uterine discharge, originating in the hydrosalpinx produced by the growth occluding the abdominal ostium of the tube. In many cases free fluid is present in the peritoneum. Diagnosis is difficult, salpingitis being closely simulated. A blood-stained discharge with ascites is suggestive. Ablation of the diseased tube, with the uterus and the rest of the adnexa, is the only treatment.

OTHER NEW GROWTHS

Myomas are very rare in the tube. Adeno-myomas have been described. They consist of an admixture of muscle fibres with epithelial tubules derived from the lining of the tube. They are of inflammatory origin. Sarcoma and hydatid cysts in this situation are also known.

THE OVARY

ABSENCE OF THE OVARY—ACCESSORY OVARY

One or both ovaries may be absent or infantile. Occasionally an accessory ovary outside the normal one may be present.

PROLAPSE

The ovary may be dragged down by a retroverted or prolapsed uterus. Not infrequently prolapse occurs with the uterus in normal position, the ligaments being relaxed from parturition or primary tissue debility.

Clinical features.—The principal symptom is dyspareunia owing to the tenderness of the prolapsed organ, though this varies enormously in different individuals. Probably some cases of chronic " ovarian " pain are due to this displacement.

Many ovaries clinically tender show at the operation filamentous adhesions previously unsuspected.

Diagnosis.—The normal ovary is not easily felt, because there is no solid background against which to feel it. Light palpation is necessary; much force pushes the organ in front of the finger, and defeats its end. Rectal examination is useful in these cases.

Treatment.—If the condition gives no trouble it should, of course, be let alone. When neurasthenia has been excluded, and the genuineness and ovarian origin of the symptoms have been established, it is proper to attempt relief.

In uncomplicated ovarian prolapse the ovarico-uterine ligament should be shortened after the method first described by me in 1907. In the more common cases associated with retroversion, rectification of the uterine displacement and the use of a pessary may succeed. This failing, ventro - suspension, combined with shortening of the ovarian ligaments, is a proper course; or, better still, intraperitoneal ligamentopexy (p. 1006), which very effectively pulls up the ovary.

INFLAMMATION (OÖPHORITIS)

Primary ovarian inflammation is rare, though it frequently arises secondarily to disease of the tube, as previously described. Occasionally a solitary abscess occurs, probably as a result of infection of a recently dehisced follicle by the *B. coli communis*. These cases are very fulminant, no symptoms being present as a rule until intraperitoneal rupture of the abscess initiates a violent peritonitis with symptoms resembling those of acute perforation of an abdominal viscus. They should be treated by oöphorectomy and peritoneal drainage.

In the condition known as " fibrotic oöphoritis," or " cirrhosis of the ovary," the organ is found much reduced in size, very hard, and devoid of follicles. The stroma shows a dense fibrosis. There is, however, no evidence that the change is inflammatory. It is met with most often in virgins, and is sometimes associated with a peculiarly violent form of dysmenorrhœa (see p. 1082).

OVARIAN GESTATION

The cause of this rare event is unknown. The oösperm embeds itself in the wall of the Graafian follicle, and the gestation sac thus formed usually ruptures at an early period into the peritoneal cavity. Cases are, however, recorded in which an apparently ovarian pregnancy endured for months, or even went nearly to term. The symptoms when rupture occurs are identical with those of ruptured tubal pregnancy, and the treatment is similar except that the ovary and not the tube claims the operator's attention (see p. 1062).

NEW GROWTHS OF THE OVARY

OVARIAN CYSTS

There is no region of the body in which such an extraordinary diversity of new growths occurs as in the ovary, and their elucidation constitutes one of the most puzzling and most interesting problems in pathology.

The ovary is developed, like the testicle, from the genital ridge which lies immediately inside the mesonephric ridge.

In the mesonephric ridge lie the mesonephric tubules and the longitudinally-running Wolffian duct, with which they are connected. The genital ridge is very early covered in embryonic life with a special layer of cells known as the germinal " epithelium." These cells are not, however, epithelial nor even ectodermic or entodermic, but probably represent certain elements early differentiated from the rest of the cells of the morula for reproductive purposes. In the development of the somatic elements of the body a progressive differentiation of the cells occurs, first into ectoderm, entoderm, and mesoderm, and later into their specialized derivatives, such as epithelium, bone, muscle, and so forth. The cells of the germinal epithelium, however, unlike those of the rest of the body, claim undifferentiated descent from the primitive blastomeres into which the dividing oösperm first splits ; from them develop the sexual elements of the new individual, in the

following manner : Certain of the cells of the germinal epithelium in-
grow into the genital ridge in a series of prolongations known as the
medullary cords. In the female these cell columns become the egg
tubes of Pflüger, and break up into a series of cell groups known as
primitive follicles ; from them the ovum and the cells of the tunica
granulosa and discus proligerus are formed. In the male these cell
cords develop into the cells lining the spermatogenic tubules ; these
tubules are subsequently brought into continuity with the mesonephric
tubules and ducts, and therefore into communication with the Wolffian
duct, which now acts as a conduit (vas deferens) for conveyance of
their secretion (spermatozoa).

In the female, continuity between the mesonephric tubules and
collecting ducts and the ingrowths from the germinal epithelium is
never established, the former remaining, together with the Wolffian
duct, as the vestiges in the mesosalpinx and ovarian hilum known as
the paroöphoron, Kobelt's tubules (epoöphoron), and Gartner's duct
respectively.

The Müllerian ducts, from which is formed the female genital
canal, are developed subsequently to the Wolffian ducts and outside
them in the mesonephros.

In the earliest stage of their existence each communicates with
the cœlom by three apertures which eventually fuse to form the
abdominal ostium of the Fallopian tube. Occasionally this fails, and
accessory ostia or cysts derived from them are found in adult life.

The ovary, therefore, besides being in immediate relation with
several vestigial structures, is the normal seat of undifferentiated
embryonic cell seclusions. The enormous growth potentialities of
these cells, as far as the ova are concerned, are held in abeyance by
the occurrence in them of a peculiar form of karyokinetic division
(maiotic mitosis) whereby the number of chromosomes contained in
each cell is reduced to one-half of those in a somatic cell.

Should this process fail to occur, the possibility of a tumour by
asexual cell division of an ovum must be admitted. The cells of the
granulosa, likewise derived from the germinal epithelium, are possibly
also the seat of initiation of such teratomatous formations, whilst others
may be derived from sequestered cells aberrant from the primitive egg
tubes, or subsequent ingrowths from the germinal epithelium. Such
an hypothesis best explains the frequency of teratomatous tumours
in the sexual glands and the fact that the ovary, though it contains
developmentally neither ectodermic nor entodermic derivatives, yet
produces enormous tumours chiefly composed of epithelium.

Cysts in the ovarian region may be divided into four groups :
(1) cysts of the ovary proper, (2) cysts of the ovarian hilum, (3) cysts
of the broad ligament, and (4) cysts of the tube.

1. **Cysts of the ovary (oöphoronic cysts).**—All ovarian cysts are at first pedunculated like the organ itself. Their walls are composed of stretched ovarian tissue, and have a characteristic pearly-white or bluish tint, according to their thickness and the character of the underlying contents.

Follicular cysts.—The simplest species are those derived by distension of the Graafian follicle in various stages of its existence. There are three varieties of follicular cyst: (a) the simple follicular cyst, (b) the follicular blood cyst, and (c) the lutein cyst.

(a) *Simple follicular cysts.*—These may be single or multiple. In the former case the whole ovary is transformed into a pedunculated, thin-walled, whitish-blue cyst, containing a thin, straw-coloured fluid. In the smaller cysts the wall is lined inside with a short columnar epithelium, but in the larger ones this is flattened out or actually disappears. Multiple follicular cyst formation is usually associated with chronic salpingo-oöphoritis, the peripheral sclerosis and adhesions preventing the dehiscence of the follicles.

(b) *Follicular blood cysts.*—After dehiscence of the follicle, bleeding normally occurs into it, producing the " corpus hæmorrhagicum." This hæmorrhage may occasionally be excessive and result in the formation of a blood cyst whose walls represent the stretched and thinned tissue of the ovary. These cysts have a very characteristic dark-red colour and are liable to rupture, with severe intraperitoneal bleeding.

(c) *Lutein cysts.*—Cystic degeneration of the corpus lutein has only been described within recent years. The cysts are usually small, and only distinguishable from the simple follicular cyst by microscopical discovery of a layer of lutein cells lining the cavity. Their significance is unknown, but they have been found with such unusual frequency in association with chorion-epithelioma that some general etiological connexion is strongly suggested.

Ovarian cyst-adenomas.—The majority of large ovarian cysts belong to this group (Fig. 615). They are multilocular, though one loculus may predominate in size. The smaller loculi are lined with a tall columnar muciniferous epithelium (Fig. 616), but in the larger ones the cells become flattened. The content of the cyst is mucin, more viscid in the smaller loculi and less so in the larger. It may be transparent, whitish-yellow, or green, or brown from blood-staining, in different cases. When large, these cysts are usually more or less adherent to the omentum or bowel.

It has been suggested that cysts of this group are derived by proliferation of certain of the cells of the follicle from sequestered aberrant remnants of the primitive egg tubes, or from subsequent ingrowths of the germinal epithelium. They may occur at any age from puberty onwards, but are commonest after 30.

Teratomatous cysts (dermoid cysts; embryomas).—The fact that the ovary is the normal seat of undifferentiated embryonic cell seclusions probably explains the extraordinary diversity of growths originating in that organ. If so, many ovarian tumours not always considered as teratomatous might be included in this category (e.g. ovarian cyst-adenomas). Setting aside these more debatable classes, there remain two whose embryonic origin is admitted by all, viz. the simple dermoid cyst and the multilocular cyst-embryoma.

Of these the *simple dermoid* is much the commoner. It is unilocular

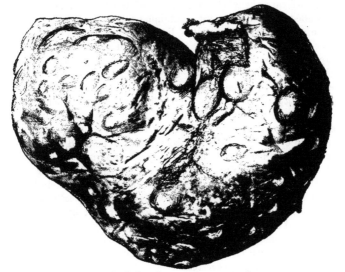

Fig. 615.—Multilocular ovarian cyst-adenoma.

as a rule, and its wall is formed of stretched ovarian tissue (Fig. 617). At one part of it the "embryonic rudiment" presents as an irregular projection into the cavity, covered by a coarse skin containing a large number of sebaceous follicles. Many hairs grow from this area, and projecting from it or embedded in it may be found one or several teeth more or less well formed, and set into an irregular plate of bone (Fig. 618). Microscopical investigation of the embryonic area, besides showing a definite skin (Fig. 619), may reveal other tissues such as cartilage, muscle bundles, or nerves. The rest of the cyst is usually lined with a flattened or definitely cubical epithelium. It contains a yellow fat, liquid when it is first removed from the body, but rapidly hardening afterwards, and then resembling cocoa butter. Embedded in it is a quantity of coarse reddish or brownish hair.

The *multilocular cyst-embryoma* is much rarer. It consists in large part of solid masses intermixed with cavities of different sizes, whose contents vary from typical dermoid material to mucus and clear serum. Those containing fat are lined with a perfect skin, coated with vernix caseosa like that of a new-born infant. Others present a mucous membrane exactly similar to that of normal bowel; whilst in some, columnar ciliated epithelium is found like that of the trachea. Microscopically, every variety of tissue characterizing the human body is found in irregular arrangement (Fig. 620), and in exceptional examples well-formed portions of the lower part of a fœtus may be present.

It is a remarkable fact that endogenous teratomas, whether occurring in the ovary or elsewhere, rarely develop before puberty, the commonest age at which they are met with being between 20 and 30.

2. Cysts of the ovarian hilum (*paroöphoronic cysts*).

— The cysts that occasionally develop in the

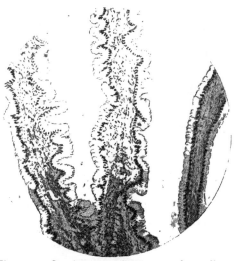

Fig. 616.—Ovarian cyst-adenoma, the loculi lined with a tall columnar muciniferous epithelium.

hilum of the ovary are probably derived from those remnants of the mesonephric tubules known as the paroöphoron and from some of the earlier ingrowths of the germinal epithelium (rete cords). They may be unilocular or multilocular; they grow into the ovary, which lies on their posterior surface, and burrow into the broad ligament in front. They are particularly prone to develop intracystic papillomas, in virtue of which they become more or less malignant (*see* Papilliferous Cysts, p. 1072). They are commonest between the ages of 30 and 50.

3. Broad-ligament cysts.

—A cyst growing in the broad ligament is covered by its peritoneal layers, and as it invades the mesosalpinx has the tube stretched across it (Fig. 621). These features are characteristic. Cysts developing in the outer third of the mesosalpinx are pedunculated; but those arising in any other position are always sessile. The ovary is at first quite separate from the cyst, but when the latter attains a large size this organ may become incorporated with its posterior wall.

Broad-ligament cysts are usually unilocular, and contain a thin straw-coloured fluid.

As regards their origin, they may be divided into two classes — (a) parovarian (epoöphoronic), and (b) inflammatory.

(a) Parovarian cysts.—Distension of the vestigial ducts of the parovarium produces cysts originating in the mesosalpinx. When developed from one of the outer

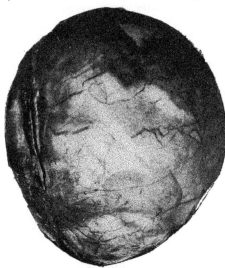

Fig. 617.—Unilocular teratomatous cyst (dermoid cyst).

group (*Kobelt's tubes*) the cyst is stalked and small. Cysts of the outer segment of Gartner's duct have a peduncle formed of the tube and the inner portion of the mesosalpinx, but those arising nearer the uterus have no pedicle and burrow downwards into the lower part of the broad ligament. Parovarian cysts have a lining of short cubical epithelium like that of the tubules from which they spring (Fig. 622). Cilia have been described, but these, if found, probably indi-

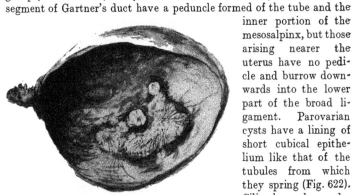

Fig. 618.—Dermoid cyst, opened to show the foetal rudiment with two well-formed teeth.

cate a Müllerian origin. Parovarian cysts contain a thin serous fluid. They are commonest between 30 and 40 years of age.

(b) **Inflammatory broad-ligament cysts.**—These cysts, originating more particularly in the deeper part of the broad ligament, are produced by lymphatic blockage (*lymphatic cysts*), and may then be multilocular, or they may be formed by encystment of a broad-ligament abscess with gradual disintegration of the pus until a thin grumous fluid results.

4. **Tubal cysts.**—Accessory fimbriated extremities of the Fallopian tube are not uncommonly found as short "anemone-like" processes, and represent the permanence of the primitive cœlomic ostia, of which there are three. Sampson Handley first pointed out that certain cysts arising in this situation are developed from such vestiges. They are unilocular, present, when small, a

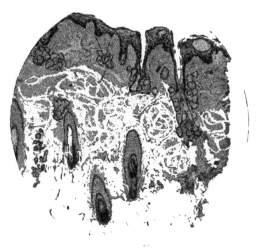

Fig. 619.—Wall of dermoid cyst.

It shows a well-formed skin containing hair-follicles, sebaceous and sweat-glands, and unstriped muscle fibres.

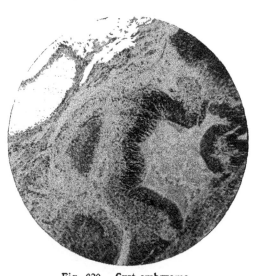

Fig. 620.—Cyst-embryoma.

Various tissues are seen embedded, in which may be noted a mass of cartilage and several spaces lined with different types of epithelium.

ciliated epithelium similar to that of the tube, and contain rudimentary plicæ. Small cysts are also found along the line of the tubo-

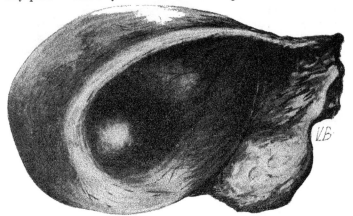

Fig. 621.—Parovarian cyst. The tube runs over it, and the ovary
is not connected with it.

ovarian fimbria. Their origin is debatable, but is probably derived
from the vestiges of the anterior end of the Wolffian duct.

Papilliferous and malignant ovarian cysts.—Intracystic papillomas may develop in any cyst lined with epithelium, and may, therefore, complicate any of the cysts
just described. The nature of the papillomatous growth
varies. Short round-topped elevations formed by fibrous
excrescence from the cyst wall are often seen. Soft villous
papillomas are particularly, but not exclusively, associated with paroöphoronic cysts. They present exu-

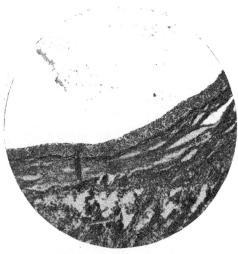

Fig. 622.—Wall of a parovarian cyst lined with
several layers of cubical epithelial cells.

berant masses growing in tufts which after a time burrow through the cyst wall and sprout on its outer surface. When large they entirely fill the cyst cavity and eventually cause rupture. They then become rapidly diffused and grafted over the whole of the surface of the peritoneum, which may be studded with thousands of little secondary growths. This change is associated with rapid effusion of peritoneal fluid.

In microscopical structure they vary. The more innocent present a single layer of columnar epithelium (Fig. 623), but in others these cells are massively arranged in many layers (Fig. 624). These latter are frankly malignant, and rapidly recur after removal, but secondary nodules of the single-layered type may spontaneously disappear after the removal of the primary growth.

Many other forms of malignant degeneration may occur in ovarian

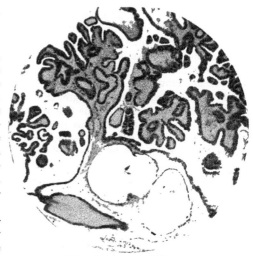

Fig. 623.—Benign papilliferous cyst.
The papillomas are covered with a single layer of epithelium.

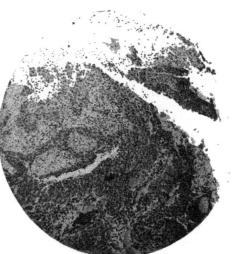

Fig. 624.—Malignant papilliferous cyst.
Large masses of epithelium cover the papillomatous outgrowths and infiltrate the cyst wall.

3 q

cysts. The cyst-adenomas not infrequently contain solid masses having the structure of spheroidal- or columnar-celled carcinoma. Squamous-celled carcinoma has been recorded arising from the skin-covered surface of a dermoid cyst, whilst the cystic embryoma may become malignant in virtue of any or all of the tissues contained in it. Thus, chorion-epithelioma and various forms of carcinoma and sarcoma may all arise in it, or the whole cyst may assume malignancy, the metastases presenting the same multiform characters as the primary growth.

A peculiar form of colloidal growth arises in some multilocular cysts. The growth perforates the cyst wall and, becoming grafted on the peritoneum, produces enormous quantities of material like painter's size, which gradually distends the peritoneal cavity. Evacuation of the contents is followed by reaccumulation, and cases are on record where this procedure has been repeated over several years. The basis of the growth is a colloid tissue containing few cells. Sarcoma of varying types may originate in a cyst wall. Secondary deposits of carcinoma in the ovary are very common, and are often partially cystic owing to the inclusion of distended follicles in the growth. They are nearly always bilateral, and are usually secondary to malignant disease of the intestine or gall-bladder.

Symptoms.—The symptoms of ovarian cysts may be divided into those due to (1) bulk, (2) pressure, (3) torsion, (4) inflammation, (5) rupture, (6) malignant degeneration.

Bulk.—The rate of growth of an ovarian cyst varies. Dermoids may grow very slowly. Cyst-adenomas attain a fair size in two years. Malignant cysts may reach a great bulk in a few months; while certain accidental occurrences such as torsion or inflammation produce very rapid increase in size.

Cysts weighing over 100 lb. have not infrequently been recorded. In the absence of complications, ovarian cysts do not at first affect the general health, but later the increasing enlargement of the abdomen is accompanied by the so-called " ovarian cachexia," characterized by extreme emaciation and an earthy or definitely pigmented colour of the skin.

Pressure.—Impaction in the pelvis may occur, with retention of urine, partial intestinal obstruction, and great pain ; but this is a much less common event than with myomas. Enormous tumours interfere with respiration and the intestinal functions, and may produce signs due to pressure on the vena cava.

Torsion.—Torsion of the pedicle is the commonest complication of an ovarian cyst. It may follow a violent effort or the emptying of a pregnant uterus, but often no cause is apparent. The first twist is usually small, but sufficient to obstruct the venous return through the pedicle. As a result, the cyst wall and the pedicle distal to the twist become œdematous and swell. This occasions a further twisting, with increased œdema; and so on, until the blood-flow through the pedicle may be entirely arrested. The cyst becomes purple or black from venous congestion, and its contents are rapidly augmented by the effusion of serum and blood into the cavity. Occasionally large quantities of blood may be thus poured out. The necrotic wall induces peritonitis around it, with the formation of adhesions through which the circulation may be re-established. Spontaneous recovery sometimes takes place, the necrotic cyst becoming sequestered by universal adhesions. More commonly, however, general peritonitis is set up, to which the patient would succumb if untreated.

A twisted cyst rapidly increases in size and becomes very tense and tender. It usually crosses the middle line to the opposite side, becomes markedly unilateral, and pulls the uterus in the same direction by the tension of the pedicle. The pain is at first spasmodic, the exacerbations coinciding with the successive twists; later on, as peritonitis is set up, the distress becomes continuous, and vomiting and flatulent distension appear.

Rupture.—Spontaneous rupture is most commonly seen with papilliferous cysts. The abdomen rapidly fills up with ascitic fluid, and some tenderness and pain may be present, owing to the secondary peritoneal implantations; these may be felt, on deep palpation, as irregular masses. The patient wastes, and often shows slight continuous fever.

Cyst-adenomas rarely rupture, owing to the early formation of adhesions. The escape of the mucous contents sets up a subacute peritonitis with pain and tenderness. Ruptured colloidal cysts present the same clinical picture as ruptured papilliferous cysts, but the distension and general deterioration are slower. The bursting of an ovarian blood cyst or profuse hæmorrhage from a corpus hæmorrhagicum almost exactly simulates a ruptured tubal gestation, but a history of preceding amenorrhœa is absent. Thin-walled follicular cysts may rupture spontaneously, or in the course of examination. The fluid is non-irritant and is soon absorbed, but the cyst re-forms after a while. Very rarely the sudden effusion of blood into the cavity of a twisted cyst has caused the wall to rupture.

Malignant degeneration.—Malignant ovarian cysts give rise to a fixed mass, ascites, and rapid emaciation. Later, metastatic masses are felt in the omentum, parietes, and liver. These secondary growths, especially those in the omentum, are often the first to attract attention. They have the bossy feel of a number of rounded nodules partially fused together, and when omental may be very movable.

Diagnosis.—If the uterus cannot be separated from the mass, absolute distinction from a myoma may be impossible. Marked fluctuation and the presence of a fluid thrill are in favour of ovarian origin, but a cystic myoma may present the same signs. Many ovarian tumours do not fluctuate, especially dermoids and multilocular cyst-adenomas, while cyst-embryomas and malignant cysts are largely solid in composition. A vascular murmur over the tumour strongly suggests a uterine origin. The history of menorrhagia usual with a myoma is rare with an ovarian cyst, unless complicated by one of these tumours.

Ovarian cysts usually grow much more quickly than myomas, while tumours first discovered under 30 or above 55 years of age are probably ovarian. The frequency with which myomas and ovarian cysts coexist must not be forgotten.

Pregnancy is distinguished from an ovarian cyst by the enlargement being uterine, by its usually greater rate of growth, by the presence over it of a vascular murmur and signs of foetal life, and by the corresponding period of amenorrhœa.

Ovarian cysts only cause amenorrhœa when they are bilateral and have totally destroyed all normal ovarian tissue. This is chiefly seen in malignant cysts, in which the rate of enlargement may be rapid and pregnancy more particularly simulated.

A distended bladder is immediately distinguished on passage of the catheter—a precaution never to be omitted in cases of doubt.

Ascites shows signs of movable fluid and produces a different shape of the abdomen, the loins particularly being bulged ; moreover, the front of the abdomen is resonant and the flanks are dull, the reverse being the case with a cyst. Encysted peritoneal fluid, as seen in some forms of tubercular peritonitis or in "encysted serous perimetritis," may closely simulate an ovarian cyst, but the swelling is fixed and the percussion note frequently partly resonant owing to adherent bowel lying over it. A large hydrosalpinx may be indistinguishable from an ovarian cyst, whilst many tense broad-ligament cysts are mistaken for broad-ligament myoma..

Retroperitoneal cysts of various kinds closely simulate ovarian cysts, but their front is resonant, and most of them (hydronephrosis, pancreatic cysts) have no connexion with the pelvis.

The diagnosis of torsion of an ovarian cyst from rupture of tubal gestation and acute salpingitis is discussed under the latter two headings. The most striking feature is *the presence of a large cystic tumour from the very outset of the symptoms.*

A ruptured papilliferous cyst or other form of cyst with ascites may be mistaken for terminal hepatic cirrhosis or acute tuberculous peritonitis. In most cases a pelvic tumour can be felt, which excludes the hepatic condition. In tuberculous peritonitis, however, a mass may also be felt per vaginam, but in this condition there is usually much more fever than in ruptured cyst.

In all cases of doubt the peritoneal cavity should be explored. Many a woman has been tapped repeatedly for an ascites due to an unsuspected papilliferous cyst.

An inflamed cyst simulates acute pyosalpinx, but the mass is from the commencement more circumscribed and defined.

Treatment.—All ovarian cysts should be removed as soon as possible, through an abdominal incision.

A pedunculated cyst is treated by excision, the pedicle being first clamped. Ligation of the pedicle should be carried out in sections, to minimize the risk of the ligatures slipping. Large unilocular cysts with clear fluid contents should be tapped before removal, but all others should be excised whole for fear of escape into the peritoneum of irritant or infected matter or transplantable tumour cells. Multilocular cysts cannot be satisfactorily tapped. Adhesions to the cyst wall should be separated as far as possible before tapping if this course be followed.

Sessile broad-ligament cysts are to be treated by enucleation from their peritoneal investment. This is often easy, the gap in the broad ligament being subsequently closed with sutures. In other cases only part of the cyst can be so removed; the remainder should be brought up to the abdominal wound and drained.

The excision of a broad-ligament cyst is sometimes facilitated by removal of the uterus. Where the cyst has burrowed deeply its removal may be a very difficult operation.

Ovarian cysts are sometimes universally adherent. In many instances the cyst wall can be readily shelled out, but in others this is impossible without serious damage to the intestines and mesentery. In this case the best course is to empty the cyst and then suture up the aperture, leaving the patient to be tapped subsequently as the fluid reaccumulates.

Cysts of the ovary or ovarian hilum burrowing into the broad ligament are treated by enucleation, like actual broad-ligament cysts.

Malignant cysts should be removed whenever possible; but great judgment must be exercised, for the bleeding in these cases may be so free that, once started, the operator may find it impossible to go back.

The operation of ovariotomy has nowadays a mortality greater than that of simple hysterectomy. This is on account of the large proportion of malignant cases dealt with, in which the death-rate is high. Excluding these, the average risk is probably 2 per cent.

FIBROMA

Fibrous tumours, many of them of large size, are occasionally met with in the ovary. They arise as (a) a diffuse fibrous overgrowth of the whole of the ovarian stroma, (b) a local encapsuled mass, or (c) a pedunculated outgrowth from the surface of the ovary. They are most frequently met with between the ages of 30 and 50. In structure they are pure fibromas, and show much less tendency to degeneration than is the ease with myomas. They take about two years to attain the size of a cricket-ball. They produce symptoms of pressure like a pedunculated subserous myoma. In most recorded cases free fluid has been present in the abdominal cavity, a circumstance that caused them to be regarded as sarcomas in the past. It is impossible to distinguish absolutely a fibroma from a subserous myoma with a long pedicle, before the abdomen is opened. The absence of menorrhagia and the detection of signs of free peritoneal fluid would suggest a fibroma. The tumour must be removed, the steps of the operation being those already described under Ovarian Cysts (p. 1077).

ADENOMA

Solid adenomas in the ovary are rare. Their nature can only be ascertained by microscopical examination, when a series of regular glandular spaces lying in a fibro-cellular stroma is revealed. Like fibromas, adenomas cause some ascites and produce pressure symptoms. They must be removed as soon as possible, and if doubt as to the innocent nature of the growth exists the uterus should be removed also.

PAPILLOMA

A rare villous type of papilloma originating in the germinal epithelium, and producing secondary peritoneal growths and ascites, is known. Removal of the primary growth is followed in some cases by spontaneous disappearance of the secondary growths in the peritoneum.

SARCOMA

Many different types of primary sarcoma occur in the ovary, the round-celled variety being the commonest. All ages are attacked, and cases have been recorded even in infancy. In children and young persons the growth is often bilateral, but in older patients only one side is usually affected.

Secondary sarcoma of the ovary is uncommon, except in the melanotic variety, in which large bilateral tumours may be found post mortem.

Ascites is early noticed, the tumour is fixed and grows rapidly, and the patient wastes. The diagnosis of malignancy is usually not difficult, but the occurrence of ascites with simple fibromas must be remembered. The histological nature of the growth can only be determined after removal. The uterus and both appendages must be totally extirpated.

CARCINOMA

Primary growths exhibit various characters in different cases, the tubular columnar-celled type being that most frequently met with.

Secondary carcinoma is much more common, and is especially associated with carcinoma of the stomach or some part of the intestines.

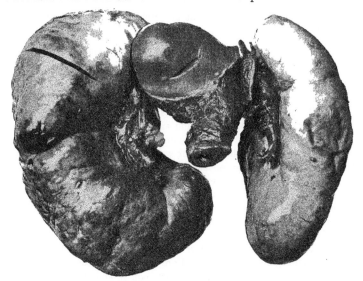

Fig. 625.—Uterus with bilateral malignant ovarian tumours.

In terminal carcinoma of the breast, surface metastases on the ovary are often found, as shown by Handley. Secondary carcinomatous tumours are nearly always bilateral, and are usually partly cystic from the inclusion of dropsical follicles in the growth (Fig. 625).

Primary carcinoma exhibits the same general symptoms and signs as primary sarcoma (*see* p. 1078). Secondary carcinomatous tumours attain a large size, and, as pointed out by Bland-Sutton, their metastatic origin may be overlooked.

Immediate removal, together with the uterus and the rest of the appendages, is the only course.

If the condition is bilateral, a very careful search should be made for a primary growth in the abdomen elsewhere.

THE PELVIC PERITONEUM AND CELLULAR TISSUE

PELVIC PERITONITIS (PERIMETRITIS)

Pelvic peritonitis is always secondary to inflammation of some of the pelvic organs. In the vast proportion of cases salpingitis is the primary cause, but occasionally this rôle is played by a solitary ovarian abscess, an infected ovarian or uterine tumour, a hæmatocele, or an inflamed appendix situated in the pelvis.

The symptoms and treatment of pelvic peritonitis, therefore, are those of the lesion to which it is secondary.

PELVIC CELLULITIS (PARAMETRITIS)

Infection of the pelvic cellular tissue is usually secondary to some lesion of the vagina, of the cervix or the body of the uterus. Thus, it is usually seen after labour or after operations upon the genital canal. Occasionally it is primary, as in cases of inflamed broad-ligament cyst, or suppuration round an intraligamentous lithopædion.

In *anterior* cellulitis the inflammatory mass is situated between the cervix and vagina and the posterior wall and base of the bladder. In *lateral* cellulitis the infection usually follows the lymphatic tract that accompanies the uterine artery and vein, and thus involves the base of the broad ligament and the paravaginal tissue. It is commonest on the left side, because parturitional laceration most often affects that side of the cervix. Where the primary lesion is in the body of the uterus or the Fallopian tube, the lymphatic tract accompanying the ovarian vessels is affected, and the mass then lies much higher. In *posterior* cellulitis the parts affected are the cellular tissue of the utero-sacral folds on either side of Douglas's pouch, and the substance of the recto-vaginal septum. The inflammation in this case invariably spreads behind the rectum, so that the gut is encircled by it.

The histological condition is one of lymphangitis and phlebitis, which may or may not suppurate. In the latter case the abscess may either (1) discharge spontaneously, above Poupart's ligament, or into the bladder, vagina, or rectum, or (2) become chronic and sequestered by fibrosis.

Symptoms.—The onset is acute, with pain, tenderness, and fever. After a few days an indurated swelling is felt per vaginam, either in front of or behind the vagina, or extending outwards from the side of the uterus to the lateral pelvic wall as a buttress-like mass.

In lateral cellulitis the swelling first appears on the abdomen as a tender induration rising above the inner third of Poupart's ligament and spreading outwards to the iliac fossa. Anterior cellulitis is less frequently felt from the abdomen, whilst posterior cellulitis does not give rise to abdominal signs. Very frequently the different varieties coexist (*complete cellulitis*). Femoral thrombosis and " white leg " often accompany lateral cellulitis.

If pus forms, the swelling becomes softer and eventually fluctuates ; large abscesses may mount under the peritoneum even as high as the loin, or sometimes they burrow under Poupart's ligament into the thigh and point at the saphenous ring. With abscess formation the temperature is markedly remittent, and heavy sweating and rapid wasting occur. If the abscess becomes chronic, an indurated fixed swelling remains, giving rise to recurring attacks of pain and fever. In anterior cellulitis more or less cystitis is always present, while in posterior cellulitis diarrhœa is common.

Diagnosis.—Acute cellulitis has to be distinguished from salpingitis and other causes of acute pelvic peritonitis.

The lateral variety is recognized by the mass extending directly outwards to the pelvic wall, and mounting upwards towards the iliac fossa. The abdominal tumour is dull on percussion, and there is a comparative absence of intestinal distension and the other signs commonly accompanying peritonitis.

Anterior cellulitis is at once distinguished by its position between the vagina and bladder, while the swelling of posterior cellulitis does not occupy the pouch of Douglas but lies lower down in the recto-vaginal septum and surrounds the bowel like a ring.

The mass formed by a chronic broad-ligament cellulitis may be mistaken for a myoma or a tense cyst, and is sometimes only distinguishable by operation. Intraligamentous gestation produces a very similar swelling, but has a distinctive history.

It is important to remember that cellulitis and salpingitis often coexist.

Treatment.—At the outset, cellulitis should be treated by fomentations applied to the lower abdomen and by frequent hot vaginal douches. In favourable eases the swelling gradually subsides, and may wholly disappear in a few weeks. If pus formation is suspected, the collection must be freely incised from its most accessible aspect, commonly just above the groin.

Where a chronic pelvic mass is formed, iodides or injections of fibrolysin may be tried to disperse it. These failing, an operation should be undertaken. Laparotomy is usually advisable because in no other way can the exact nature of the mass be ascertained. It may be found, for instance, that the tumour is really a tubo-ovarian abscess which has under-burrowed the broad ligament. Encysted broad-ligament abscesses may sometimes be enucleated whole. If not, they should be stitched to the parietal wound and drained.

FUNCTIONAL DISEASES OF THE FEMALE GENITAL ORGANS

PRURITUS

Pruritus may be due to some structural change like leucoplakic vulvitis, or to glycosuria, but cases also occur in which no gross cause can be discovered, especially at the climacteric and during pregnancy. Such cases are to be treated by sedative ointments, and by the administration of bromides internally.

DYSPAREUNIA

All abnormalities of the genital tract tend to dyspareunia, but especially senile atrophy of the vagina, kraurosis vulvæ, vaginitis, salpingitis, and fixed retroversion of the uterus. Besides these, a purely functional type exists in which, with total absence of sexual feeling, the mere idea of the act is abhorrent. In cases of both classes coitus is more or less resisted by spasmodic · contraction of the vaginal sphincters (*vaginismus*). The two types are often combined, for the actual pain due to organic deformity or disease, by abolishing sexual feeling, evolves the painful idea that is the basis of the functional affection and inhibits the flow of mucus that assists the act. Where organic deformity or disease is the sole or underlying cause of the affection it must be treated on the lines already laid down. Purely functional cases are very difficult to treat. A plastic operation enlarging the vaginal orifice may be tried.

DYSMENORRHŒA

There are four types of dysmenorrhœa—(1) " virginal," (2) obstructive, (3) congestive, and (4) "ovarian."

1. " *Virginal* " *dysmenorrhœa* (" *spasmodic* " *dysmenorrhœa*).—Virginal dysmenorrhœa begins, as a rule, a year or more after puberty. The pain starts either with or slightly before the discharge, and at first endures for a few hours only, but in the course of years it becomes more prolonged. It is of a heavy, continuous, "tearing" character, felt in the lower abdomen in the mid-line and down the vagina. When severe it is accompanied by nausea or actual sickness. Its cause is not known, but its character suggests *tension*, and it is probably due to the stretching of the tense peritoneum and rigid musculature of the virgin uterus by the menstrual congestion. It rarely persists after childbirth, and in some instances is improved by marriage. The old term "spasmodic" is misleading, for the character of the pain is continuous.

Obstructive dysmenorrhœa.—This may be actual or relative. Actual obstruction is seen in congenital or acquired atresia of the cervix or vagina. At first these conditions cause no pain, because the cervix and the vagina (especially) readily stretch to accommodate the retained blood. After a while, however, severe spasms of pain are experienced.

Relative obstruction occurs when the menstrual contents are relatively too bulky to pass easily through the cervix. The best example is a case of menorrhagia with the formation of intra-uterine clots, the expulsion of which is attended with strong colicky pain.

A less frequent cause is the shedding each month of a mucosal cast from the body of the uterus (*membranous dysmenorrhœa*), the passage of which is associated with similar distress. In some of these cases the cast-shedding appears to be a natural peculiarity. In others it is the result of inflammatory change (*exfoliative endometritis*).

Congestive dysmenorrhœa.—The pain of all uterine and appendage disease or displacement is accentuated by the monthly congestion of the parts. This accentuation of a pain more or less constantly present is termed congestive dysmenorrhœa. It is best observed in chronic endometritis or salpingitis, especially when associated with retroversion or prolapse.

"*Ovarian*" *dysmenorrhœa.*—Interference with the normal dehiscence of the Graafian follicle, as in chronic salpingo-oöphoritis, may possibly, by raising intra-ovarian tension, cause pain. Excessive hæmorrhage into the follicle after dehiscence may also produce the same effect. In certain cases of extreme dysmenorrhœa, although no obvious defect can be discovered on examination, the pain is referred constantly to the region of the ovary on one or both sides, and dilatation of the cervix has no effect. Though the term "ovarian" dysmenorrhœa is often used, monthly pain practically never occurs after hysterectomy with conservation of the ovaries.

Treatment.—Many drugs are used for dysmenorrhœa, of which the most important are phenacetin, antipyrin, phenalgin, antikamnia, guaiacum, aletris, styptol, and the bromides. Their results are uncertain, and often only temporary.

Definite organic disease, when present, must be treated appropriately. "Virginal" dysmenorrhœa is most successfully relieved by dilating the uterus up to 12–14 Hegar immediately before the period.

Membranous dysmenorrhœa is difficult to cure. Free dilatation of the cervix and curettage is the proper course, but the monthly separation of the cast is likely to recur.

In extreme cases of dysmenorrhœa, all other treatment failing, subtotal hysterectomy should be performed. Oöphorectomy is never to be recommended.

LEUCORRHŒA

Leucorrhœa implies a mucous discharge originating in the gland of the cervix. Though a functional increase in this discharge may occur during pregnancy, or for a few days after the menstrual flow, excessive and persistent leucorrhœal discharge is always due to cervicitis (*see* p. 1010).

METRORRHAGIA

Bleeding from the uterus unconnected with the menses is always due to organic disease. Carcinoma of the uterus, corporeal or cervical polyps, endometritis, and retained conception products are the commonest causes. The treatment will be found set out under these conditions.

MENORRHAGIA

Excessive loss at the periods is seen with myoma, adeno-myoma, fibrotic metritis, endometritis, and mucous or fibroid polyps.

Functional menorrhagia is sometimes seen at puberty, on the resumption of the menses after lactation, at the climacteric, and in certain circumstances unexplainable in our present state of knowledge.

With regard to menopausal menorrhagia, it is most important to remember that the excessive losses are balanced or more than balanced by periods of amenorrhœa. Constantly recurring menstrual losses are not normal to this epoch, while continuous bleeding, contrary to the public impression, is altogether abnormal, and should be immediately investigated.

Treatment.—Functional menorrhagia is to be treated by drugs, of which the most useful are ergot, hydrastis, hamamelis, cotarnin, and calcium lactate or chloride. Where an organic cause exists operative treatment is usually advisable.

AMENORRHŒA

Amenorrhœa may be due to congenital absence or operative removal of the uterus or ovaries. Occasionally, persons structurally normal and in good health never menstruate, probably as a result of deficient ovarian activity. Congenital or postoperative occlusion of some part of the genital canal produces a spurious amenorrhœa. Amenorrhœa is particularly associated with chlorosis, while certain prolonged wasting diseases, such as tuberculosis, tend to it. Acute endometritis or oöphoritis may suppress a period, while the physiological epochs of pregnancy, lactation, and the climacteric are normally accompanied by absence of the menses.

Treatment.—The menstrual flow is not a necessity to health; its absence, therefore, requires treatment on the score of its cause alone. In chlorosis, purgatives and iron give good results. In general debility the usual tonics and hygienic régime are indicated. For functional amenorrhœa, aloes and iron are useful.

INDEX TO VOL. II

3 r *

PRINTED BY
CASSELL AND COMPANY, LIMITED, LA BELLE SAUVAGE,
LONDON, E.C.
10.1113

Lightning Source UK Ltd.
Milton Keynes UK
UKHW052230291218
334411UK00014B/919/P